Principles of Drug Action:
The Basis of Pharmacology

Principles of Drug Action:
The Basis of Pharmacology

SECOND EDITION

AVRAM GOLDSTEIN, M.D.

LEWIS ARONOW, Ph.D.

SUMNER M. KALMAN, M.D.

Professors of Pharmacology
Stanford University School of Medicine
Stanford, California

A Wiley Biomedical-Health Publication

JOHN WILEY & SONS
New York   London   Sydney   Toronto

Library of Congress Cataloging in Publication Data

Goldstein, Avram.

   Principles of drug action:

  (A Wiley biomedical-health publication)

   1. Drugs—Physiological effect. I. Aronow,
Lewis, joint author. II. Kalman, Sumner M., joint
author. III. Title [DNLM: 1. Pharmacology.
QV38 G624p 1973]

RM300.G63   1974   615'.7   73-15871

ISBN 0-471-31260-6

Printed in the United States of America

10 9 8 7 6 5 4 3 2

Preface to the Second Edition

The concept that guided us in writing this textbook is embodied in the preface to the first edition, which appeared five years ago. We hoped—naively, as it turned out—that the basic principles of pharmacology were sufficiently immutable, or at least changed slowly enough, so that new editions would be required only rarely. It is true that the major principles have not needed revision. However, advances have been so rapid in certain areas that major additions were called for, especially in our selection of the illustrative material from the experimental literature. Among these areas that have "come of age" within the last few years are receptor isolation, the revolutionary advances in analytic chemistry applied to the detection and quantitation of drugs and drug metabolites, environmental toxicity, the immunochemical basis of drug allergies, and drug-drug interactions in man. Material that was not germane to the principal theme of the book has been deleted; examples are the commentaries on sources of information for selecting drugs in clinical practice and the appendix on prescription writing. On balance, more has been added than subtracted, resulting in a modest increase in the size of the book.

We have been pleased with the favorable comment and wide acceptance that greeted the first edition. We have retained the general format, except that we have eliminated all footnote material, placing references, instead, at the ends of chapters to improve the smooth flow and appearance of the text.

We are grateful to numerous colleagues for bringing errors of substance and of form to our attention. Among these we thank especially Drs. James F. Lenney and Douglas S. Riggs who, in different ways, contributed very considerably to the elimination of errors. A new edition, however, is bound to contain new errors. Again we ask readers to bring these to our attention, be they small or large.

We thank Jean Colvin and Linda Cummings for their extraordinary contribution to this book. They carried out with meticulous care and superb skill a variety of editorial tasks that were essential to the production of the finished work. We thank Chris Hulden for preparation of the new art work. We are grateful to our new publishers, John Wiley & Sons, who have seen this second edition through to publication efficiently and speedily. Specifically, we thank Alan Frankenfield of the New York office, and Bernard Scheier, Linda Riffle, and Elodie Sabankaya of the Palo Alto office.

Avram Goldstein
Lewis Aronow
Sumner M. Kalman

Stanford, California

V

Preface to
the First Edition

Pharmacology is the science of drugs, their chemical constitution, their biologic action, and their therapeutic application in man. It includes toxicology, which encompasses the harmful effects of all chemicals, whether they are used medicinally or not. The variety of new uses to which drugs are being put, and the increasing exposure of whole populations to potent chemical agents, have created a wider and more intense interest in pharmacology than has ever existed before. The time is long past when anyone can acquire a complete knowledge about all drugs. But many people in diverse fields of endeavor need a foundation, a conceptual framework, upon which may be built the specific knowledge about drugs that is most germane to their own needs.

In this book we have tried to provide a coherent, rational, and scientifically correct account of the principles underlying every aspect of this science. For physicians, medical students, and others whose aim is to acquire an up-to-date and comprehensive understanding of pharmacology, this book is intended to serve as a basic text, to be supplemented by the systematic textbooks. The fundamental concepts developed here, which ordinarily occupy but a few pages in standard texts, are meant to provide the physician and medical student with the requisite background both for understanding the basis of drug therapy, and for appraising new developments in the field. We hope the book will also be a valuable introduction to pharmacology for all those investigators and students of the natural sciences who, using drugs as research tools, wish to learn the principles of drug action but have no need of a comprehensive catalogue.

Our aim was to expose and elaborate upon the fundamentals of pharmacology in a systematic and rigorous manner. We have tried to re-examine critically those areas in which generalizations seemed to rest upon shaky foundations, and to furnish a new theory or interpretation when it seemed to be called for. The book focuses upon principles and mechanisms rather than upon drugs but a great many drugs are specifically discussed in order to illustrate and exemplify. We have drawn widely upon the published literature for pertinent examples, many of them directly relevant to the use of drugs in man. Research papers and reviews are cited in the footnotes; we have chosen principally those that will serve the student best, without regard to completeness of citation or priority of discovery.

The scope of the book is broad, reflecting the breadth of modern pharmacology. The first chapter deals with mechanisms of drug-receptor interaction and considers the theoretical basis of dose-reponse relationships. This is followed by three chapters on the fate of drugs in the body—their absorption, distribution, excretion, and metabolism—and the factors that determine the time course of drug action. Chapters 5 through 12 deal with the adverse effects of drugs and the mechanisms responsible. Dose-related toxicity is considered, along with methods for its quantitative estimation and the modes of action of specific antidotes. The pharmacogenetic basis of drug idiosyncrasy is presented as well as the immunochemical basis of drug allergy. Drug resistance in lower species is contrasted with drug tolerance and physical dependence in man and other animals. Special chapters are devoted to effects of drugs upon cell heredity—chemical mutagenesis, carcinogenesis, and teratogenesis— and some consideration is given to the public-health aspects of these phenomena in relation to the widespread exposure of human populations to drugs. The last two chapters discuss the strategy of the discovery and development of new drugs, and the methods employed to assess their potential usefulness in experimental animals and in clinical trials in humans. Guidelines are also presented for the selection of drugs in clinical practice. A concise summary of the principles of prescribing is given in Appendix I.

We have adhered, in general, to the standardized terminology and abbreviations followed by the *Journal of Biological Chemistry*. For the column headings in tables and the labeling of coordinate axes in the illustrations the convention is that units accompanied by a multiplication factor are to be understood as part of an equation: for example, under the heading "Cells $\times$ 10^{-5}" an entry of 3.0 would mean 3.0×10^5 cells, from the equation "Cells $\times$ 10^{-5} = 3.0." All temperatures are Centigrade, although the symbol C. is omitted. Logarithms to the base 10 are indicated by log, natural logarithms by ln. Nonproprietary drug names are used, without capitalization; trade names, if used at all, are capitalized, but the superscript symbol ® is not employed. The abbreviations found in this book (unless they are self-explanatory) are listed in Appendix II.

We are indebted to the Literary Executor of the late Sir Ronald A. Fisher, F.R.S., to Dr. Frank Yates, F.R.S., and to Oliver and Boyd Ltd., Edinburgh, for permission to reprint Table IX from their book *Statistical Tables for Biological, Agricultural and Medical Research*.

We are deeply indebted to our teachers, colleagues, and students who helped guide our thinking toward the outlook upon pharmacology that is embodied in this book. We are grateful to Professor Walther Wilbrandt and Dr. William B. Pratt for reading and commenting upon various chapters. We thank Mrs. Ray Jeffery for skillful and efficient typing of the manuscript, and Mrs. John Naughton for careful checking of bibliographic citations and other assistance in preparing the book for publication. It has been a pleasure to work with Paul B. Hoeber and his staff, especially Miss Claire Drullard, Miss Jo Hinkel, and Mrs. Rose Yager. The authors are responsible for any deficiences or errors that remain and would be grateful if readers would call them to our attention. We also welcome readers' suggestions for future editions concerning the inclusion of new material exemplifying principles and mechanisms.

Avram Goldstein
Lewis Aronow
Sumner M. Kalman

Palo Alto, California

Contents

CHAPTER 6

Pharmacogenetics and Drug Idiosyncrasy   437

CHAPTER 7

Drug Allergy   489

CHAPTER 14

Drug Evaluation in Man

CHAPTER 1
Molecular Mechanisms of Drug Action

RECEPTORS

Whatever effects a drug produces in a biologic system must be regarded as ultimate consequences of physicochemical interactions between that drug and functionally important molecules in the living organism. Sometimes a drug may act by combining with a small molecule or ion, as when an antacid neutralizes hydrochloric acid or a chelating agent complexes Pb^{2+} ion in the treatment of lead poisoning. In the great majority of cases, however, drugs are presumed to interact with macromolecular components of tissues. These elements with which drugs combine we call *receptors*.

The concept of receptors has its origin in two quite different lines of experimentation carried out in the early years of the 20th century. Paul Ehrlich (1845–1915) was greatly impressed by the high degree of antibody specificity against the antigenic substances that stimulated their production and imagined a stereospecific lock-and-key fit between them. He postulated specific "side chains" in protoplasm, with unique chemical and steric architecture with which only antibodies of the right shape and chemical composition could combine. Later, in his pioneering work on chemotherapy, when the phenomena under investigation were interactions between synthetic organic chemicals and parasitic protozoa, the same concepts were extended. Again a high degree of specificity was observed. On the one hand, small variations in a drug's chemical structure affected its antiparasitic potency in a dramatic way. On the other hand, several drugs with about the same antiparasitic efficacy might differ greatly in toxicity to the host. To explain these findings Ehrlich assumed that all cells had "side chains" which were essential for their life processes, but that the composition and shapes of these differed in different kinds of cells. Thus, chemotherapeutic drugs could be fashioned to combine specifically with "side chains" of the parasite, yet at the same time fit poorly the "side chains" of host tissues. From sketches in Ehrlich's notebooks it is apparent that he thought of the "side chains" as functional chemical

1

groupings such as sulfhydryl groups (–SH), amino groups (–NH$_2$), and so on, embedded in some sort of stereospecific macrostructure. To those hypothetical specific chemical groupings of protoplasm upon which chemotherapeutic drugs were assumed to act Ehrlich gave the name *receptors*.[1]

About the same time, J. N. Langley (1852–1926) was following up Claude Bernard's basic work on the South American arrow poison, curare. Bernard had found that this drug blocked transmission of impulses from motor nerves to skeletal muscles, and had localized the site of the block to the fine nerve terminals embedded in the muscle substance.[2] Langley found, however, that when a motor nerve was cut and allowed to degenerate, it was still possible to stimulate the muscle chemically by application of nicotine to the region where the nerve had formerly terminated. Moreover, curare blocked this action of nicotine. Yet even during curare blockade, either in innervated or denervated muscle, direct electrical stimulation of the muscle fibres elicited a contractile response. These observations could only mean that nicotine and curare both act upon some substance which is neither nerve nor muscle. When nicotine combines with it, this substance somehow triggers the contractile response of muscle. Curare can combine with it, yet not trigger a contractile response, thereby preventing the interaction with nicotine. To this hypothetical specialized material in muscle Langley gave the name *receptive substance*.[3–5]

Ehrlich and Langley were influential in establishing a new tradition in pharmacology. They were guided by the principle that the explanation of drug actions was to be sought not in vague "tonic" effects or poorly defined "poisonous" actions on the whole body, not in a mysterious power to combat "disease," but rather in physicochemical interactions of drugs at definite sites of action. Ehrlich's dogma that drugs cannot act unless they are bound to receptors—"corpora non agunt nisi fixata"—was controversial in his time but seems commonplace to us today. More and more receptors are being identified as specific proteins or nucleic acids. In this book we shall use the term *receptor* to describe a macromolecule with which a drug interacts to produce its characteristic biologic effect.[6–14]

BINDING FORCES IN THE DRUG-RECEPTOR INTERACTION

Bond Types[15]

The Covalent Bond.   A covalent bond is formed when two atoms share a pair of electrons. This is the familiar strong bond that holds together the atoms of organic molecules, with typical bond energy of about 100 kcal mole^{-1}. Because of the high binding energy, covalent bonds are essentially irreversible at ordinary temperatures unless a catalytic agent (e.g., an enzyme) intervenes. The covalent binding of drugs to receptors, unlike most drug-receptor interactions, results in stable long-lasting complexes.

Let us consider drugs that are alkylating agents (Table 1-1).[16–18] Such compounds form a reactive cationic intermediate, a carbonium ion, by virtue of the strong electron-attracting power of the group to which the alkyl residue is initially attached. In the case of nitrogen mustard and similar alkylating agents, the reaction proceeds by a first-order mechanism (SN1 type), since the rate-limiting step is an initial

TABLE 1-1. Structures and reaction mechanisms of some alkylating agents.

Alkylating agent	Structure	Carbonium ion form	Product of reaction with R^-
Ethyl methane sulfonate	$CH_3CH_2-O-\overset{\displaystyle O}{\underset{\displaystyle O}{S}}-CH_3$	$CH_3CH_2^+$	CH_3CH_2-R
Busulfan	$CH_3-\overset{\displaystyle O}{\underset{\displaystyle O}{S}}-O-(CH_2)_4-O-\overset{\displaystyle O}{\underset{\displaystyle O}{S}}-CH_3$	$CH_3-\overset{\displaystyle O}{\underset{\displaystyle O}{S}}-O-(CH_2)_4^+$ $R-(CH_2)_4^+$	$CH_3-\overset{\displaystyle O}{\underset{\displaystyle O}{S}}-O-(CH_2)_4-R$ $R-(CH_2)_4-R'$
Mechlorethamine (nitrogen mustard)	$CH_3N{\displaystyle \begin{array}{l} CH_2CH_2Cl \\ CH_2CH_2Cl \end{array}}$	$CH_3N{\displaystyle \begin{array}{l} CH_2CH_2^+ \\ CH_2CH_2Cl \end{array}}$ $CH_3N{\displaystyle \begin{array}{l} CH_2CH_2R \\ CH_2CH_2^+ \end{array}}$	$CH_3N{\displaystyle \begin{array}{l} CH_2CH_2-R \\ CH_2CH_2Cl \end{array}}$ $CH_3N{\displaystyle \begin{array}{l} CH_2CH_2-R \\ CH_2CH_2-R' \end{array}}$
Phenoxybenzamine			

cyclization to an unstable ethyleneimmonium cation, with release of a chloride ion, followed by strained-ring scission yielding the reactive carbonium ion. The carbonium ion then reacts avidly with an electron donor group such as carboxylate, phosphate, or sulfhydryl anion. If the nucleophilic acceptor (R^-) is a weak base, the reaction will result in a net production of hydrogen ions. Atoms of N, S, and O are

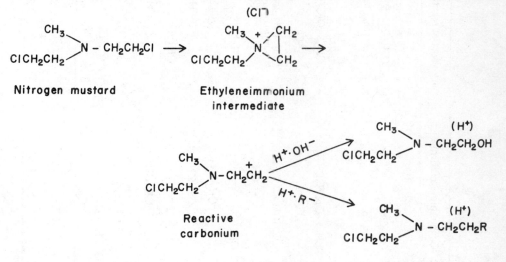

Nitrogen mustard   **Ethyleneimmonium intermediate**

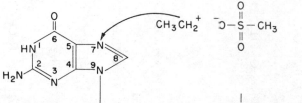

Reactive carbonium   **Products**

effective electron donors and therefore undergo alkylation reactions. Usually a proton is released from the amine, sulfhydryl, or hydroxyl group, but when a heterocyclic ring is alkylated (e.g., guanine), the positive charge can be retained (Figure 1-1).

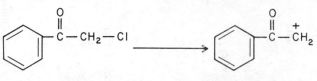

FIGURE 1-1. Alkylation of DNA guanine by a mutagen, ethyl methane sulfonate. *The carbonium ethyl group is shown making an attack on the electron-rich nitrogen atom in position 7. The deoxyribose phosphate backbone of the DNA strand is also shown, but the base attached to the neighbor deoxyribose has been omitted for clarity.*

Another type of reaction is exemplified by some of the tear gas riot control agents, such as chloroacetophenone ("CN").[19] Compounds of this type do not require any

Chloroacetophenone   **Reactive Carbonium**

initial cyclization for their activation, but form carbcnium ions rapidly. The reaction rates are therefore second-order (SN2 type), depending on the concentrations of both reactants, the carbonium ion, and the acceptor moiety.

Ethyl methane sulfonate (Table 1-1) is a potent mutagen which acts by alkylating the nitrogen atom in position 7 of guanine in the intact deoxyribonucleic acid (DNA)

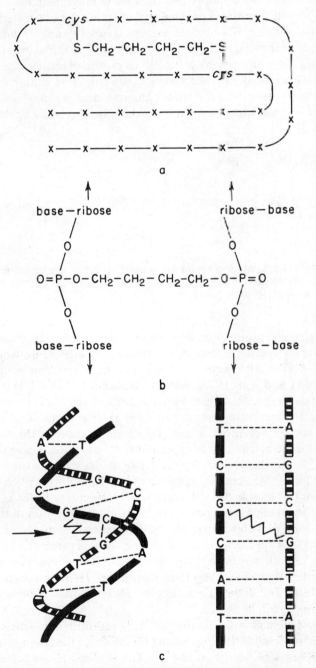

FIGURE 1-2. Postulated effects of bifunctional alkylating agents.

molecule (Figure 1-1), thereby changing the properties of the genetic material and its behavior at subsequent replications.[20]

A bifunctional alkylating agent is capable of forming two covalent bonds and thereby cross-linking two macromolecules or two parts of the same macromolecule. Such an agent is busulfan (Table 1-1), a drug used in the treatment of myeloid leukemia. This compound is seen to be simply two residues of ethyl methane sulfonate joined "back to back." Some postulated mechanisms of action are illustrated in Figure 1-2.

Another bifunctional agent used in cancer chemotherapy is mechlorethamine (nitrogen mustard) (Table 1-1). This simple molecule, as might be surmised, reacts rather nonspecifically with a variety of functional groups of proteins and nucleic acids. A bifunctional agent need not necessarily cross-link. For example, a postulated reaction with proteins involves alkylating a glutamic acid carboxyl group with mechlorethamine, the second carbonium ion formed by the alkylating agent reacting with water (Figure 1-3).

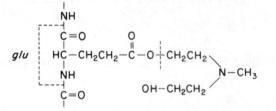

FIGURE 1-3. Postulated product of alkylation of a glutamic acid (*glu*) residue by mechlorethamine, the second carbonium ion of the alkylating agent having reacted with water.

More interesting alkylating agents are those with complex structures, which offer more possibilities for specific interaction at specialized sites. Thus, whereas nitrogen mustard reacts in vivo with water, with all sorts of protein molecules, with ribonucleic acid (RNA), and with DNA, phenoxybenzamine (Table 1-1) is an alkylating agent with a far more specific action. Vascular smooth muscle is innervated by sympathetic nerves, which release norepinephrine at their endings. The norepinephrine combines with specific receptors, which trigger contraction of the smooth muscle. In arterioles this is the mechanism for maintaining the normal degree of resistance to the blood flow. Phenoxybenzamine is remarkable in that it blocks the norepinephrine receptors with a fairly high degree of specificity.[21,22] Thus, during phenoxybenzamine blockade, the smooth muscle can still contract in response to other agents. That the blockade caused by phenoxybenzamine results from an alkylation of the receptors is suggested by its long persistence and practically irreversible character.

Another example of specificity in an alkylating agent is presented by the antibiotic mitomycin (Figure 1-4), which alkylates and cross-links the complementary strands of the DNA duplex, thus preventing their replication. Here, the original compound must first be reduced and undergo a molecular rearrangement in order to become an effective alkylating agent, as shown.[23]

One of the best understood examples of drug-receptor interaction through formation of a covalent bond is the long-lasting inhibition of the cholinesterase enzymes by organic phosphates and carbamates.[24-26] The cholinesterases belong to the class of "serine enzymes," which have a serine residue in the active center that plays an

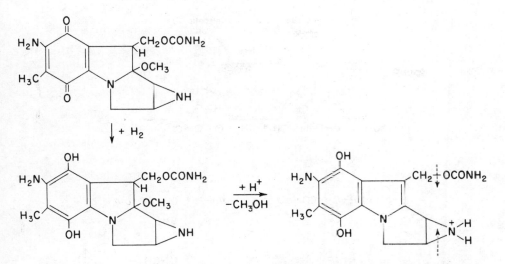

FIGURE 1-4. Mitomycin C (upper left) and its postulated reactive form (lower right). *The broken arrows show bonds that are known to be split when the reactive carbonium ions are formed. (From Iyer and Szybalski.[23] By permission of the American Association for the Advancement of Science.)*

essential role in the catalysis.[27] In alkaline phosphatase, liver aliesterase, and pseudo-cholinesterase, the amino acid sequence in the active center is *glutamic acid–serine–alanine.* In chymotrypsin, trypsin, and others it is *aspartic acid–serine–glycine.* In phosphoglucomutase it is *alanine–serine–histidine.* These enzymes have completely different substrate specificity requirements, so substrate access to the active center must, in each instance, be governed by specific features of the tertiary protein structure, dependent, in turn, upon differences in primary structure. Yet the actual catalytic steps mediated by these several enzymes are essentially the same. The enzyme carries out a nucleophilic attack upon an acyl carbon or phosphorus atom, resulting in the transient acylation of the enzyme and release of the group formerly acylated. Then the acyl group is transferred to a water hydroxyl ion (peptidases, esterases, phosphatases) or to another acceptor (phosphoglucomutase).

Figure 1-5 illustrates the mechanism of catalysis in the hydrolysis of acetylcholine by a cholinesterase and the mode of action of two inhibitors of the enzyme. Figure 1-5a represents the active center of the enzyme. Substrate specificity is determined by two sites approximately 5 A apart, an anionic site that forms an ionic bond with the cationic N of choline esters, and an esteratic site at which the ester bond is actually split. The initial interaction here is thought to be electron donation (probably from a histidine nitrogen atom) to the electrophilic carbonyl carbon atom. At a subsequent step (Figure 1-5b) this carbon atom is transferred to a serine hydroxyl group and choline is liberated. The transient acetylated enzyme then reacts with water, yielding acetic acid and regenerating the enzyme.

Diisopropylfluorophosphate (DFP) (Figure 1-5c) and similar organic phosphates are themselves esters containing a phosphorus atom that is electron deficient by virtue of the electron-attracting power of the attached halogen. Such a molecule can enter the active sites of all the "serine enzymes" and there participate in a reaction analogous to the normal acylation of enzyme by substrate. The phosphorus atom makes an electrophilic attack on the electron-rich oxygen atom of the serine residue,

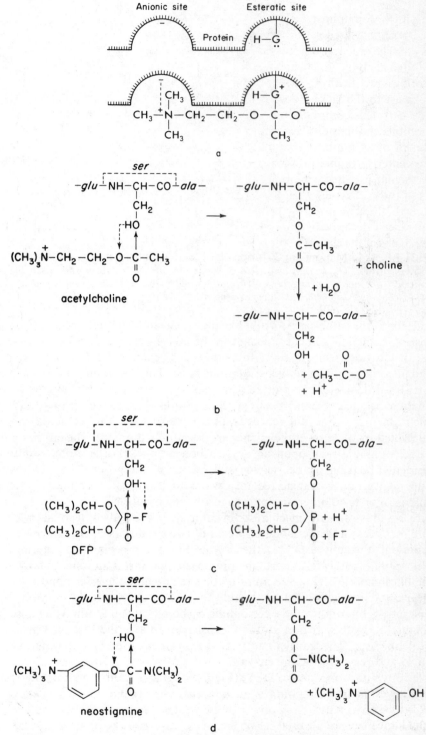

FIGURE 1-5. Substrate and inhibitor interactions with a cholinesterase. *In b, c, and d, only the reactions with the essential serine (ser) residue in the esteratic site are shown.*

yielding diisopropylphosphorylserine, and the fluoride anion and a proton are re-leased. Phosphorylated serine residues have been isolated from enzymes treated in this way.[28] The reaction is nonspecific; DFP enters the active sites of all the enzymes, even though each has its own exacting substrate specificity requirements. The phos-phorylation is practically irreversible, unlike the normal transient acylation mechanism.

A contrast to the lack of specificity of DFP is provided by the drug neostigmine (Figure 1-5d). This compound, by virtue of its close structural similarity to a choline ester, inhibits cholinesterases quite specifically. It is now known that the long-lasting component of its inhibitory action is the result of a dimethylcarbamylation of the enzyme center, presumably at the same serine residue with which DFP combines. The molecular architecture of neostigmine restricts its effective access to the active centers of those enzymes whose substrates it resembles, namely, the cholinesterases.

Although there is no real theoretical distinction, a particular kind of covalent bond has been described—the *coordinate covalent bond.* This bond is formed when both electrons of the electron pair that forms the bond between two atoms are donated by the same atom. In biologic systems the donor atom is usually nitrogen, oxygen, or sulfur, since these contain a pair of *s*-orbital electrons, usually unshared when the valence electrons have participated in bond formation. The electronic configuration of these elements is shown in Table 1-2. Consider the electron distribution in the outer orbitals of a typical carbon-bound amino group:

$$\overset{\circ}{\underset{\circ}{C}} : \overset{\bullet\bullet}{\underset{\bullet\bullet}{\overset{H}{\underset{H}{N}}}} :$$

TABLE 1-2. Electron configurations of selected atoms. (From Pauling,[15] Table 2-4.)

Atomic number		K $1s$	L $2s$	$2p$	$3s$	M $3p$	$3d$	N $4s$
H	1	1						
C	6	2	2	2				
N	7	2	2	3				
O	8	2	2	4				
Na	11	2	2	6	1			
Mg	12	2	2	6	2			
P	15	2	2	6	2	3		
S	16	2	2	6	2	4		
K	19	2	2	6	2	6	—	1
Ca	20	2	2	6	2	6	—	2
Mn	25	2	2	6	2	6	5	2
Fe	26	2	2	6	2	6	6	2
Co	27	2	2	6	2	6	7	2
Cu	29	2	2	6	2	6	10	1
Zn	30	2	2	6	2	6	10	2

The five electrons originally associated with the nitrogen atom are distinguished here from those contributed to the bonds by hydrogen and carbon, but it should be evident that all electrons are actually equivalent. The nitrogen electron octet is complete, and the valence of 3 for nitrogen is satisfied, yet the $2s$ electron pair remains unshared. (The inner, $1s$ orbital, containing two electrons, the helium core, is not shown here.) The simplest example of a coordinate covalent bond is the donation of this unshared electron pair to a proton:

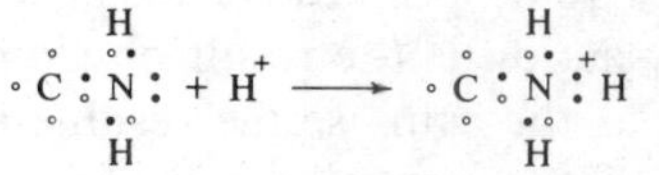

$$
\begin{array}{ccc}
\text{H} & & \text{H} \\
\overset{\cdots}{\text{C}} : \overset{\cdots}{\text{N}} : \ + \ \text{H}^+ & \longrightarrow & \overset{\cdots}{\text{C}} : \overset{\cdots}{\text{N}} : \text{H}^+ \\
\text{H} & & \text{H}
\end{array}
$$

Note that the positive charge associated with the proton is retained by the complex since there has been no net gain or loss of electrons. This type of bond formation plays a very important role in the ionization of drugs and in certain classes of drug-receptor interaction. Below we consider the formation of coordination complexes, especially chelate complexes.

Except for the coordination of a hydrogen ion, the atoms that share donated electron pairs in coordination complexes are usually metallic cations. These are the biologically important ions Na^+ and Mg^{2+} (atomic numbers 11, 12), K^+ and Ca^{2+} (atomic numbers 19, 20), Cu^+ (or Cu^{2+}) and Zn^{2+} (atomic numbers 29, 30). In addition, the transition elements have a peculiar ability to accept an electron in an unfilled inner orbital without disturbing ionic bonding involving the outer-orbital valence electrons. Transition elements of pharmacologic importance include Mn, Fe, and Co (atomic numbers 25, 26, 27). The basis of the behavior described here is evident in the electronic configurations shown in Table 1-2.

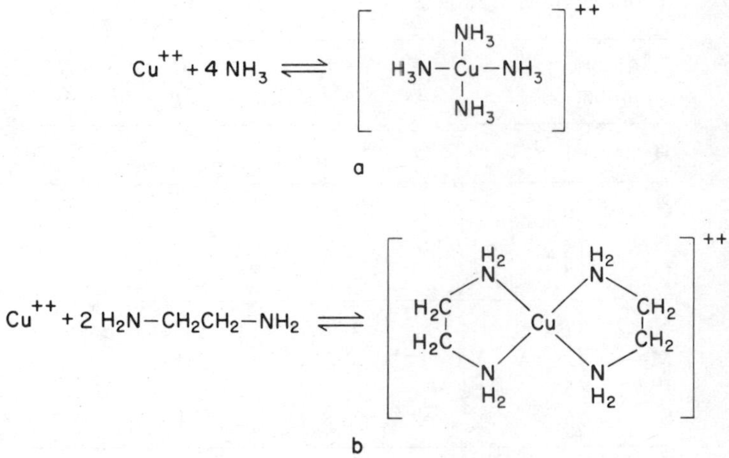

a

b

FIGURE 1-6. Copper coordination complexes.

Figure 1-6 depicts the formation of coordinate covalent bonds between four nitrogen atoms and a cupric ion (Cu^{2+}), resulting in a stable complex. Cupric ion has nine instead of ten electrons in its $3d$ orbital (cf. Table 1-2) and zero instead of one electron in its $4s$ orbital, the double positive charge reflecting the excess of protons over electrons in the whole ionized atom. The pairs of electrons contributed by the ammonia nitrogen atoms complete a stable octet for copper; but because no electrons have been gained or lost in the reaction, there is no change in net charge.

Chelation is the formation of coordination complexes through ring systems, often 5- or 6-membered rings. Such a complex is shown in Figure 1-6b, between the bidentate (i.e., containing "two teeth") chelating agent ethylenediamine and the cupric ion. The donation of electrons by four nitrogen atoms is identical to that in the copper–ammonia complex, but here the metal atom is held very much more tightly, in two 5-membered rings. A tetradentate chelating agent of considerable pharmacologic importance, ethylenediaminetetraacetate (EDTA, edetate, edathamil), is shown in Figure 1-7, together with its calcium complex.

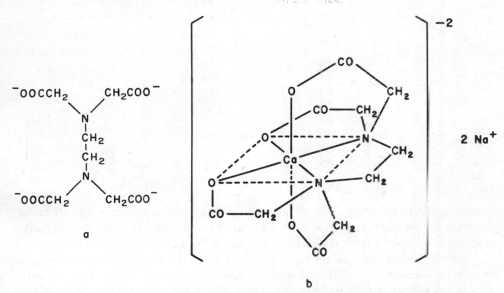

FIGURE 1-7. Ethylenediaminetetraacetate (EDTA) (a) and its salt, calcium disodium edatate (b). *In (b) bonds are shown in solid lines, a plane of reference is indicated by broken lines. (From Martell, p. 9.[29] By permission of J. B. Lippincott.)*

Chelate complexes vary greatly in stability (i.e., in the tendency to dissociate) depending upon the nature of the chelating agent and of the complexed atom. Stability is expressed quantitatively by the "stability constant" K in the mass law equation for the equilibrium relationship between free and complexed reactants, as follows:

$$\text{metal} + \text{chelating agent} \underset{k_2}{\overset{k_1}{\rightleftharpoons}} \text{complex}$$

$$\frac{(\text{complex})}{(\text{metal}) \times (\text{chelating agent})} = \frac{k_1}{k_2} = K$$

For any given chelating agent the magnitude of the stability constants is determined largely by the atomic structures of the various metals, so that the rank order of the metals remains roughly the same regardless of which particular chelating agent may be used. A typical rank order is shown in Table 1-3, for the complexing of different metals by EDTA. The very wide range of stabilities, extending over many orders of

TABLE 1-3. Stabilities of chelate complexes of various metal ions with EDTA.
(From Martell and Calvin, Appendix I.[30] By permission of Prentice–Hall.)

Metal ion	Log of stability constant of complex
Na^+	1.7
Li^+	2.8
Ba^{2+}	7.8
Sr^{2+}	8.6
Mg^{2+}	8.7
Ca^{2+}	10.6
Mn^{2+}	13.4
Fe^{2+}	14.4
Co^{2+}	16.1
Zn^{2+}	16.1
Cu^{2+}	18.3
Ni^{2+}	18.4
Cd^{2+}	16.4
Pb^{2+}	18.2

magnitude, is noteworthy. A metal with a higher stability constant would effectively compete for the chelating agent with a metal of lower stability and, given sufficient time, would displace the less tightly bound metal from complexes already formed.[30]

Naturally occurring chelate complexes are known to play important roles in biologic systems. It may well be that the principal importance of the metals essential for life lies in their ability to form functional chelate complexes. These are evidently well suited to act as bridges to facilitate electron transfer, such as must occur in the catalytic formation or cleavage of any covalent bond. In cytochrome c, for example, as in other heme proteins, an iron atom is chelated, forming four 6-membered rings containing the pyrrole nitrogen atoms of the porphyrin nucleus. Two additional coordinate covalent bonds hold the complexed iron to imidazole N of histidine residues in the associated protein. Analogous chelate complexes of biologic importance are chlorophyll (a magnesium complex) and vitamin B_{12} (a cobalt complex).

Magnesium and other divalent cations that behave as enzyme activators are thought to function by binding substrate at the active site through chelation. This role is illustrated for the zinc enzyme carboxypeptidase in Figure 1-8. The Zn^{2+} ion is bound to S^- of the single cysteine residue of the protein, and also by a coordinate covalent bond to N of the amino-terminal asparagine residue. The substrate is probably held to Zn^{2+} by coordinate bonds to carbonyl O and peptide N, thus forming a chelate ring. Binding of substrate to electron donor (B) and proton donor (A) groups of the protein is also postulated. The peptide bond could then be weakened by the tendency of the metal ion to draw electrons away from it, so that an acyl enzyme intermediate would be formed, which could then react with OH^- to regenerate $-COOH$. The ionic radius of Zn^{2+} plays a key role in determining reaction specificity. Substitution of other metals for zinc not only diminishes or abolishes the usual

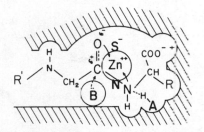

FIGURE 1-8. Postulated interaction of a terminal dipeptide with carboxypeptidase. *The zinc ion is bound to a cysteine sulfur atom and an asparagine
nitrogen atom of the enzyme; these groups are shown just above and below Zn^{2+}. B is an
electron donor group and A is a proton donor group of the enzyme. Partial ionic
character of the carbonyl oxygen and carbon is indicated in the usual way. The postulated
series of electron shifts, which weakens the peptide bond as described in the text, are
shown by arrows. (From Vallee, Figure 7.[31])*

peptidase action, but may at the same time greatly enhance a completely different
catalytic action, such as hydrolysis of ester bonds.[31,32]

Any discussion of the tight complexing of metals to receptors calls for special
consideration of sulfhydryl groups in proteins and coenzymes. Bonds between sulfur
and metal ions, which may be ionic, covalent, or of mixed type, are exceptionally
strong. This is reflected in the practically irreversible character of such metal sulfides
as AgS, HgS, CuS, and PbS. When a metal-sulfur bond is included in a chelate ring,
stability is greatly enhanced. Such chelation may involve oxygen or nitrogen in
addition to sulfur, but the most stable chelate structures of this type are those in
which two sulfur atoms participate in a 5- or 6-membered mercaptide ring (Figure 1-9).

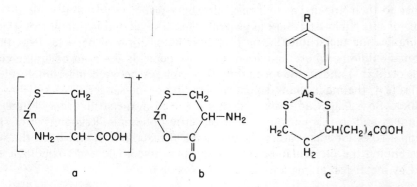

FIGURE 1-9. Two forms of a zinc-cysteine chelate (a and b) and the
probable structure of the complex between dihydrolipoic acid and organic
arsenical (c).

Thus, mercaptide formation may proceed in several ways, as depicted in Figure 1-10.
Such reactions are important because certain enzymes require –SH as part of their
active centers, and because –SH groups or specific –S–S– bonds often play key roles
in the maintenance of the correct configuration of a protein. Sulfhydryl-combining
reagents such as *p*-chloromercuribenzoate (PCMB) have long been employed as
enzyme inhibitors, and pharmacologic agents containing a heavy metal atom in an
organic molecule are quite common. For example, organic mercurials act as diuretic

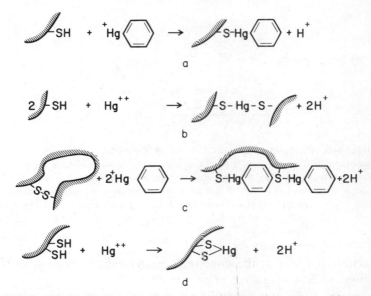

FIGURE 1.10. Four different modes of mercaptide formation with a protein (cysteine) sulfhydryl group.

agents, and organic arsenicals, antimonials, and bismuth compounds have chemotherapeutic efficacy against certain spirochetal and protozoan parasites. Organic silver compounds are effective antibacterial antiseptics. The heavy metals have toxic effects in man, particularly upon the liver, kidneys, heart, and brain.[33]

Chelation is not only important in binding substrates to their enzymes and coenzymes to their apoenzymes; it may also be a primary mechanism for the maintenance of subcellular structure in general. This is suggested by the growing body of data implicating metal ions in the reversible association of particles (e.g., the two ribosomal subunits, whose functional integrity depends upon an adequate concentration of Mg^{2+}) and in the formation of complexes between macromolecules and particles (e.g., the magnesium-dependent binding of messenger RNA to ribosomes). Metallic cations (e.g., Ca^{2+}) are evidently involved in the structure and function of membranes and in the generation of bioelectric potentials. Recognition of specific functional roles for metal atoms in biochemical reactions should open the way to understanding the molecular basis of many pharmacologic and toxicologic effects caused by metal-containing and metal-complexing drugs.[34]

The Ionic Bond and the Hydrogen Bond.   The *ionic bond* results from coulombic forces (electrostatic attraction) between oppositely charged ions. The bond strength is approximately 5 kcal mole^{-1} and the force of attraction between the ions diminishes as the square of the distance between them. Proteins and nucleic acids have many potential anionic and cationic groups, but only a restricted set of these is actually ionized in the physiological pH range. As shown in Table 1-4, the anionic groups of proteins are the terminal carboxyl groups, the carboxyl groups of aspartic acid and glutamic acid, and to some extent the sulfhydryl groups of cysteine. The anionic groups of nucleic acids are the phosphoryl residues. Cationic groups appear in lysine, arginine, histidine, amide $-NH_2$ of glutamine and asparagine, and terminal amino $-NH_2$ of proteins. Mucopolysaccharides contain anionic sulfate residues, and cationic

TABLE 1-4. Ionizing groups in proteins and nucleic acids.
For discussion of pK'_a see pp. 19–20. (Data of Jordan,[40] Cohn and Edsall,[41] and Steinhardt and Beychok,[42] Table II. By permission of Reinhold Publishing Corp. and Academic Press.)

Group	Potential charge	pK'_a
I. *Groups completely or almost completely ionized at pH 7.4*		
α-carboxyl (terminal –COOH)	−	1.8–2.4
β-carboxyl (*asp*)	−	3.7
γ-carboxyl (*glu*)	−	4.3
primary phosphoryl (terminal)	−	0.7–1.0
secondary phosphoryl	−	5.9–6.0
ε-ammonium (*lys*)	+	10.5
guanidinium (*arg*)	+	12.5
II. *Groups partially ionized at pH 7.4*		
sulfhydryl (*cys*)	−	8.2
imidazolium N (*his*)	+	6.0
α-ammonium (terminal –NH₂)	+	7.5–10.3
amide N (*gln*)	+	9.1
amide N (*asn*)	+	8.8
III. *Groups practically nonionized at pH 7.4*		
phenolic hydroxyl (*tyr*)	−	10.0
aromatic hydroxyl (uracil, thymine, guanine)	−	9.2–9.8
sugar hydroxyl	−	12.3–12.6
aromatic amino (adenine, guanine, cytosine)	+	3.3–4.6

amino sugars may occur in other macromolecules. In any particular instance the availability of charged groups for interaction will depend upon the composition and tertiary structure of the receptor macromolecule. An ionic group, for example, may be folded into a completely inaccessible location, or may already be bonded internally to another ionic group of the same protein. In the case of the nucleic acids the phosphoryl groups may serve as ionic links to an associated basic protein (e.g., a histone) and thus be unavailable for interaction.

Drugs may contain potential cationic and anionic groups of all kinds, capable of forming ionic bonds with oppositely charged receptor groups. The influence of pH upon the ionization of drugs is discussed later. Electrostatic attraction may operate between ionized receptor groups and atoms of a drug molecule that are not obviously ionized but have a partial ionic character. The carbonyl group offers a good illustration. Here, the electrons forming the C=O bond are known to be shared unequally. The oxygen atom has a relative excess, the carbon atom a relative deficit. Thus the bonded pair as a whole is a dipole, either end of which may be attracted to another ion. Interactions are known, for example, in which the carbonyl carbon atom, by virtue of its partial positive charge, combines with an anionic site of an enzyme or other receptor surface. An example has already been shown in Figure 1-5.

The *hydrogen bond*[35] is a special kind of ionic bond that arises from the ability of a proton to accept an electron pair in part from each of two electron donor atoms such as oxygen or nitrogen, and thus to form a bridge approximately 3 A in length

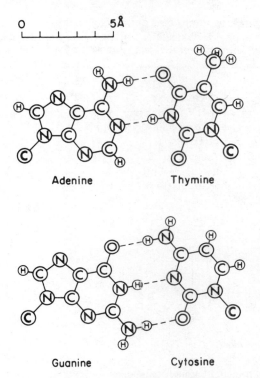

FIGURE 1-11. Specific hydrogen bonding between the complementary base pairs of DNA. *Pairing of adenine and thymine and of guanine and cytosine in the double-helical DNA molecule. Hydrogen bonds are shown as dotted lines. The 1'C atom of each deoxyribose residue is also shown. (From Stent, Figure 3-9.[36] By permission of W. H. Freeman.)*

between them. The bond strength is very much less than for a covalent bond (only about 2–5 kcal mole^{-1}) but the additive effects of several such bonds can stabilize an interaction significantly. This is best illustrated by the hydrogen bonding between complementary base pairs in the DNA helix (Figure 1-11). Here, the hydrogen bonds not only determine the specific complementarity of A-T and G-C pairs, but the total of two to three hydrogen bonds per pair, multiplied by many hundreds of base pairs in the long DNA molecule, confers a high degree of stability on the whole structure (Figure 1-12). These bonds are broken by thermal agitation at quite high "melting temperatures," usually around 80° or higher.[38] They are broken in the process of DNA replication at much lower temperatures, but it is thought that only one base pair at a time is separated as the double helix unwinds; the exact mechanism, however, is not yet known.

The ability to form hydrogen bonds underlies the specificity of those drugs which are incorporated into nucleic acids by a "counterfeit" mechanism, in place of natural bases (p.117). They can stabilize complexes between drugs and receptors which would otherwise interact only weakly. They play a major role in determining the tertiary structure of proteins by linking amino acid residues that are widely separated in the primary chain, and thus stabilizing the specific folded conformations. Finally, internal hydrogen bonds may greatly affect the physical properties of drug molecules. This is illustrated by the properties of salicylic acid, the ortho isomer of hydroxy-

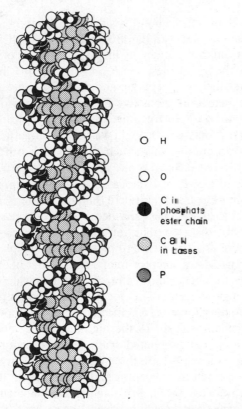

FIGURE 1-12. A segment of the DNA duplex, hydrogen bonded at each base pair. (*From Stent,*[36] *Figure 3-9, after Feughelman et al.,*[37] *Figure 1; by permission of W. H. Freeman and Macmillan Journals Ltd.*)

benzoic acid (Figure 1-13). The intramolecular hydrogen bond in this molecule effectively reduces the affinities of both the carboxyl and the phenolic hydroxyl groups for water molecules, and thus drastically alters the solubility. The para and

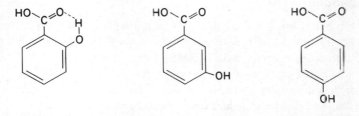

o-hydroxybenzoic acid   m-hydroxybenzoic acid   p-hydroxybenzoic acid
(salicylic acid)

FIGURE 1-13. Isomers of hydroxybenzoic acid.

meta isomers, which cannot possibly form such an intramolecular hydrogen bond, are soluble to the extent of about 1 g/100 ml water at 20°, whereas salicylic acid is soluble to less than one fifth this amount.[39]

The van der Waals Bond.   This bond is a very weak interaction between dipoles or induced dipoles, often between similar atoms. Because of their abundance in organic molecules, carbon atoms are principally involved in bonds of this type between drugs and receptors. The theory of these close-range attractive forces was developed by van der Waals, and further by Heitler and London, whose names are commonly used in describing them. The attractive forces (also known as *electron correlation attraction*[43]) arise from slight distortions induced in the electron clouds surrounding each nucleus as two atoms are brought very close together. Very weak transient atomic dipoles are produced, which then attract each other electrostatically. The bond energy is only about 0.5 kcal mole^{-1}. The force of attraction is inversely proportional to the seventh power of distance, so a very close approximation of the interacting atoms is much more important here than for ordinary ionic bonds. It might be imagined, because of their weakness and because they decrease so rapidly with slight increase of interatomic distance, that van der Waals forces would be unimportant. On the contrary, there is every reason to believe that they play a major role in determining the specificity of drug-receptor interactions. First of all, when these forces are summed over a large number of interacting atoms, a considerable binding may result albeit the individual bond is weak, as for hydrogen bonding in DNA. Second, the very fact that the binding force is so critically dependent upon interatomic distance provides a physicochemical basis for the high degree of selectivity that may be observed among a series of closely related drugs, a phenomenon ascribed to "goodness of fit." Thus, a drug molecule whose three-dimensional shape (conformation) allows a very close approximation to a receptor surface is said to "fit" that receptor better (and therefore to be more effective there) than a related molecule with slightly different conformation. As a drug molecule approaches the receptor surface, a sharp increase in binding force will be manifested quite abruptly (provided a close enough approach is possible), as many electron correlation attractions come into play simultaneously. In this situation even a minor degree of misfit could, by impeding the necessary perfect approximation of the complementary molecular surfaces, produce a major disruptive effect upon the overall binding.

Drug-Receptor Interaction as Resultant of the Several Bond Types

The binding force that holds a drug in combination with its receptor arises from the concerted operation of numerous bonds of the several types discussed. Once distributive and diffusive processes have brought a drug molecule into the vicinity of a receptor surface, random thermal agitation produces multiple collisions with that surface. The drug is usually in solution, that is to say, surrounded wholly or partly by water molecules. The receptor surface, likewise, by virtue of its polar groups, can be thought of as covered by a sheath of water molecules. The binding of the drug to the receptor must then entail the mutual squeezing out of the intervening water layers. The interaction as a whole is therefore sometimes described as the formation of hydrophobic bonds.

Let us consider the probable course of events as a drug molecule approaches its receptor. Consider the fields of force as one moves outward, away from the receptor surface, into the surrounding aqueous medium. The van der Waals attraction will fall off to a negligible value at a relatively short distance, but the coulombic forces, which diminish only as the square of the distance, will continue to be felt farther from the center of the charge density. Therefore, although usually only one or a few ionic bonds are formed, the earliest attraction that draws an approaching drug molecule toward its receptor is often an electrostatic one.

In order to result in a significant drug action, and in order for specificity to be manifested, the primary interaction has to be reinforced by accessory bonds. Indeed, the energy of thermal agitation at 37° is sufficient to disrupt a single, unreinforced ionic bond. Here, hydrogen bonds, van der Waals attractions, and covalent bonds (if any are to be formed) come into play. A good fit will allow a maximum area of close approximation between the drug and the receptor, bringing appropriate groups on both surfaces into close enough contact (1–3 A) for bond formation. Even without formation of a covalent bond, the concerted effects of ionic bonds, hydrogen bonds, and dipole-induced dipole bonds may yield quite stable complexes. One of the fascinating aspects of pharmacology is the seeming paradox that many drugs are obviously unreactive in the chemical sense, yet biologically these same inert molecules may be highly potent, extremely selective, and also bound remarkably tightly to components of living cells. With most drugs, however, the binding to receptors is not so tight as to preclude dissociation entirely. A reversible interaction is established, which obeys the law of mass action. If this were not so, most drugs would have exceedingly long persistence and duration of action in the body.

The Ionization of Drugs

An acid is a proton donor, a base is a proton acceptor. The strength of the bond between proton and base is determined by the electron-attracting or electron-repelling properties of other atoms in the molecule. This bond strength determines the extent of ionization at a given pH, as reflected in the pK'_a (negative logarithm of the acid dissociation constant). Recall that

$$\text{acid} \underset{k_2}{\overset{k_1}{\rightleftharpoons}} \text{base} + H^+$$

At equilibrium,

$$k_1(\text{acid}) = k_2(\text{base})(H^+)$$

$$(H^+) = \frac{k_1}{k_2} \cdot \frac{(\text{acid})}{(\text{base})} = K'_a \cdot \frac{(\text{acid})}{(\text{base})}$$

whence the Henderson–Hasselbalch equation:

$$pH = -\log(H^+) = pK'_a + \log\frac{(\text{base})}{(\text{acid})}$$

and at 50% ionization, log (base)/(acid) = 0, so

$$pK'_a = pH$$

Most drugs contain weak acidic or basic groups (or both), so that their states of ionization, which influence their interactions with receptors, will depend upon the pK'_a values of these groups and upon the ambient pH.

The concepts of acid and base should not be confused with those of cation and anion. They are unrelated, except that by virtue of proton dissociation a base necessarily has one less positive charge than its conjugate acid. Figure 1-14 presents a few examples.

Acid		Base			pK_a'
$CH_3\overset{\displaystyle O}{\overset{\|}{C}}-OH$	$\rightleftharpoons$	$CH_3\overset{\displaystyle O}{\overset{\|}{C}}-O^-$	$+$	H^+	4.8
NH_4^+	$\rightleftharpoons$	NH_3	$+$	H^+	9.3
H_2CO_3	$\rightleftharpoons$	HCO_3^-	$+$	H^+	6.5
H_3PO_4	$\rightleftharpoons$	$H_2PO_4^-$	$+$	H^+	2.0
$H_2PO_4^-$	$\rightleftharpoons$	$HPO_4^=$	$+$	H^+	7.1
$HPO_4^=$	$\rightleftharpoons$	$PO_4^{\equiv}$	$+$	H^+	12.3

FIGURE 1-14. Some examples of acid-base equilibria.

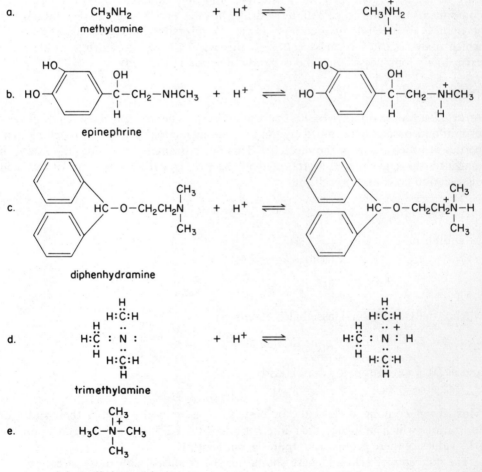

a. CH_3NH_2 methylamine $+ \; H^+ \rightleftharpoons \; CH_3\overset{+}{N}H_2$

b. epinephrine

c. diphenhydramine

d. trimethylamine

e. tetramethylammonium

FIGURE 1-15. Tertiary nitrogen compounds and their ionization (a–d), and a quaternary compound (e).

The ability of nitrogen to donate an unshared pair of electrons, already discussed in connection with the coordinate covalent bond, plays a central role in the ionization of drugs. Compounds containing trivalent nitrogen are capable of associating with hydrogen ion and thereby acquiring a positive charge. This is shown in Figure 1-15 for three different drugs. Methylamine contains a primary amino group, epinephrine a secondary amino group, and diphenhydramine a tertiary amino group, but all can become cations under acidic conditions. The mechanism, which is the same for all three, is indicated in Figure 1-15d, using trimethylamine as an example. Since the ability to neutralize a hydrogen ion resembles the behavior of alkalis, drugs of this kind that occur in plant material were called "alkaloids." Alkaloidal drugs, in the free base form, tend to be poorly soluble in water; but if they are treated with acid the acquired positive charge results in a greatly enhanced solubility. Acid salts of these compounds may be crystallized, and these will then dissolve readily in pure water. It should be understood that the particular anion, or cation, with which a drug molecule is associated has no influence upon that drug's biologic action. Just as the properties of Na^+ in solution are the same, whether derived from $NaCl$ or $(Na)_2SO_4$, so the actions of morphine sulfate are not distinguished from those of morphine hydrochloride. However, the official names of drugs as given in the United States Pharmacopeia[44] or other compendia, specify particular salts. Certain salts are so insoluble that they may influence the rate of absorption of a compound.

If a nitrogen atom donates its unshared electron pair to an atom other than hydrogen (usually a carbon atom), thus forming a coordinate covalent bond, the nitrogen atom is said to be quaternized (Figure 1-15e). Drugs containing quaternary nitrogen are not bases (although they are sometimes erroneously called that) but are permanent organic cations, for they cannot lose their positive charge at any pH. In contrast, tertiary nitrogen compounds have a pK_a that is usually near the physiologic pH range. A large fraction of their molecules may be cationic at pH 7.4, but these are in equilibrium with some nonionized free base. This difference between tertiary and quaternary nitrogen compounds has important implications for the passage of drugs across membranes (cf. Chapter 2), and it also provides a basis for investigating the role of ionic bonds in drug-receptor interactions, as illustrated below.

The physiologic substrate of the enzyme acetylcholinesterase is the quaternary ester acetylcholine. Neostigmine, an inhibitor of the enzyme, is also a quaternary ester and a structural analog of the substrate. Another inhibitor is physostigmine, a naturally occurring alkaloid and also a structural analog of the substrate; its pK_a' is 8.5. These compounds are shown in Figure 1-16. It is supposed that acetylcholine forms an ionic bond with an anionic site in the active center of the enzyme (Figure 1-5), and it is also supposed that inhibitors which are structural analogs must interact at the same anionic site.

The broad pH optimum of the enzyme permits studies to be carried out over a wide range of pH values to determine whether the efficacy of an inhibitor depends upon pH. On the hypothesis that a positive charge (as in acetylcholine) is essential for interaction with the enzyme, one would predict that inhibition by neostigmine (the quaternary inhibitor) should be independent of pH. Inhibition by physostigmine, on the other hand, should be greatest on the acid side of its pK_a', when practically all molecules are cationic, falling towards zero on the alkaline side as bound protons dissociate. The observations illustrated in Figure 1-17 were in general agreement with these predictions. However, according to the simplest model, the relationship of

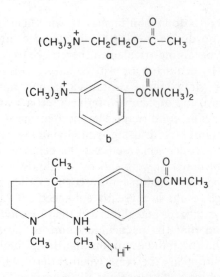

FIGURE 1-16. Acetylcholine (a); neostigmine (b); and physostigmine, cationic form (c).

inhibition to pH should be identical to a pH-ionization curve for a base with pK'_a = 8.5. The lack of strict conformity, shown in Figure 1-17, indicates that complicating factors are present.

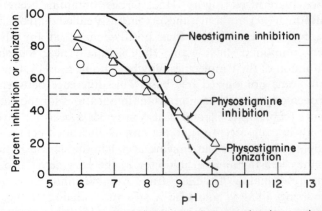

FIGURE 1-17. Inhibition of cholinesterase by neostigmine and physostigmine as a function of pH, and the ionization of physostigmine. (*Adapted from Wilson and Bergmann, Figure 1.*[45])

STRUCTURE-ACTIVITY RELATIONSHIPS AND THE CONFORMATION OF THE RECEPTOR SURFACE

Methods of Studying Receptors

There are two ways to gain information about a receptor. The first and only really satisfactory approach is to identify and isolate it. Then the investigation can follow established biochemical and physicochemical procedures. The mode of interaction with a drug can be studied by means of electron spin resonance, fluorescence, and other spectrometric techniques. Analytical ultracentrifugation and high-resolution electron micrography can yield information about size, shape, and density. Nuclear magnetic resonance and x-ray crystallography provide data from which secondary and tertiary structure may be deduced. Finally, sequence analysis can establish the primary structure of the macromolecule. These direct approaches to the study of receptors are discussed in later sections of this chapter.

The second way of obtaining information about receptors is indirect. It has dominated pharmacologic research in the past. The approach is to draw inferences about a receptor from the biologic end results caused by drugs. A powerful tool employed toward this end has been the study of structure-activity relationships (abbreviated SAR).[46-53] A suitable biologic effect of a drug is chosen for study. A prototype drug, which elicits the characteristic effect, is then modified systematically in its molecular structure. Substituents are added or subtracted at various positions and in different steric configurations. A series of such chemically related drugs is known as a congeneric series. By testing the members of a series and observing how biologic potency is affected by each molecular modification, one may ultimately draw conclusions about the precise mode of combination of a drug with its receptor surface. In the following sections we illustrate, with selected examples, the types of information that can be obtained in SAR studies, and the kinds of inference (and their limitations) that can be drawn about the nature of the drug-receptor interaction and the conformation of the receptor surface.

Acetylcholine and Congeners

Acetylcholine (AcCh) is a neurotransmitter which is released from cholinergic neurons at many locations in the body. It acts upon receptors in skeletal muscle end-plates, in smooth muscles, in cells of secretory glands, in ganglion cells of the autonomic nervous system, and probably in certain nerve cells of the central nervous system. In addition, AcCh receptors are found in smooth muscles that have no cholinergic innervation, for example, most arteriolar smooth muscles.

A convenient tissue upon which the biologic action of AcCh and its congeners can be assayed is the clam heart.[54] This organ beats spontaneously when it is suspended in a bath of sea water, and the frequency and amplitude of the contractions can be recorded, as illustrated in Figure 1-18. A drug to be tested is diluted serially in sea water. A small volume of the most dilute solution is added to the bath. If no effect is observed, a larger volume may be added, and then progressively more concentrated solutions are tried until an action is obtained. Between doses the tissue bath is flushed with sea water to remove the drug. The concentration required to produce any given effect may be estimated by interpolating between doses or by more accurate bio-statistical procedures.[55] In order to make results obtained with different clam hearts comparable, it is customary to use as criterion the concentration of drug that elicits 50% of the maximal effect obtainable; this is referred to as the ED50 (ED = "effective dose").

The characteristic action of AcCh and related compounds on the clam heart is to reduce the amplitude of contraction, as illustrated in Figure 1-19. A major advantage of the clam heart is that it does not hydrolyze choline esters rapidly. Consequently, differences in potency within this series of drugs can be detected readily, uncomplicated by differences in rates of degradation.

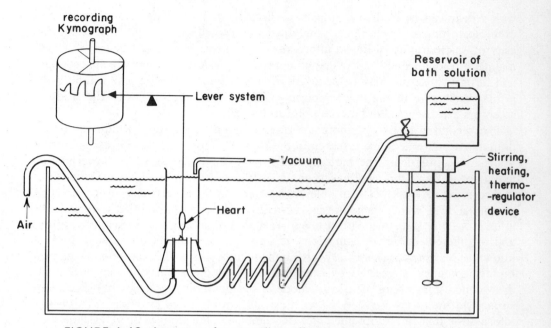

FIGURE 1-18. Apparatus for recording effects of drugs on isolated clam hearts or other muscle tissue. *Agonists, antagonists, or extracts containing unknown substances may be added directly to tissue bath and removed by flushing with several volumes of solution from the reservoir. Bath solution is aerated by a constant stream of air or oxygen.*

The chemical formula of AcCh is shown in Table 1-5 (compound 1). The salient features are: (a) a quaternary nitrogen atom bearing a positive charge and surrounded by three methyl groups; (b) a two-carbon methylene chain; (c) an oxygen atom in the main axis of the molecule; (d) a carbonyl oxygen atom about 5 A from the cationic charge; and (e) a two-carbon acyl residue. The relative importance of some of these

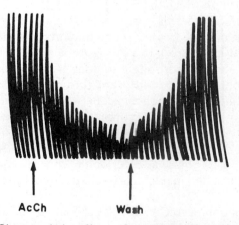

AcCh   Wash

FIGURE 1-19. Characteristic effect of acetylcholine upon spontaneously beating clam heart. *Record on kymograph drum is depicted. Contractions cause upward deflection. Addition of AcCh, and removal of AcCh by washing, are shown by arrows. (After Welsh and Taub, Figure 1.[56])*

TABLE 1-5. SAR data for AcCh and some congeners.
The trimethylammonium group remains unmodified throughout this series.
(Data of Welsh and Taub.[56,57] By permission of Williams & Wilkins.)

Compound	Relative potency (AcCh = 1000)
1. $CH_3 - {}^+N-CH_2-CH_2-O-\overset{\displaystyle O}{\overset{\|}{C}}-CH_3$ (AcCh), with CH_3 groups above and below N	1000
2. $-CH_2-CH_2-CH_2-\overset{\displaystyle O}{\overset{\|}{C}}-CH_3$	83
3. $-CH_2-CH_2-O-CH_2-CH_3$	15
4. $-CH_2-CH_2-CH_2-CH_2-CH_3$	14
5. $-CH_2-CH_2-\overset{\displaystyle O}{\overset{\|}{C}}-CH_2-CH_3$	6.2
6. $-CH_2-\overset{\displaystyle O}{\overset{\|}{C}}-CH_2-CH_2-CH_3$	1.6
7. $-CH_3$	0.05
8. $-CH_2-CH_3$	0.07
9. $-CH_2-CH_2-CH_3$	3.0
10. $-CH_2-CH_2-CH_2-CH_3$	4.3
11. $-CH_2-CH_2-CH_2-CH_2-CH_2$	21.5[a]
12. $-CH_2-CH_2-CH_2-CH_2-CH_2-CH_3$	2.9
13. $-CH_2-CH_2-CH_2-CH_2-CH_2-CH_2-CH_3$	0.05

[a] The difference between this value and that for the identical compound 4 results from the determinations being carried out on different occasions

features was explored by systematic testing of congeners on the clam heart, with the results shown in Table 1-5.

When the oxygen atom in the ester bond was replaced by a methylene group, so that this portion of the molecule became an aliphatic ketone (compound 2), potency dropped to about 8 %. When, on the other hand, the carbonyl oxygen atom alone was eliminated, leaving an ether oxygen atom in the main chain (compound 3), potency was reduced to 1.5 %. If, however, the ether oxygen in compound 3 was replaced by carbon (compound 4), there was no further change in potency. Thus, the full biologic effect of AcCh on this system requires the ester structure, but the carbonyl group itself plays a significant role. Compounds 5 and 6 show that the exact position of the carbonyl group, 5 A from the cationic nitrogen atom, is very important.

In another series of molecular modifications the length of the alkyl chain was varied, all oxygen atoms having been eliminated. Compounds 7–13 show clearly that a five-carbon chain is optimal. Choline does not differ in potency from compound 8, from which it differs only by an alcoholic $-OH$. Finally, changes in the alkyl groups attached to the nitrogen atom were tried. Starting with AcCh, one methyl group at a time was removed. The results (not shown in Table 1-5) were clear-cut. The analogous dimethylamine, which still retained a positive charge by accepting a proton, was nearly as potent as AcCh itself. The monomethylamine, however, showed a striking loss of potency, although it was still cationic, and the unsubstituted primary amine was practically inert. In the other direction, when one of the AcCh methyl groups was replaced by ethyl, there was little loss of activity. When a second group was changed to ethyl, activity was reduced drastically. When more than two groups were so replaced, an excitatory rather than inhibitory effect on the clam heart was produced. The uncharged carbon analog of AcCh, dimethylbutyl acetate,

$$CH_3-\underset{\underset{CH_3}{|}}{\overset{\overset{CH_3}{|}}{C}}-CH_2-CH_2-O-\overset{\overset{O}{\|}}{C}-CH_3$$

was wholly inert.

These findings, referred to a three-dimensional molecular model of AcCh (Figure 1-20a), permit one to draw certain conclusions about the nature of the receptor site in the clam heart (Figure 1-20b). The requirement for a cationic group at one end of

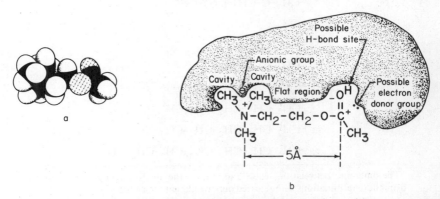

FIGURE 1.20. Acetylcholine and its postulated interaction with a receptor.

the drug molecule indicates the presence of a complementary anionic group on the receptor surface. The steric model reveals that the nitrogen atom, bearing its substituent methyl groups, is free to rotate with relation to the carbon chain. The changes in activity on methyl removal and ethyl substitution on the cationic "head" therefore suggest that the anionic site on the receptor is embedded in a cavity that will just accommodate two methyl groups. Since one of the three symmetrically disposed methyls must necessarily point away from the receptor surface, and since free rotation makes all three methyls equivalent, removing one or changing it to ethyl has little effect. We assume that the two essential methyl groups help to stabilize the AcCh-receptor complex through van der Waals forces, and that any larger substituent, not fitting properly into the cavity, seriously distorts the goodness of fit of the rest of the molecule to its complementary site. It is likely that the carbon atoms of the main chain lie in close approximation to a flat portion of the receptor surface, contributing further van der Waals attractions to the overall binding. The carbonyl oxygen atom might well participate in hydrogen bond formation with an appropriate receptor group (e.g., the −NH of a peptide bond), thus further stabilizing the interaction. Although wholly inferential, such a picture offers a consistent and reasonable explanation of the SAR data.[59]

The broad deductions from SAR data have been refined considerably through x-ray crystallographic studies on crystals of acetylcholine and its congeners,[60-62] and by measurements on scale models of the molecules.[63] Acetylcholine itself interacts at two different kinds of receptor site—the nicotinic site at neuromuscular junctions and autonomic ganglia, and the muscarinic site at parasympathetic effectors in smooth muscle and secretory glands. The pharmacologic properties of these sites are discussed elsewhere (p. 73). Each type of site is acted upon specifically by a certain set of congeners. Thus, whereas AcCh itself has the appropriate molecular structure to interact with either kind of receptor, nicotine (for example) acts only at nicotinic sites, muscarine only at muscarinic sites. Consistent with these pharmacologic observations, AcCh is relatively flexible and capable of assuming various conformations. Congeners containing ring systems, like nicotine and muscarine, have much more rigid structures, permitting unambiguous inferences about which atoms and distances are critical for the given pharmacologic action.

The essential features are shown in Figure 1-21. Nicotinic agents, including drugs that block at nicotinic sites, have a common structural pattern, shown at the top of the figure. In addition to a cationic center, there is a group 5.9 A distant that can act as an acceptor for a hydrogen bond. In AcCh and some of its congeners this is the carbonyl oxygen, but in nicotine it is the pyridine nitrogen. In the muscarinic series (bottom) the hydrogen bond acceptor is an oxygen atom at 4.4 A from the center of positive charge. This is the esteratic oxygen in AcCh, the ring oxygen in muscarine. In addition, a methyl group corresponding to the acetyl methyl in AcCh or the ring methyl in muscarine strongly reinforces the interaction.

The Polymethylene Bismethonium Series

Good examples of acetylcholine antagonist drugs are the polymethylene bismethonium compounds, which block certain classes of AcCh receptors. The prototype structure is

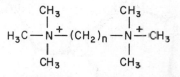

polymethylene bismethonium

These molecules are perfectly symmetrical, containing two cationic groups separated by a simple aliphatic chain. The only molecular variable to be considered here is n, the number of carbon atoms in the polymethylene chain or, in other words, the distance between the two positively charged nitrogen atoms.

Two distinct biologic effects of importance are produced by compounds in this series: *ganglionic blockade* and *neuromuscular blockade*. We shall examine SAR data for both kinds of action in a single species, the cat.[64,65] The assay system for ganglionic

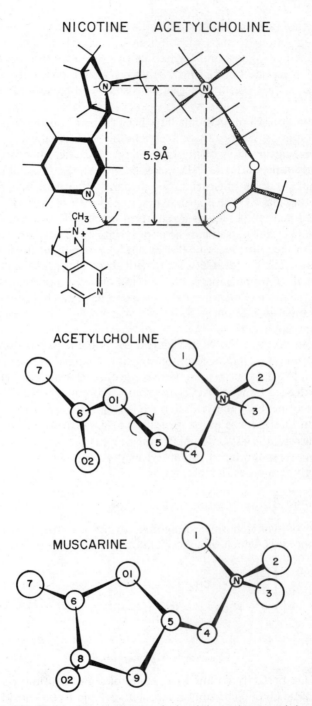

FIGURE 1-21. Molecular structures of nicotinic and muscarinic congeners of AcCh. *Top: l-Nicotine and the corresponding conformation of AcCh, with 5.9 A distance between cationic N and hydrogen bond acceptor group. Bottom: L(+)-Muscarine and the corresponding conformation of AcCh, with 4.4 A distance between cationic N and H-bond acceptor group O1. Group 7 is* CH_3. *(From Beers and Reich,*[63] *Figure 3 and Chothia and Pauling,*[61] *Figures 1 and 3.)*

blockade employs the nictitating membrane. This structure is composed largely of smooth muscle, innervated by postganglionic sympathetic nerve fibers originating in the superior cervical ganglion (Figure 1-22). The ganglion cells whose axons carry

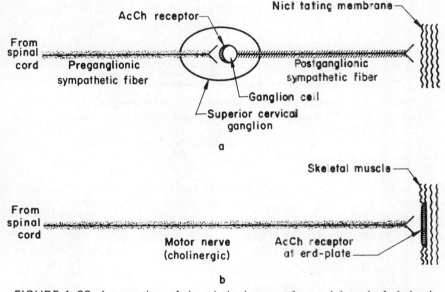

FIGURE 1-22. Innervation of the nictitating membrane (a) and of skeletal muscle (b).

impulses out to the nictitating membrane receive impulses from preganglionic sympathetic nerve fibers, which emerge in the ventral roots of the spinal cord. These preganglionic fibers are cholinergic (i.e., they liberate AcCh) and the ganglion cells upon which they impinge are called "cholinoceptive" (i.e., they contain AcCh receptors). In the assay system the nictitating membrane is attached to a lever or strain gauge for recording its contractions. A continuous train of electrical stimuli to the preganglionic fibers results in a corresponding train of impulses along the post-ganglionic fibers, and the nictitating membrane responds with a sustained contraction. If, during stimulation, synaptic transmission from the preganglionic terminals to the ganglion cells is blocked, then no impulses will arrive at the nictitating membrane, which will therefore relax. If this happens, a simple way to confirm that the blockade is at the ganglion rather than at a more peripheral site is to stimulate the postganglionic fiber electrically and elicit a normal response of the nictitating membrane. In the assay a drug to be tested is injected intravenously at appropriate dosage to produce a certain degree of blockade (Figure 1-23). The relative potencies of various drugs may then be expressed in terms of the ratios of the respective doses that produce the same degree of blockade.

The assay system for skeletal neuromuscular blockade employs any convenient muscle (e.g., tibialis anterior) and the appropriate motor nerve (e.g., sciatic). Motor nerves are cholinergic and skeletal muscle contains specialized cholinoceptive structures (end-plates) where the nerve fibers terminate. In the assay the motor nerve is stimulated at regular intervals by single shocks large enough to elicit maximal contractions from the muscle. These muscle contractions are recorded. A drug-

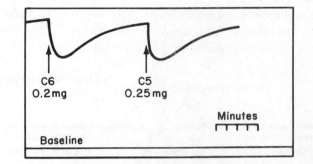

FIGURE 1-23. Typical effects of ganglionic blocking agents on the nictitating membrane of the cat. *Sustained contraction of nictitating membrane excited
by stimulation of cervical sympathetic; hexamethonium (C6) and pentamethonium (C5)
given intravenously at arrows. (From Paton and Zaimis, Figure 10.[64] By permission of
the British Medical Journal.)*

induced blockade of transmission between nerve ending and muscle end-plate
manifests itself as a decline in amplitude and ultimate disappearance of the muscle
twitches (Figure 1-24). During such neuromuscular blockade direct electrical stimulation of the muscle fibers will confirm that their intrinsic capacity for contraction is
unimpaired (arrow 2 in Figure 1-24). The procedure for determining relative drug
potencies is like that described for the cat nictitating membrane preparation.

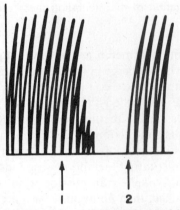

FIGURE 1-24. Typical effect of a neuromuscular blocking agent on cat
nerve-muscle preparation *in situ. Tension recording from tibialis muscle stimulated by nerve shock every 10 sec; at arrow 1, decamethonium (0.1 mg) injected intravenously; at arrow 2, muscle was stimulated directly. (From Paton and Zaimis,
Figure 2.[64] By permission of the British Medical Journal.)*

Eight different compounds were tested in both assay systems, with the results
shown in Figure 1-25. Two distinct optima were found, one at $n = 5$–6 for ganglionic
blockade, another at $n = 10$ for neuromuscular blockade. It is apparent, therefore,
that even though the ganglionic and muscle end-plate receptors both are stimulated
by local release of acetylcholine from nerve endings, these receptors cannot be identical.
One way to interpret the data is shown in Figure 1-26. We assume there is in both
receptors (as we did in the case of the clam heart) a configuration complementary to
that of acetylcholine. That the presence of a second cationic group confers blocking

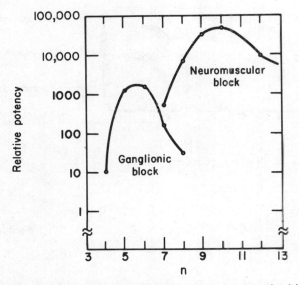

FIGURE 1-25. SAR data for ganglionic and neuromuscular block by polymethylene bismethonium compounds. *The number of* $-CH_2-$ *groups between
cationic groups is n; relative potency has logarithmic scale. (From Paton and Zaimis,
Figure 17.[64] By permission of the British Medical Journal.)*

potency leads us to deduce the presence of a second anionic site on the receptor
surface, lying outside the acetylcholine-combining region. Both anionic sites are presumed to be embedded in cavities capable of accommodating two methyl groups (the
third methyl group is then oriented away from the surface). The essential difference
between the ganglionic and muscle end-plate receptors is presumed to be in the
distance between these anionic sites. As Figure 1-26 demonstrates, the ganglionic site
would interact strongly with pentamethonium, the C5 compound shown at (b), or
with hexamethonium (C6, not shown); these drugs would then act as ganglionic
blockers by preventing the receptor from responding to acetylcholine (a). The C10
compound, decamethonium (c), is too long to fit the ganglionic receptor but would
act as a neuromuscular blocker by preventing the combination of acetylcholine (e)
with muscle end-plate receptor. Finally, succinylcholine (d), a neuromuscular blocking agent of practical importance is shown; it is obviously well endowed for specific
interaction with the muscle end-plate receptor.[66]

The qualitative and quantitative properties of receptors in the same tissue of various
species may be compared. The length of the polymethylene chain was varied, and the
resulting compounds were tested for neuromuscular blockade in the cat, rabbit,
mouse, and rat.[64] Regardless of species, the C10 compound was the most potent,
implying that the muscle end-plate receptors in all four species have anionic sites
at the same separation. The potencies differed, however, over nearly a 1000-fold range.
It has also been shown that various skeletal muscles of a single animal may have
different affinities for the same neuromuscular blocking agent.[67] These observations
are understandable if the receptors are proteins, since so many cases of species and
tissue differences in enzymes and other proteins are already known. Isozymes, for
example, are demonstrably different forms of enzyme protein, which may be present in
varying ratios in different tissues, but which have the same catalytic function. We can

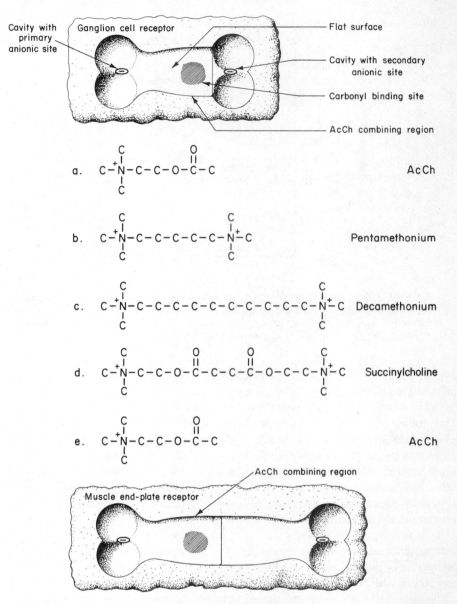

FIGURE 1-26. Hypothetical acetylcholine receptors. *Schematic visualizations of receptors in ganglion cell (above) and in muscle end-plate (below), deduced from SAR data. The structures of AcCh and several blocking agents are shown, with their various chemical groupings aligned to the receptor regions with which they are assumed to interact. A similar AcCh-combining region is shown on both receptors. Pentamethonium shows greatest selectivity for the ganglion cell receptor, decamethonium and succinylcholine for the end-plate receptor.*

speculate on the possibility that genetically determined abnormalities of receptor structure could result in defective function (as in myasthenia gravis) or in unusual sensitivity to a drug.[68,69]

The Narcotic Analgesics

We have seen how systematic variation in the structure of a drug molecule leads to alterations in potency for some specified biologic effect, and how certain inferences can be drawn about the nature of the receptor surface with which the drug must interact. Thus far we have considered only symmetric molecules or those in which free rotation about bonds would permit functional groups to assume various positions in space. We now turn our attention to stereoisomers, the study of whose biological effects has led to what is known as *conformation analysis*. Here, inferences are drawn about the three-dimensional structure of the receptor surface.

In the case of geometric isomers (e.g., *cis-trans* configurations) it is obvious why one of a pair should show preferential biologic activity. In Figure 1-27, for example,

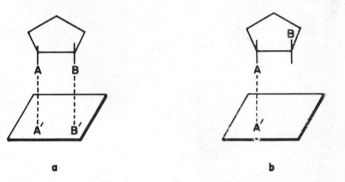

FIGURE 1-27. Geometric isomerism. *The rectangle represents a receptor surface.* (*From Beckett, Figure 2.*[70])

if functional groups A and B both have to interact with complementary groups on the receptor, only the *cis* isomer will have biologic activity. In the case of optical isomers, all interatomic distances are identical in the two enantiomorphs, which are mirror images of each other, but a receptor surface can nevertheless distinguish the two forms. As is the case in many stereospecific enzyme reactions, it is only necessary to suppose that the drug-receptor interaction involves at least three of the groups (or three regions) attached to the asymmetric carbon atom, as illustrated in Figure 1-28. If the complementary interacting regions C', D', and B' were arranged as shown on the left, the optical isomer depicted on the right could not interact properly.

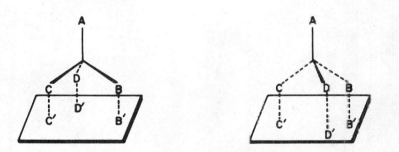

FIGURE 1-28. A pair of optical enantiomorphs, showing the different patterns of projection of three functional groups onto a receptor surface. (*From Beckett, Figure 1.*[70])

SAR studies with a series of narcotic analgesic compounds provide a wealth of material for deducing properties of the receptor that mediates their pain-relieving properties.[70–73] The methods are quite simple. Constant heating is applied to a rat's tail, so that in about 10 sec a tail "flick" is observed. After injection of an analgesic agent into the rat, the tail flick is delayed and may even be abolished. The extent of delay is dose related, so the potencies of various compounds may be compared. For example, the relative doses of different drugs may be found that prolong the tail-flick time to the same extent. It is known that narcotic analgesics act upon pain pathways

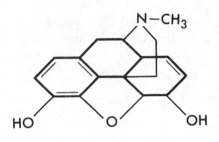

Morphine (a)

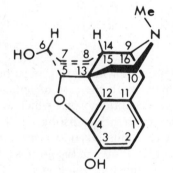

D(−)-Morphine (b)

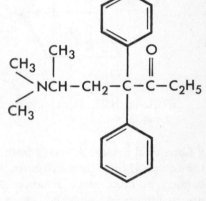

Methadone (c)

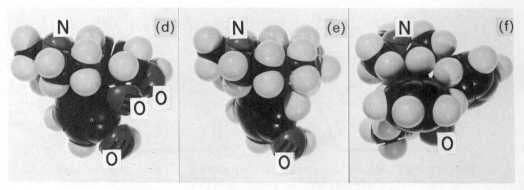

FIGURE 1-29. Structures of the narcotic analgesics.

in the central nervous system and that all the congeners investigated enter the brain and spinal cord readily. However, we have no idea how the analgesic effect is brought about, nor, in particular, what biochemical events might be implicated. It must be remembered, therefore, that the receptor, whose structural features are inferred from the SAR studies to be described, is entirely hypothetical.

Figure 1-29a depicts the morphine molecule in its usual flat representation. This compound was long regarded as a substituted phenanthrene derivative, as indeed it is; but eventually it was realized that although the phenanthrene nucleus could be modified or even eliminated without loss of analgesic activity, the piperidine ring was essential. The nitrogen atom of this ring is about 80% cationic at physiologic pH ($pK'_a = 7.9$), so it is supposed that one important element of the drug-receptor interaction may be an ionic bond to an anionic site on the receptor surface. The narcotic (morphine-like) analgesics are best thought of as N-methylpiperidine compounds with bulky ring substituents.

The naturally occurring isomeric form of morphine is D(−) (Figure 1-29b), i.e., the absolute configuration at carbon atom 13 corresponds to that in D-glyceraldehyde, and the compound is levorotatory. There are several centers of asymmetry: the correct absolute configuration at each one has been established.[74−77] A real understanding of the molecular geometry can only be had from a space-filling scale model. Such a model of D(−)-morphine is shown in Figure 1-29d. The T shape is apparent. The nitrogen atom is positioned in a flat hydrophobic surface containing nine carbon atoms, those of the piperidine ring (C9, C14, C13, C15, C16) and those of the partially unsaturated ring (C13, C5, C6, C7, C8, C14). The other two rings protrude in a perpendicular plane, with the phenolic hydroxyl group at C3 a maximum distance from the nitrogen. The oxygen atom at C3 appears to be essential for activity, suggesting that a hydrogen bond to an amino group in the receptor might stabilize the drug-receptor complex. The alcoholic −OH at C6, the C7–C8 unsaturation, and the oxygen bridge are unnecessary; a synthetic congener, levorphanol (Figure 1-29e), lacks these groups but is more potent than morphine.

It is evident from the molecular model that the two essential groups (nitrogen and phenolic −OH) could not both interact on a flat receptor site. It is surmised, therefore, that the receptor must have the shape of an irregular pouch, into which the narcotic molecule can fit, making the essential contacts on different walls of the pouch. A large part of the hydrophobic regions comprising the cross-piece and stem of the T would ideally come into close contact with hydrophobic areas on the receptor surface, to provide binding through van der Waals forces. This view is supported by the pharmacologic inertness of the L(+) enantiomers throughout the narcotic series; that they have neither agonistic nor antagonistic activity suggests that they are excluded from the receptor site by their "wrong" geometry.

Let us examine another synthetic analgesic, methadone (Figure 1-29c). Here it is astonishing that the compound should behave like morphine, because it seems to be merely an aliphatic chain bearing two benzene rings and a terminal dimethylamine group. Yet molecular models reveal not only that it is possible to arrange the atoms so that they simulate the morphine configuration, but that steric factors force such a configuration upon the compound. As seen in Figure 1-29f, a pseudopiperidine ring is formed, and the benzene rings themselves are not free to rotate about carbon atom 4 of the aliphatic chain (as might have been thought on the basis of the flat structural representation), but are restricted to a conformation like that of the corresponding rings in the phenanthrene nucleus of morphine. Again, of the two optical isomers, only D(−)-methadone, which fits the postulated receptor, is analgesic. Meperidine, a seemingly simple phenylpiperidine carboxylic acid ester, has no center of asymmetry, but one of its possible conformations corresponds to that of the D(−) compounds in the narcotic series.

Certain minor modifications of the D(−)-methadone molecule emphasize further the principle of "goodness of fit" in drug-receptor interactions. If the −CH₃ attached to the carbon atom adjacent to the nitrogen atom is removed, analgesic potency decreases but the compound is still an effective analgesic. If, instead, a second −CH₃ is attached to the same carbon atom, analgesic potency is abolished. Evidently, the groove on the receptor surface will accept

$$-CH_2-\underset{\underset{CH_3}{|}}{CH}-$$

as well as (or somewhat better than) $-CH_2CH_2-$, as would be expected from the fact that the additional methyl group is free to orient outward from the groove. The difficulty with the structure

$$-CH_2-\underset{\underset{CH_3}{|}}{\overset{\overset{CH_3}{|}}{C}}-$$

is presumably that the groove cannot accommodate the additional width at all, or that one methyl group will necessarily project downward; in either case the entire molecule will be prevented from achieving the necessary perfect fit to the receptor surface.

Finally, substitution of allyl $(-CH_2CH=CH_2)$ for methyl on the nitrogen atom produces a remarkable change. Such compounds behave as specific competitive antagonists of analgesia (and other effects) produced by any of the narcotics.[77] It is assumed, therefore, that they interact with the same receptors. When morphine itself is changed in this way, the resulting compound, nalorphine, displays a curious mixture of agonistic and antagonistic actions; it produces some analgesia and also is capable of blocking morphine-induced analgesia, depending upon the dose ratio. Pure antagonists also exist; the most widely used (and the antidote of choice for narcotic overdose) is naloxone, N-allyl oxydihydromorphinone. This compound is of theoretical interest because the complete abolition of agonistic properties (as compared with nalorphine) must be attributed to the hydroxyl group at C14. This substitution places −OH directly adjacent to the N atom, sterically blocking the opportunity for interaction with the receptor at this position.

Congeners of the Adrenal Glucocorticoid Hormones

Another illustration of conformational specificity is found in the steroid hormones of the adrenal cortex, known as glucocorticoids. The prototype structure, that of cortisol (hydrocortisone), an important adrenal hormone in man, is shown in Figure 1-30. In contrast to the morphine-like analgesics, here the active molecules contain no ionizing groups; therefore their interactions with the receptors must depend upon

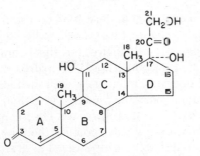

FIGURE 1-30. Cortisol (hydrocortisone, 17-hydroxycorticosterone). *As drawn here, the α surface is away from the reader, α-substituents are indicated by dotted lines; the β surface faces the reader, β-substituents are shown by solid lines.*

conformational fit (and possibly hydrogen bonds), with electron correlation (van der Waals) attractions probably playing the major role in stabilizing the hydrophobic binding.

At physiologic levels in the body these compounds promote the conversion of amino acids to carbohydrate—the glucocorticoid effect. When administered at high dosage they also suppress inflammatory reactions in tissues. The anti-inflammatory effect is not well understood, but it seems to parallel the glucocorticoid action in a large series of compounds of widely differing potencies. Considerable progress has been made in isolating a receptor that appears to be involved in the mediation of these effects (p. 67). The effects upon salt retention (the so-called mineralocorticoid action) are quite independent; cortisol itself has moderate activity of this kind, but other steroids vary widely in the ratio of glucocorticoid to mineralocorticoid activity.

We shall now consider SAR data for glucocorticoid effects only, for a limited set of compounds closely related to cortisol.[78-82] For investigating the influence of structural modifications the liver glycogen deposition test is employed. An alcoholic solution of the steroid to be tested is injected into fasting mice. Some time later (usually 7–12 hr) liver glycogen determinations are performed. Criterion of effect is the increase of liver glycogen content per gram of body weight. Although tests differ in detail, a reference compound is usually employed so that relative potencies may be estimated. Thus, in the following discussion the potency of congeners is always related to that of cortisol.

In order to appreciate the implications of some of the data one must recall that the steroid nucleus is a fairly planar structure (Figure 1-30). There is a lower edge, defined by carbon atoms 3–8, 14, and 15, and an upper edge, defined by carbon atoms 2, 1, 10, 9, 11–13, and 17. In addition, there is an α surface away from the reader (i.e., on the back side of the page), and a β surface, facing the reader. As usual, α-substituents are shown by a broken line, β-substituents by a solid line. The substituent groups in cortisol are a ketonic oxygen at C3, β-methyl groups at C13 and C19, a β-hydroxyl at C11, and a β-glycollyl side chain as well as an α-hydroxyl at C17. Besides, the bond between C4 and C5 is unsaturated. The question is, which of these features of the molecular structure are essential to the glucocorticoid effect, and what may be deduced about the surface of the receptor that mediates this effect?

As for the structural features already present in cortisol, the SAR findings may be summarized as follows. At C11, activity was abolished if the β-hydroxyl was removed or blocked by acetylation or shifted to the α configuration, or even if an α-methyl was introduced without deleting the β-hydroxyl. Also, the β-hydroxyl could be oxidized to ketonic oxygen without loss of activity; but this is not conclusive because body enzymes reduce it to hydroxyl again. Thus, 11-β-hydroxyl is essential to activity and is evidently an important point of interaction with the receptor surface.

Specific quantitative data about the β-methyl at C18 are lacking, but β-methyl at C19 could not be removed without loss of activity. The β configuration of the side chain at C17 was found to confer much greater potency than the α configuration. As to the side chain itself, reduction of C20 to an alcohol led to drastic loss of potency. At C21, oxidation to an aldehyde had no effect; but as was true of oxidation at C11, the conclusion is uncertain because the aldehyde was probably converted back to an alcohol in the body. Replacement of the alcoholic hydroxyl at C21 by halogens, in the order of increasing atomic radius, led to interesting results. With fluorine the potency was enhanced 5-fold, but the larger chlorine or bromine abolished activity. Thus, unlike the situation at C11, the hydroxyl at C21 as such is not essential, but excessive bulk is not tolerated. The adverse effect of bulk at C21 was confirmed by esterifying the hydroxyl with glycine; the resulting compound was inert.

Removal of the α-hydroxyl at C17 (corticosterone) reduced but did not abolish activity. If it was replaced by an acetonide bridge between C16 and C17, activity was enhanced some 5-fold, indicating that the alcoholic hydroxyl as such is not required.

The double bond between C4 and C5 was found to be absolutely essential; hydrogenation here abolished activity. Moreover, a second double bond, between C1 and C2, enhanced activity 5-fold. On the other hand, when ring A contained 3 double bonds, all biologic activity disappeared. Interpretation is ambiguous, however, since making the ring aromatic alters the planar structure and at the same time changes

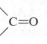

at C3 to

$$\diagdown C=O \diagup$$

$$\diagdown C-OH \diagup$$

Now we turn our attention to substituents that can be added to the cortisol molecule. At C2 we find a situation much like that at C21; a small addition (α-methyl) enhanced activity almost 10-fold, whereas a more bulky group (α-ethyl) abolished it. At C9 a complete series of α-halogen additions have been studied; fluorine enhanced activity some 10-fold, chlorine enhanced to a lesser degree, while the bulkier bromine and iodine diminished potency. Likewise, $-OH$ and $-OCH_3$ practically abolished activity. Addition of fluorine at C12 in the α configuration increased activity 10-fold, much as did the same substitution at C9. It seems, therefore, that the α surface in this region of the molecule plays a rather critical role in attaining a good fit to the receptor.

Substitutions at C16 produced no dramatic effects. An α-methyl group enhanced potency 4-fold, whereas a β-methyl reduced potency by about one-half. An α-hydroxyl here, unlike α-methyl, reduced potency somewhat. Quantitative data on the addition of substituent groups along the lower edge of the molecule are not available, except that methyl at C4 abolishes activity. Halogenation or methylation at the C6α position increases activity.

It should be recognized how difficult a task it has been, from the chemical point of view, to synthesize and prove the structures of so many steroid congeners. Yet a really thorough systematic survey, which could reveal the relative importance of every structural feature of the molecule, would require a far larger number of compounds. Two important limitations should also be noted. First, as long as assays are carried out in a whole animal, it is always possible that the effect of a molecular alteration is primarily to modify the metabolism or elimination of a drug, or its access to a site of action. Consequently, any inferences about a receptor surface must be tentative. Second, a substituent may act primarily to change the electron density at an adjacent atom, so the finding that alterations at a given location influence biologic activity does not necessarily implicate that location in the interaction with receptor.

Despite the qualified nature of the evidence, it seems possible, nevertheless, to draw some limited conclusions from the SAR data cited here. Substituents of the cortisol molecule that are essential to its glucocorticoid activity are arrayed along the upper edge (Figure 1-30) in the β configuration, and the hydroxyl group at C11 seems to play a key role in the drug-receptor interaction. As a first approximation, then, we might imagine that the β surface of the molecule has to lie flat against a complementary receptor surface. If this were the case, however, the α surface would face away from the receptor, and α-substituents should be without effect. The fact is, as we have seen, that α-substituents may either enhance activity greatly or abolish it altogether. We are forced to the conclusion, therefore, much as with the narcotic analgesics (p. 35), that the receptor must be something like a pocket into which the cortisol molecule can fit. Presumably, the upper edge of the steroid is oriented toward the bottom of the pocket, where interacting groups and recesses are spatially arranged to accommodate the essential substituents. The α and β surfaces of the hormone would each be in contact with one side of the pocket, so that substituents of both kinds would influence (for better or worse) the fit of the whole molecule to the receptor. Findings with other planar compounds suggest the possibility that steroids may interact with DNA by fitting into pockets formed by adjacent base-pair layers (intercalation).[83]

Congeners of the Pituitary Polypeptide Hormones

The polypeptide hormones oxytocin and vasopressin afford an interesting extension of the principles of biologic specificity to larger and more complex molecules.[84,85] Both hormones, products of the posterior pituitary gland, consist of 9 amino acid residues of the usual L configuration (Figure 1-31). A disulfide bridge between the

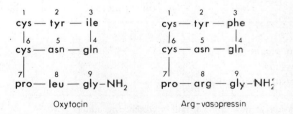

Oxytocin   Arg-vasopressin

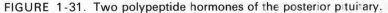

FIGURE 1-31. Two polypeptide hormones of the posterior pituitary.

cysteine residues at positions 1 and 6 creates a hexapeptide ring, and residues 7, 8, and 9 form a "tail," as shown. Oxytocin and vasopressin differ in two ways. In oxytocin residue 3 in the ring is isoleucine, whereas in vasopressin it is phenylalanine. Residue 8, in the tail, is leucine in oxytocin and arginine in most mammalian vasopressins (lysine in the pig and hippopotamus).

Oxytocin characteristically causes contraction of uterine smooth muscle. The primary action of vasopressin is antidiuretic; it acts on cells of the renal tubules, in a way not fully understood, to cause increased water reabsorption from the tubular lumen. Another action of vasopressin, from which its name is derived, is to cause contraction of arteriolar smooth muscle and thereby increase blood pressure in experimental animals (but not in man). These typical effects can be assayed quite easily. To assay oxytocic activity, for example, one horn of a rat uterus may be suspended in a tissue bath of appropriate aerated medium, and attached to a lever or strain gauge so that the magnitude of uterine contractions can be measured. Dilutions of a test compound and of oxytocin may then be compared by ascertaining the concentrations of each that are required in the tissue bath to cause equal and moderate contraction of the muscle (e.g., 50% of maximal). Vasopressin-like activity may be assayed by the blood pressure increase in the rat or cat after intravenous injection, or by the antidiuretic effect in the rat. When oxytocin was compared with arginine vasopressin in two such assay systems, the results shown on the first and third lines of Table 1-6 were obtained. Oxytocin had a strongly selective effect upon uterine smooth muscle. Arginine vasopressin, conversely, showed high potency on rat blood pressure but relatively little effect on the uterus.

Since oxytocin and vasopressin differ with respect to two amino acids, one in the ring and one in the tail, the question arises what relative role is played by each. Here nature has performed a crucial experiment for us. In the lower vertebrates a hormone is found, arginine oxytocin (vasotocin), in which the oxytocin molecule has arginine instead of leucine at position 8 in the tail. Table 1-6 shows that this single substitution in the tail somewhat reduces the oxytocic potency, but the main effect is a dramatic enhancement of vasopressin-like activity. The converse experiment has been performed by means of a synthetic analog containing the vasopressin ring but leucine instead of arginine in the tail. Table 1-6 shows that this compound, leucine vasopressin (oxypressin), is as ineffective an oxytocic agent as vasopressin

TABLE 1-6. Comparison of polypeptide hormones and congeners in two assay systems.

Figures represent relative potency in international units per milligram. (Data of Boissonnas et al.[84])

	Oxytocin-like activity on rat uterus	Vasopressin-like activity on rat blood pressure
Oxytocin	450	5
Arg-oxytocin (vasotocin)[a]	75	125
Arg-vasopressin	20	400
Leu-vasopressin (oxypressin)[b]	20	3

[a] *Arg* replaces *Leu* in position 8 of tail, oxytocin ring intact.
[b] *Leu* replaces *Arg* in position 8 of tail, vasopressin ring intact.

itself, but the vasopressin-like activity has been almost abolished. Thus, the bioassay data for both modified hormones lead to the same generalization. Oxytocin-like activity is reduced if the tail is modified, and even more so if the ring is modified. Vasopressin-like activity, on the other hand, cannot survive the substitution of a neutral leucine for a basic amino acid (arginine or lysine) in the tail, but is not greatly reduced by substitution at position 3 in the ring.

The most thorough and systematic investigations have been carried out on the oxytocin series. Any shortening of the tripeptide tail causes a drastic reduction in both kinds of biologic activity, even if a terminal amide is retained. Within the ring nearly any substitution of one amino acid for another leads to considerable loss of potency, even when the substitution is a reciprocal one (e.g., an interchange of tyrosine and phenylalanine in positions 2 and 3 of the vasopressin ring) so that the amino acid composition remains exactly the same. The importance of the phenolic hydroxyl of tyrosine in position 2 is also indicated by the effect of O-methylation of this residue; oxytocin- and vasopressin-like activities both disappear and some antagonism to vasopressin is manifested. Other instances of antagonism to one or the other hormone effect have been noted as results of small substitutions in the ring or the tail peptides.

It is instructive to note that a seemingly trivial alteration may have major effects. In oxytocin, the substitution of leucine for isoleucine at ring position 3 entails no more than shifting a side-chain methyl group to an adjacent carbon atom, yet the oxytocic potency falls to 1/10, and the pressor potency decreases even more. When valine is substituted at this position, the loss of oxytocic activity is not so great, but there is a disproportionate decrease of pressor potency. This kind of unequal influence of a substituent upon two different biologic effects may have great practical value, despite the fact that both potencies are diminished. A larger dose will still elicit the desired oxytocic action, but at that effective dosage the undesirable pressor side effects will be reduced. From a practical point of view, therefore, valine-oxytocin represents a more selectively oxytocic drug than the natural hormone. In the same way, in the vasopressin series, greater selectivity of antidiuretic action relative to pressor side effects may be obtained through appropriate molecular modifications.

The hexapeptide ring of oxytocin contain 20 atoms. Removal of the terminal amino group from the cysteine residue at position 1 yielded a crystalline compound, deamino oxytocin (Figure 1-32), which was about as potent as oxytocin itself.[86] An analog, containing an additional $-CH_2-$ at position 1 (i.e., a 21-membered ring) was practically inactive, and the corresponding compound with a $-CH_2-$ removed at position 1 (i.e., a 19-membered ring) was less than 1/20 as potent as deamino oxytocin. These observations make it plain that the 20-membered ring is necessary for biologic activity in this series, an intriguing finding in view of the presence of a 20-membered ring in the apparently unrelated pancreatic hormone insulin. Finally, a $-CH_2-$ was removed from position 1 and added at position 6, yielding a 20-membered ring that differed from deamino oxytocin in only one detail: the $-S-S-$ group was shifted about 1.5 A away from the tail. The oxytocic potency of this compound was as low as though it contained a 19-membered ring. Thus, the position of the $-S-S-$ group relative to the rest of the molecule is critical.

In summary, SAR studies with these posterior pituitary hormones permit some crude deductions to be drawn about the nature of the complementary receptor surfaces with which the hormones must interact. The cyclic polypeptide structure with its 20-membered ring is essential. This provides a fairly rigid framework from

42 Molecular Mechanisms of Drug Action

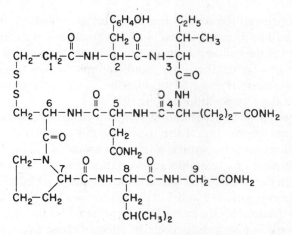

FIGURE 1-32. Deamino oxytocin. (*From Jarvis and du Vigneaud, Figure 1.*[86] *By permission of the American Association for the Advancement of Science.*)

which the amino acid side chains and the tripeptide tail project. Because of the identical L-configuration of the nine amino acids, all the side chains can form a complex "molded" contour on the same surface, which could then match the complementary surface of the correct receptor. Evidently, receptor surfaces in uterine muscle, arteriolar muscle, and renal tubule epithelium have in common certain features such as a shape and area suited to accommodate a ring-and-tail structure of this size, and a critically situated site for attachment to, or reaction with, the disulfide bridge. In addition, each kind of receptor must have differentiating features that specify optimal distances between essential functional groups on the interacting hormone. Antagonistic effects of structural analogs are probably best interpreted as resulting from reasonably good fit, without those key interactions between functional groups on the hormone and on the receptor surface that must "trigger" the characteristic biologic response.

Cycloserine and the Inhibition of Bacterial Cell Wall Synthesis

Interference with cell wall synthesis is a common mode of action of antibacterial drugs.[87] Penicillin acts in this way and causes the accumulation of complexes containing UDP and oligopeptide fragments linked to acetylglucosamine, which can be identified with known constituents of the bacterial cell wall. Evidently, penicillin blocks a cross-linking polymerization reaction that yields the completed cell wall mucopolypeptide.[88] Several other drugs interfere at other stages in this biosynthetic pathway. One of these, cycloserine, provides us with a remarkable illustration of steric specificity in drug action.

Cycloserine (Figure 1-33) is the amide of serine, closed on itself by dehydrogenation to form a 5-membered ring. It obviously resembles not only serine, but also the very similar amino acid alanine. Cycloserine inhibits the enzyme alanine racemase, which catalyzes the transformation of L-alanine to D-alanine. D-Alanine, in turn, is an essential constituent of the cell wall peptide. In the presence of cycloserine, therefore, D-alanine is depleted, the partial peptide (lacking its terminal D-*ala*–D-*ala* fragment) accumulates, new cell wall synthesis cannot proceed, and cell death results.

In this antibacterial action only D-cycloserine is effective, not its enantiomorph. Studies with purified alanine racemase[89] showed that K_i (the enzyme-inhibitor dissociation constant) for D-cycloserine was about $5 \times 10^{-5}\ M$, whereas L-cycloserine was wholly without effect even at concentrations greater than $1 \times 10^{-2}\ M$. This difference seems surprising. A racemase obviously has to interact with both stereoisomers of its substrate; thus with alanine racemase, the values for the enzyme-substrate dissociation constants were approximately $5 \times 10^{-3}\ M$ for both L-alanine

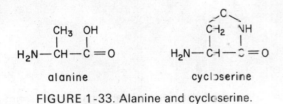

FIGURE 1-33. Alanine and cycloserine.

and D-alanine. How, then, can an enzyme that fails to distinguish between the L and D forms of its amino acid substrate nevertheless make such a sharp distinction between the L and D forms of a structural analog inhibitor? The answer is that the open chain structure of an amino acid permits free rotation about several bonds and consequently there is a high degree of flexibility in the conformation as a whole. Although D-alanine and L-alanine obviously could not occupy identical three-dimensional spaces, they can both look remarkably similar on one surface (e.g., the surface that has to interact with an enzyme). The rigid internal ring of cycloserine abolishes, in large measure, this conformational flexibility, so that the two stereoisomers cannot be forced onto the same surface.

Three-dimensional models are almost a necessity for visualizing this kind of restriction in shape. Figure 1-34 shows all four compounds. We know that D-cycloserine is the active form; so we start with the assumption that it fits the enzyme surface well. As a matter of fact, the dissociation constants given above indicate that the enzyme surface offers a substantially better fit to D-cycloserine than to either of the substrates, inasmuch as the affinity was about 100 times greater. Let D-cycloserine be placed (as in the figure at upper right) on a plane surface with its free amino group, carbonyl group, and ring —NH— from left to right. Then, as shown in the bottom row of the figure, both D-alanine and L-alanine can assume the corresponding configuration, with carboxyl —OH in the place of the homologous ring —NH— of cycloserine. L-Cycloserine (upper left) cannot be forced into the same configuration. When two of the three groups are in the plane, the third one projects upward, as shown by the free amino group in the figure. The specificity of the enzyme-inhibitory action of D-cycloserine is thus apparently accounted for.

Antibacterial Sulfonamides

In the series of antibacterial sulfonamides biologic potency is modified by substituents which do not themselves seem to partake in the combination with receptor, but rather influence the ionic character of another group on the molecule. Figure 1-35 shows the structure of *p*-aminobenzoic acid (PAB), an essential growth factor or biosynthetic intermediate in many bacteria. This compound is normally condensed

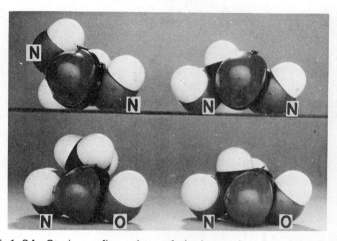

FIGURE 1-34. Steric configurations of alanine and cycloserine. *Bottom row, alanine; top row, cycloserine. The alanine structure is viewed with its −COOH grouping at front right, −NH₂ at left. In L-alanine (left) the methyl group projects upward; in D-alanine (right) it projects downward to rear and is hidden. The α-carbon atom is seen between the carbonyl O and amino N, and its H atom projects upward. The corresponding cycloserine structures are viewed at the same angle. D-cycloserine (right) assumes the same configuration as L- and D-alanine; the ring is in the viewing plane, and the ring O atom is hidden in the rear. The rigid ring structure prevents L-cycloserine (left) from assuming a similar configuration. With the carbonyl O and the ring in the same plane, the amino group is forced upward into a different plane, as shown. (After Roze and Strominger.[89])*

enzymically with a glutamylpteridine compound to form folic acid, the precursor of a coenzyme essential in the biosynthetic utilization of single-carbon units. Figure 1-35 also shows the nonionized and ionized forms of a prototype sulfonamide. In view of the close structural similarity of the sulfonamides to PAB, it is not surprising that these compounds also can combine with the condensing enzyme, thereby competitively

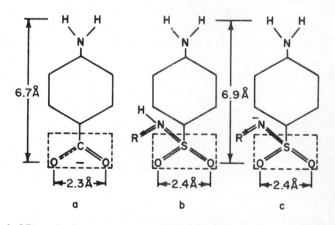

FIGURE 1-35. *p*-Aminobenzoate (PAB) and sulfonamide structures. *a, PAB ionized form; b, sulfonamide, nonionized form; c, sulfonamide, ionized form. All three rings are aromatic. Although negative charge resulting from loss of proton is shown associated with sulfonamide N atom, strict localization of the charge is not implied. (From Bell and Roblin, Figure 2.[90] By permission of the American Chemical Society.)*

inhibiting the normal entry of PAB into folic acid. The ultimate consequence is a folic acid deficiency manifested as a reversible inhibition of bacterial growth.

The simplest member of the sulfonamide series is sulfanilamide, in which both hydrogen atoms on the amide nitrogen are unsubstituted. The other sulfonamides carry substituents; a few out of the hundreds that have been synthesized and tested are shown in Table 1-7. Just as a free *p*-amino group is essential for substrate activity in PAB, so in a sulfonamide drug a free *p*-amino group is essential for antibacterial

TABLE 1-7. Some sulfonamides with different acid strengths. (Data of Bell and Roblin.[90] By permission of American Chemical Society.)

Compound	R^a	pK'_a
Sulfanilamide	–H	10.43
Sulfapyridine	(pyridine ring)	8.43
Sulfathiazole	(thiazole ring, S, N)	7.12
Sulfadiazine	(pyrimidine ring, N, N)	6.48
Sulfacetamide	$-\overset{\overset{\text{O}}{\|\|}}{C}-CH_3$	5.38

[a] Cf. Figure 1-35.

action. In contrast, there are almost no limitations to the possible substituents on the amide nitrogen compatible with antibacterial efficacy. It may be deduced that whereas the *p*-amino group combines with the enzyme surface, the amide nitrogen with its substituent probably does not.

What then is the role of substituents? A plausible explanation is suggested by the relationship between the $-SO_2-$ group in the sulfonamides and the $-CO_2^-$ group of PAB. The latter is completely ionized at neutral pH, and there is independent evidence that a negative charge here promotes combination with the enzyme. Thus it may be inferred that sulfonamides should become more potent with increasing electron density in the $-SO_2-$ region, and this property should be influenced by electron-attracting substituents on the amide nitrogen. Any tendency to draw electrons away from the N–H bond will be reflected in an increased ease of proton dissociation which can be measured by the pK'_a value of each compound. That various R substituents are capable of altering pK'_a profoundly is seen in Table 1-7. Sulfanilamide itself is a very weak acid, i.e., its proton is tightly bound; but electrophilic substituents in the other compounds increase the acid strength to varying degrees.

In order to explore the relationship between pK_a' and antibacterial potency, a great many sulfonamides were tested.[90] Cultures of *Escherichia coli* were maintained in buffered medium at pH 7. By means of a dilution series the minimum molar concentration of each sulfonamide required to inhibit growth was estimated, and the pK_a' was also determined for each compound. The observations are presented in Figure 1-36. Here, for greater clarity, the graph shows reciprocals of bacteriostatic

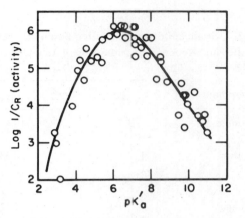

FIGURE 1-36. Relationship of antibacterial potency to acid strength in the sulfonamide series. *The logarithm of the reciprocal of the bacteriostatic concentration is the measure of potency. Each point represents a different sulfonamide. One discrepant point has been eliminated for justifiable reasons. All the testing was done at pH 7. (From Bell and Roblin, Figure 1.[90] By permission of the American Chemical Society.)*

concentrations as indices of potency (since lower effective concentration means greater potency), and in order to span several orders of magnitude in potency a logarithmic scale is used. Beginning at the extreme right with the weakest acids, and moving toward the left, antibacterial potency is seen to increase as acid strength increases. Since the tests were performed at pH 7, this portion of the curve shows that an increasing degree of ionization favors antibacterial activity. Thus, under the experimental conditions, a compound with a pK_a of 11 would be practically nonionized, whereas one with a pK_a of 6 would be 91 % ionized.

The findings, thus far, are consistent with the conclusion that the anionic form of a sulfonamide is the active form. One would predict, however, that all compounds with $pK_a' < 6$ should be maximally active, since all these would be nearly completely ionized at pH 7. Some special explanation is therefore required to account for the decreasing potency of the more acidic sulfonamides. One such explanation focuses more closely upon the charge distribution in the sulfone group itself. As the substituent R is made more electrophilic, so that the amide proton dissociates (as described above), the sulfone group shares in the electronegative character of the resulting anionic amide. Beyond a certain point, however, when complete ionization has already been attained, a still more strongly electrophilic substituent will begin to draw electrons away from the sulfone group. The altered charge distribution, with diminished electron density in the $-SO_2-$ region, will cause a diminution in antibacterial potency. Interesting attempts have also been made to explain SAR observations such as described above in terms of physicochemical properties of the various congeners.[91a–d]

CHARACTERIZATION OF DRUG–RECEPTOR INTERACTIONS

Model Interactions

Binding of Drugs to Plasma Proteins. The specific reversible binding of small organic molecules to a protein in solution can serve as a useful model of drug-receptor interactions.[92] In both the model and the real receptor in the body a specific set of bonds must be formed between the interacting molecules. The outstanding difference is, of course, that in the case of a receptor "something happens" as a consequence of the interaction, whereas in the model system only the binding itself can be observed. Thus, a wide variety of tissue proteins and nucleic acids may be thought of as "silent receptors." They display the same sorts of specific and nonspecific interactions with drugs as do functional receptors, and they also may bind sufficient drug (often far more than the actual receptors) to modify significantly the quantity available for combination with the primary receptors (p. 159). Let us consider some typical investigations in which physical binding of small molecules to a pure protein was measured.

The two principal methods that have been employed are spectrophotometry and equilibrium dialysis (or ultrafiltration).[92a] The basis of the spectrophotometric procedure is the fact that the absorption spectrum of an organic compound, which depends upon resonance within the molecule, may be altered in characteristic ways when the molecule interacts with another.[93] This is illustrated in studies with an anionic azo dye, methyl orange (Figure 1-37).[94] The compound consists of an azo-

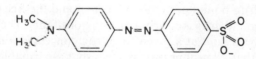

FIGURE 1-37. Structure of methyl orange.

benzene nucleus carrying a dimethyl amino group and a sulfonate ion. Figure 1-38 shows the spectral shifts induced at various pH values when the dye was mixed with solutions of albumin. These shifts, from which the extent of binding can be estimated, are similar to those observed in nonaqueous solvents. They are attributed to the formation of ionic bonds between the sulfonate group and cationic groups of the protein, which is tantamount to suppressing the dye ionization. The isoelectric point of albumin is at pH 4.9, so the interactions observed here occurred despite a net negative charge on the protein. Local electrostatic repulsion undoubtedly occurs between glutamic and aspartic acid residues of albumin and the sulfonate group of the dye. Nevertheless, because the albumin surface is so large compared with the ligand, cationic amino acid residues in favorable local environments can provide

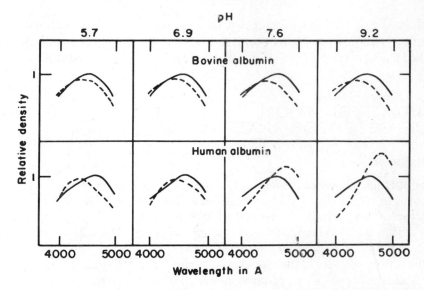

FIGURE 1-38. Spectral shifts induced by combination of methyl orange with bovine and human plasma albumin. *Solid curves, dye alone; broken curves, dye in the presence of albumin. The four panels represent different pH values, from left to right, as shown at top. (From Klotz et al., Figure 11.*[94] *By permission of the American Chemical Society.)*

suitable binding sites. The same principle presumably applies to a receptor site, which may constitute a small patch on the large surface of a macromolecule.

In equilibrium dialysis the protein and drug solutions are placed on opposite sides of a dialysis bag and the whole assembly is shaken at a constant temperature (commonly near 0°) until equilibrium is achieved. Since only the small drug molecule is freely diffusible, the difference between the drug concentration in the compartment containing protein (bound drug plus free drug) and that in the compartment containing free drug alone gives the concentration of bound drug. The relationship between the moles of drug bound per mole of protein and the free drug concentration in equilibrium with bound drug is clearly a measure of affinity. The tighter the binding, the more drug will be bound at a given free drug concentration. If the simplifying assumption is made that all groups on a protein that are capable of binding a given drug have the same affinity for that drug, then the law of mass action leads to a straightforward descriptive equation:

$$(R) + (X) \rightleftharpoons (RX)$$

$$\frac{(R)(X)}{(RX)} = K$$

where (X) is the concentration of free drug at equilibrium; (R) the concentration of free binding sites; (RX) the concentration of occupied binding sites; and K the dissociation constant. If n is the number of binding sites per protein molecule, and P the molar concentration of protein in the system, then nP, the total concentration of binding sites, is equal to $(RX) + (R)$, and

$$nP(X) - (RX)(X) = K(RX)$$

$$[K + (X)](RX) = nP(X)$$

Now let r be moles of drug bound per mole of total protein; then

$$r = \frac{(RX)}{P} = \frac{n(X)}{[K + (X)]}$$

If a series of determinations is carried out, with constant protein and varying drug concentrations, then a plot of r against (X) will have the familiar form of an adsorption isotherm, as shown in Figure 1-39a. Here, r approaches a saturation value n, the number of binding sites per molecule. If r is plotted against $\log(X)$, a symmetrical sigmoid curve will be obtained, as shown in Figure 1-39b. The value of n can be estimated from an approach to a maximum value. The position of the curve on the horizontal axis corresponds to the affinity, and the value of $\log(X)$ at half-saturation is $\log K$. For the case $n = 1$, this curve is analogous to a plot of fraction ionized against

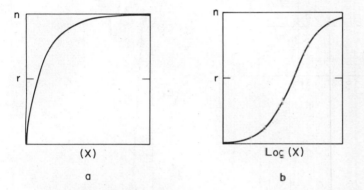

FIGURE 1-39. Two ways of plotting the adsorption isotherms for drug-protein interaction. *In (a) and (b), r is the moles drug bound per mole protein; n, the number of binding sites per molecule protein; X, drug concentration. (From Goldstein, Figures 1 and 6.*[92]*)*

pH, from the Henderson–Hasselbalch equation. For multiple binding sites ($n > 1$) with different affinities for the drug, the curve could assume a rather complex shape.

The mass action equation can be rearranged so that linear graphs are obtained, with intercepts and slopes corresponding to the parameters of the equation. The double-reciprocal plot is one example, which will be described later in the chapter (p. 84). Here we examine another very useful linear transformation:

$$Kr + r(X) = n(X)$$

$$\frac{r}{(X)} = \frac{-r}{K} - \frac{n}{K}$$

Then plotting $r/(X)$ against r should yield a straight line with two intercepts, n (on the x axis) and n/K (on the y axis), whence K is obtained. Examples of this approach, often called a "Scatchard plot,"[95] are shown in Figure 1-40. The first graph deals with the binding of calcium ions by casein. The measurements appear to conform with a straight line; from the intercepts, there are 16 binding sites per molecule, with the same apparent affinity for the ion ($K = 5 \times 10^{-3} M$).

A useful feature of this type of graph is that if there are distinct sets of binding sites with different affinities, two or more line segments may be distinguishable. The precise interpretation of the slopes and intercepts may be complicated.[98] The second example in Figure 1-40 illustrates this type of plot for the binding of acetylcholine

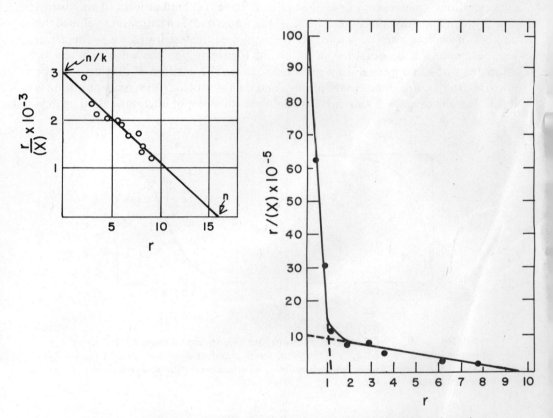

FIGURE 1-40. The Scatchard plot, another way of plotting the adsorption isotherms. *Here the intercept on the x axis gives* n; *that on the y axis gives* n/K *whence* K *is obtained. Left: Data for binding of* Ca^{2+} *to casein. Right: Binding of acetylcholine to a proteolipid extracted from electroplax tissue of the electric eel.* (*From Klotz,[96] Figure 9 and De Robertis et al.,[97] Figure 3.*)

to a proteolipid extracted from an acetylcholine-sensitive tissue. Evidently there is one binding site with high affinity, and about ten other sites where the binding is much weaker.

The results of equilibrium dialysis with methyl orange and human albumin are shown in Figure 1-41, upper curve. One mole of dye was bound per mole of protein at about 10^{-5} M free dye concentration, but the data were not extended sufficiently to permit any estimate of n. The effects of altering the dimethylamine group were studied by obtaining comparable data for modified molecules containing diethyl, dipropyl, and dibutyl instead of dimethyl on the amine nitrogen. There was a progressive loss of binding affinity, illustrated in Figure 1-41, lower curve, for the dibutyl derivative (butyl orange). This finding was remarkable inasmuch as nonspecific binding to

protein surfaces almost invariably increases with increasing length of alkyl substituents, by virtue of the hydrophobic properties of polymethylene chains. Apparently,
therefore, the site on albumin that interacted with the amine nitrogen could be regarded as embedded in a cavity that would accommodate only very short alkyl
chains.

Altering the nature of the anionic residue produced only small effects; thus, the
sulfonate (methyl orange) and carboxylate (methyl red) were bound somewhat more

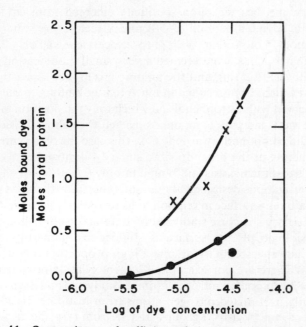

FIGURE 1-41. Comparison of affinity of human albumin for methyl
orange (X) and butyl orange (black circles). (*From Klotz et al., Figure 5.*[4]
By permisssion of the American Chemical Society.)

strongly than the phosphonate or arsonate. Changing the position of the anionic
group, on the other hand, produced major effects regardless of the nature of the group.
Although meta substituted compounds were bound about as well as para substituted
ones, the interaction no longer occurred when the anionic group was placed ortho to
the azo link. To test whether an ortho substituent disrupted the binding by steric
interference with an interaction involving the diazo group, a derivative of methyl
orange was tested in which methyl groups had been introduced ortho to both azo
nitrogen atoms. This compound was bound as strongly as methyl orange itself.
It was inferred, therefore, that the anionic group itself must interact, presumably
with a particular cationic side chain of the albumin. The results indicated that
another group on the dye molecule must also be involved in the interaction, presumably the dimethylamine (as suggested previously by the effects of substitution on
this group), and that the distance between the two receptor groups must correspond
to that between dimethylamine nitrogen and a meta or para anionic substituent,
about 12 A.

Further investigations revealed that iodination of the albumin, which specifically altered 13 of the 18 tyrosine residues in the protein, markedly reduced the extent of the binding. Implication of tyrosine in the binding strongly suggested that hydrogen bonding plays a role, since the phenolic −OH of that amino acid readily donates hydrogen to form a bond with amine nitrogen. The picture that emerged from these experiments was, therefore, of several specific binding sites on the albumin surface, at each of which a tyrosine residue is very nearly 12 A distant from a cationic group (e.g., an ϵ-amino group of lysine).

Interesting findings bearing upon specificity emerged from equilibrium dialysis experiments with bovine albumin.[99] With phenylacetate the value of n was found to be 25 moles mole^{-1} of protein. With phenoxyacetate n was only 7, but the affinity was 17 times greater. Thus, what seemed a very small modification (introducing an oxygen atom between the ring and the anionic group) abolished the binding to 18 sites previously available, but resulted in much tighter binding to the other 7. Similar effects were observed with nitrophenols, in which only the position of the nitro group was varied. The meta and para compounds reacted with about 22 sites per molecule, but with the ortho compound n was only 6. In this case the ortho substituent actually prevented interaction at the other 16 sites, since 2,4-dinitrophenol (which has both ortho and para substituents) was still bound at only 6 sites.

From the investigations described above, and others like them, we are able to form a picture of the albumin surface in relation to its drug-binding capacity. The molecule is globular, its tertiary structure stabilized by internal disulfide bonds and hydrogen bonds. At physiologic pH, its surface is studded by numerous charged groups, accounting for its water solubility despite a high proportion (about 56%) of hydrophobic residues. There are, for example, 83 carboxylate anions from aspartic and glutamic acids, 83 protonated nitrogen atoms from lysine and arginine, and an additional 16 partially protonated nitrogen atoms from histidine. In addition there are 49 serine and threonine hydroxyl groups, and 18 from tyrosine, as well as 4 cysteine sulfhydryls. There are large hydrophobic regions that can be thought of as "oily patches," composed of aliphatic and aromatic side chains from alanine, leucine, isoleucine, valine, proline, methionine, phenylalanine, and tyrosine. One can readily imagine how binding sites of different degrees of specificity could be present on such a surface, given certain spacings of ionic, hydrogen bonding, and hydrophobic groups, complementary to the various parts of a drug molecule.

Consider the case of methyl orange (Figure 1-37). Several hydrophobic regions could interact weakly with the azobenzene portion of the molecule. Only in some of these, however, would a positive charge be in a favorable position to interact with the sulfonate ion, thus increasing the binding affinity. And at only a single site might there also be, at just the right distance from the positive charge, a cavity capable of accommodating the dimethyl amino group, and a tyrosine residue capable of forming a hydrogen bond with the amino N atom. These speculations are in accord with the typical finding that there are many binding sites of poor specificity and low affinity, but only one or a few of good specificity and high affinity.

Ligand-Induced Conformational Change in Hemoglobin. The power of new technologic advances (particularly through x-ray crystallography) and their significance for pharmacology are well illustrated in the establishment of a complete three-dimensional structure for hemoglobin, at a resolution of a few angstrom units.[100–103] This molecule is the normal carrier of oxygen and it interacts specifically with the cofactor diphos-phoglycerate. It also may be regarded as a receptor for the toxic gas carbon monoxide. The scale model (Figure 1-42) shows how the two α-chains and the two β-chains, folded in an asymmetric pattern, are assembled into a compact structure containing four pockets to accommodate the heme groups and provide for the reversible

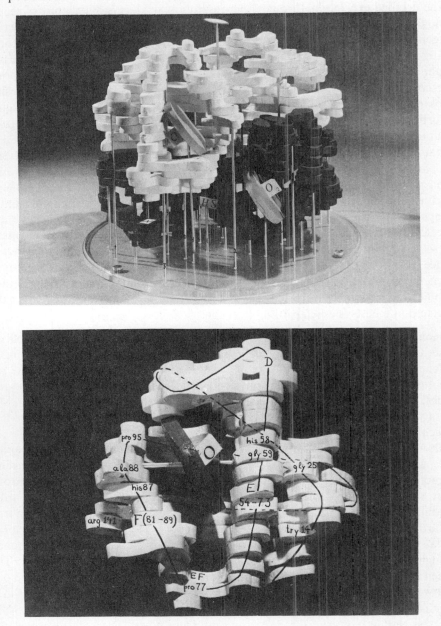

FIGURE 1-42. Tertiary structure of hemoglobin. *The upper figure illustrates the complete molecule. α-Chains are shown white, β-chains are black. Heme groups are represented by flat grey disks each carrying an oxygen molecule. The lower figure is a detail of one α-chain, showing the course of the peptide-bonded backbone and the positions of some amino acids with their sequence numbers, counting from the —NH₂ terminus. (From Cullis et al., Figs. 3 and 10;[100] prints obtained through the courtesy of M. F. Perutz.)*

attachment of four O_2 molecules. Hemoglobin has long been known as the classic example of positive cooperativity, the binding of each oxygen causing an increased affinity for the next. This phenomenon, revealed by a slope greater than unity on a Hill plot (cf. p. 110 Figure 1-87), underlies the efficiency of oxygen unloading at the tissues, where the oxygen tension is not low enough to accomplish this otherwise.

The detailed exposition, through high-resolution x-ray crystallography of reduced hemoglobin and oxyhemoglobin, of the stepwise conformational changes induced by oxygen binding, offers a beautiful illustration of what drugs may do to receptors. A small rotation (less than 1 A) of an α-chain iron atom into the plane of the heme upon combination with the first O_2 carries with it the histidine residue to which it is bound. The consequent movement of the local α-helix squeezes out a tyrosine residue, breaking ionic bonds to groups in the other α-chain. The resulting propagated disturbance in the quaternary structure, with numerous local displacements up to 7 A, result in a stepwise increase in the ease with which a subsequent O_2 can be bound at a β-chain heme. Opening of the pocket previously occupied by tyrosine permits entry and partial immobilization of cysteine β-93 (p. 63). Modification of these transitions by diphosphoglycerate accounts for the reduction of oxygen affinity by this cofactor, thus further promoting oxygen loss at the tissues. The whole sequence of conformational change typifies the wider class of reactions known as *allosteric*, which have quite general importance.[104] Thus, substrates may induce such changes in enzymes as part of the normal mechanism of catalysis, and drugs that prevent such changes or induce unfavorable steric alterations may thereby block enzyme action.[105] Allosteric effects in membrane-bound receptors probably play a major role in the generation (or blockade) of bioelectric potentials by drugs, and in the mediation of other drug effects upon membranes (cf. p.109).

Actinomycin–DNA Interaction: Stabilized Intercalation.   Advances comparable with those just discussed are taking place in establishing complete spatial structures for nucleic acids. The outstanding example that relates to drug actions was the confirmation, through a multitude of physicochemical, biochemical, and genetic techniques, of the Watson–Crick double-helical structure for DNA (Figure 1-12). More recently, complete primary sequences and conformations of several transfer-RNA molecules have been elucidated.[106]

DNA is the receptor upon which several mutagenic, growth-inhibiting, carcinogenic, and carcinolytic drugs act.[107] Among these are the antibiotics mitomycin C and actinomycin D. Actinomycin D (Figure 1-43) contains a phenoxazone chromophore, bearing two identical cyclic pentapeptide chains (L-threonine, D-valine, L-proline, sarcosine, and L-methylvaline). The interesting steric aspects of the structure are not evident in the planar diagram. The chromophore lies in a plane perpendicular to that of the cyclic pentapeptides, and there is a two-fold axis of symmetry through the chromophore, conferring a T shape upon the whole molecule. Thus, as seen in the diagram, one pentapeptide would project upward, as shown, the other downward from the chromophore. If the two pentapeptides are thought of as in the plane of the paper, the chromophore would protrude toward the reader. As will be seen, this geometry is crucial to the drug's interaction with DNA.

The story of the complete establishment of the molecular mechanism of action of this antibiotic is a remarkable one. It was early found to form a complex with DNA, and to exert a specific blocking action upon the transcription of DNA into messenger

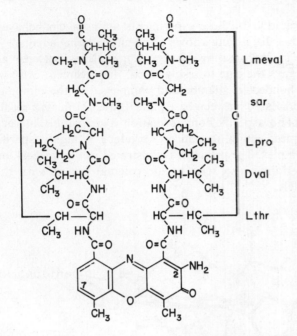

FIGURE 1-43. Structure of actinomycin D. *The chromophore is shown at bottom, the two identical pentapeptide units above.*

RNA, thereby causing growth inhibition in bacterial and mammalian cells. The drug was effective upon native DNA and also upon synthetic deoxyribonucleoside polymers containing guanine, but not upon RNA or copolymers containing only deoxyadenosine and deoxythymidine.[108] A model was therefore proposed,[109] in which the antibiotic interacted by specific hydrogen bonding with the 2-amino group of guanine, with the pentapeptide side chains lying in the minor groove of the DNA. Since other evidence had implicated the minor groove as a site of attachment of the DNA-directed RNA polymerase, the mechanism of action seemed to be well accounted for.

Subsequent studies, however, indicated quite clearly that actinomycin intercalated between base pairs of DNA.[110] This was shown by changes in spectral properties of the actinomycin chromophore, and by alterations in the viscosity and sedimentation coefficient of DNA, typical of those seen with known intercalating compounds. Strong support for this view came from an interesting technique, using supercoiled circular DNA such as the replicative form of the phage ΦX174.[111,112] Intercalation between the DNA bases necessarily produces a local distortion in the helix, since the stacked bases above and below the intercalated molecule are spread apart slightly. Obviously, this can only occur if the helix pitch in the immediate vicinity is steepened slightly. In a closed circular DNA[113] containing supercoils, each intercalated base will slightly relieve the supercoiling, through the local effect on the helix—a topologic necessity that can be demonstrated readily with twisted rope models. When a sufficient number of molecules have been intercalated, the supercoiling will be abolished, and further intercalation will induce supercoiling in the opposite direction. These effects are very easy to detect by changes in sedimentation behavior, since supercoiled circles are more compact than uncoiled ones, and therefore sediment more rapidly. In these experiments actinomycin behaved like ethidium, proflavin, and other drugs long known to be intercalating agents.

Finally, x-ray crystallography of crystal complexes between actinomycin and deoxyguanosine gave the clue to resolving the disagreement as to whether the antibiotic hydrogen-bonded to guanine and complexed in the minor groove of DNA, or whether it intercalated between base pairs. It does both. The resulting model is an elegant example of how specific bond formation, hydrophobic interaction, and stereochemical properties, acting in concert, produce a highly specific lock-and-key drug-receptor complex. The principle is illustrated in Figure 1-44, but the interested reader should certainly also refer to the original papers with their illuminating space-filling models.[114,115]

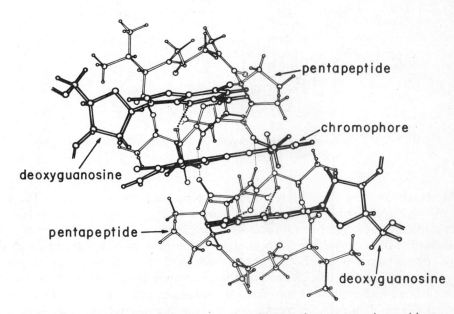

FIGURE 1-44. Interaction of actinomycin with two deoxyguanosine residues. *The diagram represents the complex as viewed in the plane of the chromophore and the two guanine residues. The T-shaped geometry of actinomycin, with its 2-fold axis of symmetry through the chromophore is evident. The cyclic pentapeptides lie in the plane of the paper, perpendicular to the plane of the chromophore, and disposed symmetrically above and below it. (From Sobell and Jain,[115] Figure 1B.)*

Figure 1-44 is a view of the complex through the plane of the chromophore. The T shape already alluded to is clearly seen here, the two identical pentapeptide chains extending symmetrically to the upper left and lower right. Two deoxyguanosine residues are shown, with the guanine bases in the plane of the chromophore, stacked above and below. The strong hydrogen bond between the 2-amino group of guanine and the carbonyl oxygen of the pentapeptide threonine residue is readily discerned as a dotted line. A weaker hydrogen bond, between the N(3) ring nitrogen of guanine and the threonine NH group, is also seen. To convert this diagram into that of a segment of DNA, one would add a deoxycytidine residue opposite each deoxyguanosine, and more base pairs to the upper left and lower right. The actinomycin pentapeptides, extending from upper left to lower right, lie exactly in what would then be the minor groove of DNA, as can be surmised from the positions and orientations of the two deoxyribose residues shown in the diagram. A large number of van der Waals contacts will then be present between the peptides and numerous atoms in the minor groove, stabilizing the complex.

An essential aspect of the actinomycin structure is its two-fold symmetry, corresponding to the two-fold symmetry of the receptor site (G-C above, C-G below). Since functionally actinomycin is a repressor (blocking transcription), albeit a rather nonspecific one, the elucidation of its molecular mode of action suggests possible analogous mechanisms for the actions of larger protein aporepressors, which must recognize a fairly long base-pair sequence on a specific operator gene.[115]

Special Techniques for Studying Drug-Receptor Interactions

Nuclear Magnetic Resonance (NMR).   Nuclear magnetic resonance offers a powerful tool for examining certain drug-protein interactions directly, rather than depending upon inferences based on the effect of substituents in the drug molecule. At fixed magnetic field strength the energy absorption by an atomic nucleus depends upon the frequency in the radiofrequency range (10^8 Hz). Absorption peaks of hydrogen and deuterium nuclei occur in entirely different spectral regions. This provides a basis for selectively examining certain protons, for example those in a drug molecule, without interference from water, by carrying out the experiment in D_2O. The local magnetic field experienced by a nucleus is determined by the electrons of the same atom. In addition, this field is affected by the magnetic moments of nearby atoms. Therefore, the absorption peaks of different protons in the same molecule can often be distinguished from one another, and a particular peak assigned unambiguously to each one. The characteristic spectral position occupied by a given peak is referred to as its "chemical shift," denoting the difference in its resonance frequency from that of protons in a reference compound. These shifts occur over a range of 1000 Hz, or 10 parts per million of the total resonance frequency. A simple example is given in Figure 1-45, showing the different chemical shifts of the methyl protons in the alcoholic and acyl radicals of methyl acetate, reflecting their different neighbors.

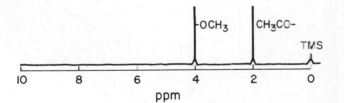

FIGURE 1-45. NMR chemical shift. *The spectrum of methyl acetate, showing downfield shift of both peaks from the tetramethylsilane (TMS) standard. (From Burgen and Metcalfe,[116] Figure 2.)*

Binding can be studied either by observing changes in chemical shift (as would be obvious from the above discussion) or by the principle of line broadening, the application of which will be presented now. The dissipation of energy by nuclei in the excited state proceeds at a certain exponential rate, with time constant T, known as the *relaxation time.* The reciprocal, $1/T$, is the *relaxation rate.* If the nucleus is tumbling very rapidly in the magnetic field, the energy dissipation is relatively slow (T approximately 0.1–1.0 sec); but if molecular motion is slowed, so that the nucleus remains oriented longer in the magnetic field (especially in relation to neighboring nuclei), the relaxation process becomes much more efficient (faster). A slow relaxation rate yields a very sharp absorption line, representing the time averaging of excited nuclei in all possible orientations during each cycle. A fast relaxation rate is characterized by a broadening of the absorption peak, since the individual contributions of nuclei in different orientations (and thus very slightly different resonance frequencies) can now be detected. The main significance of all this is that if the nuclei of interest are bound to a large macromolecule, their tumbling rate is substantially slowed—they are, as it were, "frozen" in place. Indeed, similar effects can be obtained by actual freezing or by increased viscosity of the medium. The extent of immobilization is directly proportional to the relaxation rate. By measuring relaxation rates of nuclei in different parts of the same molecule, one can obtain a remarkably detailed picture of the interactions at the binding site. For details of the theory and practice, the reader is referred elsewhere.[93,116,122]

An interesting application of this technique to sulfonamide–albumin interactions will be described.[117] The antibacterial sulfonamides are a group of compounds differing only in the substituent on the sulfonamide N atom (Figure 1-35, Table 1-7). Binding studies by spectral methods and equilibrium dialysis indicated that the serum albumin molecule had a single binding site of moderately high affinity. By NMR it was possible to distinguish clearly between protons on the benzene ring and in the

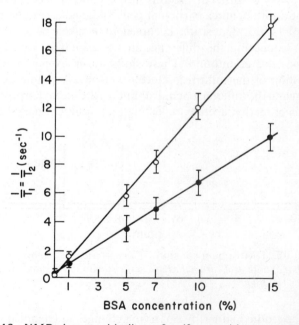

FIGURE 1-46. NMR data on binding of sulfacetamide to serum albumin. *Relaxation rates as a function of bovine serum albumin (BSA) concentration. Open circles = ring protons; solid circles = methyl protons. (From Jardetzky and Wade–Jardetzky,[117] Figure 4.)*

substituent group, e.g., the methyl protons of sulfacetamide. Then the influence of serum albumin could be studied independently upon these different portions of the molecule. The result was quite striking. Binding occurring over the entire surface of the molecule would be expected to shorten all relaxation times by the same factor, as the albumin concentration was increased. The finding, however, was that the benzene ring interaction was preferentially stabilized, as shown in Figure 1-46. The two linear plots converge on the y axis, at 0 albumin concentration, since in the absence of albumin a single relaxation rate is observed for the entire molecule, tumbling freely in solution. Interesting findings also emerged relative to the specificity of the binding site. Competition experiments showed that other aromatic compounds, such as benzene, phenol, and phenylacetate did not interfere with sulfacetamide binding. On the other hand, a sulfonamide with a bulky double-ring substituent (sulfaphenazole) was bound at two different sites—the usual sulfonamide site, and also a nonspecific hydrophobic site that interacted with the phenazole group.

As primary, secondary, and tertiary structures of receptor proteins are elucidated, we can expect to see how the general principles of drug-protein interaction revealed in the studies with serum albumin are manifested in each instance. In the remainder of this section we shall discuss an example in which such detailed understanding is already at hand.

The elucidation of primary, secondary, tertiary, and quaternary structures of proteins is proceeding rapidly.[118,119] Ribonuclease is a good example, the primary and partial secondary structure of which is shown in Figure 1-47. Here, x-ray crystallography indicates a compact structure with very little helical content. The positions

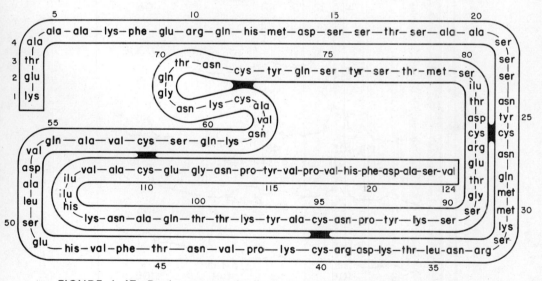

FIGURE 1-47. Bovine pancreatic ribonuclease. *Sequence numbers of the amino acids begin at the NH$_2$-terminus. The four −S−S− bonds between cys residues are shown as black regions. (From Stein, Figure 2.[120])*

of the −S−S− bridges impose a curious asymmetry upon the entire folded molecule. All the methionine residues are evidently buried inside, whereas most of the basic lysine side chains are exposed on the surface. Residues known to be involved in the catalytic action (and therefore presumed to be in the active center) prove to be far apart on the primary chain. Thus, the two histidine residues at positions 12 and 119, as well as lysine at position 41, are believed to be within about 5 A of each other in the native enzymically active state of the protein.[120,121] A three-dimensional model has been constructed.[121a]

Ribonuclease is a rather small protein (MW = 13,680) that acts as an endonuclease, hydrolyzing 3′–5′ phosphodiester bonds in RNA. The phosphate must be attached to a 3′-OH of a pyrimidine nucleoside. A particular groove in the three-dimensional structure of the enzyme has been identified as the active site. Pyrimidine mononucleotides inhibit the catalytic action, so that they may properly be considered as prototypes of drugs that interfere with normal enzymic processes.

The NMR spectrum of ribonuclease in solution, like that of most proteins, is very complex, since the different chemical shifts of the 124 amino acid residues overlap, yielding a broad nondescript envelope rather than sharp resonance lines. Fortunately, the C2 protons of the four histidine residues stand alone, downfield from the envelope attributable to the aromatic amino acids. Moreover, their chemical environments are sufficiently different from one another so that four distinct peaks are observed. These can be assigned unambiguously to residues 105, 12, 119, and 48 (Figure 1-48a). Now by the elegant technique of observing the effect of increasing concentration of an inhibitor, 3′-CMP, upon each of these peaks, conclusions may be drawn about which

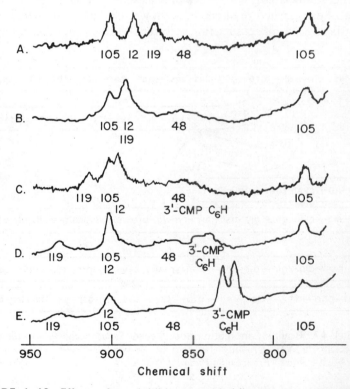

FIGURE 1-48. Effect of an inhibitor on histidine proton resonances in ribonuclease. (a) Ribonuclease alone. (b–e) With 2, 5, 10, and 30 mM 3′-CMP. The peaks are identified by His positions in the primary sequence. The C6 proton resonance of cytidine is also indicated. (From Meadows and Jardetzky,[123] Figure 1.)

(if any) histidine residues are involved in the inhibitor interaction at the active site. Figure 1-48 (b–e) shows the results. As the inhibitor concentration was increased, His-105 and His-48 were unaffected, whereas His-119 and (to a lesser extent) His-12 moved downfield.

The remarkably detailed picture reproduced in Figure 1-49 emerged His-119 forms a hydrogen bond with the nucleotide phosphate group: His-12 interacts with the

COMPLEX OF 3'-CMP WITH RNase

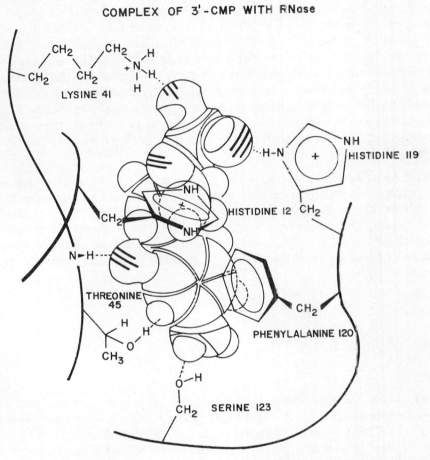

FIGURE 1-49. Structure of the complex between ribonuclease and an inhibitor. *A scale model of 3'-CMP is shown lying in the active site and interacting with various residues identified by sequence number. (From Meadows et al.,*[124] *Plate I.)*

ribose; and the 6 position of cytidine interacts with Phe-120. Other interactions stabilizing the complex involve Lys-41, Thr-45, and Ser-123. The data are entirely consistent with the assignment of amino acid residues to the active site (by folding in of widely separated portions of the primary sequence), based upon x-ray crystallographic evidence. Later extensions of this work led to postulation of a detailed sequence of steps for the catalytic process in ribonuclease action, in which His-119 and His-12 participate as reversible proton acceptors and donors.[125]

A technical refinement has opened the way for greater progress in this field by permitting selected amino acid residues to be studied, free of interference. Chemical synthesis or biosynthesis of proteins from deuterated amino acids allows one to remove most of the contents of an envelope of overlapping spectra to another spectral region, leaving protons of a single amino acid for study.[126] The most interesting application of this approach may well be to the problem of "drug"-induced conformational change in repressor proteins. Repressors, in the apoprotein form, bind specifically and firmly to DNA of an operator region. Inducers (derepressors) are small molecules that interact specifically with the repressors in their DNA-bound state, resulting in their dissociation from DNA, so that transcription can be initiated. The most plausible mechanism postulates a conformational change in the repressor protein, induced by its interaction with the derepressor. Since the *lac* repressor has been isolated and can be made in large amounts biosynthetically from deuterated amino acids,[126a] we can probably look forward to significant progress in analysis of the mechanism by NMR. A similar approach might eventually be used to elucidate the molecular mechanism of action of drugs such as neurotransmitters, which are thought to act by inducing conformational change in membrane proteins at post-synaptic receptor sites.

Electron Spin Resonance (ESR). This technique can yield information about interactions with naturally occurring molecules that contain a paramagnetic atom such as iron. The approach to be described here employs "spin labels" attached to drug or other ligand molecules, as "reporters" of the state of orientation or molecular motion of the ligand.[127,128] A spin label is a paramagnetic free radical, typically a nitroxide ring bearing an unpaired electron localized on the N–O group. A general structure is

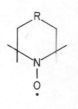

where R may be any drug or other ligand. When placed in solution in a magnetic field, at an appropriate frequency in the microwave range (typically 3200 gauss at 9000 MHz), such a free radical yields a set of very sharp resonance peaks (Figure 1-50). Immobilization by binding to a macromolecule or membrane causes peak broadening and diminished amplitude, much as described already for NMR. This phenomenon can be put to three different uses to yield information about the interaction.

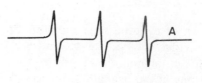

10 gauss

FIGURE 1-50. ESR spectrum of a typical nitroxide spin label free in solution. (*From Chignell,*[93] *Figure 14.*)

1. Orientation of the spin-labeled ligands with respect to a large structure (such as a membrane) oriented in the magnetic field can be deduced. In this way, for example, a long-chain hydrophobic analog of a phospholipic, spin-labeled near the polar head group, was shown to orient itself perpendicular to the long axis of a nerve.[127]

2. Changes in motion of the spin label attached to a specific site in a macromolecule can be deduced from spectral changes, as illustrated in Figure 1-51 for a nitroxide spin label attached covalently to specific cysteine residues (β-93) in horse hemoglobin.[127,129] Here conformational change in the hemoglobin on oxygenation results in restriction of mobility of the label, reflecting an alteration of the local chemical environment (cf p. 54).

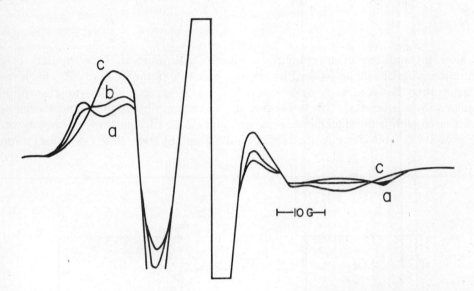

FIGURE 1-51. ESR spectra of spin-labeled horse hemoglobin. *The β-93 cysteine residues were spin labeled; (a) completely oxygenated; (b) partially oxygenated (71%); (c) completely deoxygenated. (From McConnell and Hubbell,[127] Figure 4.)*

3. Since unpaired electrons perturb the magnetic fields of nearby nuclei, spin labels may also be used in conjunction with NMR to study interactions. A spin-labeled analog of nicotinamide adenine dinucleotide (NAD) was used in this way to gain information about the active site geometry of alcohol dehydrogenase and the influence of substrate thereon.[130,131]

The principle of line broadening by immobilization of spin labels has proved extraordinarily useful in immunoassay. Here the "receptor site" is an antibody to the drug of interest. The results are not only of theoretical interest, but have led to the development of an operational "spin immunoassay" technique.[132,133] We illustrate the method for morphine assay, as might be used in a system designed to detect drugs subject to abuse, in urine or saliva. First, a morphine antibody is produced by standard immunologic procedures, using morphine as hapten, covalently coupled to BSA as antigen (b in diagram below), permitting rabbits or goats to produce the antibody. As with most drugs, quite specific antibodies can be made, with affinity constants in the range 10^6–10^7 M^{-1}. Second, a spin-labeled morphine is prepared (c in diagram); the nitroxide-free radical is attached at the same position that had served to couple morphine to albumin in the antigen.

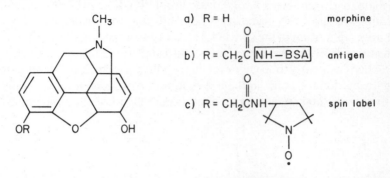

Now the spin-labeled morphine is combined with antibody in a capillary tube containing buffer and an oxidant to prevent reduction of the free radical. This is the reagent tube. If placed in the cavity of an ESR spectrometer, virtually no absorption peaks will be observed; this is because of the extreme broadening and flattening associated with firm attachment of the spin label in or adjacent to the antibody site (Figure 1-52). Consider now the effect of adding an unknown fluid containing some

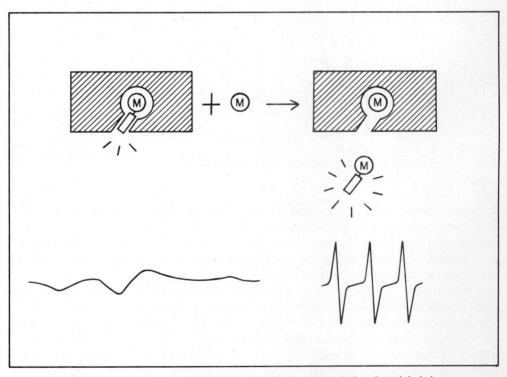

FIGURE 1-52. The principle of spin immunoassay. *Left: Spin-labeled morphine immobilized by interaction with morphine antibody. Nitroxide ESR spectrum, below, has very small amplitude because of peak broadening. Right: Competitive displacement of spin-labeled morphine by morphine. Free mobility in solution leads to appearance of sharp ESR peaks, below. (From Leute et al.,[133] Figure 1.)*

morphine. There will be a rapid competitive displacement of spin-labeled morphine from the antibody. Free spin-labeled morphine will tumble freely in solution, giving rise to sharp resonances, the amplitude of which will be a measure of the amount displaced, and therefore of the morphine concentration in the added fluid. The method has several major advantages, among them that the "readout" is almost instantaneous, that there is no need for any chemical manipulations (free spin label is measured without interference from bound spin label), and that very small volumes (about 10 μl) suffice.

Quite apart from its general applicability to drug detection and assay, the method yields interesting quantitative data about the specificity of antibody sites. For example, although the narcotic opiate receptor in brain does not distinguish well between morphine and methadone (which are isosteric, cf. p. 34), antibodies do. Evidently the antibody sites recognize shape and chemical composition in different ways than the receptor does. Thus, a morphine antibody bound morphine and methadone with affinity constants 1.3×10^6, and 4×10^2, respectively. A methadone antibody had more than 10-fold lower affinity for morphine, and 10,000-fold higher affinity for methadone.

Fluorescence Spectroscopy.   Fluorescent probes can be used for at least three distinct purposes in investigating interactions with proteins or other macromolecules: (a) as spectroscopic "rulers" to estimate distances between sites on a macromolecule; (b) to detect rotational motions related to the flexibility of a macromolecule; (c) to report on the hydrophobic character of a binding site.[134]

The use as a spectroscopic "ruler" is based on the principle of energy transfer from a fluorescent donor to a fluorescent acceptor, which can only occur efficiently over a range of approximately 10–65 A. In a typical experiment, an energy donor, m-acetylbenzenesulfonamide, was allowed to interact at the active site of carbonic anhydrase, which is specifically inhibited by sulfonamides containing an unsubstituted primary amine group. The bound sulfonamide was excited at 330 nm, a wavelength at which tryptophan residues are not excited. The emission spectrum showed tryptophan fluorescence, demonstrating that energy transfer occurred, and therefore that a tryptophan residue was present at or close to the active site of the enzyme.[135] In a similar study an acridine dye was attached covalently to the 3' end of yeast phenylalanine transfer RNA. Excitation of the dye led to emission from a naturally occurring fluorescent base adjacent to the anticodon segment of the tRNA, whence the distance between these sites (more than 40 A) could be estimated.[136]

The detection of rotational motions is based upon measurement of fluorescent emission anisotropy after very brief (nanosecond) flashes of exciting light. Here the polarization of fluorescence is determined and the emission anisotropy (ratio of fluorescence intensities in two perpendicular planes) plotted as a function of time, as in Figure 1-53. A linear decay slope indicates a rigid unit tumbling with uniform motion on a nanosecond time scale. The same technique was used to confirm a model of antibodies in which two antigen-binding sites are separated by a flexible (hinge) region.[137] It may be possible to apply the method to the problem of distinguishing conformational states of receptors with occupied and unoccupied active sites.

Finally, the intensity of fluorescence and the wavelength of maximum emission depend upon the solvent polarity. Thus, some dyes are virtually nonfluorescent in aqueous solution but become fluorescent in nonpolar solvents or when the local

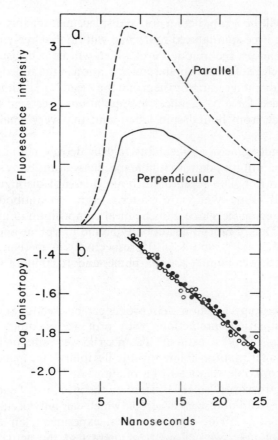

FIGURE 1-53. Fluorescence emission anisotropy in the nanosecond range.
A fluorescent anthranilic acid derivative was covalently bound at the active site of chymotrypsin. Polarization of fluorescence emission was measured in two planes (upper graph). Ratios of emissions were plotted on a log scale against time (lower graph). (From Stryer,[138] Figure 8.)

environment at a binding site is hydrophobic. Such a dye, 1-anilino-8-naphthalene, interacts with the heme-binding site on apomyoglobin or apohemoglobin. Its stoichiometric displacement by hemin, leading to progressive disappearance of fluorescence, is illustrated in Figure 1-54.

RECEPTOR ISOLATION

Steroid Hormone Receptors

Research on the identification and isolation of soluble receptors for steroid hormones began in the 1960's, when tritiated steroids of very high specific radioactivity became available. High specific radioactivity was essential because of the very small amounts of these compounds that are specifically bound at receptor sites. Nonspecific interactions usually dominate the overall binding, so that special techniques are needed to detect a small amount of specific binding in the presence of a large amount of

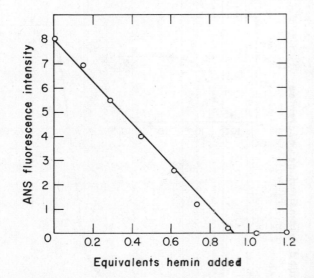

FIGURE 1-54. Fluorescent probe to detect a hydrophobic-binding site. *A naphthalene dye was allowed to interact at heme-binding site of apomyoglobin, producing intense fluorescence. As shown, the dye was stoichiometrically displaced by hemin, with concomitant loss of fluorescence. (From Stryer,[139] Figure 4.)*

nonspecific binding. By nonspecific binding we mean interaction with a variety of proteins such as plasma albumin, which occurs with many steroids and derivatives, and which is unrelated to the stereochemistry of the steroid or its biologic activity. Although it might seem possible for association constants of these nonspecific interactions to assume any value, it has been found without exception that they are smaller than those for specific interaction. Typically, nonspecific binding is characterized by low affinity and high capacity, specific receptor binding by high affinity and low capacity. Illustrations of this same principle have already been given in connection with binding to plasma albumin (p. 52).

Several kinds of protein or other macromolecule might react specifically with steroid hormones, including enzymes responsible for their synthesis or degradation, and transport systems, either systemic (e.g., the corticosteroid-binding globulin in mammalian blood plasma) or cellular. Finally, there is the hormone receptor, which binds the active steroid and initiates the sequence of events leading to the biologic response. Hormone receptors are specific, not only for the biologically active steroids, but also for the given tissue. Thus, only target tissues contain the relevant receptors. The uterus has receptors for estrogens, but not for progesterone, testosterone, or glucocorticoids. Thymus or fibroblast tissue has receptors for glucocorticoids but not for the sex hormones. And prostate or seminal vesicles contain receptors for androgens alone.

Some of the characteristics are shown in Figures 1-55 and 1-56. The system studied was a fibroblast cell culture, the growth of which is inhibited by glucocorticoids. This growth inhibition is related to the thinning of skin, muscle wasting, and thymic involution seen with high doses of these hormones in man. Fibroblasts, therefore, represent a target tissue, especially suitable for this study because they are known not to metabolize steroids to a significant extent. Figure 1-55 shows the amount of an active glucocorticoid bound by the cells, as a function of the steroid concentration in

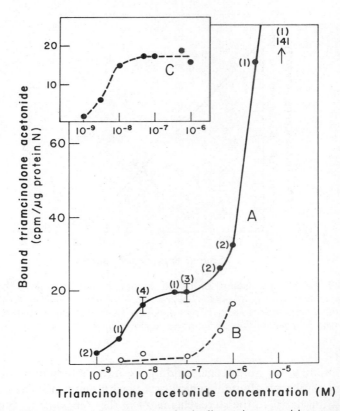

FIGURE 1-55. Binding of a pharmacologically active steroid to a soluble cell fraction. *A culture of mouse fibroblasts was incubated with* ^3H-*triamcinolone acetonide, and the bound steroid was measured as described in the text. Curve A: Binding in the absence of competing steroid. Curve B: Binding in the presence of competing steroid. Curve C: Differences between the corresponding points on curves A and B. (From Hackney et al.,*[140] *Figure 3.*)

the medium (curve A). Binding was measured by preparing a cytoplasmic extract of the cells after incubation with labeled triamcinolone acetonide, and filtering the extract through columns of Sephadex G-25. This molecular sieving procedure separates free steroid, of low molecular weight, from protein-bound steroid, which passes directly through the column in the macromolecular fraction. Two modes of binding are seen—a high-affinity type that appears to become saturated at about $10^{-8}\,M$, and a second, high-capacity type at higher steroid concentrations, which shows no sign of saturation. Only the first type of binding could be blocked by a very potent, nonradioactive glucocorticoid, fluocinolone acetonide (curve B). The difference in binding of triamcinolone acetonide in the absence and presence of the competing steroid (curve C) is shown in the insert; it presumably represents the specific receptor-like binding. The nonspecific binding is evidently not affected by the competing steroid, perhaps because the binding capacity is so large.

The conclusion that curve C represents receptor binding is strengthened by the following observations. The ability of various steroids to block this binding is exactly correlated with their potencies as glucocorticoids and growth inhibitors, over a very wide range of potencies (Figure 1-56). Closely related but inactive steroids such as

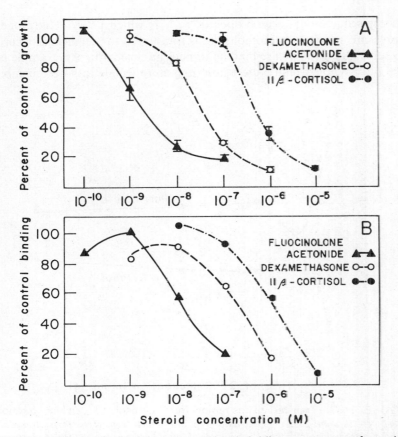

FIGURE 1-56. Relationship between growth-inhibitory potency of steroids and their ability to block the specific binding of triamcinolone acetonide. *(A) Log dose-response curves for growth inhibition of fibroblasts in cell culture. (B) Inhibition of the binding of ^{3}H-triamcinolone acetonide in the macromolecular fraction in the presence of competing nonradioactive steroids. (From Hackney et al.,[140] Figure 2.)*

11 α-cortisol, estradiol-17β, and testosterone neither block binding nor inhibit the growth of these cells. Moreover, a steroid-resistant variant of the cells, obtained by selection in the presence of low concentrations of 11β-cortisol, is cross-resistant to growth inhibition by all the active glucocorticoids. Such cell lines demonstrate drastically reduced amounts of specific binding.

Similar studies have been carried out with various steroid hormone target cells and tissues, with the aim of relating the initial binding to the ultimate biologic effect. For example, following the binding of cortisol to the soluble receptor in thymus cells, a sequence of reactions evidently occurs before the first biochemical manifestation (depressed glucose uptake) can be observed.[141] One of these steps is apparently temperature sensitive; another is inhibited by actinomycin D (implicating RNA synthesis). Evidence is mounting that the initial receptor-hormone complex is transferred from the cytoplasm to the nucleus, where it acts in some way not yet understood, to modify RNA and protein synthesis. This pattern seems to apply not only to the glucocorticoids, but also to other steroid hormones such as estradiol, testosterone, aldosterone, and progesterone in their respective target tissues.

A two step sequence has been proposed[142,143] in which a steroid hormone, bound to a cytoplasmic receptor macromolecule, is transferred to the nucleus, where it may undergo some alteration before binding to nuclear chromatin. An example is shown in Figure 1-57. Whole isolated uteri from immature female rats were incubated for

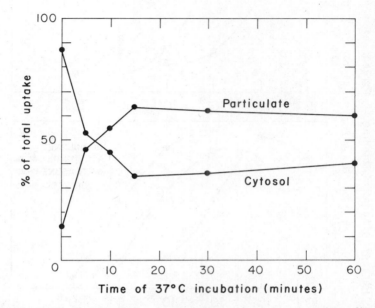

FIGURE 1-57. Transfer of estradiol from cytosol to nuclear fraction. *Uteri were incubated with* ^{3}*H-estradiol-17β, at 0°, then transferred to fresh medium without estradiol at 37°. The distribution of label between the cytosol and nuclear fractions is shown as a function of incubation time. (From Shyamala and Gorski,*[147] *Figure 4.)*

short periods in a buffer solution containing ^{3}H-estradiol-17β at 0°. When such uteri were washed, homogenized, and separated into cytosol and particulate (nuclear) fractions, about 85% of the radioactivity was found in the cytosol fraction. Continued incubation at 0° did not significantly alter this distribution. However, transfer of the uteri to fresh solution (no estradiol) at 37° caused a shift of the label into the nuclear fraction. In both the cytosol and nuclear fractions, the estradiol was bound to a macromolecule, but the sedimentation coefficients were different. Autoradiograms, both in vitro and in vivo, showed that labeled estradiol was specifically retained in the nuclei of target organs;[142] similar results have been obtained with aldosterone in toad bladder.[144] The general schema is illustrated in Figure 1-58.

Exactly how the cytoplasmic and nuclear binding of estradiol and other steroid hormones leads to the biochemical events associated with hormone action is not yet clear. The simplest hypothesis is modeled after the classical principles of derepression, with the hormone inducing messenger RNA synthesis.[145] Certainly enhanced nuclear RNA synthesis is one of the earliest detectable effects of estradiol administration; a 40% increase in ^{3}H-uridine incorporation into nuclear RNA is seen as early as 2 min after hormone administration in the ovariectomized adult rat.[146] Thus, while steroid hormone effects at the level of translation cannot be ruled out, it appears

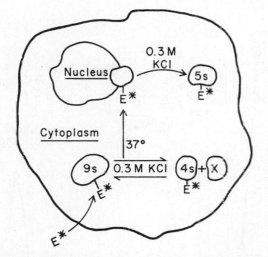

FIGURE 1-58. General scheme for the transfer of estradiol from cytoplasm to nucleus. *Interpretation of experiments like that shown in Figure 1-57 where E* is labeled estradiol. Cytoplasmic receptor is shown as a 9S particle, capable of dissociating into smaller subunits. The 4S subunit, carrying E*, enters the nucleus upon 37°C incubation, whence it can be extracted as a 5S complex. (From Mueller,[148] Figure 12.)*

that enhanced transcription, leading to increased amounts of ribosomal RNA, is an early and perhaps key response. Whether transcription of specific messenger RNA molecules occurs is not yet established. Several reports indicate that RNA extracted from hormone-stimulated target organs may be capable of causing hormone-like effects when placed in the lumen of an immature uterine horn.[149]

A potentially useful new tool for receptor isolation is *affinity chromatography*.[150] The method requires that a ligand be attached covalently to a solid matrix, usually a column of aminated polysaccharide such as Sepharose, a beaded form of cross-linked dextran (agarose). Best results are usually obtained if the ligand is connected to the matrix by a chain of atoms long enough to permit interaction with the binding site, free of steric hindrance. Simple passage of a mixture of proteins containing the complementary macromolecule may then result in retardation of the desired protein because of its high affinity for the attached ligand. Indeed, the binding may be so tight that displacement by a competing ligand is necessary, or a simple alteration of ionic strength, pH, or temperature may suffice to weaken the binding and elute the macromolecule.

The procedure is illustrated in Figure 1-59A for the corticosteroid-binding globulin from plasma, a high-affinity α-globulin that appears to serve a transport function for this class of hormone. Here 2 liters of human plasma were passed through a Sepharose column with attached cortisol. After the bulk of the proteins had passed through the column, and no more was emerging, addition of cortisol to the eluting buffer yielded another peak. A single further purification step on hydroxylapatite produced pure corticosteroid-binding globulin. An indication of the efficiency of the method is given by the yield: From the 2 liters of plasma containing 144 g of protein, 52 mg of the specific protein were obtained, i.e., less than 1 part in 2000 of the original material. Figure 1-59B represents a Scatchard plot of the binding (cf. p. 49, Figure 1-40), obtained by equilibrium dialysis. A single binding site of high affinity is evident.

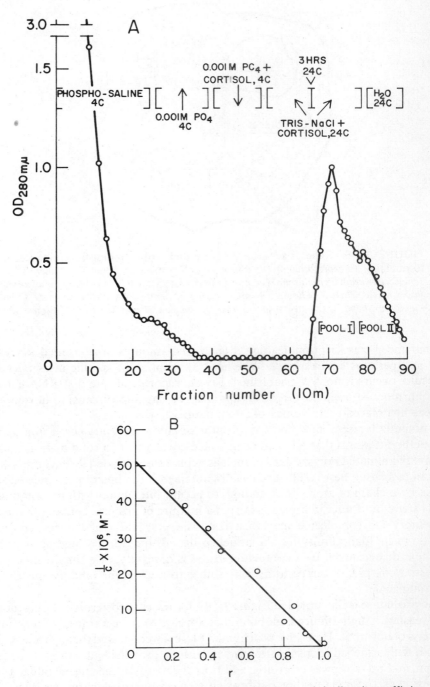

FIGURE 1-59. Isolation of corticosteroid-binding globulin by affinity chromatography. (*A*) *Elution profile of proteins from 2 liters of human plasma. First portion of the double peak eluted at right contained the specific globulin.* (*B*) *Scatchard plot of interaction between pure corticosteroid-binding globulin and cortisol, by equilibrium dialysis. The moles of cortisol bound per mole of protein* (r) *is plotted on the* x *axis. By extrapolation, a single binding site is deduced. Intercept on* y *axis yields association constant,* $5 \times 10^7 M^{-1}$. (*From Rosner and Bradlow,[151] Figures 2 and 6.*)

Affinity chromatography has been used with great success for the isolation of other soluble proteins, especially enzymes (using specific inhibitors as the attached ligands).[152] The method also shows promise for the isolation of membrane-bound receptors. Thus, for example, glucagon–agarose columns have been found to retard the passage of liver cell membrane fragments containing glucagon receptors.[153]

Acetylcholine Receptor

Some effects of AcCh on effector organs have already been described (p. 23). This neurotransmitter is released at cholinergic nerve terminals, diffuses into a synaptic cleft, and interacts with receptors in the postsynaptic membrane, causing a movement of Na^+ into the cell, and an efflux of K^+ from the cell. The result is a localized depolarization, which if it exceeds a threshold value, leads to a propagated depolarization in the postsynaptic element—another nerve cell, a muscle cell, or a modified muscle cell (electroplax) of electric eels and rays.

Acetylcholine receptors have different properties in different anatomical locations. In the neuromuscular junction or ganglia of the autonomic nervous system they are known as "nicotinic" receptors because they are stimulated by nicotine; this type is selectively blocked by agents like tubocurarine. In smooth muscle, AcCh receptors are known as "muscarinic" because they are selectively stimulated by muscarine; these are blocked by agents like atropine. Receptor isolation must necessarily entail loss of the characteristic membrane depolarization effects. The pattern of interaction with the various agonists and antagonists is therefore an important criterion for establishing the identity of a putative receptor. At the least, an AcCh receptor isolated from a nicotinic site should display specific binding of the nicotinic agonists and antagonists, i.e., the binding pattern must be consistent with the known pharmacologic properties of the ligands upon the tissue from which the receptor was obtained.

A peculiar difficulty is that acetylcholinesterase is almost always present in postsynaptic membranes acted on by AcCh. Since this enzyme obviously interacts with AcCh, it must be demonstrated that a putative receptor is not merely acetylcholinesterase. From time to time it has been proposed that acetylcholinesterase is identical to the AcCh receptor, but this has seemed highly unlikely. Irreversible inhibition of the enzyme, as by DFP, does not impede receptor function; on the contrary, the preservation of AcCh against hydrolysis may intensify the tissue response to AcCh. Conversely, receptor antagonists like tubocurarine or atropine do not affect the enzyme. Other proteins capable of interacting specifically with AcCh may also be present, for example presynaptic systems for reuptake of choline, synthesis of AcCh, or storage of AcCh in vesicles. In addition, the usual difficulties associated with nonspecific binding complicate the approach to the problem. Cholinergic agonists and antagonists are cations and therefore may be expected to interact with numerous anionic residues in macromolecules. The earliest attempts to isolate an AcCh receptor from electric organs[154,155] using tubocurarine as a tightly bound ligand, led to inconclusive results; nonspecific binding to acidic mucopolysaccharides and possibly other membrane components obscured any receptor binding.

In addition to the problem of nonspecific binding, another difficulty had to be overcome before significant progress could be made. A ligand like AcCh, which does not display a very great affinity for the receptor sites, will dissociate during the fractionation procedures, unless special precautions are taken.[156]

The difficulties cited above were circumvented by the fortunate discovery of α-bungarotoxin, a basic protein with a molecular weight of about 8000 obtained from a snake venom. This substance is a specific and irreversible blocker of AcCh receptors. It prevents the depolarizing action of AcCh at vertebrate neuromuscular junctions, thus resembling tubocurarine except for its irreversibility. Experiments with ^{3}H-tubocurarine had shown that after intravenous injection in the mouse, the radioactive label was localized in the discrete end-plate region of the diaphragm, where it could be demonstrated by autoradiography.[157,158] Figure 1-60 presents typical results of

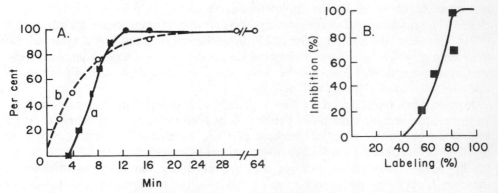

FIGURE 1-60. Autoradiography and inhibition of response of mouse diaphragm by bungarotoxin. *(A) Diaphragm stimulated electrically in tissue bath in the presence of ^{3}H-bungarotoxin (10 μg/ml). Curve a: Inhibition of twitch response. Curve b: Intensity of labeling (grain count) of end-plates. (B) Curve relating percent labeling to inhibition of response, derived from the two curves of A. The squares represent four additional experiments in which the percent labeling was measured by washing one-half of a diaphragm when the desired degree of inhibition was reached, and permitting the other half to be labeled to completion with ^{3}H-bungarotoxin. (Modified from Barnard et al.,[159] Figures 2 and 3.)*

a similar experiment with ^{3}H-bungarotoxin.[159] Diaphragms were mounted in a tissue bath in such a way that they could be stimulated electrically through the phrenic nerve. When ^{3}H-bungarotoxin was introduced, an inhibition of the muscle response developed over a period of about 10 min (panel A), reflecting the slow irreversible attachment of the toxin. At various times, in different experiments, the tissue was removed, washed, and subjected to autoradiography. After development, grain counts over the end-plates gave a measure of the intensity of labeling. A maximum labeling occurred after sufficient exposure to a high concentration of the toxin; thus, the degree of labeling in any experiment could be expressed as a percent of the maximum. Evidently, about half of the sites could be occupied without affecting the muscle response, but then further labeling led to complete inhibition. Panel B shows the same data as panel A (with four additional experiments), plotted to show the percent of inhibition of response as a function of the percent of maximal labeling. The rough agreement between pharmacologic action and physical attachment of bungarotoxin is clear. But the lack of perfect agreement requires explanation. Possibly the initial reaction of bungarotoxin is with another macromolecule, not the receptor. Possibly the inhibition of muscle response requires simultaneous occupancy of two or more receptor sites.

Receptor isolation was attempted, using electric tissue from the sting-ray, *Torpedo*, because of its high content of cholinergically innervated electroplax cells.[160] Membrane fragments prepared from a homogenate were found to bind bungarotoxin. The binding was saturable, and it was interfered with by carbamylcholine (an agonist) or tubocurarine (an antagonist). Since bungarotoxin cannot be removed from the binding sites, the preparation of ligand-free receptors required a special technique. Since the molecular weight of the toxin is low relative to that of the receptor, labeled and unlabeled receptors could be obtained in the same fractions after gel filtration and density gradient centrifugation. The procedure, therefore, was to allow membrane fragments to interact with a very small amount of ^{131}I-bungarotoxin, to label only a small fraction of the total receptor pool. Then the radioactivity served as a marker in the fractionation procedures. Extraction with a nonionic detergent (Triton X-100) solubilized about 8% of the total protein and all of the radioactivity. Further purification yielded a single labeled peak, which also contained ligand-free receptors that could be studied further. The receptor material was readily distinguished from acetylcholinesterase. It consisted of units of molecular weight of approximately 80,000, each carrying one binding site, and aggregating readily into oligomers.

Agonists and antagonists with structural relationship to AcCh have also been used to study the AcCh receptor. One such agonist is muscarone, which interacts specifically with nicotinic sites and cannot be degraded by acetylcholinesterase. Material partially solubilized from *Torpedo* electroplax was subjected to equilibrium dialysis to study the binding.[161] A dissociation constant of $7 \times 10^{-7} M$ was found, and the

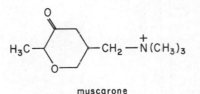

muscarone

binding was interfered with by a variety of drugs known to be nicotinic agonists or antagonists but not by those without such activity. Of numerous enzymes tried, only trypsin, chymotrypsin, and phospholipase C destroyed binding activity, suggesting that the receptor might be a phospholipoprotein.

The electric eel, *Electrophorus*, is particularly suitable for study of the AcCh receptor because individual electroplax cells are large enough to be dissected out and mounted for recording of membrane potentials with a microelectrode. Each electroplax is innervated by about 5×10^4 cholinergic nerve terminals, forming some 10^9-10^{10} synaptic contacts. The receptor protein appears to be present to the extent of about 10–20 μg gram^{-1} of fresh tissue.[162] Membrane fragments extracted with deoxycholate yielded a soluble preparation in which binding could be studied by equilibrium dialysis.[163] The ligand was ^{14}C-decamethonium, a potent reversible agonist for depolarization of the intact electroplax. Two types of binding site were found. One was the catalytic site of acetylcholinesterase, the other appeared to be the receptor. Binding at both sites was blocked by agents like hexamethonium, carbamylcholine, and phenyltrimethylammonium, which are known to affect both the enzyme and the receptor function in intact tissue. Antagonists like tubocurarine or gallamine, which block nicotinic AcCh receptors but not the enzyme, interfered with binding only at the site without acetylcholinesterase activity. Typical results are shown in Figure 1-61.

When an experiment like that shown in Figure 1-61B was carried out with a snake venom protein similar to bungarotoxin, an irreversible partial blockade of decamethonium binding resulted, much like the reversible block by tubocurarine. When the toxin was covalently attached to an agarose matrix for affinity chromatography

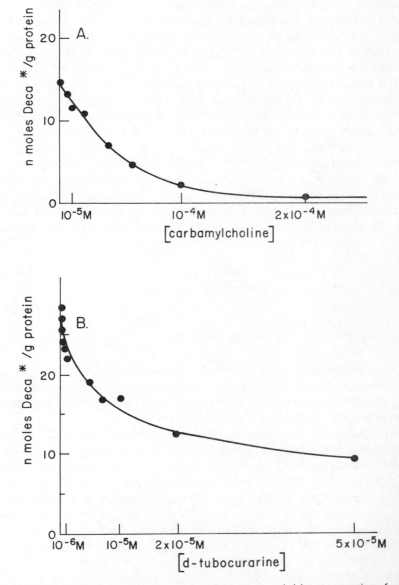

FIGURE 1-61. Binding of decamethonium to a soluble preparation from electroplax. *Two types of blocking of the binding of* ^{14}C-*decamethonium are shown.* (A) *Blocking by carbamylcholine; all sites are blocked.* (B) *Partial blocking by tubocurarine; the unaffected binding is to acetylcholinesterase sites.* (*From Changeux et al.,*[163] *Figures 2 and 5.*)

(p. 71), receptor molecules were selectively absorbed, the esterase activity being separated readily. The irreversible nature of the toxin binding, however, prevented recovery of receptor protein in an active form.

The snake-venom proteins are examples of site-directed reagents, but the molecular basis of their specificity for the AcCh receptor site is not yet understood. Classical site-directed affinity labeling reagents incorporate a reactive group into a congener of the normal ligand. Such reagents were first introduced for enzyme active site labeling; they are analogs of the substrates or inhibitors of a given enzyme.[164] The electroplax AcCh receptor has been studied with an analog of the agonist phenyltrimethylammonium, containing a reactive diazonium group.[165] This compound, p-(trimethylammonium)benzene diazonium fluoroborate (Tdf), irreversibly blocks the depolarizing action of AcCh, carbamylcholine, and other agonists. The block is prevented by reversible antagonists like tubocurarine. Irreversible cholinesterase inhibitors are without effect on the depolarizing action of the agonists, nor is the blockade by Tdf affected; thus, acylation of the esteratic site of acetylcholinesterase (p. 7) does not interfere with the binding of Tdf to the AcCh receptor.

Maleimide derivatives of phenyltrimethylammonium have also been used as site-directed reagents.[166] The electroplax receptor evidently is held in its active conformation by a disulfide bond, for it becomes insensitive to agonists after treatment with the reducing agent, dithiothreitol, and recovers fully upon reoxidation. Maleimido groups react only with reduced $-SH$, and therefore do not inactivate the receptor in its native state. However, if the reduced, inactive receptor is exposed to the maleimide reagent, it is irreversibly blocked, so the reoxidation to a functional state is no longer possible. The site-directing function of the phenyltrimethylammonium moiety is indicated by the fact that N-ethylmaleimide is about 1000 times less potent in irreversibly blocking the reduced receptor. These results confirm that a disulfide bridge is part of or close to the receptor site, and is required for receptor function. It is interesting that interaction with bungarotoxin does not require integrity of the $-S-S-$ bridge, but occurs equally well in reduced electroplax preparations.[167]

Much effort has been devoted to comparing apparent dissociation constants in pharmacologic systems with actual dissociation constants for binding to the putative receptor isolated from membranes. For such experiments a convenient model system was developed—the excitable microsac—which evidently contains the receptor in a functional state, yet is simpler than the whole electroplax cells from which it is prepared.[163] Membranes from homogenized electroplax tissue were allowed to form osmotically intact sacs (much like synaptosomes from nerve terminals) in the presence of radioactive $^{22}Na^+$. After washing and resuspension in an appropriate buffer, the spontaneous leakage of $^{22}Na^+$ was slow, but could be accelerated by addition of AcCh or other cholinergic agonists. This phenomenon evidently reflects the membrane alterations that underlie induced depolarization in the intact tissue. The dissociation constant for decamethonium (1.2 μM) was the same in the microsacs as in the isolated electroplax, and the corresponding binding constant with a deoxycholate extract was nearly the same (0.8 μM). With carbamylcholine the constants were 40, 30, and 18 μM, respectively, and with phenyltrimethylammonium 20, 13, and 13 μM. With antagonists the agreement was very good between the microsacs and electroplax, but the binding affinity was weaker by about one order of magnitude, for reasons not fully understood.

A somewhat different approach to the problem has concentrated upon the extraction of proteolipids from tissues responsive to AcCh. Proteolipids are hydrophobic proteins, as yet not well characterized, which are found in membranes in association with phospholipids and sphingolipids. The classical procedure for extracting them employs a mixture (2:1) of chloroform and methanol. A special formulation of Sephadex (LH-20) permits an empirical fractionation by increasing methanol concentration, which combines solvent partition, adsorption, and molecular sieving. Brain proteolipids extracted and fractionated in this way bound radioactive tubocurarine and atropine, while extracts from electric tissue bound tubocurarine and other nicotinic agonists and antagonists but not atropine.[168] Extracts from electric tissue were allowed to interact with radioactive AcCh, then fractionated on Sephadex LH-20.[169] The results are shown in Figure 1-62. The bound AcCh was in a single

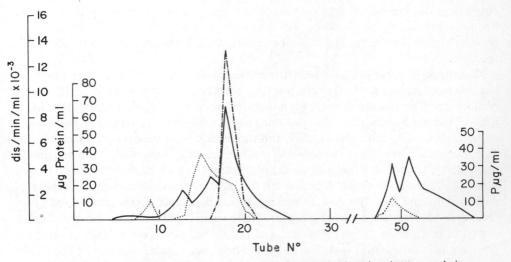

FIGURE 1-62. Fractionation of proteolipid from electric tissue and its interaction with AcCh. *Lyophilized electric tissue from the electric eel was extracted with chloroform–methanol, incubated with* ^{14}C–*AcCh, and fractionated on Sephadex LH-20. Elution was initially with chloroform, then with increasing concentrations of methanol in chloroform.* ——— = *protein;* –·–·–·–·– = *radioactivity;* ········ = *lipid P. (From de Robertis et al.,[170] Figure 1.)*

peak (peak 3), coincident with one of the proteolipid peaks but not with most of the phospholipid. Kinetic studies of the binding revealed two distinct interactions, the high-affinity binding was characterized by a dissociation constant of about $10^{-7} M$ and a single saturable site per protein molecule, assuming a molecular weight of 40,000. In addition, there were about 10 binding sites with much lower affinity ($10^{-5} M$), possibly representing nonspecific ionic interactions. These results were shown earlier (Figure 1-40), to illustrate the use of Scatchard plots.

Further evidence that the proteolipid peak described above may contain the AcCh receptor was obtained in the following experiments.[171] An artificial bilayer membrane was established in a pinhole contained in a plastic diaphragm separating two salt solutions. Such membranes are called "black lipidic membranes," from their light-reflective properties; they were made of cholesterol and phospholipid from cerebral cortex. Conductivity was measured by current flow in the nanoampere range with a very small d.c. potential across the membrane. In the normal condition conductivity is very low. Figure 1-63B shows that if an indifferent proteolipid fraction was incorporated into the membrane, neither AcCh nor choline produced significant change in conductivity; and the same result was obtained (not shown) in the absence of any proteolipid. However, when the proteolipid of peak 3 (Figure 1-63) was present at 1

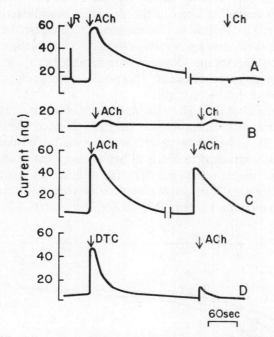

FIGURE 1-63. Effects of AcCh on conductance of artificial membranes containing specific proteolipid. *The records show nanoampere currents as measures of membrane conductance. In each case an artificial bilayer membrane was prepared, containing an added proteolipid from electric tissue. A, C, and D contained material from peak 3 (the AcCh-combining peak) of Figure 1-62; B contained material from peak 1. R = control addition without proteolipid; Ch = choline; DTC = tubocurarine. (From Parisi et al.,[171] Figure 1.)*

part to 10,000 of phospholipid—the same peak already demonstrated to interact with radioactive AcCh—the membrane became responsive to AcCh as well as to tubocurarine, but not to choline, which lacks agonistic efficacy in the electroplax. Each addition of an effective agent caused a sharp increase in membrane conductance (increased current flow), which returned to baseline in a minute or so The effect of tubocurarine was interesting because in its presence AcCh no longer was effective. These results are certainly reminiscent of those produced in intact biologic membranes, suggesting that the AcCh receptor proteolipid may be functional even in an artificial system. On the other hand, it is possible that any specific ligand–macromolecule interaction occurring within an artificial membrane would lead to the observed conductance changes, as suggested by similar experiments with antigen–antibody interactions.[172] Future research will have to clarify this point and also establish the relationship between the proteolipid characterized here and the detergent-extracted macromolecule described earlier.

Insulin Receptor

Insulin is a protein of molecular weight 5800, consisting of 51 amino acids arranged in two chains cross-linked by two disulfide bonds. One well-established effect of this hormone is to stimulate the uptake of glucose by cells. This can be measured readily in isolated fat cells incubated in vitro in the presence of radioactive glucose; since glucose is metabolized as quickly as it gains access to the glycolytic enzymes in the cell interior, the rate of production of radioactive CO_2 reflects the rate of transport of glucose across the cell membrane. Once cells are broken, of course, the characteristic biologic effect can no longer be measured. This poses special problems for the isolation and characterization of insulin receptors.

It could be surmised from the high molecular weight of this and other polypeptide or protein hormones that their receptors were probably located on the outer surface of the cell membranes, but a direct demonstration of this was undertaken at the outset.[173] Insulin was covalently attached to beads of Sepharose, as already described for the technique of affinity chromatography (p. 71). The attachment was carried out in two ways—through the terminal nitrogen of phenylalanine (residue 1 on the B chain), and through the side-chain amino group of lysine-29, the penultimate residue on the B

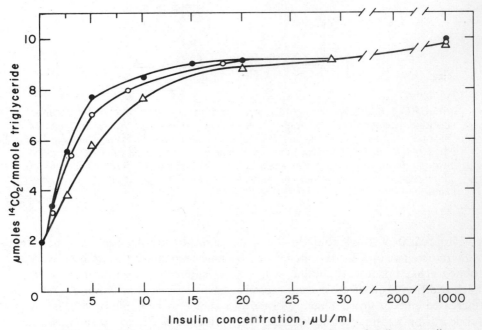

FIGURE 1-64. Effect of insulin on the exterior surface of adipose cells. *Isolated fat cells were incubated for 2 hr at 37°C with radioactive glucose and beads of Sepharose to which insulin had been covalently bound. Production of radioactive CO_2 was a measure of glucose uptake into the cells. Triglyceride content is a convenient way of expressing the number of fat cells. The 3 curves, from left to right, are for native insulin, an insulin-Sepharose complex bound through B-chain N-terminal phenylalanine, and a complex bound through B-chain lysine-29. (From Cuatrecasas,[173] Figure 2.)*

chain. The biologic activity of such polymer-bound insulin preparations was then tested as described above. Figure 1-64 shows that both forms of Sepharose-linked insulin were nearly as effective as native insulin in solution. Since the particle size of the Sepharose beads ranged from 60 to 300 μm and the fat cells had diameters of only 50–100 μm, it seemed evident that the insulin, although bound to an insoluble matrix, was able to interact with receptor sites on the outer membrane surface. The possibility that insulin was being released into solution was carefully excluded.

Further studies were carried out with ^{125}I-labeled insulin, which retained full biologic activity.[174] Now specific binding could be studied. Fat cells were incubated with labeled insulin alone and also in the presence of high concentrations of native insulin. The purpose of this maneuver, as already described for glucocorticoid binding (p. 68), was to distinguish specific (displaceable) from nonspecific binding. As Figure 1-65 shows, the binding proceeded at an easily measurable rate with the low

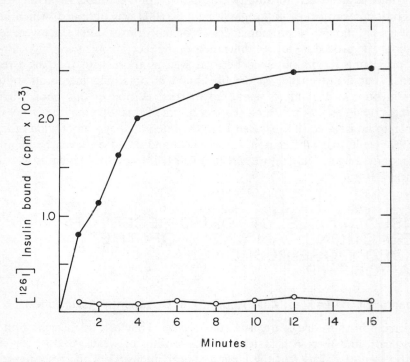

FIGURE 1-65. Rate of binding of insulin to fat cells. *Incubation at 24°C with* [125]*I-labeled insulin (6.8 × 10⁻¹¹ M) in the absence (upper curve) and presence (lower curve) of native insulin (6.9 × 10⁻⁶ M). (From Cuatrecasas,*[174] *Figure 4.)*

concentration of ^{125}I–insulin used, and virtually all of it was prevented by native insulin. Both the association and dissociation rates could be studied. The experiments showed that about 11,000 molecules of insulin could be bound to a single fat cell. The insulin–receptor interaction followed simple mass law kinetics. The association reaction was bimolecular, with a rate constant $1.5 \times 10^7 \ M^{-1} \ \text{sec}^{-1}$, while the dissociation was first-order with a rate constant $7.4 \times 10^{-4} \ \text{sec}^{-1}$. This slow dissociation of the complex results in a very low dissociation constant, $5 \times 10^{-11} \ M$. Remarkably, the concentration of insulin for half-maximal effect on glucose uptake is very nearly the same, 6.1×10^{-11} M.

Cells were next disrupted, and membrane fragments were separated from nuclei and from soluble cell components. Insulin binding was found exclusively in the membrane fragments, and all the insulin bound by the intact cell could be recovered in the membranes. Association and dissociation rates were again determined with these preparations, yielding $k_1 = 8.5 \times 10^6$ and $k_2 = 4.2 \times 10^{-4}$; thus a dissociation constant 5×10^{-11} was computed, exactly the same as before. Equilibrium dialysis gave virtually the same result.[175] It seems reasonably certain, therefore, that despite the inability to measure any biochemical response to insulin in broken cell preparations, the specific binding serves as a valid way to label the receptor for further fractionation and isolation.

Finally, material was purified from detergent extracts of liver cell membranes, which could be absorbed to affinity chromatography columns of insulin–agarose. Upon elution, a protein of molecular weight 300,000 was obtained, which bound 1 mole of insulin mole^{-1} of protein, and was virtually pure. Detergents were required throughout the procedure for solubilization of the receptor protein.[183]

The promising results obtained here, as well as those with the AcCh receptor, betoken a significant change in the likelihood of obtaining membrane-bound receptors in pure form. Only 5 years ago the first edition of this book carried the following statement: "Some think that receptors of this type may be impossible, in principle, to be isolated. If separated from the integrated system of which they are a part, they would lose all function, it is argued, and could not even be identified as receptors any longer. Only future research will tell if such pessimism is warranted." Evidently it is not.

CONSEQUENCES OF DRUG-RECEPTOR INTERACTIONS: ANALYSIS OF THE GRADED DOSE-RESPONSE RELATIONSHIP

Application of the Law of Mass Action: The Occupancy Assumption

Biologic responses to drugs are, as a rule, *graded*. They can be measured on a continuous scale, and there is a systematic relationship between the dose (or effective concentration) of a drug and the magnitude (or intensity) of the response it elicits. Application of the law of mass action to the dose-response relationship was largely the contribution of A. J. Clark (1885–1941).[176,177] An observed biologic effect was assumed to be a reflection of the combination of drug molecules with receptors, much as the rate of appearance of products in an enzyme reaction reflects the degree of combination of substrate molecules with enzyme-active centers. The magnitude of a response was postulated to be directly proportional to the occupancy of receptors by drug molecules, with a maximal response corresponding to occupancy of all the receptors. Then equations could be derived from simple mass law principles, describing the dependence of effect upon dose.

Let a drug, X, combine with a receptor site, R, to yield a complex, RX, producing a biologic response of magnitude Δ proportional to the amount (or concentration) of RX, so that

$$R + X \underset{k_2}{\overset{k_1}{\rightleftharpoons}} RX$$

$$\Delta = k_3(RX)$$

Then at equilibrium,

$$\frac{(R)(X)}{(RX)} = \frac{k_2}{k_1} = K_X$$

where K_X is the dissociation constant of the complex. Then if (R_T) is the total receptor concentration, and since $(R_T) = (R) + (RX)$,

$$\frac{(R_T - RX)(X)}{(RX)} = K_X$$

and, rearranged,

$$\frac{(RX)}{(R_T)} = \frac{(X)}{K_X + (X)}$$

Now let Δ_{max} be the maximal response of which the system is capable, obtained when all receptors are occupied; so

$$\Delta_{max} = k_3(R_T)$$

Then,

$$\frac{\Delta}{\Delta_{max}} = \frac{(RX)}{(R_T)}$$

and therefore

$$\Delta = \frac{\Delta_{max}(X)}{K_X + (X)} \tag{1}$$

This is the familiar hyperbolic function in which $\Delta = 0$ when $(X) = 0$, and Δ approaches Δ_{max} when (X) becomes very large. When half-maximal response is obtained,

$$\frac{\Delta}{\Delta_{max}} = \frac{(X)}{K_X + (X)} = \frac{1}{2}$$

so the concentration of (X) required for half-maximal response is equal to K_X.

The derivation of equation (1) is identical to that of the classical Michaelis–Menten equation, which gives the velocity v of an enzyme reaction as a function of the substrate concentration (S), the enzyme-substrate dissociation constant K_m, and the maximum velocity V_{max}:

$$v = \frac{V_{max}(S)}{K_m + (S)}$$

Here the proportionality $v = k_3(ES)$ refers to the breakdown of a steady-state intermediate, whereas the analogous proportionality $\Delta = k_3(RX)$ is assumed without reference to any particular underlying mechanism. The equations developed here are quite generally applicable; they subsume enzyme-substrate and enzyme-inhibitor interactions as special cases.

Three critical assumptions, which underlie the derivation or usual application of equation (1), may be formulated explicitly, as follows:

1. *Response is proportional to receptor occupancy.* This will be referred to as the "occupancy assumption." In the case of enzyme-substrate and enzyme-inhibitor interactions, since the observed response is determined directly by the concentration of enzyme-bound substrate or inhibitor, the assumption is soundly based. With respect to drug effects in general, however, we are as yet unable to accept or reject the assumption on experimental or theoretical grounds. In a later section we shall discuss alternatives to the "occupancy assumption."

2. *One drug molecule combines with one receptor site.* This is the simplest reaction mechanism, from which equation (1) (and also the Michaelis–Menten treatment) is derived. We shall consider later some molecular combining ratios other than unity.

3. *A negligible fraction of total drug is combined,* so that in equation (1) the term (X), which refers to uncombined drug, may be replaced by (X_T), the total drug concentration. A system in which this assumption is true is said to operate in zone A.[178] In experiments where binding is actually measured, as in equilibrium dialysis, uncombined drug is determined and equation (1) (equivalent to the equations on p. 161) can be used rigorously. However, when a biologic response is the criterion of effect, only *total* drug added to the system is known. It is then usual to assume zone A behavior, as we shall do in the following section (and as is customary in mathematical treatments of enzyme reactions based on the Michaelis–Menten approach). Later, however, we shall examine the consequences when a system does not operate in zone A.

If equation (1) is inverted, the equation of a straight line is obtained:

$$\frac{1}{\Delta} = \frac{K_X}{\Delta_{max}} \cdot \frac{1}{(X)} + \frac{1}{\Delta_{max}} \tag{2}$$

with slope K_X/Δ_{max} and intercept $1/\Delta_{max}$ when reciprocal response magnitudes $1/\Delta$ are plotted against reciprocal doses $1/(X)$, actually $1/(X_T)$, as explained above in connection with the *zone A* assumption.

This procedure is known as a double-reciprocal (or Lineweaver–Burk) plot (Figure 1-66).[179] Increasing drug concentrations are to the left, so the y axis is at $1/(X) = 0$, corresponding to infinite drug concentration, where all receptors are occupied. The y intercept gives $1/\Delta_{max}$. Since the slope, given by equation (2), is K_X/Δ_{max}, K_X could be obtained by estimating the slope; but an easier way is simply to extend the line downward and to the left, as shown. The x intercept will then be $-1/K_X$.

The double-reciprocal plot has been applied widely to the analysis of antagonisms and particularly to enzyme inhibitions, but it has limitations.[180] An antagonist Z is said to be *noncompetitive* if it inactivates the receptor so that the effective complex with agonist X cannot be formed, regardless of the concentration of X. Z might combine with R at the same site where X ordinarily combines, but so firmly that it cannot be displaced. Alternatively, Z could combine at a different site, in such a manner as to prevent a conformation change in R that is essential to its proper combination with X, or that is requisite to producing the characteristic biologic response. Yet again, Z might itself induce a conformation change in R that abolishes the reactivity of the site where X should interact. In noncompetitive antagonism the effects upon receptors

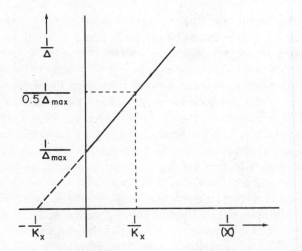

FIGURE 1-66. The double-reciprocal plot. *Symbols are defined in text. Intercept on y axis gives reciprocal of* Δ_{max}; *that on x axis gives negative reciprocal of* K_X.

may be reversible or irreversible; the essential point is that the agonist has no influence upon the degree of antagonism or its reversibility.

If the dose-response range is first explored with an agonist alone and then in the presence of a fixed dose (or concentration) of a noncompetitive antagonist, the system will behave as though the total number of available receptor sites had been reduced. Nevertheless, whatever receptors remain should display unchanged affinity for X. In the double-reciprocal plot (Figure 1-67a), since Δ_{max} is reduced proportionately

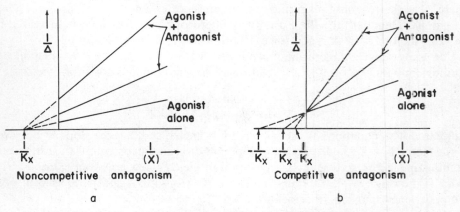

FIGURE 1-67. Analysis of antagonisms by double-reciprocal plots.

to the decrease in free receptors, the y intercept will increase. On the other hand, the x intercept $(-1/K_X)$ will remain unchanged.

An antagonist is said to be *competitive* if it combines reversibly with the same receptor sites as the agonist. In the most straightforward mechanism, Z occupies the same sites as X, but without triggering those special events that cause the biologic response.

In the case of enzyme inhibition this may simply mean that the Z molecule, although it combines with enzyme, is incapable of undergoing catalytic transformation, or that it is acted upon very slowly compared with the normal substrate. In the case of a receptor that normally undergoes a change in shape by virtue of combination with X, the Z molecule may occupy the site without producing the essential conformation change. The effect of the competition, in any case, is a reduction of the apparent affinity of X for R in the presence of Z, as predicted by the law of mass action. In competitive antagonism Δ_{max} is not altered, since a high enough ratio of $X:Z$ should force complete occupancy of receptors by X despite the presence of Z. In the double-reciprocal plot, therefore (Figure 1-67b), the y intercept remains unchanged, but the affinity ($-1/K_X$, x intercept) is reduced. It should be realized that any molecular mechanism that leads to this experimental result will be interpreted as competitive antagonism. For example, if the combination of Z with R induced a conformational change that altered the binding energy of RX, the antagonism would be classified as competitive, even if Z and X combined with R independently at different sites.

Abbreviated derivations follow for equations that apply to double-reciprocal plots of noncompetitive and competitive antagonisms.[179]

For reversible noncompetitive antagonism, where antagonist Z forms a complex RZ with dissociation constant K_Z,

$$\frac{(R)(Z)}{(RZ)} = K_Z$$

Following the same steps as in the derivation of equation (1), and then substituting, gives

$$\frac{1}{\Delta'} = \left(1 + \frac{Z}{K_Z}\right)\left(\frac{K_X}{\Delta_{max}}\right)\left(\frac{1}{X}\right) + \left(1 + \frac{Z}{K_Z}\right)\left(\frac{1}{\Delta_{max}}\right)$$

where Δ' is the response magnitude in the presence of a fixed concentration (Z) of antagonist. Thus both the slope and the y intercept of equation (2) are increased by the same factor $1 + Z/K_Z$, and since (Z) is known, K_Z can be found.

For competitive antagonism, uncombined receptors (R) must be in simultaneous equilibrium with (RX) and (RZ). Solution of the simultaneous equations yields

$$\frac{1}{\Delta'} = \left(1 + \frac{Z}{K_Z}\right)\left(\frac{K_X}{\Delta_{max}}\right)\left(\frac{1}{X}\right) + \frac{1}{\Delta_{max}}$$

Compared with equation (2), the y intercept is unchanged, but the slope is increased by the factor $1 + Z/K_Z$. In effect, the apparent dissociation constant K_X is increased by this same factor, so that the x intercept now yields a new apparent value $-1/K_X$, which is the original $-1/K_X$ times the factor $K_Z/(K_Z+Z)$. Again here, as with noncompetitive antagonism, since (Z) is known, K_Z can be found.

Often the equation for competitive inhibition of a receptor is put in the form

$$\frac{(X)_Z}{(X)_0} - 1 = K_Z(Z)$$

where the symbols have the same meanings as above. Here $(X)_0$ is the concentration of agonist to produce an arbitrarily chosen response in the graded portion of the dose-response curve, e.g., a half-maximal response. Then $(X)_Z$ is the concentration needed to produce the same response in the presence of concentration (Z) of the antagonist;

$(X)_Z/(X)_0$ is known as the *dose ratio*, the ratio of the two agonist concentrations producing the same response in the presence and absence of antagonist. Since K_X does not appear in the equation, the same dose ratio will be found regardless of what agonist is used. Determination of K_Z is simple, requiring only one concentration of the antagonist, and the determination of the dose ratio at any convenient response level.

A good example of the use of a double-reciprocal plot to establish the mechanism of an inhibitory effect is shown in Figure 1-68. The N-demethylation of a morphine

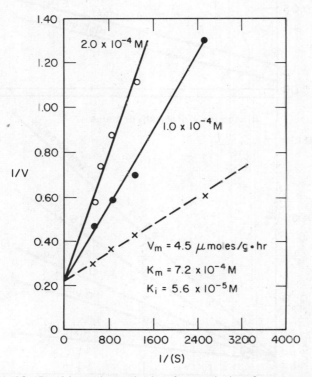

FIGURE 1-68. Double-reciprocal plot for analysis of enzyme inhibition. *Effect of chlorpromazine on* N-*demethylation of ethylmorphine by a microsomal system. Chlorpromazine concentrations are shown on the two upper curves; the lower curve was obtained in the absence of chlorpromazine;* V *is reaction velocity,* (S) *is substrate concentration. The parameters computed from the intercepts (x intercept not actually shown) are given at lower right. (From Rubin et al., Figure 2 [181])*

analog by a microsomal drug-metabolizing system was studied.[181] The rate of formation of formaldehyde, the ultimate product of the reaction, was measured at various substrate concentrations. The results shown as a broken line were obtained, whence the intercept and slope yielded $V_{max} = 4.5$ μmoles g^{-1} h^{-1} and $K_m = 7.2 \times 10^{-4}$ M. Here the symbols are those customarily used in enzymology, v for the reaction velocity (instead of Δ), V_{max} instead of Δ_{max}, (S) for substrate concentration [instead of (X)], K_m for Michaelis constant (instead of K_X), and K_i for enzyme-inhibitor dissociation constant (instead of K_Z). The experiment was repeated in the presence of chlorpromazine at two different concentrations. Clearly, chlorpromazine inhibits the reaction competitively; its K_i was found to be $5.6 \times 10^{-5} M$, i.e., its affinity for the enzyme was more than 12 times greater than that of the morphine analog.

Figure 1-69 illustrates the application of a double-reciprocal plot to biologic responses in which the nature of the receptors is unknown.[182] If histamine is injected

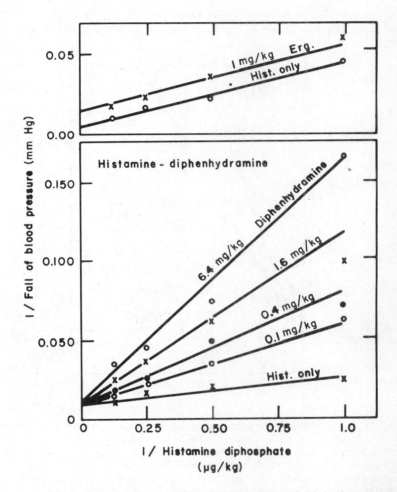

FIGURE 1-69. Double-reciprocal plot for analysis of biologic response. *Blood pressure fall caused by histamine in the dog was measured. In upper section, antagonism by ergotamine was studied; in lower section, antagonism by an antihistaminic drug, diphenhydramine, at several concentrations (doses kg^{-1}). (From Chen and Russell, Figure 4.[182])*

into the blood stream, there is a prompt fall in blood pressure, and this effect can be antagonized by pretreatment with antihistaminic drugs. In the experiments depicted, it could be concluded that diphenhydramine acts as a competitive antagonist of histamine, whereas the antagonism caused by ergotamine is noncompetitive.

The Log Dose-Response Curve

In pharmacology it is conventional to show the relationship between dose and response more directly than on a double-reciprocal plot. In Figure 1-70, two methods of graphical presentation are compared. The dose of a glucocorticoid drug was varied, as in the SAR studies described earlier, and the amount of glycogen deposited in the liver was measured. In both cases the dependent variable (amount of glycogen) is plotted on an arithmetic scale of ordinates. On the left the values of the independent variable (dose) are also plotted on an arithmetic scale on the x axis, but on the right these same data are plotted on a logarithmic scale. The curves, which are fairly typical, indicate that from a practical standpoint the logarithmic dosage scale is preferable. Line segments rather than hyperbolic curves are obtained, which are much easier to deal with in statistical analysis. Moreover, drugs that produce the same effect by the same mechanism but differ in potency yield parallel line segments, and this is very convenient. For example, in Figure 1-70b the constant horizontal separation of

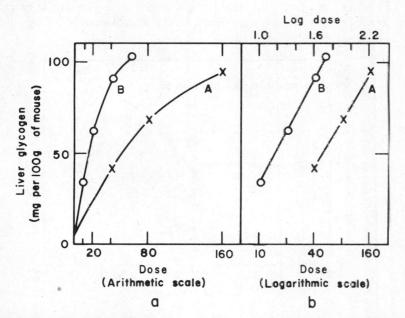

FIGURE 1-70. Linear and semilogarithmic dose-response curves. *Effects of two steroids, 11-dehydrocorticosterone (A) and cortisone (B), on liver glycogen in mice. (From Gaddum, Figure 85[184] adapted from Venning, Figure 2.[185])*

the lines is a measure of the potency ratio for the two drugs, since the difference (log dose A − log dose B) is the same as log (dose A/dose B), where the doses are those required to produce an equal response. Another practical advantage of the logarithmic dosage scale is that a wide range of doses can be presented readily in a single graph. Thus, quite apart from any theoretical considerations, there are sufficient reasons for plotting dose-response relationships on semilogarithmic coordinates, and it has become customary to do so.

Obviously, the line segments of Figure 1-70b could not extend indefinitely to both extremes of the log dose scale. There must be some dose which is so low that no perceptible response is obtained, and there must also be doses so high that the capacity of the biologic system to respond is exceeded. In the case of the glucocorticoids, there would be a maximum possible increment in the amount of liver glycogen. Thus we might predict, a priori, some kind of sigmoid curve, approaching zero response at very low doses and a maximum response at very high doses. This prediction is borne out experimentally. A typical log dose-response (LDR) curve extending over a wide dose range is shown in Figure 1-71. Here, several concentrations of histamine were added to a tissue bath in which a section of guinea pig ileum was suspended, and the amplitude of the resulting contractions was measured. The curve is seen to be sigmoid, and to approach zero and a maximum asymptotically. It is symmetrical about the point at which 50% of the maximum response is obtained, and its maximum slope and point of inflection occur at this midpoint. Line segments, such as those in Figure 1-70b, are derived from the central nearly linear portions of sigmoid LDR curves. The lower the ED50 (the dose for half-maximal response) the more potent the drug. The ED50 for histamine in Figure 1-71 is approximately 0.6 μg.

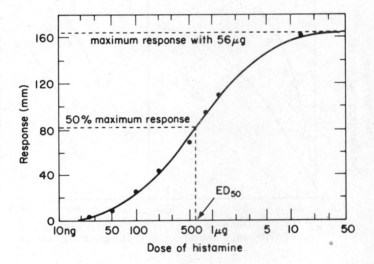

FIGURE 1-71. LDR curve for histamine acting on guinea pig ileum in a tissue bath. *Response magnitude (read directly from a kymograph tracing) is proportional to actual contraction of the ileum. Histamine dose added to constant-volume tissue bath is shown on a logarithmic scale. (Adapted from Paton, Figure 4.[186])*

The position of an LDR curve on the x axis reflects the affinity of the drug for its receptor. Since by convention the scale of dosage increases from left to right, it follows that for a series of congeneric drugs interacting with the same receptor a set of parallel LDR curves is expected. The curve for the most potent drug will be at the left, curves for drugs with poorer affinities for the receptor will lie farther to the right. An example is shown in Figure 1-72. Here, the response measured was contraction of the isolated cat spleen strip upon exposure to epinephrine or norepinephrine in a

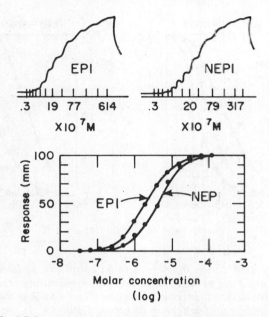

FIGURE 1-72. LDR curves for epinephrine (EPI) and norepinephrine (NEPI) action on isolated cat spleen. *Upper portion: Actual concentration activity recordings for the two catecholamines obtained in a single spleen strip. Lower portion: Semilogarithmic plot of the data in upper panel. (From Bickerton, Figure 1.*[187]*)*

tissue bath. The actual record of responses is shown on the upper line, the corresponding LDR curves below. The apparent affinity of epinephrine for the receptor that mediates the contractile response is seen to be about twice that of norepinephrine. Just as the parallelism of these two curves is regarded as consistent with an identical mechanism of action (i.e., interaction with the same receptor site), so in general would a lack of parallelism create the strong presumption that two drugs produce the same end effect by different mechanisms. Further evidence that the two drugs combine at the same receptor is the fact that the same maximum contraction was obtained.

The analysis of antagonisms in the framework of the LDR curve is straightforward.[183,188,189] In the presence of a competitive antagonist, the curve for an agonist will be shifted to the right, but neither the slope not the maximum response would be expected to change. The antagonist simply alters the effective affinity of agonist drug for receptor. Figure 1-73a gives a typical example. In the same system as described above, using the spleen strip, contractions were elicited by norepinephrine as before, and also in the presence of two different concentrations of an antagonist, tolazoline. The parallelism of the curves is not perfect, perhaps because of the modifying effect of a saturable uptake process upon the LDR curve itself,[190] but the interpretation is obvious; tolazoline occupies the receptor site competitively but cannot itself trigger a contractile response. If sufficient norepinephrine is present, the tolazoline blockade can be overcome completely.

The effect of a noncompetitive antagonist upon the LDR curve will be quite different. The agonist curve will again be shifted to the right, but the slope will be reduced and the maximum response will diminish, in relation to the degree of noncompetitive blockade established. This is nicely illustrated in the same biologic

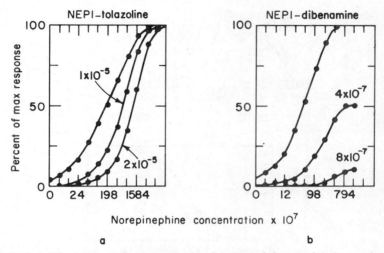

FIGURE 1-73. LDR curves in analysis of antagonisms. *Isolated cat spleen, as in Figure 1-72, stimulated by NEPI at various molar concentrations, as indicated. In (a) and (b) the curve farthest to left is the control, the others were obtained in the presence of two antagonist concentrations. (From Bickerton, Figure 3.*[187])

system (Figure 1-73b) by the effects of two concentrations of dibenamine, an alkylating agent, upon the contractile response to norepinephrine.

Now we shall examine to what extent actual LDR curves can be described by equations based on the law of mass action. Let f be the fraction of maximal response obtained at a given dose, as follows:

$$f = \frac{\Delta}{\Delta_{max}} = \frac{(RX)}{(R_T)}$$

Substituting from equation (1), and rearranging yields

$$f = \frac{(X)}{K_X + (X)}$$

$$(X) = K_X\left(\frac{f}{1 - f}\right)$$

By substituting $(X_T) - (RX)$ for (X) and $f(R_T)$ for (RX), we obtain

$$(X_T) = K_X\left(\frac{f}{1 - f}\right) + f(R_T) \tag{3}$$

Total drug = free drug + bound drug

Equation (3) is broadly applicable to dose-response relationships in which the "occupancy assumption" applies, and in which the molar combining ratio of drug to receptor is unity (our first and second assumptions); it does not presuppose any particular fraction of total drug bound to receptors (our third assumption). If in equation (3) the term $f(R_T)$, representing bound drug, is very much smaller than $K_X[f/(1 - f)]$, representing free drug, it may be ignored. For any moderate values of f this simplification can be made if (R_T) is small compared with K_X (e.g., R_T/K_X less than 1/10). We will then have the *zone A* approximation, in which practically all drug molecules are free even at receptor saturation, so that

$$(X_T) \cong (X) = K_X\left(\frac{f}{1-f}\right) \tag{3A}$$

At the other extreme, if R_T is very much larger than K_X, then the expression $K_X[f/(1-f)]$, representing free drug, becomes negligible for any moderate values of f. We will then have the *zone C* approximation, in which practically no drug molecules are free, as follows:

$$(X_T) \cong f(R_T) \tag{3C}$$

Here, because the drug-receptor dissociation constant is so small, or the receptor concentration is so large, the binding is essentially stoichiometric ("pseudo-irreversible") even though the interaction is technically a reversible one. A truly irreversible drug-receptor combination would give the same equation and corresponding LDR curve.

Behavior intermediate between these two extremes, which has to be described by the full form of equation (3), is known as *zone B* behavior. The validity of simplifying equation (3), in the cases of *zone A* and *zone C*, it should be noted, depends entirely upon the ratio R_T/K_X, i.e., upon the concentration of receptors expressed in units of the drug-receptor dissociation constant.

For the same reason equation (3) can be written more usefully in the following way:

$$\frac{(X_T)}{K_X} = \frac{f}{1-f} + f\left\{\frac{(R_T)}{K_X}\right\}$$

The three forms of this equation are plotted as LDR curves in Figure 1-74. Here the x axis shows log dose, each dose being expressed in units of the drug-receptor dissociation constant. Thus f is plotted against $\log(X_T/K_X)$.

The LDR curve for *zone A* in this graph will be recognized as the familiar symmetrical sigmoid, which inflects at $f = 0.5$. Indeed, the zone A LDR curve is identical

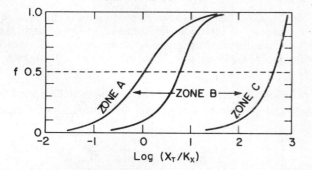

FIGURE 1-74. Theoretical LDR curves for the 3 zones of behavior. *Ordinal values f are fractions of maximal response or fractional occupancy of receptors. Abscissal values are logarithms of drug concentration (dose) normalized by expressing in units of the drug-receptor dissociation constant. In zone A practically all the drug is free. In zone C practically all the drug is combined with receptor sites. In zone B neither free nor combined drug can be neglected; only a single representative curve is shown. (Adapted from Straus and Goldstein, Figure 2.[178] By permission of Cambridge University Press.)*

to the graphic representation of the Henderson–Hasselbalch equation, and for the following reason. We may rewrite equation (3A):

$$\log(X) = \log K_X + \log\left(\frac{f}{1-f}\right)$$

which is completely equivalent to

$$\log(\text{H}^+) = \log K_a' + \log\left(\frac{\text{acid}}{\text{base}}\right)$$

$$= \log K_a' + \log\left(\frac{\beta}{1-\beta}\right)$$

where β is the nonionized fraction. Inversion yields the description of the customary plot of fraction ionized as a function of pH.

Zone A LDR curves for a congeneric drug series (like ionization-pH curves for a set of weak acids) are parallel sigmoids (Figure 1-75) with invariant slopes at their

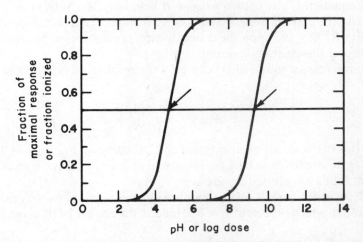

FIGURE 1-75. Zone-A LDR curves for two congeneric drugs with different affinities for receptor, or pH-ionization curves for two weak acids with different pK_a'. *Perpendiculars dropped from the intersections indicated by arrows will give ED50 (equal to K_X under zone A conditions) or pK_a', respectively.*

midpoints. The position of each curve on the x axis is determined by its K_X. The midpoint slope is found by differentiating the logarithmic form of equation (3A) (see above), as follows:

$$d\ln(X) = d\ln\left(\frac{f}{1-f}\right) = \frac{df}{f(1-f)}$$

$$\frac{df}{d\log(X)} = 2.303\,f(1-f)$$

and, at the midpoint, when $f = 0.5$,

$$\frac{df}{d\log(X)} = 0.576$$

For zone C the theoretical curve is described by the logarithmic form of equation (3C):

$$\log f = \log (X_T/R_T)$$

in which the molecular ratio of drug to receptors determines the fractional response. The LDR curve (Figure 1-74) is no longer sigmoid, and differentiation yields a midpoint slope of 1.15, just double that of the zone A curve; LDR curves for zone B are in all respects transitional between zone A and zone C; one such curve is depicted in Figure 1-74.

Figure 1-76 presents typical experimental data on enzyme-substrate and enzyme-inhibitor interactions plotted as LDR curves. The slopes of both curves at their midpoints are almost exactly 0.576, the theoretical zone A value.

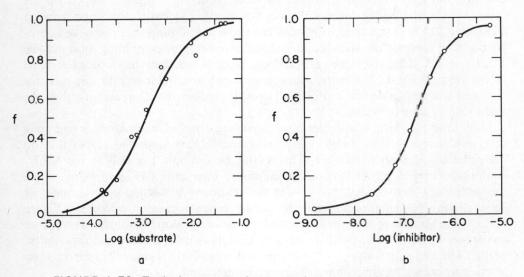

FIGURE 1-76. Typical enzyme-substrate and enzyme-inhibitor interactions plotted as LDR curves. *Both curves depict experiments with plasma cholinesterase. Fraction of maximal velocity or fractional inhibition is plotted against logarithm of substrate or inhibitor concentration. (a) AcCh as substrate; (b) physostigmine as inhibitor. Velocity measured in the presence of a saturating concentration of substrate. (Adapted from Goldstein, Figure 1,[191] and Straus and Goldstein, Figure 4.[178] By permission of Cambridge University Press.)*

In all the foregoing we have assumed that one molecule of drug combines with one receptor site, and there are good reasons to believe that this is usually the case. But other combining ratios are not out of the question. A cross-linking alkylating agent would give the reaction

$$X + 2R \rightleftharpoons XR_2$$

with drug/receptor combining ratio 1/2. Also, two substrate molecules may sometimes occupy an enzyme active center in such a way that the functional 1/1 combination is prevented ("excess substrate inhibition"), and there may be other ways in which two drug molecules could occupy one receptor site, according to the following reaction scheme:

$$2X + R \rightleftharpoons X_2R$$

with drug/receptor combining ratio 2/1. Equations for the corresponding LDR curves will not be derived, but some conclusions may be stated briefly. In zone A the midpoint slope is $0.576\,n$, where n is the drug/receptor combining ratio; so for ratios 1/2, 1/1, and 2/1 the slopes are 0.288, 0.576, and 1.15, respectively. In zone C the slope is 1.15 for all values of n.

A systematic change in the shape and symmetry of the curves is evident as one passes from zone A to zone C (Figure 1-74), but in a real biologic test system the precision of observations at near-maximum responses would not usually be good enough to distinguish between a curve that flattens at the top (zones A and B) and one that abruptly reaches maximum response (zone C). Midpoint slopes, on the other hand, can often be measured quite accurately. Evidently, any slope between 0.288 and 1.15 is compatible with mass law theory, assuming that response is proportional to receptor occupancy and that the drug/receptor combining ratio may be 1/2, 1/1, or 2/1. If the combining ratio 1/2 can be excluded, then the slope is restricted to the range 0.576–1.15. Finally, if one drug molecule combines with one receptor site, and if a negligible fraction of total drug is combined with receptors, then the slope should have the value 0.576.

In an unusually large number of cases, involving drugs of many kinds acting upon diverse biologic systems, LDR curves are found to have midpoint slopes that do not differ significantly from 0.576. This is true, for example, not only in the AcCh–cholinesterase and physostigmine-cholinesterase interactions (Figure 1-76), where the receptor is well defined, but also in the actions of histamine upon guinea pig ileum (Figure 1-71) and of norepinephrine and epinephrine upon cat spleen (Figure 1-72). In the absence of any other reason why a particular slope should be favored, the recurrence of values close to 0.576 suggests strongly that the mass law interpretation of the LDR curve (including the "occupancy assumption") is generally correct, even in cases where the receptors have not been characterized.

Alternatives to the Occupancy Assumption

Fractional Occupancy Threshold.   If the receptors with which a drug combines do not have a rate-limiting role in the overall reaction sequence leading to the characteristic biologic response, then no drug effect at all will be seen until a certain *fractional occupancy threshold* is exceeded. This alternative to the occupancy assumption demands serious consideration because it has a clear theoretical basis and is known to apply to some instances of enzyme inhibition. Consider a sequence of metabolic conversion in which the biologic response produced by a drug X is proportional to the reduction in the steady-state concentration of a product M brought about by drug inhibition of one enzyme, E_3, in the pathway as follows:

$$\xrightarrow{\quad E_1 \quad} J \xrightarrow{\quad E_2 \quad} K \xrightarrow[\uparrow]{\quad E_3 \quad} L \xrightarrow{\quad E_4 \quad} \textcircled{M} \xrightarrow{\quad E_5 \quad}$$
$$X$$

If X inhibits the enzyme E_3, and if E_3 is rate limiting for the production of M, then we should expect the "occupancy assumption" to be valid, since the fractional inhibition of E_3 will reduce the rate of production of M proportionately. If, on the other hand, E_3 is present in excess, then some degree of inhibition may occur without significant effect upon M. But with increasing inhibition a point will finally be reached when E_3 becomes rate limiting, and then further reduction in its activity will cause the onset of drug effect. The general result is to steepen the LDR curve.

For drug/receptor molecular combining ratio $1/1$, if f_0 be the *fractional occupancy threshold* below which no drug effect occurs, and if (as before) the maximal drug effect ($f = 1.0$) occurs at receptor saturation, then in zone A

$$(X_T) = K_X \left\{ \frac{f + [f_0/(1 - f_0)]}{1 - f} \right\} \tag{4A}$$

and in zone C

$$(X_T) = (R_T)\{f + (1 - f)f_0\} \tag{4C}$$

These modified equations describe LDR curves with interesting new properties. Figure 1-77 is an illustration for $f_0 = 0.5$. The curve representing fractional occupancy $(RX)/(R_T)$ is no longer identical to that representing fractional response f; the latter is displaced to the right and it will rise more steeply the greater the value of f_0.

In zone A the midpoint slope cannot exceed 1.15, twice the slope of the usual zone A curve. In zone C, however, the greater the value of f_0, the steeper the slope, without limit. For example, in Figure 1-77 with fractional occupancy threshold 0.5, the LDR

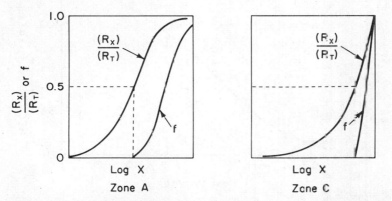

FIGURE 1-77. Theoretical LDR curves for fractional occupancy threshold 0.5. *It is assumed that no biologic response occurs until one-half the receptors are occupied ($f_0 = (RX)/(R_T) = 0.5$). As usual, f represents the fraction of maximal response, but it is no longer identical to fractional occupancy of receptors, (RX)/(R_T). Total drug concentration (X_T) is plotted logarithmically along the abscissal axis. Broken lines define f_0; up to half-saturation of the receptors there is no biologic response ($f = 0$).*

slope at $f = 0.5$ is 0.863 in zone A and 3.45 in zone C. For a very large excess of receptors (e.g., $f_0 = 0.9$) the LDR curve in zone C could be so steep as to mimic an all-or-none type of response.

An interesting consequence of the displacement of biologic response curves to the right of receptor occupancy curves is that the experimentally determined LDR will now underestimate the true affinity of drug for receptor, i.e., the ED50 will be a larger number than K_X.

A concrete example of the influence of excess receptors is found in the properties of carbonic anhydrase inhibitors.[193-195] These drugs cause diuresis by blocking hydrogen ion secretion in the kidney tubules.

$$CO_2 + H_2O \underset{X}{\overset{C.A.}{\rightleftharpoons}} H^- + HCO_3^-$$

$$\downarrow \overline{\frac{cell}{urine}}$$

The enzyme carbonic anhydrase (C.A.) catalyzes the hydration of CO_2, which is not a rapid process in the absence of the enzyme. Thus, the availability of sufficient H^+ to maintain a normal rate of acidification of the tubular urine requires the presence of C.A. As expected, if C.A. is sufficiently inhibited, the urine becomes more alkaline. Since HCO_3^- in the glomerular filtrate is no longer neutralized as completely, the effect of a C.A. inhibitor (X) can be estimated by measuring the urinary HCO_3^-.

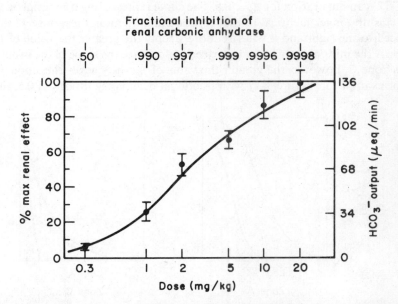

FIGURE 1-78. Fractional occupancy threshold with a carbonic anhydrase inhibitor. *Acetazolamide was given intravenously to dogs (7 to 13 animals at each dose), and urine HCO_3^- output was measured for a 30 min period. Points and vertical bars are means and their standard errors. Untreated dogs excreted only 4 μeq of HCO_3^- per minute. Fractional inhibitions of renal carbonic anhydrase were estimated from determinations of renal acetazolamide content at each dose level and the known enzyme-inhibitory properties of this drug. (From Maren, Figure 3.[193])*

Figure 1-78 shows an LDR curve for one such drug, acetazolamide, in comparison with the computed fractional inhibition of the enzyme at each drug dose. Clearly, C.A. is present in excess initially. As in the theoretical illustration (Figure 1-77) about one-half of the enzyme activity has to be abolished before any biologic response is seen (f_0 approximately 0.5). Similarly, 99.7% of the enzyme activity has to be abolished in order to achieve half of the maximum possible effect.

Efficacy (Intrinsic Activity).   According to the occupancy assumption, the magnitude of a response is determined by the number of receptors occupied. Agonist drugs are supposed to differ in affinity for the receptor, so that different doses are required to achieve the same degree of receptor occupancy, and hence the same response. A molecule of any agonist occupying a given receptor site is assumed to make the same quantal contribution to the overall response as a molecule of any other agonist.

However, instances are known in which various agonists that apparently act on the same receptor site produce maximal responses of different magnitudes, an observation not readily accounted for by the theory. Attempts have therefore been made[8,196] to modify receptor theory, by endowing every drug with two independent properties concerned with its receptor combination: affinity (as discussed already) and a new property, "efficacy," or "intrinsic activity." Affinity describes the tendency of the drug to form a stable complex with receptor. Efficacy describes the biologic effectiveness of the drug-receptor complex. The two properties are considered to be unrelated, much in the same way as are affinities and turnover rates in a series of substrates of a given enzyme. Here, for example, an agonist and an antagonist could have the same affinity for a receptor site, but the former would have a high, the latter a low efficacy. Since the biologic effect of a drug at a given dose would be determined both by the extent of receptor occupancy (determined by affinity) and by the efficacy, it follows that according to this theory equal biologic responses need not imply equal degrees of receptor occupancy, and maximal responses may vary from drug to drug. This has, indeed, been observed in numerous instances; an example is shown in Figure 1-79. A series of alkyl trimethylammonium compounds was tested

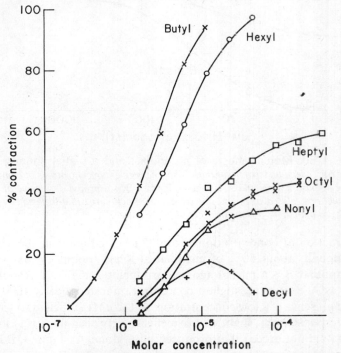

FIGURE 1-79. Agonists and partial agonists on the guinea pig ileum. *A series of alkyl trimethylammonium ions was tested. Contraction is expressed as percent of the maximum obtainable with AcCh. (From Stephenson,[196] Figure 1.)*

on the isolated guinea pig ileum. The butyl and hexyl derivatives were good agonists, producing nearly as great a maximal response as acetylcholine. But the heptyl and higher analogs had only partial agonist activity, as indicated by the reduced maximal response.

The efficacy concept implies that partial agonists should have antagonist properties. Since they occupy receptor sites, yet produce only weak effects of their own, they should prevent access of strong agonists to these sites. This proves to be generally true. In the investigation shown in Figure 1-79, for example, the octyl derivative was found to antagonize the effect of the butyl compound.

The spectrum of effects, from agonistic to antagonistic, is well displayed in Figure 1-80, a study of the interaction between two congenerically related drugs in their effects on the isolated rat jejunum. Compound A is a good agonist, producing full

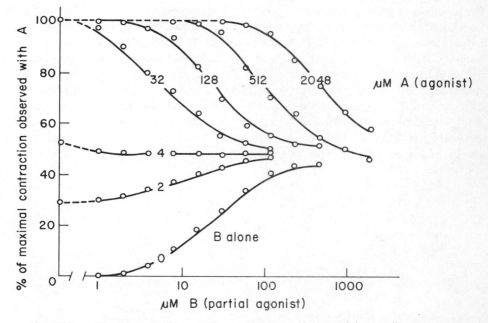

FIGURE 1-80. Mutual effects of an agonist and a partial agonist. *The rat jejunal strip was studied in a tissue bath. The x axis gives concentrations of compound* B, *a partial agonist. Compound* A *is a good agonist,* B *is a propyl derivative of* A. *Both compounds are related to muscarone (cf. p. 75). Each curve is a different concentration of* A, *as indicated. (From Ariens et al.,[198] Figure 27.)*

muscle contraction at concentrations from 32 μM or higher in the absence of the second compound, about 50% of maximal at 4 μM (points on axis of ordinates, $B = 0$). Compound B is a partial agonist, producing a maximal response less than half as great as A, even at the highest concentration tested, nearly 1000 μM (bottom curve). In the presence of a low concentration of A (2 μM), sufficient to yield only 30% of maximal response itself, slight additive effects were seen as B was increased, but the maximum did not exceed that produced by B alone. At 4 μM A, B had virtually no effect at any concentration. At higher concentrations of A, B acted as an antagonist, and at sufficiently high concentrations reduced the maximal response to that associated with B alone.

Spare Receptors.   Much of the pharmacologic data on drug-receptor interactions is derived from studies on smooth or striated muscle. Obviously, there are many steps between the interaction of a drug with a membrane receptor and the consequent changes in ion fluxes, depolarization, intracellular release of calcium, and finally the contraction of the muscle. It is certainly plausible that the limiting factor for maximal shortening of the muscle might not be the total number of receptors but rather one or more of these intervening processes. Thus a maximal response might be obtained with only a small fraction of the available receptors occupied. This would be exactly the opposite situation from that described earlier, in which no response is obtained until a considerable fraction of the receptors is occupied. Certain anomalous effects, not readily explained by simple mass law theory and the elementary occupancy assumption, led to the formulation of this alternative, known as the *spare receptor* hypothesis.[192,196,197]

The "atropine anomaly" is typical of such effects.[199] Acetylcholine reduces the amplitude of contraction of the frog heart; the LDR curve is shown in Figure 1-81,

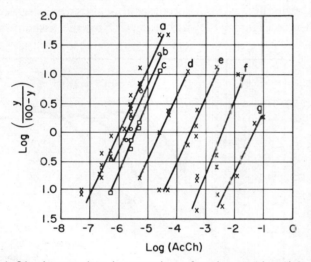

FIGURE 1-81. Antagonism by atropine of action produced by AcCh on isolated frog heart. *Abscissal scale is log molar concentration of AcCh in the tissue bath. On ordinal scale, y is percent reduction of amplitude of spontaneous contractions by AcCh, and log of y/(100 − y) is plotted. Curves show results with the following molar concentrations of atropine: (a) none; (b) 10^{-8}; (c) 10^{-7}; (d) 10^{-6}; (e) 10^{-5}; (f) 10^{-4}; (g) 10^{-3}. (From Clark, Figure 1.[199])*

curve a. The vertical axis here has been modified so that the curves are linear rather than sigmoid. If the heart, in a tissue bath, is treated with a small dose of atropine and then retested with AcCh, the entire LDR curve is shifted slightly to the right (curve b). Increasing doses of atropine shift the curve progressively further to the right (curves c–g). The set of curves is essentially parallel. Each 10-fold increment in atropine concentration makes it necessary to increase the AcCh dosage about 10-fold to obtain the same response as before. At all atropine concentrations the same maximum response can be elicited, provided the AcCh concentration is made high enough.

These effects of atropine on the AcCh LDR curve seem to fit the classical description of competitive antagonism. According to mass law theory and the "occupancy assumption," when maximal response is obtained in the presence of atropine the receptors should be fully occupied by AcCh molecules and the atropine molecules should have been displaced. Therefore, if the contents of the tissue bath are removed while a high concentration of AcCh is present, then replaced several times by solution containing the same high AcCh concentration, and finally replaced by fresh solution without AcCh or atropine, the heart should have regained its original sensitivity to AcCh. In fact, however, the decreased sensitivity produced by atropine persists. With repeated washings, the atropine effect does diminish very slowly and eventually disappears, but the rate of washout is the same whether or not AcCh is in the wash solutions. Thus, the antagonism, which is apparently competitive, is at the same time practically irreversible and is also unaffected by the presence of agonist!

A similar anomaly is observed with the alkylating agents related to dibenamine, which are thought, on grounds of chemical reactivity, to combine irreversibly with receptors.[200] A strip of guinea pig ileum was exposed to histamine at various concentrations and the amplitudes of the isotonic contractions were measured. The control LDR curve shown in Figure 1-82 was obtained. Now the tissue was exposed to a

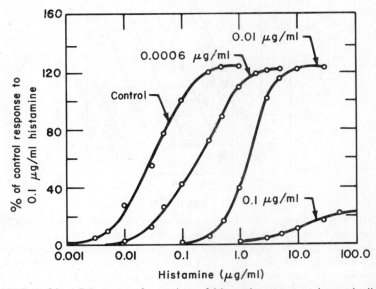

FIGURE 1-82. LDR curves for action of histamine upon guinea pig ileum, showing effects of an antagonist related to dibenamine. *Curve at far left is control, concentrations of antagonists are shown on other curves. (From Nickerson, Figure 1.[200])*

dibenamine-like drug for 5 min. The sensitivity of the tissue to histamine was markedly reduced by this treatment, and the effect was practically irreversible; repeated washing failed to remove the blockade. Higher concentrations of histamine, however, overcame the antagonism, as shown, except at the highest antagonist concentration. Again, as in the atropine anomaly, neither by eliciting maximal responses nor by repeated washing could the original sensitivity of the tissue be restored. If the data are plotted according to the double-reciprocal method, both dibenamine and atropine fulfill the criteria for competitive antagonists, despite their irreversibility.

From data of the kind shown in Figures 1-81 and 1-82, it is a straightforward matter to compute the dose ratio of agonist required to produce equivalent responses in the presence and absence of antagonist (cf. p. 87), and thus the affinity constant for the antagonist may be obtained. For smooth muscles, values of about $10^9\ M^{-1}$ are commonly found, and studies with radioactive atropine in guinea pig ileum have revealed a low-capacity high-affinity binding with just this affinity constant.[201] Such a computation, however, yields no information about the true affinity constant for the agonist. If maximal response were obtained at a very low fractional occupancy, the estimate based on the midpoint of the LDR curve with agonist alone would lead to a serious overestimate of the affinity (underestimate of the dissociation constant).

Anomalous antagonisms, such as illustrated in Figures 1-81 and 1-82, are explained as follows by the spare receptor concept. Consider the acetylcholine–atropine example (Figure 1-81). The affinity of acetylcholine for the receptors is assumed to be low, but maximal response of the muscle is obtained when only a small fraction of the total receptor pool is occupied. Let us call the total number of receptors n, and suppose that $0.01n$ in combination with AcCh is sufficient to cause a maximal muscle response, so that 99% of the receptors are "spare receptors." Suppose atropine irreversibly (or nearly so) blocks 90% of the receptors, leaving $0.10\ n$ available for interaction with AcCh. Obviously, it will now require 10% occupancy to produce the $0.01\ n$ necessary for maximal response. And since the mass law (for zone A, cf. p. 92) predicts that the fractional occupancy is determined only by the concentration of free ligand, a much higher AcCh concentration will now be required. Thus, typical shifts to the right in the LDR curve, as observed in Figure 1-81, are accounted for, giving the appearance of competitive antagonism. The process has a limit, however. When the antagonist occupies enough receptor sites, no concentration of agonist will be able to give a maximal response, because not enough free receptors are available. Such behavior is indicated in the curve at the extreme right of Figure 1-82.

The spare receptor hypothesis predicts that although potent agonists will behave as just described in the presence of antagonists, as long as spare receptors remain available, weak agonists will not. A weak agonist, by definition, is one of low efficacy; it requires a high fractional occupancy to produce a response, and even then is unable to produce the maximal response of which the tissue is capable. This means that few or no spare receptors are present, and consequently, antagonists should reduce the maximal response at once, rather than causing parallel shifts of the LDR curves. Figure 1-83 illustrates this behavior for a strong and weak agonist on the guinea pig ileum. Methylfurmethide is a compound with acetylcholine-like actions; it is very potent, and can produce the maximal development of tension of which the muscle is capable. As the figure shows, C8-TMA (n-octyltrimethylammonium) is a weak agonist, both in terms of the much higher concentrations required and the lower maximum response achievable. Hyoscine is a very slowly dissociating antagonist like atropine in this system. Just as predicted, the methylfurmethide LDR curve undergoes a parallel displacement to the right, whereas the C8-TMA curve is displaced downward at once. A similar but rather more complicated result was found by other investigators, using the irreversible alkylating agent, dibenamine, as antagonist.[202]

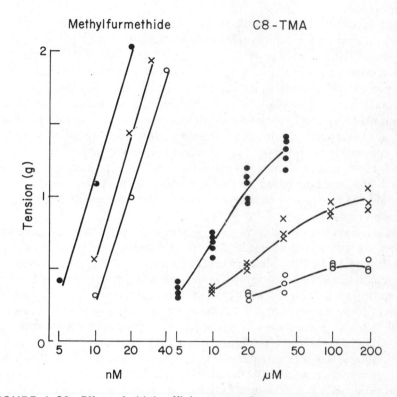

FIGURE 1-83. Effect of a high-affinity antagonist upon responses to a strong and a weak agonist. *Guinea pig ileum in tissue bath. Curve at left of each set is control with agonist alone. Methylfurmethide is a potent agonist, C8-TMA is a weak agonist. The two curves at the right, in each set, are in the presence of 0.16 nM and 0.3 nM hyoscine. (From Rang,[203] Figure 8.)*

A teleological argument can be offered in favor of spare receptors where response (as to neurotransmitters) needs to be extremely rapid in onset and termination, yet sensitive to very low transient agonist concentrations. If sensitivity were achieved by a very high affinity constant, the rate constant for dissociation (k_2) would necessarily be low, and the termination of effect would be slow. A large spare receptor capacity provides a mechanism for obtaining response at very low agonist concentrations, with a rapid dissociation rate constant and therefore a relatively low affinity.

Theory Based on the Rate of Drug-Receptor Combination (Rate Theory). The central concept here is that "instead of attributing excitation to the occupation of receptors by drug molecules, it is attributed to the *process* of occupation, each association between a drug molecule and a receptor providing one quantum of 'excitation.'"[186,204,205] The magnitude of a response is proportional to the *rate* at which drug molecules associate with receptor sites. This rate depends upon the concentration of free drug, the concentration of free receptor sites, and k_1, the rate constant for association of drug molecules with receptors. Thus, the "occupancy assumption" is abandoned, and the principle of intrinsic activity is adopted; however, "efficacy" is no longer an *ad hoc* constant but is defined by the rate constant k_1, which may differ from drug to drug. According to this theory, the distinction between an agonist and an antagonist is determined solely by the value of k_2, the rate constant for dissociation. If k_2 is large, then the rate of dissociation of the drug-receptor complex will be high, making free receptor sites available at a high rate for new effective collisions with drug molecules. Thus, drugs with high k_2 are agonists. In contrast, if k_2 is small, the drug-receptor complex, once formed, will be stable, the rate of dissociation will be low, free receptors will become available for new association events only infrequently, and consequently there will be little or no excitation. Therefore, drugs with low k_2 will display only weak agonist action or none at all. The persistent occupancy of receptor sites by such a drug will reduce the number of sites available for combination with an agonist, so that the drug will behave as an antagonist. Both for agonists and for antagonists the potency is, of course, determined by the equilibrium dissociation constant k_2/k_1, which as usual describes the affinity of drug for receptor.

According to this theory, two rate constants determine a number of different aspects of drug action, and the theory predicts certain relationships between these. Some striking examples of agreement between prediction and observation have indeed been found. It is important to note, however, that values for k_1 and k_2 are deduced from the biologic effects, in terms of the theory itself, since no way has yet been found to measure these constants independently. Under these conditions internal consistency of the data is less impressive than if these constants could have been predicted a priori from physicochemical data.

Rate theory offers a possible explanation of why some drugs are agonists, some partial agonists, and some antagonists, depending upon the value of k_2. It has been suggested that excitation (agonist action) may actually depend upon an ion displacement mechanism wherein the magnitude of response is determined by the rate of displacement of ions (e.g., K^+) from receptor sites in a membrane. Concrete supporting evidence for some such molecular hypothesis would greatly strengthen the case for rate theory, by providing a plausible basis for the crucial thesis that the *process* of occupation of receptor sites provides the excitatory stimulus.

The theory is said to explain why antagonists tend to be bulkier than agonists, since there is alleged to be greater chance for nonspecific binding of bulky molecules than of small molecules at receptor sites. It is also claimed that the theory explains why antagonists that are very potent have a slow onset of action, since the more potent they are, the lower the dose (or concentration) at which they must be used, and consequently the slower will they equilibrate. Both of these arguments apply with equal force to the mass law theory based upon the occupancy assumption; the latter argument, in particular, has long been recognized with respect to enzyme inhibitors.[206]

Rate theory offers a provocative explanation for the finding that some antagonists stimulate first then block as the stimulation fades. A good example is nicotine, which initially excites the autonomic ganglion cell, then blocks it so that it no longer responds to various agonists, including nicotine itself. According to rate theory, the stimulation is a consequence of the initial associations between drug molecules and receptors, which proceed at a high rate (much as is assumed for agonists) because at the outset all receptors sites are vacant. However, this kind of initial stimulatory behavior, which is predicted by the theory, is not observed with all antagonists.

Rate theory accounts for a phenomenon known as "fade," in which an agonist causes an immediate peak response that fades off to a lower plateau at equilibrium. The theory predicts such behavior for all agonists, since the initial rate of combination is bound to be higher than the eventual rate at the steady-state. However, numerous instances are known in which fade cannot be observed at all.

Anomalous antagonisms of the kind discussed earlier in connection with atropine are said to be accounted for by rate theory. The effect of a tightly bound antagonist occupying some receptor sites is to reduce the number of sites with which agonist molecules can combine. This will reduce the total number of association events per minute, but raising the dose of agonist may increase the rate of its association with the remaining free receptors sufficiently to restore the full response. This may be plausible, but how is the overcoming of a complete blockade to be explained? If complete blockade is interpreted to mean that all receptor sites are occupied by antagonist molecules, then no free receptors remain, and the explanation fails. The explanation, therefore, must really presuppose the notion of "spare receptors."

Rate theory has been used to predict successfully the slopes of LDR curves, which are found to depend upon the same two rate constants.[207] It is interesting to note, however, that the two uncomplicated LDR curves presented as Figures 4 and 5 in the original description of rate theory [186] fit nearly perfectly the theoretical mass law curve based upon the occupancy assumption, with slope 0.576 as predicted for zone A with molecular combining ratio 1/1. These experimental curves were obtained with histamine and AcCh acting on guinea pig ileum; the histamine curve was shown in Figure 1-71. One prominent feature of LDR curves that cannot be accounted for at all by rate theory is the common observation that for a given biologic effect, every agonist in a series of congeners yields the same maximal response, regardless of its potency. Explanations have to be sought outside the framework of the theory, in terms of hypothetical limitations in the response capacity of the contractile tissue.

Finally, whether or not rate theory proves to be valid for drug effects in contractile tissues, it is clearly inapplicable to the considerable class of drug-receptor interactions in which the occupancy assumption is known to be valid because the drug is a substrate or inhibitor of an enzyme, and also to a growing number of cases involving a functional macromolecule other than an enzyme (e.g., drugs acting upon nucleic acids).

Statistical Distribution of Receptor Sensitivities.   Another way of looking at the typical LDR curve takes no account of molecular events or mechanisms.[208] It is supposed that a receptor can exist in either of two states, dormant or activated. Every activated receptor is assumed to contribute, in the case of an agonist drug, an equal increment to the overall response (in the case of an antagonist, an equal decrement). Each receptor has its own threshold drug concentration at which activation occurs, so that the whole population of receptors in a tissue displays a range of drug sensitivities. The distribution of these sensitivities is postulated to be log normal, i.e., if the frequency in various sensitivity classes is plotted against log dose (or concentration), a Gaussian curve will be obtained whose breadth reflects the variance of the individual receptor sensitivities. When plotted instead as a cumulative frequency distribution, a typical LDR curve will result (Figure 1-84) whose slope now reflects the variance of receptor sensitivities. It is possible that receptors

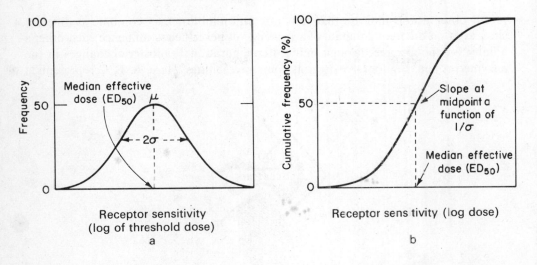

FIGURE 1-84. Statistical distribution of receptor sensitivities.

exist which are complex enough to form a heterogeneous population with respect to drug sensitivity. It is also possible that variable diffusion of drug molecules to receptor sites at different locations in the tissues might result in a range of apparent sensitivities. No such instances, however, have actually been demonstrated. On the other hand, in those numerous cases in which receptors have been identified as macromolecules, this theory is inapplicable, because macromolecules of a specified kind are identical and therefore have identical affinities for a given drug. Moreover, the observed tendency for LDR slopes in diverse systems to cluster near the single value 0.576 accords well with the mass law interpretation but finds no plausible explanation in terms of a statistical distribution of receptor sensitivities.

Allosteric Effects.   Anomalous antagonism and the phenomenon of partial agonism were discovered and demanded explanation at a time when virtually nothing was yet known about the actual physical events in drug-receptor interaction. Thus, the interpretations presented above—the spare receptor hypothesis and the efficacy concept—were necessarily *ad hoc* attempts to find consistent explanations of the observed phenomena. We are not yet able to substitute explanations based directly upon physicochemical understanding, but some progress has been made. The recognition of the general importance of allosterism[209] in metabolic regulation has been accompanied by the realization that allosteric transitions (induced conformational changes) undoubtedly play a major role in drug action,[210–212] especially for drugs acting on membrane-bound receptors—precisely the class of interaction in which departure from simple mass-law behavior has been observed.

It has long been recognized that an inhibitor could modify the function of an enzyme by combining elsewhere than at the substrate site. For example, a heavy metal could form mercaptides and thereby alter the configurational state of an enzyme in such a manner as to destroy essential functional relationships at the active center. It had been assumed that inhibition of this kind would have to be noncompetitive. However, recent observations indicate that substrate and inhibitor may combine at different sites, even on different subunits of a protein, yet nevertheless influence each other's affinity for the enzyme through induced configurational (allosteric) changes in the enzyme protein. Figure 1-85 suggests some possibilities. Here, A, B, C represents a

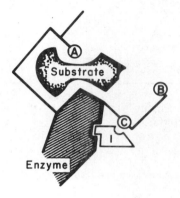

FIGURE 1-85. Conformation change at an enzyme-active site. *A flexible active site is depicted, in which groups A and B must both be in contact with substrate for catalytic action to occur. An inhibitor I attracts group C and thus prevents proper alignment of B. If this changes the affinity of substrate for enzyme, competitive inhibition will be observed. (From Koshland, Figure 9.[105])*

flexible active site, which assumes a catalytically active form under the influence of a substrate molecule. An inhibitor of an entirely different shape, combining at a different site, could impede the substrate-induced configurational change. In the model case shown here, the inhibition could appear to be competitive, if the affinity of substrate or inhibitor for their respective sites were each diminished by combination of the other with its site.

A case of allosteric inhibition that has been studied extensively is the "feedback" inhibition of aspartyl transcarbamylase by cytidine triphosphate (CTP), an end-product of the pyrimidine biosynthetic pathway in which the enzyme partici-pates.[213-215] The step catalyzed by this enzyme is the coupling of carbamyl phosphate to aspartate at the beginning of the reaction sequence.

That CTP inhibits by combining at a different site from the substrates has been shown in treatments such as heat, urea, or Hg^{2+}, which abolish the affinity of enzyme for CTP without affecting its activity toward aspartate or carbamyl phosphate. Moreover, there is no obvious chemical relationship between CTP and either of the two substrates. The enzyme, which is a hexameric aggregate, can be separated physi-cally into two subunits, a dimer that interacts with substrates but not with CTP and a tetramer that interacts with CTP alone. Despite this clear evidence for physically distinct substrate and inhibitor sites, an apparently competitive LDR curve was obtained when reaction velocity was measured in the presence of CTP (Figure 1-86). Thus, all reaction velocities up to the control V_{max} could be obtained in the presence of CTP by increasing the substrate concentration sufficiently.

Note that the scale of abscissas in Figure 1-86 is not logarithmic but linear. On a linear plot, however (cf. Figure 1-39), the enzyme–substrate saturation curve should be hyperbolic. The sigmoidal nature of the curve observed here is typical of what is seen when there are cooperative effects, i.e., when the combination of a molecule of substrate enhances the affinity of the enzyme for the next molecule of substrate. The example best studied is the oxygen–hemoglobin saturation curve, where the effect depends upon the substrate-induced interaction of the four subunits.[102] For aspartyl

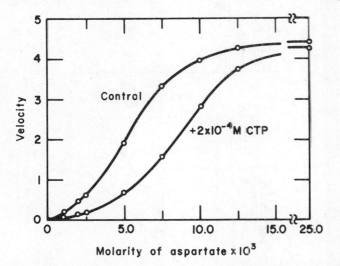

FIGURE 1-86. Reversal of CTP inhibition of ATC-ase by aspartate. *Reaction mixture contained an excess of carbamyl phosphate; aspartate was varied as indicated. Note that abscissal scale is linear, not logarithmic, so normal Michaelis–Menten kinetics should give a rectangular hyperbola. The sigmoid curve is characteristic of reactions showing cooperative effects of subunits. (From Gerhart and Pardee, Figure 3.[214])*

transcarbamylase it is thought that the substrate induces a change in the state of aggregation of the enzyme from an inactive to an active state; CTP, in turn, modifies the enzyme conformation so that the affinity for aspartate is decreased.

Studies with cholinergically innervated cells from the electric eel, *Electrophorus*, have provided experimental evidence of cooperativity in membrane-bound receptors.[216] Individual electroplax cells are large enough to be dissected out and mounted for recording of membrane potentials with a microelectrode. When data were obtained on the relationship between the extent of depolarization and the concentration of cholinergic agonists, a systematic departure from the simple mass law isotherm was observed. If the quantum of response generated by a single receptor were the result of interaction with a single agonist molecule, according to the equation

$$X + R \rightleftharpoons XR$$

a linear plot of XR on the y axis against X on the x axis would yield a hyperbolic curve, exactly as when the Michaelis–Menten relationship is observed in enzyme kinetics (cf. p. 83). If more than one molecule of agonist were required to occupy receptor sites simultaneously in order to produce a response, or if occupancy of one site facilitated occupancy of another, a sigmoid curve would result, as already shown in Figure 1-86. Figure 1-87A shows this effect with the cholinergic agonist phenyl-trimethylammonium (PTA) acting on electroplax cells to reduce the membrane potential.

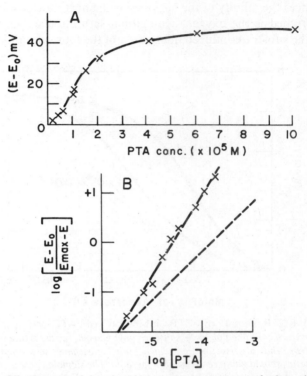

FIGURE 1-87. Cooperativity in the response curve of the electroplax. *Resting potential* (E_0) *was* −80 mV. *Data are for the agonist PTA left in contact long enough (10–20 min) to establish steady-state conditions. The depolarization is expressed as the difference* ($E − E_0$). *A. Linear plot showing sigmoid shape deviating from theoretical hyperbola. B. Hill plot of the same data. Broken line is for theoretical Hill coefficient of unity. (From Changeux and Podleski,[216] Figure 1.)*

A Hill plot is the classic way of demonstrating cooperativity, as first applied to the oxygen–hemoglobin interaction. This is a linear transformation of the general equation

$$nX + R \rightleftharpoons X_nR$$

in which the slope yields n directly. Here one plots $\log\{(X_nR)/[R_T-(X_nR)]\}$ against $\log(X)$, where R_T is the total receptor concentration. Assuming that an observed response, Δ, is proportional to occupancy of receptor sites, one plots $\log\{\Delta/(\Delta_{max}-\Delta)\}$ on the y axis. Figure 1-87B gives the Hill plot of the same data, yielding a slope of 1.7, equal to the Hill coefficient, n.

Experiments with carbamylcholine as agonist had an unexpected outcome. Antagonists did not alter the sigmoid shape of the dose-response curve; but another agonist, decamethonium, transformed it into a normal hyperbola with Hill coefficient equal to unity. In other words, the two cholinergic agonists, carbamylcholine and de-camethonium, were not merely additive but displayed mutual cooperativity. In older terminology we would describe these effects as synergistic. Other examples of synergism, and evidence of conformational change caused by antagonists, have been reported.[217,218]

The analogies between these effects on electroplax membranes and allosteric transitions in regulatory enzymes suggested the following model[216]: AcCh receptor protomers (single units) exist in two interconvertible states, a depolarized state (D) with greater affinity for agonists, and a polarized state (P) with greater affinity for antagonists. The membrane potential is governed by the relative proportions of the two states. Thus, an agonist selectively complexes with the D state, shifting the equilibrium in that direction. An antagonist selectively complexes with the P state, thus preventing the shift to the D state. Low "intrinsic activity" of a partial agonist would be determined by its ability to complex with either state, but with variable preferential affinity for the D state. Thus, differences in maximal response would be explained readily, for regardless of how high was the concentration of such a drug, it would hold a definite proportion of the total receptor pool in the inactive P state.

Cooperativity implies a mutual influence of neighboring protomers, the conformational transition of one protomer favoring a similar transition in its neighbors, possibly through a lattice matrix extending through the membrane. Anomalous antagonisms may be explained, at least in part, as follows. A high-affinity or irreversible antagonist (e.g., atropine) could combine very tightly at an allosteric site on the receptor (not at an AcCh site), thereby inducing a conformational change that reduces the affinity of AcCh for its site. Higher concentrations of AcCh would then produce maximal response despite the continued firm attachment of the antagonist.

These speculative interpretations are advanced only to emphasize the many possible ways of looking at the rather complex phenomena associated with drug actions on membrane-bound receptors. All the theories discussed here and elaborated upon so extensively in the published literature suffer from the same weakness. In the absence of concrete physicochemical evidence on drug-receptor interactions, they have a certain heuristic value, but remain inconclusive. The simple mass-law description, including the occupancy assumption, adequately describes a very large number of drug-receptor interactions in which the receptor is a soluble macromolecule. The known phenomena of allosterism illuminate the mechanism of action of a further set of drugs at the molecular level. What remains is the special class of receptors that appear to be integrally bound to membranes. These sometimes yield anomalous kinetic data, not readily explained on simple mass-law theory. Since the subject matter of pharmacology has long been dominated by studies on smooth and striated muscles, it is not surprising that theoretical attempts to explain these anomalies have commanded so much attention. It seems likely, however, that real understanding will have to await further progress in the isolation of membrane-bound receptors.

DRUG ACTIONS THAT ARE NOT MEDIATED DIRECTLY BY RECEPTORS

The earlier sections of this chapter concerned specific interactions between drugs and receptors, leading directly to a characteristic biologic response. We now consider three mechanisms of drug action that do not depend upon any drug-receptor complex, or in which a receptor is only remotely involved.

Nonspecific Effects and Membrane Perturbations

The osmotic diuretics, such as urea or mannitol, provide a good example of this mechanism. The compound, once taken into the body, is filtered at the glomeruli and thus increases the osmolarity of the tubular urine. Water must therefore be reabsorbed against a higher osmotic gradient than otherwise, so reabsorption is slower and a diuretic effect is observed. In the same category are the osmotic cathartics, such as magnesium sulfate. Neither Mg^{2+} nor SO_4^- traverses the intestinal wall readily, so that an osmotic equivalent of water is necessarily retained within the lumen of the gut. The same principle underlies the action of intravenously administered plasma substitutes (e.g., polyvinyl pyrrolidone) or blood plasma itself. In acute blood loss or other situations where it is essential to restore and maintain the blood volume, these osmotically active macromolecules remain within the vascular system together with their osmotic equivalent of water.

Certain drugs owe their actions entirely to their acidic or basic properties. The antacids, for example, comprise various inorganic and organic bases and ion exchange resins which can be administered by mouth for the purpose of neutralizing excessive acidity in the stomach. Ammonium chloride, used to acidify the urine, contributes a hydrogen ion to the body fluids when NH_4^+ is metabolized to the neutral end-product urea. Some common organic acids that function as antiseptics in the urinary tract and as topical spermicides in the vaginal canal are thought to act primarily as acidifying agents.

Several kinds of nonspecific destructive agents are used in disinfection and antisepsis, as well as in contraception. Detergents destroy the integrity of lipid membranes and also cause the dissociation of nucleoprotein complexes (e.g., ribosomes) whose integrity depends upon ionic bonds. Halogens, peroxides, and other oxidizing agents bring about a widespread destruction of organic matter. Denaturants belonging to numerous chemical classes destroy the integrity and functional capacity of cell membranes, subcellular particles, and proteins.

Perhaps the most interesting drugs in this category are the volatile general anesthetics. These are remarkable for their lack of any obvious molecular feature in common. Substances as unrelated as diethyl ether, cyclopropane, nitrous oxide, and even xenon produce very similar effects on the brain. It has long been recognized that the usual drug-receptor models would not accommodate these drugs. An observed positive correlation between oil/water partition coefficient and anesthetic potency led to the concept that volatile anesthetics dissolve in the lipid membranes of neuronal tissues and thereby somehow alter physiologic function.[219,220] It is true that, at least approximately, equimolar concentrations of the volatile anesthetics in the lipids of brain tissues would produce equal degrees of anesthesia. However, equally good correlations are also found between anesthetic potency and other physicochemical properties.[221,222] The ability of the volatile anesthetics to stabilize water clathrates has been made the basis of a theory of anesthesia,[43,223,224] the validity of which, however, has been questioned.[225]

Local anesthetics also appear to act by nonspecific alteration of the structure of neuronal membranes, and a number of aliphatic and aromatic alcohols have local anesthetic actions. Although its mode of action is unknown, it also appears likely that the effects of ethyl alcohol upon the brain may result from a nonspecific interference with membrane function. This speculation rests mainly upon the extraordinarily low potency of ethanol and the extreme simplicity of its chemical structure.

The lowest intoxicating concentration is about 0.5 mg ml^{-1}, or 0.01 M; the lethal concentration is nearly 0.1 M. Such concentrations do not suggest specific receptor sites with affinities of the usual magnitudes. And the information content of the simple structure CH_3CH_2OH is so low that one is hard pressed to imagine a specific complementary receptor site. These considerations make the study of nonspecific drug-membrane interactions relevant to the pharmacologic effects of a whole class of drugs.[226]

The NMR and ESR techniques (pp. 57, 62) are well suited to examining drug interactions with membranes, and also membrane structure as revealed by use of drugs as probes. An example of the NMR approach deals with the interaction of benzyl alcohol and erythrocyte membranes.[116] The alcohol concentration was varied, and the dependence of relaxation rate of the aromatic ring protons upon concentration was examined, as described earlier. The result at low concentrations (Figure 1-88) was as expected—a very large increase of relaxation rate over that in aqueous solution, reflecting the constraints imposed by the ordered lipid structure of the membrane upon free rotation of the benzyl alcohol molecules that had penetrated.

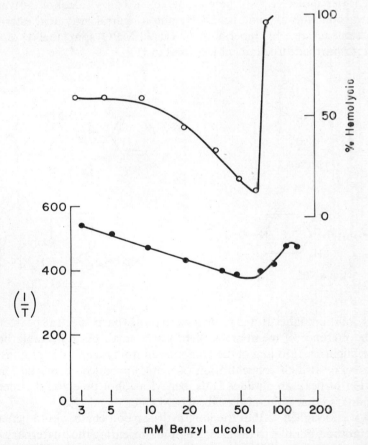

FIGURE 1-88. Benzyl alcohol in membranes by NMR. *Relaxation rate of benzyl alcohol in erythrocyte membranes is plotted against concentration in the lower curve, hemolysis of intact erythrocytes against concentration in the upper curve. (From Burgen and Metcalfe,*[116] *Figure 6.)*

With increasing concentration the relaxation rate fell progressively, indicating a disruptive action upon the membrane, leading to an ever more fluid environment. Finally, at 60 *mM*, there was an abrupt reversal of this trend, coinciding (upper curve) with the hemolytic concentration for intact erythrocytes. At this critical concentration binding sites on membrane protein, ordinarily not accessible to the alcohol, are evidently unmasked by disruption of the lipid structure, and this is thought to account for the upturn in the relaxation rate (increased binding). The concentration of benzyl alcohol required for local anesthetic actions is reasonably close to this critical value for hemolysis.

A molecule particularly well suited for NMR because of a very strong sharp resonance or a convenient chemical shift may also be used as a "reporter," i.e., as a probe to report on the state of its local environment. Thus, when benzyl alcohol was used at low concentration and another alcohol was introduced at varying concentration, the benzyl alcohol relaxation rate varied much as in Figure 1-88. This reflects the change in membrane fluidity around benzyl alcohol molecules, even though these remained at low concentration throughout the experiment.

Similar studies on erythrocyte membranes were carried out by ESR.[227] Three different reporter molecules will be considered—a benzyl alcohol derivative (II), a long hydrocarbon with cationic head (III), and a neutral fatty acid ester (IV). In II and III the same tetramethyl piperidine-1-oxyl (TEMPO) spin label (I) was attached, but a different nitroxide free radical was used in IV.

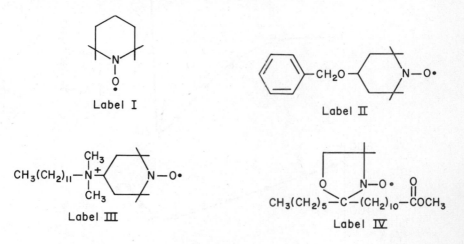

Label I

Label II

Label III

Label IV

In aqueous solution, label II (0.2 m*M*) gave typical sharp spectral peaks (cf. Figure 1-50). In the presence of membranes there was a small but detectable broadening, indicating a slight partitioning of the compound into hydrophobic regions. Addition of benzyl alcohol at high concentration (200 m*M*) produced a marked broadening and reduction of peak amplitude. Thus, benzyl alcohol fluidized the membrane in certain regions, so that more of the label could enter.

Label III was designed so that the long hydrocarbon chain would penetrate deep into the membrane, parallel to the oriented lipids, orienting the quaternary group and spin label in the plane of the polar head groups near the membrane surface. This location is supported by the finding that the spin label is readily reduced (and its resonances abolished) by reducing agents in the aqueous medium. Label III alone, in

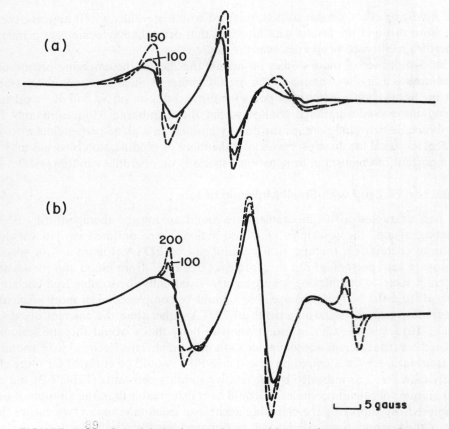

FIGURE 1-89. Spin-label interactions with erythrocyte membranes. *ESR spectra, spin label III. Solid lines = label + membranes; dotted lines = addition of benzyl alcohol (in a) or xylocaine (in b) at concentrations (mM) indicated. (From Hubbell et al.,*[227] *Figures 3 and 4.)*

aqueous solution without membranes, would give very sharp peaks. As seen in Figure 1-89 (solid curves) there was a pronounced peak broadening in the presence of membranes. This was also observed (not shown) with the separated lipid and protein components of membranes. The effect reflects a restriction of free mobility imposed by intercalation of the label in a highly structured, oriented array of hydrocarbon chains. When benzyl alcohol was added, the effect was to cause peak sharpening and increased amplitude, corresponding to increased mobility of the reporter label. Thus, as shown with NMR, benzyl alcohol fluidized the membrane structure. Here we see further that this effect extends to the membrane surface (the position of the label), which is normally much less fluid than the hydrophobic interior. Cationic local anesthetics like xylocaine competitively displaced the probe molecules, as might be expected, leading to increasing amplitude of a sharp peak corresponding to the free label in aqueous solution (Figure 1-89b).

Experiments with label IV revealed very similar effects. Peak broadening indicated strong immobilization of the label, the reporter radical in this case being buried deep in the membrane interior. Neutral local anesthetics fluidized the environment of the label very effectively. Xylocaine and other cationic local anesthetics caused only a mild fluidizing effect, similar to that obtained with benzyl alcohol. It appears, therefore, from this and the results with label III, that drugs like xylocaine act primarily to perturb membrane properties near the surface.

The significance of these studies on membranes lies in the emerging picture of a membrane as a highly dynamic structure (cf. Chapter 2). Such functions as ion transport or the reversible opening of pores for rapid diffusion of Na^+ or K^+ evidently depend upon conformational change within the membrane. Unquestionably the membrane fluidity (and perhaps the fluidity gradient in a plane perpendicular to the surface) is critical for these processes, and therefore its modification by drugs may be an important mechanism of drug action, especially on neuronal membranes.

Interaction of Drug with Small Molecule or Ion

The best examples of this mechanism are found among the therapeutically useful chelating agents, the principles of whose actions were outlined earlier. Calcium disodium edetate is a therapeutically useful salt of EDTA (Figure 1-7), a specific antidote in lead poisoning. The drug removes free Pb^{2+} from blood and tissues and renders it inert by complexing it very tightly. Eventually the soluble lead chelate is excreted from the body. Of course, Pb^{2+} could be complexed even more efficiently by administering the tetrasodium salt of EDTA rather than the calcium disodium chelate. However, the Ca^{2+} concentration of body fluids would then be seriously depleted because calcium would replace sodium in the chelate. Even in lead poisoning, the atom ratio Pb/Ca is extremely low. Thus, Pb^{2+} would be chelated far more efficiently than Ca^{2+}, as indicated by the relative stability constants (Table 1-3), but the total amount of calcium complexed would be much greater than the amount of lead complexed. By supplying the chelating agent as a calcium complex, we ensure that none of the essential body calcium will be removed, yet Pb^{2+} will effectively displace Ca^{2+} from EDTA in accordance with its 10^7-fold greater affinity.[26]

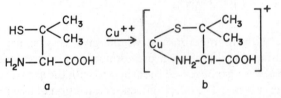

FIGURE 1-90. Penicillamine (a) and its copper chelate (b).

Another therapeutic use of a chelating agent is the employment of penicillamine (β,β-dimethylcysteine, Figure 1-90) to remove copper from body tissues in the hereditary disorder of copper metabolism known as hepatolenticular degeneration, or Wilson's disease.[228] Here there appears to be defective synthesis of the copper-binding protein ceruloplasmin, resulting in progressive accumulation of free copper in the liver and brain. The damage to these organs may be prevented, and to some extent reversed, by repeated administration of the chelating agent. The complexed and solubilized copper is excreted in large amounts in the urine.

The principle of mercaptide formation is applied in the use of dimercaprol (British anti-lewisite, BAL).[34,229] This drug is a simple glycerol derivative containing two vicinal sulfhydryl groups capable of forming a very stable mercaptide ring, as already described (p. 13).

H$_2$CSH
|
HCSH   +   Cl$_2$AsCH=CHCl   ⟶
|
H$_2$COH

Dimercaprol   Lewisite

H$_2$CS
|＼
HCS   AsCH=CHCl
|
H$_2$COH

Mercaptide complex

By virtue of its free hydroxyl group, dimercaprol remains soluble even after it has chelated a metal atom. Thus, various heavy metals (arsenic, mercury, gold, antimony, bismuth), whether present as free ions or in organic complexes (such as lewisite), may be removed from the tissues and body fluids, rendered nontoxic by combination with dimercaprol, and then excreted in the urine.

Incorporation of Drug into a Macromolecule

A "counterfeit incorporation" mechanism, wherein a drug replaces a normal metabolite in the synthesis of an important cellular constituent, certainly requires the activity of enzymes. The effect of the drug, however, is not attributable directly to interaction with an enzyme. Rather, the drug participates as a substrate; the reaction product rather than the drug produces the characteristic biologic response.[230]

A case of "counterfeit incorporation" that has been studied intensively is that of the thymine analog 5-bromouracil (BU).[231] The van der Waals radii of Br and —CH$_3$ are very nearly the same (Table 1-8), so BU resembles thymine quite closely. BU enters

TABLE 1-8. Atomic radii (van der Waals) of halogens and related groups.
(Data from *Handbook of Chemistry and Physics*, 45th edition. Cleveland, Ohio, Chemical Rubber Co., 1964–65, p. D-90.)

Atom or group	Radius (Å)
H	1.20
F	1.35
Cl	1.80
Br	1.95
CH$_3$	2.00
I	2.15

all the preliminary reactions that ordinarily lead to the synthesis of thymidine triphosphate; bromodeoxyuridine triphosphate then enters the DNA polymerase

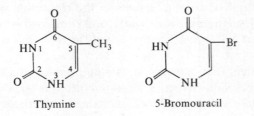

Thymine   5-Bromouracil

reaction, pairing opposite adenine. Depending upon the ratio of BU to thymine in the cellular environment, DNA can be synthesized in which up to 40% of the thymine is replaced by BU, without significant adverse effect. Under these conditions, cell populations grow and divide normally; it is obvious, therefore, that practically all the incorporated BU molecules function as though they were thymine, both at replication and at transcription. Because of the increased density of BU (compared with thymine), BU-substituted DNA has proved useful in experiments requiring density labeling of one DNA strand. Despite its generally normal function, BU-containing DNA shows an increased mutation rate, presumably because of a heightened probability that BU will pair anomalously with guanine instead of with adenine (p. 637). Other abnormalities resulting from the presence of BU and other base analogs in DNA are increased sensitivity to x irradiation, increased frequency of chromosome breakage, and mitotic abnormalities in mammalian cells.[232] These effects are discussed at greater length in Chapter 10.

5-Fluorouracil (FU) presents an interesting contrast.[231] This compound is not incorporated into DNA at all, but acts readily as a counterfeit of uracil, consistent with the small van der Waals radius of the fluorine atom.

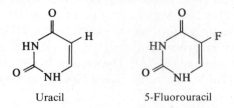

Uracil   5-Fluorouracil

There are two primary effects of FU. It is handled metabolically like uracil, forming a riboside and riboside phosphates. The monophosphate strongly inhibits the enzyme thymidine synthetase (which normally converts deoxyuridine monophosphate to thymidine monophosphate), thereby blocking the *de novo* synthesis of thymine. At the same time, FU is converted to the nucleoside triphosphate and then incorporated into messenger-RNA in place of uracil. "Miscoding" may result through misreading of codons containing FU during the assembly of polypeptide chains, so that incorrect amino acids are inserted. Phenotypically altered proteins are thus formed, which may be nonfunctional, partly functional, or even fully functional, depending upon the particular protein and the nature and position of each amino acid substitution.

An amino acid analog may be incorporated into a protein in place of a natural amino acid, provided it can serve as substrate for an amino acid activating enzyme. Once attached to a transfer RNA molecule, its addition to a growing polypeptide chain appears to be inevitable, since it has been shown that informational specificity during the stepwise assembly of the polypeptide resides only in the mRNA codon, the transfer RNA itself, and some features of the ribosomal binding site. Thus, for example, if the analog ethionine is activated and combined with the specific methionine transfer RNA, it will then be treated exactly as though it were methionine at the subsequent steps.[233]

Sometimes a protein that contains an analog in place of a natural amino acid is functional, sometimes not. When *Bacillus subtilis* was grown in the presence of ethionine, an amylase was formed that contained this analog and methionine in

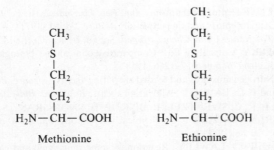

about equal amounts. The enzyme not only had normal activity, but its physical properties were indistinguishable from those of the normal amylase. When *E. coli* was grown in the presence of *p*-fluorophenylalanine, the induced enzyme β-galactosidase contained the analog in place of phenylalanine but nevertheless displayed normal

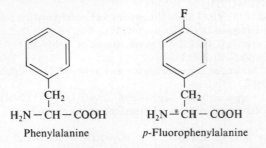

activity. In the same organism, under the same conditions, however, activities of several constitutive enzymes were absent.[234] In *Bacillus cereus* grown in *p*-fluorophenylalanine, the induced enzyme penicillinase contained the analog and had impaired activity as well as altered (but still identifiable) immunologic properties.[235]

REFERENCES

1. P. EHRLICH: Chemotherapeutics: scientific principles, methods and results. *Lancet* 2:445 (1913).
2. C. BERNARD: *Leçons sur les Effets des Substances Toxiques et Médicamenteuses.* Paris, J. B. Bailliere et Fils, Chapters 16–23 (1857).
3. J. N. LANGLEY: On nerve endings and on special excitable substances in cells. *Proc. Roy. Soc.* B78:170 (1906).
4. J. N. LANGLEY: On the contraction of muscle, chiefly in relation to the presence of "receptive" substances. Part IV. The effect of curari and of some other substances on the nicotine response of the sartorius and gastrocnemius muscles of the frog. *J. Physiol.* 39:235 (1909).
5. W. M. FLETCHER: John Newport Langley. In memoriam. *J. Physiol.* 61:1 (1926).
6. A. ALBERT: Selective Toxicity, 4th ed. London, Methuen Ltd. (1968).
7. E. J. ARIËNS: *Molecular Pharmacology.* New York, Academic Press (1964).
8. E. J. ARIËNS and A. M. SIMONIS: A molecular basis for drug action. *J. Pharm. Pharmacol.* 16:137, 289 (1964).
9. R. F. FURCHGOTT: Receptor mechanisms. *Ann. Rev. Pharmacol.* 4:21 (1964).
10. H. G. MAUTNER: The molecular basis of drug action. *Pharmacol. Rev.* 19:107 (1967).
11. D. R. WAUD: Pharmacological receptors. *Pharmacol. Rev.* 20:49 (1968).
12. S. EHRENPREIS, J. H. FLEISCH, and T. W. MITTAG: Approaches to the molecular nature of pharmacological receptors. *Pharmacol. Rev.* 21:131 (1969).

13. A. S. V. BURGEN: Receptor mechanisms. *Ann. Rev. Pharmacol.* 10:7 (1970).
14. H. P. RANG: Drug receptors and their function. *Nature* 231:91 (1971).
15. L. PAULING: *The Nature of the Chemical Bond*, 3rd ed. Ithaca, Cornell University Press (1960).
16. D. A. KARNOFSKY, Consulting Ed.: Comparative clinical and biological effects of alkylating agents. *Ann. N.Y. Acad. Sci.* 68:657–1266 (1958).
17. S. S. BROWN: Nitrogen mustards and related alkylating agents. *Advance. Pharmacol.* 2:243 (1963).
18. P. BROOKES and P. D. LAWLEY: Alkylating agents. *Brit. Med. Bull.* 20:91 (1964).
19. S. A. CUCINELL, K. C. SWENTZEL, R. BISKUP, H. SNODGRASS, S. LOVRE, W. STARK, L. FEINSILVER, and F. VOCCI: Biochemical interactions and metabolic fate of riot control agents. *Fed. Proc.* 30:86 (1971).
20. P. BROOKES and P. D. LAWLEY: Reaction of some mutagenic and carcinogenic compounds with nucleic acids. *J. Cell. Comp. Physiol.* 64:111, Supp. 1 (1964).
21. R. F. FURCHGOTT: The use of β-haloalkylamines in the differentiation of receptors and in the determination of dissociation constants of receptor-agonist complexes. *Adv. Drug Res.* 3:21 (1966).
22. S. C. HARVEY and M. NICKERSON: Reactions of dibenamine and some congeners with substances of biological interest in relation to the mechanism of adrenergic blockade. *J. Pharmacol. Exp. Therap.* 112:274 (1954).
23. V. N. IYER and W. SZYBALSKI: Mitomycins and porfiromycin: chemical mechanism of activation and cross-linking of DNA. *Science* 145:55 (1964).
24. D. R. DAVIES and A. L. GREEN: The mechanism of hydrolysis by cholinesterase and related enzymes. *Adv. Enzymol.* 20:283 (1958).
25. I. B. WILSON: Molecular complementarity and antidotes for alkylphosphate poisoning. *Fed. Proc.* 18:752 (1959).
26. J. E. CASIDA: Esterase inhibitors as pesticides. *Science* 146:1011 (1964).
27. D. E. KOSHLAND, JR.: Correlation of structure and function in enzyme action. *Science* 142:1533 (1963).
28. H. S. JANSZ, D. BRONS, and M. G. P. J. WARRINGA: Chemical nature of the DFB-binding site of pseudocholinesterase. *Biochim. Biophys. Acta* 34:573 (1959).
29. A. E. MARTELL: The Relationship of Chemical Structure to Metal-Binding Action in *Metal-Binding in Medicine*, ed. by M. J. Seven. Philadelphia, Lippincott (1960).
30. A. E. MARTELL and M. CALVIN: *Chemistry of the Metal Chelate Compounds*. Englewood Cliffs, N.J., Prentice–Hall (1952).
30a. Editorial, Today's drugs: Chelating agents in medicine. *Brit. J. Med.* 2:270 (1971).
31. B. L. VALLEE: Active center of carboxypeptidase A. *Fed. Proc.* 23:8 (1964).
32. W. N. LIPSCOMB, J. C. COPPOLA, J. A. HARTSUCK, M. L. LUDWIG, H. MUIRHEAD, J. SEARL, and T. A. STEITZ: The structure of carboxypeptidase A. III. Molecular structure at 6 A resolution. *J. Mol. Biol.* 19:423 (1966).
33. H. PASSOW, A. ROTHSTEIN, and T. W. CLARKSON: The general pharmacology of the heavy metals. *Pharmacol. Rev.* 13:185 (1961).
34. M. J. SEVEN, ed.: *Metal-Binding in Medicine*. Philadelphia, Lippincott (1960).
35. G. C. PIMENTEL and A. L. MC CLELLAN: *The Hydrogen Bond*. San Francisco, W. H. Freeman (1960).
36. G. S. STENT: *Molecular Biology of Bacterial Viruses*. San Francisco, W. H. Freeman (1963).
37. M. FEUGHELMAN, R. LANGRIDGE, W. E. SEEDS, A. R. STOKES, H. R. WILSON, C. W. HOOPER, M. H. F. WILKINS, R. K. BARCLAY, and L. D. HAMILTON: Molecular structure of deoxyribose nucleic acid and nucleoprotein. *Nature* 175:834 (1955).
38. J. MARMUR and P. DOTY: Determination of the base composition of deoxyribonucleic acid from its thermal denaturation temperature. *J. Mol. Biol.* 5:109 (1962).
39. N. V. SIDGWICK and R. K. CALLOW: Abnormal benzene derivatives. *J. Chem. Soc.* 125:527 (1924).
40. D. O. JORDAN: The physical properties of nucleic acids. In *The Nucleic Acids*, Vol. I, ed. by E. Chargaff and J. N. Davidson. New York, Academic Press (1955).
41. E. J. COHN and J. T. EDSALL: *Proteins, Amino Acids and Peptides*. New York, Reinhold (1943).
42. J. STEINHARDT and S. BEYCHOK: Interaction of proteins with hydrogen ions and other small ions and molecules. In *The Proteins*, 2nd ed., ed. by H. Neurath, New York, Academic Press (1964).
43. L. PAULING: The hydrate microcrystal theory of general anesthesia. *Anesthesia Analg. Curr. Res.* 43:1 (1964).

44. *The Pharmacopeia of the United States of America*, 18th revision. Easton, Pa., Mack Publishing Co. (1970).
45. I. B. WILSON and F. BERGMANN: Studies on cholinesterase. VII. The active surface of acetylcholine esterase derived from effects of pH on inhibitors. *J. Biol. Chem* 185:479 (1950).
46. N. ROBINSON: Molecular size and shape. *J. Pharm. Pharmacol.* 12:129, 193 (1960).
47. B. M. BLOOM and G. D. LAUBACH: The relationship between chemical structure and pharmacological activity. *Ann. Rev. Pharmacol.* 2:67 (1962).
48. J. B. VAN ROSSUM: The relation between chemical structure and biological activity. *J. Pharm. Pharmacol.* 15:285 (1963).
49. F. N. FASTIER: Modern concepts in relationship between structure and biological activity. *Ann. Rev. Pharmacol.* 4:51 (1964).
50. A. BURGER and A. P. PARULKAR: Relationships between chemical structure and biological activity. *Ann. Rev. Pharmacol.* 6:19 (1966).
51. C. J. CAVALLITO: Some relationships between chemical structure and pharmacological activities. *Ann. Rev. Pharmacol.* 8:39 (1968).
52. A. KOROLKOVAS: *Essentials of Molecular Pharmacology*. New York, Wiley-Interscience, (1970).
53. A. ALBERT: Relations between molecular structure and biological activity: stages in the evolution of current concepts. *Ann. Rev. Pharmacol.* 11:13 (1971).
54. J. H. WELSH and R. TAUB: The action of choline and related compounds on the heart of *Venus mercenaria. Biol. Bull.* 95:346 (1948).
55. A. GOLDSTEIN: *Biostatistics: An Introductory Text*. New York, Macmillan (1964).
56. J. H. WELSH and R. TAUB: Structure-activity relationships of acetylcholine and quaternary ammonium ions. *J. Pharmacol. Exp. Therap.* 99:334 (1950).
57. J. H. WELSH and R. TAUB: The significance of the carbonyl group and ether oxygen in the reaction of acetylcholine with receptor substance. *J. Pharmacol. Exp. Therap.* 103:62 (1951).
58. P. G. WASER: Chemistry and pharmacology of muscarine, muscarone, and some related compounds. *Pharmacol. Rev.* 13:465 (1961).
59. P. G. WASER: The cholinergic receptor. *J. Pharm. Pharmacol.* 12:577 (1960).
60. C. CHOTHIA and P. PAULING: The conformation of cholinergic molecules at nicotinic nerve receptors. *Proc. Nat. Acad. Sci. U.S.A.* 65:477 (1970).
61. C. CHOTHIA and P. PAULING: Conformations of acetylcholine. *Nature* 219:1156 (1968).
62. C. CHOTHIA and P. PAULING: Conformation of cholinergic molecules relevant to acetylcholinesterase. *Nature* 223:919 (1969).
63. W. H. BEERS and E. REICH: Structure and activity of acetylcholine. *Nature* 228:917 (1970).
64. W. D. M. PATON and E. J. ZAIMIS: The pharmacological actions of polymethylene bis trimethylammonium salts. *Brit. J. Pharmacol.* 4:381 (1949).
65. W. D. M. PATON and E. J. ZAIMIS: The methonium compounds. *Pharmacol. Rev.* 4:219 (1952).
66. D. GROB: Neuromuscular pharmacology. *Ann. Rev. Pharmacol.* 1:239 (1961).
67. D. B. TAYLOR, R. D. PRIOR, and J. A. BEVAN: The relative sensitivities of diaphragm and other muscles of the guinea pig to neuromuscular blocking agents. *J. Pharmacol. Exp. Therap.* 143:187 (1964).
68. D. GROB and R. J. JOHNS: Further studies on the mechanism of the defect in neuromuscular transmission in myasthenia gravis, with particular reference to the acetylcholine-insensitive block. In *Myasthenia Gravis*, Proceedings 2nd International Symposium, ed. by H. R. Viets. Springfield, Ill., Charles C. Thomas (1961).
69. G. H. GLASER: Pharmacological considerations in the treatment of myasthenia gravis. *Advance Pharmacol.* 2:113 (1963).
70. A. H. BECKETT: Stereochemical factors in biological activity. *Fortschr. Arzneimittelforsch.* 1:455 (1959).
71. A. H. BECKETT and A. F. CASY: Analgesics and their antagonists: biochemical aspects and structure-activity relationships. *Prog. Med. Chem.* 4:171 (1965).
72. R. B. BARLOW: Steric aspects of drug action. In *Steric Aspects of the Chemistry and Biochemistry of Natural Products* (Biochemical Society Symposia #19), ed. by J. K. Grant and W. Klyne. Cambridge, Cambridge University Press, (1960) p. 46.
73. P. S. PORTOGHESE: Relationships between stereostructure and pharmacological activities. *Ann. Rev. Pharmacol.* 10:51 (1970).

74. K. W. BENTLEY and H. M. E. CARDWELL: The absolute stereochemistry of the morphine, benzylisoquinoline, aporphine, and tetrahydroberberine alkaloids. *J. Chem. Soc.* (1955), p. 3252.

75. M. MACKAY and D. C. HODGKIN: A crystallographic examination of the structure of morphine. *J. Chem. Soc.* (1955), p. 3261.

76. R. S. CAHN, C. K. INGOLD, and V. PRELOG: The specification of asymmetric configuration in organic chemistry. *Experientia* 12:81 (1956).

77. W. R. MARTIN: Opioid antagonists. *Pharmacol. Rev.* 19:463 (1967).

78. I. E. BUSH: Chemical and biological factors in the activity of adrenocortical steroids. *Pharmacol. Rev.* 14:317 (1962).

79. J. FRIED and A. BORMAN: Synthetic derivatives of cortical hormones. *Vitamins and Hormones* 16:303 (1958).

80. G. W. LIDDLE and M. FOX: Structure-function relationships of anti-inflammatory steroids. In *Inflammation and Diseases of Connective Tissues*, ed. by L. C. Mills and J. H. Moyer. Philadelphia, Saunders (1961), pp. 302–309.

81. L. C. MILLS: Adrenal cortex and adrenocortical hormones, in *Drill's Pharmacology in Medicine*, 4th ed., ed. by J. R. Di Palma. New York, McGraw-Hill (1971), Chapter 73.

82. H. J. RINGOLD, J. M. H. GRAVES, A. CLARK, and T. BELLAS: Studies with the 3 α-hydroxy-steroid dehydrogenase from *Pseudomonas testosteroni*. Enzyme-substrate complementarity as the basis of selectivity and steric specificity. *Rec. Prog. in Hormone Res.* 23:349 (1967).

83. L. S. LERMAN: The structure of the DNA–acridine complex. *Proc. Nat. Acad. Sci. U.S.A.* 49:94 (1963).

84. R. A. BOISSONNAS, ST. GUTTMANN, B. BERDE, and H. KONZETT: Relationships between the chemical structures and the biological properties of the posterior pituitary hormones and their synthetic analogues. *Experientia* 17:377 (1961).

85. R. A. BOISSONAS and ST. GUTTMAN: Chemistry of the neurohypophysial hormones. In *Handbook of Experimental Pharmacology: Neurohypophysial Hormones and Similar Polypeptides*, ed. by B. Berde. Berlin, Springer–Verlag, 23:40 (1968).

86. D. JARVIS and V. DU VIGNEAUD: Crystalline deamino-oxytocin. *Science* 143:545 (1964).

87. H. R. PERKINS: Composition of bacterial cell walls in relation to antibiotic action. *Adv. Pharmacol.* 7:283 (1969).

88. E. M. WISE, JR. and J. T. PARK: Penicillin: its basic site of action as an inhibitor of a peptide cross-linking reaction in cell wall mucopeptide synthesis. *Proc. Nat. Acad. Sci. U.S.A.* 54:75 (1965).

89. U. ROZE and J. L. STROMINGER: Alanine racemase from *Staphylococcus aureus*: conformation of its substrates and its inhibitor D-cycloserine. *Mol. Pharmacol.* 2:92 (1966).

90. P. H. BELL and R. O. ROBLIN, JR.: Studies in chemotherapy. VII. A theory of the relation of structure to activity of sulfanilamide type compounds. *J. Amer. Chem. Soc.* 64:2905 (1942).

91a. C. HANSCH and T. FUJITA: ρ-σ-π Analysis. A method for the correlation of biological activity and chemical structure. *J. Amer. Chem. Soc.* 86:1616 (1964).

91b. C. HANSCH, A. R. STEWARD, and J. IWASA: The correlation of localization rates of benzene-boronic acids in brain and tumor tissue with substituent constants. *Mol. Pharmacol.* 1:87 (1965).

91c. O. R. HANSEN: Hammett series with biological activity. *Acta Chem. Scand.* 16:1593 (1962).

91d. W. B. NEELEY: The use of molecular orbital calculations as an aid to correlate the structure and activity of cholinesterase inhibitors. *Mol. Pharmacol.* 1:137 (1965).

92. A. GOLDSTEIN: The interactions of drugs and plasma proteins. *Pharmacol. Rev.* 1:102 (1949).

92a. C. F. CHIGNELL: Physical methods for studying drug-protein binding. In *Handbook of Experimental Pharmacology*, Vol. 28, No. 1. Berlin, Heffter–Heubner (1971), pp. 187–212.

93. C. F. CHIGNELL: Spectroscopic techniques for the study of drug interactions with biological systems. *Adv. Drug Res.* 5:55 (1970).

94. I. M. KLOTZ, R. K. BURKHARD, and J. M. URQUHART: Structural specificities in the inter-actions of some organic ions with serum albumin. *J. Amer. Chem. Soc.* 74:202 (1952).

95. G. SCATCHARD: The attractions of proteins for small molecules and ions. *Ann. N.Y. Acad. Sci.* 51:660 (1949).

96. I. M. KLOTZ: Protein interactions, in *The Proteins*, ed. by H. Neurath and K. Bailey. New York, Academic Press (1953), Ch. 8.

97. E. DE ROBERTIS, G. S. LUNT, and J. L. LA TORRE: Multiple binding sites for acetylcholine in a proteolipid from electric tissue. *Mol. Pharmacol.* 7:97 (1971).

98. I. M. KLOTZ and D. L. HUNSTON: Properties of graphical representations of multiple classes of binding sites. *Biochemistry* 10:3065 (1971).

99. J. D. TERESI and J. M. LUCK: The combination of organic anions with serum albumin. VI. Quantitative studies by equilibrium dialysis. *J. Biol. Chem.* 174:653 (1948).

100. A. F. CULLIS, H. MUIRHEAD, M. F. PERUTZ, and M. G. ROSSMANN: The structure of haemoglobin. IX. A three-dimensional Fourier synthesis at 5.5 A resolution: description of the structure. *Proc. Roy. Soc.* A265:161 (1962).

101. M. F. PERUTZ: *Proteins and Nucleic Acids.* Amsterdam, Elsevier (1962).

102. M. F. PERUTZ: Stereochemistry of cooperative effects in haemoglobin. *Nature* 228:726 (1970).

103. Anon: The truth about haemoglobin. *Nature* 228:806 (1970).

104. J. MONOD, J. WYMAN, and J. P. CHANGEUX: On the nature of allosteric transitions: a plausible model. *J. Mol. Biol.* 12:88 (1965).

105. D. E. KOSHLAND, JR.: Conformation changes at the active site during enzyme action. *Fed. Proc.* 23:719 (1964).

106. D. H. GAUSS, F. VON DER HAAR, A. MAELICKE, and F. CRAMER: Recent results of tRNA research. *Ann. Rev. Biochem.* 40:1045 (1971).

107. B. A. NEWTON: Chemotherapeutic compounds affecting DNA structure and function. *Adv. Pharmacol.* 8:150 (1970).

108. E. REICH: Actinomycin: Correlation of structure and function of its complexes with purines and DNA. *Science* 143:684 (1964).

109. L. D. HAMILTON, W. FULLER, and E. REICH: X-ray diffraction and molecular model building studies of the interaction of actinomycin with nucleic acids. *Nature* 198:538 (1963).

110. W. MÜLLER and D. M. CROTHERS: Studies of the binding of actinomycin and related compounds to DNA. *J. Mol. Biol.* 35:251 (1968).

111. M. WARING: Variation of the supercoils in closed circular DNA by binding of antibiotics and drugs: evidence for molecular models involving intercalation. *J. Mol. Biol.* 54:247 (1970).

112. M. WARING: Distortion of DNA structure and function by intercalating molecules. *Proc. 4th Int. Cong. Pharmacol.* Basel, Schwabe and Co., 1:308 (1970).

113. D. R. HELINSKI and D. B. CLEWELL: Circular DNA. *Ann. Rev. Biochem.* 40:899 (1971).

114. S. C. JAIN and H. M. SOBELL: The stereochemistry of actinomycin binding to DNA. I. Refinement and further structural details of the actinomycin-deoxyguanosine complex. *J. Mol. Biol.* 68:1 (1972).

115. H. M. SOBELL and S. C. JAIN: The stereochemistry of actinomycin binding to DNA. II. Detailed molecular model of actinomycin-DNA complex and its implications. *J. Mol. Biol.* 68:21 (1972).

116. A. S. V. BURGEN and J. C. METCALFE: The application of nuclear magnetic resonance to pharmacological problems. *J. Pharm. Pharmacol.* 22:153 (1970).

117. O. JARDETZKY and N. G. WADE–JARDETZKY: On the mechanism of the binding of sulfonamides to bovine serum albumin. *Mol. Pharmacol.* 1:214 (1965).

118. I. M. KLOTZ, N. R. LANGERMAN, and D. W. DARNALL: Quaternary structure of proteins. *Ann. Rev. Biochem.* 39:25 (1970).

119. L. STRYER: Implications of x-ray crystallographic studies of protein structure. *Ann. Rev. Biochem.* 37:25 (1968).

120. W. H. STEIN: Structure-activity relationships in ribonuclease. *Fed. Proc.* 23:599 (1964).

121. H. NEURATH, ed.: *The Proteins*, 2nd ed. New York, Academic Press (1963)

121a. F. M. RICHARDS: Personal communication.

122. G. C. K. ROBERTS and O. JARDETZKY: Nuclear magnetic resonance spectroscopy of proteins. *Adv. Prot. Chem.* 24:447 (1970).

123. D. H. MEADOWS and O. JARDETZKY: Nuclear magnetic resonance studies of the structure and binding sites of enzymes. IV. Cytidine 3'monophosphate binding to ribonuclease. *Proc. Nat. Acad. Sci. U.S.A.* 61:406 (1968).

124. D. H. MEADOWS, G. K. ROBERTS, and O. JARDETZKY: Nuclear magnetic resonance studies of the structure and binding sites of enzymes. VIII. Inhibitor binding to ribonuclease. *J. Mol. Biol.* 45:491 (1969).

125. G. C. K. ROBERTS, E. A. DENNIS, D. H. MEADOWS, J. S. COHEN, and O. JARDETZKY: The mechanism of action of ribonuclease. *Proc. Nat. Acad. Sci.* 62:1151 (1969).

126. O. JARDETZKY: Nuclear magnetic resonance studies of protein binding sites: The complex of staphylococcal nuclease with 3',5'-thymidine diphosphate. In *Molecular Properties of Drug Receptors*, Ciba Foundation, ed. by R. Porter and M. O'Connor. London, J. and A. Churchill, (1970) p. 113.

126a. O. JARDETZKY: Personal communication.

127. H. M. MC CONNELL and W. L. HUBBELL: Application of spin labels in pharmacology. *Proc. Fourth Int. Cong. on Pharmacol.* Basel, Schwabe & Co. 1:273 (1969).

128. H. M. MC CONNELL and B. G. MC FARLAND: Physics and chemistry of spin labels. *Quart. Rev. Biophys.* 3:91 (1970).

129. H. M. MC CONNELL: Spin label studies of cooperative oxygen binding to hemoglobin. *Ann. Rev. Biochem.* 40:227 (1971).

130. H. WEINER: Interaction of a spin labeled analog of nicotinamide-adenine dinucleotide with alcohol dehydrogenase. I. Synthesis, kinetics, and electron paramagnetic resonance studies. *Biochemistry* 8:526 (1969).

131. A. S. MILDVAN and H. WEINER: Interaction of a spin-labeled analog of nicotinamide-adenine dinucleotide with alcohol dehydrogenase. II. Proton relaxation rate and electron paramagnetic resonance studies of binary and ternary complexes. *Biochemistry* 8:552 (1969).

132. R. K. LEUTE, E. F. ULLMAN, A. GOLDSTEIN, and L. A. HERZENBERG: Spin immunoassay technique for determination of morphine. *Nature New Biol.* 236:93 (1972).

133. R. K. LEUTE, E. F. ULLMAN, and A. GOLDSTEIN: Instant determination of opiate narcotics in urine and saliva by spin immunoassay. *J. Am. Med. Ass.* 221:1231 (1972).

134. L. STRYER: Fluorescent probes of biological macromolecules. In *Molecular Properties of Drug Receptors*, Ciba Foundation Symposium, ed. by R. Porter and M. O'Connor. London, J. and A. Churchill (1970), p. 133.

135. W. C. GALLEY and L. STRYER: Triplet–triplet energy transfer in proteins as a criterion of proximity. *Proc. Nat. Acad. Sci. U.S.A.* 60:108 (1968).

136. K. BEARDSLEY and C. R. CANTOR: Studies of transfer RNA tertiary structure by singlet–singlet energy transfer. *Proc. Nat. Acad. Sci. U.S.A.* 65:39 (1970).

137. J. YGUERABIDE, H. F. EPSTEIN, and L. STRYER: Segmental flexibility in an antibody molecule. *J. Mol. Biol.* 51:573 (1970).

138. L. STRYER: Fluorescence spectroscopy of proteins. *Science* 162:526 (1968).

139. L. STRYER: The interaction of a naphthalene dye with apomyoglobin and apohemoglobin. A fluorescent probe of nonpolar binding sites. *J. Mol. Biol.* 13:482 (1965).

140. J. F. HACKNEY, S. R. GROSS, L. ARONOW, and W. B. PRATT: Specific glucocorticoid-binding macromolecules from mouse fibroblasts growing in vitro. A possible steroid receptor for growth inhibition. *Mol. Pharmacol.* 6:500 (1970).

141. K. M. MOSHER, D. A. YOUNG, and A. MUNCK: Evidence for irreversible, actinomycin D-sensitive, and temperature-sensitive steps following binding of cortisol to glucocorticoid receptors and preceding effects on glucose metabolism in rat thymus cells. *J. Biol. Chem.* 246:654 (1971).

142. E. V. JENSEN, T. SUZUKI, T. KAWASHIMA, W. E. STUMPF, P. W. JUNGBLUT, and E. R. DE SOMBRE: A two-step mechanism for the interaction of estradiol with rat uterus. *Proc. Nat. Acad. Sci. U.S.A.* 59:632 (1968).

143. E. V. JENSEN, M. NUMATA, P. I. BRECHER, and E. R. DE SOMBRE: Hormone-receptor interaction as a guide to biochemical mechanism In *The Biochemistry of Steroid Hormone Action*, ed. by R. M. S. Smellie. Biochemical Society Symposia No. 32. New York, Academic Press (1971).

144. I. S. EDELMAN and D. O. FANESTIL: Mineralocorticoids. In *Biochemical Actions of Hormones*, Vol. 1, ed. by G. Litwack. New York, Academic Press (1970), Ch. 8.

145. P. KARLSON: New concepts on the mode of action of hormones. *Perspectives in Biol. and Med.* 6:203 (1963).

146. A. R. MEANS and T. H. HAMILTON: Early estrogen action. Concomitant stimulations within 2 minutes of nuclear RNA synthesis and uptake of RNA precursor by the uterus. *Proc. Nat. Acad. Sci. U.S.A.* 56:1594 (1966).

147. G. SHYAMALA and J. GORSKI: Estrogen receptors in the rat uterus. Studies on the interaction of cytosol and nuclear binding sites. *J. Biol. Chem.* 244:1097 (1969).

148. G. C. MUELLER: Estrogen action: a study of the influence of steroid hormones on genetic expression. In *The Biochemistry of Steroid Hormone Action*, ed. by R. M. S. Smellie. Biochemical Society Symposia No. 32. New York, Academic Press (1971).

149. M. M. FENCL and C. A. VILLEE: Effect of RNA from estradiol-treated immature rats on protein synthesis in immature uteri. *Endocrinology* 88:279 (1971).

150. P. CUATRECASAS and C. B. ANFINSEN: Affinity chromatography. *Ann. Rev. Biochem.* 40:259 (1971).

151. W. ROSNER and H. L. BRADLOW: Purification of corticosteroid-binding globulin from human plasma by affinity chromatography. *J. Clin. Endocrinol.* 33:193 (1971).

152. P. CUATRECASAS, M. WILCHEK and C. B. ANFINSEN: Selective enzyme purification by affinity chromatography. *Proc. Nat. Acad. Sci.* 61:636 (1968).

153. F. KRUG, B. DESBUQUOIS, and P. CUATRECASAS: Glucagon affinity absorbents: selective binding of receptors of liver cell membranes. *Nature New Biol* 234:268 (1971).

154. C. CHAGAS: Studies on the mechanism of curarization. *Ann. N.Y. Acad. Sci.* 81:345 (1959).

155. S. EHRENPREIS: Isolation and properties of a drug-binding protein from electric tissue of electric eel. *Proc. 1st Int. Pharmacol. Meeting* 7:119 (1961).

156. A. GOLDSTEIN, L. I. LOWNEY, and B. K. PAL: Stereospecific and nonspecific interactions of the morphine congener levorphanol in subcellular fractions of mouse brain. *Proc. Nat. Acad. Sci. U.S.A.* 68:1742 (1971).

157. P. G. WASER: Autoradiographic investigations of cholinergic and other receptors in the motor end-plate. *Adv. Drug Res.* 3:81 (1966).

158. P. G. WASER: On receptors in the postsynaptic membrane of the motor endplate. In *Molecular Properties of Drug Receptors*, ed. by R. Porter and M. O'Connor. Ciba Foundation Symposium. London, J. and A. Churchill (1970), p. 59.

159. E. A. BARNARD, J. WIECKOWSKI, and T. H. CHIU: Cholinergic receptor molecules and cholinesterase molecules at mouse skeletal muscle junctions. *Nature* 234:207 (1971).

160. R. MILEDI, P. MOLINOFF, and L. T. POTTER: Isolation of the cholinergic receptor protein of Torpedo electric tissue. *Nature* 229:554 (1971).

161. R. D. O'BRIEN, L. P. GILMOUR, and M. E. ELDEFRAWI: A muscarone-binding material in electroplax and its relation to the acetylcholine receptor. II. Dialysis assay. *Proc. Nat. Acad. Sci. U.S.A.* 65:438 (1970).

162. S. EHRENPREIS, J. H. FLEISCH, and T. W. MITTAG: Approaches to the molecular nature of pharmacological receptors. *Pharmacol. Rev.* 21:131 (1969).

163. J. P. CHANGEUX, J. C. MEUNIER, and M. HUCHET: Studies on the cholinergic receptor protein of Electrophorus electricus. I. An assay in vitro for the cholinergic receptor site and solubilization of the receptor protein from electric tissue. *Mol. Pharmacol.* 7:538 (1971).

164. B. R. BAKER: Specific irreversible enzyme inhibitors. *Ann. Rev. Pharmacol.* 10:35 (1970).

165. J. P. CHANGEUX, T. R. PODLESKI, and L. WOFSY: Affinity labeling of the acetylcholine receptor. *Proc. Nat. Acad. Sci. U.S.A.* 58:2063 (1967).

166. A. KARLIN: Chemical modification of the active site of the acetylcholine receptor. N.Y. Heart Association Symposium, *J. Gen. Physiol.* 54:245s (1969).

167. E. BARTELS and T. L. ROSENBERRY: Snake neurotoxins: effect of disulfide reduction on interaction with electroplax. *Science* 174:1236 (1971).

168. E. DE ROBERTIS: Molecular biology of synaptic receptors. *Science* 171:963 (1971).

169. J. L. LA TORRE, G. S. LUNT, and E. DE ROBERTIS: Isolation of a cholinergic proteolipid receptor from electric tissue. *Proc. Nat. Acad. Sci. U.S.A.* 65:716 (1970).

170. E. DE ROBERTIS, G. S. LUNT, and J. L. LA TORRE: Multiple binding sites for acetylcholine in a proteolipid from electric tissue. *Mol. Pharmacol.* 7:97 (1971).

171. M. PARISI, E. RIVAS, and E. DE ROBERTIS: Conductance changes produced by acetylcholine in lipidic membranes containing a proteolipid from electrophorus. *Science* 172:56 (1971).

172. S. C. KINSKY, J. A. HAXLEY, D. A. ZOPF, C. R. ALVING, and C. B. KINSKY: Complement-dependent damage to liposomes prepared from pure lipids and Forssman hapten. *Biochemistry* 8:4149 (1969).

173. P. CUATRECASAS: Interaction of insulin with the cell membrane: the primary action of insulin. *Proc. Nat. Acad. Sci. U.S.A.* 63:450 (1969).

174. P. CUATRECASAS: Insulin-receptor interactions in adipose tissue cells: direct measurement and properties. *Proc. Nat. Acad. Sci. U.S.A.* 68:1264 (1971).

175. P. CUATRECASAS: Properties of the insulin receptor of isolated fat cell membranes. *J. Biol. Chem.* 246:7265 (1971).

176. A. J. CLARK: *The Mode of Action of Drugs on Cells.* London, E. Arnold Co. (1933).

177. A. J. CLARK: General pharmacology. In *Handbuch der Experimentellen Pharmakologie*, Vol. IV, ed. by A. Heffter. Berlin, Springer–Verlag (1937).

178. O. H. STRAUS and A. GOLDSTEIN: Zone behavior of enzymes. *J. Gen. Physiol.* 26:559 (1943).

179. J. L. WEBB: *Enzyme and Metabolic Inhibitors*, Vol. I. New York, Academic Press (1963).

180. J. E. DOWD and D. S. RIGGS: A comparison of estimates of Michaelis–Menten kinetic constants from various linear transformations. *J. Biol. Chem.* 240:863 (1965).

181. A. RUBIN, T. R. TEPHLY, and G. J. MANNERING: Kinetics of drug metabolism by hepatic microsomes. *Biochem. Pharmacol.* 13:1007 (1964).
182. G. CHEN and D. RUSSELL: A quantitative study of blood pressure response to cardiovascular drugs and their antagonists. *J. Pharmacol. Exp. Therap.* 99:401 (1950).
183. P. CUATRECASAS: Affinity chromatography and purification of the insulin receptor of liver cell membranes. *Proc. Nat. Acad. Sci. U.S.A.* 69:1277 (1972).
184. J. H. GADDUM: *Pharmacology*, 7th ed. London, Oxford University Press (1972).
185. E. H. VENNING, V. E. KAZMIN, and J. C. BELL: Biological assay of adrenal corticoids. *Endocrinol.* 38:79 (1946).
186. W. D. M. PATON: A theory of drug action based on the rate of drug-receptor combination. *Proc. Roy. Soc.* B154:21 (1961).
187. R. K. BICKERTON: The responses of isolated strips of cat spleen to sympathomimetic drugs and their antagonists. *J. Pharmacol. Exp. Therap.* 142:99 (1963).
188. Symposium on drug antagonism. *Pharmacol. Rev.* 9:211–268 (1957).
189. O. ARUNLAKSHANA and H. O. SCHILD: Some quantitative uses of drug antagonists. *Brit. J. Pharmacol.* 14:48 (1959).
190. S. Z. LANGER and U. TRENDELENBURG: The effect of a saturable uptake mechanism on the slopes of dose-response curves for sympathomimetic amines and on the shifts of dose-response curves produced by a competitive antagonist. *J. Pharmacol. Exp. Therap.* 167:117 (1969).
191. A. GOLDSTEIN: The mechanism of enzyme–inhibitor–substrate reactions. *J. Gen. Physiol.* 27:529 (1944).
192. R. P. STEPHENSON and R. B. BARLOW: Concepts of drug action, quantitative pharmacology and biological assay. In *A Companion to Medical Studies*, ed. by R. Passmore and J. S. Robson. Philadelphia, Blackwell Scientific Publ., Ltd., F. A. Davis Co. (1970), Ch. 3.
193. T. H. MAREN: The relation between enzyme inhibition and physiological response in the carbonic anhydrase system. *J. Pharmacol. Exp. Therap.* 139:140 (1963).
194. T. H. MAREN: Renal carbonic anhydrase and the pharmacology of sulfonamide inhibitors. In *Handbook of Experimental Pharmacology*, Berlin, Springer–Verlag, 24:195 (1969).
195. J. T. EDSALL: The carbonic anhydrases of erythrocytes. *Harvey Lectures* 62:191 (1966–67).
196. R. P. STEPHENSON: A modification of receptor theory. *Brit. J. Pharmacol.* 11:379 (1956).
197. E. J. ARIËNS, J. M. VAN ROSSUM, and P. C. KOOPMAN: Receptor reserve and threshold phenomena. I. Theory and experiments with autonomic drugs tested on isolated organs. *Arch. Int. Pharmacodyn.* 127:459 (1960).
198. E. J. ARIËNS, A. M. SIMONIS, and J. M. VAN ROSSUM: Drug-receptor interaction: interaction of one or more drugs with one receptor system. In *Molecular Pharmacology*, Vol. I., ed. by E. J. Ariëns. New York, Academic Press (1964), p. 171.
199. A. J. CLARK: The antagonism of acetylcholine by atropine. *J. Physiol.* 61:547 (1926).
200. M. NICKERSON: Receptor occupancy and tissue response. *Nature* 178:697 (1956).
201. W. D. M. PATON and H. P. RANG: The uptake of atropine and related drugs by intestinal smooth muscle of the guinea-pig in relation to acetylcholine receptors. *Proc. Roy. Soc.* B163:1 (1965).
202. A. S. V. BURGEN and L. SPERO: The action of acetylcholine and other drugs on the efflux of potassium and rubidium from smooth muscle of the guinea-pig intestine. *Brit. J. Pharmacol.* 34:99 (1968).
203. H. P. RANG: The kinetics of action of acetylcholine antagonists in smooth muscle. *Proc. Roy. Soc.* B164:488 (1966).
204. W. D. M. PATON: The principles of drug action. *Proc. Roy. Soc. Med.* 53:815 (1960).
205. W. D. M. PATON and D. R. WAUD: A quantitative investigation of the relationship between rate of access of a drug to a receptor and the rate of onset or offset of action. *Arch. Exp. Pathol. Pharmakol.* 248:124 (1964).
206. A. GOLDSTEIN: A relationship between the rate of attaining equilibrium and the velocity constant of the reverse reaction in certain enzyme-inhibitor systems. *Experientia* 8:442 (1952).
207. W. D. M. PATON: Receptors as defined by their pharmacological properties. In *Molecular Properties of Drug Receptors*, Ciba Foundation, ed. by R. Porter and M. O'Connor. London, J. and A. Churchill (1970).
208. J. H. GADDUM: Theories of drug antagonism. Symposium on drug antagonism. *Pharmacol. Rev.* 9:211 (1957).
209. J. MONOD, J. P. CHANGEUX, and F. JACOB: Allosteric proteins and cellular controls systems. *J. Mol. Biol.* 6:306 (1963).

210. B. BELLEAU: A molecular theory of drug action based on induced conformational perturbations of receptors. *J. Med. Chem.* 7:776 (1964).

211. J. P. CHANGEUX, J. THIERY, Y. TUNG, and C. KITTEL: On the cooperativity of biological membranes. *Proc. Nat. Acad. Sci. U.S.A.* 57:335 (1967).

212. A. KARLIN: On the application of "a plausible model" of allosteric proteins to the receptor for acetylcholine. *J. Theoret. Biol.* 16:306 (1967).

213. J. C. GERHART and A. B. PARDEE: The enzymology of control by feedback inhibition. *J. Biol. Chem.* 237:891 (1962).

214. J. C. GERHART and A. B. PARDEE: Aspartate transcarbamylase, an enzyme designed for feedback inhibition. *Fed. Proc.* 23:727 (1964).

215. G. MARKUS, D. K. McCLINTOCK, and J. B. BUSSEL: Conformational changes in aspartate transcarbamylase. III. A functional model for allosteric behavior. *J. Biol. Chem.* 246:762 (1971).

216. J. P. CHANGEUX and T. R. PODLESKI: On the excitability and cooperativity of the electroplax membrane. *Proc. Nat. Acad. Sci. U.S.A.* 59:944 (1968).

217. H. P. RANG and J. M. RITTER: A new kind of drug antagonism: evidence that agonists cause a molecular change in acetylcholine receptors. *Mol. Pharmacol.* 5:394 (1969)

218. E. J. ARIËNS: *Molecular Pharmacology.* New York, Academic Press (1964) Figure 25, Section IIB.

219. H. H. MEYER: Zur Theorie der Alkoholnarkose: Erste Mittheilung. Welche Eigenschaft der Anästhetica bedingt ihre narkotische Wirkung? *Arch. Exp. Pathol. Pharmakol.* 42:109 (1899).

220. E. OVERTON: Beiträge zur allgemeinen Muskel- und Nerven-physiologie. *Arch. ges. Physiol.* 92:115 (1902).

221. J. FERGUSON: The use of chemical potentials as indices of toxicity. *Proc. Roy. Soc.* B127:387 (1939).

222. B. P. SCHOENBORN and R. M. FEATHERSTONE: Molecular forces in anesthesia. *Adv. Pharmacol.* 5:1 (1967).

223. R. M. FEATHERSTONE and C. A. MUEHLBAECHER: The current role of inert gases in the search for anesthesia mechanisms. *Pharmacol. Rev.* 15:97 (1963).

224. J. F. CATCHPOOL: The Pauling theory of general anesthesia. In *Structural Chemistry and Molecular Biology*, ed. by A. Rich and N. Davidson. San Francisco, W. H. Freeman (1968), p. 343.

225. K. W. MILLER, W. D. M. PATON, and E. B. SMITH: Site of action of general anaesthetics. *Nature* 206:574 (1965).

226. A. W. CUTHBERT: Membrane lipids and drug action. *Pharmacol. Rev.* 19:59 (1967).

227. W. L. HUBBELL, J. C. METCALFE, S. M. METCALFE, and H. M. MC CONNELL: The interaction of small molecules with spin labeled erythrocyte membranes. *Biochim. Biophys. Acta* 219:415 (1970).

228. I. H. SCHEINBERG and I. STERNLIEB: Copper metabolism. *Pharmacol. Rev.* 12:355 (1960).

229. R. A. PETERS, L. A. STOCKEN, and R. H. S. THOMPSON: British Anti-Lewisite. *Nature* 156:616 (1945).

230. R. M. HOCHSTER and J. H. QUASTEL, eds.: *Metabolic Inhibitors*, Vol. I. New York, Academic Press (1963).

231. R. W. BROCKMAN and E. P. ANDERSON: Pyrimidine analogues. In *Metabolic Inhibitors*, Vol. I, ed. by R. M. Hochster and J. H. Quastel. New York, Academic Press (1963).

232. Y. MARUYAMA, G. SILINI, and H. S. KAPLAN: Studies of the LSA ascites lymphoma of C57B1 mice. II. Radiosensitization in vivo with 5-bromodeoxycytidine and combined 5-fluorodeoxyuridine and 5-bromodeoxycytidine. *Int. J. Radiat. Biol.* 7:453 (1963).

233. F. CHAPEVILLE, F. LIPMANN, G. VON EHRENSTEIN, B. WEISBLUM, W. J. RAY, and J. BENZER: On the role of soluble ribonucleic acid in coding for amino acids. *Proc. Nat. Acad. Sci. U.S.A.* 48:1086 (1962).

234. W. SHIVE and C. G. SKINNER: Amino acid analogues. In *Metabolic Inhibitors* Vol. I, ed. by R. M. Hochster and J. H. Quastel. New York, Academic Press (1963).

235. M. H. RICHMOND: Immunological properties of exopenicillinase synthesized by *Bacillus cereus* 569/H in the presence of amino acid analogues. *Biochem. J.* 77:112 (1960).

CHAPTER 2
The Absorption, Distribution, and Elimination of Drugs

INTRODUCTION

We now turn our attention to the factors that determine the access of a drug to its site of action.[1] Most drugs are distributed throughout the body in the water phase of the blood plasma. In order to act, therefore, unless it acts topically at the site of application, a drug must first enter the blood. It will then reach the tissues of each organ at a rate determined by the blood flow through that organ and by the rapidity of passage of the drug molecules across the capillary bed and into the cells of that particular organ.

Within the blood plasma some of the drug molecules may be bound to proteins and thus may not be freely diffusible out of the plasma. As a general rule the amount of any drug in the tissues where it acts is but a very small part of the total drug in the body. Most of the drug remains in the various fluid compartments in solution, or is localized by adsorptive or partition processes in subcellular particles, at macromolecular surfaces, or in fat depots. Even within the target cells themselves, cellular fractionation studies and radioautography usually reveal that most drug molecules are associated with structures having nothing to do with the specific drug effect.

Finally, even if no cell components other than the specific receptors were capable of binding drug molecules, we should nevertheless expect to find only a small fraction of the drug associated with these receptors. The reason is that approximately 80% of the cell mass is water and only a very small fraction of the cell dry weight is likely to be represented by the specific receptors. Moreover, the receptors are macromolecules of high molecular weight, each bearing only one or a few specific drug-binding sites. Thus, even at complete receptor occupancy, and even with fairly high drug-receptor affinity, provided the drug interacts reversibly, most of the drug molecules will be in

129

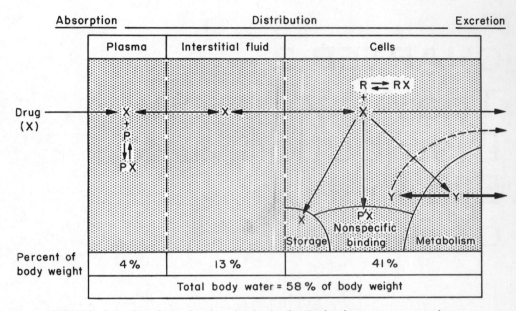

FIGURE 2-1. The fate of a drug in the body. *Broken lines represent membranes. Numbers at bottom are percentages of body weight represented by each fluid compartment in the adult male. X is free drug; PX, drug-protein complex in plasma; P'X, complex of drug with nonspecific binding sites in tissues; Y, a metabolic product of X; and RX, drug-receptor complex.*

the ambient water phase in equilibrium with those bound to the receptor. This general view of drug distribution is represented schematically in Figure 2-1.

A drug enters the circulation by being injected there directly (intravascular route) or by absorption from depots where it has been placed. The commonest such depot is the gastrointestinal tract, the drug having been taken orally or, rarely, administered by rectum. The other common routes of administration are subcutaneous and intramuscular. Several less usual routes are also employed, for example, through the skin (percutaneous) and by inhalation. Drugs are sometimes applied for their local effects, and then the aim is to *minimize* absorption into the circulation; an example is the injection of a local anesthetic agent subcutaneously or into the spinal canal.

A drug is eliminated from the circulation by metabolism, excretion, and accumulation in tissues. The rate of each of these processes that contribute to termination of the drug action is determined by the chemical and physical properties of the drug and its interaction with the specialized tissues responsible for the elimination reactions. The kidney plays the major role in drug excretion. However, other excretory routes may be of prime importance for one or another drug. An example is excretion into the gastrointestinal tract, directly from the blood or by way of the bile. The sweat may play a role in the excretion of some drugs. Volatile agents are eliminated at the lungs. The liver is of chief importance in drug metabolism, but drugs are also degraded in other tissues. Often, metabolic alteration of structure is a prerequisite to renal excretion. Accumulation at any site must obviously occur at the expense of other sites. Thus, lipid-soluble drugs may be localized in the large depots of neutral fat that comprise a significant fraction of the body weight. It is not unusual, long after administration of such a drug, to find practically all the drug molecules in the body stored in this way.

It follows from this brief review that the time course of drug action, determined by the effective concentration of drug at receptor sites, depends in a complex way upon the relative rates of all the processes cited. In this chapter we shall first examine the various routes by which drugs may be administered, and the important characteristics of each route. Then the factors influencing the distribution of drugs into the tissues will be considered, with special attention to the passage of drugs into the central nervous system and across the placenta into the fetus. Finally, routes of drug elimination will be analyzed. The principles and pathways of drug metabolism will be deferred to the next chapter. In Chapter 4 we shall consider the combined effects of absorption, distribution, and elimination upon the time course of drug action.

DRUG ABSORPTION: ROUTES OF ADMINISTRATION

The possible routes of drug entry into the body may be divided into two classes— *enteral* and *parenteral*. In enteral administration the drug is placed directly in the gastrointestinal tract by placing it under the tongue (*sublingual*), by swallowing it (*oral, p.o., per os*), or by rectal administration. In parenteral administration the gastrointestinal tract is bypassed. There are many parenteral routes. The commonest are subcutaneous (*s.c.*), intramuscular (*i.m.*), and intravascular; but drugs may also be applied to the skin or injected intradermally, for local effect or to be absorbed percutaneously; they may be inhaled for direct action on the bronchial tree or to be absorbed into blood at the alveoli; they may be injected into or near the spinal canal; they may be introduced intravaginally. We shall discuss the principal routes of administration, their peculiar advantages and disadvantages, and the various determinants of the rate of onset and the duration of drug action.

Intravascular Administration

The common method of introducing a drug directly into the blood stream is to inject it intravenously (*i.v.*), usually into the antecubital vein. The obvious advantage of this route is that the drug is placed in the circulation with minimum delay, a matter of importance when speed is essential. Another advantage is control. The injection can be made slowly, and it can be stopped instantaneously if untoward effects should develop. Large quantities of fluid can be introduced over a long time by means of a constant infusion apparatus, and thus the rate of drug administration can be held constant for indefinite periods. Sometimes it is important that the drug concentration in plasma be held within fairly narrow limits, or that it not fall below some desired minimum; in such instances the establishment and maintenance of a plasma plateau by means of continuous infusion (p. 314) necessitates use of the intravenous route.

Intravenous infusion may be the safest way to administer a drug that has a narrow margin of safety between therapeutic and toxic blood levels. This is especially true of drugs that are rapidly excreted or metabolized; excessive concentrations can be reduced rapidly by merely stopping the infusion or reducing its rate. An important practical example is the use of lidocaine to prevent dangerous ventricular arrhythmias and fibrillation in the wake of coronary occlusions.[2] The effective blood level is in the range 1 to 4 μg/ml. If this is not achieved and maintained, the patient is exposed to the risk of potentially fatal arrhythmia; if it is exceeded, serious toxicity, including convulsive seizures, may be produced. Therefore, a carefully regulated constant rate of intravenous infusion is the method of choice. As shown in Figure 2-2, there is a nearly

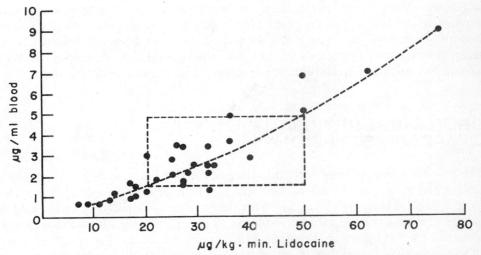

FIGURE 2-2. Relation between rate of infusion and blood level of lidocaine. *Data for 21 patients are given. Blood levels were measured after 2 hr of constant infusion. Area within rectangle is considered to be the appropriate therapeutic range. (From Gianelly et al., Figure 3.[2])*

linear relationship between infusion rate and blood level of lidocaine, but the variability between patients is considerable, indicating the desirability of individualizing the infusion rate. The principles underlying establishment of steady-state plasma levels by constant intravenous infusion are considered in Chapter 4.

The intravenous route is also suited for substances that cannot be absorbed well from tissue depots or the gastrointestinal tract, or that would be destroyed before appreciable absorption could occur (e.g., whole blood, blood plasma and plasma substitutes, and protein hormones). Finally, drugs that would be intolerably painful in the subcutaneous or muscle tissues by virtue of their irritant properties may often be injected slowly into a vein without any difficulty; an example is nitrogen mustard (p. 3), used in cancer chemotherapy.

The intravenous route has drawbacks. A drug once injected into a vein cannot be recalled, whereas a stomach pump or emetic can remove material from the stomach, and various procedures can delay absorption from a subcutaneous depot. Too rapid an injection rate may evoke catastrophic effects in the circulatory and respiratory systems. Blood pressure may fall to dangerous levels, cardiac irregularities or arrest may ensue, respiration may become shallow and irregular.

These effects may be seen even with simple salt solutions or other pharmacologically inert substances if these are injected rapidly enough. Probably the precipitating factor is a bolus of concentrated solute suddenly reaching the myocardium and the chemoreceptors in the aortic arch and carotid sinus. The possible magnitude of solute concentration to which these tissues may be exposed can be calculated readily. Let x be the total dose (in grams) of a drug to be injected intravenously in order to achieve a therapeutic concentration throughout the body water at eventual equilibrium. In a 70 kg man with about 42 liters of body water, this eventual concentration (ignoring elimination processes) will be $(x/42)$ mg/ml. Now suppose the injection is made into a vein in a period of 1 sec. The blood returning to the heart in 1 sec is 1/60 of the cardiac output (6 liters/min), or about 100 ml. Since all the injected drug will pass through the lungs, reach the heart, and be expelled into the aorta, we shall have $(x/100)$ g/ml, or $10x$ mg/ml, for a period of 1 sec in these tissues. This is a 400-fold higher concentration than the therapeutic level that will be reached eventually, at equilibrium. Even if we assume that the concentration is tolerable when the total amount of drug is dissolved in the whole volume of circulating plasma, the bolus would contain a transient 30-fold excess over this concentration after a 1 sec injection.

Safety, therefore, demands that all intravenous injections be performed slowly, preferably over a period not much less than that required for a complete circulation of the blood, i.e., 1 min. Quite apart from the need to avoid high transient drug concentrations, one wishes to be able, if necessary, to discontinue the administration if anything untoward happens; and many seconds may be required for adverse reactions to develop. The circulation time, for example, between the antecubital vein and the brain is roughly 10–15 sec. If sudden loss of consciousness or convulsions were to occur 15 sec after the start of drug injection, the difference between having emptied the syringe and having it still three-quarters full could be very significant for the patient's welfare. The same argument applies to the consequences of accidentally injecting a wrong solution, whether a wrong drug or the right drug at a wrong concentration.

Anaphylactoid reactions, caused by administration of a drug to a sensitized individual (cf. Chapter 7), may be especially severe after intravenous injection, probably because of the sudden massive antigen–antibody reaction. When the drug is given by other routes, its access to antibody molecules is necessarily slower; moreover, its further absorption can be retarded or prevented at the first sign of a serious allergic reaction.

Embolism is another possible complication of the intravenous route. Particulate matter may be introduced if a drug intended for intravenous use precipitates for some reason, or if a particulate suspension intended for intramuscular or subcutaneous use is inadvertently given into a vein. Hemolysis or agglutination of erythrocytes may be caused by injection of hypotonic or hypertonic solutions, or by more specific mechanisms. Some drugs damage the vascular wall and lead to local venous thrombosis, especially after prolonged infusions.

Infection by bacterial contaminants was commonplace until the development of aseptic technique, and the infectious hepatitis virus was sometimes spread from person to person by syringes and needles until disposable sets came into use. Self-administration of drugs, particularly by addicts, remains a cause of infection because asepsis is usually ignored. Intravenous injection of drugs was long complicated by the development of fever due to pyrogens in water, especially when large volumes were infused. The pyrogenic substances (bacterial lipopolysaccharides) are heat-stable but can be removed by special procedures; thus, solutions for injection are now prepared in pyrogen-free water. Finally, excessive amounts of fluid (e.g., salt solutions given intravenously) may lead to elevated blood pressure and cardiovascular failure, especially when renal function is deficient.

The intra-arterial route is used rarely, principally for the injection of substances used diagnostically. A typical example is the injection of a radiopaque compound into the carotid artery to visualize the circulation of the brain roentgenographically. Certain specialized techniques in cancer chemotherapy call for regional infusions of drugs by an arterial route.

Intramuscular Administration

Drugs injected into skeletal muscle (usually in the deltoid or gluteal regions) are generally absorbed rapidly. Blood flow through the muscles at rest is about 0.02–0.07 ml/min per gram of tissue, and this flow rate may increase many times during exercise as additional vascular channels open. Quite large amounts of solution can be introduced intramuscularly, and there is usually less pain and local irritation than is encountered by the subcutaneous route. Ordinary aqueous solutions of drugs are usually absorbed from an intramuscular site within 10–30 min, but faster or slower absorption is possible, depending upon the vascularity of the site, the ionization and lipid solubility of the drug, the volume of the injection, the osmolality of the solution, and probably other variables. Small molecules are absorbed directly into the capillaries from an intramuscular site, whereas larger molecules (e.g., proteins) gain access to the circulation by way of the lymphatic channels. Radiolabeled compounds of widely different molecular weights (maximum 585) and physical properties were found to be absorbed from rat muscle at virtually the same rate, about $16\% \text{ min}^{-1}$.[3] This implies that the absorption process is limited by the blood flow.

Drugs that are insoluble at tissue pH, or that are in an oily vehicle, form a depot in the muscle tissue, from which absorption proceeds very slowly. Because frequently repeated injections are inconvenient to patients and physicians alike, much ingenuity has been expended in developing *depot preparations* of various drugs for intramuscular use. For example, the procaine salt of penicillin is injected as a microcrystalline suspension that dissolves and enters the blood stream over a period of a few days. The kinetics of absorption from depots and some of the advantages and disadvantages of depot preparations are discussed fully later.

Subcutaneous Administration

Absorption of drugs from the subcutaneous tissues is influenced by the same factors that determine the rate of absorption from intramuscular sites.[4] Blood flow is said to be poorer than in muscle, so the absorption rate is often stated to be slower. Actually, there seems to be no simple way to measure blood flow in a subcutaneous area. Some drugs, at least, are known to be absorbed as rapidly from subcutaneous tissues as from muscle.

Certain drugs produce severe pain when injected subcutaneously; local necrosis and sterile abscesses may also occur. Some agents have to be administered intravenously because no solution concentrated enough to be useful can be given subcutaneously or intramuscularly.

The rate of absorption from a subcutaneous depot may be retarded by immobilization of the limb, local cooling to cause vasoconstriction, and application of a tourniquet proximal to the injection site to block the superficial venous drainage and lymphatic flow. These techniques, customarily applied to slow down venom absorption in snake bites, are also of value in the emergency treatment of adverse drug reactions after subcutaneous or intramuscular administration. Epinephrine, in minute amounts, may be incorporated with a subcutaneous injection in order to constrict the local vasculature and thereby retard absorption. This is of special value when the injected drug is meant to act locally at the injection site rather than systemically. The best example is the inclusion of epinephrine in preparations of local anesthetic agents to prolong their action on sensory nerve fibers passing through the subcutaneous tissues. Drugs may affect the rate of their own absorption if they alter the blood supply or capillary permeability locally. Methacholine, for example, causes vascular dilation as part of its cholinergic action; consequently it enters the blood stream so rapidly from a subcutaneous site that it causes systemic effects as early as 1.5 min after injection.

A prime determinant of the absorption rate from a subcutaneous depot is the total surface area over which the absorption can occur. Although the subcutaneous tissues are somewhat loose, and moderate amounts of fluid can be administered, the normal connective tissue matrix prevents indefinite lateral spread of the injected solution. These barriers may be overcome with the aid of hyaluronidase, an enzyme that breaks down mucopolysaccharides of the connective tissue matrix; the resulting spread of injected solution leads to a much faster absorption rate. Hyaluronidase is sometimes used for administering large fluid volumes to infants, in whom continuous intravenous infusions present special difficulties.

An effective way of achieving slow absorption for a long time is to incorporate a drug into a compressed pellet that can be implanted under the skin. The drug must be relatively insoluble and the pellet must resist disintegration by the subcutaneous fluid environment. These conditions have been achieved with certain steroid hormones.[5]

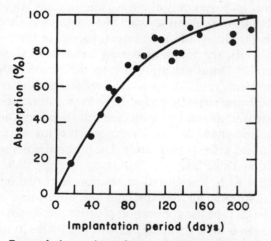

FIGURE 2-3. Rate of absorption of testosterone pellets in human subjects. *Pellets weighed 100 mg and were cylindrical (diameter 2.5 mm, thickness 4.6 mm). Implantation sites were subcutaneous. Each point represents a pellet in a single subject. Pellets were weighed initially and again after removal. The curve is a theoretical one calculated from an arbitrary rate constant of absorption and the assumption that absorption rate is proportional to surface area throughout the dissolution process. (From Bishop and Folley.[5])*

Pellets of testosterone, of a cylindrical shape, about 5 mm in diameter, 5 mm thick, and weighing 100 mg, were implanted subcutaneously into human subjects. Upon removal at different intervals for individual subjects, the pellets were weighed carefully and the weight loss thus determined. Figure 2-3 shows that the absorption rate was nearly constant at about 1 % per day for 2 months and then diminished gradually, with absorption essentially complete at 5–6 months. For spherical pellets the ratio of surface area to volume increases with decreasing diameter. Thus, when drugs are prepared as spheres of known diameter the rate of absorption can be predicted; the larger the spheres the slower the rate of absorption of a given amount of drug. This principle has been used in the design of long-acting insulin preparations; the so-called Lente insulins are small zinc insulin crystals (about 30 μm), of uniform size to provide a reproducible rate of absorption.

The ideal shape of a subcutaneous pellet for achieving a constant rate of absorption would be a flat disk. Absorption should occur almost exclusively from the two opposite surfaces, since the area of the edge is negligibly small by comparison. Moreover, the exposed area for absorption would hardly change at all as the disk becomes thinner, so that the absorption rate should be nearly constant until practically all the drug is absorbed. Studies in rats and mice have verified the correctness of these predictions. A useful experimental technique for establishing morphine tolerance and dependence in various small laboratory animals employs subcutaneously implanted pellets of morphine. The drug is released into the body at a constant rate for several days, producing a steady-state level, much as would be attained by a constant intravenous infusion.[6]

Absorption of Drugs Through the Skin

The skin efficiently retards the diffusion and evaporation of water except at the sweat glands. The epidermis, although only about 0.2 mm thick, is largely responsible. The outer, horny layer (*stratum corneum*) consists of a continuous sheet of flattened cells, densely packed with keratin, which constitutes a barrier to the penetration of water-soluble substances. Thus, the intact epidermis behaves qualitatively like cellular membranes in general.[6a] Drugs penetrate at rates determined largely by their lipid/water partition coefficients (p. 172), water-soluble ions and polar molecules (except for the very smallest) being virtually excluded.[7,8] Even substances that are very lipid soluble penetrate slowly in comparison with their rates of penetration of other, thinner, cell membranes. The underlying dermis, which consists of loosely arranged connective tissue and is vascularized, is freely permeable. The properties of the principal layers of skin are summarized in Table 2-1.

Two problems have to be considered in relation to percutaneous absorption of drugs: the use of this route for therapy, and the absorption of toxic substances through the skin. The therapeutic application of drugs presents no special problem of penetration if the action is to be upon the exposed surface (as in treatment of wounds or burns) or upon the superficial layers of the *stratum corneum*. Drugs may be incorporated into vehicles (creams, ointments) that adhere to the skin and permit local diffusion, or baths containing the drug may be employed. As would be expected from their lipid solubility, steroids such as the anti-inflammatory glucocorticoids and the sex hormones diffuse readily into the skin after topical application. They are retained in the skin for long periods, and they are also metabolized there. However, if the drug

TABLE 2-1. Stratified organization of the skin.
(From Katz and Poulsen,[8] Table 2.)

Layers	Epidermis	Dermis	Subcutaneous fat
Function	Barrier	Connective tissue support	Thermal insulation, cushion
Embryonic origin	Ectoderm	Mesoderm	Mesoderm
Thickness (mm)	0.2	3–5	Variable
pH	4.2–6.5	7.2–7.3	—
H_2O content (%)	10–25	Up to 70	Low
Cellular activity	Actively dividing cells	Mostly noncellular	Closely packed cells
Cellular contents	Keratinocytes → keratin	Fibrocytes → collagen	Lipocytes → lipids
	Melanocytes → melanin	Fibroblasts, histiocytes, mastcells	—
Vasculature	None	Blood vessels, lymphatics, sweat glands	Blood vessels

is water soluble, and if the pathologic condition is in the deeper layers of the epidermis or in the dermis, systemic administration may be necessary. Antibacterial and antifungal agents, for example, are often more effective in skin infections when given by mouth or by injection than when applied to the skin surface.

Much investigation has been directed toward developing pharmacologically inert organic solvents that might facilitate drug penetration through the skin. Dimethyl sulfoxide (CH_3SOCH_3, DMSO) is an example.[9] This liquid is miscible with water and with many organic solvents, and is capable of increasing the penetration of ionized drugs into the deeper layers of skin. Unfortunately, these effects are accompanied by (or even in part attributable to) local tissue damage, and some generalized toxicity has also been observed in animal experiments. It remains to be seen whether some nontoxic solvent of this kind could have general usefulness in dermatologic therapy, or for expanding the usefulness of the percutaneous route for drugs with systemic actions.

Toxic effects are often produced by the accidental absorption through the skin of highly lipid-soluble substances used for various industrial purposes. General experience leads people to suppose that the skin is a reliable protection against the environment; so little thought is given to the possibility of poisoning by this route. Carbon tetrachloride and other organic solvents penetrate the body in this way and can cause serious toxic effects. Organic phosphate (DFP, parathion, malathion) and nicotine insecticides have caused deaths in agricultural workers as a result of percutaneous absorption. Chlorovinylarsine dichloride (lewisite), a mustard gas, is readily absorbed through the intact skin.

Electrical gradients have been used to drive drugs into the skin in the method known as *iontophoresis*. An ionized drug in solution is placed in an absorbent material on the skin in contact with an electrode. By applying a galvanic current to this electrode and to another placed elsewhere on the body surface, the drug ions are made to migrate through the epidermis. Studies with iodine 131 have shown that this method is quite efficient, at least for introducing very small amounts of drugs into the skin and general circulation.[10] The reproducibility, however, between subjects and even between different skin areas in the same subject leaves much to be desired. The general utility of the method is obviously rather limited.

Inhalation of Drugs

Drugs may be inhaled as gases and enter the circulation by diffusing across the alveolar membranes. This is the mode of administration of the volatile anesthetics. These drugs all have relatively high lipid/water partition coefficients, and inasmuch as their atomic or molecular radii are quite small and the alveolar membrane is quite permeable, they all equilibrate practically instantaneously with blood in the alveolar capillaries. The interesting differences among these agents in the kinetics of their equilibration in whole body water and in the rates of onset and decline of their anesthetic effects depend primarily upon their aqueous solubilities (blood/air partition coefficients). This will be discussed fully elsewhere (p. 338).

Drugs may also be inhaled as *aerosols*,[11,11a] and many toxic substances enter the body in this way. Aerosols are liquid or solid particles so small that they remain suspended in air for a long time instead of sedimenting rapidly under the force of gravity. Table 2-2 gives sedimentation rate as a function of particle diameter, computed from Stokes' law for the viscous drag on a moving sphere.

TABLE 2-2. Rate of gravitational sedimentation in quiet air as a function of particle size. Sedimentation rates are computed from Stokes' law as described in the text.

Particle diameter, μm	Sedimentation rate, cm sec^{-1}
100	28.7
50	7.17
25	1.79
10	0.287
5	0.072
1	0.0029

Stokes' law:

$$f = 6\pi nrv$$

where f is force in dynes; n is viscosity of air at 20° and atmospheric pressure and is equal to 1.9×10^{-4} g sec^{-1} cm^{-1}; r is radius of sphere in centimeters; and v is constant velocity of movement when force f is balanced by the viscous drag.

For a sphere moving under the force of gravity, $f = $ mass $\times$ g, where $g = 980$ cm sec^{-2}; and assuming unit density,

$$f = \frac{4}{3}\pi r^3 g$$

When the viscous drag opposes the force of gravity so that the rate of fall is constant,

$$6\pi n r v = \frac{4}{3}\pi r^3 g$$

$$v = \frac{D^2 g}{18n}$$ where D is diameter of sphere in centimeters

$$v = 2.87 \times 10^5 D^2$$

Particles below about 10 μm in diameter are of interest for the present discussion. Examples are bacteria and viruses, smoke, industrial fumes, dust laden with fission products from nuclear explosions, pollens, insecticide dusts or sprays, and inhalant sprays used in the therapy of pulmonary disease.

Impaction is the term used to describe the deposition of aerosol particles in the respiratory tract. The degree of impaction is determined by the rates of sedimentation, diffusion, and inertial precipitation. In considering the rate of movement of substances within the respiratory tract, diffusion may be ignored, except for very small particles. Inertial precipitation arises from the tendency of a particle moving in a stream of air to continue in its original direction when the air current changes direction, and thus to impact upon some tissue. This occurs, for example, at bronchial branch points.

The extent of impaction in different parts of the respiratory tract may be computed for particles of various sizes, and such computations have been confirmed by some experimental data. In the nasal passages large particles (> 10 μm) are almost completely removed; particles 5 μm in diameter are removed to an extent of about one-half; and particles 2 μm in diameter, to an extent of about one-fifth. Below 1 μm, nasal impaction is negligible. Table 2-3 gives theoretical results for particle sizes

TABLE 2-3. Percent retention of inhaled aerosol particles in various regions of the respiratory tract.
The figures in the columns are percent retention; the column headings are particle sizes in μm. A 4 sec respiratory cycle is assumed. (From Hatch and Gross,[11] Table 3-4.)

	Percent retention									
	450 cm³ Tidal air					1500 cm³ Tidal air				
	20	6	2	0.6	0.2	20	6	2	0.6	0.2
Mouth	15	0	0	0	0	18	1	0	0	0
Pharynx	8	0	0	0	0	10	1	0	0	0
Trachea	10	1	0	0	0	19	3	0	0	0
Pulmonary bronchi	12	2	0	0	0	20	5	1	0	0
Secondary bronchi	19	4	1	0	0	21	12	2	0	0
Tertiary bronchi	17	9	2	0	0	9	20	5	0	0
Quarternary bronchi	6	7	2	1	1	1	10	3	1	1
Terminal bronchioles	6	19	6	4	6	1	9	3	2	4
Respiratory bronchioles	0	11	5	3	4	0	3	2	2	4
Alveolar ducts	0	25	25	8	11	0	13	26	10	13
Alveolar sacs	0	5	0	0	0	0	18	17	6	7
Totals	93	83	41	16	22	99	95	59	21	29

between 0.2 and 20 μm, at two extreme values of the tidal air. The following conclusions may be drawn: (a) The larger the particle the greater its tendency to impact and be retained in the upper respiratory tract. (b) At high tidal volumes and the same respiratory rate, the airstream velocity is greater, thus particles of all sizes tend to be driven deeper into the pulmonary tree before impacting. (c) As particles become smaller, their retention is primarily limited to the most peripheral parts of the pulmonary tree, beyond the terminal bronchioles, but the total retention is substantially less than for larger particles. (d) When particles become extremely small (0.2 μm), the total retention begins to increase again, probably because diffusion becomes a significant factor in the translocation of particles from the lumen to the walls of the bronchioles and alveoli.

A mucous blanket, propelled cephalad by ciliary movements, covers the upper respiratory tract down to the terminal bronchioles, and impacted aerosol particles are cleared by this mechanism. Particles that deposit in the alveolar sacs must first be transported up to the mucous layer, presumably in a fluid film covering the epithelium. Particles in the alveoli are also ingested by phagocytic cells. The efficiency of clearance of solid particles from the lungs is remarkable. For example, not more than a minute fraction of all the mineral dust inhaled during a lifetime is retained in the lungs. However, a small decrease in the clearance capacity of the lungs could cause a marked increase in the amount of retained particulate matter; this may be a factor leading to the development of pneumoconiosis in miners exposed to silica dusts.

Particle size strongly influences the rate at which material is absorbed through the alveolar epithelium, probably because of the greatly increased surface area for solubilization as particle diameter becomes smaller. For example, particles of uranium dioxide larger than 3 μm had no toxic effect whatsoever when introduced into the trachea in rats, but the same relatively insoluble material was absorbed into the circulation and caused kidney damage when smaller particles were employed.[12]

Exposure to lead in aerosol form presents a potentially serious occupational and environmental hazard, largely because of the widespread use of organic lead compounds (e.g., lead tetraethyl) in gasoline. Lead is released from motor vehicles largely as lead halides, which are converted in the atmosphere to carbonates and oxides. The median diameter of airborne lead particulates is about 0.25 μm, small enough to be absorbed with good efficiency (25–50%) from the respiratory tract.[13,14] Rural areas typically have atmospheric lead concentrations as low as 0.5 μg m^{-3}, whereas in urban centers such as Los Angeles the concentrations were found to be 5–16 μg m^{-3} and even higher during busy traffic hours. Figure 2-4 gives the observed relationship between average exposures to atmospheric lead and the mean blood level. The data are from various subjects living and working in different environments—farmers, city dwellers, traffic policemen, and so on. Also included are data from volunteers exposed to atmospheres of known lead content. Blood levels of about 100 ng ml^{-1} (at extreme left of figure) reflect the enteral absorption of about 10% of the average 300 μg dietary intake.[15] It is clear that lead aerosols, derived almost entirely from leaded fuels, can contribute significantly to the body burden of this heavy metal. An atmospheric concentration of 10 μg m^{-3}, yielding about 340 ng ml^{-1} in blood, has been considered to be a "safe" exposure level,[16] but the long-term toxic effects of chronic exposure to low concentrations have not been sufficiently studied.

Drugs in aerosol form can elicit very rapid responses when inhaled. Histamine or pilocarpine administered in this way to dogs or guinea pigs can cause bronchiolar

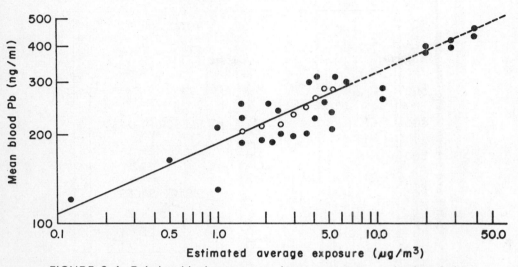

FIGURE 2-4. Relationship between respiratory exposure to lead and the mean blood level. *Open circles are epidemiologic data, solid circles are data from experimental subjects. (From Goldsmith and Hexter, Figure 1.[13])*

constriction and fatal asphyxia within 1 min. An aerosol containing atropine can reverse within a minute the bronchospasm caused by a carbachol aerosol.

Particles larger than 2 μm in diameter probably do not reach the alveolar sacs, as shown in Table 2-3. Some commercially available nebulizers apparently produce particles 1–3.5 μm in diameter, so most of the deposition will occur in the larger bronchial passages. But for most effective therapy the smallest bronchi and alveolar ducts should be reached by the drug, so particles smaller than 1 μm in diameter are desirable. A technique that promotes deposition of particles is for the subject to hold his breath after inhalation, to maximize the effective time for particle diffusion. Another technique is to add hygroscopic substances to the aerosol; the droplets then become larger as they traverse the moist respiratory tract, and the rate of impaction due to sedimentation is increased.

With aerosols of small particle size the amount of drug reaching the alveoli may be large; and since the rate of absorption into the blood stream is much more rapid at the alveolar sacs than elsewhere in the pulmonary tree, the systemic absorption of the drug may be appreciable. Hence, care must be exercised in giving drugs such as the sympathomimetic bronchodilators by aerosol to avoid side effects on the cardiovascular system. Isoproterenol, for example, in a 0.5% aerosol, is an effective bronchodilator, but a 1% aerosol is apt to cause undesirable cardioaccelerator and hypotensive actions after only a few inhalations.

Widespread unrestricted use of aerosols containing isoproterenol and related bronchodilators was apparently responsible for a large increase in mortality from asthma over a period of 7 years in England. The group principally affected was in the age range 10–14 years.[17] As shown in Figure 2-5, the death rate rose in parallel with the use of these preparations, then fell rapidly with restriction of over-the-counter sales and urgent warnings to physicians. The mechanism involved in the excess deaths remains uncertain, but overdosage leading to cardiac failure is a possibility. Experiments

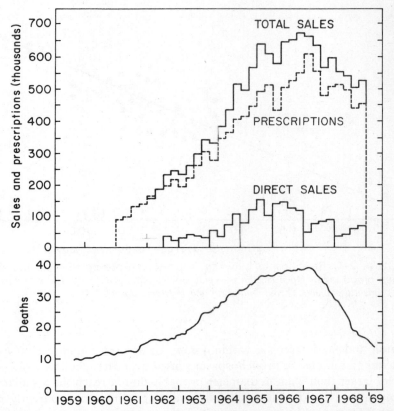

FIGURE 2-5. Increased deaths from asthma in England and Wales, 1959–
1968. *Data for people aged 5–34. Deaths are given as monthly moving averages.
Sales and prescriptions are on a quarterly basis. (From Inman and Adelstein, Figure
3.[20])*

in dogs showed that isoproterenol was far more cardiotoxic when the animals were
made hypoxic than in controls.[18] Another factor may have been related to the
finding that under normal conditions a large fraction of the inhaled isoproterenol is
swallowed rather than absorbed at the bronchial tree. The evidence is derived from
studies with radioactive drug.[19] When administered orally, about two-thirds of the
material was recovered from urine as a conjugate of isoproterenol, presumably because of direct passage via the portal system to the liver. When given intravenously,
the pattern of radioactivity in urine was entirely different; the principal metabolite
was a conjugate of the 3-*O*-methyl derivative, and about 40% of the isoproterenol
was excreted unchanged. When administered by aerosol, the pattern was the same
as by the oral route. Thus, unpredictable differences in the amount swallowed during
an acute asthmatic state could lead to large variations in the amount of free isoproterenol in the circulation. Toxicity due to the Freon propellant may also be a
contributing factor.

Under certain circumstances aerosols may be used effectively for systemic effects.
Penicillin, digitalis glycosides, diuretics, and tranquilizers have been given in this
way, but aerosol therapy has not been exploited very widely. The route has a certain
value when rapid relief is needed on an intermittent basis for acute exacerbations of a

chronic illness, especially if self-administration is desirable. For a person known to be subject to anaphylactic reactions to bee venom or allergenic foods, the self-administration of epinephrine from a nebulizer could be life-saving.

Administration of Drugs by the Enteral Route

Drugs are given most commonly by mouth. This is certainly the most convenient route, and it is the only one of practical importance for self-administration. Absorption, in general, takes place along the whole length of the gastrointestinal tract, but the chemical properties of each drug determine whether it will be absorbed in the strongly acid stomach or in the nearly neutral intestine.[20a] Gastric absorption is favored by an empty stomach, in which the drug, in undiluted gastric juice, will have good access to the mucosal wall. Only when a drug would be irritating to the gastric mucosa is it rational to administer it with or after a meal. However, the antibiotic griseofulvin is an example of a substance with poor water solubility, the absorption of which is aided by a fatty meal.[21] The large surface area of the intestinal villi, the presence of bile, and the rich blood supply all favor intestinal absorption.

The presence of food can impair the absorption of drugs given by mouth. Suggested mechanisms include reduced mixing, complexing with substances in the food, and retarded gastric emptying. In experiments with rats, prolonged fasting was shown to diminish the absorption of several drugs, possibly by deleterious effects upon the epithelium of intestinal villi.[22]

Drugs that are metabolized rapidly by the liver cannot be given by the enteral route because the portal circulation carries them directly to the liver. An example is lidocaine, already discussed for its value in controlling cardiac arrhythmias. This drug is absorbed well from the gut, but is completely inactivated in a single passage through the liver.[23,23a]

Drugs are occasionally administered by rectum, but most are not as well absorbed here as from the upper intestine. Aminophylline, used in suppository form for the management of asthma, is one of the few drugs routinely given in this way. Inert vehicles employed for suppository preparations include cocoa butter, glycerinated gelatin, and polyethylene glycol. Because the rectal mucosa is irritated by anisotonic solutions, fluids administered by this route should always be isotonic with plasma (e.g., 0.9% NaCl).

The principles governing the absorption of drugs from the gastrointestinal lumen are the same as for the passage of drugs across biologic membranes elsewhere (p. 164). Low degree of ionization, high lipid/water partition coefficient of the nonionized form, and small atomic or molecular radius of water-soluble substances all favor rapid absorption. Water passes readily in both directions across the wall of the gastrointestinal lumen. Sodium ion is probably transported actively from lumen into blood. Magnesium ion is very poorly absorbed and therefore acts as a cathartic, retaining an osmotic equivalent of water as it passes down the intestinal tract. Ionic iron is absorbed as an amino acid complex, at a rate usually determined by the body's need for iron. Glucose and amino acids are transported across the intestinal wall by specific carrier systems. Some compounds of high molecular weight (polysaccharides, neutral fats) cannot be absorbed *until* they are degraded enzymically. Other substances are not absorbed *because* they are destroyed by gastrointestinal enzymes; insulin, epinephrine, histamine are examples. Substances that form insoluble precipitates in the gastrointestinal lumen or that are not soluble either in water or in lipid obviously cannot be absorbed.

Absorption of Weak Acids and Bases.   The gastric juice is very acid (about pH 1), whereas the intestinal contents are nearly neutral (actually very slightly acid). The pH difference between plasma (pH 7.4) and the lumen of the gastrointestinal tract plays a major role in determining whether a drug that is a weak electrolyte will be absorbed into plasma, or whether it will be excreted from plasma into the stomach or intestine. We may assume, for practical purposes, that the mucosal lining of the gastrointestinal tract is impermeable to the ionized form of a weak acid or base (p. 175), but that the nonionized form equilibrates freely. The rate of equilibration of the nonionized molecule is directly related to its lipid solubility. If there is a pH difference across the membrane, then the fraction ionized may be considerably greater on one side than on the other. At equilibrium, the concentration of the *nonionized* moiety will be the same on both sides, but there will be more *total* drug on the side where the degree of ionization is greater. This mechanism is known as *ion trapping*. The energy for sustaining the unequal chemical potential of the acid or base in question is derived from whatever mechanism maintains the pH difference; in the stomach this mechanism is the energy-dependent secretion of hydrogen ions.

Consider how a weak electrolyte distributes across the gastric mucosa between plasma (pH 7.4) and gastric fluid (pH 1.0). In each compartment the Henderson–Hasselbalch equation gives the ratio of the concentrations (base)/(acid). Here, and throughout the rest of this book, we shall designate the negative logarithm of the acid dissociation constant by the symbol pK_a rather than using the more rigorously correct pK_a'.

$$pH = pK_a + \log \frac{(base)}{(acid)}$$

$$\log \frac{(base)}{(acid)} = pH - pK_a$$

$$\frac{(base)}{(acid)} = antilog\,(pH - pK_a)$$

For a weak acid with $pK_a = 3$, $pH - pK_a = 4.4$ in plasma and -2 in stomach. Thus, in plasma at equilibrium, $\log[(base)/(acid)] = 4.4$, and (base)/(acid) = 25,000. In stomach, $\log[(base)/(acid)] = -2$, and (base)/(acid) = 0.01. Now for a weak acid it is the acid moiety that is nonionized and is in free equilibrium in both compartments:

	Plasma pH 7.4			Stomach pH 1.0	
H^+ +	A^- ⇌ HA	⇌	HA ⇌	H^+ +	A^-
25,000	⇌ 1.0	⇌	1.0 ⇌		0.01

Total drug (i.e., base + acid):

	25,001	1.01
or:	24,800	1.0

For a weak base with the same pK_a, the fraction (base)/(acid) in each compartment will, of course, be exactly the same as above. The difference is that now the non-ionized form, which has to be equated on both sides, is the base:

	Plasma	Stomach
$\dfrac{\text{(base)}}{\text{(acid)}}$	$\dfrac{25,000}{1}$ $\rightleftharpoons$	$\dfrac{0.01}{1}$

Rewriting these fractions to equate the numerators, we obtain

	Plasma	Stomach
	$\dfrac{1}{4 \times 10^{-5}}$ $\rightleftharpoons$	$\dfrac{1}{100}$

	Plasma	Stomach
Total drug concentration ratio	1	101

The conclusions are obvious. Weak acids are absorbed readily from the stomach. Weak bases are not absorbed well; indeed, they would tend to accumulate within the stomach at the expense of drug in the blood stream. Naturally, in the more alkaline intestine, bases would be absorbed better, acids more poorly.

A simple general equation to describe the concentration ratios of a drug on both sides of a membrane at equilibrium, as determined by the ion-trapping mechanism, may be derived as follows:[24]

Let the two sides be at pH_I and pH_{II}. Then

$$pH = pK_a + \log \frac{\text{(base)}}{\text{(acid)}}$$

$$\log \frac{\text{(base)}}{\text{(acid)}} = pH - pK_a$$

$$\frac{\text{(base)}}{\text{(acid)}} = 10^{(pH - pK_a)}$$

and R, the ratio of total drug concentration on side I to that on side II, is given by

$$R = \frac{(\text{acid}_I) + (\text{base}_I)}{(\text{acid}_{II}) + (\text{base}_{II})}$$

Substituting base = acid $\cdot 10^{(pH - pK_a)}$, we obtain

$$R = \frac{(\text{acid}_I)[1 + 10^{(pH_I - pK_a)}]}{(\text{acid}_{II})[1 + 10^{(pH_{II} - pK_a)}]}$$

For acids, $(\text{acid}_I) = (\text{acid}_{II})$, so that

$$R = \frac{1 + 10^{(pH_I - pK_a)}}{1 + 10^{(pH_{II} - pK_a)}}$$

$$R = \frac{1 + \text{antilog}\,(pH_I - pK_a)}{1 + \text{antilog}\,(pH_{II} - pK_a)}$$

For bases,

$$(\text{acid}) = \frac{\text{(base)}}{10^{(pH - pK_a)}} = \text{base)} \cdot 10^{(pK_a - pH)}$$

$$R = \frac{(\text{base}_I)[1 + 10^{(pK_a - pH_I)}]}{(\text{base}_{II})[1 + 10^{(pK_a - pH_{II})}]}$$

and since $(base_I) = (base_{II})$,

$$R = \frac{1 + 10^{(pK_a - pH_I)}}{1 + 10^{(pK_a - pH_{II})}}$$

$$R = \frac{1 + antilog\,(pK_a - pH_I)}{1 + antilog\,(pK_a - pH_{II})}$$

It should be realized that although the principles outlined here are correct, the system is dynamic, not static. Drug molecules that are absorbed across the gastric or intestinal mucosa are removed constantly by blood flow; thus, simple reversible equilibrium across the membrane does not occur until the drug is distributed throughout the body.

Absorption from the stomach, as determined by direct measurements, conforms, in general, to the principles outlined above. Organic acids are absorbed well since they are all almost completely nonionized at the gastric pH; indeed, many of these substances are absorbed faster than ethyl alcohol, which had long been considered one of the few compounds that were absorbed well from the stomach. Strong acids whose pK_a values lie below 1, which are ionized even in the acid contents of the stomach, are not absorbed well. Weak bases are absorbed only negligibly, but their absorption can be increased, as expected, by raising the pH of the gastric fluid. All this is shown in Table 2-4, the results of experiments in which drugs were placed in the ligated stomachs of rats and the residual amounts determined after 1 hr. Especially interesting is the effect of changing the stomach pH by addition of sodium bicarbonate. Acids like salicylic and nitrosalicylic acids, with pK_a's well on the acid side of neutrality, were absorbed much more poorly when the gastric acidity had been neutralized, for they were then almost completely ionized. Very weak acids like thiopental and phenol were but little affected by the same pH change, since even at pH 8 they remained almost wholly nonionized.

The three barbituric acid derivatives studied (Table 2-4, thiopental, barbital, secobarbital) are interesting because, although they have about the same pK_a, the extent of their gastric absorption differed considerably. This is related to the difference in lipid/water partition coefficients of their nonionized forms. Measurements in a number of organic solvents have revealed that thiopental has the highest partition coefficient, secobarbital a considerably smaller one, barbital the smallest of all.

As for bases, only the weakest were absorbed to any appreciable extent (Table 2-4) at normal gastric pH, but their absorption could be increased substantially by neutralizing the stomach contents. The quaternary cations, however, which are charged at all pH values, were not absorbed at either pH.

The accumulation of weak bases in the stomach by ion trapping mimics a secretory process; if the drug is administered systemically it accumulates in the stomach. Dogs were given various drugs intravenously by continuous infusion to maintain a constant drug level in the plasma, and the gastric contents were sampled by means of an indwelling catheter. The results, representing concentrations after 30–60 min, are shown in Table 2-5. Both acids and bases behaved according to expectation. The stronger bases ($pK_a > 5$) accumulated in stomach contents to many times their plasma concentrations; the weak bases appeared in about equal concentrations in gastric juice and in plasma. Among the acids only the weakest appeared in detectable amounts in the stomach. It may be wondered why the strong bases, which are completely ionized in gastric juice, and whose theoretical concentration ratios (gastric

TABLE 2-4. Absorption of organic acids and organic bases from the rat stomach. The percent absorbed in 1 h is expressed as mean ± range, followed by the number of experiments in parentheses. (After Schanker et al.,[25] Tables I and II.)

| | | Percent absorbed in 1 hr | |
	pK_a	0.1 M HCl	NaHCO$_3$, pH 8
Acid			
5-Sulfosalicylic	(strong)	0 ± 0 (2)	0 ± 0 (2)
Phenosulfonphthalein	(strong)	2 ± 2 (3)	2 ± 1 (2)
5-Nitrosalicylic	2.3	52 ± 3 (2)	16 ± 2 (2)
Salicylic	3.0	61 ± 7 (4)	13 ± 1 (2)
Acetylsalicylic	3.5	35 ± 4 (3)	—
Benzoic	4.2	55 ± 3 (2)	—
Thiopental	7.6	46 ± 3 (2)	34 ± 2 (2)
p-Hydroxypropiophenone	7.8	55 ± 3 (2)	—
Barbital	7.8	4 ± 3 (4)	—
Secobarbital	7.9	30 ± 2 (2)	—
Phenol	9.9	40 ± 5 (3)	40 ± 5 (3)
Base			
Acetanilid	0.3	36 ± 3 (2)	—
Caffeine	0.8	24 ± 3 (2)	—
Antipyrine	1.4	14 ± 3 (4)	—
m-Nitroaniline	2.5	17 ± 0 (2)	—
Aniline	4.6	6 ± 4 (3)	56 ± 3 (2)
Aminopyridine	5.0	2 ± 2 (3)	—
p-Toludine	5.3	0 ± 0 (2)	47 ± 4 (2)
α-Acetylmethadol	8.3	0 ± 0 (4)	—
Quinine	8.4	0 ± 0 (2)	18 ± 2 (2)
Dextrorphan, levorphanol	9.2	0 ± 2 (8)	16 ± 1 (2)
Ephedrine	9.6	3 ± 3 (2)	—
Tolazoline	10.3	7 ± 2 (4)	—
Mecamylamine	11.2	0 ± 0 (2)	—
Darstine	(cation)	0 ± 0 (2)	—
Procaine amide ethobromide	(cation)	0 ± 0 (2)	5 ± 1 (2)
Tetraethylammonium	(cation)	0 ± 1 (2)	—

juice/plasma) are very large, should neverthess have attained only about 40-fold excess over plasma. Direct measurements of arterial and venous blood showed that essentially all the blood flowing through the gastric mucosa was cleared of these drugs; obviously, no more drug could enter the gastric juice in a given time than was brought there by the circulation. Another limitation comes into play when the base pK_a exceeds 7.4; now, a major fraction of the circulating base is cationic and a decreasing fraction is nonionized, so that the effective concentration gradient for diffusion across the stomach wall is reduced.

The ion trapping mechanism provides a method of some forensic value for determining the presence of alkaloids (e.g., narcotics, cocaine, amphetamines) in cases of

TABLE 2-5. Gastric secretion of drugs in the dog.
Measurements were made 30–60 min after initiation of continuous intravenous drug infusion.
(From Shore et al.,[26] Tables 1 and 3.)

	pK_a	Plasma protein binding (%)	Plasma concentration (total) (mg/liter)	Gastric juice concentration (mg/liter)	Gastric / Plasma concentration ratio	Ratio corrected for plasma binding	Theoretical ratio
Bases							
Acetanilid	0.3	0	126	126	1.0	1.0	1.0
Theophylline	0.7	15	81	118	1.5	1.3	1.5
Antipyrine	1.4	0	230	938	4.1	4.2	4.2
Aniline	5.0	25	8.5	358	42		10^4
Aminopyrine	5.0	15	24	1010	42		10^4
Quinine	8.4	75	4.7	189	40		10^6
Levorphanol	9.2	50	0.2	8.3	42		10^6
Tolazoline	10.3	23	13.2	135	10		10^6
Acids							
Salicylic	3.0	75	338	0	0	0	10^{-4}
Probenecid	3.4	75	14	0	0	0	10^{-4}
Phenylbutazone	4.4	90	195	0	0	0	10^{-3}
p-Hydroxypro- piophenone	7.8	75	5.5	0.62	0.11	0.5	0.6
Thiopental	7.6	75	20	2.0	0.10	0.5	0.6
Barbital	7.8	0	254	152	0.6	0.6	0.6

death suspected to be due to overdosage of self-administered drugs. Drug concentrations in gastric contents may be very high even after parenteral injection.

Absorption from the intestine has been studied by perfusing drug solutions slowly through rat intestine in situ and by varying the pH as desired. The principles that emerge from such studies are the same as those for stomach; the difference is that the intestinal pH is normally near neutrality. Some data are presented in Table 2-6. As the pH was increased, the bases were absorbed better, the acids more poorly. Detailed studies with a great many drugs in unbuffered solutions revealed that in the normal intestine, acids with $pK_a > 3.0$ and bases with $pK_a < 7.8$ are very well absorbed; outside these limits the absorption of acids and bases, respectively, fell off rapidly. This behavior leads to the conclusion that the "virtual pH" in the microenvironment of the absorbing surface in the gut is about 5.3; this is somewhat more acidic than is usually considered to be the pH in the intestinal lumen.

Absorption from the buccal cavity has been shown to follow exactly the same principles as described above for stomach and intestine.[28] The pH of saliva is usually about 6. The relationship between pH, pK_a, and lipid/water partition coefficient was studied in human subjects by the following simple procedure. A known amount of a drug, usually 1 mg, in 25 ml of buffer, was placed in a subject's mouth. It was circulated by means of vigorous movements of the tongue and cheeks, and with care not to

TABLE 2-6. In situ intestinal absorption of drugs from solutions of various pH values in the rat.
The percent absorbed is expressed as mean ± range: figures in parentheses indicate number of animals. (From Hogben et al.,[27] Table 1.)

| | | Percent absorbed | | | |
| | | pH of intestinal solution | | | |
	pK_a	3.6–4.3	4.7–5.0	7.2–7.1	8.0–7.8
Bases					
Aniline	4.6	40 ± 7 (9)	48 ± 5 (5)	58 ± 5 (4)	61 ± 8 (10)
Aminopyrine	5.0	21 ± 1 (2)	35 ± 1 (2)	48 ± 2 (2)	52 ± 2 (2)
p-Toluidine	5.3	30 ± 3 (3)	42 ± 3 (2)	65 ± 4 (3)	64 ± 4 (2)
Quinine	8.4	9 ± 3 (3)	11 ± 2 (2)	41 ± 1 (2)	54 ± 5 (4)
Acids					
5-Nitrosalicylic	2.3	40 ± 0 (2)	27 ± 2 (2)	<2 (2)	<2 (2)
Salicylic	3.0	64 ± 4 (4)	35 ± 4 (2)	30 ± 4 (2)	10 ± 3 (6)
Acetylsalicylic	3.5	41 ± 3 (2)	27 ± 1 (2)	—	—
Benzoic	4.2	62 ± 4 (2)	36 ± 3 (4)	35 ± 4 (3)	5 ± 1 (2)
p-Hydroxypro- piophenone	7.8	61 ± 5 (3)	52 ± 2 (2)	67 ± 6 (5)	60 ± 5 (2)

allow any to be swallowed. After 5 min, the whole volume was expectorated into a beaker, the mouth was rinsed several times with water, and the drug concentration was assayed, usually by gas-liquid chromatography. Absorption was taken to be the difference between the amount introduced and the amount remaining. These studies yielded remarkably consistent results for a given subject on different days, with more variability between subjects. The extent of absorption in 5 min varied from drug to drug as shown in Figure 2-6. Bases were absorbed only on the alkaline side of their pK_a, i.e., only in the nonionized form. At normal saliva pH only chlorpheniramine, the weakest base tested, was absorbed to a significant extent. In a series of *n*-alkyl substituted carboxylic acids (Figure 2-6B), the inverse relationship was found; all were absorbed best on the acid side of the pK_a. In addition, absorption increased with the length of the alkyl chain, reflecting the increase in lipid/water partition coefficient. The efficient buccal absorption of the lipid-soluble vasodilator, nitroglycerine, is made use of routinely in the treatment of angina pectoris; a pellet containing the drug is placed under the tongue. However, the rapid absorption of numerous other drugs, as demonstrated here, had not been documented previously. An interesting application of this technique might be to obtain estimates of the passage of various substances through biologic membranes in vivo.

Methods of Modifying Drug Delivery

Enteral Route: Drug Formulations, Bioavailability.   As pointed out earlier, although the enteral route is very convenient, the numerous factors influencing absorption make it rather unpredictable. It is subject to considerable variability from patient

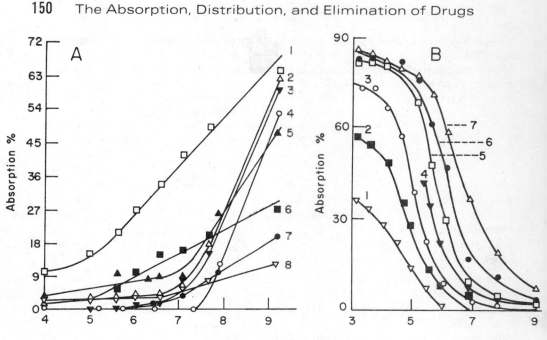

FIGURE 2-6. Buccal absorption of organic acids and bases. *The tests were performed on human subjects, as described in text. (A) Basic drugs: 1, chlorpheniramine; 2, ephedrine; 3, methylephedrine; 4, ethylephedrine; 5, pseudoephedrine; 6, nicotine; 7, norpseudoephedrine; 8, norephedrine. (B) Congeneric series of p-n-alkyl phenylacetic acids: 1, unsubstituted phenylacetic acid; 2, methyl; 3, ethyl; 4, propyl; 5, butyl; 6, pentyl; 7, hexyl. (From Beckett and Hossie, Figures 7 and 13.*[28])

to patient and even in the same patient at different times. Considerable effort has therefore been expended, especially by the pharmaceutical industry, to develop drug formulations with better absorption characteristics.[29] Enteric coatings were introduced long ago, to resist the action of gastric fluids and to disintegrate and dissolve after passage into the intestine. The purpose was to protect a drug that would be degraded in the stomach, to prevent nausea and vomiting caused by local gastric irritation, to achieve a high local concentration of a drug intended to act locally in the intestine, to produce a delayed drug effect, or to deliver a drug to the intestine for optimal absorption there. Enteric coatings are usually fats, fatty acids, waxes, shellac, or cellulose acetate phthalates. The major problem, however, is the great variability in gastric emptying time, especially on different diets; measurements in human subjects show a range from a few minutes to as long as 12 hr for passage of enteric coated tablets through the pylorus.[29a]

More complex, laminated coatings have been introduced—so-called *sustained release* medications.[30] The drug may be applied in soluble form to the outside layer of a tablet containing an insoluble core. More of the same drug is trapped inside the core so that it can dissolve in intestinal fluid that gains access through pores in the matrix. Thus an initial dose is provided in the outer coating, followed by a delayed release from the core. A variation on this theme consists of tiny pellets of drug with different coatings subject to dissolution at different rates, so that the total drug dose is released over a prolonged period.

Several variables have been shown to affect the rate of release of drugs from sustained-release preparations in vitro; for example, the size of the tablet and concentration of drug determine the surface area for solution and the actual rate at which drug will dissolve. The pore size of the inert matrix and its resistance to sloughing, the presence of water-soluble substances in the matrix, and the intrinsic solubility of the drug in an aqueous medium also affect the rate of release.[31] Obviously the rate of movement of the preparation through the gastrointestinal tract can also affect the amount absorbed.[32] If the intestinal contents move too rapidly, a portion of the drug may be wasted in the feces.

Variability in drug absorption from sustained-release preparations may be very great. A well-conducted trial compared a sustained release with a conventional dosage form of ferrous sulfate in 12 patients.[33] To estimate absorption the preparations were labeled with radioactive iron. Each subject had a 2-day trial of each regimen: standard preparation 3 times daily, sustained-release preparation once daily. All the tests were arranged in a random order. Nine patients absorbed much more (1.5–10 times more) of the conventional dosage form than of the sustained-release form. Two patients absorbed more of the sustained-release preparation. One patient absorbed less than 2% of the total dose of either preparation. Most important, the variation between subjects was much greater with the sustained-release preparation than with the conventional form.

A clear danger of sustained-release preparations is that a larger dose than usual is administered at one time, it being assumed that the sustained release will yield a continuous slow rate of absorption. If the actual rate of release should be unexpectedly high, potentially toxic levels may result; if unexpectedly low, therapeutically inadequate levels may result. Either outcome might endanger the patient. Furthermore, sustained-release preparations are invariably more expensive than ordinary dosage forms. So the choice of such preparations ought to be justified by some real need. Certainly the oral ingestion of a drug 3 or 4 times daily presents no hardship to the patient; the substitution of a single daily dose of a sustained-release preparation would not be warranted unless some advantage other than convenience had been demonstrated. Some drugs only need to be administered once daily in their ordinary dosage forms (e.g., reserpine, digitalis glycosides); with these there is no possible justification for sustained-release preparations. Federal regulations[34] require that all sustained-release preparations be regarded as new drugs; thus their safety and efficacy must be demonstrated before they may be introduced into clinical use.

The difficulties associated with reliable administration of drugs by the enteral route have raised important questions about *bioavailability*. Given that two formulations contain the same amount of a certain drug, will both actually yield the same amount at the same rate for absorption into the circulation? Two testing procedures are relevant. First, the rate of disintegration of the tablet or capsule can be measured in vitro in a medium simulating the gastric or intestinal contents. Here considerable variability has been found, attributable to differences in particle size, binders, compression of the tablet, or thickness of the capsule wall. Second, once disintegration has occurred, the rate of dissolution of the drug in the aqueous medium can be determined. Again variability has been observed, presumably related to the particle size and to the presence of substances capable of preventing the efficient wetting of drug particles. Major differences have been noted, not only between products of different manufacturers, but also between lots by the same manufacturer. Clearly, dissolution tests are more relevant than disintegration tests, but even after dissolution, substances capable of complexing with drug molecules may interfere with their efficient passage across the intestinal wall. Thus, the most satisfactory test is to measure blood or plasma levels, i.e., to determine bioavailability directly. This type of test has revealed important differences between preparations of aspirin, chloramphenicol, diphenylhydantoin, oxytetracycline, and other drugs.[35]

Sometimes, of course, large variations are tolerable. But often the consequences of too-slow or too-rapid absorption, or of greater or lesser total absorption, can be serious for the patient. Figure 2-7 illustrates the remarkable differences in serum digoxin levels achieved with four preparations of this cardiac glycoside administered

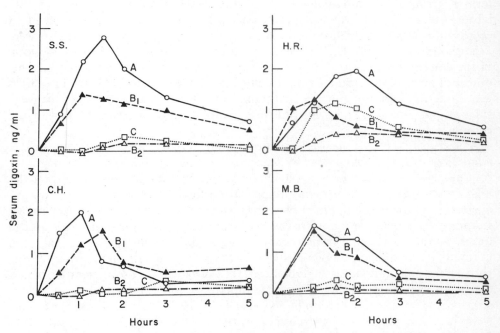

FIGURE 2-7. Differences in absorption of four digoxin products in four subjects. *Products of three manufacturers are designated A, B_1, B_2, and C. The four subjects are identified by initials, S.S., H.R., C.H., and M.B. Order of administration was varied. Interval between administrations to the same subject was 8 days to 4 weeks. All subjects received two 0.25 mg tablets of digoxin by mouth with 100 ml of water after an overnight fast. (From Lindenbaum et al., Figure 3.[36])*

on different occasions to four volunteer subjects.[36] All the preparations were technically in conformance with the standards that regulate drug content, yet preparations B_2 and C were distinctly inferior to A and B_1. It may be argued that the dosage of a cardiac glycoside has to be titrated in the individual patient anyway, and the data presented in the figure certainly show significant subject-to-subject variability. It would seem desirable, however, for all preparations of a given drug to be as good as the best from the standpoint of bioavailability. An important lesson is the potential danger of switching preparations after a patient has been stabilized on any one preparation, in view of the narrow therapeutic margin in this class of drugs.

Another example concerns the anticoagulant, bishydroxycoumarin. A manufacturer of this drug increased the size of the tablet in order to facilitate breaking it into fractional doses. This was accomplished by increasing the amount of inert filler. It was found that inadequate therapeutic effects were then obtained, and the dosage had to be increased. To overcome this difficulty, the company dispersed the drug more finely. The result was excessive anticoagulant activity, and several patients suffered hemorrhagic reactions.[37] As a result of all these findings over the past several years, increasing effort is being devoted to the development of assay procedures for standardizing bioavailability and achieving better quality control over drug formulations for enteral use. It seems unlikely, however, that the basic problem—the intrinsic unreliability of the enteral route—can be solved in this way.

Sustained Release from Parenteral Depots.   Two purposes could be served by improved forms of depot preparation: a long-sustained nearly zero-order absorption into the circulation, simulating a slow constant intravenous infusion; and a prolonged local release for drug action on tissues in the immediate vicinity, avoiding significant systemic effects as the drug is diluted in the general circulation. Experimental approaches have been made to both of these goals.

Silicon rubber ("Silastic polymer") is virtually inert, evoking no tissue reactions. It can be shaped into flexible tubes, cylindrical plugs, or membranous sacs. If the polymerization is carried out in the presence of a drug, the drug can be incorporated into the polymer matrix, from which it later diffuses, as through a molecular sieve.

Arteriovenous shunts of silicon rubber tubing were important in the development of improved renal dialysis units (artificial kidneys) for home use. An interesting application is the production of general anesthesia by diffusion of ether, nitrous oxide, halothane, etc., through a thin-walled external shunt.[38] Conceivably, such a system could provide an anesthetic or analgesic agent on demand, the rate of entry of the drug into blood being regulated by the patient.[39] There are formidable problems, however, as with any exteriorized arteriovenous shunt (leaks, infections, clotting), and even if all these were overcome, the procedure seems unlikely to have much practical application. A similar arrangement has been proposed for continuous or frequent monitoring of blood gases by manometric measurements of gas partial pressures in a glass sleeve surrounding the tubing.[40] Yet another promising application has been the use of silicon rubber arteriovenous shunts for introducing nutrients into patients with grossly defective intestinal function.[41]

A synthetic progesterone (medroxyprogesterone acetate) has been incorporated into silicon rubber rings, which could be placed intravaginally.[42] A slow release and systemic absorption of the hormone was achieved, producing typical effects on basal body temperature and on the endometrium and vaginal epithelium, and effectively preventing conception. Here the hormone actions were systemic, as with contraceptive pills taken by mouth, but the vaginal route was chosen for convenience. The medicated ring could be removed monthly, leading to prompt menstruation, then replaced by a new one.

Another promising approach has been to insert a Silastic tubing loaded with progesterone directly into the uterus. Here slow release of very small quantities led to local contraceptive action without significant systemic absorption, and ovulation was not suppressed.[43] The most dramatic demonstration of this was in rabbits. An empty Silastic tubing was inserted into one uterine horn, a tubing containing progesterone into the other. After insemination, embryos developed only in the horn not exposed to progesterone.[44] A thin Silastic membrane incorporating pilocarpine has been used successfully to treat glaucoma. The membrane is placed in the conjunctival sac, so that slow release of the drug maintains a constant degree of miosis, obviating the need for periodic application of eye drops.[45]

The principle of a diffusion-limited slow rate of drug release from a Silastic capsule should be applicable to the administration of numerous drugs at a subcutaneous implantation site, whenever very prolonged action is required.[46] If the physical properties of the polymer membrane can be standardized to yield zero-order release over periods of weeks or months, this technique may have very wide applicability. Its advantages could include not only a more constant rate of drug delivery as compared with the enteral route, but also the bypassing of human volition (and attendant errors of omission) in drug administration. In short, much of the nuisance of pill-taking or self-injection (as in diabetics) could be eliminated. The method might also have value in providing long-term protection against the effects of narcotics by continuous delivery of a narcotic antagonist (see p. 607).

New Techniques for the Intravascular Route.   As indicated by the developments recounted above, there has been increasing recognition that the time-honored methods of administering drugs are generally clumsy and inefficient, falling far short of the ideal.[47] It may be argued, of course, that no great improvement is needed over the oral ingestion of 0.5 g of aspirin to relieve a headache or the intramuscular injection of a single dose of benzathine penicillin G to cure primary syphilis. In numerous instances, however, the appropriate aim is to establish and maintain a constant plasma drug level, sufficient for the therapeutic need, yet below the toxic concentration. The narrower the margin of safety, the more rigorous is the requirement. As pointed out already, the safest and most reliable route for this purpose is the constant intravenous infusion. It is probably within reach of modern technology, especially in view of the extraordinary miniaturization of components developed in the course of space research, to assemble a small, battery-operated, infusion system. With incorporation of a sensor element, such a mechanism could possibly maintain a constant drug level by feedback regulation of the infusion rate, or even adjust drug delivery to the physiologic state of the patient. A system that adjusted an insulin infusion to the blood sugar level could mimic the homeostatic mechanisms controlling secretion of that hormone from the normal pancreas. Corticosteroid secretion in the normal person undergoes marked diurnal variation; possibly hormone replacement therapy should ideally simulate these normal fluctuations. Vigorous research and development along the lines outlined here may be expected in the coming years.

DRUG DISTRIBUTION

Apparent Volume of Distribution

The body water may be regarded as partitioned into several compartments that are functionally distinct. These are the vascular fluid, the extracellular (interstitial) fluid, and the intracellular fluid. In a normal lean 70 kg man, the whole body water comprises about 58% of the body weight, or about 41 liters. The extracellular water is about one-third of the total, around 17% of the body weight, or approximately 12 liters. Included in this is the volume of circulating plasma water, about 4% of body weight, or 3 liters. The whole blood volume, including the intracellular water of the erythrocytes, is about twice the plasma volume, or about 6 liters. These data were summarized in Figure 2-1. The volumes of the various compartments differ slightly between adult males and females. In obese people a larger fraction of the body weight is fat, so the fluid compartments all represent smaller percentages of the body weight. In infants the body water is a higher percentage of the body weight (as much as 77%), in part because the bony tissues are incompletely calcified and hence contribute less to body weight than in the adult.

The *apparent volume of distribution* (V_d) of a drug is the fluid volume in which it seems to be dissolved. The determination of V_d is simple in principle.[48] A known amount of a drug is injected intravascularly, and after sufficient time for it to distribute, a sample of blood is taken and the drug's concentration in plasma water is determined. Suppose the drug were distributed ideally, without any metabolic degradation, without being eliminated from the body, and without any binding or sequestration. The situation would then be analogous to finding the volume of fluid in a flask by adding a known amount of dye, mixing, and then determining the resulting concentration.

Let x be the amount of dye added, and c the resulting concentration; then $c = x/V_d$, or $V_d = x/c$.

A high molecular weight dye, Evans Blue, is almost wholly confined to the circulating plasma, and therefore can be used in just this way to determine the total plasma volume (and the blood volume, if the hematocrit is also known). Several minutes are needed for complete mixing of the dye with the circulating plasma. During this time the plasma concentration falls to a plateau, which then remains unchanged, whence V_d is found. A significant fraction of the circulating blood is in tissues where the blood flow is slow. The initial very fast mixing (about 1 min) distributes the dye into the volume of blood that perfuses kidney, brain, liver, lungs, and the active musculature. Over the next several minutes this solution will be diluted by the entry of dye-free blood from the more slowly perfused tissues (fat depots, skin, etc.). If 100 µg of Evans Blue were injected, the plateau concentration would be about 33 ug/liter, and $V_d = 100/33 = 3$ liters.

Many different substances distribute approximately into the extracellular fluid volume. Chloride and sodium ions, for example, are primarily extracellular, but a small fraction is always found within cell water; consequently V_d's determined with isotopes of these ions (^{24}Na is often used) tend to be a little higher than the true volume of extracellular space. Stable or radioactive bromide salts, thiocyanate, radioactive iodide, sucrose, and inulin have been used to estimate the extracellular fluid, and each V_d differs slightly from another. Actually, the ratio of extracellular fluid volume to tissue water differs from tissue to tissue, and so does the capillary permeability, so the differences in V_d probably reflect real differences in distribution. In general, with these substances, the initial very rapid fall of the plasma level due to intravascular mixing blends into a further decline, reflecting distribution into the interstitial fluid. Thus a lower plateau is reached than with Evans Blue. If 100 mg of bromide ion were injected (as NaBr), the ultimate plateau reached before significant excretion could occur would be about 8 mg/liter, whence $V_d = 100/8 = 12$ liters, the approximate volume of the extracellular fluid.

Finally, the volume of the total body water may be estimated by tracer water (D_2O or ^3H_2O) or some substances with high lipid/water partition coefficient, since these

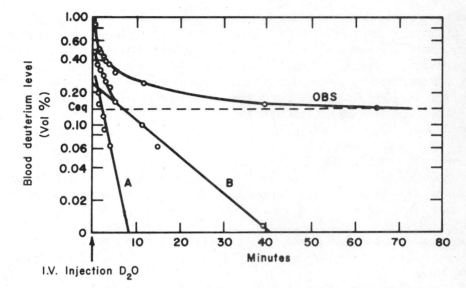

FIGURE 2-8. Distribution of deuterium oxide into total body water. D_2O, *80 ml, was given intravenously to a human subject weighing 82 kg. Samples were taken from the femoral artery. Note logarithmic scale of ordinates. Upper curve (OBS): raw observations; lower curves (A and B): analysis into kinetic components, as described in the text. C_{eq} denotes the equilibrium concentration eventually attained. (Adapted from Schloerb et al., Figure 8.[49])*

cross cell membranes readily (p. 172). Here, an hour or more may be required for all the body tissues to come to equilibrium, and various fractions of the body water may be observed to equilibrate at different rates. In Figure 2-8 an experiment with heavy water is shown. Here, 80 ml of D_2O was injected intravenously and samples of blood from the femoral artery were analyzed for their deuterium content by means of a falling-drop density determination. The standard deviation of this determination is small, about 4 parts per 1000; the final estimates of body water are accurate to ± 0.2 liters. The upper curve represents the raw data, D_2O concentration (on a logarithmic scale) plotted against time. Equilibrium was attained in about an hour, at a plateau level of about 0.16 vol%, or 1.6 g/liter; thus $V_d = 80/1.6 = 50$ liters, representing 61% of the body weight in this subject who weighed 82 kg.

In this experiment the arterial concentration curve could be analyzed into two log-linear kinetic components. The procedure is as follows: the net rate of movement of D_2O out of the blood stream should be proportional to the difference, at any moment, between the arterial concentration and the eventual concentration to be attained at equilibrium. The first step was, therefore, to subtract the equilibrium concentration (C_{eq}) from each point. This yielded the middle curve B. This curve seems to be composed of at least two processes going on at different rates. The final part is log linear, so it was assumed that whatever process it represented had gone on from the start. An extrapolation was therefore made back to time zero. Now the extrapolated part of curve B was subtracted from the actual early points on curve B, yielding another straight line (A) with a much steeper slope. In other words, the observed course of decline of the arterial plasma level could be accounted for by two simultaneous exponential decay curves with different time constants.

Despite the alluring simplicity of analyses like the above, they can be very mis-leading.[49a] The processes going on at such different rates, for example, could have nothing to do with fluid compartments but might represent the equilibration of two groups of tissues with very different vascularity. Frequently the volume of distribution of a drug is determined experimentally and (as in this example) is found to correspond reasonably well with the actual volume of some fluid compartment. Thus, any drug with V_d approximately 12 liters might be supposed to enter extracellular fluid but not to penetrate cells. Two factors may operate frequently to invalidate such direct and simple interpretations. On the one hand, if (as is commonly done) the total plasma drug concentration is determined rather than that in plasma water, then a high degree of protein binding will make the observed concentration unduly high, and the estimate of V_d will therefore be falsely low. If a substantial fraction of the drug is bound to plasma proteins in the concentration range studied, this error can be very large. For example, in the hypothetical case just proposed, where $V_d = 12$ liters, if the original dose were 100 mg, then the observed plasma concentration was about 8.0 μg/ml. If the drug is 70% bound at this total concentration, then the true equilibrium concentration in plasma water is only 2.4 μg/ml and the true volume of distribution is 42 liters, a volume greatly in excess of the extracellular fluid and close to that of the total body water. On the other hand, binding or sequestration of drug at an extra-vascular site can withdraw so much from the circulation that V_d will appear to be very large. A drug that is stored in fat depots (e.g., cyclopropane, thiopental) may have an apparent volume of distribution very much greater than the entire fluid volume of the body.

A practical problem in estimating V_d is the fact that drugs do not often display ideal behavior. They are metabolized, excreted, or sequestered, so that no real distribution plateau is ever attained. The plasma concentration falls rapidly at first, more slowly later, and then the concentration continues to fall. What is needed is an estimate of what the plasma concentration would have been in the absence of the

TABLE 2-7. Distribution of antipyrine in dog tissues.
Antipyrine (1.5 g) was given intravenously; tissues were obtained for analysis 1.5 hr later. The dog weighed 13 kg. (From Brodie and Axel-rod.[51] Table 2.)

Tissue	Antipyrine in tissue water (μg/ml)	$\dfrac{\text{Tissue water antipyrine}}{\text{Plasma water antipyrine}}$
Plasma	148	1.0
Whole blood	147	1.0
CSF	122	0.82
Brain	141	0.95
Muscle	145	0.98
Heart	145	0.98
Lung	135	0.91
Kidney	154	1.04
Liver	145	0.98
Spleen	149	1.00

process responsible for the continuous decline. This estimate is obtained by extrapolating the eventual stable rate of decline back to the time of injection. Naturally, this has to be done on a semilogarithmic plot, it being assumed that the various phases of drug disappearance from plasma are all first order. An illustration is presented in Figure 2-9. Antipyrine (1 g) was injected intravenously in four human subjects. Inasmuch as the investigators were not interested in the kinetics of approach to equilibrium but only in estimating V_d, the first venous blood samples were drawn after an hour had elapsed. The rates of plasma level decline were nearly identical in the four subjects, corresponding to the rate of metabolism of antipyrine. The extrapolated values, 28–41 μg/ml, yielded values for V_d from 25–36 liters. These volumes are rather low for total body water, but direct determinations of antipyrine in dog tissues after 1.5 hr (Table 2-7) showed that the drug does equilibrate (or nearly so) with cell water. In the subjects represented in Figure 2-9, D_2O gave slightly higher values of V_d.

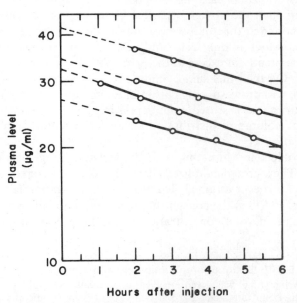

FIGURE 2-9. *Distribution of antipyrine into total body water. Antipyrine (1 g) was injected intravenously in 4 human subjects. Plasma levels are shown. The rapid fall of plasma level during the first hour (phase of distribution) was not measured. The slopes represent metabolism and excretion. (From Soberman et al., Figure 1.*[50])

The D_2O estimates are usually somewhat too high because water in the gastrointestinal tract (usually not considered part of the body water) equilibrates with the heavy water; and more important, because deuterium exchanges with hydrogen in many compounds in the body tissues, so that part of the deuterium removed from the plasma is no longer in the form of water at all. The antipyrine estimates, on the other hand, are usually low because an appreciable fraction of the plasma antipyrine is bound to plasma protein; how this affects the estimate of V_d was explained earlier.

The Binding of Drugs to Plasma Proteins

The interactions between drugs and proteins were discussed in Chapter 1 from the standpoint of the molecular mechanisms responsible. Here we shall consider how

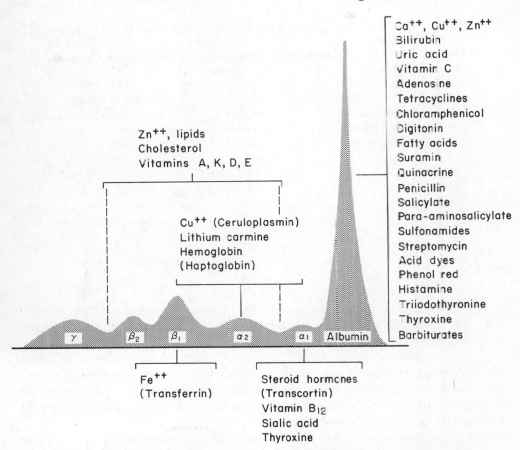

Zn^{++}, lipids
Cholesterol
Vitamins A, K, D, E

Cu^{++} (Ceruloplasmin)
Lithium carmine
Hemoglobin
(Haptoglobin)

Ca^{++}, Cu^{++}, Zn^{++}
Bilirubin
Uric acid
Vitamin C
Adenosine
Tetracyclines
Chloramphenicol
Digitonin
Fatty acids
Suramin
Quinacrine
Penicillin
Salicylate
Para-aminosalicylate
Sulfonamides
Streptomycin
Acid dyes
Phenol red
Histamine
Triiodothyronine
Thyroxine
Barbiturates

γ   β$_2$ β$_1$ α$_2$ α$_1$ Albumin

Fe^{++}
(Transferrin)

Steroid hormones
(Transcortin)
Vitamin B$_{12}$
Sialic acid
Thyroxine

FIGURE 2-10. Interactions with plasma proteins. *Plasma proteins are depicted according to their relative amounts (y axis) and electrophoretic mobilities (x axis). Some representative interactions are listed. (Adapted from Putnam, Figure 6.[52])*

interactions with plasma proteins influence the distribution of drugs in the body and their access to sites of action, of metabolism, and of excretion.

Several kinds of plasma protein interact with small molecules (Figure 2-10). The metal-binding globulins transferrin and ceruloplasmin interact strongly and specifically with iron and copper, respectively, and are essential to the transport of these ions in the body. The α- and β-lipoproteins account in large measure for the binding of lipid-soluble molecules, including those of physiologic importance, such as vitamin A and other carotenoids, vitamin D, cholesterol, and the steroid hormones. The antibody γ-globulins interact very specifically with antigens but negligibly with most drugs.

By far the most important contribution to drug binding is made by albumin, the principal protein of plasma (50% of the total). It has been crystallized and well characterized; and because it reacts with a wide variety of drugs, it is used frequently in model investigations of drug binding. Its molecular weight is about 69,000 and at its isoelectric point (pH 5) it carries about 100 each of negative and positive charges (Table 2-8). At plasma pH (7.4) it has a net negative charge, but nevertheless it can interact with anions as well as with cations. Every positively or negatively charged

TABLE 2-8. Potential binding sites for charged molecules or ions in bovine serum albumin.
(Analytical data from Tanford et al.[53] By permission of the American Chemical Society.)

Amino acid	Group	Number of residues per molecule
Aspartic and glutamic	$-COO^-$	101
Tyrosine	$-O^-$	18
Cysteine	$-S^-$	0.7
Terminal	$-COO^-$	1
Histidine	$-NH^+-$	17
Lysine	$-NH_3^+$	57
Arginine	$=NH_2^+$	22
Terminal	$-NH_3^+$	1

group could be considered a binding site for the predominant counterion species; thus, Na^+ interacts at the anionic groups, Cl^- at the cationic groups. Such single, unreinforced ionic bonds are weak. The number of binding sites for drug molecules per albumin molecule is usually much smaller than the total number of charged groups (sometimes only one or two), the affinity at these few sites is very much greater than that for the common counterions, and the binding depends strongly upon the molecular structure of the drug. Some of the methodologic aspects of studies on binding specificity were discussed elsewhere (p. 47).

The reversible binding of drugs by proteins often requires that the native configuration of the protein be intact. This has important practical consequences for the assay of bound and free drug. Most routine procedures for determination of drug concentrations in plasma or other body fluids begin with a deproteinization step. This step is invariably a precipitation (e.g., with phosphotungstic or trichloroacetic acid), followed by removal of protein by filtration or centrifugation. In such procedures the analytical data will represent *total* drug concentrations because the protein-bound drug is released into the supernatant solution or filtrate. Most bioassay procedures, on the other hand, will be sensitive only to *free* (unbound) drug if whole plasma is used for the assay. Dilution of the plasma, however, favors dissociation because it reduces the concentration of free drug in equilibrium with the protein-bound moiety; therefore, the degree of binding will usually be underestimated if a dilution step precedes the assay. At infinite dilution all reversible complexes would be completely dissociated.

If a drug is able to combine with a certain number of sites, n, on each protein molecule, and if all these sites have the same affinity for the drug, and if there are no cooperative effects on affinity (i.e., the binding of a drug molecule to one site does not influence the affinity for the next site), then simple mass-law expressions describe the relationship between binding and the concentration of free drug at equilibrium. The total number of binding sites is nP, where P is the total protein concentration; so, as in the expression for receptor binding (p. 33), we have

$$\frac{(PX)}{nP} = \frac{(X)}{K + (X)}$$

where (X) is the concentration of free drug, (PX) is the concentration of drug-protein complex, and K is the dissociation constant. Let r be the ratio $(PX)/P$, i.e., the moles of drug bound per mole of protein. Then

$$r = \frac{n(X)}{K + (X)}$$

and a plot of r against (X) (Figure 2-11a) yields a typical hyperbolic curve, identical to an adsorption isotherm. The same equation, in the familiar form of a log dose-response curve, is plotted in Figure 2-11b. The saturation of available sites (in this example, when $r = 10$) is evident.

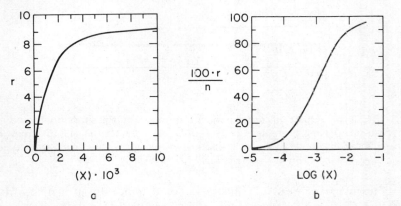

FIGURE 2-11. Relationship between drug concentration (X) and moles bound per mole of protein (r), for a drug interacting with plasma albumin.

The problem that concerns us in this chapter is not how many drug molecules can be bound to a molecule of plasma protein, but rather what *fraction* of the total drug molecules in the plasma is bound. We should like to know how the bound fraction β varies with drug concentration, protein concentration, maximum number of binding sites, and affinity constant. By definition,

$$\beta = \frac{(PX)}{(PX) + (X)} = \frac{1}{1 + (X)/(PX)}$$

But from the previous equation

$$\frac{(X)}{(PX)} = \frac{K + (X)}{nP}$$

so that

$$\beta = \frac{1}{1 + K/nP + (X)/nP}$$

This equation tells us that for a given protein concentration, and a given number of binding sites per protein molecule, if the binding affinity is very high (K very low) and the drug concentration is very low, practically all the drug present will be bound (β approaches unity). As common sense suggests, if the total number of binding sites is reduced, a greater fraction of total drug tends to become free. An exact quantitative

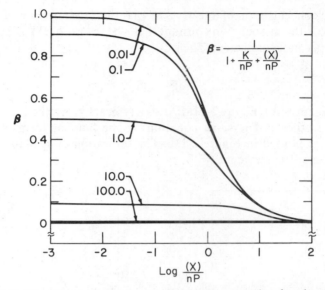

FIGURE 2-12. Effect of drug concentration upon the fractional binding of a drug to plasma proteins. *Axis of ordinates: fraction bound (β); axis of abscissas: relative scale of log concentration for a fixed protein concentration. See text for explanation. (From Goldstein, Figure 7.*[54])

analysis, shown in Figure 2-12, illustrates some important principles. Here, the horizontal scale is $\log (X)/nP$, and the individual curves are for chosen values of K/nP.

In plasma, P is fixed, and both n and K are determined by the particular drug whose distribution is under consideration; thus, nP is invariant and the whole expression K/nP is invariant. The horizontal scale becomes a measure of the logarithm of the free drug concentration. For a given drug, one particular curve (for one value of K/nP) will be relevant. We see that all drugs at high enough concentration saturate the binding sites. At still higher concentration the additional drug is all free, so that the fraction bound decreases toward zero. At high concentrations the maximum amount of drug is bound to the plasma proteins, but this maximum amount represents only a small fraction of total drug. As the drug concentration is progesssively reduced (e.g., by elimination mechanisms in the body) the fraction bound tends to increase; but the extent of the increase may be negligibly small, for some drugs have too low an affinity to be bound significantly even at very low concentrations. In those cases where the fraction bound does increase at low drug concentration, a maximum fraction bound is always approached. If the affinity is high enough or the concentration of binding sites is high enough, or both, then this maximum fractional binding may approach unity, i.e., practically all the drug is bound. But it need not do so, and many drugs are only partially bound even under the most favorable conditions.

It follows that reports about the fractional binding of drugs in plasma (usually expressed as "percent of drug bound to plasma protein") are not useful unless qualified by a statement of the free drug concentration at the equilibrium actually measured. Interactions should be measured at therapeutic drug concentrations if conclusions relating to these concentrations are to be drawn; investigations carried out at higher concentrations may provide greater convenience or accuracy in the assay procedures, but the degree of fractional binding may be underestimated seriously.

The effects of protein binding upon drug distribution can be deduced readily from the same principles.[55,56] At equilibrium the concentration in the extravascular water will be the same as the unbound concentration in plasma water, i.e., usually lower than the total plasma level. The difference in total drug concentration between plasma and cerebrospinal fluid in patients led to the initial observation of reversible drug-protein interaction.[57] Several sulfonamide drugs were found to reach levels in cerebrospinal fluid that were always below that in plasma, sometimes as low as one-quarter the plasma concentration. Yet the sulfonamides were very effective in bacterial meningitis, so the low concentrations were obviously adequate. It was found that the concentrations in cerebrospinal fluid were the same as in plasma water; these, indeed, were the true bacteriostatic concentrations.

Only free drug is available for glomerular filtration; therefore the persistence of a drug that is excreted in this way can be influenced by the fractional binding. Moreover, the rate of disappearance from the body tends to be self-limiting, at least through the range in which fractional binding increases with falling drug concentration; the lower the concentration, the smaller the fraction subject to filtration at the glomeruli.

On the other hand, active processes like secretion at the renal tubules, or carrier-mediated transport across other cell membranes, are not restricted to free drug. The reversibility of the drug-protein interaction is so rapid that free drug molecules withdrawn from the water phase by one of these active processes are replaced instantly by more free drug derived by dissociation of the bound complex. Penicillin and p-aminohippuric acid (PAH) are examples; even at concentrations where they are bound as much as 90% to plasma protein they are cleared almost completely from the blood by renal secretory mechanisms during a single passage through the kidney.

The rate of transfer of drug molecules from the blood stream into the tissues, by diffusion across capillary membranes, depends upon the concentration gradient of free drug. Thus, protein binding can slow the disappearance of drug from the circulation and also provide a reservoir of bound drug, which will replenish (by dissociation) some of the drug that is lost by metabolism and excretion. A striking example is suramin, a polycyclic sulfonated compound used in the prophylaxis of trypanosomiasis. Some of this drug is bound very tightly to plasma protein,[58] and it is apparently not metabolized in the body. Effective plasma levels persist for weeks after a single intravenous injection. Another example of retention by the plasma proteins is the dye Evans Blue, mentioned earlier. It is useful in estimating the plasma volume only because the high fractional binding to plasma proteins minimizes the escape of dye at the capillaries.

A most remarkable example of tight binding to plasma albumin is presented by an iodinated contrast medium, 3-hydroxy-2,4,6-triiodo-α-ethylhydrocinnamic acid (Figure 2-13). The compound was used some years ago for the purpose of visualizing the gallbladder with x rays. The determination of serum protein-bound iodine (PBI)

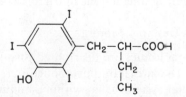

FIGURE 2-13. 3-Hydroxy-2,4,6-triiodo-α-ethylhydrocinnamic acid.

is a valuable procedure in the assessment of thyroid function. When the PBI procedure was attempted in patients who had received the iodinated contrast medium, absurdly high PBI values were obtained. This led to the discovery that a metabolic derivative of the iodinated contrast medium was retained in the plasma for years; determinations in patients at various intervals after they received the drug yielded an estimate of about 1 year for the half-life of the complex with plasma albumin (Figure 2-14).

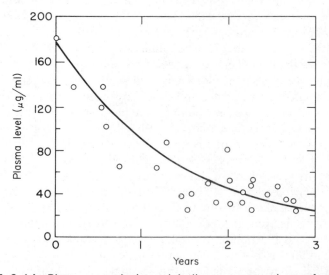

FIGURE 2-14. Plasma protein-bound iodine concentrations after administration of an iodinated contrast medium (3-hydroxy-2,4,6-triiodo-α-ethylhydrocinnamic acid). *Data are shown for 15 patients who presumably received the same standard dose. Iodine levels are shown as functions of time after administration of the contrast medium. (From Astwood, Figure 5.[58a])*

Differences in the drug-binding capacity of plasma proteins are found between species. Such differences have also been noted occasionally among people (e.g., in the extent of digitoxin binding) and in a few instances a genetic basis has been demonstrated (cf. Chapter 6). People vary greatly in the dosage of many drugs that is required to produce a therapeutic action. Possibly a part of this variability might be accounted for by differences in protein binding.

Competition between two drugs for the same binding sites on plasma proteins may lead to large increases in the free concentration of one of them in the plasma water, thus enhancing its therapeutic effect, producing unexpected toxicity, or increasing its rate of metabolism or excretion. On the other hand, one drug may enhance the affinity of plasma albumin for another drug. These phenomena will be considered at length in the discussion of drug interactions in Chapter 14.

Passage of Drugs across Biologic Membranes

Blood Capillaries. Drug molecules are distributed throughout the body by means of the circulation of blood. The cardiac output (about 6 liters min^{-1}) is equivalent to the whole volume of the vascular system. Thus, within a minute or so after a drug enters the blood stream it is largely diluted into the total blood volume as a result of turbulent mixing and of unequal flow rates through the various vascular beds. This initial phase of dilution is best observed with a drug that passes only slowly, or not at all, out of the blood stream. With such a drug the volume of distribution in the first few minutes should approach 6 liters if the drug permeates erythrocytes freely, or about 3 liters (the approximate plasma volume) otherwise. If a drug can leave the capillaries readily, its concentration may fall so fast that the initial phase of dilution is obscured, and a much larger volume of distribution is then approached (p. 154).

The rate of entry of a drug into the various tissues of the body obviously depends upon the relative rates of blood flow through the respective capillary beds and the permeability of the capillaries for the particular drug molecules. Blood flow varies within wide limits, from the brain, for example, which is richly supplied, to cartilage, tendons, and joints, which are much more poorly vascularized. Blood flowing through the kidneys is ultrafiltered at the capillaries of the renal glomeruli, and most of the ultrafiltrate is reabsorbed by the renal tubules. Drug molecules, to the extent to which they are free in the plasma, and filterable, will also appear in the glomerular filtrate, whence they may be reabsorbed or excreted in the urine. A small fraction of the cardiac output gives rise, at the choroid plexus of the brain, to cerebrospinal fluid; and this protein-free solution, circulating over the tissues of the central nervous system, may contain some of the drug. The aqueous humor too may contain filterable drug derived from the blood. The bile may serve as a route for passage of drug out of the circulation into the intestinal tract, and drug molecules also pass directly from the blood across the gastrointestinal mucosa. At all the capillaries some ultrafiltration occurs, driven by high hydrostatic pressure at the arterial end; and there is some reabsorption of interstitial fluid at the venous end, driven primarily by the colloid osmotic pressure of plasma. Depending upon their molecular size and other properties, drug molecules may move with this bulk flow of solvent. Some of the drug in the interstitial fluid will remain in lymph and return to the circulation by way of the lymphatic channels. Since drug molecules that pass out of the circulation have first to traverse the capillary walls, we shall consider what is known about capillary permeability.

The functional anatomy of capillaries has been studied by direct microscopic observation of living tissue; quantitative data about permeability have been obtained chiefly by perfusion of isolated regions such as the cat hindlimb.[59-61] Blood was perfused through the femoral artery, and the rate of disappearance of various solutes was studied. One method was to measure the "osmotic transient," i.e., the change in osmotic pressure as the solute passed into the interstitial fluid. This was accomplished by suspending the limb in a delicate balance and opposing the osmotic movement of fluid by adjustments of the hydrostatic venous and arterial pressures so as to maintain isogravimetric (constant weight) conditions. This procedure sufficed to measure a wide range of transfer rates with half-times from a few minutes to more than an hour. Another method was to measure directly the arteriovenous concentration difference; this method would be useful for transfer rates not much slower than the flow rates employed.

Lipid-soluble molecules like urethane, paraldehyde, or triacetin left the blood almost instantaneously in its passage through the tissue, and so did gases of physiologic or pharmacologic interest (oxygen, carbon dioxide, nitrogen, and the anesthetic gases). For all the substances in this class, the most important determinant of the rate of transcapillary movement was the lipid/water partition coefficient. The *partition coefficient* is the ratio of concentration in lipid phase to concentration in aqueous phase when a substance is allowed to come to equilibrium in a two-phase system. The conditions of measurement (e.g., temperature, pH) must be specified. Glycerol derivatives, for example, passed through capillary walls at rates that varied with their lipid/water partition coefficients, but in the opposite order to what would be expected from their aqueous diffusion coefficients. In the glycerol series increasing molecular size is achieved by increasing the length of hydrophobic substituents, so that partition coefficients and aqueous diffusion coefficients tend to vary inversely. The rapid rates of movement of all lipid-soluble compounds indicated that practically the entire capillary endothelial surface must be available for their diffusion.

For water-soluble molecules of various sizes, the results were quite different, as indicated in Table 2-9. Here, the smaller the molecule the more rapidly did it pass out

TABLE 2-9. Permeability of muscle capillaries to water-soluble molecules.
Data for radius of equivalent sphere are calculated from viscosity or diffusion measurements, taking into account the degree of hydration. The diffusion coefficient across the capillary is the rate of movement for unit molar concentration difference as given by the Fick equation. $dM/dt = (C_1 - C_2)P$. (Data from Pappenheimer[59] and Renkin.[60])

			Diffusion coefficient	
	Molecular weight	Radius of equivalent sphere (A)	In water, D (cm^2/sec) $\times$ 10^5	Across capillary, P (cm^3/sec · 100 g)
Water	18		3.20	3.7
Urea	60	1.6	1.95	1.83
Glucose	180	3.6	0.91	0.64
Sucrose	342	4.4	0.74	0.35
Raffinose	594	5.6	0.56	0.24
Inulin	5,500	15.2	0.21	0.036
Myoglobin	17,000	19	0.15	0.005
Hemoglobin	68,000	31	0.094	0.001
Serum albumin	69,000		0.085	<0.001

of the capillary. Even the smallest molecules (including water itself) behaved as though only a very small fraction of the capillary wall (about 0.2%) was available for their filtration or diffusion. Moreover, the impediments to free diffusion (i.e., discrepancies between theoretical diffusion coefficients and transcapillary diffusion coefficients) were greater as molecular size increased. It appeared that a system of pores about 30 A in radius must be present to account for the restricted diffusion as molecular radii approached 30 A (corresponding to a molecular weight of approximately 60,000), and for the sharp cutoff above this.

Improved quality and special staining techniques have revealed electron microscopic evidence consistent with these conclusions.[62] The capillary membrane is composed of an interlocking mosaic of endothelial cells with slits (junctions) between them that could function as the postulated pores. Water-soluble compounds introduced into the capillary lumen can be observed to extravasate through these slits.[62a] In addition, a system of vesicles continuous with the inner and outer surfaces of the capillary membrane may transport larger molecules at slow rates by a process of pinocytosis, as described below.

The relatively small water-soluble molecules traverse the capillary membrane largely by diffusion in aqueous medium; their rates of movement are nearly independent of the perfusion pressure but are directly proportional to the concentration gradient across the capillary. Molecules the size of proteins penetrate only very slowly, and their rate of movement is strongly dependent upon the pressure difference between the arterial and venous ends of the capillary. Since the actual passage of large molecules across the capillary is so slow, the methods described above cannot be employed. Instead, studies were carried out by labeling proteins or polysaccharides in the perfusion inflow, then analyzing the lymph drainage from the perfused limb. Contrary to earlier concepts that considered interstitial fluid as an ultrafiltrate of blood, the protein content of lymph was found to be nearly one-half that of blood plasma. This lymph protein undoubtedly originated in the blood and crossed the capillary wall. There is still doubt about the precise mechanism whereby macromolecules traverse the capillary endothelium, albeit very slowly. Pinocytosis (the engulfing of fluid by cell processes) has been suggested as a possible mechanism, and computations based upon microscopic study of the formation and movement of pinocytotic vesicles indicate that the known rates of transcapillary passage of macromolecules could be accounted for by this mechanism.

It follows from all the above that the rate at which a drug leaves the blood stream will depend upon its lipid solubility, its molecular weight, and its physical state of aggregation. If it is bound to macromolecules, then its rate of transcapillary passage will be determined by that of the protein or other substance to which it is bound. Capillaries differ widely in their permeability characteristics; those of the glomeruli, for example, are very much more permeable to molecules of all sizes than are those of the muscles (hindlimb). The sinusoidal capillaries of the liver appear to lack any endothelial wall and therefore permit the passage of large molecules quite readily. Thus, capillaries in the various organ systems display wide variation in their permeability to drugs. Nevertheless, all the capillaries except those of the brain permit drugs to pass with relative ease compared with cell membranes, and thus all drugs of small or intermediate molecular size that are free in the circulation gain access readily to the interstitial fluid. In brain, on the other hand, a special histologic feature (investment of the capillaries by a cellular sheath, p. 186) drastically reduces the permeability to water-soluble molecules of all sizes.

The capillaries are not rigid tubes with invariant properties. They too are subject to the actions of drugs as well as to effects of tissue metabolites and hormones. Capillary permeability can be enhanced by such agents as histamine and estrogens, and by decreased tissue pH associated with lactic acid production. Humoral agents like norepinephrine affect the passage of substances across capillaries by constricting arterioles, thus reducing capillary blood flow and hydrostatic pressure in the capillary lumen.

Cell Membranes

Membrane structure.[63-73]   Cell membranes are of importance to pharmacology for two principal reasons. First, many drugs owe their pharmacologic effects to a primary action at the outer membrane surface. Second, drugs that act inside cells must obviously pass through the cell membrane first. An adequate picture of cell membrane structure must therefore account not only for the known bioelectric properties and biochemical functions, but must also include surface receptors and mechanisms for the passage of drugs to the cell interior. For secretory cells and neurones the movement of substances out of the cell must also be explained.

It has long been recognized that cell membranes contain a bimolecular layer of phospholipid molecules, oriented perpendicular to the plane of the membrane, with polar head groups aligned at both surfaces, and long hydrocarbon chains extending inward. Electron micrographs confirm this general picture, showing a usual thickness of about 100 A. Physical measurements, especially by free-radical probes (cf. p. 114), have established the existence of a fluidity gradient. The outer and inner surfaces have a fairly rigid structure, with restricted molecular motion, as would be expected from the interaction of tightly packed polar groups. The interior of the membrane, in contrast, is quite fluid, with a high degree of molecular motion of loosely ordered hydrophobic chains.

At one time it was thought that sheets of unfolded protein covered the inner and outer membrane surfaces, and that an additional layer of globular proteins (e.g.,

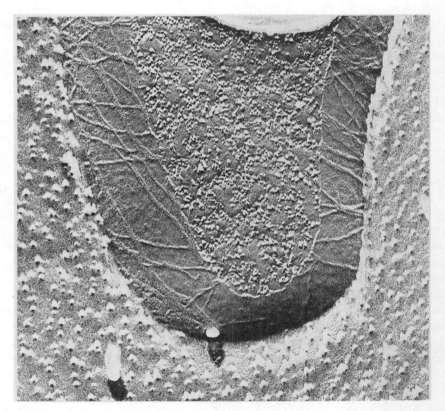

FIGURE 2-15. External surface and cleaved interior of a human red cell membrane. *Platinum-carbon replica of freeze-cleaved membrane covered with fibrous actin. The actin strands are sharply cut off at the junction of the smooth outer face and particle-covered interior. See text. (From Tillack and Marchesi, Figure 4.[74])*

enzymes) was localized at the inner surface. Recent advances in electron microscopy and analytic data on membrane proteins have led to a different concept, the *fluid mosaic* model. Erythrocytes were exposed to fibrous actin, a molecule that adheres to the outer membrane surface and is readily identified in electron micrographs. Hemolysis yielded membranes, which were then frozen and fractured by a technique that splits them along a cleavage plane within the fluid interior. The water was sublimated away, and the preparations were then shadowed with platinum-carbon, and photographed in the electron microscope. Figure 2-15 shows the outer membrane surface clearly marked with actin fibers. The surface itself is smooth. The inner plane revealed by the freeze-fracture is quite different in appearance, and not at all consistent with the simple lipid bilayer model. A random array of globular units, about 85 A in diameter, is seen protruding. These are evidently proteins, not lined up along the outer and inner surfaces, but embedded in the substance of the membrane, as shown diagrammatically in Figure 2-16.

Investigations into the nature of such proteins have yielded results of extraordinary interest. Antigenic determinants on the exterior of the red cell membrane have been known to be glycoprotein in nature. Amino acid sequence analysis of one class of protein extracted from the erythrocyte membrane revealed many carbohydrate residues along the N terminal portion—evidently at the external membrane surface. There follows a segment of 34 amino acids, all nonpolar lipophilic residues, presumably occupying the membrane interior. Finally, the C terminal portion contains

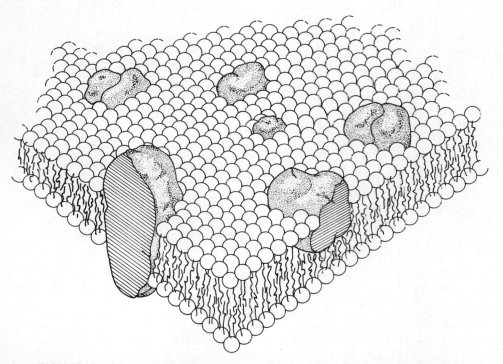

FIGURE 2-16. Lipid-globular protein mosaic model of the cell membrane. *The circles represent ionic and polar head groups of the phospholipid molecules. Wavy lines represent the fatty acid chains. Solid bodies with stippled surfaces represent the globular integral proteins. (From Singer and Nicholson, Figure 4.[73])*

a mixture of polar and nonpolar residues, possibly associated with or extending beyond the inner membrane surface. It is possible to imagine, therefore, that such proteins, traversing the entire thickness of the membrane, could transduce drug effects from external receptors to metabolic processes in the cell interior, could trans-

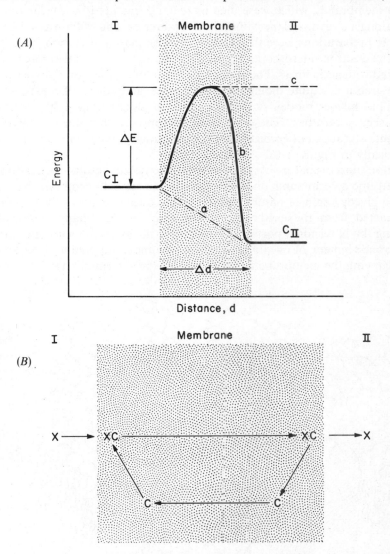

FIGURE 2-17. Schematic representations of drug movement through membranes. (A) Energy levels. C_I represents concentration at surface I; C_{II}, concentration at surface II. Thickness of membrane is Δd. Simple downhill diffusion is represented by broken line a. Downhill diffusion after overcoming an energy barrier, ΔE, is represented by solid curve b. Uphill transport, as in a "pump" mechanism, is indicated by uphill portion of curve b, then by broken line c. (B) Carrier transport system. X is a drug insoluble in the substance of the membrane; C is a lipid-soluble carrier molecule, freely diffusible in the membrane; and XC is a drug-carrier complex. A modified version of this scheme would utilize a coupled energy-yielding process to form or cleave XC, and a counter-transport of another ion or molecule, Y, to the outer membrane surface, as in Figure 2-24.

port ions or small molecules through the membrane, or could aggregate or disaggregate in a manner that would open or close aqueous channels through the membrane.

Membranes of different cells vary considerably in structural detail and in function. For example, liver and pancreas cells, because they produce proteins for use elsewhere in the body, require a mechanism for secreting macromolecules. This seems to be accomplished by packaging the proteins in vesicles that become confluent with the cell membrane; the contents are thus extruded and enter the extracellular spaces or gland ducts. This process is known as *exocytosis*. At the synaptic terminals of neurones a similar mechanism operates to release neurotransmitters from storage vesicles into the synaptic cleft. Calcium ions evidently play an important part in these events.[75]

Entry of drugs into cells.   The entry of drugs into cells depends upon many of the same mechanisms already considered for transcapillary movement. Very small water-soluble molecules and ions (e.g., K^+, Cl^-) evidently diffuse through aqueous channels of some kind. Lipid-soluble molecules of any size diffuse freely through the cell membranes. Water-soluble molecules and ions of moderate size, including the ionic forms of most drugs, cannot enter cells readily except by special transport mechanisms. Finally, since proteins do gain access to cell interiors, it may be that pinocytosis plays some role here.

Figure 2-17A depicts the cell membrane as a barrier to the passage of drug molecules. An analogy is made to chemical reactions, which may proceed (a) spontaneously "downhill," (b) "downhill," but only after first surmounting an energy barrier, or (c) "uphill" to a higher energy level through utilization of energy from a coupled energy-yielding system. Here, mechanism (a) corresponds to the diffusion of drug molecules through aqueous channels in a membrane (if the molecules are small enough) or through the substance of the membrane, in accordance with Fick's law, down a chemical potential gradient. Mechanism (b) is illustrated by the example of a drug that is too large to pass through any pores that may be present, and is also practically insoluble in the membrane, but can form a lipid-soluble complex at the membrane surface (Figure 2-17B). The complex then moves by diffusion within the membrane, down a gradient with respect to *its* chemical potential, to the other wall, where free drug can be released. Finally, mechanism (c) is represented by an active concentrating or secreting mechanism, in which a coupled system furnishes energy for driving ("pumping") the drug to a region of higher concentration, also, presumably, by means of a carrier complex intermediate.

Diffusion.   Rates of diffusion of substances across biologic membranes can be measured in many ways. The most reliable method is to sample the solutions on both sides of the membrane at intervals, and thus determine the concentrations of a substance as it diffuses into the cell from the medium. More than 30 years ago an elegant series of experiments was performed on the penetration of nonelectrolytes into the large cells of the marine plant *Chara ceratophylla*. The findings turned out to be generally relevant to penetration of other kinds of cells by non-electrolytes.

The entrance rates conformed to the diffusion equation of Fick, i.e., they were proportional to the concentration gradients. However, a distinctive diffusion coefficient had to be assigned to each substance because the membrane (as in the case of capillaries, p. 165) offered different degrees of resistance to the passage of each substance. There was no polarity; diffusion rates were the same for influx and efflux of a given substance.

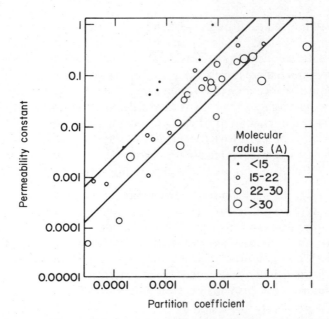

FIGURE 2-18. Relationship between oil/water partition coefficient and cell membrane permeability. *Abscissas: partition coefficient, olive oil/water; ordinates: permeability rate constant in* Chara ceratophylla. *Each circle represents a single compound; radius of circle symbolizes the molecular radius, in angstroms, as indicated.* (*From Collander and Bärlund.*[77])

There was a good correlation between partition coefficients (olive oil/water) and penetrating ability. This is shown in Figure 2-18, where molecular size is indicated by the size of the symbol used for each compound. Except for very small or very large molecules, there was a fairly direct proportionality between the rate of penetration (permeability constant) and the partition coefficient. Molecules below about 15 A radius penetrated faster than their partition coefficients would lead one to predict. Very large molecules with high partition coefficients were retarded somewhat. More recent studies with red cell membranes have refined these principles. The ether/water partition coefficient was found to correlate better with permeability constants than did other solvent/water partition coefficients. Lipophilic molecules capable of forming hydrogen bonds were found to interact in this way during passage through the membrane.[76]

The influence of partition coefficient upon the diffusion of drugs into cell membranes has an important bearing upon certain biologic actions. Various nonelectrolytes of wholly unrelated structures produce general anesthesia (formerly called "narcosis") when they are present in sufficient concentration in the central nervous system. Ether (diethyl ether), cyclopropane, nitrous oxide, the primary alcohols, carbon disulfide, and chloroform are examples. The diversity of molecular structure among these drugs has always been puzzling. A systematic relationship is found, however, between anesthetic potency and oil/water partition coefficient. One of the earliest examples studied is summarized in Table 2-10, showing the concentration of four alcohols required in the aqueous medium in order to produce equivalent degrees of anesthesia in tadpoles immersed in that medium. As the length of the hydrophobic

TABLE 2-10. Anesthesia produced by primary alcohols in tadpoles.
(Data of Overton[78] and Meyer and Hemmi.[79])

Alcohol	Anesthetic concentration in aqueous medium (M)	Partition coefficient (cottonseed oil/water)
CH_3OH	0.57	0.00966
C_2H_5OH	0.29	0.0357
C_3H_7OH	0.11	0.156
iso-C_4H_9OH	0.045	0.588

chain increases, so does the oil/water partition coefficient, and also the anesthetic potency, the required aqueous concentration becoming lower and lower. Thus, the effective concentration in a lipid biophase would be the same for a wide variety of compounds. This has led to the concept that a certain amount of anesthetic drug, physically dissolved in the membranes of nerve cells, suffices to alter the functional properties of those membranes. The excitability of nerve cells arises from the ability of their membranes to become depolarized quite suddenly by the inrush of Na^+ ions. Possibly the dissolved molecules of anesthetic prevent this reversible permeability change.

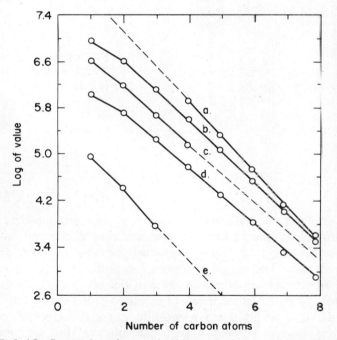

FIGURE 2-19. Properties of normal primary alcohols. (c) Solubility (moles × 10^{-6} liter^{-1}); (b) toxic concentration for typhoid bacillus (moles × 10^{-6} liter^{-1}); (c) concentration reducing surface tension of water to 50 dynes cm^{-1} (moles × 10^{-6} liter^{-1}); (d) vapor pressure at 25° (mm Hg × 10^4); (e) partition coefficient between cottonseed oil and water (× 10^3). (From Ferguson, Figure 1.[80])

Arguments based upon correlation between a biologic effect and a particular molecular property, such as lipid/water partition coefficient, must be regarded with caution. Examination of other properties may also reveal good correlation, as in Figure 2-19 for a congeneric series of alcohols. Here antibacterial potency is indeed correlated very well with oil/water partition coefficient. But with increasing length of the carbon chain, the biologic action is seen also to be correlated with decreasing water solubility, increasing effect on aqueous surface tension, and decreasing vapor pressure.

Even when unrelated compounds are compared with respect to some physical property, good correlation with biologic potency may be found. Table 2-11 illustrates

TABLE 2-11. Concentrations of gases and vapors producing the same degree of anesthesia in mice at 37°.
Thermodynamic activity is expressed as the ratio of the partial pressure p_t of the agent to its saturation vapor pressure p_s. (Data of Ferguson,[80] Table V.)

	Saturation pressure at 37° (p_s) (mm Hg)	Anesthetic concentration (% by volume)	Activity (p_t/p_s)
Nitrous oxide	59,300	100	0.01
Acetylene	51,700	65	0.01
Methyl ether	6,100	12	0.02
Methyl chloride	5,900	14	0.01
Ethylene oxide	1,900	5.8	0.02
Ethyl chloride	1,780	5.0	0.02
Diethyl ether	830	3.4	0.03
Methylal	630	2.8	0.03
Ethyl bromide	725	1.9	0.02
Dimethylacetal	288	1.9	0.05
Diethylformal	110	1.0	0.07
Dichlorethylene	450	0.95	0.02
Carbon disulfide	560	1.1	0.02
Chloroform	324	0.5	0.01

such a correlation for volatile anesthetic agents in mice, anesthesia being used as a measure of entry of the agents into neuronal membranes. The second column gives the concentration of each agent required to produce the same moderate degree of anesthesia at equilibrium. The partial pressures, computed from these concentrations, varied over a 20-fold range. But the chemical activities, estimated as ratios of anesthetic partial pressure (p_t) to saturation pressure (p_s), varied over a very much smaller range. In other words, equal chemical activities produced equal degrees of anesthesia.

Thus, correspondence between a particular physical property and anesthetic potency cannot be assigned a cause-and-effect relationship, for some colligative property could equally well play the principal role.[81] The fact that high oil/water partition coefficient is associated with high anesthetic potency does not necessarily mean that the anesthetic acts in the lipid phase of cell membranes. The very same hydrophobic groups that make a molecule "prefer" the lipid to the water phase would also give it a high affinity for the surface of a protein or other macromolecule in preference to the ambient aqueous solution.

For weak acids and bases the ionized and nonionized forms have completely different lipid/water partition coefficients. The ionized groupings (usually $-COO^-$ or $-NR_2H^+$, see p. 19) interact strongly with water dipoles and consequently penetrate only poorly or not at all into the lipoidal cell membranes. Thus, drugs that are partially ionized at body pH enter cells at rates that are strongly pH dependent. For all practical purposes the diffusion rate can usually be ascribed to the concentration gradient for the nonionized form alone.

Figure 2-20 shows this typical pH dependence for an acridine dye with a pK_a of 9.65. Here, the rate of entry into cultured human conjunctival cells was measured by a

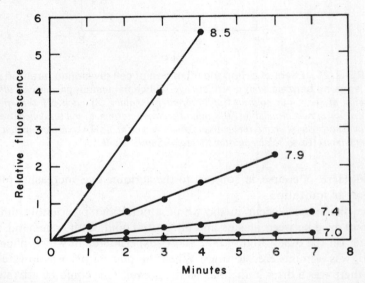

FIGURE 2-20. Effect of pH on entry of an acridine dye into cultured human conjunctival cells. *Intracellular dye concentration was measured by a fluorometric technique. The dye, proflavin, has $pK_a = 9.65$. The pH value of the surrounding medium is given on each curve. (After Robbins, Figure 5.*[82] *By permission of the Rockefeller University Press.)*

quantitative fluorescence technique. At pH 8.5 about 8% of the dye is in the nonionized form, the remainder having a proton associated to a nitrogen atom in the acridine ring. At the more acidic pH values, an ever smaller fraction is nonionized. The penetration rates are seen to vary as though only the nonionized form crossed the cell membrane.

Figure 2-21 illustrates the same principle for benzoic acid. The concentration required to inhibit cell division by 50% in fertilized sand dollar eggs was ascertained at various values of pH in the medium. The graph shows these 50% inhibitory concentrations as a function of pH. Although diffusion rate is not measured directly here, the result is similar. Increasing concentrations of the ionized form are required to achieve the same end-point, but always the same concentration of the nonionized

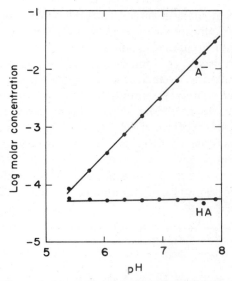

FIGURE 2-21. Effect of pH on the inhibition of cell division in fertilized sand dollar eggs by benzoic acid. *Fertilized eggs of* Echinarachnius parma *were allowed to develop in sea water solutions of different pH values. At each pH the effective concentration of benzoic acid for 50% inhibition was determined, and the concentrations of the benzoate ion* (A^-) *and the undissociated benzoic acid* (HA) *were computed from the Henderson–Hasselbalch equation.* (Data of Smith, Table 5.[83])

benzoic acid. Here, of course, in contrast to the acridine dye, increasing pH causes a greater degree of ionization.

The same phenomena occur in the whole animal and profoundly influence the distribution of drug between plasma and interstitial fluid on the one hand, and intracellular water on the other. Figure 2-22 shows experiments in which phenobarbital, a weak acid, was administered to dogs. When the plasma pH was lowered by CO_2 inhalation, there was a drop in the plasma drug level. This could be attributed to the fact that a greater fraction of the total phenobarbital in the blood assumed the nonionized acid form. The plasma concentration of undissociated diffusible phenobarbital was thus increased, and a larger amount of the drug moved across the cell

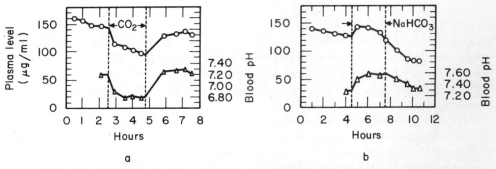

FIGURE 2-22. Effects of acidosis and alkalosis on phenobarbital plasma levels in dogs. *Phenobarbital concentrations are designated by circles, blood pH values by triangles.* (From Waddell and Butler, Figures 2 and 3.[84])

membranes and into cells, where the pH remains relatively stable. Plasma alkalosis produced the opposite shift. These shifts occurred in all the tissues studied, including brain, where the depth of anesthesia paralleled the tissue concentrations. In other words, administration of acid deepened the anesthesia, while alkalosis lightened it. To promote just such a shift of drug out of the tissues (and also for a similar effect at the kidneys, see p. 397), alkalosis is induced therapeutically in the treatment of barbiturate poisoning.

Membrane transport.[85,86]   Substances that are insoluble in the cell membrane may nevertheless pass into the cell interior by forming a complex with a "carrier." The process is represented schematically in Figure 2-17B. The carrier complex XC is assumed to be freely diffusible in the membrane. Since XC is formed at surface I and cleaved at surface II, its concentration gradient will run down from I to II, but that of free carrier will run down in the opposite direction. Thus, diffusion can provide the means for cycling (or shuttling) the carrier across the membrane. If the concentration of X remains lower at II than at I (as when it is metabolized inside a cell), then the transport is "downhill" and requires no net expenditure of energy by the cell. Glucose in erythrocytes is a good example; because it moves down a concentration gradient into the cells, the process has been described as "facilitated diffusion," but the high degree of substrate specificity makes it evident that some kind of carrier is involved. A system of acceptor-donor macromolecules, in fixed positions across the membrane, and operating in the manner of a bucket brigade, could possibly serve as the carrier mechanism, but a diffusible carrier is easier to imagine.

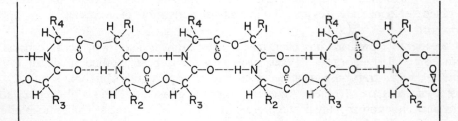

FIGURE 2-23. Structure of valinomycin. $R_1 = CH_3$; $R_2 = R_3 = R_4 = CH(CH_3)_2$. *Thus, the sequence is (L-lactic acid, L-valine, D-α-hydroxyisovaleric acid, D-valine), repeated three times. The molecule is cyclic; the conformation is represented by bending the left and right edges down into the plane of the paper and joining the vertical lines. (From Ohnishi and Urry, Figure 1.[87])*

An interesting example of carrier-mediated diffusion is provided by the antibiotic valinomycin (Figure 2-23). This is a cyclic peptide containing 12 residues arrayed as three identical sequences of four residues each: L-lactic acid, L-valine, D-α-hydroxy-isovaleric acid, D-valine, with alternating peptide and ester linkages. The structure is stabilized by internal H-bonds, as shown. The eight carbonyl oxygens of the valine residues face inward, forming a cage, within which a K^+ ion can be held by coordinate bonds.[87] The external surface of the ring presents a mosaic of hydrophobic side chains. The valinomycin molecule therefore can function as an ion carrier (ionophore), transporting K^+ through the hydrophobic interior of membranes.[88] This effect has been demonstrated in bacterial cells and also in artificial phospholipid bilayers.

Quantitative measurements have shown that the rate of diffusion of K^+ through such membranes is the same as that of ligand-free valinomycin, whereas free hydrated K^+ is virtually unable to penetrate the membrane.[89,90] Although this antibiotic provides a plausible model for carrier transport, it is not yet clear if analogous compounds serve this function in normal membrane transport systems.

Referring again to Figure 2-17B, if the concentration of X is higher at II, the transport is "uphill"; chemical energy must then be expended to drive the unidirectional transport, for otherwise the same system would operate to move X in the opposite direction, from II to I. Transport requiring energy is also called "active transport" because of the active coupling of energy-yielding reactions needed to drive the transport; work is done by the cell at the expense of energy derived from metabolism. Examples of active transport are the secretion of H^+ into the stomach and into the renal tubular urine, the accumulation of iodide ions in the thyroid gland, the absorption of glucose and amino acids in the intestine, and their reabsorption in the kidney, and the secretion of numerous organic anions and cations by the proximal renal tubules. The "sodium pump" is discussed at length in a later section.

A number of drugs appear to be moved across cell membranes by transport systems. Examples are the renal tubular secretion of penicillin, phenol red, and tetraethylammonium ion; the secretion of penicillin or sulfobromophthalein (BSP) into the bile; and the transport of some drugs from cerebrospinal fluid into blood (p. 195). Membrane transport systems can be blocked by drugs that interfere with energy production. They display a high degree of steric specificity, and they are subject to competitive inhibition by compounds that bear a close structural relationship to the normal transport substrates. For these reasons it is supposed that proteins are somehow involved; enzymes are obviously required for activation of a carrier in an uphill transport.

Considerable progress has been made in isolating transport proteins, especially from bacterial membranes.[91] One system that has been studied in detail is the bacterial sugar transport system, which can transport nine different sugars.[92] At least 2 enzymes are involved: An energy supplying protein (HPr) is phosphorylated from phosphoenolpyruvate in the presence of Mg^{2+} by enzyme I. Then phosphate is transferred to a specific sugar by enzyme II, and the sugar is simultaneously translocated across the membrane. The phosphorylated sugar is trapped inside the cell, since it cannot diffuse across the membrane. A small protein (9400 daltons), HPr has no affinity for the sugar substrates. Enzyme II is specific for each sugar. The mechanism of the translocation step is unknown. It could involve a "revolving door" mechanism, in which the transport protein actually rotates, carrying the sugar from outside to inside of the membrane, or a conformational change could have the same consequence. Such mechanisms are plausible in the context of the fluid-mosaic model of the cell membrane (p. 167). Bacterial proteins serving to transport sulfate, D-galactose, and various amino acids have also been isolated.[93,94] Mutants lacking a transport protein show greatly diminished entry of a specific substrate.[91]

Similar transport systems have been identified in mammalian cells. An example is the system for calcium transport in small intestine, which requires vitamin D for its continued function, calcium absorption being greatly impaired in rachitic animals.[95] Vitamin D itself is inactive; it must first be transformed to a polar metabolite (e.g., 25-hydroxycholecalciferol) in the liver. Thus, infusion of the polar metabolite into the intestinal arterial tree of a rachitic animal causes an increase of calcium transport within an hour. Vitamin D itself is without effect in the isolated perfused intestine, and acts only after a lag of about 12 hr when given systemically. Actinomycin D (or puromycin) blocks the enhanced calcium absorption if given simultaneously with vitamin D, but has no effect once the enhanced absorption has developed.[96] It appears, therefore, that the response to the vitamin involves the stimulation of synthesis or prevention of degradation of a protein with a high turnover rate. A likely candidate is a calcium-binding protein, which has been identified.[97] Its molecular weight is about 24,000, and it binds one atom of calcium with an affinity constant of $2.6 \times 10^5 \ M^{-1}$. This protein is virtually absent in rachitic animals, but appears soon after vitamin D administration. Its role in the translocation mechanism is not yet understood.

Modification of membrane function by drugs.   It is now evident that many drugs exert their actions by combining with receptors on the outer surface of cell membranes. The effect, probably by an allosteric mechanism, is to change the permeability of the membrane ("opening pores") to ions, or to modify carrier transport systems, or to influence the activity of an enzyme on the inner membrane surface. Vasopressin (p. 39) and other polypeptide hormones are thought to act in this way. That the action of vasopressin cannot be a nonspecific one upon membranes in general is shown by the great differences in sensitivity of different cells to the hormone. Cells of the distal and collecting tubules, for example, respond by a great increase in permeability to water, whereas proximal tubules do not seem to be affected. Such findings imply the presence of specific receptors on the surfaces of sensitive cells. Evidence has already been reviewed (p. 80), showing that insulin can act even when bound to a polymer matrix that would certainly prevent its penetration into the membrane. Neurotransmitters act upon the postsynaptic membrane without having to penetrate into the neurone. And according to the "second messenger" hypothesis, several different hormones and neurotransmitters act by combining, each with a specific receptor, on the external surface of a cell membrane, thereby activating adenyl cyclase on the inner surface and causing an increase in the intracellular 3'-5'-adenosine monophosphate.[98]

Microelectrode techniques have established the presence of a potential difference across cell membranes, generally around 60–90 millivolts (mV). The inside of the cell is negative with respect to the outside. The Gibbs–Donnan equilibrium predicts an unequal distribution of other ions when any ion is prevented from equilibrating across the membrane. The resulting concentration gradients produce a potential difference whose magnitude is given by the Nernst equation.[99] Analysis of the ion concentrations in intracellular and interstitial fluids of mammalian muscle cells reveals that whereas K^+ and Cl^- are in equilibrium with the membrane potential, Na^+ is not. The observed excess of external over internal Na^+ concentration would be in equilibrium with a membrane potential of $+65$ mV, in contrast to the actual -90 mV. Thus, the membrane behaves as though it is largely impermeable to Na^+, but freely permeable to the other small ions. The great excesses of internal over external K^+ and of external over internal Cl^- are seen as the expected consequence of the Na^+ impermeability, as predicted by the Gibbs–Donnan equilibrium. Studies with radioactive Na^+, however, revealed that this ion does indeed cross the membrane, at a sufficient rate so that equal concentrations would soon be established inside and outside the cell, unless Na^+ were being extruded continually. The conclusion generally accepted today is that a "sodium pump" operates to exclude Na^+ from the cell interior. This, of course, is tantamount to making the membrane selectively impermeable to Na^+.

The physical basis of the sodium pump is a sodium and potassium-activated adenosine triphosphatase, widely distributed in cell membranes, and especially abundant in secretory cells and excitable tissue such as nerve and muscle.[100] The good correlation between the activity of this enzyme and the cation flux in a variety of tissues is shown in Table 2-12. The enzyme has proved difficult to isolate from other

TABLE 2-12. Comparison of cation fluxes and Na–K ATPase activities. Standard error of the mean and the number of determinations are given in parentheses. (From Bonting,[100] Table 4.)

Tissue	Temperature (°C)	Cation flux (10^{-14} mole cm^{-2} sec^{-1})	Na–K ATPase activity (10^{-14} mole cm^{-2} sec^{-1})	Ratio
Human erythrocytes	37	3.87	1.38 (± 0.36; 4)	2.80
Frog toe muscle	17	985	530 (± 94; 4)	1.86
Squid giant axon	19	1200	400 (± 79; 5)	3.00
Frog skin	20	19,700	6640 (± 1100; 4)	2.97
Toad bladder	27	43,700	17,600 (± 1640; 15)	2.48
Electric eel, non-innervated membrane	23	86,100	38,800 (± 4160; 3)	2.22

components of membranes, but partial purification has been achieved after solubilization with a nonionic detergent followed by chromatography on agarose.[101] A single peak with apparent molecular weight 670,000 was obtained—a lipoprotein molecule of sufficient size to span the entire thickness of the membrane. A model has been proposed for the transport function, based upon a conformational change induced by phosphorylation (Figure 2-24).[102] The enzyme is phosphorylated by ATP at the inner membrane surface. It is thereby converted to a form with a high affinity for Na^+. The cation binding sites are translocated to the outer membrane surface, where dephosphorylation results in decreased Na^+ affinity and increased K^+ affinity. The conformational change leads to translocation of the sites to the inner surface, where K^+ ions are discharged, and the cycle repeats. The model is supported by the finding that the phosphorylation step, in vitro, is dependent on Na^+, while dephosphorylation requires K^+.[103]

It has been known for some time that ouabain and other cardiac glycosides inhibit cation transport and also inhibit Na^+–K^+-activated ATPase.[104] The nearly perfect quantitative agreement between these two effects of ouabain are shown in Figure 2-25. The transport of Na^+ was inhibited only when the drug was added to the external, serosal surface of the membrane; there was no effect at the mucosal surface. The ability of cardiac glycosides to act by combining with a receptor on the outer surface of the cell membrane was confirmed with another cardiac glycoside, digoxin.[105] A sensitive technique was used to record the amplitude of contraction of single, isolated cardiac cells from young rats. Digoxin, covalently attached to serum albumin, caused increased rates and amplitudes of contraction. The response was obtained

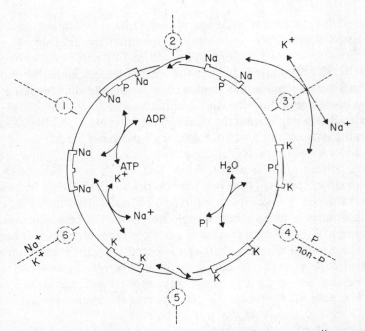

FIGURE 2-24. Membrane Na^+–K^+ ATPase operating as a sodium pump.
*Circle represents cell membrane. Sequence of reactions reads clockwise from 1. At 2,
phosphorylation translocates cation binding sites outward; at 5, dephosphorylation
translocates sites inward. (From Bonting, Figure 33.[100])*

instantaneously, and was abolished when the chamber was washed out. Control
experiments eliminated the possibility that the drug-protein complex was dissociated
to any extent, and contamination with free drug was excluded.[105a]

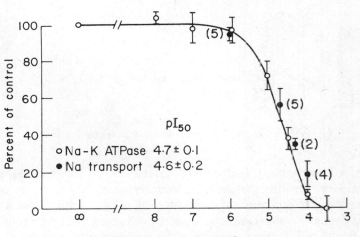

FIGURE 2-25. Effect of ouabain on Na–K ATPase activity and short circuit
current (Na^+ transport) in toad bladder. *Enzyme activity (open circles) was
determined in homogenates, short-circuit current (solid circles) was measured with
ouabain added to the serosal side of the chamber containing the toad bladder. Number
of experiments indicated in parentheses. (From Bonting, Figure 18.[100])*

The molecular mechanism of action of the cardiac glycosides is still unclear. The K^+-dependent dephosphorylation step is inhibited by ouabain. The binding of ^{3}H-digoxin to the ATPase requires ATP and Mg^{2+}, is stimulated by Na^+, and is depressed by K^+,[106] suggesting that the drug interacts with the phosphorylated intermediate, perhaps preventing dephosphorylation and thus blocking the cycle by preventing discharge of Na^+ ions at the surface.

Further evidence implicating the ouabain-sensitive Na–K ATPase as the essential element in the sodium pump was obtained with sheep red blood cells.[107] Most sheep have erythrocytes with low K^+ concentration, about 13 mM (called LK cells), but in some the concentration is about 80 mM (HK cells), more like the usual value in other mammalian species. These two phenotypes are determined by two alleles at a single genetic locus. For complete inhibition of the sodium flux, HK cells have to bind about 6 times as many ouabain molecules as do LK cells. The normal ratio of Na^+ fluxes or of K^+ concentrations in the two cell types is about 6. It appears, therefore, that the essential difference between HK and LK cells is the number of Na–K ATPase molecules per cell; as judged by the number of ouabain molecules bound, there are 42 and 8 pump sites, respectively (about 1 μm^2 membrane surface). The value for HK cells is about one-half that reported for human red cells. A given site, whether HK or LK, transported about 50–60 ions sec^{-1}.

An unusual effect of drugs upon membranes underlies the action of a class of antibiotics, the polyenes, including several antifungal agents such as amphotericin B, nystatin, and filipin.[108] The structure of filipin is shown in Figure 2-26. The salient

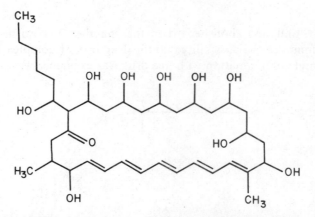

FIGURE 2-26. Structure of filipin, a polyene antibiotic.

features are a hydroxylated, hydrophilic surface and an unsaturated, conjugated, lipophilic surface. Sensitive fungal cells, when exposed to antibiotics of this type, display a functional disturbance of membrane integrity, resulting in loss of ions and various small water-soluble molecules from the cell interior. The polyene antibiotics are bound only to cells that are sensitive to their killing action, and the site of binding is the cell membrane. Sterols are required for this binding; extraction of sterols abolishes the binding capacity and the antibiotic sensitivity. Incubation with sterols can restore the binding capacity and the sensitivity. This is shown in Table 2-13 for *Mycoplasma*. Cholesterol-grown cells were killed by amphotericin B, whereas cholesterol-free cells were not. When sensitive cells were incubated in cholesterol-free

TABLE 2-13. Effect of cholesterol on sensitivity of cells to a polyene antibiotic.

M. laidlawii were grown in medium with cholesterol (S cells) or without cholesterol (R cells). Both cell types were washed and suspended in cholesterol-free medium. Samples were removed for viable counts with and without exposure to amphotericin B for 2 hr. Cholesterol was added to the R cells. After incubation for 2 hr at 4° or 37°, the cells were washed, and sensitivity to amphotericin B was tested as before. (From Feingold,[109] Table 1.)

Cell type	Survivors after 2 hr exposure to amphotericin B (%)
Cholesterol-grown cells (S cells)	2
Cholesterol-free cells (R cells)	200
S cells incubated in cholesterol-free medium for 2 hr at:	
37°C	150
4°C	5
R cells incubated in cholesterol-containing medium for 2 hr at:	
37°C	3
4°C	180

medium at low temperature, their sensitivity to the antibiotic did not change; but when the incubation was carried out at 37°, they lost cholesterol and their sensitivity was abolished. The converse results were obtained with resistant, cholesterol-free cells.

Intact cells were not required for the demonstration of these effects. Artificial membranes were prepared from lecithin and dicetyl phosphate in the presence of glucose. Under the proper conditions, such artificial phospholipid membranes form small vesicles (liposomes) bounded by many concentric phospholipid bilayers and containing aqueous interiors. In this case glucose was trapped inside the liposomes. Exposure of the liposomes to filipin (Figure 2-27) produced a concentration-dependent damage, manifested as increased permeability to glucose, and this process was greatly augmented by the prior incorporation of cholesterol into the membrane structure. The polyene antibiotics are known to form a complex with sterols, but how this disrupts the membrane integrity is not known.

An interesting example of how, by increasing membrane permeability, one drug may potentiate the action of another, is shown in Figure 2-28. Rifampicin is an antibiotic that binds to bacterial RNA polymerase, inhibiting RNA synthesis and thus blocking cell growth. It is poorly effective against fungi but becomes fungicidal in the presence of amphotericin B.[111] Evidently, the cell membrane is made permeable to rifampicin. Similar effects of amphotericin B have been demonstrated with 5-fluorocytosine, another inhibitor of bacterial RNA synthesis. This phenomenon might conceivably have therapeutic value in increasing the selectivity of antifungal agents by potentiating the desired actions at concentrations that are nontoxic to the mammalian host.

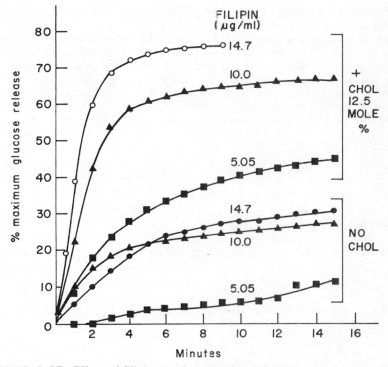

FIGURE 2-27. Effect of filipin on glucose release from liposomes.   *Lipo-somes were prepared from lecithin and dicetyl phosphate in the presence of glucose. Cholesterol was present (upper curves) or absent (lower curves). The rate of release of glucose from the interior of the liposomes was measured. (From Kinsky et al., Figure 8.[110])*

Passage of Drugs into the Central Nervous System

The Capillaries and the Cerebrospinal Fluid. The brain constitutes only 2% of the body weight, yet receives about 16% of the cardiac output. The average blood flow is about 0.5 ml g^{-1} min^{-1}, compared with approximately 0.05 in resting muscle. One might expect, therefore, that drugs would equilibrate very rapidly between blood and brain. And indeed some do, but many substances enter brain tissue only very slowly, and some practically not at all.[111a]

A drug may gain access to the tissues of the central nervous system by two distinct routes: the capillary circulation and the cerebrospinal fluid (CSF). The internal carotid and vertebral arteries come together at the base of the brain to form the circle of Willis, from which major vessels issue to supply each side of the brain, including the choroid plexuses of the lateral and third ventricles where the CSF is formed. Blood flow rates to various parts of the brain have been estimated by measuring the rate of transfer of radioactive krypton (^{79}Kr) from blood to tissues. Table 2-14 reveals wide differences. For example, cerebral white matter has a much lower blood supply than several parts of the cortex. This corresponds to the observed density of capillaries, about 300 mm^{-2} cross section in the cerebral white matter, as compared with about 1000 in cortex. Radioautographic studies (p. 189) showed that drugs penetrate into cortex more readily than into white matter, probably because of the greater delivery

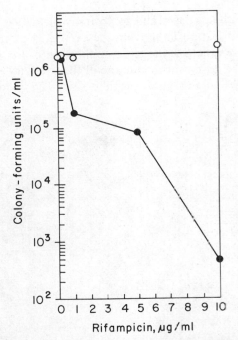

FIGURE 2-28. Effect of amphotericin B on sensitivity of a fungus to rifampicin. *Cell suspensions were inoculated into tubes containing rifampicin in the presence (solid circles) and absence (open circles) of 30 ng ml⁻¹ of amphotericin B. Viability after 7 days incubation was measured by the colony-forming capacity of the cells,* S. cerevisiae. (*From Medoff et al., Figure 2.*[111])

rate of drug to the tissues. The lateral nuclei of the hypothalamus receive a particularly rich blood supply, and here again drugs enter quite rapidly. Certain specialized areas are also found to be penetrated unusually well by dyes and other substances, but whether because of a rich blood supply or exceptionally permeable capillaries, or both, is not clear. These include the area postrema in the roof of the fourth ventricle (containing the chemoreceptor trigger zone for emesis, an important site of drug action), the pineal body, and the posterior lobe of the hypophysis.

It has already been stated that some capillaries in the body (e.g., those of the glomeruli and liver) are more permeable than those of muscle. In the brain, however,

TABLE 2-14. Blood flow in representative areas of the brain of the unanesthetized cat. (From Kety,[112] Table 2.)

	Mean blood flow ($ml^{-1} g \, min^{-1}$)		Mean blood flow ($ml^{-1} g \, min^{-1}$)
Inferior colliculus	1.80	Caudate	1.10
Sensorimotor cortex	1.38	Thalamus	1.03
Auditory cortex	1.30	Association cortex	0.88
Visual cortex	1.25	Cerebellar nuclei	0.87
Medial geniculate	1.22	Cerebellar white matter	0.24
Lateral geniculate	1.21	Cerebral white matter	0.23
Superior colliculus	1.15	Spinal cord white matter	0.14

the capillaries are much less permeable to a variety of water-soluble substances. The outstanding structural feature underlying the decreased permeability of capillaries in the central nervous system is the close application of the glial connective tissue cells (astrocytes) to the basement membrane of the capillary endothelium. Electron micrographs indicate that this glial sheath is about 85% complete (Figure 2-29).

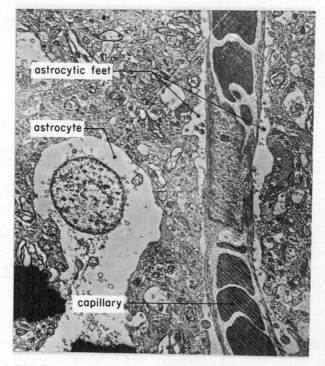

FIGURE 2-29. Electron micrograph of the vascular bed of rat cerebral cortex. *Longitudinally sectioned capillary showing its sheath of astrocytic processes and a nearby astrocyte. The cellular sheath, a unique feature of brain capillaries, impedes the passage of water-soluble drugs and accounts for the "blood-brain barrier." (From Maynard et al., Plate I.[113])*

Beneath this sheath the basement membrane is homogeneous, relatively dense, and about 300–500 A thick. The endothelium appears to be a continuous sheet of cells without visible pores. A drug leaving the capillaries in the central nervous system has therefore to traverse not only the capillary endothelium itself but also the membranes of glial cells in order to gain access to the interstitial fluid. Estimates of the volume of this fluid are as low as 5–15% of the brain volume. Its composition differs strikingly from that of interstitial fluid elsewhere by the nearly complete absence of protein; there are also some differences in the ionic composition.

One would predict from their investment by a cellular sheath that the permeability characteristics of brain capillaries should be rather like those of cell membranes elsewhere in the body, and not like the permeability characteristics of the usual, porous capillary structure. This is, in general, true. Ionized or nonionized water-soluble substances may be practically excluded, unless they are quite small, but lipid-soluble compounds enter the brain easily and rapidly. Misconceptions about an absolute "blood-brain barrier" arose from early studies showing the failure of certain dyes to enter the brain after their intravenous administration. These observations failed to take into account the strong binding of dyes to plasma proteins, reducing the concentration of free dye available for diffusion; they failed to consider the degree of ionization, a major determinant of diffusion into brain; and they failed to control the possible decolorizing of dyes by metabolic processes in brain tissue. Results obtained by modern techniques, described below, indicate that the "blood-brain barrier" really represents a quantitative rather than a qualitative difference in capillary permeability, as compared with other tissues.

The CSF is formed at the choroid plexus by a process of active secretion in which Na–K ATPase plays an essential role. Inhibitors of this enzyme, such as ouabain, cause a diminution of the flow rate that is closely correlated with the degree of enzyme inhibition.[100] The CSF flows through the ventriculocisternal system, bathes the surfaces of the brain and spinal cord, and then flows into the venous blood sinuses through a system of large channels and valves in the arachnoid villi.[114] In man its rate of formation is about 0.3 ml min^{-1} and its total volume about 200 ml, so the rate of turnover is approximately 10% hr^{-1}. Drugs may enter CSF by way of the choroid plexus or by diffusion directly across the capillaries into the interstitial fluid. Drugs may leave the CSF by bulk flow into the venous sinuses, by diffusion back into the capillaries, by absorption at the choroid plexus, or by diffusion into the neuronal cells. One consequence for drug equilibration is that brain cells, brain interstitial fluid, and CSF may come to equilibrium with plasma water at quite different rates. It is even possible for a drug entering CSF to be "washed out" continually by the bulk flow of water, so that equilibrium between its concentration in plasma water and in CSF is never attained. Let us begin with no drug in CSF, and abruptly establish a constant plasma level of drug. Then the net rate of entry of drug into CSF is given by $Q(c_p - c_c)$, where Q is a constant with the dimensions of clearance (milliliters of plasma water cleared of drug per minute), determined by the permeability for the drug; c_c is the drug concentration in CSF; and c_p is the drug concentration in plasma water. The rate of exit of drug from CSF is given by Fc_c, where F is the bulk flow rate. Then

$$\frac{dc_c}{dt} = \frac{1}{V}[Q(c_p - c_c) - Fc_c]$$

where V is the volume of CSF. This equation can be integrated to give the exponential approach of c_c to its steady-state level. The steady state itself is found directly by setting $dc_c/dt = 0$, whence

$$\frac{c_c}{c_p} = \frac{Q}{(Q + F)} = \frac{1}{(1 + F/Q)}$$

Evidently, the ratio of drug concentration in CSF to that in plasma water approaches unity (true equilibrium) as the rate of bulk flow becomes small relative to the "clearance" of drug from blood into brain; but the steady-state ratio can become indefinitely low at the other extreme.

In addition to its almost complete lack of protein, CSF differs from plasma water by having lower concentrations of K^+, Ca^{2+}, and phosphate, and a higher concentration of Cl^-. The glucose level is lower, but this is not necessarily remarkable in view of the rapid metabolic utilization of glucose in CSF. The pH of CSF is about 0.1 unit more acid than plasma.[115] Interpretation of these differences in ionic concentrations requires a knowledge of the electrochemical potential difference. Fragmentary data suggest that CSF may be about 10 mV positive with respect to plasma; this would be sufficient to explain the cation and anion inequalities (by the Gibbs–Donnan equilibrium), provided Na^+ were actively secreted into CSF. Other evidence also points to a "sodium pump" in the choroid plexus, intimately associated with the mechanism of formation of CSF. Moreover, the choroid plexus has been demonstrated to be a site of active transport of iodide and thiocyanate, and also of phenol red, penicillin, and other organic acids from CSF into blood. This mechanism accounts for the fact that the normal CSF concentration of iodide is very low compared with that in plasma water.[116]

Systematic studies of the functional permeability of membranes separating blood from CSF were carried out in goats.[117] The ventriculocisternal system was perfused with a solution approximating the normal composition of CSF, under controlled pressure and flow rate. The perfusate entered the lateral ventricle and was collected at the cisterna magna. The difference between the concentration of a substance added to the perfusion fluid and its effluent concentration could be ascribed to loss by bulk flow into the venous system and to diffusion across the ependymal lining into the capillary system. The clearance of inulin was found to be proportional to the CSF hydrostatic pressure, falling to zero when the pressure was reduced slightly below that in the venous sinuses. It was concluded that inulin was cleared only by bulk flow; this was entirely consistent with the previous finding that inulin and dextran (a very much larger polymer) were cleared at the same rate. Thus, the normal rate of bulk flow (i.e., rate of formation of CSF) could be estimated from the rate of disappearance of inulin at normal CSF pressure.

Knowing the rate of bulk flow, and the conditions for abolishing it entirely, made it possible to estimate the diffusional components of clearance of various molecules. For water, measured by means of tritiated water, the diffusional component predominated, even at high rates of bulk flow (i.e., at high hydrostatic pressures). As molecular size of various solutes was increased, the diffusion rate became restricted. As compared with muscle capillaries (p. 166) where the observations on restricted diffusion were consistent with a system of pores with radius about 30 A, here it was concluded that the equivalent pore radius was no larger than about 8 A. Thus, inulin (15 A) was completely excluded, whereas sucrose (4.4 A) diffused across, but more slowly than predicted from its diffusion coefficient in free solution. Even molecules as small as fructose and creatinine showed some restriction in their diffusion. The general picture was that of a porous membrane with aqueous channels very much smaller than those in muscle capillary endothelium.

Differences in the rates of penetration into various parts of the brain have been revealed by the injection of radioactive substances.[118,118a] Studies with the hydrophilic small molecule ^{14}C-urea showed that after intravenous injection in the rat there was much faster entry into cerebellar cortex than into cerebellar white matter of CSF. Other studies indicate that the heavy myelinization of white matter significantly impedes the entry of drugs. For example, in newborn kittens, where myelinization is still incomplete, ^{14}C-urea achieved equal penetration into cerebral white and grey matter within 1 hr, but the same experiment in an adult cat revealed a marked impediment to penetration of the white matter. This may possibly be relevant to the problem of kernicterus in infants (p. 821). In addition to the explanations advanced earlier, it may be that incomplete myelinization permits bilirubin to penetrate brain cells in abnormally large quantities.

Autoradiograms have furnished visual evidence about the routes of entry of drugs into brain and of differences in drug distribution and binding among the various brain areas. When such studies were performed in the cat with lipid-soluble substances like thiopental, which penetrate into brain extremely fast, the observed pattern of labeling corresponded to the relative vascularity of the different areas. Thus, at 1 min the label appeared in cortex, geniculate bodies, and inferior colliculi; and in 30 min the entire brain became uniformly labeled.

The entry of lipophilic volatile anesthetics into brain was studied by autoradiography in squirrel monkeys.[119] Figure 2-30 shows a typical result with ^{14}C-halothane. An anesthetic dose was injected intravenously, the animal was killed after 2 or 5 min,

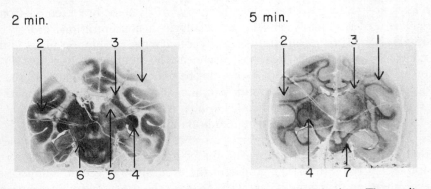

FIGURE 2-30. Distribution of ^{14}C-halothane in monkey brain. *The radio-active anesthetic was injected intravenously. Animals were killed 2 or 5 min later and the heads were frozen immediately in liquid nitrogen. Coronal sections were left in contact with film in liquid nitrogen for 8–12 weeks. 1 = subcortical white matter; 2 = cerebral cortex; 3 = caudate nucleus; 4 = lateral geniculate nucleus; 5 = posterior thalamus; 6 = reticular formation; 7 = optic chiasm. (From Cohen et al., Figure 1.[119])*

and the head was frozen immediately in liquid nitrogen to minimize redistribution of the anesthetic by diffusion postmortem. At 2 min, the halothane is seen to be concentrated in grey matter, largely reflecting the vascularization pattern. By 5 min, the anesthetic is largely redistributed into the white matter of cerebral and cerebellar cortex and the major fiber tracts. Certain interesting exceptions are noted, however, such as the retention of label in the reticular formation when other well vascularized areas such as hypothalamus have largely lost the drug. This finding is provocative because the reticular formation is known to be an important site of anesthetic action, but it remains to be shown that the localization of anesthetic agents there is more than coincidental.

A contrast to the pattern of distribution of volatile anesthetics is that seen in Figure 2-31, where ^{35}S-acetazolamide was injected intravenously in cats. The earliest labeling observed, at 1 hr, clearly outlines the ependymal lining of the ventricles and the surrounding tissue, suggesting that this drug first gains access to the CSF. The choroid plexus was found to be a primary site of entry of acetazolamide into CSF.

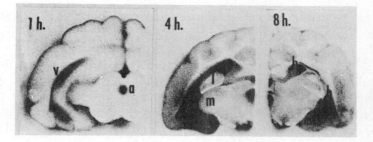

FIGURE 2-31. Autoradiograms of cat brain after intravenous injection of
^{35}S-acetazolamide. *Transverse sections from cats sacrificed at 1, 4, and 8 hr after
injection.* V *is lateral ventricle;* h *is hippocampus.* (*From Roth et al., Figure 1.*[120])

Much later, at 4 hr, the drug has evidently entered areas of the brain remote from the
ventricular borders. Finally, at 8 hr, especially high concentrations are observed
(presumably bound) in the caudate nucleus, hypothalamus, and hippocampus, whereas
drug concentrations in other areas have declined. The binding of a drug to a discrete
area of the brain, as in this instance, may not be uncommon. For example, the anticonvulsant diphenylhydantoin reaches a total concentration in brain 10 times that
in plasma water, persisting more than 24 hr after a single injection.

In these studies, the entry of a drug into brain initially by secretion at the choroid
plexus and then across the ependymal linings of the ventricles raises the question
how the subsequent passage of drug into brain structures is mediated. Does a slow
diffusion out of the capillaries throughout the brain finally become manifest, as in
the autoradiogram in Figure 2-31 at 4 hr? Or does the drug continue to enter brain
tissue primarily across the ventricular walls? Intraventricular injections of brom-
phenol blue in cats showed that intense staining occurred that penetrated deep into the
brain, even to the outer surfaces.[121] Moreover, this penetration did not occur if the
intraventricular injection was made after death. There appears, therefore, to be a
transfer of substances across the ependymal borders of the ventricles, perhaps (it is
thought) mediated by metabolically active glial cells. Such an indirect route of
entry into brain cells may explain why the central actions of some drugs may be slower
in onset and last much longer than the peripheral actions.

Factors that Determine Rates of Drug Penetration into Brain and CSF.   The very
wide range of penetration rates observed for substances passing from the blood stream
into the brain and CSF seemed to defy rational explanation and led to the convenient
but rather mysterious concept of a "blood-brain barrier." Evidence amassed in
recent years[122-124] has provided the basis for understanding how the physical
properties of each drug determine how readily it will cross the membranes that
separate the cerebral blood supply from the brain cells or CSF. In order to obtain
valid data in this field one must, of course, be able to measure drug concentrations in
blood, CSF, and brain at short time intervals and accurately. The method of determination has to be specific, distinguishing the drug from any of its metabolic products.
Otherwise, one might measure drug plus metabolite in plasma and drug alone in
brain or CSF, and thus arrive at completely false relative concentrations. In addition,
the following criteria have to be satisfied:

Protein binding.   Since only free drug molecules pass across the membranes under
study, the drug concentrations should ideally be measured in the water phase of all

tissues. Determination of drug concentration in whole brain (the common procedure) presupposes that a negligible fraction is bound, but instances are known in which binding to cellular sites is considerable. Certainly the degree of binding to plasma proteins must be ascertained; because the rate of diffusion across a membrane is proportional to the *free* drug concentration, the measured rates will be determined by this concentration, and not by the total drug concentration in plasma. At equilibrium, the concentration in CSF will be equal to the free drug concentration in plasma (i.e., in plasma water). CSF contains practically no protein, so corrections do not have to be made for free drug concentrations in this fluid. Since the fraction of drug that is bound to protein depends upon the drug concentration (p. 161), the relevant information is the fraction bound at the concentration actually studied in the experiment. If the plasma drug level falls during an experiment, the fraction bound may increase, and it is therefore best to maintain a constant plasma level throughout the whole experimental period. Obviously, binding to plasma protein should be measured at normal plasma pH and, if possible, at normal body temperature.

Ionization.   For drugs that are weak electrolytes the pK_a must be known so that the degree of ionization at pH 7.4 can be computed from the Henderson–Hasselbalch equation. The permeability of membranes to the nonionized form of a weak electrolyte is so much greater than to the ionic form that for all practical purposes the latter may be considered not to penetrate at all. This major influence of ionization is illustrated by a study[125] in which sulfonamides were injected intraperitoneally into rats. One hour later the animals were decapitated and the concentrations of drug compared in brain and in whole blood. Despite the fact that no corrections were made for protein binding or binding to brain tissue, there was a clear-cut result. For 12 different sulfonamides with pK_a's in the range of 2.9–7.8, the brain/blood ratio at 1 hr was approximately 0.1, and actually may have been 0 since blood trapped in the brain was included in the brain drug analyses. With pK_a greater than 7.8, there was a systematic increase in the brain/blood ratio, to nearly unity at pK_a 10.4. Inasmuch as the plasma pH is 7.4, and sulfonamides dissociate as acids, those compounds whose pK_a values lay below 7.4 would be largely ionized as anions at plasma pH. Sulfonamides with pK_a values much above 7.4 would be almost completely nonionized at plasma pH. Thus, the results are tantamount to saying that the sulfonamide anion did not penetrate into brain at all, even in an hour, so that the rate of transfer from plasma to brain was proportional to the concentration of the nonionized moiety. Ideally, the pH should be measured, not only in plasma but in all the compartments under study, since relatively small pH differences on the two sides of a membrane may appreciably influence the distribution ratio through an ion-trapping effect (p. 144).

Partition coefficient.   The lipid solubility of a drug plays a major role in determining the rate at which it penetrates into brain and CSF. Because the only meaningful measurement here is that for the nonionized form of the drug, the determination of a solvent/water partition coefficient should be performed with a strongly acid aqueous phase when the drug is an acid and a strongly alkaline aqueous phase when the drug is a base. If (as frequently done) partition coefficients are measured at pH 7.4, relationships between drugs may be obscured by simultaneous changes in the degree of ionization and in the partition coefficient of the nonionized form. Unfortunately, there is no way to decide which organic solvent most resembles cell membranes. In general, when compounds are ranked according to their partition coefficients in one solvent, there is approximate correspondence to the rank order in a different solvent, although minor discrepancies do occur. Good correlations with rates of passage across biologic membranes are obtained with nonpolar solvents like *n*-heptane or benzene, but ether has also proved useful.[76] The absolute values of the partition coefficients have not proved useful; it is the rank order in a series of compounds that one tries to relate to the rates of penetration into brain or CSF.

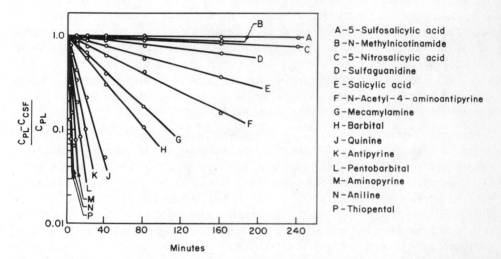

FIGURE 2-32. Kinetics of entry of various drugs into CSF. C_{PL} *is concentration of drug in plasma water.* C_{CSF} *is concentration in cerebrospinal fluid. The drug level in plasma was held constant. Note that the ordinal scale is logarithmic. (From Brodie et al., Figure 1.[126])*

Figure 2-32 presents the results of a series of experiments in which rates of drug entry into CSF were measured in dogs. The plasma drug levels were held constant by means of a continuous intravenous infusion. The data are plotted on logarithmic ordinates as the difference between the plasma level and the CSF level, divided by the plasma level at each sampling. For plasma levels the free drug concentrations in plasma water were used. A penetration process that was exponential (as expected from the Fick equation) would yield a family of straight lines with slopes representing the penetration rate constant for each drug. Conformity to the expectation is obvious in Figure 2-32. According to Fick's law, the rate of diffusion is proportional to the concentration gradient. Thus, the rate at which the concentration *difference* $c_p - c_c$ decreases is proportional to that difference.

$$\frac{d(c_p - c_c)}{dt} = -P(c_p - c_c)$$

Here P is a penetration rate constant with the dimension of reciprocal time. If the drug level in plasma water is held constant, as by a continuous infusion, we may divide both sides of the equation by c_p, as follows:

$$\frac{d(c_p - c_c)/c_p}{(c_p - c_c)/c_p} = -P \, dt$$

and integrating, we obtain

$$\ln\left(\frac{c_p - c_c}{c_p}\right) = -Pt$$

The constant of integration is 0, since when $t = 0$, $c_c = 0$, and $\ln[(c_p - c_c)/c_p] = 0$.

It follows that semilogarithmic plots of $[(c_p - c_c)/c_p]$ against time should yield a family of straight lines whose negative slopes are the penetration (permeability) rate constants. The dimensions of P are $\min^{-1}$, and the half-times to equilibrium are given by $t_{1/2} = 0.693/P$.

From experiments of this kind the penetration rate constants for many drugs have been obtained. Table 2-15 presents such data for some of the drugs included in Figure 2-32, and for others. The tabulation includes all three parameters that should influence the rate of drug penetration, if that process is purely a physical diffusion of nonionized drug through a lipid barrier: the fraction bound to plasma protein, the nonionized fraction, and the n-heptane/water partition coefficient of the nonionized moiety. In column (f) an "effective partition coefficient" has been computed by multiplying together the fraction not ionized and the partition coefficient. The observed values of P, the penetration rate constant, were obtained by considering only that fraction of drug in the plasma which is not bound to protein; the actual data showing fraction bound are given in column (b). The semiquantitative agreement between the rank orders in columns (f) and (g) is noteworthy.

Some prototype data in Table 2-15 may be examined profitably. Compounds like thiopental and aniline penetrate into CSF very quickly because they are largely nonionic at plasma pH and have very high partition coefficients. Pentobarbital, although it is even less ionized than thiopental has a very much lower partition coefficient, and therefore penetrates more slowly. Barbital, although its nonionized fraction is about the same as that of thiopental, and although it is much less bound to plasma protein, has so low a partition coefficient that its penetration is very slow. Sulfaguanidine is the extreme example of a compound whose very poor lipid solubility retards its penetration into CSF. Salicyclic acid is largely bound to plasma protein, and the free fraction is nearly all ionized; it would hardly penetrate at a measurable rate were it not for the fact that the partition coefficient of its nonionic form is so high. Similar considerations apply to mecamylamine. Its nonionized form has a much higher partition coefficient than any other compound listed, so on these grounds alone it would be expected to penetrate extremely fast. However, it is a basic compound with pK_a well above the physiologic range, so that a negligibly small fraction is nonionic at pH 7.4. The diffusion gradient for the lipid-soluble form of the drug is therefore extremely small compared with the total drug concentration present in plasma. The unfavorable ionization effectively cancels out the highly favorable partition coefficient, to yield a moderately low rate constant of penetration.

Pharmacologic Consequences of the Diverse Rates of Entry of Different Drugs into the Central Nervous System.   The most obvious consequence of the very slow rate of entry of water-soluble and ionized drugs into the brain and spinal cord is that systemic administration of such substances may be useless if the intended site of action is the central nervous system. Penicillin, for example, is a water-soluble cyclic peptide bearing a carboxyl group that is completely ionized at plasma pH. On the basis of its structure alone one would expect it to enter brain and CSF very slowly.

TABLE 2-15. Correlation of physical properties of weak electrolyte drugs with their rates of penetration into cerebrospinal fluid. The penetration rates into CSF were determined in dogs as in Figure 2-32. Data for plasma protein binding may not always have been obtained at the same concentrations used in the in vivo experiments on penetration rate. The entries in column (f) are obtained by multiplying the nonionized fraction (d) by n-heptane/water partition coefficient (e). The letters (A) and (B) after drug names indicate *acid* and *base*, respectively. (Data from Brodie et al.,[26] Tables 1 and 2 and text, and from Hogben et al.,[27] Table 3.)

(a) Drug	(b) Fraction bound to plasma protein at pH 7.4	(c) pK_a	(d) Fraction nonionized at pH 7.4	(e) Partition coefficient n-heptane/ water of nonionized form	(f) Effective partition coefficient (d) × (e) ($\times 10^3$)	(g) Penetration rate constant P (min^{-1})	(h) Penetration half-time (min)
Thiopental (A)	0.75	7.6	0.613	3.3	2000	0.50	1.4
Aniline (B)	0.15	4.6	0.998	1.1	1100	0.40	1.7
Aminopyrine (B)	0.20	5.0	0.996	0.21	210	0.25	2.8
Pentobarbital (A)	0.40	8.1	0.834	0.05	42	0.17	4.0
Antipyrine (B)	0.08	1.4	>0.999	0.005	5.0	0.12	5.8
Barbital (A)	<0.02	7.5	0.557	0.002	1.1	0.026	27
Mecamylamine (B)	0.20	11.2	0.016	>400	>4.8	0.021	32
N-Acetyl-4-aminoantipyrine (B)	<0.03	0.5	>0.999	0.001	1.0	0.012	56
Salicyclic acid (A)	0.40	3.0	0.004	0.12	0.48	0.006	115
Sulfaguanidine (A)	0.06	>10.0	>0.998	<0.001	<1.0	0.003	231

In addition, this drug is actively removed from CSF at the choroid plexus. Thus the drug, despite its general efficacy as a systemic antibacterial and spirocheticidal agent, cannot be relied upon in infections of the central nervous system like meningitis or syphilis. In meningeal infections the restrictions to passage of drugs into the CSF are often lessened as a result of the inflamed abnormal state of the membranes, but this cannot be counted upon.

The converse proposition is also true. Drugs that act upon the central nervous system after systemic administration must obviously have a suitable combination of those properties that confer ready penetration, namely, low ionization at plasma pH, low binding to plasma protein, and fairly high lipid/water partition coefficient. These correlations of physicochemical properties with entry into brain can be taken advantage of. Atropine, for example, is a tertiary amine that penetrates brain readily and has significant pharmacologic actions there; its quaternized derivative, atropine methyl sulfate, is effectively excluded from the central nervous system, yet it produces the same anticholinergic effects in the periphery as does atropine. Neostigmine, a quaternary ammonium cholinesterase inhibitor (p. 21), acts only peripherally; in contrast, the very lipid-soluble organic phosphate insecticides and nerve gases penetrate into the brain, causing convulsions and central respiratory depression as well as the usual array of intensified acetylcholine actions in the peripheral autonomic and neuromuscular systems. Norepinephrine and other amine neurotransmitters are unable to enter the brain when administered intravenously in tolerated doses.

Some drugs are virtually excluded from the central nervous system when they are administered systemically but have striking actions when injected directly into the CSF.[121] Often, these central effects are unlike any peripheral effects produced by the same drugs, and sometimes they are quite opposite. Penicillin, practically devoid of any toxicity by the usual routes of administration (except in allergically sensitized individuals), causes convulsions if brought into direct contact with spinal cord or brain. Intravenous epinephrine has cardiovascular and hyperglycemic actions and it also produces arousal; injected into a lateral ventricle, on the other hand, it brings about a sleep-like state. Tubocurarine has been studied thoroughly. In the periphery this drug causes paralysis through neuromuscular blockade. When injected into a lateral ventricle in the cat, it initiated a symptom complex that strikingly resembled an epileptic seizure in man: tremor, myoclonic contractions, loud calling, and generalized convulsions associated with spiking activity in the electroencephalogram. These effects did not occur when the drug was injected into the cisterna magna, whence the CSF flows into the subarachnoid space, indicating that the drug acts on deep structures, not surface ones bathed by subarachnoid fluid. Moreover, the discharge was most pronounced on the side of the injection, suggesting a local action on areas in the vicinity of the lateral ventricles. Other experiments localized this effect of tubocurarine to the hippocampus. Acetylcholine, which certainly cannot enter brain from the capillaries (both because it is a quaternary ammonium cation, and because it is hydrolyzed so rapidly by plasma and tissue cholinesterases), caused a curious catatonic stupor when injected intraventricularly in cats. Cholinesterase inhibitors evoked the same symptom complex when administered by the same route.

An interesting consequence of the relationship between ionization and penetration into brain is the effect of acidosis or alkalosis upon the distribution of drugs between brain and plasma. The general effect, insofar as it applies to all body tissues, has already been discussed (p. 176). Here, the practical importance is that toxic amounts of such central nervous depressants as the barbiturates can be removed from the brain by establishing a pH gradient, as illustrated earlier in Figure 2-22. If the plasma is made temporarily more alkaline than the CSF (as by sodium bicarbonate infusion), the fraction of ionized barbiturate in plasma increases and the nonionized fraction decreases. A concentration gradient is thus established for the diffusible (nonionized) form of the drug, and a net movement ensues from brain to plasma. Were the drug not excreted or metabolized, this shift would eventually be reversed, as the CSF itself became more alkaline, or the plasma alkalosis was compensated. A second and important effect of the alkalosis, however, is to promote renal excretion of the drug, since ionized compounds are reabsorbed very poorly from the tubular urine (p. 211). As the urine becomes alkaline as well as the blood, an enhanced urinary output results from the ion-trapping effect. Obviously, for all drugs whose range of ionization is near pH 7.4, alkalosis will favor the removal of acidic ones from the central nervous system and passage of basic ones into the central nervous system; acidosis will have the opposite effects.

A dramatic result of the rapid penetration of lipid-soluble substances into the brain is the quick onset of anesthesia caused by gases such as cyclopropane and nitrous oxide, which diffuse very readily through lipid membranes. A less apparent instance of high lipid solubility affecting the onset and duration of drug action is the behavior of thiopental as an intravenous anesthetic agent. Thiopental is unique among the commonly used barbiturates in its very high partition coefficient and extremely rapid passage into the brain. Its oxygen homolog, pentobarbital, has a lower partition coefficient and therefore enters brain somewhat more slowly (Table 2-15). The structures and physical constants for these two drugs are given in Table 2-16. A single intravenous injection of thiopental can produce an almost instantaneous state of anesthesia that lasts for only about 5 min, followed by rapid and complete recovery. If the single dose is made very much larger, the anesthesia will be too deep and respiratory arrest will occur. Pentobarbital has about the same potency as thiopental, i.e., approximately the same concentration in brain is required to produce anesthesia. But no dose can be found that will mimic the ultrashort duration of action of thiopental.

TABLE 2-16. Comparison of structures and properties of thiopental and pentobarbital.

	Thiopental	Pentobarbital
Structure	$\begin{array}{c} O \\ \parallel \\ HN \underset{S}{\overset{}{\diagdown}} \underset{N}{\overset{}{\diagup}} \underset{H}{\overset{}{}} O \end{array}$ CH$_2$CH$_3$, CHCH$_2$CH$_2$CH$_3$, CH$_3$	$\begin{array}{c} O \\ \parallel \\ HN \underset{O}{\overset{}{\diagdown}} \underset{N}{\overset{}{\diagup}} \underset{H}{\overset{}{}} O \end{array}$ CH$_2$CH$_3$, CHCH$_2$CH$_2$CH$_3$, CH$_3$
pK_a	7.6	8.1
Fraction nonionized at pH 7.4	0.61	0.83
Partition coefficient of nonionized form (heptane/water)	3.3	0.05

If the same intravenous dose is given that was effective in the case of thiopental, no anesthesia results. If the dose is raised, any desired depth of anesthesia can be attained, but the onset will be slow (several minutes) and the duration long (an hour or more).

At first the ultrashort duration of thiopental action was ascribed to a rapid rate of metabolism, since the drug disappeared eventually from the blood without being accounted for in the urine. Then it was found that thiopental becomes localized in the fat depots, so that after several hours practically all of a single dose is found there. This manifestation of the drug's high lipid/water partition coefficient was then made responsible for its ultrashort duration of action. However, the blood supply to the fat depots is insufficient to transfer more than a fraction of the total body thiopental there within the 5 min period that concerns us. What data are available show clearly that the rate of sequestration of thiopental in fat is relatively slow, extending over a period of hours. What, then, is the real explanation of thiopental's ultrashort duration of action?

Experiments were performed with rats administered thiopental or pentobarbital intravenously, and decapitated at 30 sec and periodically thereafter. The results, shown in Figure 2-33, were quite clear. Thiopental entered the brain extremely

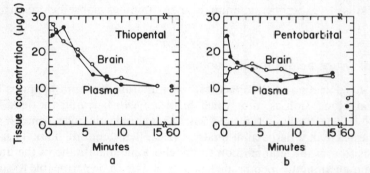

FIGURE 2-33. Plasma and brain concentrations of thiopental (a) and pentobarbital (b) after intravenous injection in rats. *The dose for both drugs was 15 mg kg^{-1}. The threshold anesthetic concentration for both drugs was about 20 µg g^{-1} of brain tissue. Each point represents the mean value for 4 male rats. (From Goldstein and Aronow, Figure 1.*[127])

rapidly, while the blood level was still very high shortly after the injection. Then, as the blood level fell rapidly as a result of the distribution of thiopental into all the tissues, the drug moved rapidly out of the brain to maintain equilibrium. The time course of this inflow and outflow of thiopental corresponded with the course of onset and offset of anesthesia. In contrast, because pentobarbital equilibrated with brain relatively slowly, the rapid fall in the plasma level was already complete by the time equilibrium was attained; for, during the few minutes the brain concentration was rising, the plasma level was falling fast. Finally, after equilibration, the rates of fall of the brain concentration and of the plasma concentration were determined by the rate of metabolism and excretion of pentobarbital. Here, since the doses of the two drugs were the same, the rats receiving pentobarbital were not anesthetized. The significant point here is the time course of the changes in brain concentration; these show why a higher dose (as compared with thiopental) would be needed to produce anesthesia, why the onset of anesthesia would be slow, and why the duration of anesthesia would be protracted. Thiopental eventually, of course, becomes localized in fat depots, but this has no influence upon the duration of anesthesia after a single small dose. If multiple doses of thiopental are administered, however, or a continuous infusion of the drug is given, then equilibrium may be attained between an anesthetic concentration in the brain and the same concentration throughout the body fluids. Under these conditions thiopental has an extremely long duration of action, and the drug effect is terminated primarily by its sequestration in fat depots, its subsequent very low rate of metabolism, and consequent gradual lowering of the concentration in all the body tissues, including the brain. The ultrashort duration of action of thiopental, therefore, is a consequence of its high lipid solubility, but only because this confers upon it the ability to enter and leave brain tissue very rapidly.

Finally, the rate of onset of barbital anesthesia presents an illustrative contrast. Although the rate of penetration of thiopental was shown to be much faster than that of pentobarbital, the latter enters brain considerably faster than many other drugs. Table 2-15 indicates that barbital has an extremely unfavorable partition coefficient, and that it penetrates very much more slowly than either thiopental or pentobarbital. This is reflected very well in its slow onset of action, which renders the drug useless as an anesthetic or hypnotic agent in man; even after intravenous administration of an anesthetic dose to experimental animals, many minutes elapse before any effects are seen.

Passage of Drugs across the Placenta

Structure and Function of the Placenta.   The mature placenta contains a network of maternal blood sinuses into which protrude villi carrying the fetal capillaries (Figure 2-34). These villi are covered with a trophoblastic layer beneath which is a layer of mesenchymal tissue and, finally, the capillary endothelium. There is also a close apposition of the fetal amnion to the chorionic membrane of the uterine wall. Isolated human amniotic membrane has been shown to be permeable to such diverse substances as Na^+, Cl^-, I^-, creatinine, quinine, Fe^{2+}, and serum albumin. In the early stages of gestation the passage of substances directly into the amniotic sac may be significant, but later the amniotic fluid is only in contact with the fetal epidermis. The exchange of foodstuffs, oxygen and carbon dioxide, and drugs must occur primarily across the placenta, from the maternal arterial supply by way of the intervillous spaces into the fetal capillaries in the villi, and thus into umbilical venous blood.

The membranes separating fetal capillary blood from maternal blood in the intervillous spaces resemble cell membranes elsewhere in their general permeability behavior. Lipid-soluble substances diffuse across readily, water-soluble substances less well the greater their molecular radii, and large organic ions very poorly or not at all. Very few detailed and systematic quantitative measurements have been made at various times throughout gestation. It is known that the tissue layers interposed between the fetal capillaries and maternal blood become progessively thinner, from about 25 μm early in pregnancy to only 2 μm at term. Permeability to sodium ions has been found to increase greatly over the same period of time, and it is likely that comparable permeability changes to other substances also occur.

The mature placenta is far more than a semipermeable membrane.[129,130] It contains energy-coupled specific transport systems for amino acids; L-histidine, for

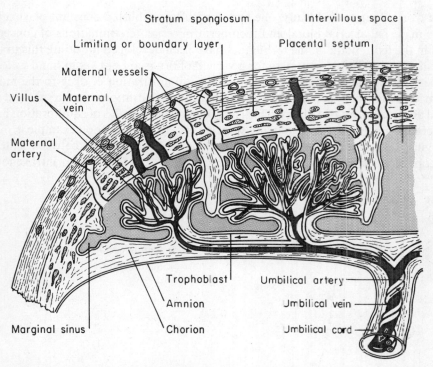

Stratum spongiosum   Intervillous space

Limiting or boundary layer   Placental septum

Maternal vessels

Villus   Maternal vein

Maternal artery

Trophoblast   Umbilical artery

Amnion   Umbilical vein

Marginal sinus   Chorion   Umbilical cord

FIGURE 2-34. Scheme of placental circulation. (*From Gray. Figure 45.*[128])

example (but not D-histidine) is transported from maternal blood to the fetal blood by an active placental transport system, by a mechanism not unlike that found in human erythrocytes; [131]I⁻ is transferred much more rapidly from mother to fetus than in the reverse direction. ^{32}P-Orthophosphate accumulates in placenta to many times its concentration in maternal blood, presumably serving as a reservoir to supply the large requirements for fetal growth. Monoamine oxidase, cholinesterase, and other enzymes are present in placenta; these may play a role in protecting the fetus against substances for which fetal tissues have not yet developed metabolic pathways (cf. p. 289). Throughout pregnancy the placenta synthesizes gonadotropins, estrogens, progesterone, and other steroid hormones. It also metabolizes both maternally and fetally derived steroids. Steroid hormone precursors are synthesized in the fetus and utilized by placental biosynthetic hormones, the resulting products appearing in the maternal circulation. Moreover, a wide variety of drugs can be metabolized by placental tissue,[131] and the placental microsomal drug-metabolizing system appears to be similar or identical to that in liver. The drug-metabolizing capacity of placenta is increased by administration of certain drugs to the mother,[132] as described in Chapter 3 for the liver.

Transplacental Passage of Various Drugs.[133-136] Study of the transplacental passage of drugs has been hampered by a number of special circumstances. Kinetic data are difficult to obtain because the fetal concentration can usually only be measured once—at the moment the fetus is delivered or (in an experimental situation) removed surgically. No methods have been developed yet for cannulating the fetal circulation in utero in small animals in a nondestructive way so that measurements could be made over a long time. Ideally, one would wish to establish a constant plasma level in the maternal arterial blood and then perform serial determinations of concentrations in the fetal blood. Some techniques have been developed for doing this in large animals (lamb, goat),[137] but data for a variety of drugs are not yet at hand.

The typical study in the human entails the administration of drug to the mother just prior to delivery, then determination of drug concentrations in maternal and cord blood at the moment of delivery. Thus, information about rates of equilibration has to be pieced together from a great many separate experiments. A good example is shown in Figure 2-35. Here, the equilibration of two sulfonamide drugs between maternal and cord blood was studied. The same dose was given to all the mothers intravenously.

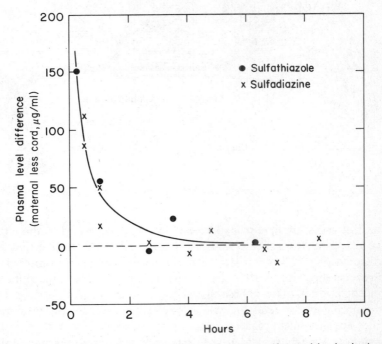

FIGURE 2-35. Maternal-fetal equilibration of two sulfonamides in the human. *Sulfonamide, 5 g, was given to mothers intravenously as the sodium salt, at zero time. Maternal and cord blood was drawn for analysis at delivery. Each point represents one subject mother and infant. Data are for unconjugated drug. (Data from Speert, Tables II and IV.[138] By permission of C. V. Mosby.)*

Whenever delivery occurred, the maternal and cord blood samples were taken simultaneously. Thus, each point on the curve represents one mother and her infant. Despite the scatter it is apparent that these sulfonamides require about 2 hr to reach complete equilibrium.

A critical comment is in order about the practice of sampling cord blood without distinguishing between umbilical venous and umbilical arterial blood, and then supposing that the concentration found represents that in the fetal tissues. When the fetus has come into complete equilibrium with maternal blood this will be true, but at all earlier times it will be false. At the outset only the umbilical vein carries any drug at all, and the umbilical artery is essentially drug-free. If the sample is taken from the cut end of the cord with placenta still in situ, it is likely to be pure umbilical venous blood, at the placental drug concentration, regardless of the amount of drug in the fetus. In general, at any time during the equilibration process, the highest levels will be found in cord venous blood, the next highest in fetal arterial blood (including cord arterial blood), and the lowest in the fetal tissues as a whole, especially those tissues with a poor blood supply. The importance of this point is illustrated by a study of the distribution of lidocaine administered to mothers just before delivery (Figure 2-36). During the first 30 min, but especially during the first 15 min, the umbilical venous blood contained considerably more drug than did the umbilical arterial blood, reflecting the dilution of the drug in the fetal circulation and the uptake of lidocaine by fetal tissues.

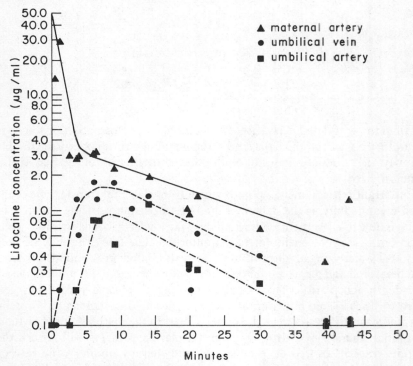

FIGURE 2-36. Lidocaine concentrations in maternal arterial, umbilical venous, and umbilical arterial plasma at delivery. *Data from human subjects following a single intravenous injection of lidocaine (2 mg kg^{-1}) in 16 mothers just before delivery. (From Shnider and Way, Figure 1.*[139])

The necessity of distinguishing between a drug and its metabolite is shown in Table 2-17. Here, sulfanilamide was administered to rabbits near term and the fetal and maternal blood samples were obtained several hours later. The total sulfanilamide concentrations give the impression that equilibrium has not yet been established, but the concentrations of unconjugated sulfanilamide are seen to be about the same in maternal and fetal blood. The experiment did not reveal why the conjugated (acetylated) product was in excess in maternal blood. It might have crossed the placenta more slowly than the parent drug because of its more polar structure; thus free sulfanilamide (the therapeutically active drug) would have attained equilibrium

TABLE 2-17. Maternal-fetal equilibration of sulfanilamide and acetylsulfanilamide in rabbits.
Sulfanilamide was administered to rabbits near term in a single oral dose and the fetal and maternal blood sampled about 3.5–5.5 hr later. Total sulfanilamide includes unchanged drug and the acetylated derivative. Figures represent mg/100 ml plasma. (From Lee et al.,[140] Table I.)

Rabbit number	Total sulfanilamide		Unconjugated sulfanilamide	
	Maternal	Fetal	Maternal	Fetal
1	26.5	18.1	15.7	14.6
2	24.7	16.7	13.7	12.1
3	21.0	12.5	2.6	2.7
4	29.2	—	9.8	6.2
5	35.2	10.3	6.3	6.4
6	11.5	7.3	4.4	3.1
7	22.0	20.0	20.3	16.9

earlier than the acetylated derivative. If a metabolic transformation proceeds rapidly in the mother but not in the fetus, and if the metabolic product crosses the placenta very slowly, the product might not equilibrate until after all of the parent drug has been metabolized.

An important measurement, without which transplacental transfer rates cannot be assessed meaningfully, is the degree of binding to plasma proteins. Obviously, only free drug is able to cross membranes, and only the free drug concentration need be the same on both sides of a membrane at equilibrium. The free drug may be measured directly (as by analyzing an ultrafiltrate); or the total (free plus bound) concentration may be measured and a correction then applied for the fraction bound, as determined independently (cf. p. 161). The extent of binding to plasma proteins is generally assumed to be the same in maternal and fetal blood, inasmuch as the protein composition of plasma appears to be the same, at least in the mature fetus. The binding of a substantial fraction of a drug to maternal plasma proteins will reduce the concentration gradient of free drug molecules and thereby diminish the rate of their passage across the placenta. It may be argued that only free drug matters anyway, since that is the pharmacologically active form. But every unit of free drug transferred to the fetus will itself undergo binding in the same proportions as in maternal blood. The fetal plasma proteins act as a sink for the drug molecules after they cross the placenta; therefore a relatively large amount of drug may have to be transferred, at a relatively low concentration gradient, in order to establish maternal-fetal equilibrium. Thus, protein binding can considerably retard the passage of drugs across the placenta.

Substances that are very lipid soluble (e.g., the anesthetic gases) diffuse across the placental membranes so rapidly that their overall rates of equilibration are probably limited only by the placental blood flow. Inasmuch as dissociation of the complexes between drugs and plasma proteins is practically instantaneous, equilibration rate would not be affected significantly by protein binding in this group of substances. For drugs transferred at moderate rates or slowly, however, diffusion is rate limiting, and protein binding can play a role.

Consider two drugs, X and Y, both therapeutically effective at the same *free* concentrations (X), (Y). Drug X is 90% bound to plasma protein [so its total concentration is $10(X)$]; Y is not bound at all. Since the volume of maternal body water is so much greater than that of the fetus, we may assume, roughly, that after equilibration the maternal plasma level remains unchanged. The net transfer of Y will be (Y) times the volume of fetal body water, and initially this will take place at a concentration gradient $(Y) - 0 = (Y)$. As for X, at equilibrium the fetus will contain (X) times the volume of fetal body water; in addition, there will be a bound component, $9(X)$ times the fetal plasma volume. The initial concentration gradient is $(X) - 0 = (X)$, so that relative to the total amount that has to be transferred the transfer rate will be much lower than it was for Y.

This dependence of the rate of equilibration of free drug upon plasma protein binding is probably unique for transplacental transfer; elsewhere (e.g., brain, renal glomeruli), the fluid on the other side of the membrane contains very little protein, so the sink effect is not operative.

Studies on fetal drug levels at various times during gestation are obviously out of the question in the human, with a few exceptions. Occasionally, data have been obtained at the time of delivery of a nonviable deformed fetus (e.g., an anencephalic monster) or a fetus killed by a drug taken suicidally by the mother. And rarely, advantage has been taken of a therapeutic abortion, usually in the first trimester, to gain information about passage of a drug into the early embryo. Under such conditions it was shown[141] that caffeine, which distributes freely into all the body water, also equilibrated with the fetal tissues when it was administered to women at the seventh or eight week of gestation.

Despite the difficulties cited above, considerable qualitative and semiquantitative information has been obtained in human and animal studies about which drugs cross readily into the fetal circulation and which do not.[142,143] Among drugs that enter the fetus at all, two extreme equilibration rates are indicated in Table 2-18. Tubocurarine, a quaternary ammonium compound that is excluded completely from the

TABLE 2-18. Maternal-fetal equilibration of tubocurarine and thiopental in humans.
Thiopental, 125 mg, was given as single rapid intravenous injection. Tubocurarine was given intravenously over a 1 min period, usually a total dose of 30–36 mg. Blood values are micrograms per milliliter of plasma. (Data of Cohen,[143] Tables 5 and 6.)

Time after drug administration (min)	Tubocurarine		Thiopental	
	Maternal	Fetal	Maternal	Fetal
5	3	0	8.5	5.5
5	2.4	0		
6	3.2	0	8.0	3.5
9	1.1	0.1	4.8	2.5
10			1.9	1.1
11	2.1	0.1	2.0	1.2
12			3.0	2.0

brain, had barely reached a detectable level in fetal blood at 9 min. Thiopental, in contrast, which equilibrates with brain as fast as the blood delivers it, had attained about half-equilibration with fetal blood at 9 min, and had reached a considerable concentration earlier than 5 min. The wide range of transplacental transfer rates is reminiscent of the kinetics of equilibration between blood and brain (or CSF). The principles, indeed, are the same, except that the placental membranes are obviously more permeable to water-soluble molecules and ions than are the brain capillaries. Moreover, as discussed in detail below (p. 205), the fastest equilibrium possible between maternal and fetal blood is a great deal slower than that between blood and brain, primarily because the blood flow to the placenta limits the rate of delivery of drug to the fetal circulation.

Of the agents (besides thiopental) that would be expected to equilibrate at the maximum rate, trichloroethylene attained nearly equal concentration in fetal and maternal blood within 16 min; other anesthetics (ether, cyclopropane, halothane) equilibrated in about the same time. Data showing unequal distribution of nitrous oxide even after 30 min are difficult to accept at face value in view of the universal finding that this gas equilibrates rapidly and completely in other tissues, including brain. Oxygen and carbon dioxide, the lipid-soluble respiratory gases, also pass rapidly across the placenta.

Narcotic analgesics have been found near equilibrium values in fetal blood plasma after several hours, but rates of transfer are not available. Some effects of morphine (e.g., depressed respiration, pinpoint pupils) have been observed in newborn infants of mothers given morphine during labor; and the occurrence of withdrawal symptoms in infants born of addicted mothers makes it plain that morphine and heroin have free access to the fetus during gestation. The tranquilizers of the phenothiazine and reserpine classes evidently cross the placenta, as judged by typical drug effects observed in newborn infants.

Steroids, as might be expected, cross the placenta readily (e.g., cholesterol, progesterone, estradiol, estriol), but the more water-soluble glucuronides of these compounds penetrate at much reduced rates. Antibiotics, including penicillin, chloramphenicol, tetracyclines, streptomycin, and erythromycin all appear in fetal blood, but rather slowly and at very different rates. Penicillin attains near equilibrium in about 10 hr, streptomycin in about 18 hr. The tetracyclines crossed the placenta extremely slowly and never reached equal concentrations, in fetal and maternal blood, but this might have been explained by the fact that the conjugated form of the drug (formed only in the mother's liver) could not pass the placental barrier. After erythromycin had been given in adequate dosage to a mother over a 16 hr period, barely detectable amounts were found at the end of this period in cord blood at delivery.

Teratogenic agents of diverse chemical structure obviously cross the placenta; numerous studies have implicated a direct action of such drugs on the tissues undergoing embryogenesis (Chapter 12). Of especial concern is the ease with which hazardous products of nuclear fission (e.g., ^{137}Cs, ^{45}Ca, ^{90}Sr, ^{131}I) cross the placental membranes and localize in vulnerable fetal tissues. Not only viruses (e.g., the teratogenic rubella virus) but cellular pathogens (e.g., spirochetes) may cross the placenta and infect the fetus.

Antibody globulins pass from the mother's circulation into that of the fetus, although slowly; but evidently some selective mechanism operates inasmuch as albumins, with lower molecular weights, penetrate the placental barrier much more slowly. More remarkable is the passage of erythrocytes in both directions across the placenta, even in late pregnancy. This used to be attributed to gross breaks in the placental continuity, but electron micrographs offer no support to such an explanation.

It is an obvious clinical fact that a mother deeply anesthetized with a barbiturate can give birth to a fairly alert infant who scores well on the Apgar test, a crude but rapid and exceedingly useful scoring system for evaluating several vital indices immediately after birth. Unfortunately, follow-up has often been haphazard, so that no reliable data are to be found on the longer-lasting and delayed effects of maternal medication on the infant. If adequate records were available, a relationship might even be sought between the extent of drug use at delivery and the overall neonatal mortality. It is clear that infants of mothers who were delivered under deep anesthesia often show depression over the next 24 hr compared with those delivered without benefit of drugs or with short-acting volatile anesthetics. "Although the youngster at birth cries vigorously and, it is true, has an arterial plasma level of thiopental lower than the mother, there is still enough drug within the child for 12 and possibly 24 hr to make this newborn infant much more drowsy than the other child. We feel that the observations at birth and at delivery do not tell the entire story.... Although you can arouse the child, the newborn can readily go back into drowsiness and practically not move for several hours."[144] The unmedicated infant, although born with a respiratory acidosis caused by CO_2 accumulation, rapidly eliminates the excess CO_2 by vigorous respiration, and the plasma pH rises to a normal level with the first hour. In the infant of the medicated mother this may not occur. With many drugs the difficulty imposed upon the infant by the unwanted drug effect and by acidosis is compounded by the absence of drug-metabolizing enzymes and by poor renal function in the neonatal period.

That a wakeful infant should be born of an anesthetized mother is not surprising when one considers what is known and can be calculated (p. 207) about the rates of equilibration of maternal and fetal tissues with respect to an anesthetic drug. What is confusing and difficult to interpret are findings indicating that fetal and maternal blood have the same concentration of a barbiturate (or other anesthetic agent) at the time of delivery, and yet the mother is anesthetized, the fetus awake. Everything we know indicates that infants should be *more* depressed than adults at a given barbiturate concentration, and should be in still further trouble because of their immature liver microsomal drug-metabolizing system (p. 289). As shown in the next section, data indicating complete equilibration of secobarbital in 3–5 min, of pentobarbital in 1 min, of thiopental in 3 min, and even of barbital (usually the slowest to penetrate cell membranes) in 4 min must be discounted.[145–147] The most likely source of error would be that the analyses were done principally on umbilical venous blood carrying a drug concentration nearly the same as the placenta but greatly in excess of that in fetal brain and body water.

Theory of Maternal-Fetal Equilibrium Rates.   The kinetics of equilibration of the fetal tissues with drugs in the maternal circulation depend upon the rates of delivery of drug to the placenta and of its removal and circulation on the fetal side, and upon the rate of permeation at each membranous interface in the system. We shall compute *maximum* rates by assuming instantaneous equilibration at every membrane, as might nearly be true of such agents as thiopental or the anesthetic gases. We shall assume at the outset that a constant drug concentration is maintained in the maternal plasma water. Later we shall postulate various rates of decline of the maternal drug level.

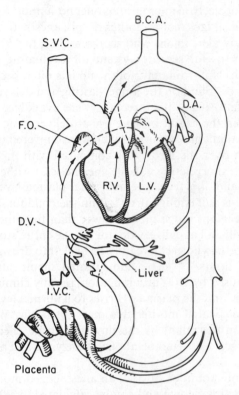

FIGURE 2-37. Plan of the fetal circulation. *I.V.C., Inferior vena cava; R.V., right ventricle; D.V., ductus venosus; D.A., ductus arteriosus; S.V.C., superior vena cava; L.V., left ventricle; F.O., foramen ovale; B.C.A., brachiocephalic artery (in man, the common carotid artery). (Adapted from Dawes, Figure 1.[148] By permission of the British Council and the Long Island Biological Association.)*

The plan of the fetal circulation is presented in Figures 2-37 and 2-38. Blood from the placental villi, which are bathed in the intervillous maternal blood, enters the fetus by way of the umbilical vein, is mixed with the venous return from the lower body of the fetus, and enters the inferior vena cava through the ductus venosus. Most of this blood, instead of entering the right heart (as it will do after birth), passes directly through the foramen ovale in the atrial septum and into the left heart. The left cardiac output supplies the fetal brain and upper extremity; a part of this blood passes into the aorta to supply the remaining fetal tissues, and a part returns to the placenta via the umbilical artery. Blood returning from the head in the superior vena cava enters the right heart. Some passes through the inactive lungs and back to the left atrium, but most bypasses the pulmonary circulation through the ductus arteriosus and enters the aorta directly. The unusual feature of this circulation is, as shown schematically in Figure 2-38, that both sides of the heart work in parallel rather than in series.

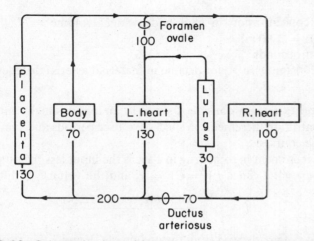

FIGURE 2-38. Schematic view of fetal lamb circulation. *This shows that both sides of the fetal lamb heart work in parallel. Approximate data for blood flow (milliliters per kilogram per minute) are shown in each portion of the circuit. (From Dawes, Figure 3.[148])*

Using the best estimates available for the blood flows and blood volumes in the human,[148–151] we derived expressions for the changes to be expected in each compartment at successive 1 sec intervals. These expressions were then evaluated by an iterative process on a digital computer to obtain the time course of drug transfer. The following diagram is a schematic representation of the placental and fetal circulations.

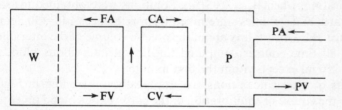

The symbols in the diagram and in the calculations below have the following meanings:

PA = drug concentration in maternal arterial blood to the placenta: flow = 8.33 ml sec^{-1}

P = drug concentration in placental intervillous blood; volume = 250 ml

PV = drug concentration in maternal venous blood draining the placenta, assumed to be equilibrated with P

CA = drug concentration in umbilical artery; flow = 8.33 ml sec^{-1} = 57% of fetal cardiac ouput

CV = drug concentration in umbilical vein, assumed to be equilibrated with P

FA = drug concentration in fetal arterial blood; flow = 6.28 ml sec^{-1} = 43% of fetal cardiac output

FV = drug concentration in fetal venous return other than umbilical vein, assumed to be equilibrated with W

W = drug concentration in fetal body water; volume = 77% of 3.5 kg fetal weight = 2700 ml

t = time in seconds

k = rate constant (sec^{-1}) for decline in maternal arterial drug level, so that

$$PA_t = PA_{t-1} - k \cdot PA_{t-1}$$

For our purposes we may consider 1 sec to be an infinitesimally small Δt. We shall solve for concentration increments in successive 1 sec periods and sum these to obtain the desired time courses.

In P, the net increment in total drug in 1 sec is the input less the output, $8.33(PA - PV) + 8.33(CA - CV)$. Since $PV = CV = P$, and the volume of dilution is 250 ml,

$$P_t = P_{t-1} + \frac{8.33(PA + FA - 2P_{t-1})}{250}$$

Since FA and CA are derived from the mixing of CV and FV in proportion to their respective flows, and since $FV = W$,

$$FA = \frac{(8.33P_t + 6.28W)}{(8.33 + 6.28)}$$

Finally, the increment in W is given by $6.28(FA - FV)/2700$, so that

$$W_t = W_{t-1} + \frac{6.28(FA - W_{t-1})}{2700}$$

When $t = 0$, then $PA = 1$, and all other concentrations are 0. The above equations were evaluated on a high-speed digital computer for all values of t until attainment of 95% equilibration, when $W_t = 0.95PA_t$. Solutions were obtained for selected values of k. Flow rates and volumes were taken from references 148–150, fetal body water from reference 151. Uncertainty about the precise volume of the intervillous space has little effect; all time courses computed for 125 ml intervillous blood are identical to those for 250 ml except within the first minute.

The results of these calculations are graphically represented in Figure 2-39. The curves show the course of equilibration of the cord venous blood (in equilibrium with placental intervillous blood), of the fetal arterial blood (such as would bathe the fetal brain), and of the fetal tissue water in general. All the assumptions on which the calculations were based would lead to an overestimate of the speed of equilibration. For example, no permeability barrier was assumed to be present in the placenta; so substances whose rates of transfer are diffusion limited may equilibrate very much more slowly than shown. Also, the entire tissue water in the fetus has been supposed to equilibrate as a homogeneous mass, with the whole of the blood traversing the nonplacental circuit, while, in fact, the poorly perfused components of the fetal tissue mass will come to equilibrium more slowly. With these qualifications we may examine the theoretical course of drug transfer.

Consider first what happens if the maternal arterial drug concentration remains constant (Figure 2-39a). Half-equilibration of the fetal tissues (shown by the curve FW) requires at least 13 min; 90% equilibration would take about 40 min. Throughout the equilibration process, but especially in the first few minutes, cord venous blood contains a much higher concentration than fetal arterial blood; and the drug concentration in fetal tissue water lags well behind that in the fetal arteries. If an

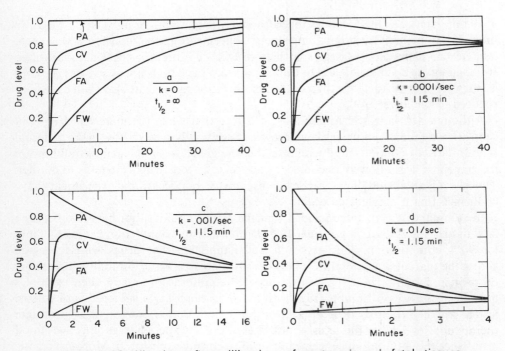

FIGURE 2-39. Kinetics of equilibration of maternal and fetal tissues. *Theoretical curves, computed as described in the text. Four time courses are shown (a, b, c, and d), representing four different elimination rate constants (k) and the corresponding biologic half-lives ($t_{1/2}$) in maternal plasma. In each case are shown the drug levels in maternal (placental) arterial blood (PA), cord venous blood (CV), fetal arterial blood (FA), and fetal body water (FW). Note change in time scale in c and d. All drug levels are expressed as fractions of the initial maternal arterial level. Absorption and distribution in the maternal circulating blood are assumed to be instantaneous.*

infant were delivered a few minutes after establishment of a constant maternal drug level, the cord venous blood would only poorly reflect the fetal drug concentration; even mixed cord blood would give a very false impression. Moreover, as long as the drug concentration in fetal arterial blood exceeds that in fetal tissue water, interruption of the cord at delivery would lead to a rapid redistribution of drug within the fetus; drug would leave organs having a rich blood supply (like the brain), which have equilibrated rapidly, and enter those of greater mass and poorer blood supply, which are still far from equilibrium. It is obvious, then, why anesthetic drugs can affect the mother and not the fetus in many common circumstances.

If the maternal blood level is falling rather than constant, then fetal equilibration is speeded; but the more rapid the disappearance of drug from maternal blood, the lower will be the actual drug level attained in the fetus at equilibrium. Figures 2-39b, c, and d show this effect quite clearly (note change of time scale in c and d). Figure 2-39c could nearly represent the administration of thiopental to a mother at delivery. During the course of the intravenous injection the arterial blood (to brain and to placenta) carries a high enough drug concentration to anesthetize the mother. Immediately after the injection is completed, thiopental leaves the circulation, equilibrating rapidly with the maternal body water, with a half-time probably not too different from the 11.5 min represented in the diagram. Suppose the infant is delivered

5–10 min later. The figure shows that although the mother's brain is still exposed to more than one-half the original anesthetic concentration, the fetal brain was never (and never will be) exposed to an anesthetic drug level. Moreover, the fetal tissue water, still lagging far behind, will accept thiopental from the fetal brain as soon as the cord is cut; very shortly, then, the thiopental concentration in the fetal brain will have been reduced to the lower level.

Although not shown in Figure 2-39, it is true that when the maternal drug concentration is falling rapidly, the fetal levels may eventually exceed those in the maternal blood. This overshoot simply reflects the sluggishness of the fetal equilibration mechanisms; it is followed, of course, by a reverse flow of drug from fetus to mother. This effect is small and of no practical consequence, but occasional experiments have confirmed that it may indeed occur.

In summary, it may be concluded that the fastest equilibration possible between fetal tissues and a *constant maternal blood level* of a drug would require at least 40 min for 90% equilibration. This makes it understandable that drugs whose passage across the placental membranes is impeded by their size, water solubility, ionization, or protein binding should require hours for equilibration; many such examples have been presented. Equilibration with a *falling maternal blood level* is, of course, faster; but if the initial drug concentration in the mother was at an appropriate therapeutic level, then the fetus is not likely ever to experience an effective blood level, since the equilibrium concentration will be considerably lower. More systematic kinetic studies in animal fetuses in utero are badly needed, as well as more critical quantitative data and long-term follow-up in humans.

DRUG ELIMINATION: THE MAJOR ROUTES

Metabolism, storage, and excretion are the three mechanisms whereby drugs are ultimately removed from their sites of action. Drug metabolism will be considered in detail in another chapter. Deposition and storage of drugs in fat depots, in the reticulo-endothelial system, and in bone play significant roles in the removal of lipid-soluble agents, colloidal substances, and heavy metals, respectively; examples of each process are dealt with elsewhere. Excretion at the kidneys, biliary system, intestine, and sometimes the lungs accounts for most drug elimination, and renal excretion is by far the most important of these routes.

Renal Excretion of Drugs

The kidney is admirably suited to the task of drug elimination.[152] About 130 ml of plasma water is filtered each minute (190 liters per day) through the glomerular membranes. Of this volume only about 1.5 liters are excreted as urine, the remainder is reabsorbed in the renal tubules. A drug will be filtered if its molecular size is not excessively large; since even some plasma albumin appears in the filtrate, most drugs, being smaller, will encounter no difficulty. The glomerular capillaries contain large pores readily visible in electron micrographs, and filtration constants derived experimentally reveal the glomerulus to be far more permeable to solutes than are the capillaries of muscle (cf. p. 165). Only free drug in plasma water (not drug that is bound to plasma proteins) can be filtered. The principles governing passage back from the glomerular filtrate across the tubular epithelium into the blood (reabsorption) are the familiar ones that relate to any trans-membrane passage. Drugs with high lipid/water partition coefficients will be reabsorbed readily: polar compounds and ions will be unable to diffuse back and therefore will be excreted, unless reabsorbed by a carrier transport system.

The kidney receives a very large blood supply (25 % of the cardiac output) through wide, short renal arteries that permit blood to enter the tissue with but little drop in hydrostatic pressure. The afferent arterioles bring blood to the glomeruli for filtration; the efferent arterioles carry about four-fifths of the same blood (one-fifth having been filtered) to the tubules, and thence to the venous collecting system. The epithelial cells of the proximal tubules are rich in mitochondria and are supplied with a "brush border" of very large area lining the tubular lumen. These epithelial cells carry on active energy-dependent reabsorption. About 80 % of the NaCl and water are isosmo-tically reabsorbed here, and so are glucose and amino acids. The proximal tubule is also the site of active secretion of various metabolites and drugs from plasma into the tubular urine. Further down the nephron, especially in the loop of Henle, attenuated squamous epithelium is seen. Still further along, the distal tubular cells again resemble those of the proximal tubule, with many mitochondria and a large luminal surface; acidification of the urine occurs here. The distal tubules and collecting ducts are sites of water reabsorption, subject to control by the pituitary hormone vasopressin (p. 39).

The renal excretory mechanisms (glomerular filtration, renal reabsorption, renal secretion, or any combination thereof) have the net effect, under most conditions, of removing a constant fraction of the drug presented to the kidneys by the renal arterial blood. A simplified nomenclature has grown up, describing the quantitative aspects of the excretory process in terms of a hypothetical "clearance" of a certain volume of plasma each minute. Let c be the concentration of a drug in the plasma water, U its concentration in urine, V_u the volume of urine, and t the time of urine collection in minutes. Then UV_u/t is the *amount* of drug excreted per minute, and obviously UV_u/tc is the volume of plasma in which this amount of drug was contained. We may imagine, then, that such a volume of plasma water was actually "cleared" of its drug per minute, and so we speak of the term UV_u/tc as the *clearance* of a drug; its units are milliliters per minute. The symbol P is often used to denote the plasma drug concentration in clearance calculations. For consistency in this book we use c for drug concentrations in plasma. Clearance is usually stated to be UV/P rather than UV_u/tc. UV being defined as the urinary excretion *per minute*.

The polymeric carbohydrate inulin (in the dog, also creatinine) is not bound appreciably to plasma proteins; it is filtered at the glomeruli and neither reabsorbed nor secreted at the tubules. Its clearance is therefore a measure of the glomerular filtration rate, about 130 ml min^{-1} in man. The clearance of glucose under normal conditions is 0, since it is completely reabsorbed in the tubules. If there were a substance so vigorously secreted by the tubules that the renal arterial plasma was completely cleared in a single passage through the kidney, that substance would serve as a measure of the renal plasma flow. Penicillin and p-aminohippurate (PAH) approach this ideal; their clearance is about 650 ml min^{-1}. Since the plasma volume is about one-half the blood volume, the renal blood flow through both kidneys, as estimated from the PAH clearance, would be about 1300 ml min^{-1}, or 25 % of the cardiac output. Of course, drugs that are actively secreted are also filtered. However, since secretion is so much more effective than filtration, it is customary to say that a certain drug is "excreted by tubular secretion" even though it is understood that a certain fraction (the *filtration fraction*, about one-fifth) is removed from the blood by filtration before that blood is even presented to the tubules.

The clearance tells us the amount of a drug that is excreted into the urine per minute, as follows:

$$\frac{dx}{dt} = clearance \times c = (\text{ml min}^{-1}) \times (\text{mg ml}^{-1}) = \text{mg min}^{-1}$$

But it tells us nothing about the extent to which the plasma drug concentration is decreased by the renal excretory process. For this we have to know the apparent volume of distribution V_d. Clearly, for a given renal clearance, the greater the volume of distribution the more total drug will have to be eliminated from the body, and the more slowly will the plasma drug level fall.

The relationship between renal clearance and the overall elimination rate, for various values of V_d, is of general interest. Let k_e be the rate constant of elimination, defined by the first-order equation $dc/dt = k_e c$. The units of k_e are reciprocal time (e.g., min^{-1}). Then

$$k_e = \frac{clearance}{V_d}$$

and since the half-time of an exponential process is given by $0.693/k$ (p. 303), the elimination half-time for a drug excreted by the kidneys will be

$$t_{1/2} = 0.693 \frac{V_d}{clearance}$$

The general relationships between clearance, rate constant of elimination, and elimination half-time are shown in Table 2-19 for several possible volumes of distribution. The fastest possible elimination half-time would be for a drug that was wholly contained in the plasma water and was cleared by tubular secretion; half the amount of the drug would be eliminated in 3 min. More usual values would lie between 13 and 44 min, depending upon the degree to which the drug had entered into body cells. The corresponding range of half-times for a drug cleared by glomerular filtration alone is seen to be 64–219 min, i.e., 1–4 hr. There is no upper limit on elimination half-times, since renal clearances may be as low as 0, and apparent volumes of distribution can exceed the body water volume if extensive tissue binding occurs. The first line of the table represents an arbitrarily selected illustration of partial reabsorption; a clearance of 30 ml min^{-1} is assumed, but any clearance between 0 (complete reabsorption) and 650 ml min^{-1} is possible.

The dependence of the elimination rate constant upon the volume of distribution is illustrated nicely by a study on the adrenergic blocking agent, tolazoline, a tertiary amine, in the dog.[153] This drug was shown in renal clearance studies to be secreted actively by the renal tubules, at a rate practically identical to that of PAH, which is cleared completely from the plasma passing through the kidney. The very high pK_a of tolazoline means that, at body pH, it is almost entirely present as the ionized moiety, and it is therefore possible that it is confined to the extracellular space, that is, to about 18% of the body weight. We can see from Table 2-19 that a drug with these properties

TABLE 2-19. Relationships between clearance, rate constant of elimination, and elimination half-time.
Entries are values for k_e, the rate constant of elimination (units = min^{-1}); parenthetic entries are corresponding values of the elimination half-time. The clearance given under "partial reabsorption" is arbitrary; any clearance between 0 (complete reabsorption) and 650 ml/min^{-1} is possible.

	Drug distributed in:		
Clearance	Plasma water (3000 ml)	Extracellular fluid (12,000 ml)	Body water (41,000 ml)
Partial reabsorption e.g., 30 ml min^{-1}	1.00×10^{-2} (69 min)	2.50×10^{-3} (277 min)	7.32×10^{-4} (947 min)
Glomerular filtration 130 ml min^{-1}	4.33×10^{-2} (16 min)	1.08×10^{-2} (64 min)	3.17×10^{-3} (219 min)
Tubular secretion 650 ml min^{-1}	2.17×10^{-1} (3 min)	5.42×10^{-2} (13 min)	1.59×10^{-2} (44 min)

should be eliminated with a half-life of about 13 min. The experiment depicted in Fig. 2-40, on the contrary, shows a measured half-life of nearly 2 hr. The discrepancy is accounted for by the fact that a large fraction of the administered drug (as shown by tissue analyses) was sequestered in liver, spleen, kidney, and other organs. The high lipid solubility of the nonionized moiety favors entry into cells, leading to a high

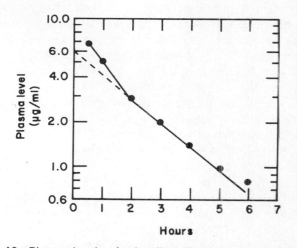

FIGURE 2-40. Plasma levels of tolazoline after intravenous administration.
The drug was given as a single injection (13 mg kg^{-1}) to a dog, and plasma levels were measured periodically. (From Brodie et al., Figure 1.[153])

tissue/plasma concentration ratio, by a principle similar to that explained for ion trapping (p. 144). Thus, the apparent V_d of such a drug is much larger than the extracellular space, and it accounts well for the surprisingly long half-life. The actual magnitude of the apparent V_d cannot be determined by extrapolation back to zero time in Figure 2-40, as one could do with the simple equilibration of a virtually closed system (cf. Figure 2-8). Here, where material is being excreted from the body at a rapid rate, extrapolation leads to serious over-estimation of V_d.[49a]

The availability of a drug for glomerular filtration is strictly dependent upon its concentration in plasma water. Meaningful clearance values can therefore not be obtained unless the degree of protein binding is determined at the relevant drug concentrations. For drugs cleared by tubular secretion, however, it makes no difference what fraction is bound to plasma protein, provided the binding is reversible. All the drug, bound as well as free, becomes available for active secretion. Then, as free drug is removed by the tubular cells, bound drug dissociates very rapidly to maintain the equilibrium with plasma water.

The tubular secretory process handles organic anions and cations by separate transport mechanisms. The group of anions has been studied most thoroughly. The process is energy dependent and is blocked by metabolic inhibitors. The secretory transport capacity can be saturated at high concentrations of the anions, so each substance has its characteristic maximum secretion rate, called "tubular maximum" (T_m). The anionic group is often a carboxyl group, but sulfones (like phenol red or chlorothiazide) carrying partial negative charges are transported equally well. The various anionic compounds compete with one another for secretion, and this can be put to practical use. Thus, probenecid will block the otherwise rapid renal secretion of penicillin and thereby prolong its duration of action in the body. Evidently, the same (or a similar) mechanism mediates the tubular reabsorption of the uric acid anion, for this is also blocked by probenecid; the uricosuric action finds some therapeutic use in gout, since uric acid excretion is thereby promoted. The normal function of the anion secretion system is apparently to eliminate from the body metabolites that have been conjugated with glycine, with sulfate, or with glucuronic acid.

Organic cations are secreted by a different pathway, also energy dependent and stereospecific. The organic cations compete with each other but not with anions. Their secretion is blocked by metabolic inhibitors, but only at inhibitor concentrations much higher than needed to interfere with anion secretion. Tetraethylammonium secretion, for example, is not interfered with by malonate at a concentration that blocks PAH secretion almost completely. On the other hand, organic mercurials (e.g., mersalyl) inhibit secretion of tetraethylammonium much more effectively than they block PAH secretion. Both of these transport-secretion systems evidently depend upon high-energy phosphate compounds, for they are equally sensitive to the "uncoupling" agent 2,4-dinitrophenol. In addition, complete, or nearly complete, clearance of these drugs means passage into the tubular lumen against a concentration gradient. Thus, renal elimination of the organic anions and cations fulfills the criteria outlined earlier (p. 178) for an active transport process.

In newborn infants, especially premature infants, the renal tubular secretory mechanisms are incompletely developed and inefficient.[154–157] Confusion is often introduced by the practice of "correcting" the clearance values on the basis of surface area. From the standpoint of drug elimination, the relevant measure is the actual clearance, relative to the volume of distribution of the drug. Experimental data on clearances in infants are presented in Table 2-20. The elimination half-time for inulin (glomerular filtration) is about three times longer in the infant, suggesting some partial impermeability of the glomerular membrane, or more likely a smaller renal blood flow relative to the body water volume. More striking is the deficiency in PAH

TABLE 2-20. Comparison of newborn and adult renal clearances.
Computations are for a drug distributed in the whole body water, but any other V_d would give the same relative values. (Data for average infant from West et al.[156] By permission of Charles C. Thomas and Cambridge University Press.)

	Average infant	Average adult
Body weight (kg)	3.5	70
Body water		
(%)	77	58
(liters)	2.7	41
Inulin clearance		
$(ml \cdot min^{-1})$	approx. 3	130
$k \, (min^{-1})$	$3/2700 = 0.0011$	$130/41,000 = 0.0032$
$t_{1/2}$ (min)	630	220
PAH clearance		
$(ml \cdot min^{-1})$	approx. 12	650
$k \, (min^{-1})$	$12/2800 = 0.0043$	$650/41,000 = 0.016$
$t_{1/2}$ (min)	160	43

excretion (tubular secretion); here, the elimination half-time is nearly 4 times longer than in the adult.

The effects of such immaturity of a major renal excretory pathway will depend upon the circumstances of drug administration. Suppose a drug that is excreted by tubular secretion is given to a premature infant intravenously, or by another route with fast absorption. If the dosage is appropriate, then the usual initial drug level will be established; the only effect of the renal secretory deficiency will be to make the slope of the elimination curve less steep than in the adult. This in itself might be beneficial, inasmuch as the duration of action of the single dose is extended. Difficulties ensue, however, with repeated dosage, for the residual drug level just before each successive dose will be higher than would have been expected in the adult. Succeeding doses may therefore build up the drug concentration to excessive levels. The likelihood of cumulation to toxic levels (cf. p. 326) will be greatly increased if the drug is one that is usually given by a slow-absorption route. Here, the customary magnitude and spacing of the doses takes into account both the absorption rate and the elimination rate. If the usual dosage schedule is employed, but the elimination rate is substantially diminished, cumulative buildup to potentially toxic levels will be inevitable. Although several of the recently discovered drug toxicity syndromes in infants have been attributed to defective drug metabolism (cf. p. 289), it is not unlikely that inefficient renal secretory mechanisms are also involved.

The acidity of the urine is maintained within fairly strict limits, usually pH 4.5–8.0. The acidification of urine, which takes place in the distal tubules and collecting ducts, may have a profound effect upon the rate of drug excretion. Since the nonionized form of a weak acid or base tends to diffuse readily from the tubular urine back across the tubule cells, it should be obvious that acidification will increase the reabsorption (and thus diminish the excretion) of weak acids whose pK_a is in the neutral range, and promote the excretion of weak bases with pK_a in the same range. What is not so obvious is that the same effects will occur even when the ionization ranges are several pH units away. This seems surprising. Salicylic acid, for example, with $pK_a = 3$, is more than 99.9% ionized at pH 7.4 and still 99% ionized at pH 5.0. One might suppose, therefore, that acidification of the distal tubular urine to pH 5.0 could have only negligible effect. On the contrary, the rate of reabsorption is greatly enhanced, as shown in the following illustration (cf. p. 144).

At pH 7.4, the ratio of base (ionized) to conjugate acid (non-ionized) is calculated from

$$7.4 = 3.0 + \log \frac{(A^-)}{(HA)}$$

$$\frac{(A^-)}{(HA)} = \frac{25,000}{1} = \frac{1000}{0.04}$$

At pH 5.0,

$$5.0 = 3.0 + \log \frac{(A^-)}{(HA)}$$

$$\frac{(A^-)}{(HA)} = \frac{100}{1} = \frac{990}{9.9}$$

	Plasma	Urine
	pH 7.4	pH 7.4
Proximal tubule	$\dfrac{1000}{0.04} \rightleftarrows$	$\dfrac{1000}{0.04}$
	pH 7.4	pH 5.0
Distal tubule	$\dfrac{1000}{0.04} \leftarrow$	$\dfrac{990}{9.9}$

With respect to the diffusible, nonionized form, acidification of the urine creates a very large diffusion gradient from urine to plasma. Consequently, the excretion of salicylate (or other weak acid) is promoted in an alkaline urine, retarded in acid urine. The opposite relationship holds for weak bases. These effects of urine pH have significant practical applications. For example, the elimination of barbiturates may be hastened by administering bicarbonate to alkalinize the urine (cf. p. 397).

Extracorporeal Dialysis

The "artificial kidney" is now widely used for the long-term maintenance of patients with chronic renal failure, or for the support of such patients until renal transplantation can be carried out. Another application is in the treatment of drug overdosages. Collapse of the blood pressure and consequent renal failure are common results of poisoning with barbiturates, tranquilizers, narcotic analgesics, and other drugs. Extracorporeal dialysis can reduce the high plasma drug level and simultaneously remove nitrogenous waste products until normal renal function is restored. The patient's blood is made to flow across cellophane membranes permeable to water and to solutes of low molecular weight. The membranes are bathed on the other side by an aqueous solution of the same ionic composition as plasma water. Thus, by simple diffusion an artificial process resembling glomerular filtration is established. Frequent changes of the dialysate bath hasten the elimination of drug from the plasma. The capacity of the apparatus depends upon the surface area of the membranes, the hydrostatic pressure difference across the membranes, the pore size, and the particular solute being removed. Substances that ordinarily are largely reabsorbed by back-diffusion may be eliminated very effectively in the "artificial kidney." Thus, a urea clearance of 140 ml min^{-1} can be achieved, about twice the normal value in man.

Several factors determine whether or not it is practicable to use this method.[158-160] Formerly artificial kidneys were available only at the larger hospitals, but technical advances have now made the procedure much less formidable; units suitable for home use are on the market. Indwelling exteriorized arteriovenous shunts made of silicon rubber tubing make it easy to connect and disconnect the apparatus as required. For the removal of drug overdoses, however, in the treatment of poisoning, extracorporeal dialysis has intrinsic limitations. A major fraction of the drug must be free in the plasma, and that portion of the total drug that is in tissues must be able to diffuse sufficiently rapidly into the plasma. The reason is that only the concentration gradient of free drug in a given extracorporeal dialysis unit determines the rate of removal from the circulation. Thus, a drug with high fractional binding to plasma proteins is a poor candidate for this method. For the same reason, significant storage of the drug in tissue depots diminishes the usefulness of the procedure. For drugs that are rapidly metabolized, so that metabolic disposition plays the major role in their removal, the artificial kidney is unlikely to accelerate the removal rate significantly. Salicylates, bromides, and the poorly metabolized barbiturates (e.g., phenobarbital) are examples of good candidates, but only if the poisoning is so severe that other methods of supportive treatment will not suffice. Ethanol and methanol poisoning are very well handled by extracorporeal dialysis; considerable acceleration of the removal rates is possible, and in the case of methanol this can prevent accumulation of the dangerously toxic metabolite, formaldehyde (cf. p. 412).

In the absence of an artificial kidney unit, peritoneal lavage (p. 397) may be employed. This technique consists of washing out the peritoneal cavity with isotonic solutions in order to remove metabolites or drugs that can diffuse readily across the peritoneal membranes. It is a relatively simple procedure, but it is much less efficient than extracorporeal dialysis.

Biliary Excretion of Drugs

A drug may be excreted by the liver cells into the bile and thus pass into the intestine.[161,162] Often the drug is conjugated in the liver first, and then passes into bile as a glucuronide, sulfate, glycinate, or glutathione conjugate. If the properties of the drug or metabolite happen to be favorable for intestinal absorption (cf. p. 143), a cycle may result (*enterohepatic cycle*) in which biliary secretion and intestinal reabsorption continue until renal excretion finally eliminates the drug from the body. Sometimes the enterohepatic cycle may be largely responsible for a drug's long persistence in the body, and a major fraction of the total drug may be trapped in this circuit. This is typically the case for some cardiac glycosides, where as much as 20% may be in the enterohepatic cycle, and the amount excreted in the feces (i.e., that portion not reabsorbed) may be as great as that appearing in the urine.

The biliary route of excretion plays a major role in the elimination of three kinds of compound with molecular weights greater than about 300: Anions, cations, and nonionized molecules containing both polar and lipophilic groups. Small molecules are, in general, excreted only in negligible amounts in the bile, perhaps because they are reabsorbed from the primary bile as it passes through the smallest canaliculi. Several findings show three distinct and independent carrier-mediated active transport processes. First, secretion into bile occurs against a high concentration gradient;

bile/plasma concentration ratios of 50/1 and higher are not unusual. Second, if the drug concentration in plasma is raised progressively, a limiting rate of drug secretion is reached, which cannot be exceeded (transport maximum) (Figure 2-41). Third, various members of the same class (anion, cation, nonionized) compete, one depressing the biliary excretion of another, but there is no competition between members of different classes.

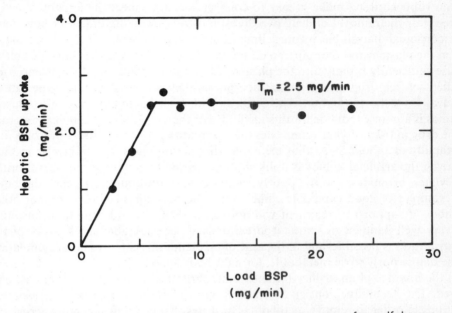

FIGURE 2-41. Saturation of the biliary excretory system for sulfobromo-phthalein. *Sodium sulfobromophthalein (Bromsulphalein, BSP) was infused intra-venously in a 26 kg dog. Plasma levels and hepatic uptake of dye were measured, and hepatic blood flow was also determined. Hepatic uptake is shown as function of varying rates of BSP presentation to liver. Transport maximum at about 2.5 mg min^{-1} is evident. (From Combes et al., Figure 3.[163])*

The organic anions that are excreted well in bile include phenol red, fluorescein, penicillin, and the bile acids. The prototype of this group is sulfobromophthalein (Bromsulphalein, BSP), which has long been used as a test of liver function. In the normal subject after an intravenous dose of 5 mg kg^{-1}, 90–100 % of the dye is removed from the blood within 30 min. The maximum rate of removal of such a dye may be depressed in liver damage, and return to normal as other aspects of liver function recover. As with renal tubular secretion, protein-bound drug is fully available for biliary secretion by virtue of its rapid dissociation; BSP itself is very largely bound to plasma proteins under the conditions of the liver function test.

Significant advances have been made in identifying proteins within the cystosol fraction of liver cells that participate in the excretion of the organic anions.[164,165] Two such proteins, designated Y and Z, have been isolated by gel filtration. These appear to play a role in bilirubin excretion, and the bilirubin binding sites may be occupied competitively by other anions such as BSP. Aquatic vertebrates that lack the capacity for biliary excretion of such compounds also lack these specific proteins. The conjugation of bilirubin and related compounds is also essential for their biliary excretion. Here the microsomal enzyme uridine diphosphate (UDP) glucuronyl-transferase is involved; its heritable deficiency leads to clinical disorders of bilirubin excretion.

There is a distinct mechanism for the biliary excretion of organic cations. Procaine amide ethobromide, a quaternary derivative of procaine amide, is a good example. The secretion of this drug is competitively depressed by other quaternary ammonium compounds (mepiperphenidol, benzomethamine, oxyphenonium, N^1-methylnicotin-amide), and these drugs are themselves secreted into the bile. Tubocurarine is also secreted by this mechanism, but not all quaternary ammonium derivatives are. Neither the small tetraethylammonium ion nor the large decamethonium ion are secreted, nor do they affect the secretion of other organic cations. Similar systems for the excretion of cations operate in the renal tubules (p. 214) and in the choroid plexus.

A major component of bile is the bile acid anion taurocholate. The bile pigments are also anions and presumably are handled by the specific secretory pathway for anions. The alkaloids strychnine and quinine appear in bile as conjugates of the bile acids, although their major excretory pathway is the kidney. The steroid hormones are partially excreted in bile, but are largely reabsorbed in the intestine. Penicillin, strepto-mycin, and the tetracyclines, as well as the organic mercurial diuretic mercuhydrin, are found in very high concentrations in bile.

The biliary secretion of large nonionized compounds is not thoroughly understood. Some molecules of this type can be conjugated to anions like glucuronate or sulfate in the hepatic cells, then transported directly across the luminal cell membrane into the smallest bile ducts; the anion transport mechanism appears to be involved. In these instances conjugation has been shown to be essential for secretion. Thus, in-hibition of the conjugation enzymes blocks biliary secretion, and animals with deficient conjugating systems secrete such drugs poorly or not at all. Many drugs and hormones, on the other hand, are secreted into the bile unchanged, despite the fact that they contain no ionizing groups. Some of the cardiac glycosides are typical. Here biliary secretion is favored by a molecular asymmetry with respect to hydrophilic and lipo-philic groups, e.g., a large steroid nucleus attached to sugar moieties at one position. Little is known about the mechanism of secretion of the nonionized molecules.

REFERENCES

1. B. N. LA DU, H. G. MANDEL, and E. L. WAY, eds.: *Fundamentals of Drug Metabolism and Drug Disposition*. Baltimore, Williams and Wilkins, (1971).
2. R. GIANELLY, J. O. VON DER GROEBEN, A. P. SPIVACK, and D. C. HARRISON: Effect of lidocaine on ventricular arrhythmias in patients with coronary heart disease. *New Eng. J. Med.* 277:1215 (1967).
3. J. BEDERKA, A. E. TAKEMORI, and J. W. MILLER: Absorption rates of various substances administered intramuscularly. *Europ. J. Pharmacol.* 15:132 (1971).
4. J. SCHOU: Subcutaneous and intramuscular injection of drugs. In *Handbook of Experimental Pharmacology*, ed. by B. B. Brodie and J. R. Gillette. Berlin, Springer–Verlag (1971). Ch. 4.
5. P. M. F. BISHOP and S. J. FOLLEY: Implantation of testosterone in cast pellets. *Lancet* 1:434 (1944).
6. C. MAGGIOLO and F. HUIDOBRO: Administration of pellets of morphine to mice; abstinence syndrome. *Acta Physiol. Lat. Amer.* 11:70 (1961).
6a. R. J. SCHEUPLEIN and I. H. BLANK: Permeability of the skin. *Physiol. Rev.* 51:702 (1971).

7. R. D. GRIESEMER: Protection against the transfer of matter through the skin. In *The Human Integument, Normal and Abnormal*, ed. by S. Rothman. Washington, D.C., Publication No. 54 of the American Association for the Advancement of Science (1959), p. 25.

8. M. KATZ and B. J. POULSEN: Absorption of drugs through the skin. In *Handbook of Experimental Pharmacology*, ed. by B. B. Brodie and J. R. Gillette. Berlin, Springer–Verlag (1971). Ch. 7.

9. R. B. STOUGHTON and W. FRITSCH: Influence of dimethylsulfoxide (DMSO) on human percutaneous absorption. *Arch. Dermatol.* 90:512 (1964).

10. R. GHYS: La résorption cutanée de l'iode radioactif introduit par iontophorèse chez l'homme. *Strahlentherapie* 105:457 (1958).

11. T. F. HATCH and P. GROSS: *Pulmonary Deposition and Retention of Inhaled Aerosols*. New York, Academic Press (1964).

11a. L. T. GREENE: Aerosols. In *Handbook of Experimental Pharmacology*, ed. by B. B. Brodie and J. R. Gillette. Berlin, Springer–Verlag (1971). Ch. 6.

12. H. P. DYGERT, C. W. LA BELLE, S. LASKIN, U. C. POZZANI, E. ROBERTS, J. J. ROTHER-MEL, A. ROTHSTEIN, C. J. SPIEGL, G. F. SPRAGUE, JR., and H. E. STOKINGER: Toxicity following inhalation. In *Pharmacology and Toxicology of Uranium Compounds*, ed. by C. Voegtlin and H. C. Hodge, New York, McGraw-Hill (1949). Ch. 10.

13. J. R. GOLDSMITH and A. C. HEXTER: Respiratory exposure to lead: epidemiological and experimental dose-response relationships. *Science* 158:132 (1967).

14. G. L. TER HAAR and M. A. BAYARD: Composition of airborne lead particles. *Nature* 232:553 (1971).

15. R. A. KEHOE: The metabolism of lead in man in health and disease. I. The normal metabolism of lead. *J. Roy. Inst. Pub. Health* 24:81 (1961).

16. G. J. STOPPS: Symposium on air quality criteria—lead. *J. Occup. Med.* 10:550 (1968).

17. F. E. SPEIZER, R. DOLL, P. HEAF, and L. B. STRONG: Investigation into use of drugs preceding death from asthma. *Brit. Med. J.* 1:339 (1968).

18. R. G. SHANKS and J. G. SWANTON: Changes in the pharmacological response to isoprenaline under conditions of hypoxia in dogs. In *The Correlation of Adverse Effects in Man with Observations in Animals*, Proc. Europ. Soc. Study Drug Toxicity, Uppsala, June 1970. Vol. 12. Amsterdam and London, Excerpta Medica Foundation (1971), Int. Cong. Series, No. 220, p. 147.

19. E. W. BLACKWELL, M. E. CONOLLY, D. S. DAVIES, and C. T. DOLLERY: The fate of isoprenaline administered by pressurized aerosols. *Brit. J. Pharmacol.* 39:194P (1970).

20. W. H. W. INMAN and A. M. ADELSTEIN: Rise and fall of asthma mortality in England and Wales in relation to use of pressurized aerosols. *Lancet* 2:279 (1969).

20a. L. S. SCHANKER: Absorption of drugs from the gastrointestinal tract. In *Handbook of Experimental Pharmacology*, ed. by B. B. Brodie and J. R. Gillette. Berlin, Springer–Verlag (1971). Ch. 2.

21. R. G. CROUNSE: Human pharmacology of griseofulvin: The effect of fat intake on gastrointestinal absorption. *J. Invest. Dermatol.* 37:529 (1961).

22. J. T. DOLUISIO, G. H. TAN, N. F. BILLUPS, and L. DIAMOND: Drug absorption II: effect of fasting on intestinal drug absorption. *J. Pharmaceut. Sci.* 58:1200 (1969).

23. R. N. BOYES, D. B. SCOTT, P. J. JEBSON, M. J. GODMAN, and D. G. JULIAN: Pharmacokinetics of lidocaine in man. *Clin. Pharmacol. Ther.* 12:105 (1971).

23a. R. E. STENSON, R. T. CONSTANTINO, and D. C. HARRISON: Interrelationships of hepatic blood flow, cardiac output, and blood levels of lidocaine in man. *Circulation* 43:205 (1971).

24. M. H. JACOBS: Some aspects of cell permeability to weak electrolytes. *Cold Spring Harbor Symp. Quant. Biol.* 8:30 (1940).

25. L. S. SCHANKER, P. A. SHORE, B. B. BRODIE, and C. A. M. HOGBEN: Absorption of drugs from the stomach. I. The rat. *J. Pharmacol. Exp. Therap.* 120:528 (1957).

26. P. A. SHORE, B. B. BRODIE, and C. A. M. HOGBEN: The gastric secretion of drugs: a pH partition hypothesis. *J. Pharmacol. Exp. Therap.* 119:361 (1957).

27. C. A. M. HOGBEN, D. J. TOCCO, B. B. BRODIE, and L. S. SCHANKER: On the mechanism of intestinal absorption of drugs. *J. Pharmacol. Exp. Therap.* 125:275 (1959).

28. A. H. BECKETT and R. D. HOSSIE: Buccal absorption of drugs. In *Handbook of Experimental Pharmacology*, ed. by B. B. Brodie and J. R. Gillette. Berlin, Springer–Verlag (1971). Ch. 3.

29. L. LACHMAN, H. A. LIEBERMAN, and J. L. KANIG: *The Theory and Practice of Industrial Pharmacy*. Philadelphia, Lea and Febiger (1970).

29a. L. C. SCHROETER: Coating of tablets, capsules, and pills. In *Remington's Pharmaceutical Science*, ed. by E. Martin. Easton, Pa., Mack Publishing Co. (1965). Ch. 40.

30. B. E. BALLARD and E. NELSON: Prolonged-action pharmaceuticals. In *Remington's Pharmaceutical Science*, ed. by E. Martin. Easton, Pa., Mack Publishing Co. (1965). Ch. 41.

31. J. LAZARUS, M. PAGLIERY, and L. LACHMAN: Factors influencing the release of a drug from a prolonged-action matrix. *J. Pharm. Sci.* 53:798 (1964).

32. T. M. FEINBLATT and E. A. FERGUSON, JR.: Timed-disintegration capsules. An in vivo roentgenographic study. *New Eng. J. Med.* 254:940 (1956).

33. P. CROSLAND-TAYLOR, D. H. KEELING, and B. M. CROMIE: A trial of slow-release tablets of ferrous sulphate. *Curr. Therap. Res.* 7:244 (1965).

34. U.S. Department of Health, Education and Welfare; Food and Drug Administration: Code of Federal Regulations, Title 21, Part 1, p. 64, para. 3.512. Washington, D.C., January 1965.

35. D. C. BLAIR, R. W. BARNES, E. L. WILDNER, and W. J. MURRAY: Biological availability of oxytetracycline HCl capsules. *J. Am. Med. Ass.* 215:251 (1971).

36. J. LINDENBAUM, M. H. MELLOW, M. O. BLACKSTONE, and V. P. BUTLER, JR.: Variation in biologic availability of digoxin from four preparations. *New Eng. J. Med.* 285:1344 (1971).

37. E. LOZINSKI: Physiological availability of dicumarol. *Can. Med. Ass. J.* 83:177 (1960).

38. J. FOLKMAN, D. M. LONG, JR., and R. ROSENBAUM: Silicone rubber: a new diffusion property useful for general anesthesia. *Science* 154:148 (1966).

39. J. FOLKMAN, W. REILING, and G. WILLIAMS: Chronic analgesia by silicone rubber diffusion. *Surgery* 66:194 (1969).

40. J. FOLKMAN, S. WINSEY, and J. H. PORTER: New method for rapid blood gas determination without blood sample. *J. Pediat. Surg.* 4:42 (1969).

41. B. H. SCRIBNER, J. J. COLE, T. G. CHRISTOPHER, J. E. VIZZO, R. C. ATKINS, and C. R. BLAGG: Long-term total parenteral nutrition. The concept of an artificial gut. *J. Am. Med. Ass.* 212:457 (1970).

42. D. R. MISHELL, JR., M. TALAS, A. F. PARLOW, and D. L. MOYER: Contraception by means of a Silastic vaginal ring impregnated with medroxyprogesterone acetate. *Am. J. Obstet. Gynecol.* 107:100 (1970).

43. A. SCOMMEGNA, G. N. PANDYA, M. CHRIST, A. W. LEE, and M. R. COHEN: Intrauterine administration of progesterone by a slow releasing device. *Fertility and Sterility* 21:201 (1970).

44. B. SESHADRI, Y. GIBOR, and A. SCOMMEGNA: Antifertility effects of intrauterine progesterone in the rabbit. *Am. J. Obstet. Gynecol.* 109:536 (1971).

45. ANON: New delivery systems may recast drug therapy. *Chem. Eng. News* 49 20 (1971).

46. A. S. LIFCHEZ and A. SCOMMEGNA: Diffusion of progestogens through Silastic rubber implants. *Fertility and Sterility* 21:426 (1970).

47. A. ZAFFARONI: A new approach to drug administration. *Proc. 31st Int. Cong. Pharm. Sci.* Washington, September 7–12, 1971.

48. S. CHIEN and M. I. GREGERSEN: Determination of body fluid volumes. In *Physical Techniques in Biological Research*, Vol. IV, ed. by W. L. Nastuk. New York, Academic Press (1962). Ch. 1.

49. P. R. SCHLOERB, B. J. FRIIS-HANSEN, I. S. EDELMAN, A. K. SOLOMON, and F. D. MOORE: The measurement of total body water in the human subject by deuterium oxide dilution. *J. Clin. Invest.* 29:1296 (1950).

49a. D. S. RIGGS: *The Mathematical Approach to Physiological Problems*. Baltimore, Williams and Wilkins (1963). Ch. 8.

50. R. SOBERMAN, B. B. BRODIE, B. B. LEVY, J. AXELROD, V. HOLLANDER, and J. M. STEELE: The use of antipyrine in the measurement of total body water in man. *J. Biol. Chem.* 179:31 (1949).

51. B. B. BRODIE and J. AXELROD: The fate of antipyrine in man. *J. Pharmacol. Exp. Therap.* 98:97 (1950).

52. F. W. PUTNAM: Structure and function of the plasma proteins. In *The Proteins*, Vol. III, 2nd ed., ed. by H. Neurath. New York, Academic Press (1965). Ch. 14.

53. C. TANFORD, S. A. SWANSON, and W. S. SHORE: Hydrogen ion equilibria of bovine serum albumin. *J. Amer. Chem. Soc.* 77:6414 (1955).

54. A. GOLDSTEIN: The interactions of drugs and plasma proteins. *Pharmacol. Rev.* 1:102 (1949).

55. B. K. MARTIN: Potential effect of the plasma proteins on drug distribution. *Nature* 207:274 (1965).

56.   P. KEEN: Effect of binding to plasma proteins on the distribution, activity and elimination of drugs. In *Handbook of Experimental Pharmacology*, ed. by B. B. Brodie and J. R. Gillette. Berlin, Springer–Verlag (1971). Ch. 10.

57.   B. D. DAVIS: The binding of sulfonamide drugs by plasma proteins. A factor in determining the distribution of drugs in the body. *J. Clin. Invest.* 22:753 (1943).

58.   H. OTT and C. SEEGER: Untersuchungen zur Frage der Germaninbindung an die Serumproteine. *Z. Gesamte Exp. Med.* 125:455 (1955).

58a. E. B. ASTWOOD: Occurrence in the sera of certain patients of large amounts of a newly isolated iodine compound. *Trans. Ass. Amer. Physicians* 70:183 (1957).

59.   J. R. PAPPENHEIMER: Passage of molecules through capillary walls. *Physiol. Rev.* 33:387 (1953).

60.   E. M. RENKIN: Transport of large molecules across capillary walls. *The Physiologist* 7:13 (1964).

61.   J. R. PAPPENHEIMER, E. M. RENKIN, and L. M. BORRERO: Filtration, diffusion and molecular sieving through peripheral capillary membranes: a contribution to the pore theory of capillary permeability. *Amer. J. Physiol.* 167:13 (1951).

62.   J. H. LUFT: The ultrastructural basis of capillary permeability. In *The Inflammatory Process*, ed. by B. W. Zweifach, L. Grant, and R. T. McCluskey, New York, Academic Press (1965). Ch. 3.

62a. M. J. KARNOVSKY: The ultrastructural basis of capillary permeability studied with peroxidase as a tracer. *J. Cell. Biol.* 35:213 (1967).

63.   H. DAVSON and J. F. DANIELLI: *The Permeability of Natural Membranes*, 2nd ed. Cambridge, Cambridge University Press (1952).

64.   L. S. SCHANKER: Passage of drugs across body membranes. *Pharmacol. Rev.* 14:501 (1962).

65.   A. M. SHANES, ed.: *Biophysics of Physiological and Pharmacological Actions*. Washington, D.C., Publication No. 69 of the American Association for the Advancement of Science (1961).

66.   E. OVERTON: Beiträge zur allgemeinen Muskel-und Nervenphysiologie. *Arch. ges. Physiol.* 92: 115 (1902), esp. p. 264.

67.   A. J. DALTON and F. HAGUENAU, eds.: *The Membranes*. New York, Academic Press (1968).

68.   D. CHAPMAN, ed.: *Biological Membranes*. New York, Academic Press (1968).

69.   D. C. TOSTESON, ed.: *The Molecular Basis of Membrane Function*. New York, Prentice–Hall (1969).

70.   W. D. STEIN: *The Movement of Molecules Across Cell Membranes*. New York, Academic Press (1967).

71.   L. A. MANSON, ed.: *Biomembranes*, Vol. I. New York, Plenum Press (1971).

72.   L. I. ROTHFIELD, ed.: *Structure and Function of Biological Membranes*. New York, Academic Press (1971).

73.   S. J. SINGER and G. L. NICOLSON: The fluid mosaic model of the structure of cell membranes. *Science* 175:720 (1972).

74.   T. W. TILLACK and V. T. MARCHESI: Demonstration of the outer surface of freeze-etched red blood cell membranes. *J. Cell. Biol.* 45:649 (1970).

75.   R. P. RUBIN: The role of calcium in the release of neurotransmitter substances and hormones. *Pharmacol. Rev.* 22:389 (1970).

76.   R. I. SHA'AFI, C. M. GARY–BOBO and A. K. SOLOMON: Permeability of red cell membranes to small hydrophilic and lipophilic solutes. *J. Gen. Physiol.* 58:238 (1971).

77.   R. COLLANDER and H. BÄRLUND: Permeabilitätsstudien an Chara ceratophylla. II. Die Permeabilität für Nichtelektrolyte. *Acta Bot. Fenn.* 11:1 (1933).

78.   E. OVERTON: *Studien über die Narkose zugleich ein Beitrag zur allgemeinen Pharmakologie*. Jena, Gustav Fischer (1901), p. 101.

79.   K. H. MEYER and H. HEMMI: Beiträge zur Theorie der Narkose. III. *Biochem. Z.* 277:39 (1935), esp. p. 45.

80.   J. FERGUSON: The use of chemical potentials as indices of toxicity. *Proc. Roy. Soc.* B127:387 (1939).

81.   T. C. BUTLER: Theories of general anesthesia. *Pharmacol. Rev.* 2:121 (1950).

82.   E. ROBBINS: The rate of proflavin passage into single living cells with application to permeability studies. *J. Gen. Physiol.* 43:853 (1960).

83.   H. W. SMITH: The action of acids on cell division with reference to permeability to anions. *Amer. J. Physiol.* 72:347 (1925).

84.   W. J. WADDELL and T. C. BUTLER: The distribution and excretion of phenobarbital. *J. Clin. Invest.* 36:1217 (1957).

85.   W. WILBRANDT and T. ROSENBERG: The concept of carrier transport and its corollaries in pharmacology. *Pharmacol. Rev.* 13:109 (1961).

86.   J. H. QUASTEL: Molecular transport at cell membranes. *Proc. Roy. Soc.* B163:169 (1965).

87.   M. OHNISHI and D. W. URRY: Solution conformation of valinomycin–potassium ion complex. *Science* 168:1091 (1970).

88.   E. F. GALE: "Don't talk to me about permeability." The Tenth Marjory Stephenson Memorial Lecture. *J. Gen. Microbiol.* 68:1 (1971).

89.   G. STARK, B. KETTERER, R. BENZ, and P. LAUGER: The rate constants of valinomycin-mediated ion transport through thin lipid membranes. *Biophys. J.* 11:981 (1971).

90.   S. M. JOHNSON and A. D. BANGHAM: Potassium permeability of single compartment liposomes with and without valinomycin. *Biochim. Biophys. Acta* 193:82 (1969).

91.   A. B. PARDEE: Membrane transport proteins. *Science* 162:632 (1968).

92.   S. ROSEMAN: The transport of carbohydrates by a bacterial phosphotransferase system. *J. Gen. Physiol.* 54:138S (1969).

93.   L. A. HEPPEL: The effect of osmotic shock on release of bacterial proteins and on active transport. *J. Gen. Physiol.* 54:95S (1969).

94.   C. F. FOX and E. P. KENNEDY: Specific labeling and partial purification of the M protein, a component of the β-galactoside transport system of *Escherichia coli. Proc. Nat. Acad. Sci. U.S.A.* 54:891 (1965).

95.   H. F. DE LUCA and J. W. SUTTIE, eds.: *The Fat-Soluble Vitamins.* Madison, University of Wisconsin Press (1970).

96.   J. E. ZULL, E. CZARNOWSKA–MISZTAL, and H. F. DE LUCA: Actinomycin D inhibition of vitamin D action. *Science* 149:182 (1965).

97.   R. H. WASSERMAN, R. A. CORRADINO, and A. N. TAYLOR: Vitamin D-dependent calcium-binding protein: Purification and some properties. *J. Biol. Chem.* 243:3978 (1968).

98.   E. W. SUTHERLAND: On the biological role of cyclic AMP. *J. Am. Med. Ass.* 214:1281 (1970).

99.   J. W. WOODBURY: The cell membrane: ionic and potential gradients and active transport. In *Medical Physiology and Biophysics*, 18th edition, ed. by T. C. Ruch and J. F. Fulton. Philadelphia, W. B. Saunders Co. (1960).

100. S. L. BONTING: Sodium-potassium activated adenosine triphosphatase and cation transport. In *Membranes and Ion Transport*, Vol. 1, ed. by E. E. Bittar. New York, Wiley-Interscience (1970). Ch. 8.

101. F. MEDZIHRADSKY, M. H. KLINE, and L. E. HOKIN: Studies on the characterization of the sodium-potassium transport adenosinetriphosphatase. I. Solubilization, stabilization, and estimation of the apparent molecular weight. *Arch. Biochem. Biophys.* 121:311 (1967).

102. L. E. HOKIN: On the molecular characterization of the sodium-potassium transport adenosine triphosphatase. *J. Gen. Physiol.* 54:327S (1969).

103. R. L. POST, S. KUME, T. TOBIN, B. ORCUTT, and A. K. SEN: Flexibility of an active center in sodium-plus-potassium adenosine triphosphatase. *J. Gen. Physiol.* 54:306S (1969).

104. J. C. SKOU: Further investigations on a Mg^{2+} + Na^+-activated adenosintriphosphatase, possibly related to the active, linked transport of Na^+ and K^+ across the nerve membrane. *Biochim. Biophys. Acta* 42:6 (1960).

105. T. B. OKARMA, P. TRAMELL, and S. M. KALMAN: The surface interaction between digoxin and cultured heart cells. *J. Pharmacol. Exp. Ther.* 183:559 (1972).

105a. E. WATSON and S. M. KALMAN: Assay of digoxin in plasma by gas chromatography. *J. Chromatog.* 56:209 (1971).

106. H. MATSUI and A. SCHWARTZ: Mechanism of cardiac glycoside inhibition of the ($Na^+ K^+$)-dependent ATPase from cardiac tissue. *Biochim. Biophys. Acta* 151:655 (1968).

107. P. B. DUNHAM and J. F. HOFFMAN: Active cation transport and ouabain binding in high potassium and low potassium red blood cells of sheep. *J. Gen. Physiol.* 58:94 (1971).

108. S. C. KINSKY: Antibiotic interactions with model membranes. *Ann. Rev. Pharmacol.* 10:119 (1970).

109. D. S. FEINGOLD: The action of amphotericin B on *Mycoplasma laidlawii. Biochem. Biophys. Res. Communic.* 19:261 (1965).

110. S. C. KINSKY, J. HAXBY, C. B. KINSKY, R. A. DEMEL, and L. L. M. VAN DEENEN: Effect of cholesterol incorporation on the sensitivity of liposomes to the polyene antibiotic, filipin. *Biochim. Biophys. Acta* 152:174 (1968).

111. G. MEDOFF, G. S. KOBAYASHI, C. N. KWAN, D. SCHLESSINGER, and P. VENKOV: Potentiation of rifampicin and 5-fluorocytosine as antifungal antibiotics by amphotericin B. *Proc. Nat. Acad. Sci. U.S.A.* 69:196 (1972).

111a. D. P. RALL: Drug entry into brain and cerebrospinal fluid. In *Handbook of Experimental Pharmacology*, ed. by B. B. Brodie and J. R. Gillette. Berlin, Springer–Verlag (1971). Ch. 12.

112. S. S. KETY: The cerebral circulation. Vol. III. In *Handbook of Physiology*, ed. by J. Field, H. W. Magoun, and V. E. Hall. Washington, D.C., American Physiological Society (1960). Ch. 71.

113. E. A. MAYNARD, R. L. SCHULTZ, and D. C. PEASE: Electron microscopy of the vascular bed of rat cerebral cortex. *Amer. J. Anat.* 100:409 (1957).

114. K. WELCH and V. FRIEDMAN: The cerebrospinal fluid valves. *Brain* 83:454 (1960).

115. H. DAVSON: Intracranial and intraocular fluids. Vol. III. In *Handbook of Physiology*, ed. by J. Field, H. W. Magoun, and V. E. Hall. Washington, D.C., American Physiological Society (1960). Ch. 72.

116. K. WELCH: Active transport of iodide by choroid plexus of the rabbit in vitro. *Amer. J. Physiol.* 202:757 (1962).

117. S. R. HEISEY, D. HELD, and J. R. PAPPENHEIMER: Bulk flow and diffusion in the cerebrospinal fluid system of the goat. *Amer. J. Physiol.* 203:775 (1962).

118. L. J. ROTH and C. F. BARLOW: Drugs in the brain. *Science* 134:22 (1961).

118a. K. ASGHAR and L. J. ROTH: Entry and distribution of hexamethonium in the central nervous system. *Biochem. Pharmacol.* 20:2787 (1971).

119. E. N. COHEN, K. L. CHOW, and L. MATHERS: Autoradiographic distribution of volatile anesthetics within the brain. *Anesthesiology* 37:324 (1972).

120. L. J. ROTH, J. C. SCHOOLAR, and C. F. BARLOW: Sulfur-35 labeled acetazolamide in cat brain. *J. Pharmacol. Exp. Therap.* 125:128 (1959).

121. W. FELDBERG: *A Pharmacological Approach to the Brain, from Its Inner and Outer Surface.* Baltimore, Williams and Wilkins Co. (1963).

122. D. P. RALL and C. G. ZUBROD: Mechanisms of drug absorption and excretion: passage of drugs in and out of the central nervous system. *Ann. Rev. Pharmacol.* 2:109 (1962).

123. D. P. RALL, J. R. STABENAU, and C. G. ZUBROD: Distribution of drugs between blood and cerebrospinal fluid: general methodology and effect of pH gradients. *J. Pharmacol. Exp. Therap.* 125:185 (1959).

124. B. B. BRODIE: Physico-chemical factors in drug absorption. In *Absorption and Distribution of Drugs*, ed. by T. B. Binns and C. Dodds. Baltimore, Williams and Wilkins (1964), p. 16.

125. P. D. GOLDSWORTHY, R. B. AIRD, and R. A. BECKER: The blood-brain barrier—the effect of acidic dissociation constant on the permeation of certain sulfonamides into the brain. *J. Cell. Comp. Physiol.* 44:519 (1954).

126. B. B. BRODIE, H. KURZ, and L. S. SCHANKER: The importance of dissociation constant and lipid-solubility in influencing the passage of drugs into the cerebrospinal fluid. *J. Pharmacol. Exp. Therap.* 130:20 (1960).

127. A. GOLDSTEIN and L. ARONOW: The durations of action of thiopental and pentobarbital. *J. Pharmacol. Exp. Therap.* 128:1 (1960).

128. H. GRAY: *Anatomy of the Human Body*, 28th ed., ed. by C. M. Goss. Philadelphia, Lea and Febiger (1966). Figure 2-51, p. 40.

129. A. A. PLENTL, ed.: Symposium on the placenta. *Amer. J. Obstet. Gynecol.* 84:1535–1798 (1962).

130. J. ASLING and E. L. WAY: Placental transfer of drugs. In *Fundamentals of Drug Metabolism and Drug Disposition*, ed. by B. N. La Du, H. G. Mandel, and E. L. Way. Baltimore, Williams and Wilkins Co. (1971). Ch. 6.

131. B. L. MIRKIN: Development pharmacology. *Ann. Rev. Pharmacol.* 10:255 (1970).

132. R. M. WELCH, Y. E. HARRISON, B. W. GOMMI, P. J. POPPERS, M. FINSTER, and A. H. CONNEY: Stimulatory effect of cigarette smoking on the hydroxylation of 3,4-benzpyrene and the *N*-demethylation of 3-methyl-4-monomethylaminoazobenzene by enzymes in human placenta. *Clin. Pharmacol. Ther.* 10:100 (1969).

133. K. W. CROSS, ed.: Symposium on foetal and neonatal physiology. *Brit. Med. Bull.* 17:79–174 (1961).

134. Symposium: maternal and fetal physiology in the perinatal period. *Anesthesiology* 26:377–549 (1965).

135. F. MOYA and V. THORNDIKE: Passage of drugs across the placenta. *Amer. J. Obstet. Gynecol.* 84:1778 (1962).

136. M. FINSTER and L. C. MARK: Placental transfer of drugs and their distribution in fetal tissues. In *Handbook of Experimental Pharmacology*, ed. by B. B. Brodie and J. R. Gillette. Berlin, Springer–Verlag (1971). Ch. 15.

137. A. M. RUDOLPH and M. A. HEYMANN: The circulation of the fetus in utero. Methods for studying distribution of blood flow, cardiac output, and organ flow. *Circulation Res.* 21:163 (1967).

138. H. SPEERT: Placental transmission of sulfathiazole and sulfadiazine and its significance for fetal chemotherapy. *Amer. J. Obstet. Gynecol.* 45:200 (1943).

139. S. M. SHNIDER and E. L. WAY: The kinetics of transfer of lidocaine across the human placenta. *Anesthesiology* 29:944 (1968).

140. H. M. LEE, R. C. ANDERSON, and K. K. CHEN: Passage of sulfanilamide from mother to fetus. *Proc. Soc. Exp. Biol. Med.* 38:366 (1938).

141. A. GOLDSTEIN and R. WARREN: Passage of caffeine into human gonadal and fetal tissue. *Biochem. Pharmacol.* 11:166 (1962).

142. C. A. VILLEE: Placental transfer of drugs. *Ann. N.Y. Acad. Sci.* 123:237 (1965).

143. E. N. COHEN: Thiopental-curare-nitrous oxide anesthesia for cesarean section, 1950–1960. *Anesthesia Analg.* 41:122 (1962).

144. P. LEIF: in Villee, ref. 142, discussion, p. 243.

145. J. FEALY: Placental transmission of pentobarbital sodium. *Obstet. Gynecol.* 11:342 (1958).

146. F. B. MC KECHNIE and J. G. CONVERSE: Placental transmission of thiopental. *Amer. J. Obstet. Gynecol.* 70:639 (1955).

147. C. E. FLOWERS: The placental transmission of barbiturates and thiobarbiturates and their pharmacological action on the mother and the infant. *Amer. J. Obstet. Gynecol.* 78:730 (1959).

148. G. S. DAWES: Changes in the circulation at birth. *Brit. Med. Bull.* 17:148 (1961).

149. C. B. MARTIN, JR.: Uterine blood flow and placental circulation. *Anesthesiology* 26:447 (1965).

150. D. E. REID: *A Textbook of Obstetrics*. Philadelphia, W. B. Saunders Co. (1962).

151. I. S. EDELMAN, H. B. HALEY, P. R. SCHLOERB, D. B. SHELDON, J. E. FRIIS-HANSEN, G. STOLL, and F. D. MOORE: Further observations on total body water. I. Normal values throughout the life span. *Surg. Gynecol. Obstet.* 95:1 (1952).

152. I. M. WEINER: Excretion of drugs by the kidney. In *Handbook of Experimental Pharmacology*, ed. by B. B. Brodie and J. R. Gillette. Berlin, Springer–Verlag (1971). Ch. 18.

153. B. B. BRODIE, L. ARONOW, and J. AXELROD: The fate of benzazoline (Priscoline) in dog and man and a method for its estimation in biological material. *J. Pharmacol. Exp. Therap.* 106:200 (1952).

154. H. L. BARNETT: Kidney function in young infants. *Pediatrics* 5:171 (1950).

155. R. F. A. DEAN and R. A. MC CANCE: Inulin, diodone, creatinine and urea clearances in newborn infants. *J. Physiol.* 106:431 (1947).

156. J. R. WEST, H. W. SMITH, and H. CHASIS: Glomerular filtration rate, effective renal blood flow, and maximal tubular excretory capacity in infancy. *J. Pediat.* 32:10 (1948).

157. W. W. MC CRORY: The excretory system. Anatomic and physiologic considerations. In *The Biologic Basis of Pediatric Practice*, ed. by R. E. Cooke. New York, McGraw–Hill (1968). Section 13.

158. G. E. SCHREINER, J. F. MAHER, W. P. ARGY, JR., and L. SIEGEL: Extracorporeal and peritoneal dialysis of drugs. In *Handbook of Experimental Pharmacology*, ed. by B. B. Brodie and J. R. Gillette. Berlin, Springer–Verlag (1971). Ch. 21.

159. G. E. SCHREINER and B. P. TEEHAN: Dialysis of poisons and drugs—Annual review. *Trans. Am. Soc. Artif. Int. Org.* 17:513 (1971).

160. G. E. SCHREINER: Dialysis of poisons and drugs. *Drug Intell. Clin. Pharm.* 5:322 (1971).

161. R. L. SMITH: Excretion of drugs in bile. In *Handbook of Experimental Pharmacology*, ed. by B. B. Brodie and J. R. Gillette. Berlin, Springer–Verlag (1971). Ch. 19.

162. G. L. PLAA: Biliary and other routes of excretion of drugs. In *Fundamentals of Drug Metabolism and Drug Disposition*, ed. by B. N. La Du, H. G. Mandel, and E. L. Way. Baltimore, Williams and Wilkins (1971). Ch. 9.

163. B. COMBES, H. O. WHEELER, A. W. CHILDS, and S. E. BRADLEY: The mechanisms of bromsulfalein removal from the blood. *Trans. Ass. Amer. Physicians* 69:276 (1956).

164. G. FLEISCHNER and I. M. ARIAS: Recent advances in bilirubin formation, transport, metabolism, and excretion. *Am. J. Med.* 49:576 (1970).

165. I. M. ARIAS: Inheritable and congenital hyperbilirubinemia. Models for the study of drug metabolism. *New Eng. J. Med.* 285:1416 (1971).

CHAPTER 3
Drug Metabolism

INTRODUCTION

Since most drugs undergo metabolic transformation, the biochemical reactions that have to be considered under the heading of drug metabolism are numerous and diverse. The main site of drug metabolism is the liver, although other tissues may also participate. A feature characteristic of nearly all these transformations is that the metabolic products are more polar than the parent drugs. This has an important consequence for renal and biliary excretion, and it may also have evolutionary significance. Substances with high lipid/water partition coefficients, which pass easily across membranes, also diffuse back readily from the tubular urine through the renal tubular cells into the plasma, and such substances therefore tend to have a very low renal clearance and a long persistence in the body. If such a drug is metabolized to a more polar compound, one with a much lower partition coefficient, its tubular reabsorption will be reduced greatly. Moreover, as we have seen in Chapter 2, the specific secretory mechanisms for anions and cations in the proximal renal tubules and in the parenchymal liver cells operate upon highly polar substances. Oxidation of a methyl group to carboxyl, for example, could make a drug suitable for the renal or biliary secretory pathway; that single metabolic alteration could reduce the biologic half-life of the drug from many hours to a few minutes. Conjugation of a relatively nonpolar drug with sulfate anion could have a similar effect. The evolutionary implication is that drug metabolizing systems have developed as adaptations to terrestrial life. Fish and other marine organisms commonly lack some of the major drug-metabolizing systems found in mammals, but they can excrete lipid-soluble exogenous and endogenous compounds directly into the surrounding water across the gill membranes.[1]

Decreased lipid solubility of a drug metabolite does not necessarily mean increased water solubility. The antibacterial sulfonamides, for example, are metabolized to more polar, less lipid-soluble acetyl derivatives, but some of these are less water soluble than their parent compounds. Sulfathiazole, for example, is transformed to acetylsulfathiazole, which is much less soluble in water than sulfathiazole itself:

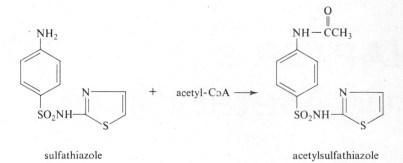

At pH 5.5 the water solubility of sulfathiazole is 960 μg ml^{-1}, that of the acetylated derivative only 60 μg ml^{-1}. The reduced water solubility of acetylsulfathiazole led to such serious toxicity from precipitation in the renal tubules that sulfathiazole was abandoned in favor of sulfonamides with more favorable properties.

A comment is in order concerning the representation of drug metabolic pathways in this chapter. All intermediates, even if they are known, will not necessarily be shown. For the sake of simplicity, weak electrolytes will be represented in their nonionized forms; it will be understood that, depending on their pK_a values, they may actually be ionized to a substantial degree at physiologic pH.

Sometimes a polar drug yields a less polar product. An example is the deacetylation of acetanilid to aniline, to be discussed shortly. Another example is the reduction of the hypnotic drug chloral hydrate to the pharmacologically active trichloroethanol, with the participation of the reduced form of nicotinamide adenine dinucleotide (NADH):

$$
\begin{array}{c}
\text{H} \\
| \\
Cl_3C-C-OH + NADH + H^+ \longrightarrow Cl_3C-C-OH + NAD^+ + H_2O \\
| \\
OH
\end{array}
\qquad
\begin{array}{c}
\text{H} \\
| \\
\\
| \\
\text{H}
\end{array}
$$

chloral hydrate   trichloroethanol

Usually, however, the same enzyme (alcohol dehydrogenase) would mediate the oxidation of an alcohol to a more polar aldehyde, passing electrons to NAD$^+$, the reverse of the reaction shown here.[2,3]

Although the duration of drug action tends to be shortened by metabolic transformation, as described above, it is not correct to think of drug metabolism as "detoxication." Very frequently, the metabolic product has greater biologic activity than the drug itself. Indeed, the desirable pharmacologic actions of some drugs are wholly attributable to their metabolites, the drugs themselves being inert; and likewise the toxic side effects of some drugs may be due in whole or in part to metabolic products.

Some typical and atypical features of drug metabolism are illustrated in Figure 3-1. Acetophenetidin (phenacetin) and acetanilid are mild analgesic and antipyretic agents that have been in clinical use for over half a century. Studies within recent years have revealed that both compounds are transformed in the body to a more polar metabolite, p-hydroxyacetanilid (acetaminophen).[4,5] As shown in the figure, acetanilid undergoes hydroxylation at the para position on the benzene ring, whereas acetophenetidin undergoes O-dealkylation.

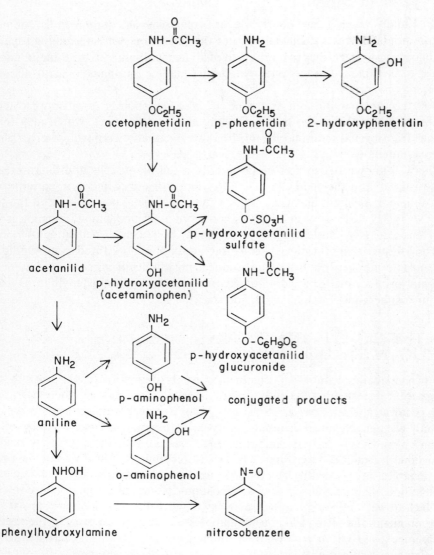

FIGURE 3-1. Metabolism of acetanilid and acetophenetidin.

The major metabolite, acetaminophen, is an antipyretic analgesic in its own right. It was possible, therefore, that this metabolite was the only active compound, and that the two older, established drugs were inert. This has been tested by inhibiting the metabolism of acetophenetidin by means of SKF 525A (p. 267). The results indicated that the unmetabolized acetophenetidin did have antipyretic activity.[6]

The further metabolism of acetaminophen entails typical conjugation reactions, yielding a sulfate ester and a glucuronide, both highly polar compounds. The conjugates appear in the urine and are pharmacologically inert. When a dose of acetanilid is given to a person, the successive metabolites peak and decay in the plasma sequentially. During the first hour, acetanilid is the principal plasma component. In the second hour, as the acetanilid level falls, the acetaminophen concentration reaches a peak. Finally, after a few hours, the principal plasma component is conjugated acetaminophen. This sequence illustrates the importance of determining separately the plasma concentrations of a drug and of all its metabolites, if meaningful information is to be obtained, since some metabolites may be pharmacologically active and some may be inert.

Both acetophenetidin and acetanilid are also metabolized to a minor extent by deacetylation of the amino group, yielding aniline derivatives, which may then be further transformed to aminophenols (that are eventually conjugated) or to phenylhydroxylamine.

The well-known toxic effect of acetanilid on red blood cells affords an excellent illustration of how the main pharmacologic action of a drug and its apparent toxicity may inhere in different chemical entities, the one a metabolic product of the other. After ordinary doses of acetanilid a small amount of methemoglobinemia is often seen, and after large doses of the drug there may be extensive methemoglobin formation and destruction of erythrocytes. This toxic action is not caused by acetanilid itself or by acetaminophen, but by aniline produced metabolically in the body. Aniline itself does not produce methemoglobin in vitro, but its metabolites, phenylhydroxylamine and nitrosobenzene (Figure 3-1), can do so.[7]

METHODS OF STUDYING DRUG METABOLISM

The principal aim in studies of drug metabolism is to identify the pathways by which drugs are transformed in the body, and to ascertain quantitatively the importance of each pathway and intermediate. Since a metabolite generally differs from its precursor by only a single chemical grouping, a typical pathway consists of a series of compounds very closely related chemically and therefore difficult to assay individually by ordinary chemical procedures. The newest technology, based on mass spectrometry, enables one to identify metabolites rapidly and with certainty in a single step; this method will be discussed later in the chapter. Sometimes a metabolic conversion can be followed directly in biologic material by virtue of some unique property of the drug or metabolite. Ring scission may abolish an absorption peak in the visible or ultraviolet spectrum; or removal of an amino group may abolish reactivity in a color reaction such as the ninhydrin reaction. Usually, however, some procedure is needed first, to separate the metabolites from each other and from the parent drug. Once separated, the various compounds can be measured by a relatively nonspecific procedure like ultraviolet spectrophotometry. The most useful methods for separating metabolites are based upon differences in their polarities and charges, which determine their relative hydrophilic or lipophilic properties. These characteristics usually change in a systematic way through a metabolic sequence.

Separation of Metabolites

Solvent extraction[8,12] is the simplest of the procedures. If the compound to be separated is a lipid-soluble base, it can be extracted from an alkaline aqueous solution into an organic solvent, because in alkali its ionization (which would make it water soluble) is suppressed. Also, a lipid-soluble acid can be extracted from acid solution into an organic solvent.

What is an appropriate organic solvent? Solvents can be arranged according to their dielectric constant; for example, heptane–benzene–chloroform–isobutanol is a series with increasing polarizability. Heptane is a pure hydrocarbon that will extract none but the most lipid-soluble, nonpolar substances. Isobutanol, on the other hand, although not as polar as water, will nevertheless extract many polar compounds that would not be extracted into heptane. Since compounds that are extractable from an aqueous phase by a nonpolar solvent are also extractable by the more polar ones, the analyst usually chooses the least polar solvent that will extract the compound he is interested in. In this way he increases the specificity of the method, and he will also be less likely to extract extraneous substances that might interfere with the subsequent assay procedure. Useful lists of solvents, arranged according to dielectric constant, have been published.[9]

Assume that drug A is metabolized to B, which in turn is conjugated, forming a product C, and that the usual order applies—B more polar than A, and C more polar than B. Suppose further that the method of assay cannot distinguish between these three compounds, so that we have to depend entirely upon a separation based on differences in partition coefficient to determine how much of each is present. First, we assay for A in a heptane extract prepared under conditions known to extract A, and only A, essentially completely. Then we might extract another sample with chloroform, under conditions that will extract A and B both, and determine A + B; subtracting the known amount of A gives the amount of B. Finally, another sample could be hydrolyzed under conditions known to release the conjugated group. Extraction with chloroform would then yield A + B + C, and by difference, C. It is noteworthy that in this procedure the solvent extractions based upon partition coefficients are sufficiently selective so that a nonspecific reaction can be used for the quantitative determinations.

The pathways illustrated in Figure 3-1 were worked out in much this way. The problem was to estimate the amounts of acetanilid, *p*-hydroxyacetanilid, conjugated *p*-hydroxyacetanilid, and aniline when all of these were present in blood, tissue, or urine. Aniline alone is extracted into benzene from an alkaline solution; it can be returned to an aqueous phase merely by shaking the benzene solution with $0.1N$ HCl. Aniline is determined in the acid solution by reacting it with nitrous acid to form a diazonium salt, which then couples readily with an amine (*N*-(1-naphthyl)-ethylenediamine), forming an azo dye, a method applicable to many aromatic amines.[10]

Acetanilid is not extracted into benzene, but can be extracted from an alkaline solution into the more polar solvent ethylene dichloride together with any aniline that may be present. After re-extraction into acid, heating will hydrolyze the *N*-acetyl bond, and the resulting aniline (that originally present plus that produced by hydrolysis) can be assayed as before. The other compounds can be assayed by similar manipulations.

Partition coefficients may be used for identification as well as for separation. How do we know that what we assay and call "aniline" in biologic material is really aniline? One could actually isolate and crystallize the substance, or a derivative, determine its melting point, infrared spectrum, and so on, but such procedures are very costly in time and effort, especially if the quantities are small. Presumptive evidence of identity is behavior identical to that of an authentic standard in various tests. For example, the substance isolated from biologic material could be compared with authentic aniline by measuring its benzene/water partition coefficient at different pH values.

Procedures like this, however, have been rendered largely obsolete by thin-layer chromatography, gas chromatography, and mass spectrometry, discussed below.

Countercurrent distribution[11] is a powerful application of the principle of differential migration, in this case liquid-liquid differential migration. At the outset, a series of tubes is set up, each containing the same volume of an aqueous buffer, and the mixture to be separated is introduced into the first tube. A volume of an organic solvent, immiscible with water, is shaken with the first tube, then transferred to the second, and a fresh volume of the organic solvent is added to the first tube. After equilibration of tubes 1 and 2, the organic upper layer of each is passed on to the next tube in sequence, fresh solvent is added to tube 1, and so on. The effect is to make the aqueous and organic phases "flow" in opposite directions. The actual successive transfers are performed simultaneously and automatically for the entire series of tubes, which may number in the hundreds when a high resolution is to be achieved. Solutes will distribute at each extraction according to their partition coefficients; the more lipophilic compounds will be carried rather quickly to the farthest tubes in the series, while hydrophilic compounds lag behind. The larger the number of extractions, the more efficiently can compounds with rather close partition coefficients be separated from each other. The precise distribution of material in the tubes can be predicted mathematically,[12] so one can compute the number of transfers required to separate two or more metabolites with known partition coefficients. Countercurrent distribution has been largely superseded by less cumbersome methods such as thin-layer, gas, or high-pressure liquid chromatography, but it remains useful as a preparative procedure, when large amounts of the separated compounds are desired.

Chromatography is a general term describing the separation of compounds by differential migration between a fixed and a mobile phase. Adsorption chromatography is similar in principle to countercurrent distribution, with a fixed column of alumina or silica gel instead of the organic phase. The surface properties of such materials favor the binding of organic molecules by van der Waals forces, ionic bonds, or hydrogen bonds. The mobile phase containing the mixture to be separated flows through the column, and compounds are retarded according to their tendency to interact with the gel or other matrix material in preference to solvent molecules. Selective elution of individual compounds may be obtained by manipulating such variables as pH, salt concentration, solvent polarity, and temperature.

Paper chromatography is an application of liquid-liquid differential migration in which an organic solvent front moves over a hydrated paper. Solutes are partitioned continuously between the phases, and thus the rate of migration is positively correlated with the organic solvent/water partition coefficient. In some instances the paper serves as more than an inert support; it contributes adsorption properties, as described above. A typical application to the separation of drug metabolites is shown in Figure 3-2. A dog was given pentobarbital labeled with ^{14}C. The urine was concentrated, and a sample was chromatographed on filter paper. The dried chromatogram was placed against a sheet of photographic film, and after sufficient exposure the film was developed. Dark areas result from ^{14}C disintegrations. Evidently, at least nine metabolic products of pentobarbital were separated in this system. Paper chromatography is very convenient, but it is not suitable for handling large quantities. The procedure is most useful for establishing a presumptive identification. If

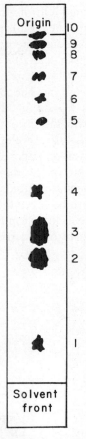

FIGURE 3-2. Separation of metabolites of ^{14}C-pentobarbital by paper
chromatography and radioautography. *The urine of a dog given pentobarbital-
2-^{14}C was chromatographed in a butanol–ammonia system. Solvent movement was
downward. Component 1 is unaltered pentobarbital. Nine metabolites, all more polar
(and therefore moving less rapidly), are shown in the radioautogram. (From Titus and
Weiss, Figure 2.[13])*

"apparent" and authentic compounds behave identically in several different solvent
systems, they may be presumed to be identical.

Thin-layer chromatography[14–17] is a form of adsorption chromatography in which a
slurry of an adsorbent like silica gel is spread over a glass plate or a plastic film and
dried. Then the sample is spotted at one end and the plate is placed vertically with its
end immersed in a shallow layer of a suitable solvent. The solvent rises by capillary
action, and the various components in the sample distribute themselves along the
plate according to their relative interactions with the adsorbent and the solvent. The
procedure is quite rapid, often being completed in less than an hour. After the plate
has been dried, the resolved spots can be visualized by indicator sprays, ultraviolet
absorption, or fluorescence; or radioactivity can be measured in appropriate ways.
The procedure is popular because of its speed, and because the separated compounds
can be recovered by simply scraping the adsorbent from the plate. Thin-layer chromatography has largely supplanted paper chromatography.

Gas chromatography[17,18] (gas-liquid chromatography, GLC) uses a nonvolatile liquid film as stationary phase, while the mobile phase is a carrier gas like nitrogen or helium. The liquid film may be coated on the walls of a long capillary tube, or on a column bed containing an inert support material of large surface area. Any compound having a significant vapor pressure in the temperature range available ($-70°$ to $400°$) can be partitioned in such a system. The materials to be resolved, in an appropriate solvent, are injected into the gas stream. They are retarded to varying extents, depending on their interaction with the liquid phase. The time from injection to emergence at a detector (the *retention time*) is characteristic of each compound, much as Rf values would be in thin-layer or paper chromatography. A wide choice of stationary phases is available, some of the most useful being silicone derivatives. Choice of column temperature, gas phase, liquid phase, and detector system is largely empirical, but broad guidelines have been established.[19-21]

A simple example of the use of GLC in a drug metabolism study is shown in Figure 3-3. Here it was shown that dogs breathing carbon tetrachloride metabolized a very

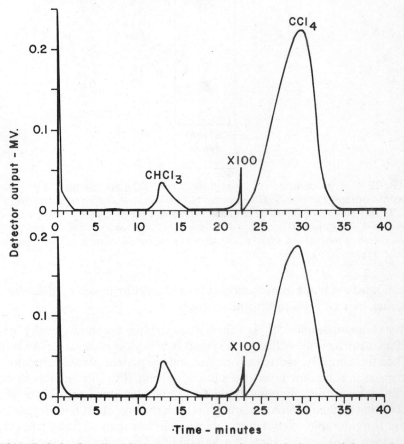

FIGURE 3-3. Gas-liquid chromatography of expired air containing carbon tetrachloride and a metabolite. *Lower record: Distillate from a solvent through which passed expired air of a dog that had received CCl_4. Upper record: Known mixture of CCl_4 and $CHCl_3$ in the ratio 3000:1. Note change of sensitivity of detector by a factor of 100 just before emergence of CCl_4 from columns. The solvent (trimethylpentane) had a retention time of 68 min. (From Butler, Figure 2.[22])*

small amount of the agent to chloroform. Expired air was passed through a trapping solvent at low temperature, the halogenated compounds were concentrated by distillation, and a small sample was introduced into a column of hexadecane on crushed firebrick. The column was operated at 40°, using a hot wire thermal conductivity detector and helium as carrier gas. The result is shown in the lower record; a small peak is observed with a shorter retention time than the major component. In the upper record an identical result is shown with a synthetic mixture of 1 part chloroform to 3000 parts carbon tetrachloride. In this instance, identification of the metabolite as chloroform rested on the identical retention times of the presumptive and known materials, and the fact that closely related derivatives had entirely different retention times. In more complicated cases, additional proofs of identity would be required. As in all chromatographic separations, if a completely unknown peak is observed, it can only be identified—even presumptively—by guessing at what compound it might be, and testing an authentic sample of that compound, to see if an identical retention time is obtained.

High-pressure liquid chromatography[23] is a refinement of simple column chromatography, incorporating some features of gas chromatography. The column bed is composed of extremely small particles (e.g., 5–10 μm) coated with a thin layer of adsorbent. A liquid solvent is forced to flow through the column by a pump at high pressure. Separations can be obtained, at high resolving power, within a few minutes. Effluent fractions can be collected for analysis, or an automatic detector can be inserted into the effluent stream. Figure 3-4 presents an early example of the application of this procedure, which will obviously find increasing application in studies of drug metabolism. Important advantages in addition to speed and high resolving power are the ability to analyze compounds of low vapor pressure (high molecular weight) and those that would be destroyed by heat. One can use gradient elution with different solvents, to achieve separations of substances with very different polarities in the same run.

Methods of separation based on electric charge include paper and gel electrophoresis and ion exchange chromatography. In *electrophoresis* the mixture to be separated is placed on a paper strip or a gel saturated with buffer at an appropriate pH. A voltage is applied and each compound then migrates toward anode or cathode at a rate proportional to its charge. *Ion exchange chromatography* employs resins carrying fixed anionic (carboxyl or sulfate) or cationic (amine or quaternary ammonium) groups. The resin is usually packed into a column and the material to be resolved is applied at the top. Compounds that carry an opposite charge will be retained on the column. To elute, the pH can be changed so as to suppress the ionization of the adsorbed compound or of the resin. Alternatively, an ion of the same charge may be used to displace the adsorbed compound competitively; for example, to separate cations on an anionic ("cation exchange") resin, elution might be accomplished with increasing concentrations of Na^+ or K^+ as salts, or H^+ as mineral acid. As the concentration of eluting cations increased (either stepwise or by a continuous gradient), more weakly charged cations would be displaced first, more strongly charged ones later, and an elution pattern could be obtained with the aid of a fraction collector. Figure 3-5 is an example of a chromatographic separation on an anion exchange resin. The pyrimidine analog 5-fluorouracil was incubated with Ehrlich ascites cells. Metabolic products were separated by applying an extract to the column and eluting with increasing concentrations of formate ion. First to emerge were the least acidic

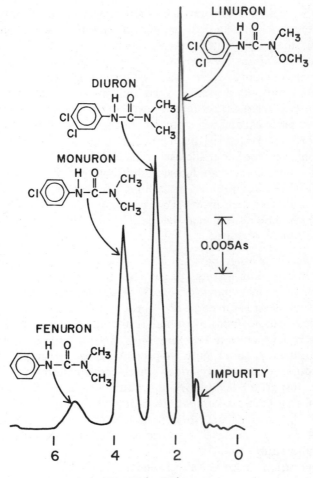

FIGURE 3-4. High-pressure liquid chromatogram of a mixture of urea herbicides. *Peak intensities represent optical densities in the ultraviolet region. Mobile phase was dibutyl ether. Note rapidity of the separation and sharp resolution of the peaks. (From Done et al., Figure 1.[23])*

products—the pyrimidine bases and nucleosides. Next, in order, were the nucleoside mono-, di-, and triphosphates. This procedure resolved at least 19 different ultraviolet-absorbing compounds, and 6 major metabolites derived from the radioactive fluorouracil. Methods based upon ion exchange columns are obviously useful for identification and quantitative assay of metabolites (as in this example) because of their high resolving power. They are also suitable for preparative procedures because columns can be adapted to handling large amounts of material.

Detection, Identification, and Quantitative Estimation of Metabolites

After metabolites have been separated, the procedures used most often for quantitative estimation are spectrophotometry, fluorometry, and the measurement of radioactivity.

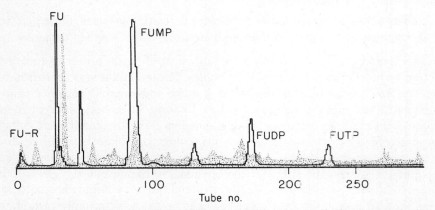

FIGURE 3-5. Separation of metabolites of fluorouracil-2-^{14}C on an anion exchange resin. *Labeled 5-fluorouracil was incubated with Ehrlich ascites cells. After 90 min the cells were harvested, and acid-soluble components were placed on an anion exchange (Dowex-1) column, then progressively eluted with increasing concentrations of formate. Stippled pattern represents optical density at 260 mµ (i.e., purines and pyrimidines and their derivatives); solid lines represent radioactivity (i.e., substances derived from the fluorouracil). FU, Fluorouracil; FU-R, fluorouracil riboside; FUMP, fluorouridylic acid; FUDP, fluorouridine diphosphate; FUTP, fluorouridine triphosphate. (From Chaudhuri et al., Chart 8.*[26] *By permission of the American Chemical Society.)*

Mass spectrometry is being used increasingly for detection, identification, and assay. Biologic assays may also be employed (cf. p. 737).

Spectrophotometry[24,25] depends upon measuring the absorption of light at a specified wavelength, usually the absorption maximum for the compound in question, and relating the optical density to the concentration. Sometimes a drug or its metabolite is intensely colored or has a very strong absorption peak in the ultraviolet range, so that it can be assayed directly in urine, plasma, or tissue extracts. Often a direct determination of optical density can be carried out after the removal of interfering substances of biologic origin by means of solvent extraction or other separative procedures. Sometimes the compound of interest has to be treated first with a reagent in order to form a light-absorbing product, which can then be measured. Infrared spectrometry, like nuclear magnetic resonance spectrometry, has not been useful primarily for quantitative assay, but rather for yielding a wealth of detailed chemical information relating to molecular structure of pure compounds.

Fluorometry[26] has proved especially useful in studies of drug metabolism because slight metabolic alterations can produce major changes in the fluorescence spectrum, the activation spectrum, or both. The method depends upon the ability of certain molecules to absorb light at one wavelength and re-emit the energy as light at another (longer) wavelength. It is inherently more sensitive than spectrophotometry because, in measuring light emitted from a sample, the sensitivity is limited only by the capabilities of the photomultiplier devices, and the "blank" is practically dark. In spectrophotometry, the assay depends upon accurate measurement of the fraction of incident light that is absorbed; at low concentration of absorbing material, this measurement of a small difference becomes increasingly imprecise. Use of the double-monochromator spectrophotofluorometer permits a high degree of specificity in the fluorometric assay; compounds not activated at the chosen activating wavelength or that do not emit at the chosen fluorescence wavelength are simply "not seen" in the assay.

Mass spectrometry[27-29] is proving to be an extraordinarily powerful tool for the detection and identification of drug metabolites. The method is very sensitive, so that extremely small quantities of substances can be measured. Norepinephrine and dopamine, for example, in amounts below 1 pmole, have been assayed in tissue samples of 0.1 mg.[30] In addition to high sensitivity, the outstanding advantage of mass spectrometry is that structures of metabolites can often be deduced directly from the mass spectra of their ion fragments, without the need for pure reference compounds. The mass spectrometer can be linked to the output of a gas chromatographic column or (possibly in the future) to a high-pressure liquid chromatographic column, and to a computer (as described below), to yield virtually instantaneous assays of drugs and their metabolites in tissues or excreta.

The sample is placed in a vacuum chamber, where it is vaporized in an electron beam. A number of products are formed, including molecular cations formed by loss of electrons; these immediately fragment into smaller ions in a manner determined by the chemical structure of each molecule. These various ions are accelerated and then sorted according to their mass-to-charge (m/e) ratios by an electromagnetic field. The resulting fan of ion trajectories can impinge on a photographic plate, or by systematically varying the field, one after another of the ion species can be focused upon a fixed photomultiplier detector. The photomultiplier tubes have very rapid responses, so that a complete mass spectrum takes less than a second. Thus, mass spectra can be obtained as fast as compounds emerge from a chromatographic column.

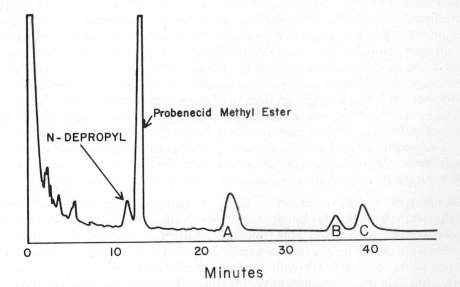

FIGURE 3-6. Gas-liquid chromatogram of probenecid methyl ester and its metabolites. *Probenecid was given to rats. Bile was treated with diazomethane to convert —COOH groups to methyl esters, then with β-glucuronidase to hydrolyze conjugates. Probenecid methyl ester and its N-depropyl derivative emerged at 13 and 12 min, respectively. Three unknown metabolites are designated A, B, and C. (From Guarino and Fales, Figure 4.[29])*

The effluent from a GLC column is composed of carrier gas at atmospheric pressure, whereas the ionization chamber of the mass spectrometer operates at high vacuum. Some device is therefore required to match the two devices. One such is a silicone membrane that permits organic compounds to pass through, while the carrier gases are excluded.

The revolutionary advances in the study of drug metabolism that have been brought about by the combination of gas chromatography and mass spectrometry (gc-ms) are illustrated by an analysis of the metabolism of probenecid.[29] Bile from rats that had received this drug was treated with diazomethane to convert —COOH groups to methyl esters; these derivatives are easier to separate by GLC. The bile was also treated with β-glucuronidase to release conjugated drug and metabolites in their free forms, soluble in organic solvents. The GLC elution pattern of an ethyl acetate extract is shown in Figure 3-6. Probenecid was known to emerge at 13 min, and the expected N-depropyl probenecid just before it, so the first two peaks could be identified readily. Metabolites A, B, and C, on the other hand, were completely unknown. The positions of A and C were different prior to treatment with β-glucuronidase, whence it was concluded that these compounds were excreted in bile as glucuronides, and therefore probably contained a hydroxyl group.

The mass spectra settled the structure of each metabolite conclusively; here we shall only consider metabolite A. The mass spectrum of probenecid methyl ester is given in the upper part of Figure 3-7, where m/e ratios are on the x axis, and the y axis is a scale of percent intensity relative to the most abundant ion. The heaviest mass ion, representing the starting material, is at m/e 299, but so little of it is present that the sensitivity had to be increased 10-fold to detect it at all. This is not unusual; often the

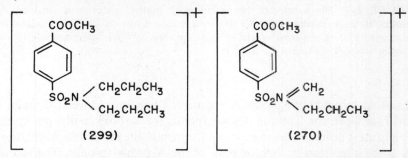

molecular ion first formed is extremely unstable. Here the N-propyl group undergoes cleavage very easily, giving rise to the abundant ion at m/e 270, because an ethyl group (Et = 29 mass units) is split off. Further cleavage results in an ion at m/e 199, consistent with rupture of the S—N bond, since this is exactly the mass of the aryl sulfate fragment alone. Finally, the fragment at m/e 135 clearly represents the carboxymethylphenyl ion.

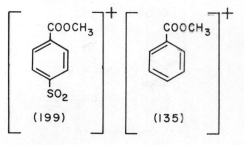

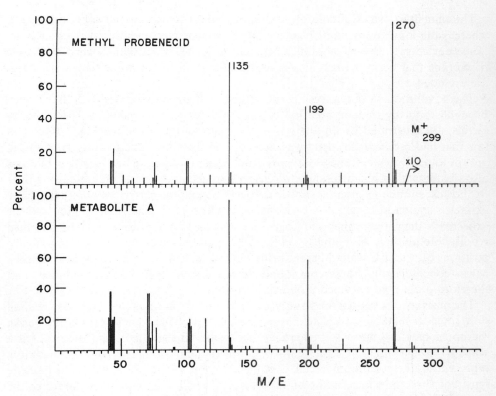

FIGURE 3-7. Mass spectra of probenecid methyl ester and one of its metabolites. *Mass/charge ratio is shown on* x *axis. Units on* y *axis are intensities relative to that of the most abundant mass ion. See text for interpretation. (From Guarino and Fales, Figures 5 and 7.[29])*

The mass spectrum of metabolite A (Figure 3-7, bottom) showed the major ions at 135 and 199 still present. Thus, in the metabolite, the carboxymethyl phenyl sulfonamide moiety must be intact. In other words, the metabolite must differ from the original drug by some alteration on one or both of the N-propyl groups. The ion at mass 270 showed that one propyl group was intact. The initial molecular ion was detected only with great difficulty, at m/e 315 (not shown), exactly 16 units greater than probenecid methyl ester. The metabolite was therefore a hydroxyl derivative; the only question was which of the propyl C atoms had been oxidized. The virtual absence of the molecular ion 315 indicated an extraordinary ease of fragmentation (to the ion

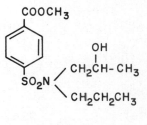

metabolite A

with mass 270), which is characteristic of adjacent C atoms bonded to heteroatoms (here N and O, respectively). Thus, metabolite A was deduced to be a hydroxy derivative on the β carbon atom of one N-propyl group; this structure was confirmed by synthesis. In a similar manner, metabolite C was shown to be an isomer of A, with a hydroxy group on the terminal carbon of the propyl group. Metabolite B proved to be the carboxylic acid resulting from further in vivo oxidation of C.

A given compound gives rise to a unique fragmentation pattern, both with respect to the masses of the various fragments and their abundance ratios. This fact has been the basis for the technique called *mass fragmentography*.[27] A computer linked to the mass spectrometer output can be programmed to pick up the specific set of masses and abundances characteristic of any particular compound (or few compounds) one wishes to detect. For probenecid methyl ester, for example, the instrument might be set to detect the fragments at m/e 270, 199, and 135, in the correct ratios; then the compound, if present even in a complex mixture, would be identified positively. The great sensitivity of mass spectrometry permits such a preprogrammed device to be used as a "sniffer," incorporating a silicone membrane such as described earlier, and thereby detecting any desired compound in ambient air.

The power and precision of mass fragmentography can be improved greatly by using internal standards.[31-33] For example, an analog of the drug to be detected is prepared, containing deuterium instead of hydrogen at specific positions in the molecule. This analog, in known quantity, is added as internal standard. Its fragmentation pattern will be identical to that of the parent drug, except that ions containing the two deuterium atoms will be shifted by 2 mass units. Thus, the peak height of each appropriate ion of the analog serves as a basis for quantitation of the corresponding peak derived from the drug. A real advantage of this method is that since the internal standard is chemically identical to the unknown compound to be assayed, no special corrections are required for losses during extraction and fractionation procedures prior to the mass spectrometry.

Radioactivity is used extensively to study drug metabolism. A radioactive isotope, often ^{14}C or ^3H, is introduced into a drug molecule by chemical or biologic synthesis. Plant alkaloids and glycosides, for example, have been prepared by growing the plants in an atmosphere containing $^{14}CO_2$. It might be thought that methods employing radioactivity should be highly specific, since only the drug and its metabolites (but no naturally occurring compound) will be radioactive. To the extent, however, that the drug is transformed to compounds that can enter normal metabolic pathways, the specificity is lost. Thus, ^{14}C in a methyl group of a drug that undergoes demethylation may enter the single-carbon pool and become incorporated into compounds wholly unrelated to the drug or its metabolites. Usually the whole gamut of separation procedures is carried out, as described above, and radioactivity counting (or radioautography, as in Figure 3-2) is used for the quantitative estimations. These are not only obtained more simply and accurately by counting than by chemical determinations, but there is also a very important increase in the sensitivity of the assays, especially when starting materials of high specific radioactivity are available.

Isotope dilution analysis[34] may be illustrated by the study of pentobarbital metabolism described earlier (Figure 3-2). One of the spots on the paper chromatogram was eluted, and a known amount of radioactivity from this "tracer" synthesized in vivo was added to pooled urine from several dogs that had received large amounts of unlabeled pentobarbital. The urine was then subjected to extraction and countercurrent separations, during which the radioactive material acted as a tracer for isolation of the same metabolite from the urine. Thus, large amounts of the metabolite could be obtained—sufficient for identification by standard chemical techniques (infrared spectroscopy, elemental analysis, melting point, etc.). The metabolite was shown to be a carboxylic acid derivative of pentobarbital.

In the method known as double isotope dilution,[35,36] two radioactive elements are present. First, a trace amount of a radioactive isotope of the drug to be detected is added to the biologic sample. For example, tritium-labeled digitoxin of high specific radioactivity was added to a plasma sample containing an unknown amount of digitoxin. The material was then extracted with organic solvents, and converted to a triacetate derivative, using ^{14}C-acetic anhydride as the reagent. This step allows the quantitation of the digitoxin triacetate finally isolated by chromatography, since the drug must be present at a molar ratio of $1:3$ relative to the ^{14}C-acetate. The recovery of ^3H radioactivity, representing the ^3H-digitoxin internal standard, serves to correct for all losses of biologically derived digitoxin during the various procedures.

CHEMICAL PATHWAYS OF DRUG METABOLISM

Drugs undergo 4 types of reaction in the body. These are oxidative, reductive, hydrolytic, and synthetic (conjugation) reactions. The oxidative reactions include aliphatic oxidation, aromatic hydroxylation, *N*-dealkylation, *O*-dealkylation, *S*-demethylation, deamination, sulfoxide formation, desulfuration, *N*-oxidation, and *N*-hydroxylation. The detailed pathways and mechanisms will be presented later. First we shall consider the properties and characteristics of the microsomal drug-metabolizing system that catalyzes the oxidative transformations.

The Liver Microsomal Drug-Metabolizing System

The oxidative metabolism of many drugs and also of steroid hormones is mediated by enzymes located in the microsomal fraction of mammalian liver, consisting of fragments of endoplasmic reticulum.[37-40] Liver is homogenized and the homogenate is centrifuged at 9000–12,000 × g for 30 min. Then the supernatant solution is centrifuged at 105,000 × g for 1 hr, and the sediment is collected. The microsome fraction thus obtained contains a hemoprotein (or family of closely related hemoproteins) known as cytochromes P450, which acts as terminal oxidase for a variety of oxidative reactions that drugs undergo. The term P450 refers to the ability of the reduced form of the hemoprotein to react with carbon monoxide, yielding a complex with absorption peak at 450 nm.

In an in vitro system containing liver microsomes, various drugs can be oxidized, provided the following components are present: NADPH, O_2, Mg^{2+}.[41] The requirement for reduced pyridine nucleotide and for molecular oxygen categorizes the enzyme system as a mixed function oxidase (also called monooxygenase).[42] One molecule of O_2 is consumed for each molecule of substrate oxidized, one atom of O is introduced into the substrate, the other is reduced, forming H_2O. The overall reaction may be formulated as follows,[43] where A is the oxidized form and AH_2 is the reduced form of cytochrome P450.

1. $NADPH + A + H^+ \rightarrow AH_2 + NADP^+$
2. $AH_2 + O_2 \rightarrow$ "active oxygen complex"
3. "active oxygen complex" + drug substrate $\rightarrow$ oxidized drug + A + H_2O

$NADPH + O_2 +$ drug substrate $+ H^+ \rightarrow NADP^+ +$ oxidized drug $+ H_2O$

The electron flow pathway has been partially worked out, and may be provisionally represented as seen in Figure 3-8. Here NADPH is oxidized by the flavoprotein, NADPH-cytochrome c reductase, forming $NADP^+$, and resulting in transfer of an

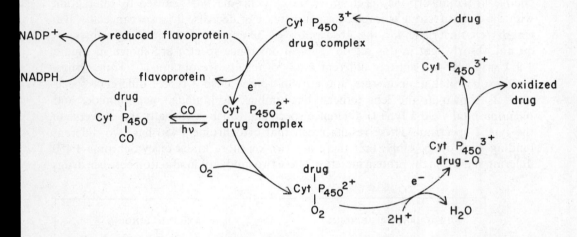

FIGURE 3-8. Electron flow pathway in the microsomal drug-oxidizing system. (*Adapted from Hildebrandt and Estabrook, Figure 14.*[44])

electron through the flavoprotein to the oxidized form of cytochrome P450, which has already interacted with the drug substrate. Since cytochrome c is not present in microsomes and plays no role in drug oxidations, a better name for the flavoprotein would be P450 reductase. The flavoprotein is able to transfer electrons to cytochrome c or other electron acceptors (methylene blue, menadione) if they are added to the incubation mixture. Such electron acceptors therefore inhibit drug oxidations while leaving NADPH oxidation unaffected or even accelerating it. The essential role of NADPH-cytochrome c reductase is also indicated by the fact that antibodies to this enzyme will block aniline hydroxylation by liver microsomes.[45] It has been postulated that another electron transport protein functions between the cytochrome c reductase and cytochrome P450. Such a protein has, indeed, been identified in an adrenal cortical mitochondrial system that oxidizes steroids[46] but probably is not present in the liver microsomal system.

The reduced $(2+)$ form of cytochrome P450 drug complex can bind O_2 to form a ternary complex. Alternatively, CO can bind instead of O_2, inhibiting drug oxidation. The reaction with CO is dependent on the ratio O_2/CO, and it is reversed upon exposure to light. Another electron must be introduced into the $P450^{2+}$-drug-O_2 complex at this point, to generate H_2O and oxidized drug. The source of this second electron could be another molecule of NADPH, but NADH and cytochrome b5 are not excluded. The "active oxygen" form of cytochrome P450 decomposes into oxidized drug, oxidized P450, and an equivalent of H_2O.

As indicated above, cytochrome P450 is found not only in liver microsomes but also in adrenal cortex, intestinal mucosa, and kidney. In adrenal cortex it functions in mitochondria to hydroxylate steroids, and most drugs are also oxidized by adrenal cortical preparations. It also appears to have an important physiologic role in the metabolism of various fatty acids to their ω and ω-1 hydroxy derivatives.

Interaction of drug substrates with cytochrome P450 has been studied by difference spectra. In this method, both cuvettes of a split-beam spectrophotometer contain microsomes in the oxidized form. A drug substrate is introduced into one cuvette. Any change in the absorption spectrum of the cytochrome P450 caused by interaction with the drug substrate is revealed as an increase or decrease in absorbance at wavelengths characteristic for the absorption of hemoproteins. The drug substrates do not absorb light in this region. Typical difference spectra are shown in Figure 3-9. Curiously, two entirely different kinds of results are obtained.[40] Some drugs, like hexobarbital, aminopyrine, and ethylmorphine yield a type I difference spectrum, as shown at the left. Others, like aniline, acetanilide, nicotinamide, and phenobarbital yield a type II difference spectrum, which is virtually the converse of the type I spectrum. These results mean that cytochrome P450 has two different binding sites or, possibly, that there are two or more kinds of cytochrome P450 differing slightly in the protein moieties. These two modes of interaction between drugs

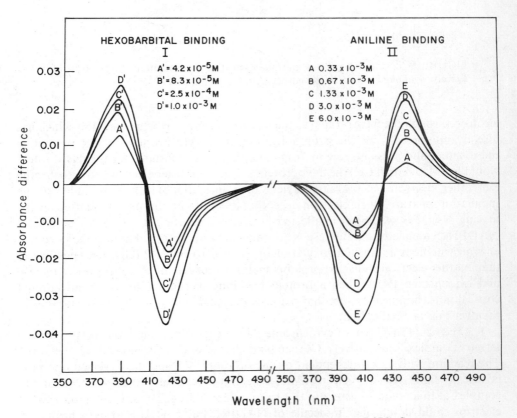

FIGURE 3-9. Difference spectra for binding of drugs to P450. *Spectra represent differences in absorption at each wavelength between ligand-free and ligand-bound cytochrome P450 at various drug concentrations. Type I binding spectra are typified by hexobarbital (at left), type II by aniline (at right). (From Mannering, Figure 12-6.*[40]*)*

and cytochrome P450 appear to have some functional significance, for the rate of reduction of cytochrome P450 by NADPH is accelerated by type I substrates but is slowed by type II substrates.[46a]

Although it has not yet proved possible to solubilize the enzyme system located in the liver microsomal fraction,[47,48] it is now known that the enzyme activity is associated with the so-called smooth-surfaced endoplasmic reticulum. The rough-surfaced variety, studded with ribosomes,[49] can be separated from the less dense, smooth-surfaced microsomes by means of sucrose density gradient centrifugation. NADPH oxidizing action and drug-oxidizing activities are both much higher in the smooth-surfaced microsomes than in the denser fraction.

Now we shall examine typical examples of the oxidative transformations catalyzed by the liver microsomal enzyme system.

Side Chain (Aliphatic) Oxidation.   The principal metabolites of pentobarbital in dog and man are alcoholic derivatives, formed by side chain oxidation:

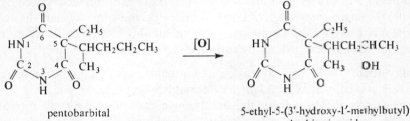

pentobarbital

5-ethyl-5-(3'-hydroxy-1'-methylbutyl)
barbituric acid

Carboxylic acids may also occur as minor metabolites:

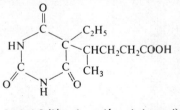

5-ethyl-5-(3'-carboxy-1'-methylpropyl)
barbituric acid

In aliphatic oxidations the products of the microsomal system are alcohols. Further oxidation to aldehydes and carboxylic acids requires the soluble enzymes alcohol dehydrogenase and aldehyde dehydrogenase (p. 251).[50]

Side chain oxidation of a slightly different kind is seen with the N_1-methylated barbiturate, hexobarbital.[51] This compound, which has a cyclohexenyl ring attached to position 5, is oxidized to a keto derivative:

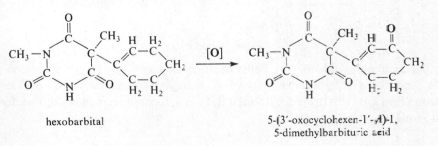

hexobarbital

5-(3'-oxocyclohexen-1'-yl)-1,
5-dimethylbarbituric acid

This was the only metabolite found in an in vitro system consisting of rabbit micro-somes, NADPH, and oxygen.[51a] In the dog, several additional metabolites are formed, including the N_1-demethylated compound and its keto derivative.

Aromatic Hydroxylation.   The conversion of acetanilid to p-hydroxyacetanilid illustrates this reaction:

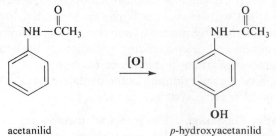

acetanilid p-hydroxyacetanilid

Steroid hormones like testosterone and estradiol-17β are also hydroxylated by a liver microsomal system requiring NADPH,[52] probably the same system that oxidizes drugs. Hydroxylations of nonlipid-soluble metabolic intermediates (e.g., phenyl-alanine, tyrosine) are carried out by entirely different enzyme systems.

N-Dealkylation.   N-Methyl, N-ethyl, and N-alkyl groups in general can be removed oxidatively and converted to aldehydes (formaldehyde, acetaldehyde, etc.). The reac-tions are clearly different from the usual single carbon transfers in intermediary metabolism, which involve either S-adenosylmethionine or a folic acid derivative. The conversion of aminopyrine to monomethyl-4-aminoantipyrine, and its further conversion to 4-aminoantipyrine, illustrate the reaction sequence:

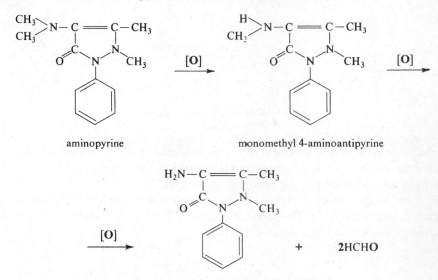

aminopyrine   monomethyl 4-aminoantipyrine

4-aminoantipyrine

Another example would be the demethylation of morphine to normorphine. The prefix "nor," referring to products of N-dealkylation, comes from the German "N ohne Radikal" ("Nitrogen without a radical"), meaning a primary amine derived from N-alkyl.

O-Dealkylation.   Aromatic ethers are cleaved, as in the following two reactions:

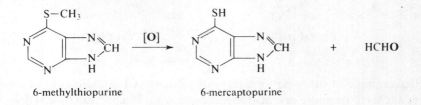

acetophenetidin   p-hydroxyacetanilid

codeine (methylmorphine)   morphine

S-Demethylation.   An oxidative reaction similar to *N*- or *O*-demethylation occurs with certain methyl thioethers:

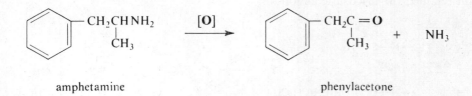

6-methylthiopurine   6-mercaptopurine

Oxidative Deamination.   The metabolism of amphetamine to phenylacetone by rabbit liver is an example of this type of oxidation:

amphetamine   phenylacetone

In the dog and rat, however, amphetamine undergoes *p*-hydroxylation of the benzene ring rather than deamination. Oxidative deamination, and *N*-oxidations in general, turn out to be more complex than the mere introduction of oxygen would suggest. When amphetamine oxidation was studied in rabbit microsomes in an $^{18}O_2$ atmosphere, two metabolites were found: phenylacetone oxime containing about 95% ^{18}O, and phenylacetone, containing about 30% ^{18}O.[53] The results imply the following reaction sequence:

$$
\text{1. } R_2CH\text{-}NH_2 \xrightarrow{[O]} \underset{\displaystyle R_2\overset{\displaystyle OH}{\underset{|}{C}}\text{-}NH_2}{} \qquad \text{(Carbinol amine)}
$$

$$
\text{2. } R_2\overset{\displaystyle OH}{\underset{|}{C}}\text{-}NH_2 \xrightarrow{-NH_3} R_2C{=}O \qquad \text{(Ketone)}
$$

$$
\xrightarrow{-H_2O} R_2C{=}NH \qquad \text{(Imine)}
$$

$$
\text{3. } R_2C{=}NH \xrightarrow{[O]} R_2C{=}NOH \qquad \text{(Oxime)}
$$

$$
\text{4. } R_2C{=}NOH \xrightarrow{+H_2O} R_2C{=}O \qquad \text{(Ketone)}
$$

Thus the initial intermediate formed is a carbinol amine; this is the same reaction thought to initiate dealkylation of tertiary amines. The carbinol amine can lose ammonia to form the ketone, retaining ^{18}O, or it can lose water to form an imine. The imine in turn is oxidized by the microsomal enzyme system[54] to the oxime. This, in turn, is partially hydrolyzed to the ketone, but now the oxygen is derived from water, not from the atmospheric ^{18}O.

Sulfoxide Formation. Thioethers in general are oxidized to sulfoxides, as below:[55]

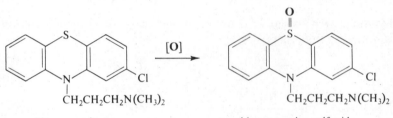

chlorpromazine   chlorpromazine sulfoxide

Another example of sulfoxide formation was discovered in the course of a search for better agents to promote uric acid excretion in gout. Phenylbutazone, a drug with antirheumatic, antipyretic, analgesic, and sodium-retaining activity, also blocks the renal tubular reabsorption of uric acid. An alcoholic metabolite that arises by side chain oxidation of phenylbutazone was found to have little antirheumatic effect but still retained the uricosuric action:

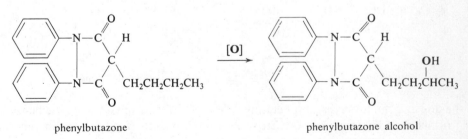

phenylbutazone   phenylbutazone alcohol

Manipulations of the side chain of phenylbutazone alcohol led to the discovery that sulfur-containing derivatives had marked uricosuric action. One of these, the 4-phenylthioethyl analog of phenylbutazone, was found to be metabolized by sulfoxide formation, to yield an even more potent uricosuric drug, sulfinpyrazone:[56]

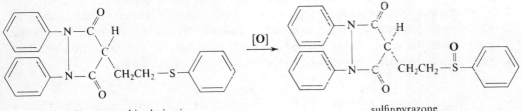

phenylbutazone thio derivative   sulfinpyrazone

Sulfinpyrazone came into therapeutic use as a selectively uricosuric drug, practically devoid of antirheumatic, analgesic, and sodium-retaining activity.

Desulfuration. The replacement of sulfur by oxygen has been reported in thiopental and related thiopyrimidines:[57]

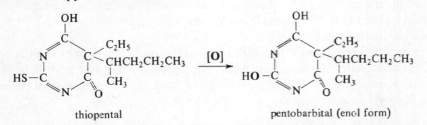

thiopental   pentobarbital (enol form)

Another example of this reaction is the conversion of parathion to its oxygen analog, paraoxon.[58,59] Parathion is used as an insecticide, but it is biologically inert; it depends for its effectiveness upon oxidative desulfuration in the insect, and for its toxicity to mammals upon oxidative desulfuration in the liver:

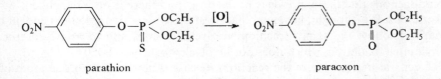

parathion   paraoxon

This reaction is reported to require NADH rather than NADPH, but otherwise it resembles the usual drug oxidations; the system is found in the microsomes, requires oxygen, and is stimulated by Mg^{2+}. The requirement for NADH is so unusual that it is deserving of more intensive investigation.

N-Oxidation and N-Hydroxylation. N-Oxidation is exemplified by the oxidative conversion of trimethylamine to its N-oxide:[60]

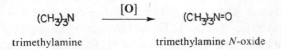

trimethylamine   trimethylamine N-oxide

Secondary and tertiary amines are oxidized by microsomal enzymes that require NADPH and molecular oxygen; but it is becoming clear that there is a special amine oxidase present (a flavoprotein distinct from NADPH-cytochrome c reductase), which is responsible for these oxidations.[61] The amine oxidase is a mixed-function oxidase, and cytochrome P450 appears not to be involved. Secondary amines are converted to hydroxylamines and tertiary amines to amine oxides.

When the carcinogenic compound 2-acetylaminofluorene is administered to rabbits or other animal species in which it produces cancer, a N-hydroxy metabolite is found in the urine. There is good evidence showing that this oxidation product, rather than the parent compound, is the actual carcinogen:[62]

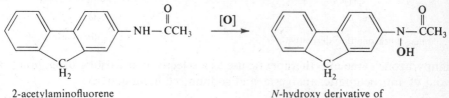

2-acetylaminofluorene

N-hydroxy derivative of
2-acetylaminofluorene

Formation of the N-hydroxy derivative of aniline, phenylhydroxylamine (p. 229), is another example of N-hydroxylation by the liver microsome system.[63,64] Imines can also be hydroxylated.[54]

In steroid hydroxylation,[65] acetanilid hydroxylation,[66] and trimethylamine oxidation,[60] studies with ^{18}O have shown that the oxygen introduced into the substrate molecule is derived from air, not from OH^- of water. In the oxidation of trimethylamine, the overall stoichiometry was shown to be:

$$(CH_3)_3N + NADPH + H^+ + O_2 \rightarrow (CH_3)_3N{=}O + NADP^+ + H_2O$$

It has not been easy to establish the stoichiometry of the cytochrome P450-dependent microsomal oxidations because the endogenous rate of NADPH oxidation is so high. As noted earlier, for example, addition of a type I drug substrate accelerates this rate, but quantitation of this increase requires knowledge about what happens to the endogenous rate in the presence of the drug, and there is no independent way to measure this. It is thought, however, that most mixed function P450-dependent drug oxidations follow the same stoichiometric relationships shown above for the trimethylamine oxidation, which does not involve cytochrome P450.[67]

The general mechanism of the reactions discussed here, in which one atom of O_2 is incorporated into a substrate, while the other is simultaneously reduced to water, may be depicted as follows:

$$AH + O{=}O + 2e \rightarrow AOH + [O^{2-}]$$
$$[O^{2-}] + 2H^+ \rightarrow H_2O$$

The nature of the actual hydroxylating intermediate, undoubtedly an oxygenated form of reduced P450, remains uncertain; it may be a superoxide, represented as the complex drug-$P450^{2+}$-O_2^{2-}. For our purposes, the protein P450 may be considered an oxygen transferase, and many of the oxidative reactions discussed above may be written as hydroxylation reactions. The subsequent steps (e.g., conversion of alcohols to aldehydes, and aldehydes to acids) may be catalyzed by other enzymes (e.g., alcohol or aldehyde dehydrogenases) or may proceed nonenzymatically.

The initial hydroxylation reactions can be written as follows:

$$R{-}CH_3 \xrightarrow{[P_{450}O]} R{-}CH_2OH$$

Aliphatic oxidation

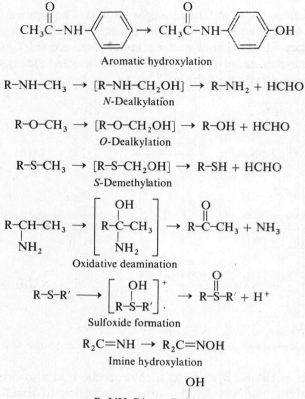

$$CH_3\overset{\overset{\textstyle O}{\|}}{C}-NH-\!\!\bigcirc\!\!\longrightarrow CH_3\overset{\overset{\textstyle O}{\|}}{C}-NH-\!\!\bigcirc\!\!-OH$$

Aromatic hydroxylation

$$R-NH-CH_3 \rightarrow [R-NH-CH_2OH] \rightarrow R-NH_2 + HCHO$$

N-Dealkylation

$$R-O-CH_3 \rightarrow [R-O-CH_2OH] \rightarrow R-OH + HCHO$$

O-Dealkylation

$$R-S-CH_3 \rightarrow [R-S-CH_2OH] \rightarrow R-SH + HCHO$$

S-Demethylation

$$R-\underset{\underset{\textstyle NH_2}{|}}{C}H-CH_3 \rightarrow \left[R-\overset{\overset{\textstyle OH}{|}}{\underset{\underset{\textstyle NH_2}{|}}{C}}-CH_3 \right] \rightarrow R-\overset{\overset{\textstyle O}{\|}}{C}-CH_3 + NH_3$$

Oxidative deamination

$$R-S-R' \longrightarrow \left[R-\overset{\overset{\textstyle OH}{|}}{S}-R' \right]^{+}_{\cdot} \rightarrow R-\overset{\overset{\textstyle O}{\|}}{S}-R' + H^{+}$$

Sulfoxide formation

$$R_2C=NH \rightarrow R_2C=NOH$$

Imine hydroxylation

$$R-NH-R' \rightarrow R-\overset{\overset{\textstyle OH}{|}}{N}-R'$$

N-Hydroxylation

In the oxidative desulfuration reactions, the oxygen atom replaces a sulfur atom, and the latter appears as sulfate, but the mechanism remains obscure.

Drug Oxidations that Are Not Mediated by the Liver Microsomal System

Aromatization of Cyclohexane Derivatives. A good example is the formation of benzoic acid from hexahydrobenzoic acid by a mitochondrial enzyme system in guinea pig and rabbit liver. Mitochondria from rat liver are less active, and those from cat, mouse, dog, monkey, and man are completely inactive.

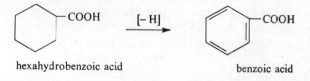

$$\bigcirc\!\!-COOH \xrightarrow{\;[-H]\;} \bigcirc\!\!-COOH$$

hexahydrobenzoic acid   benzoic acid

The system requires magnesium ions, coenzyme A, ATP or an ATP-generating system, and oxygen.[68] The first step appears to be the formation of hexahydrobenzoyl-CoA, which is then dehydrogenated to the aromatic product. Glycine stimulates the reaction, probably by removing benzoic acid through conjugation to form hippuric acid.

Alcohol and Aldehyde Oxidation. Alcohol dehydrogenase and aldehyde dehydrogenase are rather nonspecific enzymes found in the soluble fraction of liver, which catalyze several important oxidative transformations. The substrates include some compounds normally found in the body, for example, the alcohol vitamin A and the aldehyde retinene. Ethyl alcohol and its metabolite, acetaldehyde, are oxidized by this pair of enzymes, as are a variety of other alcohols and aldehydes, for example, p-nitrobenzyl alcohol and its aldehyde:[50]

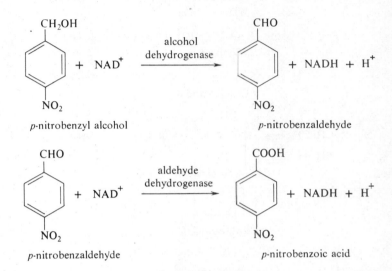

The oxidation of chloral hydrate to trichloroacetic acid also occurs,[69] although the major metabolic pathway for this drug is reduction to trichloroethanol. The enzyme responsible appears to be different from ordinary liver aldehyde dehydrogenase, although it is also found in the soluble fraction of liver and requires NAD^+ :

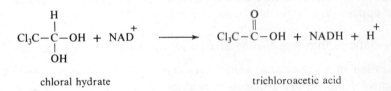

Claims have been made that a microsomal ethanol oxidizing system (MEOS) also exists, and is responsible, at least in part, for ethanol oxidation in man and rats.[70] However, most of the studies purporting to show the existence of such a pathway can probably be explained by slight contamination with alcohol dehydrogenase and a small amount of catalase activity which cannot be removed from microsomes.[71,71a]

Purine Oxidation. Several purine derivatives (e.g., 6-mercaptopurine, theophylline, caffeine) are known to undergo oxidation in vivo,[72] and it seems likely that xanthine oxidase (which normally interacts with hypoxanthine and xanthine) could participate in some of these reactions. The metabolism of the methylated xanthines is complex;[73] theophylline is largely oxidized to methyl- and dimethyluric acid, while theobromine is demethylated to 3- and 7-methylxanthines, as shown in Figure 3-10. Caffeine (1,3,7-trimethylxanthine) is metabolized both by demethylation and by oxidation; thus, 1,3-dimethyluric acid, 1-methyluric acid, 1,7-dimethylxanthine, 1-methyl-

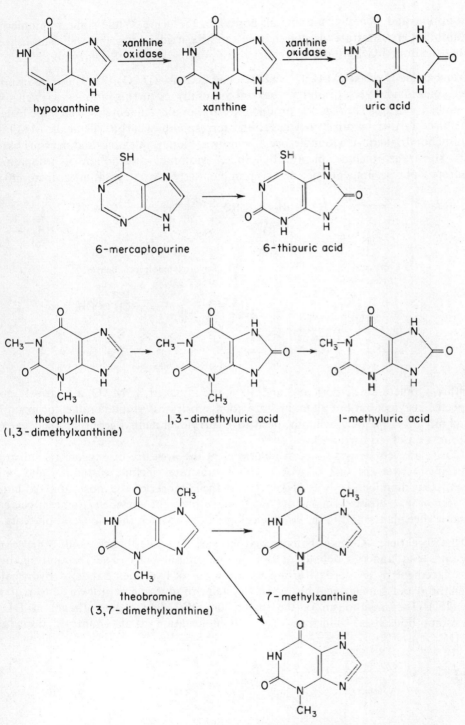

FIGURE 3-10. Pathways of purine metabolism. (*Adapted from Cornish and Christman.*[73])

xanthine, and 7-methylxanthine all appear in the urine. While some monomethyl-xanthines are substrates for the enzyme xanthine oxidase, it seems well established[74] that the dimethylxanthines and caffeine are not oxidized by this enzyme.

Monoamine Oxidase (MAO)[75] and Diamine Oxidase (DAO).[76]   These two similar enzymes oxidatively deaminate several naturally occurring amines as well as a number of drugs. The reaction products are aryl or alkyl aldehydes, which are usually oxidized further by other enzymes to the corresponding carboxylic acids. MAO is a mitochondrial enzyme found especially in liver, kidney, intestine, and nervous tissue. Its substrates include phenylethylamine, tyramine, catecholamines (dopamine, norepinephrine, epinephrine), and tryptophan derivatives (tryptamine, serotonin):

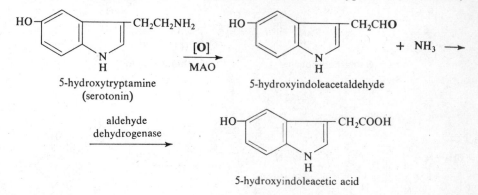

5-hydroxytryptamine
(serotonin)

5-hydroxyindoleacetaldehyde

5-hydroxyindoleacetic acid

Other simple amines, both aryl and alkyl, are attacked by MAO, a relatively non-specific enzyme, but not all amines are good substrates. Amphetamine, for example, and any other phenylethylamine derivative carrying a methyl group on the α carbon atom, are not oxidized well.

DAO also converts amines to aldehydes in the presence of oxygen. Its substrate specificity overlaps that of MAO. Good substrates include histamine and poly-methylene diamines, $H_2N-(CH_2)_n-NH_2$. In the latter series, the most rapid oxidation is seen at $n = 4$ (putrescine) and $n = 5$ (cadaverine). The enzyme is found in bacteria and higher plants, and in the soluble cell fractions of liver, intestine, and placenta.

Dehalogenation.   Certain halogenated insecticides, anesthetics, and other compounds can undergo dehalogenation in the animal body. The reactions include displacement by a hydroxyl group, splitting out of hydrogen halide (dehydrohalogenation) and displacement by an acetylcysteine residue (mercapturic acid formation, p. 261). The metabolism of the insecticide DDT (chlorophenothane) in DDT-resistant houseflies[77] illustrates dehydrohalogenation to the nontoxic derivative DDE:

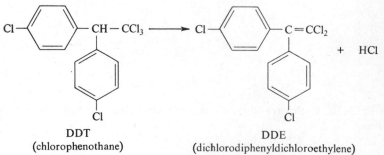

DDT
(chlorophenothane)

DDE
(dichlorodiphenyldichloroethylene)

TABLE 3-1. DDT-dehydrochlorinase activity in homogenates of different strains of DDT-resistant and DDT-sensitive flies.

The reaction mixture consisted of 2 ml of homogenized flies (equivalent to 12 flies), 0.003 M glutathione, 200 μg DDT in 50 μl alcohol, and 1 ml of 0.137 M phosphate buffer, pH 7.4. The reactions were run under a nitrogen atmosphere at 37°, and the amount of DDE formed was measured. Strain D was formerly resistant but had reverted back to nearly normal sensitivity. The actual strain designations have been deleted here; they may be found in the original publication. (Data of Sternburg et al.,[77] Table 6.)

Strain	Median lethal dose (μg DDT)	DDT converted to DDE in 4 hr (μg)
A	0.25	0
B	0.3	0
C	1.5	8
D	1.85	12
E	25.0	24
F	50.0	46
G	75.0	63

The enzyme system requires glutathione. Table 3-1 shows that resistant flies (strains E, F, G) have this enzyme, but sensitive flies (strains A, B, C, D) do not; its presence enables the insect to destroy the insecticide and thus to be immune to its action. More sensitive methods of assay reveal a small amount of enzyme activity even in sensitive flies.[78] In higher animals, the final product appearing in the urine after DDT ingestion is dichlorodiphenylacetic acid, presumably a metabolic product of DDE.

The halogenated anesthetics are not as resistant to metabolic conversion as was thought at one time. While the metabolism of some of them may be, in quantitative terms, very small—see, for example, the appearance of trace amounts of chloroform after carbon tetrachloride administration (p. 234)—in other instances the metabolism may be very extensive indeed.[79] Halothane, fluroxene, and methoxyflurane (Figure 3-11) have been shown to be metabolized to the extent of 10–20% or more in man and experimental animals.[80]

Generally the carbon–fluorine bond has been found to be more stable than the carbon–chlorine bond. Nevertheless, substantial amounts of free fluoride ion have been found in man and experimental animals after methoxyflurane administration, sufficient to implicate the fluoride ion as responsible for instances of renal toxicity (polyuric renal insufficiency).[81]

The metabolites of methoxyflurane have been reported[82] to include dichloroacetic acid, methoxydifluoroacetic acid, inorganic fluoride, CO_2, and oxalic acid. In man, about 10–20% of the methoxyflurane administered underwent ether cleavage, and as much as 40% was dechlorinated. It is obvious that extensive dehalogenation occurs, but the metabolic pathways are not completely worked out. Evidence available[83] strongly suggests that the familiar NADPH, O_2-dependent, P450 microsomal system

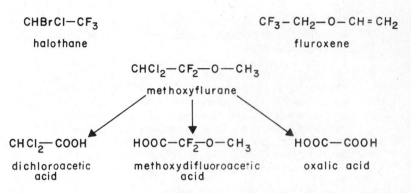

CHCl$_2$—COOH
dichloroacetic
acid

HOOC—CF$_2$—O—CH$_3$
methoxydifluoroacetic
acid

HOOC—COOH
oxalic acid

FIGURE 3-11. Halogenated anesthetics and some metabolic products.

may be involved in these dehalogenation reactions. While the toxic potential of the volatile anesthetics in patients was long a matter of concern, the adverse effects upon an occupationally exposed group—anesthetists—was recognized only recently.[84] A metabolite of the anesthetic is often implicated in these toxic reactions—liver and kidney damage, miscarriages, reduced fertility, or even cancer. It is not safe to dismiss any metabolite as "unimportant" merely because it is generated in very small amounts.

Reduction

Azo and Nitro Reduction.[85]   Azo reduction is illustrated by an important historical example. The era of specific antibacterial chemotherapy began with the introduction of Prontosil, an azo dye, for the treatment of streptococcal and pneumococcal infections. Subsequently it was discovered[86] that the active drug was not Prontosil itself but a metabolite, sulfanilamide (*p*-aminobenzenesulfonamide):

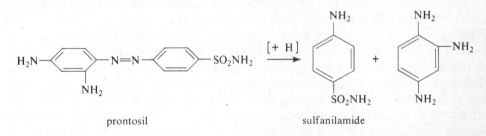

Nitro reduction is also illustrated well by an antibacterial agent, the antibiotic chloramphenicol, which is transformed in part to an amine by bacterial and mammalian nitro reductase systems:[87]

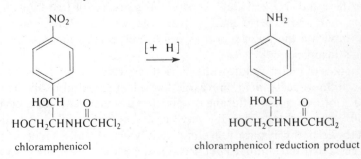

Azo and nitro reductions occur in rabbit and rat liver homogenates. At first the activity was thought to be present in the soluble cell fraction as well as in the microsomes. Later reports[49] indicated that the activity of the "soluble" supernatant fraction was actually in a class of light microsomes that sedimented unusually slowly. In contrast to the microsomal drug-oxidizing system, which is confined to the liver, these reductases are found in other tissues too. Although some differences have been noted between the azo and nitro reductase systems, they have many features in common. Both involve anaerobic reactions, require NADPH, and are stimulated by flavins (flavin mononucleotide, flavin adenine dinucleotide, riboflavin).[87] However, the reduced flavins might be acting simply as nonenzymic electron donors for the nitro group; thus any enzyme that reduced FAD would appear to be a nitro reductase.[88]

The capacity to reduce azo bonds may be rather weak in mammalian tissues, for in those instances where extensive reduction occurs (e.g., Prontosil), intestinal bacteria appear to be largely responsible.[89] A good example is the metabolism of salicylazosulfapyridine in the rat. The intestinal microflora cleave the azo bond, yielding 5-aminosalicylate and sulfapyridine, both of which (in contradistinction to the original drug) could be absorbed and further metabolized.[90] Germ-free animals fed this same drug excreted none of the normal metabolites in urine or feces; instead, virtually all the drug was recovered unchanged in the feces.

Alcohol dehydrogenase functions as a reductase when it catalyzes the conversion of chloral hydrate to trichloroethanol (p. 228).

Hydrolysis

Drug metabolism by hydrolysis[91] is restricted to esters and amides. The numerous hydrolytic enzymes (esterases and amidases) are found in blood plasma and other tissues, including the liver, usually in the soluble fraction of the cells. Enzymes prepared from different tissues or different species can have widely differing substrate specificities. The hydrolysis of the local anesthetic procaine by liver and plasma cholinesterase is illustrative:

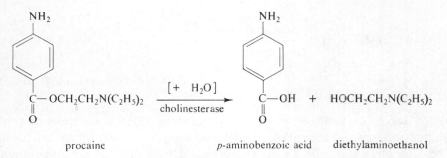

procaine   *p*-aminobenzoic acid   diethylaminoethanol

When the amide bond −CONH− is hydrolyzed, an acid and an amine are formed instead of an acid and an alcohol (as in the hydrolysis of an ester). Procaine amide, the amide analog of procaine, is hydrolyzed in the tissues much more slowly than procaine, and not at all in plasma. Most amides are hydrolyzed more slowly than the corresponding esters.

Not all esters undergo hydrolysis in the body. Atropine, for example, is hydrolyzed to an insignificant extent in mouse and man,[92,93] but very rapidly by some rabbits (cf. p. 287). Enzymes responsible for hydrolysis of esters include acetylcholinesterase, plasma cholinesterase, and even carbonic anhydrase, which has been shown to catalyze the hydrolysis of esters of α- and β-naphthol[94] in addition to its better known role in the hydration of CO_2. The hydrolysis of succinylcholine by plasma cholinesterase is an important example of rapid termination of drug effect by metabolic cleavage; some interesting examples of genetic variation in plasma cholinesterase, leading to altered drug responses, will be discussed in Chapter 6.

Addition (Conjugation) Reactions

Several kinds of small molecules normally present in the body can react with drugs or with drug metabolites. Glucuronic acid combines with phenols, alcohols, aromatic amines, and carboxylic acids to form the corresponding glucuronides. Addition of ribose and phosphate converts purine and pyrimidine analogs to nucleosides and nucleotides. Amines and carboxylic acids can be acylated. Other examples are the synthesis of mercapturic acids and of sulfuric acid esters, transsulfurations, and methylations.

Synthesis of Glucuronides.[95]   The soluble fraction of liver contains enzymes that catalyze the synthesis of uridine diphosphate-glucuronic acid (UDPGA):

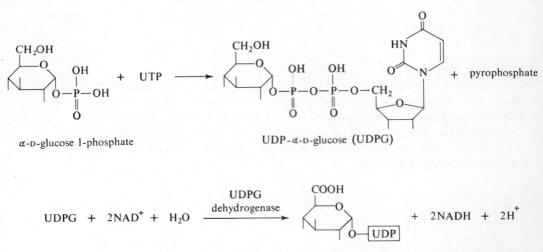

α-D-glucose 1-phosphate   UDP-α-D-glucose (UDPG)

UDP-α-D-glucuronic acid (UDPGA)

UDPGA serves as a donor of glucuronic acid to various acceptors. Enzymes mediating this process are called *transferases*. They are found in the microsomes of liver and other tissues.[96] As shown above, UDPGA has the α configuration at the glucuronic acid-phosphate link; the compound is not affected by the enzyme β-glucuronidase. However, the glucuronides that are formed invariably have the β configuration. Thus, the transfer reaction must proceed by a "backside attack" (Walden inversion).

The hydroxyl group in phenols and aliphatic alcohols is conjugated with glucuronic acid to form a hemiacetal glucuronide. Compounds of this type are often called "ether glucuronides":

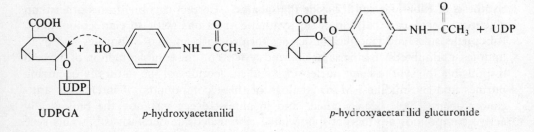

UDPGA   *p*-hydroxyacetanilid   *p*-hydroxyacetanilid glucuronide

Carboxylic acids are conjugated through the carboxyl group to form ester glucu-ronides:

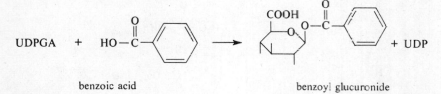

benzoic acid   benzoyl glucuronide

In all these reactions, there is a nucleophilic attack by the electron-rich atom (oxygen, nitrogen, or sulfur) on carbon atom 1 of the glucuronic acid in UDPGA.[97] Glucuronides of naturally occurring compounds (e.g., steroid alcohols, thyroxine, bilirubin) appear to be formed by the same pathways as glucuronides of foreign compounds.

A glucuronyl transferase has been solubilized and partially purified from rabbit liver microsomes.[98] The enzyme, which required no cofactors other than UDPGA, was active in forming ethereal and ester glucuronides but completely lacked the ability to form *N*-glucuronides. This indicates that a different enzyme is responsible for amine glucuronide formation. Moreover, the Gunn rat (p. 821), a strain that is genetically incapable of forming bilirubin glucuronide or other ester or ether glucu-ronides, is able to form aniline glucuronide in normal amounts.[99]

Aromatic amines[100] and even occasionally a sulfhydryl group[101] can be conju-gated. The nitrogen and sulfur glucuronides are acid labile, in contrast to the oxygen-linked glucuronides.

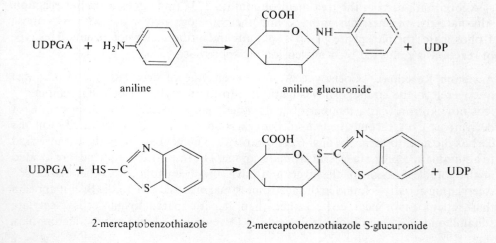

aniline   aniline glucuronide

2-mercaptobenzothiazole   2-mercaptobenzothiazole S-glucuronide

Synthesis of Ribosides and Riboside Phosphates.   Certain carbohydrates other than glucuronic acid can participate in synthetic reactions with foreign compounds. Ribonucleosides and ribonucleotides are formed with analogs of purines and pyrimidines, undoubtedly by the same enzyme systems (in the soluble fraction of the cell) responsible for synthesizing nucleosides and nucleotides of the naturally occurring purines and pyrimidines. Many analogs of these compounds, of interest as anticancer agents, have been studied; and in almost every instance, the biologically active compounds are the phosphorylated ribonucleoside derivatives.[102] This type of reaction is exemplified by conversion of 6-mercaptopurine to a ribonucleotide[103] by reaction with PRPP, catalyzed by a purine phosphoribosyl transferase:

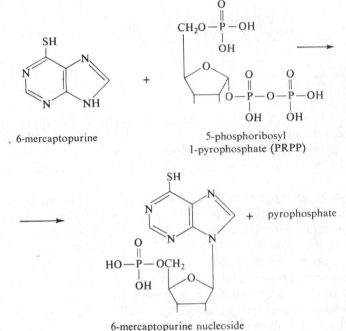

6-mercaptopurine

5-phosphoribosyl
1-pyrophosphate (PRPP)

6-mercaptopurine nucleoside
monophosphate

Allopurinol, used in the treatment of gout (p. 273), undergoes a similar reaction. Alternatively, purines, pyrimidines, and their analogs may react with α-D-ribose 1-phosphate; the phosphate group is split out and a ribonucleoside results. This type of reaction is catalyzed by a nucleoside phosphorylase.

Acylation Reactions.   Coenzyme A (for "coenzyme of acetylation") (CoA) was discovered in the course of investigations into the acetylation of sulfanilamide.[104] It is now known that a number of acids other than acetic acid can also form CoA derivatives. CoA, through its free sulfhydryl group, reacts with an activated form of a carboxylic acid to form the acyl-CoA derivative. The acyl group is then transferred to a suitable acceptor, such as an aromatic amine. The responsible enzymes are located in the soluble fraction of the liver, and have also been found in other tissues.[105] Acetylating activity is found in the gastrointestinal mucosal cell. In the liver it appears that reticuloendothelial cells, rather than hepatic parenchymal cells, acetylate sulfanilamide and p-aminobenzoic acid.[106] Developmental and genetic factors play

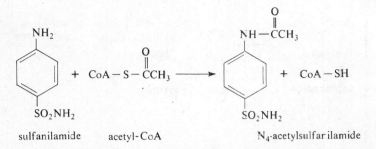

sulfanilamide   acetyl-CoA   N₄-acetylsulfarilamide

an important role in acetylation reactions. Individuals of both human and rabbit species can be classified as "rapid" or "slow" acetylators of isoniazid. This genetic polymorphism will be discussed in detail in Chapter 6.

The mechanism of acetylation of isoniazid by the enzyme N-acetyltransferase has been studied using purified enzyme preparations.[107,108] It was shown that the enzyme mediated two exchange reactions—one between acetyl-CoA and CoA, the other between isoniazid and acetylisoniazid. The enzyme could catalyze each exchange reaction in the absence of the other. While each reaction was reversible, the overall reaction (acetylation of isoniazid) was not reversible. This reaction sequence is characteristic of what has been called a "ping-pong Bi-Bi" mechanism, in which the overall reaction proceeds in two steps, with the formation of an acylated enzyme intermediate. It may be depicted as follows:

$$\text{enzyme} + \text{AcCoA} \rightleftharpoons \text{Ac-enzyme} + \text{CoA}$$
$$\underline{\text{Ac-enzyme} + \text{substrate} \rightleftharpoons \text{Ac-substrate} + \text{enzyme}}$$
$$\text{AcCoA} + \text{substrate} \xrightarrow{\text{enzyme}} \text{Ac-substrate} + \text{CoA}$$

The reaction sequence may also be depicted as a process, from left to right. as follows:

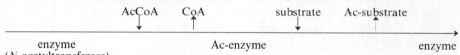

Here, a foreign amine is conjugated with the naturally occurring acetic acid. The converse also occurs, a foreign carboxylic acid forming a CoA derivative, which is then conjugated with a naturally occurring amine, such as glycine, ornithine (in birds and reptiles), or glutamine (in man and chimpanzee).

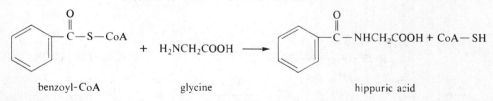

benzoyl-CoA   glycine   hippuric acid

Mercapturic Acid Formation.[109]   A few aromatic hydrocarbons, halogenated aromatic hydrocarbons, and halogenated nitrobenzenes are excreted in the urine as conjugates with an acetylated cysteine residue. The likely reaction mechanism is shown in Figure 3-12, for naphthalene as substrate. It is thought that an activated substrate first reacts with peptide-bound cysteine (probably glutathione). The conjugations are mediated by a number of enzymes, collectively called glutathione

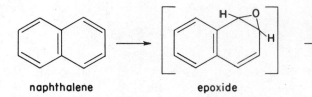

naphthalene   epoxide   activated glutathione

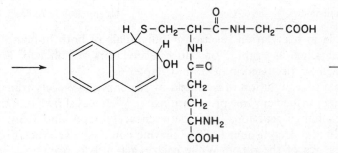

S-(1,2-dihydro-2-hydroxy-1-naphthyl)glutathione

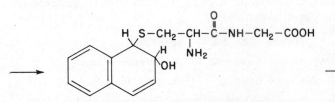

S-(1,2-dihydro-2-hydroxy-1-naphthyl)cysteinylglycine

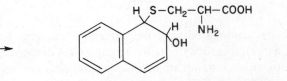

S-(1,2-dihydro-2-hydroxy-1-naphthyl)cysteine

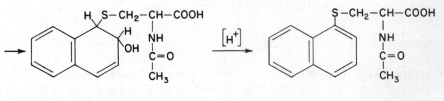

N-acetyl-S-(1,2-dihydro-2-hydroxy-   1-naphthylmercapturic acid
1-naphthyl)cysteine

FIGURE 3-12. Mercapturic acid formation. (*Adapted from Boyland et al.*[111])

S-transferases, found in supernatant fractions of rat liver homogenate.[110] The resulting glutathione conjugate is hydrolyzed to form an arylcysteine intermediate, and the cysteine amino group is then acetylated to form the final mercapturic acid. Most of the intermediates shown in Figure 3-12 have been isolated from rat bile after naphthalene administration.[111] Epoxide formation may be the first step in activation of substrates of this type,[112] especially since the hydroxy derivatives (1- and 2-naphthols) appear in the bile. All the 2-hydroxynaphthyl intermediates undergo spontaneous dehydration at acid pH, yielding the corresponding mercapturic acids. The hydroxy compounds are therefore sometimes called "premercapturic acids"; the mercapturic acids themselves (including the end-product shown) probably arise by deomposition of these precursors in acid urine.[113] It is not known which (if any) physiologic substrates are ordinarily metabolized by this pathway.

A curious reaction sequence involving mercapturic acid formation leads to the apparent reduction of certain sulfonamides. This unusual pathway is illustrated by the fate of a carbonic anhydrase inhibitor, 2-benzothiazolesulfonamide.[101] In most sulfonamides, which do not undergo this type of reaction, the sulfonamide group is attached to an aromatic ring, but here the sulfonamide sulfur atom is bound to a heterocyclic ring:

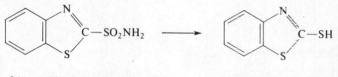

2-benzothiazolesulfonamide   2-mercaptobenzothiazole

Further investigation led to the remarkable finding that the sulfur in the −SH group of the product was not derived from the sulfur of the sulfonamide group, but was contributed by glutathione. The pathway is shown in Figure 3-13.

Synthesis of Sulfuric Acid Esters.   These compounds, often called "ethereal sulfates," are formed by the reaction of phenolic and aliphatic hydroxyl groups, and of certain amino groups, with an activated form of sulfate. The enzymes responsible for sulfate activation, and for the transfer of sulfate to the acceptor, are found in the soluble fraction of the liver.[115] The system is normally concerned with the synthesis of sulfated polysaccharides like chondroitin sulfate and heparin. The initiating reaction is the formation of adenosine 5′-phosphosulfate (APS) from the sulfate ion and adenosine triphosphate (ATP), followed by a further reaction with ATP to form 3′-phosphoadenosine 5′-phosphosulfate (PAPS). The sulfate group is then transferred to a phenolic acceptor (e.g., *p*-hydroxyacetanilid) in the presence of an appropriate transfer (sulfotransferase) enzyme:

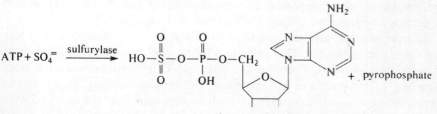

adenosine 5′-phosphosulfate (APS)

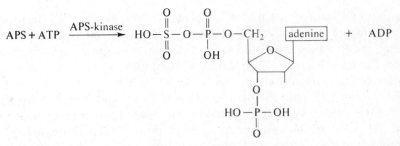

$$\text{APS} + \text{ATP} \xrightarrow{\text{APS-kinase}}$$

3'-phosphoadenosine 5'-phosphosulfate (PAPS)

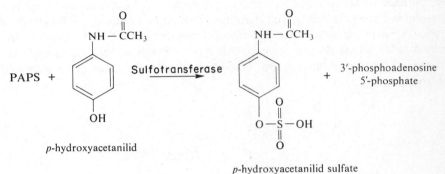

p-hydroxyacetanilid

p-hydroxyacetanilid sulfate

There are a number of different sulfotransferases specific for different acceptor molecules. In liver, for example, simple phenols, phenolic steroids, alcoholic steroids, chloramphenicol, and aromatic amines are all handled by different enzymes.[116]

N-, O-, and S-Methylation.   Methylations proceed by a pathway in which S-adenosylmethionine serves as methyl donor. There are a number of methyltransferase enzymes. One of these, catechol O-methyltransferase (COMT), is found in the soluble supernatant fraction of rat liver and other tissues. It can catalyze the transfer of a methyl group to a phenolic −OH of epinephrine, norepinephrine, and other catechol derivatives (e.g., dihydroxyphenylethylamine, dihydroxybenzoic acid).[117] Methylation occurs in the meta position. The reaction is dependent upon magnesium ions; S-adenosylmethionine is required, but ATP and methionine can substitute, in which case S-adenosylmethionine is formed in the presence of rat liver supernatant fraction.

COMT activity is found in all species, and is widely distributed in mammalian tissues. This enzyme is involved in the physiologic inactivation of the adrenergic neurotransmitter norepinephrine, as well as of other catechol amines, whether of endogenous or exogenous origin. The reaction is shown on p. 265.

A different enzyme catalyzes the O-methylation of N-acetylserotonin, to form the pineal hormone melatonin. This enzyme is found only in the pineal gland. It utilizes S-adenosylmethionine, but unlike the catechol O-methyltransferase, it does not require Mg^{2+}. It is known as hydroxyindole O-methyltransferase, since it can methylate various hydroxyindole compounds such as serotonin, bufotenine, and 5-hydroxyindoleacetic acid; however, the best substrate is N-acetylserotonin.[118]

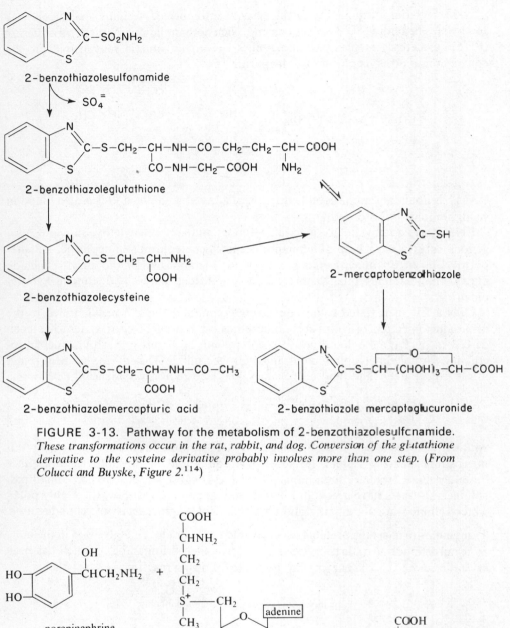

2-benzothiazolesulfonamide

$SO_4^=$

2-benzothiazoleglutathione

2-benzothiazolecysteine

2-mercaptobenzothiazole

2-benzothiazolemercapturic acid

2-benzothiazole mercaptoglucuronide

FIGURE 3-13. Pathway for the metabolism of 2-benzothiazolesulfonamide. *These transformations occur in the rat, rabbit, and dog. Conversion of the glutathione derivative to the cysteine derivative probably involves more than one step. (From Colucci and Buyske, Figure 2.[114])*

norepinephrine

S-adenosylmethionine

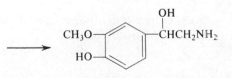

normetanephrine

S-adenosylhomocysteine

N-Methylation of numerous amines has been reported. A highly specific enzyme methylates histamine.[119] Another enzyme, phenylethanolamine *N*-methyltransferase (PNMT), methylates phenylethanolamine derivatives, and is responsible for the conversion of norepinephrine to epinephrine:[120]

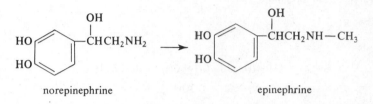

norepinephrine   epinephrine

PNMT is abundant in the soluble fraction of adrenal medulla, and it is also found in small amounts in heart and brain.

PNMT can methylate phenylethanolamines but not phenylethylamines. Endogenous substrates include norepinephrine, normetanephrine, epinephrine, metanephrine, and octopamine. Foreign compounds metabolized by the enzyme include phenylethanolamine, phenylephrine, norephredrine, para- and dihydroxynorephedrine.[121]

Only a few methylated sulfur-containing compounds have been identified in the urine after injection of sulfhydryl compounds,[122] but an in vitro system has been described[123] that methylates such –SH compounds as dimercaprol (BAL), mercaptoethanol, *O*-methylmercaptoethanol, and hydrogen sulfide. The enzyme has been found in rat liver, kidney, and lung microsomes, and also requires *S*-adenosylmethionine.

$$\text{HS–CH}_2\text{CH}_2\text{OH} \xrightarrow{\text{\textit{S}-adenosylmethionine}} \text{CH}_3\text{–S–CH}_2\text{CH}_2\text{OH}$$
Mercaptoethanol   *S*-Methylmercaptoethanol

Although a wide range of exogenous sulfhydryl compounds are methylated by this microsomal enzyme system, no sulfhydryl compound of physiologic importance (homocysteine, cysteine, glutathione) will serve as substrate. Apparently, only lipid-soluble substrates have access to the microsomal system. Just how the highly polar, water-soluble *S*-adenosylmethionine participates in the reaction is not yet understood.

Transsulfuration and the Metabolism of Cyanide.   Cyanide is metabolized in the body by a mitochondrial sulfurtransferase (formerly called "rhodanese"), which has been crystallized.[124,125] The enzyme catalyzes the following reaction:

$$\text{CN}^- + \text{S}_2\text{O}_3^{2-} \rightarrow \text{CNS}^- + \text{SO}_3^{2-}$$
cyanide thiosulfate thiocyanate sulfite

The thiosulfate-cyanide sulfurtransferase is found in liver, kidney, and other tissues, but blood has very little. Small amounts of cyanide are normally ingested in some foods, so the enzyme may possibly have a physiologic protective role in inactivating cyanide.

Another sulfurtransferase in liver, kidney, and blood cells utilizes β-mercaptopyruvic acid as sulfur donor rather than thiosulfate:

$$\text{CN}^- + \text{HS–CH}_2\overset{\overset{\textstyle O}{\|}}{\text{C}}\text{–COOH} \rightarrow \text{CNS}^- + \text{CH}_3\overset{\overset{\textstyle O}{\|}}{\text{C}}\text{–COOH}$$
β-mercaptopyruvic acid   pyruvic acid

This enzyme is present in the soluble fraction rather than in the mitochondria, and exhibits a high degree of substrate specificity for mercaptopyruvic acid; however, several compounds besides cyanide can serve as sulfur acceptors. For example, the enzyme can generate thiosulfate from sulfite:

$$HS-CH_2-\overset{\overset{\displaystyle O}{\|}}{C}-COOH + SO_3^{2-} \rightarrow S_2O_3^{2-} + CH_3-\overset{\overset{\displaystyle O}{\|}}{C}-COOH$$

The thiosulfate can then serve as sulfur donor for thiocyanate sulfurtransferase in cyanide detoxication.

Both enzymes could be involved in the inactivation of cyanide. In cyanide poisoning, cyanide becomes bound to iron atoms in the cytochromes, destroying the electron transport capacity. The immediate removal of this cyanide, in the treatment of cyanide poisoning, is achieved (as described fully on p. 410) by promoting its binding to methemoglobin. The subsequent conversion of cyanide to the nontoxic thiocyanate is promoted by furnishing thiosulfate (or mercaptopyruvate) as substrates for the above reactions.

INHIBITION OF DRUG METABOLISM

SKF 525A

Because the substrate specificity of the microsomal P450 system is so poor, numerous drugs compete with each other for oxidation.[126] Thus, any particular substrate is likely to inhibit the metabolism of another. It has been shown typically that for a given drug, the K_m (determined from its rate of metabolism) is nearly identical to the K_I (determined from its inhibition of the metabolism of another drug), implying that the inhibitory action is due to occupancy of a substrate site. However, the exact significance of kinetic constants is debatable in complex systems like this, which include particulate enzymes and, very likely, permeability barriers.

One of the most thoroughly investigated of these substrate inhibitors of drug metabolism is β-diethylaminoethyl diphenylpropylacetate, more usually known by

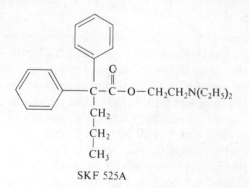

SKF 525A

its commercial code number SKF 525A. The action of this compound upon microsomal drug oxidations was discovered in the course of routine studies of its pharmacologic properties. The drug had little effect of its own, but when administered prior to hexobarbital, it caused a dramatic prolongation of the hypnotic action. The plasma half-life of hexobarbital was greatly increased, whereas the intrinsic sensitivity of the brain to hexobarbital (measured as the plasma level at the moment of awakening) remained unchanged. Moreover, when animals that had received hexobarbital alone were given SKF 525A at the instant of awakening, they did not go back to sleep, as they ought to have done if SKF 525A had made them more sensitive to the barbiturate.[127]

SKF 525A affects the metabolism of a great many drugs in the same way as it does that of hexobarbital; for example, the durations of action and biologic half-lives of other barbiturates, amphetamine, numerous analgesics, aminopyrine are also prolonged. In every such case the rate of metabolism in vitro by a liver microsomal preparation is also inhibited. Curiously, not all microsomal oxidative reactions are inhibited; N-dealkylation of N-methyl aniline, O-dealkylation of phenacetin, and hydroxylation of acetanilide by rabbit microsomes are relatively unaffected.[126] Even more surprising, SKF 525A inhibits the hydrolysis of procaine, a reaction in which microsomes are not involved at all, and also some glucuronidation reactions, which require microsomes but are not oxidative.

The kinetics of the SKF 525A inhibition are a subject of controversy. Certainly, simple competitive kinetics are observed in some instances, indicating that SKF 525A interacts at the drug-binding site.[128] This is consistent with its known affinity for the type I binding site of cytochrome P450 (cf. p. 244). Moreover, SKF 525A is metabolized by N-dealkylation to the secondary and primary amines, both of which are capable of inhibiting drug metabolism. On the other hand, in some laboratories, and with some substrates, noncompetitive kinetics have been observed.[129]

Disulfiram

Another important inhibitor of drug metabolism is disulfiram (tetraethylthiuram disulfide, Antabuse):

$$\begin{array}{c} C_2H_5 \\ C_2H_5 \end{array} > N - \overset{\overset{\displaystyle S}{\|}}{C} - S - S - \overset{\overset{\displaystyle S}{\|}}{C} - N < \begin{array}{c} C_2H_5 \\ C_2H_5 \end{array}$$

disulfiram

This compound has virtually no pharmacologic effects of its own. If, after its administration, however, ethyl alcohol is ingested, a violently unpleasant syndrome develops, including flushing, dyspnea, nausea, vomiting, and hypotension. These remarkable effects are specific for alcohol, and they occur even a day or two after disulfiram is taken. The drug was introduced for the treatment of chronic alcoholism. The alcoholic takes disulfiram regularly; thus, his resolve to abstain from alcohol is reinforced by the knowledge of how ill he will inevitably become if he drinks. If he drinks nevertheless, serious toxicity may ensue. The hypotension may be severe enough to produce shock, and myocardial damage has been reported. These potentionally dangerous effects limit the use of disulfiram to selected patients under strict medical supervision, who are also usually receiving psychotherapy.

Disulfiram inhibits aldehyde dehydrogenase, the enzyme that normally oxidizes acetaldehyde to acetic acid in the pathway ethanol → acetaldehyde → acetic acid.

This accumulation of acetaldehyde is thought to be responsible for the characteristic physiologic disturbances in humans, since the syndrome can be reproduced, at least in part, by acetaldehyde infusion. When ethanol is ingested under normal conditions, the acetaldehyde level does not exceed a few micrograms per milliliter. This level is virtually independent of the dose of ethanol, since (cf. p. 305) the alcohol dehydrogenase, which catalyzes formation of acetaldehyde, is saturated at ethanol concentrations in the mildly intoxicating range. When an identical dose of ethanol is given after disulfiram pretreatment, the ethanol blood level curve is the same, but acetaldehyde concentrations reach levels severalfold higher.[130]

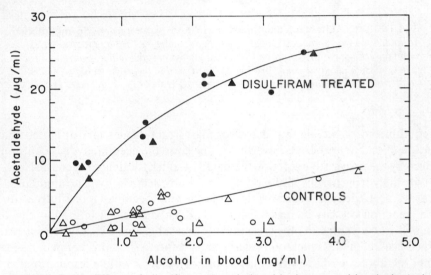

FIGURE 3-14. Effect of disulfiram on relationship between blood alcohol and acetaldehyde concentrations in rabbits. *Groups of rabbits were given ethanol after pretreatment with disulfiram, others were given same dose of alcohol without pretreatment. At 1 hr (circles) and again at 2 hr (triangles), blood ethanol and acetaldehyde levels were determined. Each point represents a single animal. (Modified, from Hald et al., Figure 3.[131])*

Figure 3-14 shows, in rabbits, how the relationship between blood ethanol concentration and blood acetaldehyde concentration is changed by disulfiram. At any given concentration of ethanol, the corresponding acetaldehyde level was increased severalfold by disulfiram.

Acetaldehyde itself can be metabolized just as rapidly by disulfiram-treated livers as by normal livers, provided a high enough concentration of acetaldehyde is present. At low concentrations of acetaldehyde, however, the rate of metabolism is greatly depressed (Figure 3-15). The finding of a normal rate of metabolism of ethanol, a normal rate of metabolism of acetaldehyde, but a higher steady-state level of acetaldehyde can all be explained on the basis of inhibition of aldehyde dehydrogenase:

$$CH_3CH_2OH \underset{}{\overset{\text{alcohol dehydrogenase}}{\rightleftharpoons}} CH_3CHO \overset{\text{aldehyde dehydrogenase}}{\longrightarrow} CH_3COOH$$

$$\underset{\text{ethanol}}{} \qquad \underset{\text{acetaldehyde}}{} \qquad \underset{\text{acetic acid}}{}$$

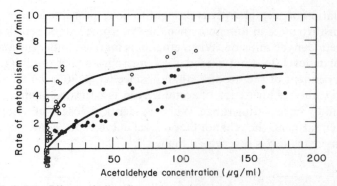

FIGURE 3-15. Effect of disulfiram upon rate of acetaldehyde metabolism. *Acetaldehyde was perfused through the livers of untreated rabbits (open circles) and rabbits pretreated with disulfiram (solid circles). Six treated and six untreated rabbits were used. Acetaldehyde concentration was measured in the perfused blood, and rate of metabolism was simultaneously determined. (From Hald et al., Figure 1.[132])*

The equilibrium of the alcohol dehydrogenase reaction lies far to the left, but the oxidation of ethanol proceeds nevertheless, because the acetaldehyde is continuously removed by the irreversible reaction mediated by aldehyde dehydrogenase. Now, if the aldehyde dehydrogenase is inhibited by disulfiram, acetaldehyde accumulates. With increasing acetaldehyde concentration, the enzyme becomes more fully saturated, and the reaction velocity increases. More acetaldehyde is also excreted by the kidney and lungs, or consumed in other reactions. Eventually, a new steady-state is reached, at which acetaldehyde is metabolized as fast as before. When this happens, the rate of ethanol metabolism will be normal. The only difference will be a much higher acetaldehyde level.

Disulfiram inhibits aldehyde dehydrogenase competitively with respect to NAD^+ but noncompetitively with respect to the substrate. This inhibition is evidently irreversible, for the recovery of enzyme activity is very slow (half-time about 24 hr), and it is prevented by cycloheximide, suggesting that new enzyme has to be synthesized.[133,134]

Some effects of disulfiram on other enzymes are important. Acting as a copper chelating agent, its reduced metabolite (diethyldithiocarbamate) inhibits dopamine-β-hydroxylase, the enzyme responsible for conversion of dopamine to norepinephrine.[135] It also acts as a nonspecific inhibitor of microsomal drug metabolism.[136,137]

Another inhibitor of the metabolism of ethanol is known. Pyrazole is quite a potent competitive inhibitor of liver alcohol dehydrogenase ($K_I = 2.6 \times 10^{-6} M$). It reacts with the enzyme and NAD^+ to form a ternary complex.[138] Pyrazole itself is too toxic to be useful therapeutically, but a less toxic derivative might possibly be valuable in treating methanol poisoning by blocking the formation of formaldehyde.

Monoamine Oxidase Inhibitors

Research on synthetic antibacterial agents led to the introduction of iproniazid, a hydrazide, for the chemotherapy of tuberculosis:

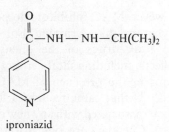

iproniazid

Unexpectedly, mood-elevating effects (euphoria) and other stimulatory actions on the central nervous system were seen. Iproniazid and related compounds were found to be MAO inhibitors. Since amines (e.g., norepinephrine, serotonin) are normally present in the brain, it was thought that inhibition of their metabolism might underlie the psychopharmacologic actions of these drugs. Related hydrazides were introduced for the treatment of severe depressions, for example, phenelzine and isocarboxazid:

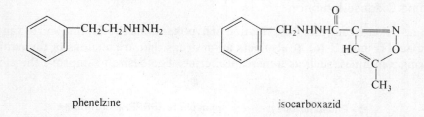

phenelzine   isocarboxazid

Several nonhydrazide inhibitors of MAO have also been developed, such as tranylcypromine and pargyline:

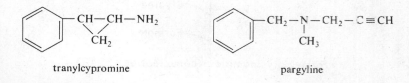

tranylcypromine   pargyline

All these MAO inhibitors act in vitro as well as in vivo. The administration of iproniazid (5×10^{-5} moles kg^{-1}) to rats resulted in complete inhibition of their liver mitochondrial MAO for 24 hr and normal activity did not return for 5 days.[139] In vitro, the onset of the inhibition by iproniazid (5×10^{-5} M) takes about 10 min. Tyramine, a substrate, can protect the enzyme and delay the development of inhibition; but once inhibition develops, it is practically irreversible.

The MAO inhibitors have complex pharmacologic actions, which are not thoroughly understood. They certainly cause elevations in the norepinephrine and serotonin levels in the central nervous system; but exactly how this action is related to their mood-elevating action is uncertain. They also may produce a variety of toxic effects, including hypotension, liver damage and jaundice, nausea, vomiting, constipation, dry mouth, and psychic disturbances (delusions, hallucinations). The hypotensive effect has been explored for possible therapeutic application.

The MAO inhibitors have little or no potentiating action upon the cardiovascular effects of the natural catecholamines, presumably because O-methylation and tissue uptake rather than oxidative deamination are primarily responsible for terminating their peripheral actions. However, MAO inhibitors do potentiate the cardiovascular effects of simple phenylethylamines like tyramine. For example, patients receiving tranylcypromine, who also took drugs of the phenylethylamine class, showed exaggerated hypertensive effects, including fatal cerebral hemorrhages.[140,141] Even foods can become dangerous in the presence of MAO inhibitors. A remarkable incident of cheese toxicity[142,143] that came to light a few years ago highlights the unexpected dangers that may be associated with any new drug. Some cheeses (Camembert, Brie, Stilton, New York Cheddar) are rich in tyramine. Ordinarily harmless because it is oxidized so rapidly by MAO, tyramine was markedly toxic in patients who had received tranylcypromine. Hypertensive crises occurred, and in a few instances, fatal cerebral hemorrhage. Consequently, tranylcypromine was removed from the market by the Food and Drug Administration, but eventually was admitted to use again provided appropriate warnings were included on the label and in the promotional literature.

Xanthine Oxidase Inhibitors

Xanthine oxidase catalyzes the oxidation of hypoxanthine to xanthine and of xanthine to uric acid (Figure 3-16). It also acts upon drugs that are analogs of the naturally occurring xanthines, such as 6-mercaptopurine. The desire to improve the efficacy

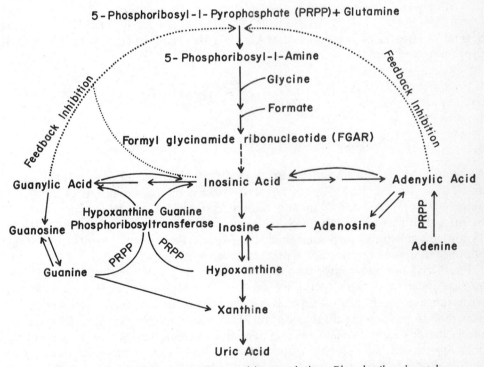

FIGURE 3-16. Purine metabolism and its regulation. *Phosphoribosylpyrophosphate (PRPP) amidotransferase catalyzes the first reaction in this sequence. It is the rate-limiting step of purine synthesis, and the activity of this enzyme is controlled by the purine nucleotide concentration through feedback inhibition. (From Kelley et al., Figure 2.[148])*

of 6-mercaptopurine in cancer therapy by blocking its metabolism to 6-thiouric acid led to the synthesis and testing of allopurinol.[144-146] This drug proved to be an effective xanthine oxidase inhibitor in vivo, and it did enhance both the therapeutic and

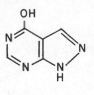

allopurinol

toxic actions of 6-mercaptopurine. The effect of greatest clinical significance, however, turned out to be its efficacy in the treatment of gout. The rate of production of uric acid in this disease is excessively high, and since the urates are poorly soluble in water, urate crystals deposit in kidney, joints, and various soft tissues. Allopurinol, by inhibiting xanthine oxidase, decreases the rate of urate synthesis, and consequently the steady-state urate level, permitting gouty deposits to redissolve.

The action of allopurinol in inhibiting xanthine oxidase would in itself be expected to raise hypoxanthine and xanthine levels (since these are the precursors of uric acid) but not necessarily to alter the total rate of synthesis and excretion of all the purines. Purine biosynthesis, however, is under feedback regulation, as shown in Figure 3-16. Blocking xanthine oxidase tends to increase the levels of hypoxanthine and guanine. In the presence of normal activity of hypoxanthine guanine phosphoribosyltransferase, levels of the corresponding nucleotides, inosinic and guanylic acids, increase. These, in turn, inhibit the first step in purine biosynthesis, the combination of PRPP with glutamine. The result of this mechanism is that allopurinol not only reduces the rate of uric acid formation from xanthine, but indirectly decreases the rate of biosynthesis of the purines.[147] In the Lesch–Nyhan syndrome (cf. Chapter 6), characterized by hypoxanthine guanine phosphoribosyltransferase deficiency, allopurinol reduces urate excretion, as usual. However, since conversion of the purine bases to nucleotides is deficient, the feedback inhibition of purine synthesis does not occur, and hypoxanthine and xanthine are excreted in increased amounts.

Allopurinol itself is converted to a nucleotide by hypoxanthine guanine phosphoribosyltransferase, and this allopurinol derivative acts directly as a feedback inhibitor of the PRPP–glutamine reaction. A further complexity is the oxidation of allopurinol by xanthine oxidase to a product, alloxanthine, which is itself a xanthine oxidase inhibitor.

STIMULATION AND DEPRESSION
OF DRUG METABOLISM

A number of drugs cause an increase in the activity of the liver microsomal drug-metabolizing enzymes of treated animals.[149-156] Among these drugs, phenobarbital, the carcinogenic hydrocarbon 3,4-benzpyrene, and the steroid hormones have been studied most thoroughly. Typically, the activities toward different substrates are differentially stimulated; thus, phenobarbital and 3,4-benzpyrene each have their own typical spectrum of stimulation. Figure 3-17 shows the characteristic response to

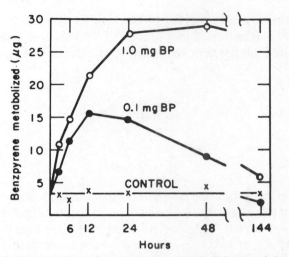

FIGURE 3-17. Stimulation of benzpyrene-metabolizing activity of rat liver by administration of benzpyrene. *Weanling rats were given a single intraperitoneal injection of benzpyrene at the doses indicated. Animals were sacrificed periodically, and benzpyrene-metabolizing activity of liver samples was measured for a 12 min period. Each point is the average from 2 rats. (From Conney et al., Figure 1.[157])*

benzpyrene in rats. The animals were treated with benzpyrene at two different doses, and then the benzpyrene hydroxylase activity of their livers was tested in vitro at intervals for 6 days. At the higher dose a 7-fold stimulation was seen, with a half-time of about 6 hr. At 6 days (144 hr), the stimulation caused by both doses had subsided. Similar results were obtained with another carcinogen, 3-methylcholanthrene. Activity toward azo dyes (reduction and demethylation) was also stimulated by these hydrocarbons.

Stimulation of drug metabolism may produce a state of apparent drug tolerance. For example, rabbits pretreated with pentobarbital for 3 days slept a much shorter time after an intravenous test dose than did controls (Table 3-2). Inasmuch as the blood concentrations of pentobarbital were about the same in both groups at the moment of awakening, all the effect is accounted for by an increased rate of metabo-

TABLE 3-2. Effect of pentobarbital pretreatment on duration of pento-barbital action.
Rabbits were pretreated with 3 daily doses of pentobarbital ($60 \, \text{mg kg}^{-1}$) subcutaneously, then given a single challenging dose of $30 \, \text{mg/kg}^{-1}$ intra-venously. Sleeping times and pentobarbital levels in plasma were measured. (Data of Remmer,[158] Table I.)

Pretreatment	Sleeping time (min)	Plasma level of pentobarbital on awakening ($\mu g \, ml^{-1}$)	Pentobarbital half-life in plasma (min)
None	67 ± 4	9.9 ± 1.4	79 ± 3
Pentobarbital	30 ± 7	7.9 ± 0.6	26 ± 2

lism; there was no significant change in the animals' sensitivities to given drug concentrations.

An abundance of evidence indicates that the stimulation of activity of microsomal enzymes involves new protein synthesis. The stimulating agents are without effect in vitro; animals have to be pretreated, and a period of time has to elapse that corresponds to known rates of protein synthesis. Phenobarbital, which stimulates a great many enzyme activities, produces a detectable increase in the amount of microsomal

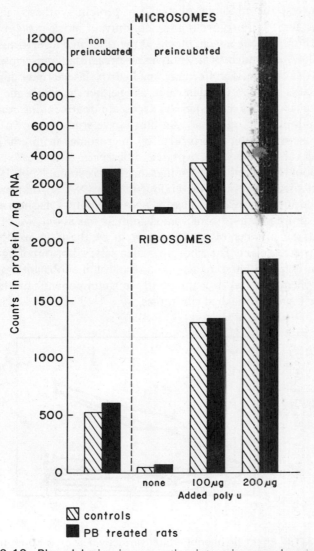

FIGURE 3-18. Phenylalanine incorporation into microsomal and ribosomal preparations from livers of treated and untreated rats. *Upper figure: Microsome preparations. Hatched columns are controls, black columns are rats pretreated with phenobarbital. At left are results with fresh preparations; at right, after preincubation to destroy endogenous mRNA. All experiments contained 3.5 mg protein. Experiments with and without added polyU are shown. Lower figure: Same experiments with ribosomes, after detergent removal of endoplasmic reticulum. (From Gelboin, Figure 2.*[164])

protein per gram of liver; but 3-methylcholanthrene, which stimulates fewer enzymes, does not. Electron micrographs show[159] that after phenobarbital treatment there is an increase in the amount of smooth endoplasmic reticulum in liver cells, and it will be recalled that the microsomal drug-metabolizing enzymes are associated with this structure. It has also been found that the kinetic properties (substrate affinities, etc.) of the various drug-metabolizing enzymes after phenobarbital stimulation are indistinguishable from those of control enzymes.[159a] The amino acid antimetabolite, ethionine, blocks the stimulatory response to phenobarbital; and methionine, which is known to reverse the ethionine blockade of protein synthesis, also prevents the ethionine effect here.[160] Puromycin and actinomycin block protein synthesis more directly than ethionine; puromycin blocks at the ribosome level (translation), actinomycin at the DNA-dependent RNA polymerase reaction (transcription). Both these agents prevent the stimulation of benzpyrene hydroxylase activity in rat liver.[161–164]

Protein synthesis may be studied in vitro, using either the whole microsome fraction from liver or the ribosomes only, after deoxycholate treatment has removed attached fragments of endoplasmic reticulum. An illustrative study is shown in Figure 3-18. Phenylalanine incorporation into protein by microsomes from control and phenobarbital-treated rats showed the expected differences—the treated rats could incorporate at about twice the rate per milligram of microsomal RNA. Preincubation of the microsomes digests away all the endogenous mRNA, so that protein synthesis then requires the addition of an artificial mRNA like polyU, as shown at upper right. Again, the rate in preparations from treated animals was about twice that of controls, suggesting that the number of sites for protein synthesis is greatly increased by phenobarbital pretreatment. The ribosomes themselves (bottom of figure) showed no differences in protein synthetic capacity as a result of phenobarbital pretreatment, so the effects of phenobarbital are apparently on components of the endoplasmic reticulum other than the attached ribosomes.

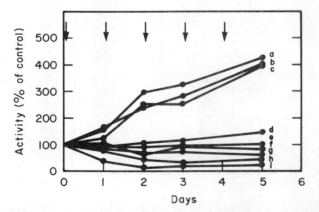

FIGURE 3-19. Effect of phenobarbital on activities of various microsomal enzymes in the rat. *Rats were injected intraperitoneally with phenobarbital (100 mg kg^{-1}) once daily as shown by arrows. Various enzyme activities of liver were measured. (a) Demethylation of aminopyrine; (b) amount of the CO-binding pigment (P-450); (c) NADPH-cytochrome c reductase; (d) amount of liver microsomal protein; (e) inosine diphosphatase; (f) NADH-cytochrome c reductase; (g) amount of cytochrome b_5; (h) glucose-6-phosphatase; (i) ATPase. Protein content is per gram liver, other data are calculated per milligram of protein. (From Orrenius and Ernster, Figure 1.*[165])

It has become clear that the stimulation produced by phenobarbital is quite specific for the essential components of the microsomal drug-oxidizing system, namely, the NADPH-cytochrome c reductase and cytochrome P450 (cf. p. 242). Figure 3-19 shows a remarkable parallelism in the time course of stimulation of demethylating activity in rat liver with repeated injections of phenobarbital, and the increase in the amounts of these two components. There was also a slight increase in total microsomal protein in liver (usually more striking in experiments like this), but no change whatsoever in a number of unrelated enzymes.

The increase in cytochrome P450 seen after phenobarbital treatment is preceded by a sharp rise in Δ-aminolevulinic acid (ALA) synthetase, the initial and rate-limiting enzyme in heme biosynthesis (see Figure 6-11). This is shown in Figure 3-20, for a single injection of phenobarbital.

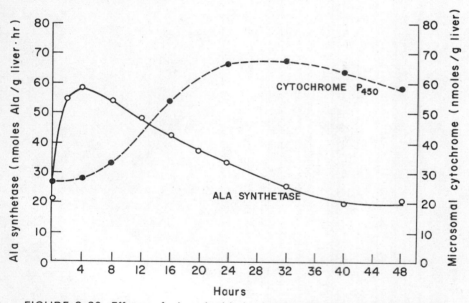

FIGURE 3-20. Effects of phenobarbital administration on ALA synthetase and cytochrome P450. *Groups of rats were given a single injection of phenobarbital (125 mg kg^{-1}) intraperitoneally at zero time, then killed at various times thereafter. Liver enzyme activities are shown. (From Marver, Figure 4.[166])*

The synthesis of heme is regulated by feedback of free heme on the formation of ALA synthetase; thus, decreased heme levels derepress synthesis of the enzyme, and heme levels are restored. Could the induction of cytochrome P450 by phenobarbital and other drugs involve this mechanism? If so, it might be expected that free heme would block all the effects related to microsomal enzyme induction by phenobarbital. This is demonstrated to be true in Table 3-3. Intraperitoneal injection of soluble heme preparations prevented the phenobarbital mediated increases in liver microsomal protein, liver phospholipid (a measure of the amount of endoplasmic reticulum), NADPH cytochrome c reductase, cytochrome P450, aminopyrine-demethylating capacity, hexobarbital-oxidizing capacity, and sleeping time following hexobarbital administration.

TABLE 3.3 Effects of heme on induction of microsomal drug metabolizing enzymes.
(Constructed from Marver; Figure 5, Tables 3 and 4.[166])

Heme[a]	Phenobarbital	Microsomal protein μg g⁻¹ liver	Phospholipid μg P g⁻¹ liver	NADPH cytochrome c reductase	P450	Sleeping time (min)	nmoles/mg protein in 10 min	
							Aminopyrine demethylase	Hexobarbital oxidation
–	–	18.0	238.0	85	75	65 ± 8	47 ± 4	24 ± 3
–	+	31.2	506.0	148	190	20 ± 3	133 ± 11	54 ± 4
+	–	19.8	261	78	60	136 ± 19	29 ± 3	17 ± 3
+	+	20.2	286	89	80	128 ± 14	36 ± 4	21 ± 4

[a] As heme albumin.

There has been a great deal of confusion about just what is proved by the fact that stimulation of an enzyme activity requires concomitant protein synthesis. The initial, unstimulated level of microsomal enzyme activity has to be regarded as a steady-state, determined by balanced rates of synthesis and degradation. The stimulation represents a change in this steady-state, but it could be brought about either by an increased rate of synthesis or a decreased rate of degradation, or both. Some instances of "enzyme induction" (for example, the stimulation of tryptophan pyrrolase activity by tryptophan) can be attributed to the stabilization of enzyme by its substrate; stimulation of the same enzyme activity by steroids is apparently a true induction.[167] Suppose the drug-induced enhancement of an enzyme activity is prevented by treatments (ethionine, puromycin) that block protein synthesis. It may be concluded that the drug-induced stimulation did not represent direct activation of an already-formed enzyme. But no conclusion can be drawn as to whether the drug caused an increased rate of enzyme synthesis or a decreased rate of enzyme degradation; no matter which of these two mechanisms is responsible for the shift of a steady-state, continued protein synthesis would be required for its manifestation. Judicious use of actinomycin may yield more decisive information about mechanism. This drug should block stimulation that depends upon the synthesis of new messenger-RNA. Provided that existing messenger-RNA continues to function, actinomycin ought not to block stimulation due to enzyme stabilization.

To see if inducers act primarily by increasing protein synthesis or by decreasing protein degradation, the incorporation of ^{3}H-leucine was followed in NADPH cytochrome c reductase and in total microsomal protein of liver.[168] Phenobarbital caused increased incorporation within 90 min, presumably reflecting a stimulation of protein synthesis. Prelabeled protein of control animals turned over (loss of label) with half-time about 3 days, and twice-daily injections of phenobarbital resulted in much longer retention of label. However, the disappearance of label from a prelabeled protein depends strongly upon the unknown efficiency of immediate reutilization of the component amino acids for new protein synthesis, before they are diluted in the general (nonradioactive) pool. Thus, the method tends to overestimate protein half-life to an uncertain degree. One study used ^{14}C-guanidino-L-arginine, which breaks down so quickly in the active urea cycle of liver that reutilization is minimized. No difference was found in the rate of microsomal protein breakdown between livers from control and phenobarbital treated animals.[169] However, another study with the same radioactive amino acid gave evidence of reduced breakdown after phenobarbital pretreatment.[170] Thus, although it is reasonably certain that inducers stimulate new microsomal protein synthesis, the question whether they also stabilize proteins against degradation remains open.

Mammalian cells growing in vitro offer an opportunity to distinguish inducer effects on transcription from those on translation in protein synthesis.[171,172] The cells can be exposed to various agents for definite periods of time, and the culture medium can be changed at will. In hamster fetal cells, benzpyrene hydroxylase (also known as aryl hydroxylase) was increased by exposure to benz(α)anthracene or other polycyclic hydrocarbons. The enzyme is a mixed function oxidase requiring molecular oxygen and NADPH. In this system, neither phenobarbital nor corticosteroids will act as inducers. Actinomycin D, puromycin, and cycloheximide all block the enzyme induction. If protein synthesis is shut off with puromycin, or if the inducer is omitted, enzyme activity decays with half-time about 3 hr. When cells were preincubated in the presence of inducer and cycloheximide for 10 hr, there was no increase in benz-pyrene hydroxylase activity. When the cells were then washed, and the medium replaced with control medium, there was an immediate sharp rise in enzyme activity, despite the fact that no inducer was present. Moreover, this occurred even in the presence of actinomycin D, but not if the cells have been exposed to actinomycin D during the preincubation. If, on the other hand, cells were preincubated in actino-mycin D, washed, and then exposed to inducer in control medium, there was only a slow increase of enzyme activity, just as observed with cells never exposed to actino-mycin. All these findings are compatible with the hypothesis that the inducer acts at the level of transcription (blocked by actinomycin) increasing mRNA synthesis for this enzyme. The subsequent translation of the mRNA (blocked by cycloheximide) appears to be an independent cytoplasmic process.

Several lipid soluble compounds that contain an allyl group but are otherwise unrelated have the capacity to destroy cytochrome P450.[173] Allyl barbiturates (allobarbital, secobarbital, aprobarbital), for example, have this action, whereas their ethyl analogs do not.[174] One of the most potent agents of this type is 2-allyl-2-iso-propylacetamide, the effect of which is shown in Figure 3-21. After a single oral dose in the rat, the content of cytochrome P450 in liver declined greatly for about 10 hr, then returned to a level much higher than normal, comparable with that attained after typical inducers like phenylbutazone (shown in figure) or phenobarbital.

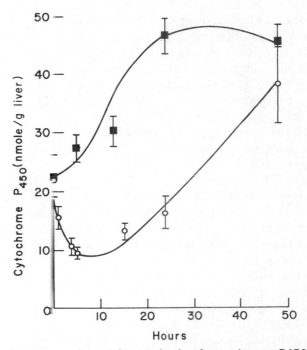

FIGURE 3-21. Destruction and resynthesis of cytochrome P450 after allyl isopropyl acetamide in the rat. *A single dose of 2-allyl-2-isopropyl-acetamide or of phenylbutazone was given to rats. Animals were killed at various times, and cytochrome P450 in livers was determined. Upper curve shows usual induction by phenylbutazone; lower curve, the destruction, followed by resynthesis after the allyl compound. Points are means and standard deviations. (From De Matteis, Figure 1.[173])*

The mechanism appears to be a kind of "suicide reaction," in which the cytochrome P450 catalyzes the metabolism of the allyl compound to a metabolite. In the course of this reaction, the heme pigment is converted to an irreversibly altered brown-green derivative. The reduction of cytochrome P450 content leads in some way (possibly through decreased levels of free heme) to induction of δ-aminolevulinic acid synthetase, and thus eventually to higher levels of cytochrome P450, as in the usual induction of the drug-metabolizing system. SKF 525A, by blocking the initial metabolism of the allyl compounds, also blocks their ability to destroy cytochrome P450. Cycloheximide, on the other hand, does not prevent the destruction of cytochrome P450, but by blocking protein synthesis it prevents the subsequent induction of increased drug-metabolizing capacity.[175]

The allyl compounds are also implicated in hepatic porphyria, a condition characterized by excessive production of heme and its precursors, δ-aminolevulinic acid and porphobilinogen. This genetic abnormality is discussed in Chapter 6.

The phase of transient decrease in cytochrome P450 produced by the allyl compounds will obviously be associated with decreased capacity to metabolize all the drugs that depend on the liver microsomal system. Depression of this system can be produced in other ways, most significantly by procedures or illnesses that have a deleterious effect on liver function. This may account for the clinical impression that drugs are liable to have enhanced or prolonged effects in patients with liver disease.[176] However, the effects are usually not striking. Moreover, patients receiving several medications simultaneously may have their deficient drug-metabolizing capacity compensated by induction effects.[177]

Starvation has prominent effects. Table 3-4 gives the results of an experiment in which mice were starved for 36 hr and then tested for their response to a standard dose of hexobarbital. The livers of these animals were homogenized, and microsomal enzyme activities were determined. All the mice were classified into groups according to how long they had slept. The animals that slept the longest oxidized hexobarbital and certain other drugs more slowly than controls; however, nitro and azo reductions were unaffected or increased. Besides starvation and parenchymal liver damage, other conditions that impair microsomal drug-metabolizing activity are obstructive jaundice, liver tumors, and alloxan diabetes.

If the drug-metabolizing system is depressed, excessive responses or prolonged responses may occur to ordinary doses of drugs. On the other hand, should a suitable maintenance dose be instituted under these abnormal conditions, it might prove inadequate later on when the rate of drug metabolism increases to normal. Or conversely, a patient using barbiturate sedatives regularly is likely to have an unusually high activity of the drug-metabolizing enzymes, as discussed already; if another drug is given simultaneously, at customary dosages, it may prove wholly ineffective. If an appropriately higher dosage of the second drug is established for this patient, the drug levels may become excessive later on, should the barbiturate be discontinued. Figure 3-22 illustrates effects of this sort in a human subject. The patient was on a maintenance dosage of 75 mg daily of the anticoagulant drug bishydroxycoumarin. Plasma levels of the drug were followed, as well as prothrombin time, a measure of the drug effect in delaying blood clotting. During periods of regular phenobarbital administration the plasma level of bishydroxycoumarin fell, and the therapeutic action of the drug was significantly diminished. This illustration points up dramatically how drugs may interact.

TABLE 3-4. Effects of starvation on drug metabolism by mouse liver microsomes. Mice were starved for 36 hr, then given hexobarbital (80 mg kg^{-1}) intraperitoneally. Normal animals usually slept less than 10 min, but sleeping time varied greatly in starved mice. The mice were sacrificed 12 hr later (48 hr starvation), and the liver microsomes were tested for their drug-metabolizing ability. Figures represent drug metabolized in a fixed incubation time (From Dixon et al.,[178] Table I.)

	Drug metabolized (μ moles g^{-1} liver)		
	Normal mice	Starved mice	
Substrate	Sleeping time (5–15 min)	Sleeping time (20–40 min)	Sleeping time (>80 min)
Hexobarbital (aliphatic oxidation)	4.46	2.79	0.77
Chlorpromazine (sulfur oxidation)	2.80	1.98	1.19
Aminopyrine (N-dealkylation)	1.48	1.11	0.46
Acetanilid (aromatic hydroxylation)	2.03	2.22	0.93
p-Nitrobenzoic acid (nitro reduction)	8.22	17.03	8.43
Neoprontosil (azo reduction)	15.55	17.65	12.59

For drugs whose effectiveness or toxicity is enhanced by a metabolic transformation, other drugs that stimulate the rate of metabolism will cause an increase in potency and toxicity. This has been demonstrated experimentally with the organic thiophosphate insecticide guthion (dimethoxybenzotriazine dithiophosphoric acid ester).

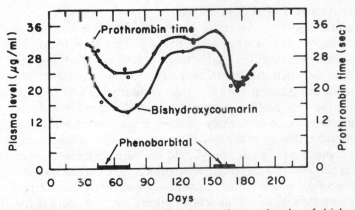

FIGURE 3-22. Effect of phenobarbital on plasma levels of bishydroxycoumarin. *A human subject was treated with bishydroxycoumarin (75 mg daily). Drug plasma levels and prothrombin times were determined periodically. Phenobarbital was administered (65 mg once daily) during periods indicated by heavy marks on abscissal axis. (From Cucinell et al., Figure 3.[179] By permission of C. V. Mosby.)*

This compound depends for its activity as a cholinesterase inhibitor upon its oxidative desulfuration at a microsomal site (cf. p. 249). Pretreatment of rats with benzpyrene or methylcholanthrene substantially increased the rate of that conversion; consequently, a given dose of guthion caused greater inhibition of brain and salivary gland cholinesterase. The median lethal dose of guthion was lowered by about half (i.e., the toxicity was doubled) in pretreated animals.[180] The same investigation revealed that pretreating the animals with SKF 525A, the inhibitor of the drug-metabolizing microsomal system, resulted in a lower toxicity of guthion.

While a large number of drugs, insecticides, and other chemicals can cause increases in rates of drug metabolism, as already described, only a few are known to depress the microsomal oxidative system on chronic long-term use. This has been shown with methylphenidate, oxyphenylbutazone, methandrostenolone, phenyramidol, nortriptyline, allopurinol, and disulfiram. For example, the half-life of bishydroxycoumarin in 6 volunteers was found to be 51 ± 3.7 hr; after 14 days of allopurinol treatment, in ordinary doses, the half-life had increased to 152 ± 30 hr.[181]

The ability of drugs to stimulate or depress the microsomal drug metabolizing system dictates great caution in multiple drug therapy of any kind.[182] And since many commercial drug preparations include more than a single drug, real problems may be encountered frequently. Amphetamine, for example, was sometimes used for diet control because it depresses the appetite. Some proprietary appetite control formulations included a barbiturate in the same capsule with amphetamine, supposedly to counteract excessive central excitation. The barbiturate could be expected to stimulate drug metabolism and thus enhance the destruction of the amphetamine. So perhaps the same end result could have been achieved with a lower dose of amphetamine and no barbiturate at all! Another problem of consequence, but not yet sufficiently investigated, is the possible influence of drugs upon the metabolism of endogenous steroid hormones. There is real cause for concern about this because these physiologically important substances are evidently metabolized by the microsomal drug-oxidizing system.

On the other hand, it may prove possible to exploit the stimulatory effect of phenobarbital on drug metabolism for a therapeutic purpose. For example, genetic disorders of glucuronide formation occur in man, much as in the Gunn rat mentioned previously; afflicted individuals, because of their impaired ability to conjugate bilirubin, have elevated bilirubin levels (unconjugated bilirubinemia) with jaundice. Administration of low doses of phenobarbital on a chronic basis can induce an increase in the low glucuronide transferase level, and thus alleviate the symptoms.[183] The insecticide DDT, which is also an inducer of microsomal enzymes, has been used successfully for the same purpose, at doses far below the toxic range, and with lasting effect due to the prolonged storage of this compound in tissues (cf. p. 361).[134]

SPECIES DIFFERENCES AND GENETIC VARIATION IN DRUG METABOLISM

Investigations into the phylogenetic aspects of drug metabolism[1] suggest that drug-metabolizing systems may have developed in response to the special needs of terrestrial life. In fish, lipid-soluble compounds can pass readily across the gills into the aquatic environment; and fish (with some exceptions) lack oxidative drug-metabolizing enzymes, neither can they form glucuronides or sulfuric acid esters. Aquatic amphibia are also unable to oxidize foreign compounds, but they can form glucuronides and sulfuric acid esters. Reptiles, birds, and mammals have the necessary enzymic machinery for increasing the polarity of lipid-soluble compounds and thus achieving their more rapid excretion (cf. p. 227). Insects have enzymes with analogous function but different in many ways from those of the vertebrates.

Azo and nitro reductase enzymes have a somewhat different distribution through the phylogenetic series than the microsomal oxidative enzymes. They (like the oxidative enzymes) are present in land-dwelling reptiles, birds, and mammals. Unlike the oxidative enzymes, they are also found in teleost fish. Amphibia and elasmobranch fishes have the azo reductase activity alone.[185]

Among the mammals there are wide differences in drug metabolism by different species, but no rationale for these differences is apparent. Rates of metabolism may differ, even when the pathways are the same, and different species may also have entirely different metabolic pathways for dealing with the same drug. An example of variation in metabolic rate is afforded by a study of a bromocyclohexenyl derivative of barbituric acid. This compound was originally synthesized in an attempt to obtain a barbiturate that would be rapidly metabolized in man. Testing was carried out in dogs, with very promising results, but it turned out that in man the compound was metabolized very slowly (Figure 3-23). This experiment illustrates a major pitfall in the use of animal screening programs for drug development. The compound selected on the basis of animal screening turned out to be useless in man. One wonders how many compounds have been discarded because of results in the dog, which would have been satisfactory in the human. The antirheumatic agent phenylbutazone presents another example. Its biologic half-life is only 3 hr in the rabbit, and less than 6 hr in the rat, guinea pig, and dog, yet in man its half-life is 3 days.

The metabolism of hexobarbital was shown to be responsible for species differences in its duration of action (Table 3-5). Determinations of plasma levels at various times following intravenous administration of the compound permitted estimation of the biologic half-life in each species. There was a direct relationship between duration of

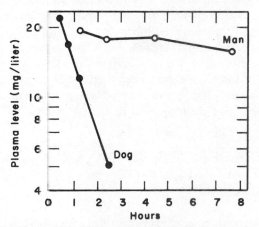

FIGURE 3-23. Metabolism of a barbiturate derivative in dog and man. *5-Allyl-5-(2-bromo-2-cyclohexenyl)-2-barbituric acid (15 mg kg^{-1}) was administered intravenously at time zero. Plasma concentrations were measured periodically, as shown, and plotted on a logarithmic scale. (From Burns, Figure 4.[186])*

TABLE 3-5. Species differences in metabolism of hexobarbital. Dose of barbiturate $100 \, \text{mg kg}^{-1}$ ($50 \, \text{mg kg}^{-1}$ in dogs). Figures in parentheses refer to number of animals in each species. Data are given $\pm$ standard deviation. The half-life in man is a crude estimate. (Data of Quinn et al.,[187] Table 2.)

	Sleeping time (min)	Hexobarbital half-life (min)	Enzyme activity (μg/g · hr)
Mice (12)	12 ± 8	19 ± 7	598 ± 184
Rabbits (9)	49 ± 12	60 ± 11	196 ± 28
Rats (10)	90 ± 15	140 ± 54	134 ± 51
Dogs (8)	315 ± 105	260 ± 20	36 ± 30
Man	—	360 (approx.)	—

action (sleeping time) and biologic half-life. In addition, the in vitro activity of microsomes prepared from livers of these animals correlated well with the drug metabolism rate in vivo. Thus, mice with the shortest sleeping time and shortest barbiturate half-life, had the highest liver microsomal enzyme activity. Presumably these species all metabolized hexobarbital by aliphatic side chain oxidation, although direct proof of this is lacking.

The sympathomimetic amine L-ephedrine can be metabolized by N-demethylation, aromatic hydroxylation, and conjugation:

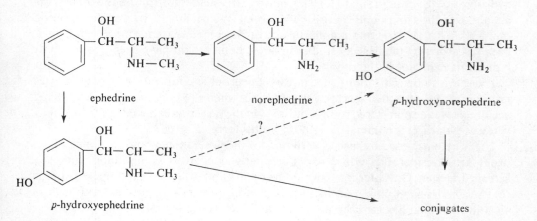

Table 3-6 shows that, in the dog, most of an administered dose of ephedrine appeared in urine as norephedrine, a potent sympathomimetic agent in its own right. When norephedrine itself was given to dogs, 72% of it was excreted unchanged. Thus, in the dog, the major route of metabolism is by N-demethylation. The guinea pig resembled the dog in this respect, but the rat excreted ephedrine largely unchanged and as hydroxylated derivatives. The rabbit, on the other hand, degraded these compounds still further, since none of the metabolites appeared in significant quantity in rabbit urine after ephedrine administration. When p-hydroxyephedrine was given, about 65% of it was excreted in the urine; but when norephedrine was given, only 3% of it

TABLE 3-6. Fate of ephedrine in several species.
Each animal received L-ephedrine (50 mg kg^{-1}) intraperitoneally. Urine was collected over a period of 24 hr. Figures in parentheses refer to number of animals in each species. (Data of Axelrod,[188] Table IV.)

		Percent of administered dose accounted for as:	
	Ephedrine	Norephedrine	Total hydroxyephedrine and hydroxynorephedrine
Dog (5)	6.5	57.8	1.5
Guinea pig (3)	2.0	38.5	0.9
Rat (4)	32.0	7.5	12.8
Rabbit (4)	0.1	1.8	1.9

was excreted. These results suggest that ephedrine is demethylated in the rabbit to norephedrine, which is then further metabolized to products not yet identified. The further metabolism does not, apparently, involve hydroxylation of the benzene ring, for in that case, the hydroxylated derivatives would have appeared in the urine. Available data for the metabolism of ephedrine in man suggest that in this species the drug is excreted almost entirely unchanged.[189]

Ethylbiscoumacetate, an anticoagulant drug, is metabolized rapidly (about 20% per hr) in both man and rabbit. Man metabolizes it by ring hydroxylation, the rabbit by hydrolysis of the ester group to form an inactive free acid. The dog, on the other hand, metabolizes the compound more slowly, about 3% per hr.[190] In a screening program seeking a short-acting coumarin derivative, ethylbiscoumacetate would have been discarded on the basis of studies in dogs; but it would have been chosen on the basis of its behavior in the rabbit.

There are some indications that in cats glucuronide conjugation is relatively less important than in other species. For example, when the carcinogen N-2-fluorenylacetamide was administered to cats, only 3% of the dose was excreted as glucuronides, whereas guinea pigs eliminated 60–80% in this form.[191]

The problems posed by species variation for the development and screening of new drugs are considerable. Obviously, potentially dangerous compounds cannot be screened in man. One alternative would be to find and utilize an experimental animal that resembles man closely in its handling of all foreign compounds; although no such ideal animal has yet been found, primates are probably most suitable.

Since drug metabolism is mediated by specific enzymes, genetic variations might be expected to occur among individuals of a species. Table 3-7 illustrates pronounced strain differences in the oxidative metabolism of one drug in mice. The data are sleeping times after a single dose of hexobarbital, but it is well known that in mice the duration of action of this drug is determined by the rate of its oxidation. Besides the highly significant differences between strains, another point is evident. The one strain that was not inbred has a much greater variability between animals (as measured by the standard deviation) than did the inbred strains. This is just what one would expect for a trait under genetic control.

TABLE 3-7. Strain differences in duration of action of hexobarbital in mice

Male mice, 70–80 days old, given hexobarbital ($125 \ mg \ kg^{-1}$) intraperitoneally. Figures in parentheses are number of mice in each strain. (Data of Jay,[192] Table 1.)

Strain	Mean sleeping time $\pm$ standard deviation (min)
A/NL (25)	48 ± 4
BALB/cAnN (63)	41 ± 2
C57L/HeN (29)	33 ± 3
C3HfB/HeN (30)	22 ± 3
SWR/HeN (38)	18 ± 4
Swiss (non-inbred) (47)	43 ± 15

An interesting example of strain difference in drug metabolism in rats concerns the volatile anesthetic methoxyflurane (p. 255), which has on occasion caused renal damage in humans. An investigation with five strains of rats revealed in one strain an unusually high rate of methoxyflurane metabolism, yielding very high levels of free fluoride ion in the blood, and thus producing renal toxicity. The renal damage could be reproduced by equivalent dosage of fluoride alone.[193] It is thought possible that the toxicity observed rarely in people may have a similar genetic basis. The genetic basis of variation in the rates of drug metabolism in man is discussed in Chapter 6.

In rats, strain differences are not usually very great, but sex differences in drug metabolism are very prominent.[194] Females sleep considerably longer than males after a given dose of hexobarbital, and they metabolize the drug more slowly. The male-female difference in the rat is seen readily with in vitro systems as well as in vivo. Females pretreated with testosterone show an increase in drug-metabolizing activity, and males pretreated with estradiol show a decrease. Similar differences between male and female rats have been demonstrated for N-demethylation of morphine congeners by microsome preparations in vitro. Curiously, sex differences in the rates of drug metabolism have not been observed in species other than the rat.

Another good example of genetically determined variation in drug metabolism occurs in rabbits. Certain individuals of this species have an unusual plasma esterase that is capable of hydrolyzing the plant ester alkaloid atropine.[195] In rabbits, the gene that controls production of this enzyme is autosomal and autonomous. Thus, each representation of the gene in the diploid organism appears to be expressed independently, so that animals homozygous for the trait have about twice as much enzyme activity as heterozygotes. However, gene expression is delayed: atropine esterase does not appear in the blood of rabbits that have the trait until they are 1–2 months old. The absence of the enzyme appears to be absolute in animals that lack the trait.[196] There is no immunologically related protein in their blood plasma, and such animals can even be sensitized to purified atropine esterase, further confirming the prior absence of any protein with similar antigenic properties.

The induction of drug-metabolizing capacity has been shown to be under genetic control in the mouse. As described earlier, phenobarbital and 3-methylcholanthrene act as inducers in quite different ways. Induction by phenobarbital leads to increased liver protein, cytochrome P450, and NADPH cytochrome c reductase, and the metabolism of a wide variety of drugs is enhanced. Hydrocarbons, on the other hand, induce formation of a spectrally distinct CO-binding cytochrome, the quantitative change in liver components is much less marked, and the metabolism of only a narrow range of substances is affected.[197]

One strain of mice (C57) responds to administration of 3-methylcholanthrene with increased formation of aryl hydrocarbon hydroxylase, but another strain (DBA) does not; yet phenobarbital is a good inducer in both strains.[198] The response of hepatic aryl hydrocarbon hydroxylase activity as a function of age with and without methylcholanthrene treatment is shown in Figure 3-24. In both strains, the constitutive levels of enzyme appeared shortly after birth and remained fairly constant

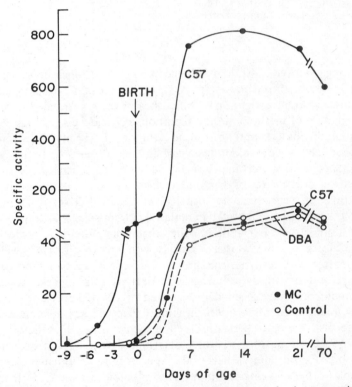

FIGURE 3-24. Genetic differences in induction of drug-metabolizing enzymes. *Two strains of mice were used, C57 and DBA. Open circles were untreated controls, solid circles are methylcholanthrene treated animals. Hepatic levels of aryl hydrocarbon hydroxylase activity were measured at various ages before and after birth. For experiments with fetuses, pregnant rats were treated with the inducer, all fetuses in a litter were pooled. The y axis gives specific activity of enzyme as units per milligram of liver homogenate protein. (From Nebert and Gielen, Figure 3.[199])*

after the first week of life. In the C57 strain but not in DBA, administration of inducer during pregnancy caused a pronounced increase in the fetal enzyme. Induction by 3-methylcholanthrene was especially marked during the first week after birth. DBA mice never responded to the inducer throughout the time period under study.

The mode of inheritance of the capacity for induction of this enzyme was studied in crosses between DBA and C57, as shown in Figure 3-25. The first and second rows show that all C57 mice responded to inducer, whereas no DBA mice did. In the F1 generation (C57 × DBA), all offspring were inducible (row 3). In the backcross of F1

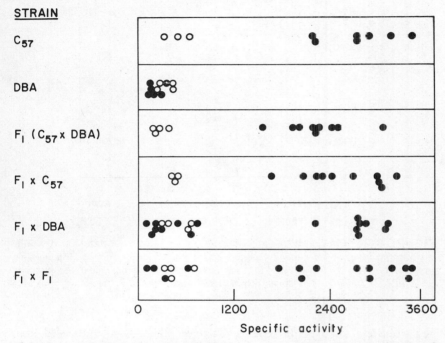

FIGURE 3-25. Genetic crosses and response to inducer. *Crosses of C57 and DBA mice were studied for their response to methylcholanthrene. Open circles represent controls, solid circles represent rats treated with methylcholanthrene. Specific activity indicates units of aryl hydrocarbon hydroxylase activity per milligram of liver microsomal protein. (From Nebert et al., Figure 2.[200])*

to C57, all mice were inducible (row 4), but in the back cross of F1 to DBA, only half the progeny were inducible (row 5). Finally, in F2 (F1 × F1), about three-fourths of the progeny were inducible. These results are all consistent with inheritance of the inducible trait as an autosomal dominant.

EFFECTS OF AGE UPON DRUG METABOLISM

It has long been recognized that the young of humans and other animals may be more sensitive to drugs than are adults. Many enzyme systems change greatly in activity during early life.[201,203]

This was shown in Figure 3-24 for one drug-metabolizing enzyme in mouse liver. A similar investigation of the activity of glucuronyl transferase in the microsomes of guinea pig livers revealed some striking differences with age (Figure 3-26). Enzyme activity for phenolphthalein conjugation was absent or very low in microsomes

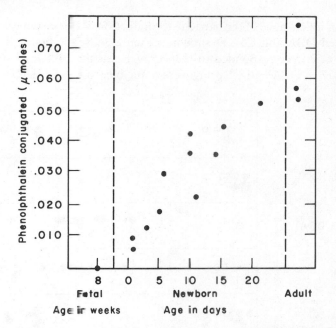

FIGURE 3-26. Phenolphthalein conjugation by fetal, neonatal, and adult guinea pig liver. *A microsome fraction was prepared from 200 mg liver, UDP-glucuronic acid was added, with 0.15 μmoles of phenolphthalein, and the mixture incubated for 30 min at 37°. (From Brown and Zuelzer, Figure 3.[202])*

obtained from fetal or neonatal guinea pig liver. The activity increased markedly during the postnatal period. Similar results were obtained with other substrates, such as *o*-aminophenol and bilirubin.

These studies have been extended to other drug-metabolizing microsomal enzymes, all of which have been found to be absent, or present in negligible amounts, in early life. The following in vitro reactions have been shown not to occur in liver microsomal preparations obtained from 1 day old guinea pigs or rabbits: *N*-demethylation (monomethyl-4-aminoantipyrine), *O*-dealkylation (phenacetin), side chain oxidation (hexobarbital), deamination (amphetamine), aromatic hydroxylation (acetanilid), sulfur oxidation (chlorpromazine), and nitro reduction (*p*-nitrobenzoic acid).[204] The drugs in parentheses were used as indicators for the presence or absence of detectable metabolic activity for each particular pathway.

In vivo studies support these conclusions. For example, when acetanilid was administered to newborn infants and to older children, and the plasma levels of *N*-acetyl-*p*-aminophenol and its glucuronide were measured, it became apparent that the oxidation and conjugation proceeded more slowly in the newborns.[205] Elevated blood bilirubin levels in the newborn (icterus neonatorum) result from deficiency of the enzymes responsible for the formation of bilirubin glucuronide.

Further evidence of the correlation between defective drug metabolism in early life and duration of drug action is presented in Table 3-8. In this study, microsomes obtained from 1 day old guinea pigs failed to metabolize hexobarbital, but there was a progressive increase in the oxidation rate in microsomes of older animals. Mice of various ages were injected with hexobarbital, and after 3 hr they were assayed in order

TABLE 3-8. Effect of age on metabolism and duration of action of hexobarbital.
In vitro experiments were done with a guinea pig liver microsome system, appropriately fortified
with cofactors. In vivo metabolism was measured by giving hexobarbital (1 mg) intraperitoneally
to a mouse and then homogenizing the entire animal and determining the residual amount of
unchanged drug. Sleeping times were measured in mice only. The number of experiments or
animals used are shown in parentheses. (Data of Jondorf et al.,[206] Tables 1, 2, and 3.)

Age (days)	Hexobarbital metabolized in vitro in 1 hr by guinea pigs (%)	Hexobarbital metabolized in vivo in 3 hr by mice (%)	Sleeping time in mice (min)		
			10 mg kg^{-1}	50 mg kg^{-1}	100 mg kg^{-1}
1	0 (3)	0 (6)	> 360 (12)	Died (12)	Died (12)
7	2.5–3.5 (3)	11–24 (6)	107 ± 26 (12)	243 ± 30 (10)	> 360 (12)
21	13–21 (3)	21–33 (6)	27 ± 11 (11)	64 ± 17 (10)	94 ± 27 (12)
Adult	28–39 (5)		< 5 (12)	17 ± 5 (12)	47 ± 11 (12)

to determine how much drug remained. The newborn animals failed to metabolize
any of the injected drug over the 3 hr period, 7 day old mice metabolized about 18%,
and 3 week old mice, about 22%. Paralleling this finding, it was observed that sleeping
times were much longer in newborn and young mice than in adult animals. However,
impaired metabolism alone will not account for the greater sensitivity of young mice
to hexobarbital; they seem also to be more sensitive to given tissue and plasma concentrations. Furthermore, very young animals have depressed renal function (p. 214)
and an unusually permeable blood-brain barrier.[207]

These findings have some important clinical implications. Infants are likely to be
more sensitive to some drugs than are adults, and to show more prolonged effects,
even after weight or surface area has been taken into account in arriving at an estimated
dosage schedule. There is also special danger in using drugs in obstetrical practice. A
drug that is relatively harmless to the mother may cross the placenta and have an
adverse effect on the fetus. After parturition, the newborn no longer has the use of a
maternal liver system to metabolize the drug, so that very long-lasting effects may then
be seen.

The tragic experience with chloramphenicol in newborn infants[208] highlights the
serious consequences that can result from deficient drug metabolism. The therapeutic
or prophylactic use of chloramphenicol in hospital nurseries led to cases of cyanosis
("gray syndrome"). Some deaths occurred, especially in premature infants, after
cardiovascular and respiratory collapse. In the adult human, about 90% of a dose of
chloramphenicol is excreted as the monoglucuronide derivative, about 8% as free
drug, and traces as the hydrolyzed deacetylated derivative. In newborn infants (and
in cats) a small amount of a dehalogenated product is also found.[209–211] In premature
infants, and during the first week or two of life in normal infants, the mechanism for
glucuronide conjugation is grossly deficient. At the same time, renal function (both
glomerular filtration and tubular secretion) is also very inefficient. Consequently, an
ordinary dose of chloramphenicol leads to a high and prolonged plasma level of the
free drug. Plasma glucuronide levels also increase because of the defective tubular
secretory mechanism; but, at least in the adult, chloramphenicol monoglucuronide is

nontoxic. Repeated doses at intervals that would be suitable in the older infant cause a progressive buildup of the plasma level of chloramphenicol into the range of severe hematologic toxicity.

The production of neonatal kernicterus by bilirubin through depressed glucuronide formation, aggravated by displacement of bilirubin from plasma albumin by certain sulfonamides and vitamin K, is discussed in Chapter 14 (p. 821).

Effects of old age on drug metabolism have not been extensively studied. An investigation of hexobarbital sleeping times in male and female rats of different ages revealed some interesting effects of age that could be attributed to the sexual status.[212] Rats begin producing sex hormones (estrogen, testosterone) at about 2 months of age. It is just at this time that sex differences in sleeping times appear. Thus, male and female rats both slept about 40 min at 1 month of age, but at 2 months the males slept 15 min on the average, while females slept 55 min. These differences persisted throughout the period of sexual maturity. Sex hormone production in rats declines at about 2 years of age. In this experiment, the sex differences in sleeping time disappeared at the same time. In another study rats 30 days of age showed a maximal rate of drug-metabolizing activity; then the activity declined progressively until 250 days of age.[213] Age effects are not prominent in mice.[214]

REFERENCES

1. B. B. BRODIE and R. P. MAICKEL: Comparative biochemistry of drug metabolism. In *Metabolic Factors Controlling Duration of Drug Action*. Proceedings of First International Pharmacological Meeting, vol. 6, ed. by B. B. Brodie and E. G. Erdös. New York, Macmillan Co. (1962) p. 299.

2. P. J. FRIEDMAN and J. R. COOPER: The role of alcohol dehydrogenase in the metabolism of chloral hydrate. *J. Pharmacol. Exp. Therap.* 129:373 (1960).

3. F. J. MAC KAY and J. R. COOPER: A study on the hypnotic activity of chloral hydrate. *J. Pharmacol. Exp. Therap.* 135 271 (1962).

4. B. B. BRODIE and J. AXELROD: The fate of acetanilide in man. *J. Pharmacol. Exp. Therap.* 94:29 (1948).

5. B. B. BRODIE and J. AXELROD: The fate of acetophenetidin (phenacetin) in man and methods for the estimation of acetophenetidin and its metabolites in biological material. *J. Pharmacol. Exp. Therap.* 97:58 (1949).

6. A. H. CONNEY, M. SANSUR, F. SOROKO, R. KOSTER, and J. J. BURNS: Enzyme induction and inhibition in studies on the pharmacological actions of acetophenetidin. *J. Pharmacol. Exp. Therap.* 151:133 (1966).

7. M. KIESE: Relationship of drug metabolism to methemoglobin formation. *Ann. N. Y. Acad. Sci.* 123:141 (1965).

8. B. B. BRODIE: Basic principles in development of methods for drug assay. In *Concepts in Biochemical Pharmacology*, ed. by B. B. Brodie and J. R. Gillette, Handb. Exp. Pharm. 28, Part 2, p. 1. Berlin, Heidelberg, New York, Springer–Verlag (1971).

9. L. C. CRAIG and D. CRAIG: Extraction and distribution. In *Techniques of Organic Chemistry*, Vol. 3, ed. by A. Weissberger, 2nd edition, New York, Interscience (1956) pp. 172–311.

10. A. C. BRATTON and E. K. MARSHALL, JR.: A new coupling component for sulfanilamide determination. *J. Biol. Chem.* 128:537 (1939).

11. L. C. CRAIG: Countercurrent distribution. *Methods in Medical Research*, 5:3 (1952).

12. E. O. TITUS: Isolation procedures—liquid extraction and isolation techniques. In *Fundamentals of Drug Metabolism and Drug Disposition*, ed. by B. N. LaDu, H. G. Mandel, and E. L. Way, Baltimore, Williams and Wilkins (1971) p. 419.

13. E. TITUS and H. WEISS: The use of biologically prepared radioactive indicators in metabolic studies: metabolism of pentobarbital. *J. Biol. Chem.* 214:807 (1955).

14. R. TRUHAUT, C. BOUDENE, and J. R. CLAUDE: Application of thin-layer chromatography to analytical toxicology. *Ann. Biol. Clin.* 26:93 (1968).

15. E. STAHL: *Thin-layer chromatography, a laboratory handbook*, 2nd ed., translated by M. R. F. Ashworth. Berlin, Heidelberg, New York, Springer–Verlag (1969).

16. E. O. TITUS: Isolation and identification of drug metabolites. See p. 123 in ref. 8, Part 2.

17. G. R. WILKINSON: Qualitative and quantitative applications of thin-layer, gas-liquid, and column chromatography. See p. 458 in ref. 12.

18. M. W. ANDERS: Gas chromatography. See p. 63 in ref. 8, Part 2.

19. H. P. BURCHFIELD and E. E. STORRS: *Biochemical Applications of Gas Chromatography.* New York, Academic Press (1962).

20. L. S. ETTRE and A. ZLATKIS: *The Practice of Gas Chromatography.* New York, Wiley–Interscience (1967).

21. H. S. KROMAN and S. K. BENDER: *Theory and Applications of Gas Chromatography in Industry and Medicine.* New York, Grune and Stratton (1968).

22. T. C. BUTLER: Reduction of carbon tetrachloride in vivo and reduction of carbon tetrachloride in chloroform in vitro by tissues and tissue constituents. *J Pharm. Exp. Therap.* 134:311 (1961).

23. J. N. DONE, G. J. KENNEDY, and J. H. KNOX: Revolution in liquid chromatography. *Nature* 237:77 (1972).

24. H. M. FALES: Isolation and identification procedures—spectral methods. See p. 437 in ref. 12.

25. P. BOMMER and F. M. VANE: The application of various spectroscopies to the identification of drug metabolites. See p. 209 in ref. 8, Part 2.

26. N. K. CHAUDHURI, B. J. MONTAG, and C. HEIDELBERGER: Studies on fluorinated pyrimidines. III. The metabolism of 5-fluorouracil-2-C^{14} and 5-fluoroorotic-2-C^{14} acid in vivo. *Cancer Res.* 18:318 (1958).

27. C. G. HAMMAR, B. HOLMSTEDT, J. E. LINDGREN, and R. THAM: The combination of gas chromatography and mass spectrometry in the identification of drugs and metabolites. *Adv. Pharmacol. Chemother.* 7:53 (1969).

28. B. J. MILLARD: Mass spectrometry in drug research. *Adv. Drug Res.* 6:157 (1971).

29. A. M. GUARINO and H. M. FALES: Gas chromatography—mass spectrometry. See p. 178 in ref. 8, Part 2.

30. S. H. KOSLOW, F. CATTABERI, and E. COSTA: Norepinephrine and dopamine: assay by mass fragmentography in the picomole range. *Science* 176:177 (1972).

31. C. G. HAMMAR and R. HESSLING: Novel peak matching technique by means of a new and combined multiple ion detector-peak matcher device. *Anal. Chem.* 43:298 (1971).

32. T. E. GAFFNEY, C. G. HAMMAR, and R. E. Mc MAHON: Ion specific detection of internal standards labeled with stable isotopes. *Anal. Chem.* 43:307 (1971).

33. O. BORGÅ and B. HOLMSTEDT: Mass fragmentography as a means of identification and quantitation of drugs in biological fluids. *Proc. 5th Int. Congr. Pharmacol.* San Francisco (1972).

34. V. T. OLIVERIO and A. M. GUARINO: Isotope dilution analysis. See p. 160 in ref. 8, Part 2.

35. B. KLIMAN and R. E. PETERSON: Double isotope derivative assay of aldosterone in biological extracts. *J. Biol. Chem.* 235:1639 (1960).

36. D. S. LUKAS and R. E. PETERSON: Double isotope dilution derivative assay of digitoxin in plasma, urine, and stool of patients maintained on the drug. *J. Clin. Invest.* 45:782 (1966).

37. J. R. GILLETTE, D. C. DAVIS, and H. A. SASAME: Cytochrome P-450 and its role in drug metabolism. *Ann. Rev. Pharmacol.* 12:57 (1972).

38. *Microsomes and Drug Oxidations*, ed. by J. R. Gillette, A. H. Conney, G. J. Cosmides, R. W. Estabrook, J. R. Fouts, and G. J. Mannering. New York, Academic Press (1969).

39. E. S. VESELL, ed.: Drug metabolism in man. *Ann. N.Y. Acad. Sci.* 179:43 (1971).

40. G. J. MANNERING: Microsomal enzyme systems which catalyze drug metabolism. See p. 206 in ref. 12.

41. J. R. GILLETTE, B. B. BRODIE, and B. N. LA DU: The oxidation of drugs by liver microsomes: on the role of TPNH and oxygen. *J. Pharmacol. Exp. Therap.* 119:532 (1957).

42. H. S. MASON: Oxidases. *Ann. Rev. Biochem.* 34:595 (1965).

43. B. B. BRODIE, J. R. GILLETTE, and B. N. LA DU: Enzymatic metabolism of drugs and other foreign compounds. *Ann. Rev. Biochem.* 27:427 (1958).

44. A. HILDEBRANDT and R. W. ESTABROOK: Evidence for the participation of cytochrome b_5 in hepatic microsomal mixed function oxidation reactions. *Arch. Biochem. Biophys.* 143:66 (1971).

45. T. OMURA: See p. 160 ref. 38.

46. J. BARON, W. E. TAYLOR, and B. S. S. MASTERS: Immunochemical studies on electron transport chains involving cytochrome P450. The role of the iron–sulfur protein, adrenodoxin, in mixed-function oxidation reactions. *Arch. Biochem. Biophys.* 150:105 (1972).

46a. P. L. GIGON, T. E. GRAM, and J. R. GILLETTE: Studies on the rate of reduction of hepatic microsomal Cytochrome P-450 by reduced nicotinamide adenine dinucleotide phosphate: effect of drug substrates. *Mol. Pharm.* 5:109 (1969).

47. Y. IMAI and R. SATO: Solubilization of aromatic hydroxylase system of liver microsomes and requirement of lipid-like factor. *Biochim. Biophys. Acta* 42:164 (1960).

48. K. KRISCH: Discussion, p. 25, in *Metabolic Factors Controlling Duration of Drug Action*, Proceedings of First International Pharmacological Meeting, Vol. 6, ed. by B. B. Brodie and E. G. Erdös. New York, Macmillan Co. (1962).

49. J. R. FOUTS: The metabolism of drugs by subfractions of hepatic microsomes. *Biochem. Biophys. Res. Commun.* 6:373 (1961).

50. J. R. GILLETTE: Side chain oxidation of alkyl substituted ring compounds. I. Enzymatic oxidation of *p*-nitrotoluene. *J. Biol. Chem.* 234:139 (1959).

51. M. T. BUSH, T. C. BUTLER, and H. L. DICKISON: The metabolic fate of 5-(1-cyclohexen-1-yl)-1,5-dimethyl barbituric acid (hexobarbital, "Evipal") and of 5-(1-cyclohexen-1-yl)-5-methyl barbituric acid ("Norevipal"). *J. Pharmacol. Exper. Therap.* 108:104 (1953).

51a. J. R. COOPER and B. B. BRODIE: The enzymatic metabolism of hexobarbital (Evipal). *J. Pharmacol. Exp. Therap.* 114:409 (1955).

52. R. KUNTZMAN, M. JACOBSON, K. SCHNEIDMAN, and A. H. CONNEY: Similarities between oxidative drug-metabolizing enzymes and steroid hydroxylases in liver microsomes. *J. Pharmacol. Exp. Therap.* 146:280 (1964).

53. C. J. PARLI, N. WANG, and R. E. Mc MAHON: A new cytochrome P-450-dependent reaction catalyzed by hepatic microsomal monooxygenases. *J. Biol. Chem.* 246:6953 (1971).

54. C. J. PARLI, N. WANG and R. E. Mc MAHON: The mechanism of the oxidation of *d*-amphetamine by rabbit liver oxygenase. Oxygen-18 studies. *Biochem. Biophys. Res. Comm.* 43:1204 (1971).

55. N. P. SALZMAN and B. B. BRODIE: Physiological disposition and fate of chlorpromazine and a method for its estimation in biological material. *J. Pharmacol. Exp. Therap.* 118:46 (1956).

56. J. J. BURNS, T. F. YU, A RITTERBAND, J. M. PEREL, A. B. GUTMAN, and B. B. BRODIE: A potent new uricosuric agent, the sulfoxide metabolite of the phenylbutazone analogue, G-25671. *J. Pharmacol. Exp. Therap.* 119:418 (1957).

57. E. SPECTOR and F. E. SHIDEMAN: Metabolism of thiopyrimidine derivatives: thiamylal, thiopental and thiouracil. *Biochem. Pharmacol.* 2:182 (1959).

58. A. N. DAVISON: The conversion of Schradan (OMPA) and Parathion into inhibitors of cholinesterase by mammalian liver. *Biochem. J.* 61:203 (1955).

59. A. N. DAVISON: Conversion of Schradan and parathion by an enzyme system of rat liver. *Nature* 174:1056 (1954).

60. J. R. BAKER and S. CHAYKIN: The biosynthesis of trimethylamine-*N*-oxide. *J. Biol. Chem.* 237:1309 (1962).

61. D. M. ZIEGLER and C. E. MITCHELL: Microsomal oxidase. IV. Properties of a mixed function amine oxidase isolated from pig liver microsomes. *Arch. Biochem. Biophysics* 150:116 (1972).

62. J. W. CRAMER, J. A. MILLER, and E. C. MILLER: *N*-Hydroxylation: a new metabolic reaction observed in the rat with the carcinogen 2-acetylaminofluorene. *J. Biol. Chem.* 235:885 (1960).

63. M. KIESE and H. UEHLEKE: Der Ort der *N*-Oxydation des Anilins im höheren Tier. *Arch. exper. Pathol. Pharmakol.* 242:117 (1961).

64. M. KIESE and H. UEHLEKE: Zwei Wege der Entmethylierung von *N*-Methylanilin durch Mikrosomen aus Rattenlebern. *Naturwissenschaften* 48:379 (1961).

65. H. S. MASON: Mechanisms of oxygen metabolism. *Advance. Enzymol.* 19:79 (1957).

66. H. S. POSNER, C. MITOMA, S. ROTHBERG, and S. UDENFRIEND: Enzymic hydroxylation of aromatic compounds. III. Studies on the mechanism of microsomal hydroxylation. *Arch. Biochem. Biophys.* 94:280 (1961).

67. B. STRIPP, N. ZAMPAGLIONE, M. HAMRICK, and J. R. GILLETTE: An approach to measurement of the stoichiometric relationship between hepatic microsomal drug metabolism and the oxidation of reduced nicotinamide adenine dinucleotide phosphate. *Mol. Pharmacol.* 8:189 (1972).

68. C. MITOMA, H. S. POSNER, and F. LEONARD: Aromatization of hexahydrobenzoic acid by mammalian liver mitochondria. *Biochim. Biophys. Acta* 27:156 (1958).

69. J. R. COOPER and P. J. FRIEDMAN: The enzymic oxidation of chloral hydrate to trichloroacetic acid. *Biochem. Pharmacol.* 1:76 (1958).

70. C. S. LIEBER and L. M. DE CARLI: Hepatic microsomal ethanol-oxidizing system: In vitro characteristics and adaptive properties in vivo. *J. Biol. Chem.* 245:2505 (1970).

71. K. J. ISSELBACHER and E. A. CARTER: Ethanol oxidation by liver microsomes: evidence against a separate and distinct enzyme system. *Biochem. Biophys. Res. Comm.* 39:530 (1970).

71a. I. E. HASSINEN and R. H. YLIKAHRI: Mixed function oxidase and ethanol metabolism in perfused rat liver. *Science* 176:1435 (1972).

72. G. B. ELION, S. CALLAHAN, R. W. RUNDLES, and G. H. HITCHINGS: Relationship between metabolic fates and antitumor activities of thiopurines. *Cancer Res.* 23:1207 (1963).

73. H. H. CORNISH and A. A. CHRISTMAN: A study of the metabolism of theobromine, theophylline and caffeine in man. *J. Biol. Chem.* 228:315 (1957).

74. V. H. BOOTH: The specificity of xanthine oxidase. *Biochem. J.* 32:494 (1938).

75. H. BLASCHKO: Amine oxidase. *The Enzymes*, 3rd ed., Vol. 8, ed. by P. D. Boyer, H. Lardy, and K. Myrbäck. New York, Academic Press (1973) pp. 337–351.

76. E. A. ZELLER: Diamine oxidases. *The Enzymes*, 3rd ed., Vol. 8, ed. by P. D. Boyer, H. Lardy, and K. Myrbäck. New York, Academic Press (1973) pp. 313–335.

77. J. STERNBURG, C. W. KEARNS, and H. MOORFIELD: DDT dehydrochlorinase, an enzyme found in DDT-resistant flies. *Agr. Food Chem.* 2:1125 (1954).

78. H. LIPKE and C. W. KEARNS: DDT dehydrochlorinase. I. Isolation, chemical properties, and spectrophotometric assay. *J. Biol. Chem.* 234:2123 (1959).

79. E. N. COHEN: Metabolism of the volatile anesthetics. *Anesthesiology* 35:193 (1971).

80. H. F. CASCORBI, D. A. BLAKE, and M. HELRICH: Halothane biotransformation in mice and man. In *Cellular Biology and Toxicity of Anesthetics*, ed. by B. R. Fink, Baltimore, Williams and Wilkins (1972).

81. R. I. MAZZE, J. R. TRUDELL, and M. J. COUSINS: Methoxyflurane metabolism and renal dysfunctions. *Anesthesiology* 35:247 (1971).

82. D. A. HOLADAY, S. RUDOFSKY, and P. S. TRUEHAFT The metabolic degradation of methoxyflurane in man. *Anesthesiology* 33:579 (1970).

83. R. A. VAN DYKE and M. B. CHENOWETH: The metabolism of volatile anesthetics. II. In vitro metabolism of methoxyflurane and halothane in rat liver slices and cell fractions. *Biochem. Pharmacol.* 14:603 (1965).

84. E. N. COHEN, J. W. BELLVILLE, and B. W. BROWN: Anesthesia, pregnancy, and miscarriage. *Anesthesiology* 35:343 (1971).

85. J. R. GILLETTE: Reductive enzymes. See p. 349 in ref. 8, Part 2.

86. J. ET MME. TRÉFOUËL, F. NITTI, and D. BOVET: Activité du *p*-aminophénylsulfamide sur les infections streptococciques expérimentales de la souris et du lapin. *Compt. Rend.* 120:756 (1935).

87. J. R. FOUTS and B. B. BRODIE: The enzymatic reduction of chloramphenicol, *p*-nitrobenzoic acid and other aromatic nitro compounds in mammals. *J. Pharmacol. Exp. Therap.* 119:197 (1957).

88. J. J. KAMM and J. R. GILLETTE: Mechanism of stimulation of mammalian nitro reductase by flavins. *Life Sci.* 2:254 (1963).

89. R. GINGELL, J. W. BRIDGES, and R. T. WILLIAMS: Gut flora and the metabolism of Prontosils in the rat. *Biochem. J.* 114:5 (1969).

90. M. A. PEPPERCORN and P. GOLDMAN: The role of intestinal bacteria in the metabolism of salicylazosulfapyridine. *J Pharmacol. Exp. Ther.* 181:555 (1972).

91. B. N. LA DU and H. SNADY: Esterases of human tissues. See p. 477 in ref. 8, Part 2.

92. J. D. GABOUREL and R. E. GOSSELIN: The mechanism of atropine detoxication in mice and rats. *Arch. Int. Pharmacodyn.* 115:416 (1958).

93. R. E. GOSSELIN, J. D. GABOUREL, and J. H. WILLS: The fate of atropine in man. *Clin. Pharmacol. Therap.* 1:597 (1960).

94. C. R. SHAW, F. N. SYNER, and R. E. TASHIAN: New genetically determined molecular form of erythrocyte esterase in man. *Science* 138:31 (1962).

95. G. J. DUTTON: Glucuronide-forming enzymes. See p. 378 in ref. 8, Part 2.

96. G. J. DUTTON: Uridine diphosphate glucuronic acid as glucuronyl donor in the synthesis of "ester," aliphatic and steroid glucuronides. *Biochem. J.* 64:693 (1956).

97. J. AXELROD, J. K. INSCOE, and G. M. TOMKINS: Enzymatic synthesis of *N*-glucuronic acid conjugates. *Nature* 179 533 (1957).
98. K. J. ISSELBACHER, F. CHRABAS, and R. C. QUINN: The solubilization and partial purification of a glucuronyl transferase from rabbit liver microsomes. *J. Biol. Chem.* 237:3033 (1962).
99. I. M. ARIAS: Ethereal and *N*-linked glucuronide formation by normal and Gunn rats in vitro and in vivo. *Biochem. Biophys. Res. Commun.* 6:81 (1961).
100. J. AXELROD, J. K. INSCOE, and G. M. TOMKINS: Enzymatic synthesis of *N*-glucosyluronic acid conjugates. *J. Biol. Chem.* 232:835 (1958).
101. J. W. CLAPP: A new metabolic pathway for a sulfonamide group. *J. Biol. Chem.* 223:207 (1956).
102. J. A. MONTGOMERY: On the chemotherapy of cancer. *Prog. Drug Res.* 8:431 (1965).
103. L. N. LUKENS and K. A. HERRINGTON: Enzymic formation of 6-mercaptopurine ribotide. *Biochim. Biophys. Acta* 24:432 (1957).
104. F. LIPMANN: Acetylation of sulfanilamide by liver homogenates and extracts. *J. Biol. Chem.* 160:173 (1945).
105. D. J. HEARSE and W. W. WEBER: Evidence for genetic and enzymic heterogeneity in the "slow" INH acetylator. *Fed. Proc.* 29:803 (1970).
106. W. C. GOVIER: Reticuloendothelial cells as the site of sulfanilamide acetylation in the rabbit. *J. Pharmacol. Exp. Ther.* 150:305 (1965).
107. W. W. WEBER and A. N. COHEN: *N*-Acetylation of drugs: Isolation and properties of an *N*-acetyltransferase from rabbit liver. *Mol. Pharmacol.* 3:266 (1967).
108. W. W. WEBER and S. N. COHEN: The mechanism of isoniazid acetylation by human *N*-acetyltransferase. *Biochim. Biophys. Acta (Amst.)* 151:276 (1968).
109. E. BOYLAND: Mercapturic acid conjugation. See p. 584 in ref. 8, Part 2.
110. J. BOOTH, E. BOYLAND, T. SATO, and P. SIMS: Metabolism of polycyclic compounds. 17. The reaction of 1:2-dihydronaphthalene and 1:2-epoxy-1:2:3:4-tetrahydronaphthalene with glutathione catalysed by tissue preparations. *Biochem. J.* 77:182 (1960).
111. E. BOYLAND, G. S. RAMSAY, and P. SIMS: Metabolism of polycyclic compounds. 18. The secretion of metabolites of naphthalene, 1:2-dihydronaphthalene and 1:2-epoxy-1:2:3:4-tetrahydronaphthalene in rat bile. *Biochem. J.* 78:376 (1961).
112. D. M. JERINA, J. W. DALY, B. WITKOP, and P. ZALTZMAN-NIRENBERG: The role of arene oxide–oxepin systems in the metabolism of aromatic substrates: III Formation of 1,2-naphthalene oxide from naphthalene by liver microsomes. *J. Amer. Chem. Soc.* 90:6525 (1968).
113. E. BOYLAND and P. SIMS: Metabolism of polycyclic compounds. 12. An acid-labile precursor of 1-naphthylmercapturic acid and naphthol: an *N*-acetyl-*S*-(1:2-dihydrohydroxynaphthyl)-L-cysteine. *Biochem. J.* 68:440 (1958).
114. D. F. COLUCCI and D. A. BUYSKE: The biotransformation of a sulfonamide to a mercaptan and to mercapturic acid and glucuronide conjugates. *Biochem. Pharmacol.* 14:457 (1965).
115. P. W. ROBBINS and F. LIPMANN: Isolation and identification of active sulfate. *J. Biol. Chem.* 229:837 (1957).
116. Y. NOSE and F. LIPMANN: Separation of steroid sulfokinases. *J. Biol. Chem.* 233:1348 (1958).
117. J. AXELROD and R. TOMCHICK: Enzymatic *O*-methylation of epinephrine and other catechols. *J. Biol. Chem.* 233:702 (1958).
118. J. AXELROD and H. WEISSBACH: Purification and properties of hydroxyindole-*O*-methyl transferase. *J. Biol. Chem.* 236:211 (1961).
119. D. D. BROWN, R. TOMCHICK, and J. AXELROD: The distribution and properties of a histamine-methylating enzyme. *J. Biol. Chem.* 234:2948 (1959).
120. N. KIRSHNER and M. C. GOODALL: The formation of adrenaline from noradrenaline. *Biochim. Biophys. Acta* 24:658 (1957).
121. J. AXELROD: Purification and properties of phenylethanolamine *N*-methyl transferase. *J. Biol. Chem.* 237:1657 (1962).
122. E. J. SARCIONE and J. E. SOKAL: Detoxication of thiouracil by *S*-methylation. *J. Biol. Chem.* 231:605 (1958).
123. J. BREMER and D. M. GREENBERG: Enzymic methylation of foreign sulfhydryl compounds. *Biochim. Biophys. Acta* 46:217 (1961).
124. B. H. SÖRBO: On the properties of rhodanese: Partial purification, inhibitors and intracellular distribution. *Acta Chem. Scand.* 5:724 (1951).

125. B. H. SÖRBO: Crystalline rhodanese. I. Purification and physiochemical examination. *Acta Chem. Scand.* 7:1129 (1953).

126. G. J. MANNERING: Inhibition of drug metabolism. See p. 452 in ref. 8, Part 2.

127. J. AXELROD, J. REICHENTHAL, and B. B. BRODIE: Mechanism of the potentiating action of β-diethylaminoethyl diphenylpropylacetate. *J. Pharmacol. Exp. Therap.* 112:49 (1954).

128. M. W. ANDERS, A. P. ALVARES, and G. J. MANNERING: Inhibition of drug metabolism. II. Metabolism of 2-diethylaminoethyl 2,2-diphenylvalerate HCl (SKF 525-A). *Mol. Pharmacol.* 2:328 (1966).

129. S. JENNER and K. J. NETTER: On the inhibition of microsomal drug metabolism by SKF 525A. *Biochem. Pharmacol.* 21:1921 (1972).

130. J. HALD and E. JACOBSEN: The formation of acetaldehyde in the organism after ingestion of Antabuse (tetraethylthiuramdisulphide) and alcohol. *Acta Pharmacol. Toxicol.* 4:305 (1948).

131. J. HALD, E. JACOBSEN, and V. LARSEN: Formation of acetaldehyde in the organism in relation to dosage of Antabuse (tetraethylthiuramdisulphide) and to alcohol concentration in blood. *Acta Pharmacol. Toxicol.* 5:179 (1949).

132. J. HALD, E. JACOBSEN, and V. LARSEN: The rate of acetaldehyde metabolism in isolated livers and hind limbs of rabbits treated with Antabuse (tetraethylthiuramdisulphide). *Acta Pharmacol. Toxicol.* 5:298 (1949).

133. W. D. GRAHAM: In vitro inhibition of liver aldehyde dehydrogenase by tetraethylthiuramdisulphide. *J. Pharm. Pharmacol.* 3:160 (1951).

134. R. A. DEITRICH and V. G. ERWIN: Mechanism of inhibition of aldehyde dehydrogenase in vivo by disulfiram and diethyldithiocarbamate. *Mol. Pharmacol.* 7:301 (1971).

135. J. M. MUSACCHIO, M. GOLDSTEIN. B. ANAGNOSTE, G. POCH, and I. J. KOPIN: Inhibition of dopamine-β-hydroxylase by disulfiram in vivo. *J. Pharmacol. Exp. Ther.* 152:56 (1966).

136. B. STRIPP, F. E. GREENE, and J. R. GILLETTE: Disulfiram impairment of drug metabolism by rat liver microsomes. *J. Pharmacol. Exp. Ther.* 170:347 (1969).

137. E. S. VESELL, G. T. PASSANANTI, and C. H. LEE: Impairment of drug metabolism by disulfiram in man. *Clin. Pharmacol. Ther.* 12:785 (1971).

138. T. K. LI and H. THEORELL: Human liver alcohol dehydrogenase: inhibition by pyrazole and pyrazole analogs. *Acta Chem. Scand.* 23:892 (1969).

139. E. A. ZELLER, J. BARSKY, and E. R. BERMAN: Amine oxidases. XI. Inhibition of monoamine oxidase by 1-isonicotinyl-2-isopropylhydrazine. *J. Biol. Chem.* 214:267 (1955).

140. L. I. GOLDBERG: Monoamine oxidase inhibitors. Adverse reactions and possible mechanisms. *J. Amer. Med. Ass.* 190:456 (1964).

141. A. MASON: Fatal reaction associated with tranylcypromine and methylamphetamine. *Lancet* 1:1073 (1962).

142. A. M. ASATOOR, A. J. LEVI, and M. O. MILNE: Tranylcypromine and cheese. *Lancet* 2:733 (1963).

143. B. BLACKWELL: Tranylcypromine. *Lancet* 2:414 (1963).

144. G. B. ELION, S. CALLAHAN, R. W. RUNDLES, and G. H. HITCHINGS: Relationship between metabolic states and antitumor activities of thiopurines. *Cancer Res.* 23:1207 (1963).

145. R. W. RUNDLES, J. B. WYNGAARDEN, G. H. HITCHINGS, and G. B. ELION: Drugs and uric acid. *Ann. Rev. Pharmacol.* 9:345 (1969).

146. T. SPECTOR and D. G. JOHNS: Stoichiometric inhibition of reduced xanthine oxidase by hydroxypyrazolo[3,4-d]pyrimidines. *J. Biol. Chem.* 245:5079 (1970).

147. W. N. KELLEY, M. L. GREENE, F. M. ROSENBLOOM, J. F. HENDERSON, and J. E. SEEGMILLER: Hypoxanthine–guanine phosphoribosyltransferase deficiency in gout. *Ann. Int. Med.* 70:155 (1969).

148. W. N. KELLEY, F. M. ROSENBLOOM, J. MILLER, and J. E. SEEGMILLER: An enzymatic basis for variation in response to allopurinol. *New Eng. J. Med.* 278:287 (1968).

149. A. H. CONNEY and J. J. BURNS: Factors influencing drug metabolism. *Ad. Pharmacol.* 1:31 (1962).

150. A. H. CONNEY and J. J. BURNS: Metabolic interactions among environmental chemicals and drugs. *Science* 178:576 (1972).

151. A. H. CONNEY: Pharmacological implications of microsomal enzyme induction. *Pharmacol. Rev.* 19:317 (1967).

152. A. H. CONNEY: Drug metabolism and therapeutics. *New Eng. J. Med.* 280:653 (1969).

153. W. SETTLE, S. HEGEMAN, and R. M. FEATHERSTONE: The nature of drug–protein interaction. See p. 175 in ref 5, Part 1.

154. A. H. CONNEY: Environmental factors influencing drug metabolism. See p. 253 in ref. 12.

155. H. V. GELBOIN: Mechanisms of induction of drug metabolism enzymes. See p. 279 in ref. 12.

156. G. J. MANNERING: In *Selected Pharmacological Testing Methods*, ed. by A. Burger. New York, Dekker (1968).

157. A. H. CONNEY, E. C. MILLER, and J. A. MILLER: Substrate-induced synthesis and other properties of benzpyrene hydroxylase in rat liver. *J. Biol. Chem.* 228:753 (1957).

158. H. REMMER: Drugs as activators of drug enzymes. In *Metabolic Factors Controlling Duration of Drug Action,* Proceedings of First International Pharmacological Meeting, vol. 6, ed. by B. B. Brodie and E. G. Erdös. New York, Macmillan Co. (1962), p. 235.

159. H. REMMER and H.-J. MERKER: Enzyminduktion und Vermehrung von endoplasmatischem Reticulum in der Leberzelle während der Behandlung mit Phenobarbital (Luminal). *Klin. Wochensch.* 41:276 (1963).

159a. K. J. NETTER and G. SEIDEL: An adaptively stimulated *O*-demethylating system in rat lever microsomes and its kinetic properties. *J. Pharmacol. Exp. Therap.* 146:61 (1964).

160. A. H. CONNEY, C. DAVISON, R. GASTEL, and J. J. BURNS: Adaptive increases in drug-metabolizing enzymes induced by phenobarbital and other drugs. *J. Pharmacol. Exp. Therap.* 130:1 (1960).

161. H. V. GELBOIN and N. R. BLACKBURN: The stimulatory effect of 3-methylcholanthrene on benzpyrene hydroxylase activity in several rat tissues: inhibition by actinomycin D and puromycin. *Cancer Res.* 24:356 (1964).

162. R. KATO, W. R. JONDORF, L. A. LOEB, T. BEN, and H. V. GELBOIN: Studies on the mechanism of drug-induced microsomal enzyme activities. *Mol. Pharmacol.* 2:171 (1966).

163. R. KATO, L. LOEB, and H. V. GELBOIN: Microsome-specific stimulation by phenobarbital in amino acid incorporation in vivo. *Biochem. Pharmacol.* 14:1164 (1965).

164. H. V. GELBOIN: Mechanisms of induction of drug metabolizing enzymes. See p. 431 in ref. 8, Part 2.

165. S. ORRENIUS and L. ERNSTER: Phenobarbital-induced synthesis of the oxidative demethylating enzymes of rat liver microsomes. *Biochem. Biophys. Res. Commun.* 16:60 (1964).

166. H. S. MARVER: The role of heme in the synthesis and repression of microsomal protein. In *Microsomes and Drug Oxidations,* ed. by J. R. Gillette, A. H. Conney, G. J. Cosmides, R. W. Estabrook, J. R. Fouts, and G. J. Mannering. New York, Academic Press (1969).

167. R. T. SCHIMKE, E. W. SWEENEY, and C. M. BERLIN: An analysis of the kinetics of rat liver tryptophan pyrrolase induction: the significance of both enzyme synthesis and degradation. *Biochem. Biophys. Res. Commun.* 15:214 (1964).

168. H. JICK and L. SCHUSTER: The turnover of microsomal reduced nicotinamide adenine dinucleotide phosphate-cytochrome c reductase in the livers of mice treated with phenobarbital. *J. Biol. Chem.* 241:5366 (1966).

169. R. T. SCHIMKE, R. GANSCHOW, D. DOYLE, and I. M. ARIAS: Regulation of protein turnover in mammalian tissues. *Fed. Proc.* 27:1223 (1968).

170. Y. KURIYAMA, T. OMURA, P. SIEKEVITZ, and G. E. PALADE: Effects of phenobarbital on the synthesis and degradation of the protein components of rat liver microsomal membranes. *J. Biol. Chem.* 244:2017 (1969).

171. D. W. NEBERT and H. V. GELBOIN: Substrate inducible microsomal aryl hydroxylase in mammalian cell cultures. *J. Biol. Chem.* 243:6250 (1968).

172. D. W. NEBERT and H. V. GELBOIN: The role of ribonucleic acid and protein synthesis in microsomal aryl hydrocarbon hydroxylase induction in cell culture. *J. Biol. Chem.* 245:160 (1970).

173. F. DE MATTEIS: Loss of haem in rat liver caused by the porphyrogenic agent 2-allyl-2-isopropylacetamide. *Biochem. J.* 124:767 (1971).

174. W. LEVIN, E. SERNATINGER, M. JACOBSON, and R. KUNTZMAN: Destruction of cytochrome P450 by secobarbital and other barbiturates containing allyl groups. *Science* 176:1341 (1972).

175. F. DE MATTEIS: Mechanisms of induction of hepatic porphyria by drugs. *Proc. 5th Internat. Congr. Pharmacol.*, p. 198, San Francisco (1972).

176. H. REMMER: The role of the liver in drug metabolism. *Am. J. Med.* 49:617 (1970).

177. A. J. LEVI, S. SHERLOCK, and D. WALKER: Phenylbutazone and isoniazid metabolism in patients with liver disease in relation to previous drug therapy. *Lancet* 1:1275 (1968).

178. R. L. DIXON, R. W. SHULTICE, and J. R. FOUTS: Factors affecting drug metabolism by liver microsomes. IV. Starvation. *Proc. Soc. Exp. Biol. Med.* 103:333 (1960).

179. S. A. CUCINELL, A. H. CONNEY, M. SANSUR, and J. J. BURNS: Drug interactions in man. I. Lowering effect of phenobarbital on plasma levels of bishydroxycoumarin (Dicumarol) and diphenylhydantoin (Dilantin). *Clin. Pharmacol. Therap.* 6:420 (1965).

180. S. D. MURPHY and K. P. DU BOIS: The influence of various factors on the enzymatic conversion of organic thiophosphates to anticholinesterase agents. *J. Pharmacol. Exp. Therap.* 124:194 (1958).

181. E. S. VESSELL: Genetic and environmental factors affecting drug response in man. *Fed. Proc.* 31:1253 (1972).

182. J. J. BURNS, S. A. CUCINELL, R. KOSTER, and A. H. CONNEY: Application of drug metabolism to drug toxicity studies. *Ann. N.Y. Acad. Sci.* 123:273 (1965).

183. S. J. YAFFE, G. LEVY, T. MATSUZAWA, and T. BALIAH: Enhancement of glucuronide-conjugating capacity in a hyperbilirubinemic infant due to apparent enzyme induction by phenobarbital. *New Eng. J. Med.* 275:1461 (1966).

184. R. P. H. THOMPSON, G. M. STATHERS, C. W. T. PILCHER, A. E. M. McLEAN, J. ROBINSON, and R. WILLIAMS: Treatment of unconjugated jaundice with dicophane. *Lancet* 2:4 (1969).

185. R. H. ADAMSON, R. L. DIXON, F. L. FRANCIS, and D. P. RALL: Comparative biochemistry of drug metabolism by azo and nitro reductase. *Proc. Nat. Acad. Sci. U.S.A.* 54:1386 (1965).

186. J. J. BURNS: Species differences and individual variations in drug metabolism. In *Metabolic Factors Controlling Duration of Drug Action,* Proc. 1st Internat. Pharmacol. Meet., vol. 6, ed. by B. B. Brodie and E. G. Erdös. New York, Macmillan Co. (1962) p. 277.

187. G. P. QUINN, J. AXELROD, and B. B. BRODIE: Species, strain and sex differences in metabolism of hexobarbitone, amidopyrine, antipyrine, and aniline. *Biochem. Pharmacol.* 1:152 (1958).

188. J. AXELROD: Studies on sympathomimetic amines. I. The biotransformation and physiological disposition of *l*-ephedrine and *l*-norephedrine. *J. Pharmacol. Exp. Therap.* 109:62 (1953).

189. D. RICHTER: Elimination of amines in man. *Biochem. J.* 32:1763 (1938).

190. J. J. BURNS, M. WEINER, G. SIMSON, and B. B. BRODIE: The biotransformation of ethyl biscoumacetate (Tromexan) in man, rabbit, and dog. *J. Pharmacol. Exp. Therap.* 108:33 (1953).

191. J. H. WEISBURGER, P. H. GRANTHAM, and E. K. WEISBURGER: The metabolism of *N*-2-fluorenylacetamide in the cat: evidence for glucuronic acid conjugates. *Biochem. Pharmacol.* 13:469 (1964).

192. G. E. JAY, JR.: Variation in response of various mouse strains to hexobarbital (Evipal). *Proc. Soc. Exp. Biol. Med.* 90:378 (1955).

193. R. I. MAZZE, M. J. COUSINS, and J. C. KOSEK: Strain differences in metabolism and susceptibility to the nephrotoxic effects of methoxyflurane in rats. *J. Pharmacol. Exp. Ther.* 184:481 (1973).

194. R. KATO, K. I. ONODA, and A. TAKANAKA: Strain differences in the metabolism and action of drugs in mice and rats. *Jap. J. Pharmacol.* 20:562 (1970).

195. P. B. SAWIN and D. GLICK: Atropinesterase, a genetically determined enzyme in the rabbit. *Proc. Nat. Acad. Sci.* 29:55 (1943).

196. F. MARGOLIS and P. FEIGELSON: Genetic expression and developmental studies with rabbit serum atropinesterase. *Biochim. Biophys. Acta* 90:117 (1964).

197. D. W. NEBERT: Microsomal cytochromes b_5 and P_{450} during induction of aryl hydrocarbon hydroxylase activity in mammalian cell culture. *J. Biol. Chem.* 245:519 (1970).

198. J. E. GIELEN, F. M. GOUJON, and D. W. NEBERT: Genetic regulation of aryl hydrocarbon hydroxylase induction. *J. Biol. Chem.* 247:1125 (1972).

199. D. W. NEBERT and J. E. GIELEN: Genetic regulation of aryl hydrocarbon hydroxylase induction in the mouse. *Fed. Proc.* 31:1315 (1972).

200. D. W. NEBERT, F. M. GOUJON, and J. E. GIELEN: Aryl hydrocarbon hydroxylase induction by polycyclic hydrocarbons: simple autosomal dominant trait in the mouse. *Nature New Biol.* 236:107 (1972).

201. N. KRETCHMER: Developmental biochemistry—a relevant endeavor. *Pediatrics* 46:175 (1970).

202. A. K. BROWN and W. W. ZUELZER: Studies on the neonatal development of the glucuronide conjugating system. *J. Clin. Invest.* 37:332 (1958).

203. P. HAHN and J. SKALA: Development of enzyme systems. *Clin. Obstet. Gynecol.* 14:655 (1971).

204. J. R. FOUTS and R. H. ADAMSON: Drug metabolism in the newborn rabbit. *Science* 129:897 (1959).

205. M. F. VEST and R. R. STREIFF: Studies on glucuronide formation in newborn infants and older children. *J. Dis. Childre* 98:688 (1959).

206. W. R. JONDORF, R. P. MAICKEL, and B. B. BRODIE: Inability of newborn mice and guinea pigs to metabolize drugs. *Biochem. Pharmacol.* 1:352 (1958).

207. S. G. DRISCOLL and D. Y. HSIA: The development of enzyme systems during early infancy. *Pediatrics* 22:785 (1958).

208. C. F. WEISS, A. J. GLAZKO, and J. K. WESTON: Chloramphenicol in the newborn infant: a physiologic explanation of its toxicity when given in excessive dose. *New Eng. J. Med.* 262:787 (1960).

209. A. J. GLAZKO, L. M. WOLF, W. A. DILL, and A. C. BRATTON, JR.: Biochemical studies on chloramphenicol (Chloromycetin). II. Tissue distribution and excretion studies. *J. Pharmacol. Exp. Therap.* 96:445 (1949).

210. A. J. GLAZKO, W. A. DILL, and M. C. REBSTOCK: Biochemical studies on chloramphenicol (Chloromycetin). III. Isolation and identification of metabolic products in urine. *J. Biol. Chem.* 183:679 (1950).

211. W. A. DILL, E. M. THOMPSON, R. A. FISKEN, and A. J. GLAZKO: A new metabolite of chloramphenicol. *Nature* 185:535 (1960).

212. E. STREICHER and J. GARBUS: The effect of age and sex on the duration of hexobarbital anesthesia in rats. *J. Gerontol.* 10:441 (1955).

213. R. KATO, P. VASSANELLI, G. FRONTINO, and E. CHIESARA: Variation in the activity of liver microsomal drug-metabolizing enzymes in rats in relation to the age. *Biochem. Pharmacol.* 13:1037 (1964).

214. R. KATO, A. TAKANAKA, and K. I. ONADA: Studies on age difference in mice for the activity of drug-metabolizing enzymes of liver microsomes. *Jap. J. Pharmacol.* 20:572 (1970).

CHAPTER 4
The Time Course of Drug Action

RATE OF DRUG ABSORPTION

The rate of drug absorption is either constant and independent of the amount of drug to be absorbed (*zero-order kinetics*) or diminishing and always in proportion to the amount of drug still to be absorbed (*exponential, or first-order kinetics*). If a drug is injected intravascularly, one cannot really speak of absorption, although in a formal sense we may regard the entire dose as being "absorbed" into the blood stream instantaneously. As we shall see (p. 307), it is convenient to analyze *the kinetics of elimination* under these conditions because no simultaneous absorption process complicates matters.

The most straightforward example of constant-rate absorption is that seen with a continuous intravenous infusion, in which the rate of entry of the drug into the vascular system is fixed and maintained at will. Two types of apparatus are employed. The simplest is a gravity-flow intravenous drip, commonly used at the bedside in hospitals. The apparatus is employed to administer blood, plasma, physiologic saline solutions, glucose, and other nutrients. It is a simple matter to add a drug in appropriate concentration. The flow rate is maintained approximately constant by a simple adjustable clamp on the tubing, and the rate is monitored by counting drops in a glass bulb designed for the purpose. A more precise apparatus is the infusion pump, calibrated to deliver solution at a constant rate. The method of continuous infusion has been used for the administration of oxytocin at term to induce labor; here, the exact regulation of dosage is of critical importance.[1] As will be discussed (p. 314), if a constant-rate infusion delivers new drug at a rate that just replaces drug eliminated from the body, a steady-state constant drug level will be maintained throughout the volume of distribution in the body.

Constant-rate absorption may be approximated by various techniques for sustained-release medication. As already shown (p. 135), a subcutaneous pellet in the shape of a flat disk may yield drug into solution at a practically constant rate until it

301

is nearly all dissolved. If the dissolution of the drug can be made the rate-limiting process for absorption (i.e., if the rate of absorption is fast compared with the rate of solution), then the overall absorption rate will be practically constant. The same principle applies to some extent to any insoluble drug in a subcutaneous or intramuscular depot during an initial period, before the total surface area exposed for solution diminishes by much. Protamine zinc insulin and procaine penicillin are examples of drugs whose absorption from depots may proceed at a nearly constant rate for some time after their administration. In sustained-release medications for oral administration, the aim of the manufacturing process is to achieve a nearly constant rate of liberation into the gastrointestinal lumen (cf. p. 150). Generally, in any solution where a supply (or reservoir) of available drug can replace what is absorbed, a constant rate of absorption may be expected. An example would be the application to the skin of a large amount of ointment or cream containing a drug; as the drug penetrates into the deeper layers of the corium, and eventually into the blood stream, it is replaced by diffusion of fresh drug; thus, a continuous gradient of drug concentration is maintained throughout the thickness of the skin, and a constant absorption rate continues as long as drug persists on the surface. Another example is found in the administration of anesthetic gases (p. 338). Here, drug absorbed into the pulmonary blood at the alveoli during each breath is replaced at the next breath from the unlimited supply maintained in the anesthetist's breathing bag.

Except for the rather special cases cited above, both for enteral and parenteral routes of administration most drug absorption follows first-order kinetics; i.e., a constant fraction of the total drug present is absorbed in each equal interval of time. After subcutaneous or intramuscular injection of a drug solution, for example, the probability that a given drug molecule will enter a nearby capillary in a given short period of time depends upon the intrinsic vascularity of the tissue (i.e., how near the capillary is), the permeability of the capillaries to the drug, the local blood flow, and the diffusion rate of the drug. The rate of absorption (molecules per minute) will be the product of this probability times the total number of drug molecules present. As the total amount of drug diminishes, the rate of absorption will obviously decrease proportionately, and the time course of the absorption process can be described by the following equations:

$$\frac{dM}{dt} = -k_a M$$

$$M = M_0 e^{-k_a t}$$

$$\ln \frac{M}{M_0} = -k_a t$$

$$\ln M = \ln M_0 - k_a t$$

$$\log M = \log M_0 - \frac{k_a t}{2.30}$$

where M_0 is the amount of drug placed initially at the absorption site, M is the amount remaining at the absorption site at time t, and k_a is the rate constant for absorption. The last two equations give straight lines, so if the amount of unabsorbed drug is plotted against time on semilogarithmic coordinates, a line should be obtained with the negative slope $k_a/2.30$ and intercept M_0 on the y axis. In this treatment back-diffusion from the blood into the depot is neglected. Figure 4-1 presents a good

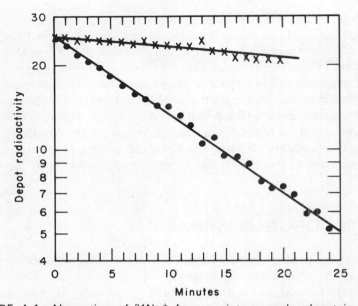

FIGURE 4-1. Absorption of $^{24}Na^+$ from an intramuscular depot in man. *The radioisotope (5 μc) was injected deep into the gastrocnemius muscle. Residual radioactivity was determined by a Geiger counter at the skin. Ordinates represent counts per minute on logarithmic scale but the scale factor (which is irrelevant to the purpose of the graph) is not given. The slope is a measure of* k_a, *the fraction removed per minute. Lower curve, control resting muscle,* $k_a = 0.064$ min^{-1}; *upper curve, epinephrine incorporated in the injection,* $k_a = 0.010$ min^{-1}. (From Kety, Figure 4.[2] By permission of C. V. Mosby.)

example. Radioactive sodium, as NaCl, was injected intramuscularly in man, and the residual radioactivity was determined for 25 min with a Geiger counter at the skin surface. The exponential course of the absorption is clearly demonstrated by the data. Incorporation of epinephrine into the injection markedly reduced the absorption rate (by reducing the local blood flow), but the residual absorption was still first order.

The rate constant of absorption tells us the instantaneous rate of absorption as a fraction of the amount still present. For the experiment of Figure 4-1, this rate constant, k_a, was 0.064 min^{-1} in the control resting muscle, meaning that the remaining sodium ions were absorbed at a rate of 6.4% min^{-1}.

Another useful measure, directly related to k_a, is the *absorption half-time,* $t_{1/2}$, the time when the drug content of the depot has been reduced to half its initial value. As shown above,

$$\ln \frac{M}{M_0} = -k_a t$$

Substituting $M/M_0 = 1/2$, we obtain

$$\ln \frac{1}{2} = -k_a t_{1/2}$$

$$t_{1/2} = \frac{0.693}{k_a}$$

For sodium absorption, where $k_a = 0.064$ min^{-1}, $t_{1/2} = 11$ min.

Very similar results were obtained in rats with several radioactive compounds.[3] Here the method was to excise the injection site at various times in different animals, and assay the remaining drug by liquid scintillation counting. The substances chosen for study were ouabain, benzylpenicillin, hexamethonium, glucose, urea, and water. Despite a range of 30-fold in molecular weight and 5-fold in diffusion coefficient, and considerable differences in ionic state and lipid solubility, the absorption rates were virtually the same—about 0.16 min^{-1} (half-time 4.4 min). This result, like that with $^{24}Na^+$, suggests that the blood flow at the injection site is the rate-limiting factor for absorption. Confirmatory evidence was a marked slowing of absorption by epinephrine (as seen also in Figure 4-1) and a speeding of absorption by the vasodilator, prostaglandin E_2.

RATE OF DRUG ELIMINATION

Elimination refers to all the processes that operate to reduce the effective drug concentration in the body fluids. Depending upon the mechanism of elimination, the course of disappearance of a drug from the body (or the decay of its plasma level) may be zero-order (constant rate) or first-order (exponential). First-order elimination is the general rule, but if an elimination mechanism can become saturated, then at drug concentrations above the saturation level the elimination will be zero-order. An excellent example already discussed is the renal tubular secretion of drugs, for which there is a maximum tubular transport capacity (T_m). If the plasma level of a drug is so high that T_m is exceeded, zero-order kinetics will obtain until the concentration falls below the saturation level, and then subsequently the elimination rate will decrease with decreasing concentration; at a low enough concentration the elimination will always be first order i.e., proportional to the concentration. The same principle applies to the secretion of drugs into the bile (p. 217), a process also characterized by a T_m for each drug.

Substrates for drug-metabolizing enzymes may be degraded or conjugated at a constant rate when their concentrations are above saturation levels, or when a coupled reaction is rate limiting. As with renal tubular and biliary transport systems at concentrations just below saturation, complex kinetics apply; then, at low saturation of enzyme (i.e., when most of the enzyme is not in combination with substrate) the reaction becomes first-order. From p. 83,

$$v = \frac{dS}{dt} = \frac{S}{(K + S)} V_{max}$$

and when $v \ll V_{max}$, so that $S \ll K$, we have approximately

$$\frac{dS}{dt} = \frac{V_{max}}{K} S$$

which is obviously the equation of a first-order process, since V_{max}/K is a constant. This is often called a *pseudo-first-order* reaction because, although two reactants (substrate and enzyme) have to combine, the latter remains constant and only the changing substrate concentration influences the reaction rate. Initially, therefore, the metabolic elimination of drugs may be zero-order or first-order, depending upon the drug concentration and the affinity of the particular drug for its metabolizing enzymes. Eventually, as drug levels fall, drug metabolism will become first order.

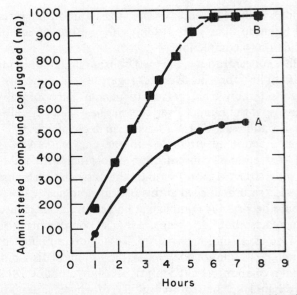

FIGURE 4-2. Examples of zero-order and first-order kinetics in drug metabolism. *Urinary excretion of glycine conjugates was followed in the rabbit after administration of 1 g doses of two different compounds: (A) anisic acid + glycine (4 g); (B) p-fluorobenzoic acid. (A) is exponential because excess glycine is supplied; the drug is also metabolized by other pathways. (B) is linear because the endogenous glycine supply is rate limiting, nearly to the end of the reaction. (From Bray et al., Figure 2.[4])*

Figure 4-2 presents an example of metabolic elimination in the same species by different kinetics. In both cases the metabolic reaction under study was the conjugation of a substituted benzoic acid with endogenous glycine by the mechanism presented on p. 261. In *A*, the drug was anisic acid (*p*-methoxybenzoic acid) and a large excess of glycine was administered simultaneously. The excretion of glycine conjugate in the urine followed a typical exponential course; the rate declined progressively as the level of unconjugated drug in the body declined. In *B*, the drug was *p*-fluorobenzoic acid and no exogenous glycine was furnished. The rate of conjugation of this compound is very much faster than that of anisic acid, but it proceeds at a constant rate (zero-order) until very little unconjugated drug remains. The reason is that because endogenous glycine cannot be made available at a sufficient rate, the glycine supply is rate limiting, so that the overall conjugation rate remains constant. When exogenous glycine was administered simultaneously with *p*-fluorobenzoic acid (not shown in the figure), the initial rate of conjugation was much faster, but it slowed progressively according to first-order kinetics.

An interesting example of zero-order metabolism is the oxidation of ethanol in man and other animals.[5-8] Ethanol is converted to acetaldehyde by the liver alcohol dehydrogenase in a NAD-coupled reaction:

$$CH_3CH_2OH + NAD^+ \rightleftharpoons CH_3CHO + NADH + H^+$$

The acetaldehyde is further metabolized to acetic acid by aldehyde dehydrogenase. The equilibrium for the oxidation of ethanol to acetaldehyde lies far to the left; with equal concentrations of NAD^+ and NADH, the equilibrium ratio of ethanol to acetaldehyde will be more than 1000:1. Only the continuous removal of acetaldehyde forces the reaction to completion.

Except at very low concentrations, the metabolism of ethanol in man is essentially constant (about 10 ml hr^{-1} on the average) regardless of concentration; the rate, however, differs considerably from person to person. Alcohol dehydrogenase has been studied extensively the human liver enzyme has been crystallized, and all the equilibrium constants and reaction rates have been determined.[9-14] The dissociation constant for the interaction of ethanol with the enzyme–NAD^+ complex is 1.2 $\times 10^{-3} M$. The blood ethanol concentration associated with mild intoxication is about 1 mg ml^{-1} ($2 \times 10^{-2} M$), or 17 times the dissociation constant. Thus, the enzyme would be 94% saturated even at this pharmacologically low level of ethanol, and saturation would be virtually complete at higher levels in the intoxicating range.

Some well-known facts about drinking are logical consequences of the zero-order kinetics and slow rate of ethanol metabolism. To achieve a mildly intoxicating level of 1 mg ml^{-1} throughout 41 liters of body water (the volume of distribution for ethanol) will require an intake of about 41 g (55 ml) of absolute ethanol. Most strong liquor contains 40–50% ethanol, so the required intake of whiskey, gin, vodka, or similar drink will be approximately 120 ml, or 4 ounces. This "priming" amount (cf. p. 320) is often ingested quite rapidly in order to obtain the desired effect. However, the maximum that can be metabolized is 10 ml hr^{-1}, so that 5 hr would be required to eliminate the 55 ml taken at the outset. It follows that continuation of the same dosing rate would very soon lead to progressively higher and more toxic blood levels. The safe maintenance dose (after priming), to maintain a constant level of mild intoxication, will be just 10 ml of ethanol (about 20–25 ml of liquor) per hour.

Most elimination mechanisms are approximately first-order; a constant fraction of the drug in the body disappears in each equal interval of time. Typical is the excretion of drugs by glomerular filtration at the kidneys, as discussed already (p. 210). Other first-order processes are the excretion of drugs by diffusion and ion trapping at the gastric or intestinal mucosa, the elimination of volatile drugs at the lungs, and the sequestration of drugs in various tissues. All these are first-order because every drug molecule has a fixed probability of being excreted within a given time; the total rate of excretion is therefore equal to that probability times the total number of drug molecules present. In the case of removal of drugs from the plasma by sequestration, as in fat depots, this probability is determined by the blood flow to the tissue concerned and the physicochemical properties of the drug that determine its sequestration.

For first-order (exponential) elimination the familiar equations apply, where X denotes total drug in the body at time t, X_0 the drug present at time zero, and k_e the rate constant for elimination:

$$X = X_0 e^{-k_e t}$$

$$\log X = \log X_0 - \frac{k_e t}{2.30}$$

$$t_{1/2} = \frac{0.693}{k_e}$$

The half-time for elimination is also called the *biologic half-life*. The meaning of $t_{1/2}$ is easily grasped, but the first-order rate constants (both for absorption and elimination) may be misunderstood. Consider a drug that is eliminated with $k_e = 0.5$ day^{-1}. This does not mean that half the initial amount will be present after one day. The rate constant, k_e, describes the instantaneous rate of elimination at any time. Thus, initially, the elimination is at such a rate that if the absolute rate continued, one-half of the drug would be gone in one day. But that absolute rate does not continue. It starts to diminish immediately, as soon as the total amount of drug starts to decrease, and it continues to diminish. Thus, the biologic half-life of such a drug is not one day, but rather $0.693/0.5 = 1.39$ days.

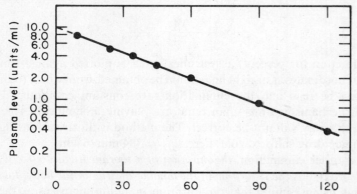

FIGURE 4-3. First-order elimination of penicillin from plasma. *Penicillin G (50,000 units, 30 mg) was injected intravenously at time zero in a dog weighing about 18 kg. Plasma levels of penicillin were determined periodically, as shown. (Adapted from Beyer et al., Figure 2.[15])*

Figure 4-3 shows a typical first-order elimination curve after intravenous injection of penicillin into a dog. The decline in the plasma level is almost perfectly linear on semilogarithmic coordinates, i.e., a constant fraction was eliminated in each equal interval of time. The biologic half-life is found by measuring the time required for a given plasma level to decline by one-half, here 25 min. The elimination rate constant k_e equals $0.693/25 = 0.028$, or about 3% per minute. The elimination rate is consistent with the renal tubular secretion of a drug whose V_d is somewhat larger than the extracellular fluid volume (cf. Table 2-19 for comparable data in man), and the first-order kinetics indicate that even at the highest concentration observed here, 8 units ml^{-1}, the T_m was not exceeded. Note that it would not be valid to compute a volume of distribution by extrapolating this elimination curve back to zero time, since errors are introduced in instances where rapid elimination is occurring (p. 213).

Another way of portraying the course of first-order elimination is based upon measurements of cumulative drug excretion in the urine. Let Y' be the total amount of drug eventually excreted, and Y the cumulative excretion to any time t. Then the rate of excretion at any moment will be proportional to the difference between the total amount to be excreted and the amount already excreted at that time, i.e., proportional to the unexcreted fraction. As we have seen,

$$\frac{X}{X_0} = e^{-k_e t}$$

where X/X_0 is the fraction of initial drug still remaining in the body. Then obviously, the fraction excreted is

$$\frac{Y}{Y'} = 1 - \frac{X}{X_0}$$

since the total drug X_0 is identical to the total amount Y' to be excreted. (If routes of elimination other than excretion play a significant role, then Y' will be smaller than X_0, but if all the mechanisms are first-order, their sum will also be first-order.) Hence,

$$\ln\left(1 - \frac{Y}{Y'}\right) = -k_e t$$

$$\log\left(1 - \frac{Y}{Y'}\right) = -\frac{k_e t}{2.30}$$

When the fraction (or percent) as yet unexcreted is plotted against time on semi-logarithmic coordinates, a straight line should be obtained, from which the half-time for excretion can be read and the elimination rate constant computed. However, if elimination mechanisms other than renal are playing a significant role, the result obtained in this way will not be correct. The method is illustrated in Figure 4-4 for the sulfonamide drug sulfisoxazole; here, $t_{1/2} = 384$ min (6.4 hr).

For a first-order elimination, *the duration of a therapeutically effective drug concentration increases as the logarithm of the amount of drug in the body fluids.* In many instances this means simply that the duration of action increases as the logarithm of the dose. This would be true, for example, if the dose were given intravenously; and

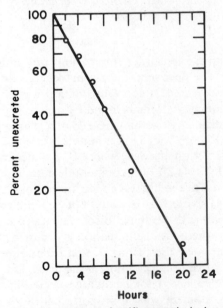

FIGURE 4-4. Kinetics of excretion of sulfisoxazole in human urine. *Note that vertical scale is logarithmic. The percent of unexcreted drug* $[100(1 - Y/Y')]$ *is plotted against time* $k = 0.108 \, hr^{-1}$ *and the biologic half-life is 6.4 hr. (From Nelson and O'Reilly,*[16] *Figure 1, redrawn by Nelson, Figure 3.*[17] *By permission of Williams and Wilkins and C. V. Mosby.)*

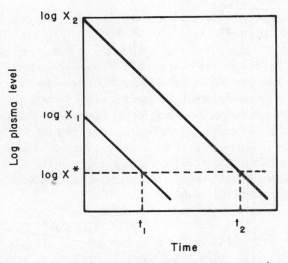

FIGURE 4-5. Schematic first-order elimination curves for two doses. *Concentration x* is the threshold concentration for therapeutic effect; x_1 and x_2 are the initial concentrations established by the two doses. It is assumed that absorption is very rapid, or that the doses were administered intravenously.*

it would be nearly true whenever the drug is absorbed very rapidly in comparison with its rate of elimination. It is easy to see from the schematic diagram of Figure 4-5 why this relationship should hold. Let x^* be the threshold concentration for therapeutic effect, established by the distribution of a just-effective dose X^* in its volume of distribution V_d. Let x_1 and x_2 be plasma levels established by the doses X_1 and X_2. Since V_d is independent of dose, $X_1 = x_1 V_d$, $X_2 = x_2 V_d$, and $X^* = x^* V_d$. The durations of effective concentrations of the two doses are t_1 and t_2; and the slopes of the elimination curves, also independent of dose, are $-k_e/2.30$. If the ordinates are natural logarithms, $\ln x$, the slopes are simply $-k_e$. If logarithms to the base 10 are used, the slope becomes $-k_e/2.30$ because $\log x = (\ln x)/2.30$.

The fundamental equation for first-order elimination (p. 306) and the geometry of Figure 4-5 yield equations describing the relationship between duration of effective concentration and dose. First we find t^*, the time required for the concentration to fall from any initial level x_0 to the threshold level x^*, as follows:

$$\log \frac{x^*}{x_0} = -\frac{k_e t^*}{2.30}$$

and, substituting $x = X/V_d$, cancelling V_d, and inverting, we obtain

$$t^* = \frac{2.30}{k_e} \log \frac{X_0}{X^*}$$

Also, obviously, for the ratio of effective times after two doses,

$$\frac{t_2}{t_1} = \frac{\log X_2 - \log X^*}{\log X_1 - \log X^*}$$

and for the increment in time with the larger dose compared with the smaller,

$$\Delta t^* = t_2 - t_1 = \frac{2.30}{k_e}(\log X_2 - \log X_1)$$

These equations, especially the one that gives t^* as a function of dose, have practical importance. The duration of a therapeutic level of a drug depends upon the *ratio of administered dose to the just-effective dose*, and also upon the rate constant of elimination. Evidently, the longer the biologic half-life (i.e., the smaller the value of k_e), the longer the duration for a given dose ratio. Whatever the duration may be at a particular ratio X_1/X^*, geometric increments in the dose will produce only linear increments in the duration of effective drug levels. Suppose, for example, that doubling the threshold dose would result in an effective drug level for 1 hr, i.e., the biologic half-life is 1 hr. Then (Figure 4-5) the dose would have to be doubled again to achieve an effective level for 2 hr, and doubled yet again to achieve a 3 hr duration. The tolerable limit of geometric increases in drug dosage will be determined by the dose-related toxicity of the particular drug.

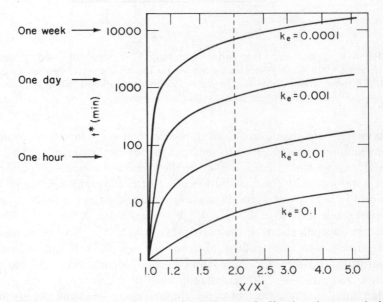

FIGURE 4-6. Relationship between duration of effective therapeutic levels and dose. *Administered dose X is assumed to be absorbed very rapidly, or to be administered intravenously; X' is the just-effective dose; t* is the time (in minutes) during which the drug concentration in the body fluids exceeds the threshold level. Each curve is for a different value of the rate constant of elimination, as indicated; biologic half-lives are (from top to bottom) 6930, 693, 69, 6.9 min. Note that both axes have logarithmic scales.*

Figure 4-6 presents a graphic summary of these relationships for realistic ranges of dose ratio and of k_e. Whatever a just-effective dose may be, it is unlikely, as a general rule, that a dose more than 5 times greater can be given without grave danger of toxicity; certainly few drugs have this large a margin of safety, although penicillin and some of the vitamins are notable exceptions. Usually one would be restricted to a smaller excess over the just-effective level, perhaps only 2- or 3-fold. Dose ratios X/X^* greater than 5 are therefore not considered here. Values of k_e spanning four orders of magnitude are indicated on the curves. Values in the range 0.01–0.001 min^{-1} are encountered frequently (biologic half-lives about 1–10 hr), since so many drugs are eliminated primarily at the kidneys without significant tubular reabsorption (cf.

Table 2-19). Figure 4-6 is shown as a log-log plot in order to encompass the wide range of durations and dose ratios. Note that if twice the just-effective dose is administered (vertical broken line), the duration of therapeutic level will be simply the biologic half-life. This leads to a useful and practical rule: If a drug's effect is to last several hours, to avoid repeated administration at shorter intervals, then that drug must be one whose biologic half-life is at least several hours; i.e., it must not be metabolized rapidly or secreted by the renal tubules. Penicillin is a good example of a drug whose biologic half-life is too short (because of its rapid renal tubular secretion), so that ordinary parenteral routes of administration (i.v., i.m.), in which absorption is rapid, may not be practical; sustained-release depot preparations[17] or orally effective forms have to be employed instead.

We have referred to the duration of effective therapeutic concentration of a drug as though it were identical to duration of action. Often it is. But there are many exceptions, instances in which a drug's therapeutic action may far outlast its presence in the body fluids. Certain bactericidal drugs kill pathogenic organisms rapidly and then need not be present at all for a certain interval, during which the pathogens are unable to recover. Alkylating agents usually produce their irreversible chemical effects very quickly, and they may also be quickly destroyed, so that they are not present at all during the subsequent period when the biologic effects develop. Organic phosphate cholinesterase inhibitors are degraded rapidly, but the consequences of their irreversible alkylation of the enzyme persist until new enzyme is synthesized. Barbiturates and other centrally acting agents may produce typical actions at a certain threshold concentration, but recovery from these actions may occur at a different concentration; thus, the duration of drug action and the time during which drug concentrations exceed the original threshold may not be the same. Finally, reserpine depletes catecholamines at nerve terminals peripherally, and in brain; the effects are long lasting, until the catecholamine stores can be replenished.

ZERO-ORDER ABSORPTION, FIRST-ORDER ELIMINATION; THE PLATEAU PRINCIPLE

Derivation of the Principle and Its Application to Constant Infusions

We shall show the derivation of an elementary principle about steady states that has direct application to the kinetics of drug accumulation in the body, and that also has much broader application to fundamental biologic, chemical, and physical processes. If the rate of input into a system is constant and the rate of output from the system is exponential, then the content of the system (here designated by X) will accumulate until a steady-state is reached:

$$\xrightarrow{k_{in}} X \xrightarrow{k_{out}}$$

$$\text{constant input rate} = k_{in}$$

$$\text{output rate} = k_{out}X$$

At the steady-state, X will have increased to X', a level at which the output rate is equal to the input rate:

$$k_{out}X' = k_{in}$$

$$X' = \frac{k_{in}}{k_{out}}$$

In such a system, the steady-state can be altered by changing the input rate k_{in} or by changing the output rate constant k_{out}, or both. Any such change will cause a *shift* to a new steady state.

According to the plateau principle, regardless of how a shift is brought about from one steady-state to another, *the time course of the shift* (i.e., the rate at which the new plateau level is reached) *is determined solely by* k_{out}, the first-order rate constant of the output process that is operative during the shift. Thus, if the shift is caused by an alteration of k_{in} without change in k_{out}, the sole determinant is the unchanged k_{out}. If the shift is caused wholly or in part by a change in k_{out}, then the sole determinant is the *new* value of k_{out}. In any case, *the rate constant for the shift is equal to k_{out}, so the shift half-time is identical to the half-time of the output process*, $0.693/k_{out}$. The same principle applies when the initial value of X is zero and k_{in} is abruptly changed from zero to some finite value; then the shift is simply the establishment of a steady-state. And the principle also applies when a steady-state value of X is in effect and k_{in} is abruptly changed to zero (i.e., the input is stopped); then the shift is simply the exponential disappearance of X, resulting in the new "steady-state" where $X = 0$.

The plateau principle is fundamental to understanding constant infusions, drug accumulation, dosage regimens, chronic toxicity by drug accumulation, and enzyme induction and stabilization. We shall derive it first, then show its specific applications. (Much of the work that led to an explicit formulation of the plateau principle was carried out collaboratively with D. B. Goldstein.) For the change in X,

$$\frac{dX}{dt} = k_{in} - k_{out}X$$

and at the initial steady-state

$$X'_1 = \frac{k_{in_1}}{k_{out_1}}$$

Now change k_{in_1} to a new value k_{in_2}, and also change k_{out_1} to a new value k_{out_2}, and consider the time course of the change in X from X'_1 to its new steady-state value X'_2. Accordingly,

$$\frac{dX}{dt} = k_{in_2} - k_{out_2}X$$

and at the new steady-state,

$$X'_2 = \frac{k_{in_2}}{k_{out_2}}$$

To find X as a function of time after the shift, differentiate with respect to time:

$$\frac{dX}{k_{in_2} - k_{out_2}(X)} = dt$$

Rearranging,

$$-\frac{1}{k_{out_2}} \frac{d[k_{in_2} - k_{out_2}(X)]}{[k_{in_2} - k_{out_2}(X)]} = dt$$

and integrating, we obtain

$$\ln [k_{in_2} - k_{out_2}(X)] = -k_{out_2}t + C$$

When $t = 0$, $X = X'$, and the constant of integration, C, is found to be

$$C = \ln [k_{in_2} - k_{out_2}(X'_1)]$$

Then substituting, and taking antilogarithms,

$$\frac{k_{in_2} - k_{out_2}(X)}{k_{in_2} - k_{out_2}(X'_1)} = e^{-k_{out_2}t}$$

Now we are concerned with the *shift* from one steady-state to the other. The total extent of the shift is $(X'_2 - X'_1)$ and the amount by which X has changed from its initial steady-state value is given by $(X - X'_1)$. Thus, the fraction f of the total shift that has been accomplished at any value of X is given by

$$f = \frac{(X - X'_1)}{(X'_2 - X'_1)}$$

and

$$X = fX'_2 + X'_1 - fX'_1$$

Substituting this value of X into the equation obtained above, and substituting for k_{in_2} its equivalent value $k_{out_2}(X'_2)$, we obtain

$$\frac{X'_2 - fX'_2 - X'_1 + fX'_1}{X'_2 - X'_1} = e^{-k_{out_2}t}$$

which simplifies to

$$1 - f = e^{-k_{out_2}t}$$

This equation makes it evident that the kinetics of the shift are the exponential kinetics of a process with rate constant k_{out_2}. The half-time of the shift is found by setting $f = 0.5$:

$$\ln (0.5) = -k_{out_2}t$$

$$t_{1/2} = \frac{-\ln (0.5)}{k_{out_2}} = \frac{0.693}{k_{out_2}}$$

Simply, $t_{1/2}$ is the half-time of the output process.

It may seem paradoxical for the time course of the establishment of a steady-state, or of a shift from one steady-state to another, to be determined by the output rate constant and to be independent of the input rate. A physical analogy may help to clarify this relationship. Consider a water reservoir with outlet at bottom and outflow rate proportional to the outlet size and the head of water pressure. What are the conditions for establishing a specified steady-state water level? Since the inflow and outflow rates will be equal at the steady state, the inflow rate cannot be chosen at will; only one particular inflow rate will yield the specified level at steady-state.

A higher inflow rate will, of course, produce a faster rise of the water level, but then the specified level will be exceeded. A slower inflow rate will produce a slower rise, but then the specified level will not be attained. Only if the outlet size is changed will it become possible to alter the inflow rate so that the specified steady-state is approached at a different rate; and clearly, the larger the outlet the more rapidly can the specified steady-state be approached.

The same principle applies when no particular steady-state level has been specified. With a given outlet the actual rate of rise of the water level will obviously be greater at high than at low inflow rate, but the steady-state level to be attained will also be proportionately greater. The *relative* rate of rise, measured as fraction of the ultimate level approached (f, as defined earlier), will be the same for all inflow rates. In a given reservoir this relative rate of approach to any steady-state will be directly proportional to the outlet size, which is analogous to the rate constant of the drug output process.

Now let us apply the plateau principle to constant infusions. Let V_d be the volume of distribution of a drug (ml); Q a constant rate of infusion of the drug $(mg \cdot min^{-1})$; k_e the first-order rate constant for elimination of the drug (min^{-1}), the rate of change of concentration being given by $k_e x$, where x is the drug concentration in plasma $(mg \cdot ml^{-1})$; and t the elapsed time (min) from the start of the infusion, from the stopping of the infusion, or from any abrupt change in the input or output rate.

Since the elimination rate is expressed in terms of the plasma concentration of the drug rather than of the total drug in the body, k_{in} is represented by Q/V_d, the rate of input per volume of body fluid. Then the equation describing the change in x with time is

$$\frac{dx}{dt} = \frac{Q}{V_d} - k_e x$$

The change in x from the start of the infusion ($x = 0, t = 0$) is given by

$$x = \frac{Q}{k_e V_d}(1 - e^{-k_e t})$$

This equation shows that with a constant infusion a plasma plateau is eventually reached; for when t becomes infinite, $1 - e^{-k_e t}$ becomes unity, and at the steady-state, $x' = Q/k_e V_d$. Rearranging, we have $k_e(x' V_d) = Q$. Here, $x' V_d$ is the total amount of drug in the body, therefore $k_e(x' V_d)$ is the elimination rate, equal to the infusion rate Q.

For any drug administered by constant infusion, therefore, if its total plasma clearance $(k_e V_d)$ is known, its plateau level can be predicted. The kinetics of attaining the plateau or of shifting from one plateau to another, or of the die-away when the infusion is stopped, are given by the general expression

$$f = 1 - e^{-k_e t}$$

where, in the general case

$$f = \frac{x - x'_1}{x'_2 - x'_1}$$

For starting an infusion ($x'_1 = 0$),

$$f = \frac{x}{x'}$$

and for stopping an infusion $(x'_2 = 0)$,

$$f = 1 - \frac{x}{x'}$$

In summary, if the rate of a constant infusion is increased or decreased, or if an infusion is started or stopped, or if the elimination rate constant is increased or decreased, the half-time of the shift to the new steady-state is the new elimination half-time (i.e., the biologic half-life of the drug). For discontinuance of an infusion, the time course of the shift is the normal die-away curve of drug concentration.

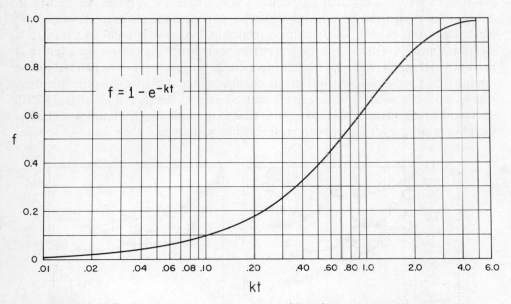

FIGURE 4-7. Generalized kinetics for shifting from one steady-state to another. *This is a graph of equation* $f = 1 - e^{-kt}$, *where f is defined as the fractional attainment of the total shift from one steady-state to another, for any system with zero-order input and first-order output ; k is the output rate constant, t is time in the same units as k. To obtain real time, divide the value of* kt *read from the graph by* k.

Figure 4-7 is the generalized graph of the equation for shifting a steady-state $(f = 1 - e^{-kt})$. The y axis is a scale of f, defined as the fraction of the total shift that has been attained. The time axis is generalized to show units of kt rather than of t, and the units themselves are immaterial (minutes, hours, days, etc.) provided k and t are expressed in the same way. To encompass the wide range of times, the x axis is logarithmic. An example will illustrate the use of this graph. Suppose a drug with elimination $k_e = 0.5 \, \text{hr}^{-1}$ is being infused at a constant rate, a steady-state plasma concentration having been established. The infusion rate is now abruptly reduced by one-half. How long will it take to accomplish 75 % of the shift to the new and lower steady-state drug level? Observe that k_e has not been changed, so the amount by which the infusion rate was changed is immaterial. The time course of approach to the new steady-state will be the same for all changes in the infusion rate. However, the actual level of the new plateau will be determined by the change in the infusion rate. Consulting the graph at $f = 0.75$, we find $kt = 1.4$; and so $t = 1.4/0.5 = 2.8$ hr. The half-time of the shift ($f = 0.5$) would be $0.693/0.5 = 1.4$ hr.

The plateau principle can be applied to experimental constant infusions in order to gain information about the way a drug is disposed of in the body. The rate of infusion is set by the investigator. By periodic determinations of the drug plasma level, the rate of attaining a plateau can be found, and this rate yields an estimate of the elimination rate constant k_e. The actual concentration at the plateau is $Q/k_e V_d$, as we have seen, from which V_d can also be estimated. By exploring a range of infusion rates leading to widely differing plateau concentrations, it is possible to see whether or not the overall elimination follows first-order kinetics, and it is also possible to see what different mechanisms play the major roles in elimination at different drug concentrations. For example, any experimental procedure that alters k_e will change the plateau level during a constant infusion. If renal excretion is a significant mechanism and the renal arteries are clamped, the plasma drug level will promptly rise, and if other first-order mechanisms are present a new plateau will be attained. By the plateau principle the time course of the shift gives an estimate of the *new* k_e, as does also the new plateau concentration (provided V_d did not change). If all elimination pathways are blocked or saturated, then continuing the infusion will cause the plasma drug level to rise without limit until toxicity and then death supervene.

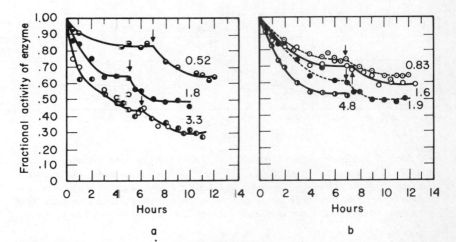

FIGURE 4-8. Constant intravenous infusions of neostigmine in dogs. *Vertical scale is activity of plasma cholinesterase, used as a measure of the concentration of neostigmine, an inhibitor of that enzyme. Since the relationship between inhibitor concentration and observed enzyme activity is complex, curves may only be interpreted semiquantitatively. Each curve represents a different infusion rate; values given are to be multiplied by 10^{-10} moles kg^{-1} min^{-1}. In graph a, renal pedicles were ligated at times shown by arrows; in graph b, infusion was started in hepatic portal vein instead of femoral vein, then shifted at arrow to femoral vein. (From Goldstein et al., Figures 8 and 11.[18])*

An application of this technique is illustrated in Figure 4-8. Here, neostigmine, a cholinesterase inhibitor, was given to dogs by constant infusion. The plasma neostigmine levels were measured periodically by a method that makes use of the degree of inhibition of the plasma cholinesterase—a given depression of enzyme activity signifies a certain concentration of neostigmine, although the relationship is not one of simple proportionality. The data shown on the figure are measurements of enzyme activity, plotted as fractions of the initial uninhibited activity. In Figure 4-8a we see that plateau levels were established at three different infusion rates into the femoral vein; and in Figure 4-8b, that infusions into the hepatic portal vein led to a lesser degree of inhibition of the enzyme (i.e., a lower drug concentration) at comparable infusion rates. Qualitatively, this indicates that the liver is a significant site of elimination of neostigmine, a conclusion that was confirmed by shifting the infusion from the portal vein to the femoral vein after the plateau levels were established (Figure 4-8b); a greater plateau concentration of neostigmine resulted. The effect of tying the renal pedicles (Figure 4-8a) indicates, in the same way, that the kidneys play a significant role in the overall elimination. The investigators used the difference between the two plateau levels, with and without the kidneys functioning, to obtain a quantitative estimate of the rate constant of renal excretion. This corresponded to a renal clearance for neostigmine of about 100 ml min^{-1}, a value consistent with elimination by glomerular filtration in the dog. The renal clearance estimate was confirmed directly by measurements of neostigmine in the urine.

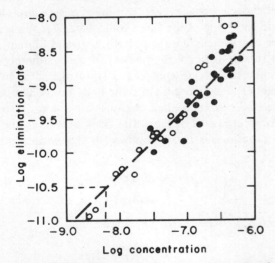

FIGURE 4-9. Relationship of elimination rate to the steady-state plasma level of neostigmine. *Solid circles, myasthenia gravis patients, for whom neostigmine is the drug of choice. Open circles, dogs. Note that this is log-log plot. Broken line has a slope of 1. Elimination rate is expressed as moles kilogram per minute, neostigmine concentration as moles per liter. (From Goldstein et al., Figure 18.*[18]*)*

Neostigmine was also administered by constant infusion to human patients suffering from myasthenia gravis, a disease for which it is the drug of choice. Figure 4-9 shows the relationship between the rate of drug infusion at the steady-state (equal to the rate of elimination at the steady-state) and the neostigmine concentration at the steady-state. The data from the experiments with dogs are also shown on the same graph. The method used by the investigators to express the infusion rate is the common one of relating dosage to body weight, since weights of experimental animals or patients vary widely. To be applicable here, the steady-state equation has to be rewritten, dividing both sides by body weight:

$$\frac{Q}{W} = k_e x' \frac{V_d}{W} = k_e x' \alpha$$

where W is the body weight and α is the volume of distribution expressed as a fraction of the body weight. Then

$$\log \frac{Q}{W} = \log x' + \log \alpha + \log k_e$$

$$\log k_e + \log \alpha = \log \frac{Q}{W} - \log x'$$

And for any two infusion rates, since α and k_e do not change,

$$\log \frac{Q_1}{W} - \log \frac{Q_2}{W} = \log x_1 - \log x'_2$$

$$\text{slope} = \frac{\log(Q_1/W) - \log(Q_2/W)}{\log x'_1 - \log x'_2} = 1$$

These equations show that if the elimination is first-order throughout the range examined, the relationship between log elimination rate and log concentration should be linear, and the slope of the line should be unity. We see from Figure 4-9 that this seems to be true of neostigmine in both dogs and humans, within the limits of the experimental errors. Since all the points fall approximately on the same line, it follows that the elimination rate constant is about the same in both species, assuming the same manner of distribution into the body fluids. This k_e can be found by applying to Figure 4-9 the equation $\log k_e + \log \alpha = \log(Q/W) - \log x'$, then making the subtractions indicated by the dotted lines, and assuming that neostigmine, a quaternary ammonium derivative, is confined to the extracellular fluid ($\alpha = 0.18$, $\log \alpha = -0.74$):

$$\log k_e - 0.74 = -10.5 - (-8.2)$$
$$k_e = \text{antilog}(-1.56) = 0.0275 \text{ min}^{-1}$$

Thus, a little less than 3% is eliminated per minute, and

$$t_{1/2} = \frac{0.693}{0.0275} = 25 \text{ min}$$

Dosage Regimens

The plateau principle also provides a fundamental basis for understanding the rationale of dosage schedules and of drug accumulation in the body. When we give a drug we are attempting to establish a certain therapeutic concentration in the body fluids, or a certain total amount of drug in the body. This *effective drug concentration* (EDC) is a characteristic biologic property of the drug, over which we have no control. If the drug level is much below this EDC, the desired drug actions will not occur. If the level is much higher, toxic effects may well become manifest.

Although the EDC has been defined here as a concentration, the argument to follow would apply equally well if EDC were the total amount of drug in the body or the amount of drug fixed at some site of action.

Dosage schedules entail two variables: the magnitude of the single dose and the frequency with which that dose is repeated, usually expressed as a *dosing interval*. For any given dose, the extent to which the drug level in the body will fluctuate within a dosing interval is determined by several factors. For a given rate of elimination, the faster the absorption, the greater the fluctuation. With rapid absorption, the bulk of the drug will enter the circulation rapidly and the drug level will be high at first, then fall relatively fast; whereas with slower absorption, the buildup to a peak will be less rapid and the drug level more sustained, as seen with sustained-release medications. For a given rate of absorption, the fluctuation is obviously greater the more rapid the elimination. No generalization will reliably answer the question just how much the drug level may be permitted to fluctuate above and below the desired level; this will depend entirely upon the particular drug. Detailed analysis of the kinetics of the establishment and decay of drug levels after single doses will be deferred to a later section (p. 333).

Here, we shall begin by ignoring the fluctuations. We assume, as a first approximation, that the absorption of a dose proceeds at a practically constant rate throughout each dosing interval, and that it is complete at the end of the dosing interval. In other words, we suppose that the conditions are practically equivalent to those of a constant infusion. Our aim is to establish and maintain the EDC as a steady-state. Obviously, if the individual dose were large enough and the dosing interval short enough, the EDC would be reached quickly; but the drug concentration would continue to increase. There must be some lower rate of drug input that would just establish but not exceed the desired EDC; this rate is defined as the *maintenance dose rate*.

A good illustration is found in the use of digitoxin to maintain cardiac compensation in a patient with congestive heart failure; the dose of about 0.1 mg daily, given day after day indefinitely, is the maintenance dose rate for this drug. What determines the maintenance dose rate of a drug, in general? The familiar equation for a constant infusion provides the answer:

$$Q = \text{maintenance dose rate} = k_e(EDC)V_d$$

where $(EDC)V_d$ is the total amount of drug required in the body at the EDC, determined by the drug's biologic potency and by its distribution in the body. Alternatively, since $(k_e V_d)$ is the total clearance, we may write

$$Q = \text{(total clearance) (EDC)}$$

The equations show that the maintenance dose rate will have to be higher the more rapidly the drug is eliminated.

The time required to establish the EDC with any drug, under the conditions specified, is given by the plateau principle; the half-time will simply be the elimination half-time. Thus, a drug with short biologic half-life can come to the EDC quickly when the maintenance dose is administered from the start. But a drug that is eliminated slowly will necessarily achieve its EDC slowly. If k_e is known, then the whole time course of approach to the EDC is simply that shown in Figure 4-7.

Once it has been decided to administer a drug, the therapeutic effect is invariably wanted quickly, certainly within a few hours. Yet this is impossible if the drug's half-life is longer than a few hours. The solution to the dosage problem for drugs that are eliminated slowly is to administer relatively large doses initially in order to establish the EDC quickly, and then to continue with the maintenance dose rate thereafter.

The large initial doses are called *priming doses*. Note especially that if the priming dose rate were continued, the EDC would be greatly exceeded, at the risk of serious toxicity. A theoretical illustration of this principle is shown in Figure 4-10. Here, the fluctuations due to the individual doses are shown also; clearly, the fluctuations can be minimized by subdividing the doses and administering them more frequently, the limit of such dose fragmentation being a constant infusion. In practice it is inconvenient to administer medication more often than once every few hours, and the desirability of uninterrupted sleep at night further demands that the dosing interval be as long as possible. A certain amount of fluctuation is therefore inevitable; and it will be more extreme the more rapidly the drug is eliminated.

Figure 4-10 is based upon a rigorous theoretical treatment of repeated drug administration leading to attainment of the EDC.[19] Whereas our application of the

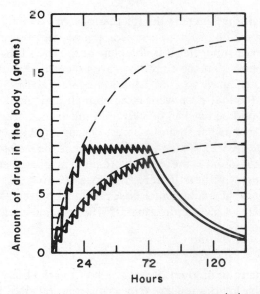

FIGURE 4-10. Curves of accumulation with repeated dosage at constant intervals. *Elimination constant* $k_e = 0.0289 \, hr^{-1}$, *elimination half-time* = 24 hr, *dosing interval* = 4 hr. *In lower curve, dose is 1 g; in upper curve, 2 g for the first six doses, then 1 g. Solid curves are computed from the given parameters; zig-zag portions represent fluctuations during period of drug administration. Broken curves indicate course of continued accumulation if drug administration were continued. Drug stopped at 72 hr. Elimination curve is seen to be identical to accumulation curve, but inverted. (From Geddum, Figure 1.[19])*

plateau principle entailed the assumption that drug absorption is continuous, this approach takes into account the fluctuations resulting from drug elimination during the intervals between doses. It assumes, however, that each single dose is absorbed instantaneously. Let M_0 be the dose of a drug, X_0 the resulting drug level in the body (X_0/V_d would be the plasma concentration), and t^* the dosing interval. Now we give M_0, at $t = 0$, repeat after $t^*, 2t^*, 3t^*, \ldots, nt^*$. At $t = 0$, just after the first dose, $X = X_0$. At $t = t^*$, just before the second dose,

$$X = X_0 e^{-k_e t^*}$$

because of the exponential elimination of the drug during the interval t^*. To simplify the algebra, denote $e^{-k_e t^*}$ by the symbol p. Then just before the second dose, at $t = t^*$,

$$X = X_0 p$$

and just after the instantaneous absorption of the second dose, still at $t = t^*$,

$$X = X_0 + X_0 p = X_0(1 + p)$$

At $2t^*$, just before the third dose,

$$X = X_0(1 + p)p$$

and just after the third dose,

$$X = X_0 + X_0(1 + p)p = X_0(1 + p + p^2)$$

Just after the nth dose,

$$X_n = X_0(1 + p + p^2 + \cdots + p^{n-1})$$

Solving the series, we obtain

$$X_n = X_0 \frac{(1 - p^n)}{(1 - p)}$$

and eventually, as $n \to \infty \cdot p^n \to 0$, since $p < 1$,

$$X_\infty = X_0/(1 - p).$$

Here X_∞ is the drug level ultimately established immediately after each dose. As shown in Figure 4-10, the "plateau" established in this model is a fluctuating one, but the peak levels do become constant, when steady-state conditions have been attained. For attainment of a certain fraction of the eventual plateau,

$$f = \frac{X_n}{X_\infty} = \frac{X_0(1 - p^n)}{(1 - p)} \cdot \frac{(1 - p)}{X_0} = (1 - p^n)$$

$$f = 1 - e^{-k_e t^* n}$$

Since $t^* n$, the dosing interval times the number of doses, is the same as the total time t, this equation is identical to that derived previously (p. 314) in connection with the plateau principle.

Suppose we wish to compute how many doses will be required at a certain dosing interval to attain a given fraction of the eventual plateau drug level. Rewriting the equation to solve for n, we obtain

$$n = \frac{\ln(1 - f)}{-k_e t^*} = \frac{2.3 \log(1 - f)}{-k_e t^*}$$

As an example, suppose $k_e = 0.1 \text{ hr}^{-1}$ and $t^* = 4 \text{ hr}$, and we wish to calculate the number of doses needed to achieve 90% of the plateau. Then

$$n = \frac{2.3 \log(1 - 0.9)}{(-0.1)(4)} = 6 \text{ doses}$$

Suppose we wish to fix the level of drug in the body and maintain that level. Obviously there will be a direct relationship between the dosing interval and the maintenance dose required. Since the maintenance dose has to replace drug that was eliminated during the dosing interval, the longer the interval, the greater the required dose and the greater also the fluctuation. As shown above,

$$X_\infty = \frac{X_0}{(1 - p)}$$

$$\frac{X_0}{X_\infty} = 1 - e^{-k_e t^*}$$

This expression gives the fraction of total drug in the body that has to be replaced in each dosing interval. Thus, immediately after the maintenance dose is given (assuming instantaneous absorption), the plateau level is restored. Just before the next dose, the fraction $(1 - e^{-k_e t^*})$ has been eliminated and must be replaced. This fraction therefore, represents the maximum fluctuation below the plateau level. Evidently, the smaller the value of k_e and the shorter the dosing interval t^*, the smaller will be the fluctuation.

As an example, suppose we wish to establish and maintain a plasma level of $10 \mu g \, ml^{-1}$ with a drug whose volume of distribution is the extracellular fluid, and whose elimination rate constant is $0.001 \, min^{-1}$. If the dosing interval is to be 3 hr, what maintenance dose is required, how long will it take to attain 90% of the desired EDC, and what will be the maximum fluctuation below the EDC?

$$V_c = 12 \times 10^3 \, ml$$

$$X_\infty = V_d(EDC) = 12 \times 10^3 \times 10 = 120 \, mg$$

$$k_e = 0.001 \, min^{-1}$$

$$t^* = 3 \times 60 = 180 \, min$$

$$\frac{X_0}{X_\infty} = 1 - e^{(-0.001)(180)} = 1 - 0.835 = 0.165$$

$$X_0 = 20 \, mg$$

The EDC will fluctuate 16.5% below its appropriate level, in other words, from 10 $\mu g \, ml^{-1}$ to 8.4 $\mu g \, ml^{-1}$ in each 3 hr interval.

The time required to attain 90% of the EDC if the maintenance dose is administered from the beginning is found readily from the number of doses needed at the fixed 3 hr interval:

$$n = \frac{2.3 \log (1 - 0.9)}{(-0.001)(180)} = \frac{-2.3}{-0.18} = 13 \, doses$$

and the time required to administer them is 39 hr. This is an undesirably long time. Obviously, the preferable procedure would be to administer the total amount required in the body (120 mg) as a single priming dose or a series of closely spaced priming doses, and then continue with the 20 mg maintenance dose.

Given a drug with $k_e = 0.2 \, hr^{-1}$ and some important reason for minimizing fluctuation. What dosing interval would be required in order to ensure that the drug level does not fall below 90% of the EDC? As shown above, fluctuation is given by the term $(1 - e^{-k_e t^*})$, and here we require

$$1 - e^{-k_e t^*} = 0.10$$

$$e^{-k_e t^*} = 0.9$$

$$t^* = \frac{2.3 \log 0.9}{-k_e} = \frac{-0.106}{-0.2} = 0.53$$

Then the required dosing interval is about 1/2 hour.

The use of priming doses to overcome the otherwise slow buildup to the EDC with drugs that have long biologic half-lives is exemplified by the procedure known as *digitalization*. One of the commonly used digitalis glycosides, digitoxin, is eliminated very slowly from the body, at a rate of approximately 10 % per day; half-life is about 7 days. Then if the daily maintenance dose were given from the start, the EDC would not nearly be achieved for weeks, an intolerable situation for a drug whose rapidity of action in congestive heart failure is potentially life saving. Moreover, drugs of this class have a very narrow range between therapeutic and toxic levels, so that large fluctuations cannot be tolerated. Digitalization consists of giving priming doses until the electrocardiographic and clinical signs confirm that the EDC is just being reached, then continuing with the much smaller maintenance dose rate.

An elegant example of the use of priming doses concerns the treatment of malaria with quinacrine. This drug was considered virtually useless for years because of its apparently poor efficacy in acute clinical attacks of malaria, and its seemingly capricious toxicity. During World War II, however, carefully conducted studies[20] of plasma levels and of elimination rates showed clearly that without priming doses the EDC could not be attained quickly enough to be effective in terminating attacks of acute malaria in the erythrocytic phase of the disease. The slow elimination rate of the drug was largely attributable to an extraordinary degree of tissue binding, especially in liver, spleen, skin, and leukocytes (Table 4-1). The binding to leukocytes produced

TABLE 4-1. Tissue levels of quinacrine in the dog.
A dog was given quinacrine, 20 mg kg^{-1} for 14 days, then sacrificed, and tissue concentrations were determined. [Data of Shannon et al.[20] By permission of Williams & Wilkins.)

Tissue	Quinacrine concentration $(mg\,kg^{-1})$
Plasma	0.061
Muscle	55
Lung	310
Spleen	571
Liver	1306

concentrations at least 1000 times those in plasma water, making whole-blood determinations of quinacrine concentration completely misleading. The fractional binding of the drug to plasma proteins was also high—from 0.75 to 0.90. Figure 4-11 shows that when the drug was given to human volunteers at a daily dose of 50 mg, many weeks were required to attain a plasma plateau. When a priming dose was given (200 mg daily for the first five days), an EDC plateau was established (actually somewhat exceeded) at the outset and then maintained by the smaller daily dose.

An interesting calculation can be made, using knowledge of the just-effective priming dosage to estimate V_d. The computation is based upon the excess of the

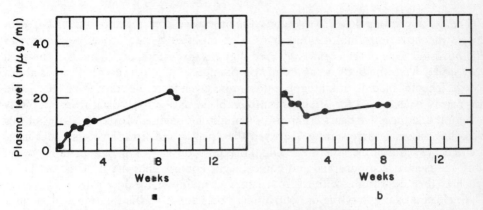

FIGURE 4-11. Establishment of quinacrine plasma levels in human subjects.
*Vertical scale is plasma quinacrine concentration in μg liter^{-1}, horizontal scale gives time
in weeks. The points are average values in groups of 7 to 9 subjects. Drug was given by
mouth, 50 mg on each of 6 successive weekdays, 100 mg on Sundays, total dose 400 mg
wk^{-1}. In graph a, this regimen was pursued from the start. In graph b, priming doses were
given on the first 5 days (200 mg daily). (Adapted from Shannon et al., Figure 1.[20])*

priming amount over the maintenance dose, and on the plateau concentration of
drug in the plasma. Figure 4-11 shows that during the priming period an excess of
150 mg was given daily for 5 days, or 750 mg excess. This established a concentration
of about 20 μg liter^{-1}. Then, assuming negligible elimination during this period of
time,

$$V_d = \frac{X}{x} = \frac{750 \times 10^3}{20} = 3.8 \times 10^4 \text{ liters (sic!)}$$

and applying the general plateau equation,

$$k_e = Q/xV_d$$
$$= \frac{50 \text{ mg day}^{-1}}{(0.02 \text{ mg liter}^{-1})(3.8 \times 10^4 \text{ liters})}$$
$$= 0.07 \text{ day}^{-1}$$

For the half-time of attaining the plateau without priming doses,

$$t_{1/2} = \frac{0.693}{0.07} = 10 \text{ days}$$

and to attain 90% of the desired plateau, from Figure 4-7, $kt = 2.3$, so that

$$t_{0.9} = \frac{2.3}{0.07} = 33 \text{ days}$$

These calculations make it obvious why quinacrine therapy was so ineffective before
the introduction of priming doses.

Obviously, for any drug the dosage during the priming period has to be larger
than during the maintenance period. But how much larger? And when maintenance
dosage is given from the start, the plateau eventually reached will obviously be higher
than the drug level after the first dose. But how much higher? In order to answer
these questions we must now specify more rigorously a rational dosage schedule that

can be applicable to all drugs, regardless of their rates of elimination. We begin by determining the *dosing interval t**. This is dependent upon the amount of fluctuation that is tolerable once the steady-state has been established. For illustrative purposes let us limit the range of fluctuation to 10% of the EDC, a reasonable figure for many drugs. This means that t^* must be equal to the time in which one-tenth of the drug amount will be eliminated. Reference to Figure 4-7 reveals that for $f = 0.1$, $k_e t = 0.1$, and so $t^* = 0.1/k_e$. Also, since $t_{1/2} = 0.693/k_e$, it follows that t^* is almost exactly one-seventh of the elimination half-time, 0.1/0.693. Now the maintenance dose rate is given by M/t^*, where M is the single dose; and thus, as shown on p. 319,

$$\frac{M}{t^*} = (\text{EDC})V_d k_e$$

$$M = (\text{EDC})V_d k_e t^* = (\text{EDC})\frac{V_d}{10}$$

This means that if no priming dosage is employed, but the maintenance dosage is used from the start, then the plateau level ultimately established will be ten times that attained during the first dosing interval. Actually somewhat more than 10-fold, because some of the first dose will have been eliminated before all of it is absorbed. For oral or parenteral sustained-release medication, the "single dose" will mean the amount of drug that is absorbed in the interval t^*, even though the nominal dosing interval may be longer.

On this dosage schedule we may also estimate, from Figure 4-7, how many doses will be required to attain 90% of the EDC without priming dosage. For $f = 0.9$, we find $k_e t = 2.3$, $t = 2.3/k_e$. But, as shown above, $1/k_e = 10t^*$; therefore $t = 23t^*$, and 24 doses will be required. If priming dosage is to be used, then, of course, the priming doses have to furnish the total amount of drug needed in the body at the EDC, i.e., $(\text{EDC})V_d$. Therefore, in the present example, the total drug given as priming doses will have to be at least 10 times the maintenance dose. (*At least*, because unless the whole priming dosage is given intravenously, some will be eliminated in each dosing interval.)

It is interesting to examine the customary dosage schedules for drugs in common use to see whether or not they conform to these rational principles; and if not, to consider why not. Clinical experience alone has served to shape a very suitable dosage schedule for the digitalis glycosides. Digoxin is the most widely used drug of this family. Here $k_e = 0.50$, one-third of the amount present is eliminated each day, and $t_{1/2} = 1.4$ days.[21] As shown above, if the fluctuation is to be held within 10% of the EDC, the rational dosing interval t^* will be $0.1/k_e$, which is equal to 5 hr. Also, as shown above, 24 doses would be required (5 days) to attain 90% of the EDC, if priming dosage were not used. A typical procedure for rapid digitalization with digoxin in a normal 70 kg man employs 1.0 mg i.v. initially, for priming. Then a maintenance dose of 0.25–0.50 mg is given. In practice, this can be given as a single daily dose, rather than dividing it, i.e., greater fluctuation of the plasma level can be tolerated than the 10% assumed above.

Now let us consider a hypothetical drug that is eliminated primarily by glomerular filtration, without extensive tissue binding. Here (cf. Table 2-19), if the drug is distributed in body water, $k_e = (0.13 \text{ liter} \cdot \text{min}^{-1})/41 \text{ liters} = 0.0032 \text{ min}^{-1}$. Applying the same criteria as before, that fluctuation is to be held to 10% of the EDC, we find $t^* = 0.1/0.0032 = 31$ min. Now as a matter of fact, such a drug would not be given parenterally every 1/2 hr, but more likely every 4 hr. Thus, as in the previous example, a far greater degree of fluctuation is tolerated for the sake of convenience, a dosing interval shorter than several hours for parenteral administration being regarded as impractical. This means either that large fluctuations are tolerable because the EDC can safely be exceeded by a large amount, or that the EDC is simply not maintained continuously and some of the therapeutic effect is sacrificed. Such a drug could, however, be given orally or in a sustained-release form parenterally, if the absorption could be smoothed out over several dosing intervals. Thus, the nominal dose interval might be 4 hr, and the nominal dose would contain eight times as much medication as was required in each 30 min dosing interval; then if the total administered dose were absorbed evenly over the whole 4 hr, the desired dose rate would be achieved.

There is a limit to the usefulness of periodic dosing. When k_e becomes much larger than 0.003 min^{-1} (e.g., when the drug is rapidly metabolized), then no dosing interval is practical and the method of constant infusion must be adopted. A good example is the administration of the polypeptide hormone oxytocin to induce labor at term; this drug is destroyed by a peptidase in the blood. Another example is succinylcholine, a neuromuscular blocking agent used in anesthesia. This drug is hydrolyzed rapidly by plasma and liver cholinesterases. Its elimination rate in vivo can be estimated from the increment in duration of effect that is produced by logarithmic dose increments. Thus, for example, in a large number of patients[22] an intravenous dose of 1000 mg caused apnea by paralyzing the muscles of respiration for 17.8 min on the average. A dose of 500 mg caused apnea for only 11.9 min. The difference, 5.9 min, represents the time required for 1000 mg to be decreased by metabolism to only 500 mg, i.e., it is the biologic half-life. Then $k_e = 0.12$ min^{-1}, a much faster rate of elimination than even renal secretory mechanisms could accomplish. Drugs are metabolized at widely varying rates, some even faster than succinylcholine. In all such cases the EDC will be established very soon after starting a constant infusion and can be maintained readily, and the drug effect will disappear within minutes after discontinuing the infusion. Complete elimination of fluctuation and excellent control are the two important advantages gained by the constant infusion of drugs with high k_e values.

Drug Accumulation and Toxicity

The plateau principle also explains why cumulative toxicity sometimes occurs. If a drug's elimination rate is slow, and one attempts nevertheless to achieve a therapeutic effect with a constant dosage schedule (i.e., without priming doses), toxicity is the likely outcome. The reason for this is that if one seeks to obtain the therapeutic action quickly, and the dose rate is chosen to give that result, then the eventual steady-state will greatly exceed the EDC. Let us suppose, for the sake of argument, that a dose rate will be chosen that suffices to attain one-half the EDC in some convenient time t_1, less than the drug's biologic half-life $t_{1/2}$. One-half the eventual plateau will be reached in $t_{1/2}$ if the same constant dose rate is continued. The question is, how much higher than the EDC will the eventual steady-state plateau be? Figure 4-7 provides the answer. At $t_{1/2}$, $kt = 0.693$. We can find the point on the horizontal scale corresponding to kt_1, since we know what fraction t_1 is of $t_{1/2}$; and thus we can determine the value of f at this point. We know that the actual drug level corresponding to this f is one-half the EDC. So $2f$ corresponds to the EDC, and the excessive drug level eventually established will be $1/2f$ times the EDC.

To illustrate, suppose a drug with a half-life of 5 days is given at a dose rate that gives one-half the EDC in 16 hr (0.67 days). Then $kt_1 = (0.693/5)(0.67) = 0.0929$; and from Figure 4-7, $f = 0.09$. Therefore the level reached at this dose rate in 16 hr is only 0.09 of the eventual plateau, which will be EDC/0.18, or 6 times the EDC. The half-time of cumulation to this probably toxic level will, of course, be 5 days.

A very good example of cumulative toxicity with repeated drug administration is seen with bromide ion in man. Bromide used to be relied upon heavily in the chronic treatment of epilepsy, and it was also used as a mild sedative. It is still found in sedative preparations sold across the counter to the general public. The EDC for this drug is about 12 meq liter^{-1}. Psychotic symptoms and neurological signs occur at concentrations above 20 meq liter^{-1}. The bromide ion is distributed in approximately the same volume as the chloride ion, a volume somewhat greater than that of the extracellular fluid, or about 15 liters in the average man. It is handled at the kidneys in much the same way as chloride—filtered at the glomeruli and largely reabsorbed in the tubules. Bromide is actually reabsorbed somewhat more efficiently than chloride; the chloride clearance is about 1.2 liters daily, the bromide clearance about 0.9 liters daily.[23] From the clearance and the volume of distribution we find $k_e = 0.9/15 = 0.06$ day^{-1}; thus, half-life $= 0.693/0.06 = 12$ days. An experimental investigation using radioactive ^{82}Br in ten human subjects and measuring plasma levels twice daily gave exactly this theoretical value for the half-life.[24]

Two conclusions may be drawn from k_e and the half-life. The half-time for achieving the steady-state on a constant daily dosage of bromide will be 12 days. And the steady-state level will be about 1/0.06 (or about 16) times the level established on the first day. To use the drug properly, one would compute the maintenance dosage as follows:

$$EDC = 12 \text{ meq liter}^{-1}$$
$$V_d = 15 \text{ liters}$$
$$\text{required amount in body at EDC} = 12 \times 15 = 180 \text{ meq}$$

The maintenance dosage is designated by Q, and

$$Q = k_e(EDC)V_d$$
$$Q = 0.06 \times 180 = 11 \text{ meq} \cdot \text{day}^{-1} \text{ or about } 0.9 \text{ g} \cdot \text{day}^{-1}$$

This dose could be given daily for an indefinite period without harm, but it will require 12 days to attain half the EDC, and 40 days (3.3 times the half-time) to achieve 90% of the EDC. Alternatively, the required 180 meq (15 g) could be given within the first few days as a priming dose to establish the EDC, followed by the maintenance dosage thereafter. The reason why toxicity develops so frequently and so insidiously with this drug is that sufficient dosage to produce any sedation at all within a day or two must necessarily be higher than the maintenance dose rate, and so it will inevitably, if continued, produce plasma bromide levels much higher than the EDC.

The bromide half-life can be shortened to 3 or 4 days by chloride administration at about 200 meq day^{-1} in excess of normal intake. The reason for this is simply that chloride and bromide are treated very much alike at the renal tubules. Increasing the chloride level in the plasma and glomerular filtrate leads to a diminution in the fraction of (chloride + bromide) that is reabsorbed, and thus to an increased bromide clearance.[25]

For the same reasons, cumulative toxicity may develop insidiously with various substances that are not employed therapeutically but to which people may be exposed chronically. Often such poisons are bound tightly at specialized sites in the body. This accumulation in vulnerable tissues causes toxic manifestations, and the low elimination rate associated with extensive binding is responsible for the slow time course of the accumulation. Poisoning by heavy metals follows this pattern. Lead, for example, is present in the urban environment as a result of the combustion of leaded gasoline, and city dwellers breathe it constantly. Because lead is stored in many tissues and deposited in bones, it has a very long half-life in the body. When a human subject was given 2 mg per day of a soluble lead salt, the blood concentration of lead increased from 0.29 μg ml^{-1} to 0.72 μg ml^{-1} with a half-time of about two months.[26] The blood level then remained fairly constant for two years during which the daily intake was maintained. Despite the steady state in the blood and body fluids, a continuous accumulation went on during the whole period of the experiment, as indicated by a persistent small discrepancy between daily intake and daily output (positive lead balance). When the daily dose was discontinued after two years, the blood level fell with a half-time of two months, but an elevated urine output persisted for much longer. Clearly we are dealing here with complex kinetics. Tissue binding and deposition in bone continue after the fluid compartments are at a steady state, and loss of lead from its sites of very light binding or deposition continues after the body fluids have nearly eliminated their lead (cf. p. 351 for analogous kinetics concerning the elimination of anesthetic gases). The symptoms of lead poisoning are, initially at least, rather vague; irritability and other mood changes predominate in the early stages, frank psychosis and encephalopathy later. The long biologic half-life results in so slow a buildup of toxic levels in the body that no connection may seem evident between the beginning of exposure to a chronically noxious environment and the development and progression of the symptoms of lead poisoning.

The kidney shows a high affinity for the organic mercurial diuretics. There is good correlation between the renal content of these drugs and the magnitude of diuretic response. Excessive binding, however, leads to typical mercuric ion toxicity, characterized primarily by impaired renal tubular function and ultimately by damage to tubule structure as well. Studies with mercurial diuretics containing ^{203}Hg have shown that after distribution is complete, the concentration in kidney is about 100 times that in plasma.[27] The mercury in the kidney is for the most part bound very tightly to sulfhydryl groups. Bismuth compounds also interact strongly with −SH groups in the kidney and cause toxic effects there; but arsenicals, which also form strong bonds with −SH, deposit largely in liver and skin, causing toxicity in those tissues. The reasons for such tissue-specific differences in binding and accumulation are unknown.

An important site of cumulative storage and toxicity is the widely distributed reticuloendothelial system, which takes up colloidal substances of many kinds. Thorium dioxide was formerly given as a colloidal solution intravenously; its opacity to x rays made it useful for roentgenographic visualization of the liver, spleen, and blood vessels. However, it is bound so tightly in the reticuloendothelial cells that its excretion is extremely slow. Since thorium is a radioisotope with a very long radioactive half-life, its clinical use has now been abandoned, for the hazards of tissue destruction and of radiation-induced carcinogenesis are increased greatly by the long biologic half-life.

Somewhat similar hazards of cumulative toxicity involving a combination of radioactivity and long biologic half-life are presented by the fallout of debris from nuclear explosions. For example, ^{90}Sr is handled like calcium by the body; it is deposited in bone, and only a minute fraction of the total is excreted daily (cf. p. 415). Therefore, with constant exposure, there is a slow buildup of the body burden. Once the element is stored in the bones, its radioactive decay subjects the erythroblastic tissues and the bone cells to continuous bombardment. Another fallout product of importance is ^{131}I, found widely in milk from cows that have grazed on lands contaminated with fallout debris. This element is concentrated in the thyroid gland by an active transport mechanism and is there incorporated into thyroid hormone. The uptake and incorporation are responsible for the long biologic half-life of iodine, and again the combination of radioactivity, accumulation, and tissue storage intensifies the risk of serious toxicity. For these reasons the potential hazard in the use of ^{131}I for the diagnosis and treatment of thyroid disease is still a matter of controversy among clinicians. Extreme hazards, for similar reasons, are presented by ^{14}C and ^3H in chemical forms that permit their incorporation into nucleic acids. A molecule of DNA containing ^{14}C atoms may persist without turnover throughout a person's life, while the radioactivity of this isotope barely diminishes in a human lifetime. If the DNA in question is contained in the germinal cells, mutations resulting from the radioactive distintegrations will present a threat to that person's progeny. Radioactive carbon or tritium present in drugs, intermediate metabolites, or even proteins are far less hazardous because of the relatively short biologic half-lives, in contrast to DNA.

Slow accumulation of drugs and poisons is also seen in the fat depots of the body. The lipid-soluble insecticide DDT has been found regularly in human fat at autopsy, even in people having no known direct contact with it. This is typical of the environmental contamination that affects everyone in cases where continuous exposure can cause slow accumulation over a period of years. Likewise, estrogenic compounds used to promote weight gain in beef cattle have been found in human fat depots at autopsy.

Kinetics of Changes in Enzyme Levels

As pointed out in Chapter 3, the enzyme content of an animal tissue is maintained at its normal level by equal rates of enzyme synthesis and enzyme degradation. A drug may increase this steady-state amount of enzyme by speeding its production or slowing its breakdown. Continuous protein synthesis is essential for both of these mechanisms. Therefore, if an enzyme "induction" is abolished by blocking protein synthesis, it cannot be concluded that increased synthesis rather than stabilization was responsible (although activation of existing enzyme can be ruled out as the mechanism of drug action). The "induction" of tryptophan pyrrolase by its substrate, for example, is prevented by puromycin, ethionine, and other inhibitors of protein synthesis; but it is now clear that tryptophan stabilizes the enzyme rather than increasing its rate of synthesis.[28]

The time course of a shift from one steady-state level of enzyme to another is given by the plateau principle; its half-time is simply the turnover half-time (half-life) of the enzyme. Consequently, if an enzyme is to respond quickly to regulatory influences, it must be degraded rapidly. The more rapidly degraded it is. the more rapidly can its level change in response to changes in either the synthesis rate or the degradation rate.[29]

Much confusion has resulted from failure to recognize this application of the plateau principle. Consider enzymes A and B, both subject to regulation by steroid hormones. Enzyme A is rapidly degraded, B is quite stable. Suppose that both rates of synthesis are increased 5-fold by hormone treatment. Then both enzyme activities will also have increased 5-fold when the new steady-state is reached, since (p. 312)

$$X' = \frac{k_{in}}{k_{out}}$$

and we have increased k_n by a factor of 5 in both cases. But the rates of increase in enzyme activity will be very different for A and for B. One day after hormone administration is begun, A may already have increased nearly 5-fold, whereas B may have changed but little. If the enzyme determinations are performed at this time, therefore, the false conclusion may be drawn that steroid hormones have a much greater effect upon the synthesis of A than upon the synthesis of B. One should always refrain from drawing negative conclusions unless sufficient data are available to be certain that the shift from one steady-state to another has been completed.

If a drug that causes increase or decrease in the steady-state level of an enzyme is given as a single injection, interpretation is usually impossible, because there is no way to assess whether or not new steady-states have been reached. Figure 4-12 presents

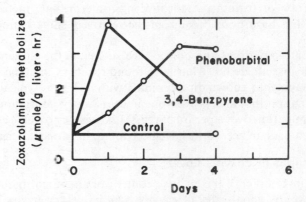

FIGURE 4-12. Stimulation of zoxazolamine metabolism by benzpyrene and phenobarbital. *Weanling rats were injected once with 3,4-benzpyrene (25 mg kg^{-1}) or with phenobarbital (33 mg kg^{-1}) twice daily for the duration of the experiment. Zoxazolamine metabolism by liver was determined in vitro at the times shown. (From Conney and Burns, Figure 1.[30])*

an illustrative example. The capacity of rat liver to metabolize zoxazolamine was followed after injections of 3,4-benzpyrene or phenobarbital. The rats that received benzpyrene had a single injection, but those that were given phenobarbital had two injections daily for the duration of the experiment. Evidently, the enzyme activity was stimulated by phenobarbital to an increase of about 4-fold over the starting level, and a new plateau was reached. The half-time of this shift was about 40 hr, whence it may be concluded that in the presence of phenobarbital the half-time of enzyme degradation was 40 hr. There is no way to decide, from these data alone, whether phenobarbital increases the rate of enzyme synthesis or decreases the rate of enzyme degradation. One might also be tempted to conclude that benzpyrene stimulates the increase in enzyme activity faster than phenobarbital does, but that would not be justified on the basis of the limited data shown. Continuous administration of benzpyrene might have increased the activity to a much higher level, so the shift half-time could well be identical to that produced by phenobarbital.

The plateau principle can be used as a practical test to distinguish between increased enzyme synthesis and decreased enzyme breakdown as mechanisms underlying a drug-induced increase in enzyme level, assuming that enzyme activation has been ruled out.[31] The following preconditions must be established: The "inducing" drug must become fully effective quickly and must remain present continuously until the new steady-state enzyme level is clearly established; and the "inducing" action must cease quickly when drug administration is discontinued. Then the half-time of the initial shift is the degradation half-time of the enzyme in the presence of the drug. The half-time of return to the original steady-state after the drug is withdrawn is the degradation half-time of the enzyme in the absence of drug. If these two time courses are the same, the drug did not stabilize the enzyme but must have acted by increasing the rate of enzyme synthesis. If the rise is slower than the fall, the drug must have acted, at least in part, by stabilizing the enzyme. The quantitative contributions of the two mechanisms may be estimated from the relationship between the initial and elevated enzyme levels, E'_1 and E'_2, respectively, as follows:

$$\frac{E'_2}{E'_1} = \frac{Q_2}{Q_1} \cdot \frac{k_1}{k_2}$$

where Q_1 and Q_2 are the respective rates of enzyme synthesis (analogous to k_{in}, p. 311), and k_1 and k_2 are the degradation rate constants in the absence and presence of the drug, respectively.

The plateau principle has been applied recently in the manner described above to the problem of analyzing the mechanism whereby continuous administration of phenobarbital increases the amount of liver microsomal barbiturate-oxidizing enzyme.[32] Phenobarbital was administered daily to rats in dosage sufficient to produce a maximal and sustained shift of the enzyme level. Then the drug was withdrawn and the enzyme level was permitted to return to the original level. The half-time of the shift up was 2.2 days, that of the shift down was 2.6 days. Thus, the enzyme turnover was essentially unaffected by the drug; the main cause of the increase in enzyme level was therefore increased rate of synthesis.

A special case of importance in pharmacology would be the stabilization of an enzyme by its inhibitor, leading to expansion of the total enzyme level at the steady-state without any change in the rate of enzyme synthesis. Stated more generally, if the interaction between a drug and its receptor stabilizes that receptor against a normal process of turnover, there will be a compensatory expansion of the steady-state level of receptor molecules. The possible relationship of such a process to drug tolerance and physical dependence is described in Chapter 9.

The quantitative description of enzyme expansion by inhibitor interaction is as follows:

Let X be the inhibitor concentration
E the free enzyme concentration
EX the concentration of inhibited enzyme
E_T the total enzyme concentration ($= E + EX$)
i the fractional inhibition ($= EX/E_T$)

and assume that the reaction of inhibitor with enzyme is very rapid relative to the rate of enzyme degradation.

In the absence of inhibitor,

$$E'_1 = E'_T = \frac{Q_1}{k_E}$$

as already shown, where k_E is the rate constant of degradation of free enzyme. The rate of change in total enzyme after introduction of inhibitor is given by

$$\frac{dE_T}{dt} = Q_1 - k_E E - k_{EX}(EX)$$

where k_{EX} is the rate constant of degradation of EX.

Then substituting $E = (1 - i) \cdot E_T$ and $EX = i \cdot E_T$,

$$\frac{dE_T}{dt} = Q_1 - k_E \left\{ 1 - \left[1 - \frac{k_{EX}}{k_E} \right] \cdot i \right\} E_T$$

At the steady-state,

$$E'_{T_2} = \frac{Q_1}{k_E \{ 1 - [1 - (k_{EX}/k_E)] \cdot i \}}$$

For the factor of change in *total* enzyme,

$$\frac{E'_{T_2}}{E'_{T_1}} = \frac{1}{1 - [1 - (k_{EX}/k_E)] \cdot i}$$

For the factor of change in *free* enzyme, substituting for E'_{T_2} its equivalent $E'_2/(1 - i)$,

$$\frac{E'_2}{E'_1} = \frac{1}{1 + (k_{EX}/k_E)[i/(1 - i)]}$$

Now if the stabilization by inhibitor is considerable, so that k_{EX}/k_E is very small, then the equation for total enzyme becomes, approximately,

$$\frac{E'_{T_2}}{E'_{T_1}} = \frac{1}{1 - i}$$

and the equation for free enzyme becomes, approximately,

$$\frac{E'_2}{E'_1} = 1$$

In other words, the free enzyme returns nearly to its original steady-state level in the presence of the inhibitor, but the total enzyme at the new steady-state is expanded to a level determined by the fractional inhibition. If, at the other extreme, the stabilization by inhibitor is insignificant (k_{EX} nearly equal to k_E), then the enzyme is simply inhibited and not expanded:

$$\frac{E'_{T_2}}{E'_{T_1}} = 1, \quad \frac{E'_2}{E'_1} = 1 - i$$

For intermediate degrees of stabilization the steady-state level of total enzyme will increase, and at the same time that of free enzyme will decrease.

FIRST-ORDER ABSORPTION, FIRST-ORDER ELIMINATION: KINETICS OF DRUG LEVELS AFTER SINGLE DOSES

We have examined the kinetics of elimination after a drug is introduced intravenously, and the time course of attaining a plateau when a drug is administered at a constant rate. We considered the constant rate to be achieved either rigorously, by a constant infusion, or approximately, by the repetition of a dose at regular intervals. In the latter case we assumed that relative to the whole time course under consideration no serious error would be introduced by ignoring fluctuations due to rapid absorption just after drug administration and progressively slower absorption between doses. Now we shall examine the detailed kinetics of the rise and fall of drug plasma levels after single doses. As is usually found to be the case (cf. p. 302), we assume the absorption process to be first-order, and we again assume overall elimination to be first-order.

Let M_0 be the dose of a drug, i.e., the amount of drug placed at the site of administration at time zero, and let k_a be the rate constant of absorption. Then at any time t thereafter, the drug remaining at the site of administration is (cf. p. 302):

$$M = M_0 e^{-k_a t}$$

Now let X be the amount of drug that has been absorbed into the circulation and let k_e be the rate constant of elimination; then

$$\frac{dX}{dt} = k_a M - k_e X$$

and, substituting for M,

$$\frac{dX}{dt} + k_e X = k_a M_0 e^{-k_a t}$$

This linear first-order differential equation yields the following solution for the case $k_a \neq k_e$, as first shown many years ago in a classical theoretical study of this problem.[33]

$$X = \frac{k_a M_0}{(k_e - k_a)}[e^{-k_a t} - e^{-k_e t}]$$

And for the case $k_a = k_e$, the following equation is obtained:

$$X = k_e M_0 t\, e^{-k_e t}$$

These equations are derived as follows:

$$\frac{dX}{dt} = k_a M - k_e X$$

and

$$M = M_0 e^{-k_a t}$$

Equation

$$\frac{dX}{dt} + k_e X = k_a M_0 e^{-k_a t}$$

is of the form

$$Y' + P(t)Y = Q(t)$$

Multiply by integrating factor $e^{dPdt} = e^{dk_e dt} = e^{k_e t}$, we obtain

$$\frac{d(e^{k_e t} X)}{dt} = e^{k_e t}\left[\frac{dX}{dt} + k_e X\right] = e^{k_e t} \cdot k_a M_0 e^{-k_a t}$$

Then we integrate both sides:

$$e^{k_e t} \cdot X = k_a M_0 \int e^{(k_e - k_a)t} \cdot dt$$

$$e^{k_e t} \cdot X = k_a M_0 \frac{e^{(k_e - k_a)t}}{(k_e - k_a)} + C$$

When $t = 0$, $X = 0$:

$$C = \frac{-k_a M_0}{(k_e - k_a)}$$

$$e^{k_e t} \cdot X = \frac{k_a M_0 \, e^{(k_e - k_a)t}}{(k_e - k_a)} - \frac{k_a M_0}{(k_e - k_a)}$$

$$X = \frac{k_a M_0}{(k_e - k_a)}[e^{-k_a t} - e^{-k_e t}]$$

and for the purpose of graphing, as in Figure 4-13,

$$\frac{X}{M_0} = \frac{1}{(k_e/k_a) - 1}[e^{-k_e t/(k_e/k_a)} - e^{-k_e t}]$$

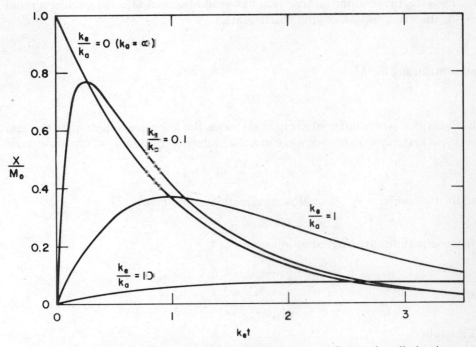

FIGURE 4-13. Kinetics of first-order absorption and first-order elimination. *This graph shows the amount of drug in the body (X) as fraction of total drug (M_0) placed at an absorption site at time zero. The family of curves is for different ratios of the rate constant of elimination (k_e) to the rate constant of absorption (k_a). The scale on the x axis includes k_e; to convert its values to actual time t, divide by k_e. See text for complete description.*

If $k_a = k_e$ then $\int e^{(k_e - k_a)t} \cdot dt = t$, and we proceed as follows from a point midway through the derivation:

$$e^{k_e t} \cdot X = k_a M_0 \int e^{(k_e - k_a)t} \cdot dt$$

Substituting $k_e = k_a$, we obtain

$$e^{k_e t} \cdot X = k_e M_0 t$$
$$X = k_e M_0 t \, e^{-k_e t}$$

Figure 4-13 presents a generalized plot of these equations. Certain normalizing procedures have been followed in order to make a single graph represent all possible relationships between dose administered, rate constant of absorption, and rate constant of elimination. The vertical scale shows X/M_0 rather than X; i.e., regardless of what the actual dose may be, we are following the fractional absorption of that dose into the body tissues from the site of administration. The above equations, showing that the time course of absorption is independent of the dose M_0, justify this procedure. The equations have been solved for various chosen values of the ratio of rate constants, k_e/k_a, and the time scale has consequently been generalized to include one of the rate constants.

For any given drug the transformed scale of time, although not reading directly in minutes, is nevertheless proportional to actual time. Some important conclusions about the kinetics of drug levels in the body may be drawn from inspection of this diagram. The curve for $k_a = \infty$ depicts the limiting case of intravenous injection, "absorption" being instantaneous. This shows the usual exponential decay of the drug level. As absorption becomes slower (k_a smaller) relative to elimination, curves are obtained that rise to a peak and then fall again. The slower the absorption relative to elimination, the later is the peak attained and the lower is its actual value.

In order to transform the time scale to real time, it is only necessary to divide the values by the elimination rate constant k_e. An example will serve to illustrate how Figure 4-13 can be used to predict real behavior of drugs. Suppose a drug is absorbed from a subcutaneous depot at a rate of 0.1 min^{-1} and eliminated by excretion and metabolism at a rate of 0.01 min^{-1}. Then $k_e/k_a = 0.1$ and every value on the $k_e t$ scale has to be divided by 0.01 (so that the scale will read 100, 200, 300 min, etc.). We see that the peak circulating drug level will be attained in about 25 min and at that time about 75% of the dose will be distributed into whatever its V_d may be.

Differentiation of the equations yields expressions for the time at which the maximum drug level is attained. For $k_a \neq k_e$,

$$t_{max} = \frac{2.30}{k_a - k_e} \log \frac{k_a}{k_e}$$

and for $k_a = k_e$,

$$t_{max} = \frac{1}{k_e}$$

These equations show that the time in which the maximum drug level is achieved is the same regardless of what dose is administered. Substitution of the values of t_{max} into the original equations yield solutions for the maximum amount of drug in the body. For $k_a \neq k_e$, the peak level is given by

$$\frac{X_{max}}{M_0} = \left[\frac{k_a}{k_e}\right]^{k_e/(k_e - k_a)}$$

and for $k_a = k_e$

$$\frac{X_{max}}{M_0} = 0.368$$

i.e., when the rate constants for absorption and elimination are equal, the peak level in the body is 37% of the dose.

These relationships are derived as follows: For $k_a \neq k_e$,

$$\frac{X}{M_0} = \frac{k_a}{(k_e - k_a)}[e^{-k_a t} - e^{-k_e t}]$$

$$t_{max} = \frac{1}{(k_a - k_e)}\ln\frac{k_a}{k_e}$$

Multiplying and dividing by $e^{-k_e t}$, we obtain

$$\frac{X_{max}}{M_0} = \frac{k_a}{(k_e - k_a)}e^{-k_e t_{max}}[e^{-(k_a - k_e)t_{max}} - 1]$$

$$= \frac{k_a}{(k_e - k_a)}e^{-[k_e/(k_a - k_e)]\ln(k_a/k_e)}[e^{-[(k_a - k_e)/(k_a - k_e)]\ln(k_a/k_e)} - 1]$$

$$= \frac{k_a}{(k_e - k_a)}\left[\frac{k_a}{k_e}\right]^{-k_e/(k_a - k_e)}\left[\frac{k_e}{k_a} - 1\right]$$

$$= \left[\frac{k_a}{k_e}\right]^{k_e/(k_e - k_a)}$$

For $k_a = k_e$,

$$\frac{X}{M_0} = k_e t\, e^{-k_e t}$$

$$t_{max} = \frac{1}{k_e}$$

$$\frac{X_{max}}{M_0} = k_e 1/k_e\, e^{-k_e(1/k_e)}$$

$$= e^{-1} = 0.368$$

These basic equations, transformed in various ways, have been used by several investigators to develop rational approaches to dosage regimens, or to examine how closely observation and theory conform in experimental animals or man.[34-37] An illustration of unusual interest concerns the precursor-product relationship for drugs that are metabolized. If a precursor W is transformed metabolically to a product X, which in turn is further transformed or excreted, then we have

$$W \rightarrow X \rightarrow \text{elimination}$$

with a rate constant $k_{W \rightarrow X}$ for the first-order transformation reaction, and a rate constant k_e for the first-order elimination of X. Then the kinetics of the rise and fall of

X are formally identical to those of sequential first-order absorption and first-order elimination. The same equations apply, and the same characteristic family of curves will be found as in Figure 4-13. This is illustrated in Figure 4-14 for anisole (methoxy-benzene) transformed to its hydroxylation product p-methoxyphenol, in the rabbit. It can be seen that administration of the precursor will have the same effect as though the product itself had been given by a slow-absorption technique. The curve labeled "Precursor administered" is determined by the relative rate constants, 0.11 hr^{-1} for the hydroxylation and 0.54 hr^{-1} for the elimination (here actually a sulfate conjugation). The curve is simply that predicted by Figure 4-13 for $k_e/k_a = 5$, and time in hours is $k_e t/0.54$.

Ideally, every drug should be given in such a way as to establish its EDC very rapidly and then maintain it with as little fluctuation as possible. Rapid establishment of the

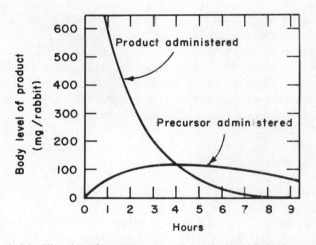

FIGURE 4-14. Kinetics of precursor-product relationship in drug metabolism. *Theoretical diagram of the body level of a product, p-methoxyphenol, in the rabbit, when its precursor, anisole, is administered, and when it is administered itself in equimolar amount. For the O-methylation, k = 0.11 hr^{-1}. Subsequent conjugation with sulfate proceeds with k = 0.54 hr^{-1}. (From Bray et al., Figure 1.[38])*

EDC, as we have seen, requires priming dosage if the rate constant of elimination is low. Practically speaking, if the drug level rises quickly and falls quickly, fluctuation can only be smoothed by repeating the dose very frequently; and this may be considered too inconvenient. Patients do not welcome parenteral administration more often than every few hours; and even oral medication is unlikely to be taken reliably more often than that, especially by ambulatory patients. Thus, if a considerable "overshoot" above the EDC is tolerable, fluctuations may be preferred to an inconvenient dose schedule. To what extent it may be safe to exceed the EDC periodically cannot be stated as a general rule; this will depend upon the range between EDC and toxic levels for each particular drug. It is absurd, therefore, to administer all drugs on arbitrary fixed schedules (e.g., with each meal, every 4 hr, etc.). Appropriate dosage schedules need to be developed for each drug, determined by its k_a, its k_e, its EDC, and the level at which its toxic effects manifest themselves. If it is important to obtain a drug's maximum benefit, then it may also be important to override considerations of convenience and to administer doses as often as necessary to maintain an effective drug level and at the same time minimize fluctuations.

KINETICS OF THE UPTAKE AND DISTRIBUTION OF DRUGS ADMINISTERED BY INHALATION

Introduction

The administration of gases, especially anesthetic gases, is characterized by two interesting new features, as compared with the drugs discussed earlier in this chapter. First, the rate of entry is controlled by a cyclic process, the respiration, so that the drug is presented for absorption at the alveoli in an interrupted fashion, about 20 times per minute. Second, many of these agents are not metabolized or excreted to any significant extent by the usual routes. They are eliminated almost entirely at the lungs, the site of their absorption. Thus, the eventual plateau at the "steady-state" is really an equilibrium. The net transfer rate from alveoli to blood is rapid at first, then progressively slower as the blood concentration builds up, until finally, at the plateau blood level, the rate of transfer from blood to alveoli equals the rate of transfer from alveoli to blood.

At equilibrium, the concentration in blood (x_b') is related to the concentration in alveolar air (x_a') by the expression

$$\frac{x_b'}{x_a'} = S,$$

where S is simply the solubility of the gas in blood. The solubility of a gas in a fluid is defined as the ratio of the concentration of dissolved gas to the concentration in the gas phase, at equilibrium. This solubility is also known as the Ostwald coefficient. The definition of solubility is often confusing to the student, but it should be remembered that, unlike solids, gases distribute themselves between a fluid and gas phase so that the amount dissolved increases without limit (theoretically, at least) as the concentration in the gas phase is increased. The only reasonable way to define solubility is, therefore, to relate the amount of gas dissolved in a given volume of fluid to the gas phase concentration required to hold it in solution.

Anesthetic gases vary widely in their solubilities, as shown in Table 4-2. Since the solubility is a ratio of concentrations, it does not matter in what units these are expressed provided they are the same for both phases. The solubility equation $x_b' = S(x_a)$ is simply another way of stating Henry's law, which relates the concentration of dissolved gas to the partial pressure in the gas phase at equilibrium. The transformation of gas concentration to partial pressure is accomplished most simply by means of the gas law,

$$pV = nRT$$

If the concentration is expressed as moles per liter (n/V), and the partial pressure p is to be obtained in mm Hg, then the gas constant R has the value 62, the temperature T being in absolute degrees.

TABLE 4-2. Properties of volatile anesthetics.
The data of this table are approximate; they are assembled from several sources, and obtained by methods of differing reliability. The expression III_{2-3} means stage III, plane 2–3 anesthesia, a typical depth for abdominal surgery. Most of the data are summarized in Larson et al.[39,40]

	Molecular weight	(S) Solubility in blood at 38°	(x'_b) mM blood at III_{2-3}	(x'_a) mM alveolar air at III_{2-3}	(p) mm Hg at III_{2-3}	$mg\ ml^{-1}$ blood at III_{2-3}	(S_L) Oil/water partition co-efficient
(Ethanol)	46	1100	88	0.080	1.5	4.0	—
Ether	74	15	20	1.3	25	1.5	3.2
Chloroform	119	7.3	1.8	0.25	4.8	0.21	100
Ethyl chloride	64	2.5	4.6	1.8	35	0.29	—
Halothane	197	2.3	1.0	0.43	8.3	0.21	220
Vinyl ether	70	1.5	2.6	1.7	33	0.18	41
Acetylene	26	0.82	22	27	520	0.57	—
Cyclopropane	42	0.47	4.1	8.7	170	0.17	34
Nitrous oxide	44	0.47	29	61	1200	1.3	3.2
Propylene	42	0.22	4.8	22	420	0.20	—
Ethylene	28	0.14	5.7	41	790	0.16	14

Example: What is the partial pressure exerted by a gas at 38° (311° Abs.) whose concentration is 8.70 millimoles liter^{-1}?

$$p = (n/V)RT = (8.7 \times 10^{-3})(62)(311) = 168 \text{ mm Hg}$$

For present purposes we will not distinguish between vapors and gases. Any substance in the gaseous state obeys the gas laws sufficiently well, regardless of whether its boiling point is above or below room temperature. The principal difference arises from the fact that while the concentration of a gas in the inspired air can be varied at will up to 100%, the maximum concentration of a vapor is limited by its vapor pressure at ambient temperature. As this vapor pressure is by definition the partial pressure in equilibrium with the liquid, it follows that no higher partial pressure can exist, any tendency to further evaporation being balanced by re-entry of vapor molecules into the liquid phase. If a liquid is to be a useful volatile anesthetic, it must therefore be potent enough, or volatile enough, so that surgical anesthesia can be produced with a partial pressure (in the inspired air) below its vapor pressure at room temperature. Throughout this section, *surgical anesthesia* means stage III, plane 2–3 anesthesia, a suitable level for major surgery without adjuvant muscle relaxants. In actual practice it is common to use many different levels of anesthesia, supplemented by the use of preanesthetic medications, muscle relaxants, and pain-relieving drugs. The reader is referred to textbooks of anesthesiology for details.

Example: The vapor pressure of ether at 20° is 442 mm Hg. This is the maximum partial pressure of ether vapor that could be attained. But the partial pressure required to produce surgical anesthesia is only about 25 mm Hg. Establishing a sufficient alveolar ether concentration therefore presents no problem.

Equilibrium in Clinical Anesthesia

The various stages of anesthesia are associated with definite concentrations of each anesthetic agent in the brain and (provided equilibrium has been attained) with definite concentrations in the circulating blood. With a number of anesthetic agents the concentrations in blood and in whole brain have been found to be approximately equal. Because of the precise relationship between depth of anesthesia and blood anesthetic concentration, and because it is impractical to measure the anesthetic concentration in the brain, we shall concern ourselves with blood anesthetic concentration. We shall further limit the discussion by considering that particular blood concentration which, at equilibrium, will produce surgical anesthesia. For any given anesthetic agent there is one and only one such blood concentration, namely, the EDC (effective drug concentration, see p. 318). If the agent is very potent, this required blood concentration will be low; if not very potent, the required blood concentration will be high. Anesthetists sometimes think of potency in connection with the effective concentration in the alveolar air, but this is a very restricted meaning. Rigorously defined, potency refers to the effective molecular concentration of a drug at its site of action, and we use the word in this sense. Low or high, the EDC is determined by the physicochemical properties of the agent on the one hand and the behavior of the central nervous system on the other, both of which are beyond the control of the anesthetist.

At equilibrium there will be a predictable relationship between this concentration in blood (the EDC) and that in the alveolar air, a relationship defined by the solubility of the agent, already discussed above. Because the solubility of any agent in blood at body temperature is a fixed physical property, also beyond the control of the anesthetist, it follows that the concentration of anesthetic required in the alveolar air in order to just reach and then maintain surgical anesthesia is also absolutely fixed and beyond control. If a lower concentration is used, we shall not achieve surgical anesthesia when equilibrium is reached; if a higher concentration is employed, we shall exceed the safe levels of surgical anesthesia and cause respiratory paralysis. The situation is exactly the same as that described for dosage regimens in general, on p. 318.

When equilibrium has been reached, the partial pressure of anesthetic in the alveolar air will obviously be the same as that in the inspired air (for example, in the anesthetist's breathing bag). The concentration in the inspired air, in equilibrium with the EDC in blood, is called the *safe anesthetic gas concentration*. If the anesthetist employs this concentration from the start, then at equilibrium a safe depth of anesthesia will be reliably achieved, and there will be no danger of exceeding this depth. In most of the subsequent discussion we shall assume that the anesthetist makes use of the safe anesthetic concentration from the beginning of the anesthesia, even though for some agents (as we shall see) such a procedure would be impractical.

Example 1: The solubility of ether at 38° is 15. If the concentration in the alveolar air is kept constant at 1.3 mM, what will be the concentration in blood at equilibrium?

$$S = 15$$
$$x'_a = 1.3 \text{ m}M$$
$$x'_b = S(x'_a) = 15 \times 1.3 = 20 \text{ m}M$$

Example 2: At equilibrium, the concentration of chloroform is found to be 1.8 mM in blood (38°), with partial pressure 4.8 mm Hg in the inspired air (20°). What is the solubility of chloroform?

The partial pressure exerted by a gas in a mixture does not change with temperature, provided the sum of all the partial pressures remains the same (i.e., 760 mm Hg at sea level). Thus, $p = 4.8$ mm Hg also at 38° in alveolar air, and

$$\frac{n}{V} = \frac{p}{RT} = \frac{4.8}{62 \times 311} = 0.25 \, \text{m}M$$

$$S = x_b'/x_a' = \frac{1.8}{0.25} = 7.3$$

Example 3: At equilibrium, the concentration of cyclopropane in the inspired air (20°) is found to be 9.2 mM and its solubility is 0.47. What is the blood concentration?

$$p = (n/V)RT = (9.2 \times 10^{-3})(62)(293) = 167 \, \text{mm Hg}$$

In the alveoli, at 38°, this same partial pressure exists, but because of expansion with increased temperature, the concentration of all gases is lower than in the inspired air. Here,

$$\frac{n}{V} = \frac{p}{RT} = \frac{167}{(62)(311)} = 8.7 \, \text{m}M$$

or, more simply,

$$\frac{n}{V} = (9.2)\frac{293}{311} = 8.7 \, \text{m}M$$

whence

$$x_b' = S(x_a') = (0.47)(8.7) = 4.1 \, \text{m}M$$

Rate of Equilibration of Blood and Body Water

Equilibration at the Blood-Alveolar Membrane. Let us now consider the factors determining the rate at which the EDC is attained when the anesthetic in the inspired air is maintained at the safe anesthetic gas concentration from the start. As the gaseous anesthetics are all relatively small molecules, they diffuse very rapidly from the blood into all the tissues of the body, and as they are generally lipid soluble, they are able to cross cell membranes rapidly and distribute themselves in intracellular as well as extracellular fluid. Thus, for an average-sized man (70 kg) we shall have to consider the equilibration not of 6 liters of circulating blood but of 41 liters of total body water.

Gas in the alveoli equilibrates almost instantaneously with blood passing through the pulmonary capillary bed. This has been established by careful physiologic studies, most recently by the use of radioactive gases. Let us assume for the moment that it were possible by some kind of special pump to maintain the safe anesthetic concentration in the alveolar air, i.e., to replace continuously all anesthetic that passes over into the pulmonary blood. In that case, all the blood coming from the lungs would continuously carry an equilibrium concentration of anesthetic, namely, the EDC, which will be reached ultimately in all the body water. The entire cardiac output passes through the pulmonary capillary bed, so if the cardiac output is 5 liters min^{-1} and the body water is 41 liters, it follows, as a first approximation, that the total body water could be brought to equilibrium in about 8 min. Actually, this is an underestimate of the time, since the equilibration is asymptotic. As soon as blood returning to the lungs contains some anesthetic, blood leaving the lungs will begin to contribute less toward equilibration of the total body water, because the anesthetic brought to the lungs by blood will simply be carried away again, and the net transfer of anesthetic will be diminished by this amount.

The asymptotic nature of the equilibration process can perhaps best be understood in relation to the total amount of anesthetic needed to bring the body water to equilibrium. If the equilibrium concentration to be achieved is x'_b and the body water amounts to 41 liters, then $41x'_b$ is the amount of anesthetic that must be transferred from the alveoli into the blood in order to reach equilibrium. At the start, when no anesthetic is yet in the blood, the net transfer will be at the rate of $5x'_b$ min^{-1}, as stated above. But now suppose the concentration in the blood and body water has already reached $0.1x'_b$. This will be the concentration in blood arriving at the lungs, while the blood leaving the lungs will always contain the concentration x'_b. The net transfer rate at this point is therefore no longer than $5x'_b$ but $5(x'_b - 0.1x'_b)$, or $4.5x'_b$ min^{-1}. Obviously then, the approach to equilibrium will continue to slow down as greater fractions of equilibrium are achieved. Complete equilibrium is only achieved in an infinite time; we can only measure the attainment of a specified *fraction* of equilibrium. The correct estimate of the time required to attain 90% equilibration of body water under these hypothetical conditions is approximately 21 min instead of our rough estimate of 8 min. The derivation of equations describing this rather complex process is an interesting exercise in the application of mathematics to physiologic problems.[41-44]

Lung "Washout."   We assumed above that it was somehow possible to establish at once and then to maintain the safe anesthetic concentration in the alveoli. As a matter of fact, respiration is a cyclic process. The amount of anesthetic inhaled in the first breath will be diluted in a considerable lung volume containing no anesthetic whatsoever. The alveolar ventilation is about 0.3 liters. The total effective lung volume after normal inspiration is equal to this volume plus the functional residual capacity and end-expiratory volume, comprising, in all, some 2.8 liters.

Now suppose the inspired gas mixture contains x'_a, the alveolar concentration in equilibrium with the EDC (i.e., x'_b). Anesthetic taken into the lungs at the first breath $(0.3x'_a)$ is diluted immediately so that the alveolar concentration during the interrespiratory pause is only $(0.3/2.8)x'_a$ or $0.11x'_a$. Some of the alveolar anesthetic passes into the blood and is carried away, while the rest remains in the lungs to be added to the amount inhaled during the next breath. If very little passes into the blood at each breath, the alveolar concentration will quickly build up in stepwise fashion toward x'_a. But if nearly all the anesthetic in the alveoli passes into the blood at each breath, the alveolar concentration after the second, third, and subsequent breaths will not be appreciably greater than after the first breath.

In general, the repeated addition of air carrying anesthetic concentration x'_a to the total lung volume containing a lower concentration causes anesthetic to accumulate in the alveoli with each successive breath. Soon, however, each inspiration replaces exactly the amount of anesthetic that passed into the blood during the previous breath. When this state is reached, the alveolar concentration would have risen but little higher than $0.11x'_a$ in the case of an agent of very high S, since nearly $0.3x'_a$ passes into the blood during each breath, and $0.3x'_a$ is the most that can be replaced by a normal inspiration. But the steady-state alveolar concentration would be nearly x'_a in the case of an agent of very low S, where very little passes into the blood during each breath. The process whereby the alveolar anesthetic concentration reaches a steady-state is termed *lung "washout."* It is virtually complete within less than 2 min.

Agents of Very Low Solubility.   We have seen that with an agent of very low solubility the alveolar concentration at the end of the washout period is practically the same as that of the inspired air (namely, the safe anesthetic concentration x_a). This anesthetic will distribute itself instantaneously and continuously between alveoli and blood in accordance with its solubility. For example, the anesthetic in 1 ml of alveolar air will bring the same volume of blood to equilibrium without appreciable change in the alveolar concentration. As shown in Figure 4-15, an agent of solubility 0.1 will have

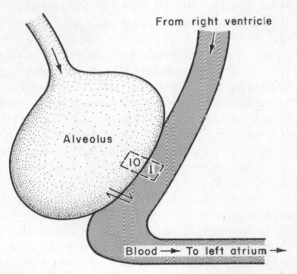

FIGURE 4-15. Diagram showing momentary equilibrium between equal volumes of blood and air at blood-alveolar membrane, for an anesthetic agent of solubility 0.1.

accomplished this when only 1/11 of the total anesthetic in the given volume of alveolar air has passed into an equal volume of blood.

The blood flowing through the lungs during each breath (respiratory rate 20 min^{-1}) is 1/20 of the cardiac output, or 0.25 liters. All this blood leaves the lungs in equilibrium with the alveolar concentration, which is practically x'_a. The blood, therefore, carries away a concentration $x_b = S(x'_a)$, or an amount equal to $(0.25)(S)(x'_a)$ per breath. For an agent of solubility 0.1, this would be $0.025x'_a$ per breath, or less than 1% of the total anesthetic in the lungs, an amount that can readily be replaced at the next inspiration.

Because the blood is already carrying all the anesthetic it can, increasing the respiratory rate or minute volume could not significantly increase the transfer of anesthetic into the blood and therefore could not shorten the equilibration time significantly.

On the other hand, increasing the cardiac output would markedly increase the rate of removal of anesthetic from the lungs. In fact, doubling the cardiac output would nearly double the rate of removal and thereby nearly halve the equilibration time. Thus, for agents of very low solubility, the cardiac output (and not the respiration) is the major physiologic factor limiting the rate of equilibration. At each breath only a small fraction of the anesthetic in the lungs is removed, and after 3 seconds even this is replenished at the next inspiration. The alveoli continuously contain nearly the safe anesthetic gas concentration, the arterial blood contains the corresponding x_b' (the EDC), and the situation is very much like the hypothetical one discussed earlier (p. 342), where 21 min was shown to be a reasonable estimate of the time required to bring the body water to nine-tenths of its equilibrium anesthetic concentration.

Agents of Very High Solubility.   We have already seen that with an agent of very high solubility so much is transferred to the blood during each breath that little if any remains in the alveoli just before the next inspiration (cf. Figure 4-15 as it would apply to an agent of solubility 10). The alveolar concentration established at the first inspiration $(0.11x_a')$ is re-established again and again (without appreciable increment) at every succeeding inspiration, and falls practically to zero before the next breath. The arterial anesthetic concentration closely reflects this fluctuating pattern, never exceeding $0.11x_b'$ initially and falling off nearly to zero during every breath. Naturally, the time required to equilibrate the body water with the inspired air will be very much longer than with low-solubility agents. Assuming that the lungs are wholly depleted at each breath, we have $0.3x_a' \times 20$, or $6x_a'$ entering the blood every minute. Since $S = 10$, this is equal to $0.6x_b'$ min^{-1}, and it would take 68 min (at the very least) to carry away from the lungs the $41x_b'$ needed to equilibrate the 41 liters of body water. This calculation ignores the asymptotic nature of the process and is therefore a considerable underestimate, as in the similar example given on p. 342.

The mean alveolar anesthetic concentration (and consequently the arterial concentration) begins to rise only as blood returning from the body tissues to the lungs carries more and more anesthetic. Slightly less is removed from the alveoli during each breath (for the reasons explained before), and the remainder gradually accumulates. With an agent of high solubility, the mean alveolar anesthetic concentration approaches that of the inspired air (x_a') at essentially the same rate as the venous blood approaches equilibrium.

Here, respiration is the principal factor that limits attainment of equilibrium. Because the blood is already removing virtually all anesthetic from the lungs, increasing the cardiac output could not materially shorten the equilibration time. But equilibration can be very substantially hastened by furnishing anesthetic to the alveoli more rapidly (i.e., by increasing the respiratory rate or depth). This is precisely what is accomplished by inhalation of CO_2, a procedure that is primarily useful in accelerating equilibration (and also de-equilibration) with agents of high solubility like ether and chloroform (Table 4-2).

The Transition Zone Between Low- and High-Solubility Behavior.   We have said a good deal about agents of "very low" and "very high" solubility. But what values of S are we justified in regarding as high or low in this connection? As S determines the relative roles of respiratory minute volume and cardiac output in limiting the equilibration rate, it follows that at an intermediate value of S these physiologic parameters will have equal importance. This critical solubility, which proves to be about

1.2, marks the center of a transition zone between the two types of extreme behavior described. Actually, this zone is fairly broad but as S becomes much smaller or much greater than 1.2, the behavior of the anesthetics will approach more closely that of the prototype low- and high-solubility agents examined in the foregoing discussion. It should be noted that the value $S = 1.2$ is arrived at on the basis of average physiologic data; namely, respiratory rate 20 min^{-1}, alveolar ventilation 0.3 liters, cardiac output 5 liters min^{-1}. A substantial change in any of these values will shift the transition zone toward higher or lower solubilities.

Figure 4-16 shows an arrangement of volatile and gaseous anesthetics according to solubility, on a scale indicating their behavior with respect to equilibration rate. As S increases, the equilibration time becomes longer, without limit. As S decreases,

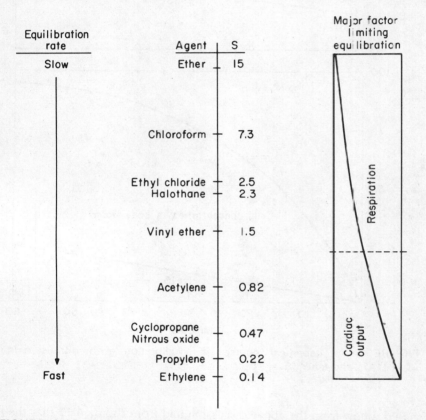

FIGURE 4-16. Relation of solubility S to equilibrium rate, showing relative limitation by respiration and cardiac output.

however, a minimum equilibration time is approached (approximately 21 min for 90% equilibration as shown earlier). Thus, agents of very low solubility do not differ materially among themselves in their rates of equilibration.

Figure 4-17 represents the calculated course of equilibration with two agents of different solubility. The change in alveolar anesthetic concentration is plotted in the upper half, the change in anesthetic concentration in body water (or venous blood) in the lower half.

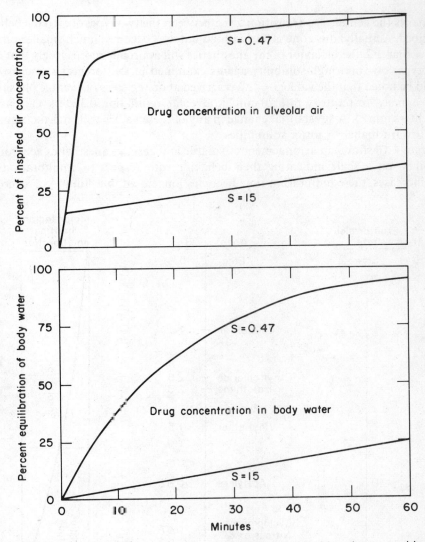

FIGURE 4-17. Theoretical course of equilibration with nitrous oxide ($S = 0.47$) and ether ($S = 15$).

It should follow from the above discussion and from Figure 4-17 that the rate of equilibration is independent of the concentration of the anesthetic agent. But at very high concentrations this is not so. Rather, the rate of approach of alveolar concentration to inspired concentration is faster, the higher the inspired concentration. This phenomenon is called the *concentration effect*.[45,46] The principle is apparent if one imagines a concentration of 100% of an anesthetic gas in the inspired air. Regardless of how much passes across the alveoli, the remaining concentration will still be 100%. And the gas drawn in to replace the volume of anesthetic agent that passes into the blood at each breath will also contain 100%. Thus, even with a high-solubility agent, the alveolar concentration will approach 100% very quickly. The concentration effect will be significant whenever the anesthetic agent comprises a significant fraction of the total inspired gas volume, as illustrated in Figure 4-18. Theoretical curves for nitrous oxide and for ether are given in Figure 4-19. As would be expected, the concentration effect is theoretically greatest for agents of high solubility. As a practical matter, however, only nitrous oxide ($S = 0.47$) is used at concentrations high enough to comprise a major fraction of the total gas volume.

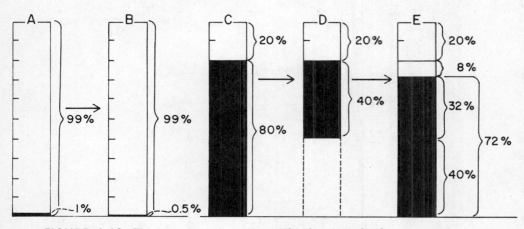

FIGURE 4-18. The concentration effect. *The change in alveolar concentration when one-half of a 1.0% concentration is taken up is shown at A and B. The decrease in concentration is proportional to the amount taken up. C, D, and E show the change when one-half of an 80% concentration is taken up. The reduction is to $40/(20 + 40) = 67\%$, which is not proportional to the amount taken up. When more gas is added at the same concentration, the final concentration (at E) is 72%. Were the reduction proportional to uptake, the final concentration would be 40%. (From Eger, Figure 1.[45])*

An interesting corollary of the concentration effect is the *second gas effect*. If an agent like halothane, used at low concentration, is present in a gas mixture with another agent like nitrous oxide at high concentration, the additional inflow of gas mixture to replace the absorbed nitrous oxide will also raise the alveolar concentration of halothane. This effect is small but significant, and it has been demonstrated in vivo.[47]

De-Equilibration.   If the anesthetic intake is abruptly stopped, after the EDC has been established, anesthetic begins to be eliminated from the blood into the lungs. The factors affecting de-equilibration of the body water are the same as those already considered in connection with equilibration. An agent of very low solubility can be eliminated almost as fast as the blood delivers it to the lungs. The elimination of an agent of very high solubility is limited by the respiratory rate and minute volume, only a small fraction being removed from the blood during a single passage. Obviously, CO_2 inhalation will be effective in hastening de-equilibration of high-S agents, but will be of no use for this purpose with low-S agents. The curves of de-equilibration are essentially inverted equilibration curves.

Potency and the Availability of Oxygen.   The potency of an anesthetic is inversely proportional to the EDC. Table 4-2 shows that potency varies widely, and quite independently of solubility. There is a relationship, which is the basis of the Meyer–Overton hypothesis (p. 173), between potency and *lipid solubility*. Anesthetics of

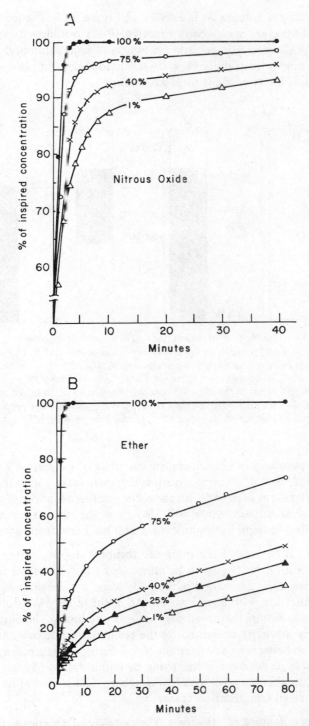

FIGURE 4-19. The concentration effect for nitrous oxide and ether. *Theoretical curves for approach of alveolar concentration to inspired concentration in man. (A) Nitrous oxide (S = 0.47). (B) Ether (S = 15). (From Eger, Figures 8-2 and 8-3.[46])*

high potency (i.e., those that act at low EDC) are generally very soluble in lipid, so that the effective concentrations of all volatile anesthetics in the lipid material of the central nervous system are thought to be approximately the same.

Potency has no bearing on the rates of equilibration or de-equilibration, which depend on S alone. This is a point about which the student is often confused. We can only reasonably compare rates of equilibration when the safe anesthetic gas concentration is consistently employed with all agents. Under these conditions, S represents the relation between how much anesthetic must be transferred into a given volume of blood (i.e., x'_b) and what "driving force" is available to accomplish the transfer (i.e., x'_a). Naturally, if we arbitrarily increase the alveolar anesthetic concentration, we can force anesthetic into the blood as fast as we wish, but the patient will be dead if we persist. The following tabular summary will illustrate why, when the safe anesthetic gas concentration is used, potency is irrelevant to the rate of equilibration.

	EDC $= x'_b$	S	$x'_a (= x'_b/S)$
Gas A	1	1	1
Gas B	1	10	0.1
Gas C	10	1	10

Gas A and gas B are equipotent. Yet, because B is 10 times more soluble than A, the "driving force" available for achieving the same x'_b is 10 times lower with B than with A, and the rate at which x'_b is approached must obviously be considerably lower.

Gas C is 10 times less potent than gas A, so the x'_b to be attained is 10 times higher. Yet, because S is the same, the "driving force" of C is just 10 times greater than that of A, and equilibrium will be reached at the same rate.

The potency of a gaseous anesthetic is immaterial except in one respect that has nothing to do with equilibration rate. If the potency is very low relative to the solubility, the safe anesthetic gas concentration may be so high that there is no room (at ordinary atmospheric pressure) for sufficient oxygen. The minimum O_2 requirement in the inspired air is about 15%, or 114 mm Hg. It follows that the partial pressure of an anesthetic gas may not exceed 646 mm Hg (33.5 mM at 38°). Reference to Table 4-2 will show that by this criterion neither ethylene nor nitrous oxide are suitable agents for producing surgical anesthesia (although they may be useful for lesser degrees of anesthesia), since both require partial pressures greater than 646 mm Hg. The only way to induce surgical anesthesia with either of these agents alone is to employ *total* pressures greater than 760 mm Hg, thereby incorporating oxygen at a partial pressure of at least 114 mm Hg. To the extent it may be thought desirable to furnish oxygen in excess of the minimum 114 mm Hg, other agents may also be found deficient. Acetylene, for example, permits only about 25% of oxygen in the anesthetic mixture. In contrast, anesthesia can be produced with a mixture of 0.7% chloroform and 99.3% oxygen.

It follows from the above discussion that after discontinuation of anesthesia with an agent like nitrous oxide, of relatively low solubility and used at high concentration, a very large amount of the gas will be delivered to the alveoli from the blood. This may result in *diffusion anoxia*, i.e., the alveoli are effectively filled with nitrous oxide diffusing from the blood, and the alveolar oxygen tension is reduced. Suppose the blood has been equilibrated with a mixture of 80% nitrous oxide and 20% oxygen. If the anesthesia is simply discontinued and the patient is allowed to breathe air, the alveoli will, for some time, contain 80% nitrous oxide, the concentration in equilibrium with the blood perfusing the lungs, and the remaining 20% (even ignoring carbon dioxide and water vapor), since it is air, will provide only one-fifth the adequate amount of oxygen. Especially in conditions of marginally sufficient oxygenation, therefore, significant anoxemia may result unless pure oxygen is administered during the early recovery phase.[48]

Influence of Body Fat

The Anesthetic Content of the Body at Equilibrium.   Up to this point we have examined the equilibration of body water as though the anesthetics did not dissolve appreciably in other components of the body. However, some of the agents are quite soluble in lipid, and fat constitutes an important fraction of the body weight. In an average person, without prominent fat depots, the fat of the organs and subcutaneous tissues amounts to not less than 15% of the body weight, while it is obvious that in very obese people this fraction may be much higher.[49]

The solubility of an anesthetic in lipids (often estimated approximately from measurements with a vegetable oil) is expressed as a partition coefficient between lipid and blood at 38°:

$$S_L = \frac{x_L}{x_b}$$

To distinguish between lipid solubility and blood solubility in this section, we shall use the symbol S_b instead of S to denote the latter, S_L to denote lipid solubility.

When the blood and body water attain their equilibrium concentration, x_b', fat will contain $x_L' = S_L(x_b')$. What volume of blood will contain the same amount of anesthetic as a given volume of fat? Obviously this "blood equivalent" of fat is simply S_L. Suppose, for example, $S_L = 10$. This means that any volume of fat at equilibrium will contain 10 times as much anesthetic as the same volume of blood, or, in other words, a liter of fat is the equivalent of 10 liters of blood. The effect of body fat is, therefore, to increase the apparent volume of distribution of an anesthetic agent to an extent that depends on S_L and the volume of fat, and thus to increase the total amount of anesthetic in the body at equilibrium. An agent of very high lipid solubility may be distributed largely in the fat depots at equilibrium, and the total anesthetic content of obese patients may be surprisingly high.

Example: The blood concentration of cyclopropane during surgical anesthesia is 4.1 mM. Molecular weight = 42, $S_L = 35$. What weight of the gas is contained in a 90 kg man, of whom 20 kg is fat?

Approximately 20 liters fat is equivalent to (20 × 35) liters blood. Total blood equivalent = 700 liters blood + 50 liters body water = 750 liters. Then the weight of gas is: 4.1 mM × 750 = 3.08 moles, or (3.08 × 42) g = 129 g. Note that of this total weight of cyclopropane, 700/750, or 93.%, is in the fat.

Rate of Uptake of Anesthetic by Fat Depots.   Let us assume that all the arterial blood arriving at a fat depot contains x_b', that the fat contains no anesthetic, and that S_L is high. A high S_L means that a great deal of anesthetic has to be transferred from blood to fat, relative to the concentration available in blood. Consequently the blood will be practically depleted of anesthetic in the proximal portion of the capillaries, and equilibration will be prolonged until, with the arrival of more and more blood carrying x_b', enough is finally transferred to bring the whole fat depot to its equilibrium concentration x_L'. This process will be reflected in the anesthetic content of venous blood draining the fat depot; initially containing practically no anesthetic, its concentration will gradually increase to x_b' when the fat depot has reached equilibrium. The word "saturate" is very often misused in this connection. There is never any question of "saturating" the body or fat depots with anesthetic, but only of equilibrating with a given alveolar anesthetic concentration.

Effect of Depot Fat Upon Rates of Equilibration and De-Equilibration of Body Water.
The rate of uptake of anesthetic by fat depots is of little interest in itself, but the question is naturally raised whether fat depots modify the rate of equilibration (or de-equilibration) of blood and body water. The maximum effect of depot fat would be observed under circumstances where all the blood flowing through all the fat depots was cleared of anesthetic in a single passage. This would be the case initially, as has already been noted, with agents of high S_L. However, the blood flow through all the fat depots represents so small a fraction of the cardiac output (approximately 3%) that the anesthetic concentration in mixed venous blood would not be substantially lowered even in this extreme case. This conclusion is confirmed by experimental data on nitrogen elimination, showing that the fat depots do not appreciably influence the main course of de-equilibration, but only come into the picture as a slow component after the concentration in mixed venous blood has fallen to a low level.[50,51]

Whatever amount of anesthetic is transferred in a given breath from lungs to blood must be distributed to various organs and tissues in proportion to their respective blood flows. Thus, the rate of uptake by fat cannot exceed a small fraction of the rate of entry from lungs into blood, except in very obese patients, where a larger fraction of the cardiac output flows through fat. The blood, brain, and body water reach near-equilibrium while fat is still far from equilibrium. Anesthetic is then transferred slowly from arterial blood to fat, and replaced at the same rate in the pulmonary capillary blood, without appreciable change in the blood concentration. Thus, once the blood and body water have been practically equilibrated, the anesthetist will be supplying anesthetic to the fat depots, by way of the alveoli and blood, whose anesthetic concentrations remain essentially constant (x_a' and x_b', respectively).

When the anesthetic is discontinued, fat depots have just as little influence on the main course of de-equilibration, and for the same reason (anesthetic flow from fat to blood being similarly limited by the total blood flow through fat). However, after the blood and body water are largely cleared of anesthetic, we should expect a continued leakage from the fat depots, slowest and most prolonged in the case of agents with high S_L. Mixed venous blood should show traces of anesthetic long after the body water is essentially de-equilibrated. Such persistence in the venous blood is observed with cyclopropane (S_b 0.47, S_L 34) and chloroform (S_b 7.3, S_L 100), but not, apparently, with nitrous oxide (S_b 0.47, S_L 3.2) or ether (S_b 15, S_L 3.2).

Speed of Induction and Recovery in Clinical Anesthesia

Induction. The progressive deepening of anesthesia reflects the increasing concentration of anesthetic agent at the sites of action in the brain. By measuring the rate of increase of the concentration in internal jugular (venous) blood as it approaches that of common carotid (arterial) blood, it has been found that when the anesthetic concentration of arterial blood is kept constant, the brain reaches 90% of equilibrium in about 7 min. The rate of blood supply to brain tissue is reported[52] to be 350 ml kg^{-1} min^{-1}, while the mean figure for the rest of the body water is approximately 100 ml liter^{-1} min^{-1}. One would therefore expect an equilibration rate about 3.5 times faster for brain than for body water as a whole. This conclusion based on the blood-flow/volume ratio agrees pretty well with the theoretical prediction of 21 min for 90% equilibration of body water, and the observed time of about 7 min for the same fraction of equilibrium in brain, both data for agents of low solubility.

The relative rates of equilibration for both the brain and body water should be the same, regardless of the blood solubility of the anesthetic agent, i.e., regardless of whether the equilibration rate is slow or fast. The rate of induction of anesthesia is therefore determined by the same factors as govern the equilibration of body water, but it is faster. A patient will reach surgical anesthesia while the venous blood and body water are still far from equilibrium, and the fat depots farther still. Thereafter, anesthetic leaves the brain at the same rate it arrives, and the patient remains at the same depth of anesthesia while the venous blood and body water (and ultimately the fat depots) come to equilibrium. If a perfect, closed system is being used, one will find that early in anesthesia new anesthetic has to be furnished at a considerable rate. As time goes on, however, less and less has to be added to the system until, eventually, no new anesthetic is required. When the whole body is at equilibrium, the patient can rebreathe the same anesthetic gas while O_2 is supplied and CO_2 is absorbed.

Practical Induction with High-Solubility Agents.   For agents of high solubility, like ether and chloroform, the theoretical induction time on our premise of maintaining the safe anesthetic gas concentration from the start would be so long (as shown earlier) that even the use of CO_2 would not make it a practical proposition. The only alternative (and that universally adopted) is to induce with higher gas concentrations, i.e., concentrations that are unsafe in the sense that continued administration would invariably lead to respiratory paralysis and death. At an appropriate time the concentration in the inspired air must be reduced to the safe anesthetic concentration. What the procedure accomplishes is to force large amounts of anesthetic rapidly into the arterial blood and thus establish a desired level of clinical anesthesia quickly. The rest of the body can then equilibrate over a long period of time while the depth of anesthesia is held constant. The procedure is exactly analogous to the use of priming doses (p. 320); it is illustrated diagrammatically in Figure 4-20 (cf. Figure 4-10).

Recovery.   The speed of recovery from surgical anesthesia to full consciousness, reflecting the progressive de-equilibration of the brain, will be influenced by the same factors that determined the speed of induction. When a low-S agent is discontinued, the arterial blood concentration falls very quickly as venous blood is almost completely cleared of anesthetic at the lungs. A steep concentration gradient is thus provided which, with the high blood-flow/brain-volume ratio, favors rapid transfer of brain anesthetic to the cerebral capillary blood, and consciousness is quickly regained.

When a high-S agent is discontinued after equilibration of the body water, the arterial concentration falls only slowly, and the de-equilibration of the brain tends to be limited by the rate of elimination of anesthetic from the whole of the body water. The way to accelerate the otherwise slow recovery from prolonged anesthesia with a

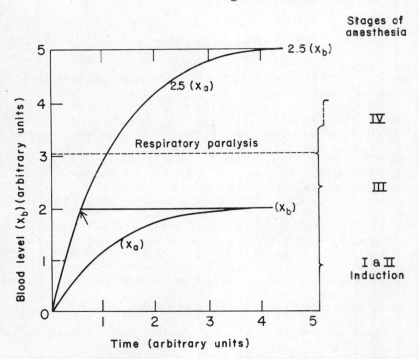

FIGURE 4-20. Approach to equilibrium in stage III ($x_b = 2$) when safe anesthetic gas concentration is employed from start is shown by curve x_a. *By using $2.5(x_a)$, the upper curve would theoretically be obtained, approaching $x_b = 5$, but respiratory failure would occur. If at arrow the anesthetic concentration in the inspired air is reduced to x_a, blood level $x_b = 2$ can be maintained. Thus, induction time can be reduced greatly.*

high-S agent is to stimulate the respiration by administering CO_2: this procedure proves highly effective in practice.

An excessive concentration of a high-S anesthetic in the blood, causing too deep an anesthesia, has very different implications depending upon the circumstances. If anesthesia has just been induced with concentrations greater than the safe anesthetic gas concentration, and the anesthetic is stopped abruptly as soon as the condition is recognized (e.g., by depressed respiration), there will be a rapid outflow of drug from the brain into the blood, whose concentration is still much lower. Because the bulk of the brain is so small compared with the body water, such a redistribution will readily reduce the danger; indeed, the patient may return toward consciousness with surprising speed. This ability of the body water to act as a "sink" for anesthetic before equilibrium is established serves as a useful safety factor. For the same reason, however, it complicates induction because the depth of anesthesia responds quickly to transient fluctuations in the alveolar anesthetic concentration (e.g., those caused by breath-holding). On the other hand, as the blood and body water approach equilibrium, recovery takes ever longer. Control of the depth of anesthesia becomes easier, but respiratory paralysis late in anesthesia presents a far more serious problem, since now the whole of the body water acts as a buffer opposing outflow of anesthetic from the brain.

REFERENCES

1. R. CALDEYRO–BARCIA and J. J. POSEIRO: Oxytocin and contractility of the pregnant human uterus. *Ann. N.Y. Acad. Sci.* 75:813 (1959).
2. S. S. KETY: Measurement of regional circulation by the local clearance of radioactive sodium. *Amer. Heart J.* 38:321 (1949).
3. J. BEDERKA, JR., A. E. TAKEMORI, and J. W. MILLER: Absorption rates of various substances administered intramuscularly. *Europ. J. Immunol.* 15:132 (1971).
4. H. G. BRAY, B. G. HUMPHRIS, W. V. THORPE, K. WHITE, and P. B. WOOD: Kinetic studies on the metabolism of foreign organic compounds. 6. Reactions of some nuclear-substituted benzoic acids, benzamides and toluenes in the rabbit. *Biochem. J.* 59:162 (1955).
5. E. K. MARSHALL, JR. and W. F. FRITZ: The metabolism of ethyl alcohol. *J. Pharmacol. Exper. Therap.* 109:431 (1953).
6. I. CAMPOS, W. SOLODKOWSKA, E. MUNOZ, N. SEGOVIA–RIQUELME, J. CEMBRANO, and J. MARDONES: Ethanol metabolism in rats with experimental liver cirrhosis. I. Rate of combustion of labeled ethanol and rate of decrease of blood ethanol levels. *Quart. J. Stud. Alcohol* 25:417 (1964).
7. K. J. ISSELBACHER and N. J. GREENBERGER: Metabolic effects of alcohol on the liver. *New Eng. J. Med.* 270:351, 402 (1964).
8. F. LUNDQUIST and H. WOLTHERS: The kinetics of alcohol elimination in man. *Acta Pharmacol. Toxicol.* 14:265 (1958).
9. E. NEGELEIN and H. J. WULFF: Disphosphopyridinproteid, alkohol, acetaldehyd. *Biochem. Z.* 293:351 (1937).
10. E. RACKER: Crystalline alcohol dehydrogenase from baker's yeast. *J. Biol. Chem.* 184:313 (1950).
11. H. THEORELL: Kinetics and equilibria in the liver alcohol dehydrogenase system. *Adv. Enzymol.* 20:31 (1958).
12. M. M. KINI and J. R. COOPER: Biochemistry of methanol poisoning. III. The enzymic pathway for the conversion of methanol to formaldehyde. *Biochem. Pharmacol.* 8:207 (1961).
13. J. P. VON WARTBURG, J. L. BETHUNE, and B. L. VALLEE: Human liver alcohol dehydrogenase. Kinetic and physicochemical properties. *Biochemistry* 3:1775 (1964).
14. N. MOURAD and C. L. WORONICK: Crystallization of human liver alcohol dehydrogenase. *Arch. Biochem. Biophys.* 121:431 (1967).
15. K. H. BEYER, H. F. RUSSO, E. K. TILLSON, A. K. MILLER, W. F. VERWEY, and S. R. GASS: "Benemid," p-(di-n-propyl-sulfamyl)-benzoic acid: its renal affinity and its elimination. *Amer. J. Physiol.* 166:625 (1951).
16. E. NELSON and I. O'REILLY: Kinetics of sulfisoxazole acetylation and excretion in humans. *J. Pharmacol. Exper. Therap.* 129:368 (1960).
17. E. NELSON: Pharmaceuticals for prolonged action. *Clin. Pharmacol. Therap.* 4:283 (1963).
18. A. GOLDSTEIN, O. KRAYER, M. A. ROOT, G. H. ACHESON, and M. E. DOHERTY: Plasma neostigmine levels and cholinesterase inhibition in dogs and myasthenic patients. *J. Pharmacol. Exper. Therap.* 96:56 (1949).
19. J. H. GADDUM: Repeated doses of drugs. *Nature* 153:494 (1944).
20. J. A. SHANNON, D. P. EARLE, JR., B. B. BRODIE, J. V. TAGGART, and R. W. BERLINER: The pharmacological basis for the rational use of atabrine in the treatment of malaria. *J. Pharmacol. Exper. Therap.* 81:307 (1944).
21. J. E. DOHERTY: The clinical pharmacology of digitalis glycosides: a review. *Am. J. Med. Sci.* 255:382 (1968).
22. W. KALOW and D. R. GUNN: The relation between dose of succinylcholine and duration of apnea in man. *J. Pharmacol. Exper. Therap.* 120:203 (1957).
23. J. W. PALMER and H. T. CLARKE: The elimination of bromides from the blood stream. *J. Biol. Chem.* 99:435 (1933).
24. R. SÖREMARK: The biological half-life of bromide ions in human blood. *Acta Physiol. Scand.* 50:119 (1960).
25. O. BODANSKY and W. MODELL: The differential excretion of bromide and chloride ions and its role in bromide retention. *J. Pharmacol. Exper. Therap.* 73:51 (1941).

26. R. A. KEHOE, J. C. CHOLAK, O. M. HUBBARD, K. BAMBACH, and R. R MC NARY: Experimental studies on lead absorption and excretion and their relation to the diagnosis and treatment of lead poisoning. *J. Indust. Hyg. Toxicol.* 25:71 (1943).

27. R. R. M. BORGHGRAEF and R. F. PITTS: The distribution of chlormerodrin (Neohydrin ®) in tissues of the rat and dog. *J. Clin. Invest.* 35:31 (1956).

28. R. T. SCHIMKE, E. M. SWEENEY, and C. M. BERLIN: The roles of synthesis and degradation in the control of rat liver tryptophan pyrrolase. *J. Biol. Chem.* 240:322 (1965).

29. C. M. BERLIN and R. T. SCHIMKE: Influence of turnover rates on the responses of enzymes to cortisone. *Mol. Pharmacol.* 1:149 (1965).

30. A. H. CONNEY and J. J. BURNS: Factors influencing drug metabolism. *Adv. Pharmacol.* 1:31 (1962).

31. H. L. SEGAL and Y. S. KIM: Glucocorticoid stimulation of the biosynthesis of glutamic-alanine transaminase. *Proc. Nat. Acad. Sci.* 50:912 (1963).

32. I. M. ARIAS and A. DE LEON: Estimation of the turnover rate of barbiturate side chain oxidation enzyme in rat liver. *Mol. Pharmacol.* 3:216 (1967).

33. T. TEORELL: Kinetics of distribution of substances administered to the body. I. The extravascular modes of administration. II. The intravascular modes of administration. *Arch. Int. Pharmacodyn.* 57:205, 226 (1937).

34. E. NELSON: Kinetics of drug absorption, distribution, metabolism, and excretion. *J. Pharmaceut. Sci.* 50:181 (1961).

35. E. NELSON: Kinetics of the excretion of sulfonamides during therapeutic dosage regimens. *J. Theoret. Biol.* 2:193 (1962).

36. E. KRÜGER-THIEMER and P. BÜNGER: The role of the therapeutic regimen in dosage design. *Chemotherapia* 10:61 (1965/66).

37. E. KRÜGER-THIEMER and P. BÜNGER: Kumulation und Toxität bei falscher Dosierung von Sulfanilamiden. *Arzneimittel-Forsch.* 11:867 (1961).

38. H. G. BRAY, W. V. THORPE, and K. WHITE: Kinetic studies of the metabolism of foreign organic compounds. 5. A mathematical model expressing the metabolic fate of phenols, benzoic acids and their precursors. *Biochem. J.* 52:423 (1952).

39. C. P. LARSON, JR., E. I. EGER, II, and J. W. SEVERINGHAUS: The solubility of halothane in blood and tissue homogenates. *Anesthesiology* 23:349 (1962).

40. C. P. LARSON, JR., E. I. EGER, II, and J. W. SEVERINGHAUS: Ostwald solubility coefficients for anesthetic gases in various fluids and tissues. *Anesthesiology* 23:686 (1962).

41. D. S. RIGGS: *The Mathematical Approach to Physiological Problems.* Baltimore, Williams and Wilkins Co. (1963).

42. D. S. RIGGS and A. GOLDSTEIN: Equation for inert gas exchange which treats ventilation as cyclic. *J. Appl. Physiol.* 16:531 (1961).

43. S. S. KETY: The physiological and physical factors governing the uptake of anesthetic gases by the body. *Anesthesiology* 11:517 (1950).

44. S. S. KETY: The theory and applications of the exchange of inert gas at the lungs and tissues. *Pharmacol. Rev.* 3:1 (1951).

45. E. I. EGER: Effect of inspired anesthetic concentration on the rate of rise of alveolar concentration. *Anesthesiology* 24:153 (1963).

46. E. I. EGER: Applications of a mathematical model of gas uptake. In *Uptake and Distribution of Anesthetic Agents*, ed. by E. M. Papper and R. J. Kitz. New York, McGraw-Hill (1963), Ch. 8.

47. R. M. EPSTEIN, H. RACKOW, E. SALANITRE, and G. L. WOLF: Influence of the concentration effect on the uptake of anesthetic mixtures: the second gas effect. *Anesthesiology* 25:364 (1964).

48. B. R. FINK: Diffusion anoxia. *Anesthesiology* 16:511 (1955).

49. P. R. SCHLOERB, B. J. FRIIS–HANSEN, I. S. EDELMAN, A. K. SOLOMON, and F. O. MOORE: The measurement of total body water in the human subject by deuterium oxide dilution. *J. Clin. Invest.* 29:1296 (1950).

50. H. B. JONES: Respiratory system: nitrogen elimination. *Med. Phys.* 2:855 (1950).

51. J. S. ROBERTSON, W. E. SIRI, and H. B. JONES: Lung ventilation patterns determined by analysis of nitrogen elimination rates; use of the mass spectrometer as a continuous gas analyzer. *J. Clin. Invest.* 29:577 (1950).

52. S. S. KETY: Quantitative determination of cerebral blood flow in man. *Methods in Medical Research* 1:204 (1948).

CHAPTER 5
Drug Toxicity

INTRODUCTION

Long before the birth of modern pharmacology, Paracelsus (1493–1541) observed that "All things are poisons, for there is nothing without poisonous qualities. It is only the dose which makes a thing a poison."[1] The first formal lectures that could be said to constitute a course in pharmacology were given at Paris in 1856 by Claude Bernard under the title "Lectures on the Effects of Toxic and Medicinal Substances."[2] These dealt with noxious gases and arrow poisons (curare). Today, that branch of pharmacology known as toxicology encompasses a broad field of investigation concerning a vast array of toxic chemicals used in industry as well as the potentially toxic drugs in therapeutic use.

The variety and availability of effective and potentially toxic drugs has increased sharply since the close of the 19th century. With the intensive development of synthetic organic chemistry, new kinds of drugs come into use each year, while a bewildering array of minor modifications are introduced into existing drugs. At the same time, the expanding availability of medical care in all countries results in an increasing exposure of large population groups to drugs. This is most dramatically exemplified by the prophylactic use on a mass scale of such drugs as the antimalarials and the steroid contraceptives.

The increased medical use of drugs leads inevitably to a greater number of toxic reactions. All drugs are toxic in overdosage, and people vary greatly in their sensitivity to drugs; so what may be a safe and appropriate dosage for one person can prove to be an overdose for another. Moreover, even in the therapeutic dose range many drugs have unavoidable toxic side effects. As a consequence, a great deal of drug toxicity is inevitably produced by physicians, who must be constantly alert to recognizing such iatrogenic (i.e., physician-caused) disease and treating it properly.[3]

The widespread distribution of drugs is also accompanied by increased hazards of accidental poisoning and suicide. Accidental poisoning is seen primarily in children; about 70% of the reported cases in the United States involve children under 5 years of age.[4] Small children are apt to ingest whatever they find, particularly drugs that are disguised as candy or made up in a sweet-tasting liquid vehicle. The leading cause of drug poisoning in children has been aspirin, which accounts for one-fifth of all the cases and a large fraction of the deaths. Vitamins, iron preparations, and chocolate-covered laxatives account for a significant but smaller number. The operation of poison control centers and a national system for collecting data from such centers exposed this hazard to public view,[5] and soon led to some effective countermeasures. Aspirin, for example, was packaged in smaller containers, containing less than a lethal dose. The medical profession and the public became more aware of the dangers of candy-coated medications. A major advance was the introduction of "child-proof" bottle closures; these are caps that can only be removed by pressing strongly with the palm of the hand and simultaneously turning.[6] These measures resulted in a significant reduction of aspirin poisonings in children.

About one-fifth of all suicide deaths are attributable to drugs, and about 90% of these are due to barbiturates. Barbiturates have long held a commanding lead over other drugs in suicide attempts, and they are second only to firearms among all methods employed for suicide.[7] Moreover, data on actual deaths by suicide certainly underestimate the use of barbiturates relative to other methods, for suicide attempts with these drugs often fail. No one knows if reducing access to lethal amounts of barbiturates would have any effect upon the overall suicide rate due to all causes, but it is likely. The ready availability of a suitable and painless means of death makes it easy for a person to take his life in a period of depression that might otherwise be transient. This places a heavy burden of responsibility on physicians and pharmacists not to dispense these hazardous agents in lethal quantities. There is really no justification for prescribing hypnotic medication at all, except on a short-term basis, when it is clearly indicated to tide the patient over some acute crisis. And then it would be appropriate not to give more than a few doses at a time into a patient's keeping. Another partial solution to this problem may lie in using the newer hypnotic agents, like the benzodiazepines (e.g., flurazepam), which evidently have a very wide margin of safety between the hypnotic and lethal dose.

Beyond the restricted range of several hundred drugs in common clinical use is a much larger array of toxic chemicals that are an integral part of our industrial society. More than 10,000 different chemicals are employed industrially in the United States, and production of new chemicals has been increasing at an annual rate of about 7%.[8] These are incorporated into more than 300,000 potentially toxic trade-marked products on the consumer market.[9]

The most intense exposure is suffered by workers who manufacture or otherwise handle such substances. Certainly things have changed greatly since the sensational radium poisoning case of 1929, when, through ignorance of the dangers, and total lack of regulation, factory girls painting watch dials with a radium solution were permitted to moisten the brushes with their lips.[10] In many countries safety precautions in industry, enforced by law and regulated by inspection, have reduced the gross hazards considerably. Today's laws require adequate protection of the worker against contact with injurious chemicals, by means of adequate clothing and suitable ventilation. Despite increased concern with worker safety, occupational toxicity continues to be a problem.

Laws alone cannot suffice, unless workers and employers really understand the reasons. Protective devices have to be practical and comfortable, or they will not be used. And there must be no economic incentive for a worker to break the prescribed rules. A face mask, for example, that increases airway resistance to the point of discomfort, will simply not be worn, nor will heavy protective clothing that impedes movement on the job.

The alert physician must be aware of the possible illnesses, some bizarre, some commonplace, that afflict workers in the various industries.

Although not as seriously at risk as the worker in industry. the average person is now exposed to an extraordinary number and variety of toxic substances in his own household. Accidental or suicidal poisonings with such materials pose difficult problems for the physician.[11-13] Not so long ago, manufacturers were not even required to list all ingredients on the label, so that optimal treatment of acute poisonings was often delayed pending a frantic search for information about the nature of the responsible chemicals.[11] Now such listing of ingredients is mandatory.[14] Again, as with accidental ingestion of drugs, children under 5 are often the victims of poisoning by household chemicals. The agents responsible are chlorine bleaches, kerosene (commonly a solvent for polishes), lye, ammonia, and phenolic disinfectants. Kerosene and the strong alkalis account for the greatest number of hospitalizations.[4]

Accidental poisoning is a significant problem for every community. There are more than 4000 fatal accidental poisonings each year in the United States.[15] About one-quarter of these are due to drugs, an increasing number of these among drug addicts. The number of nonfatal poisonings is estimated to exceed one million per year, or about one per 200 of the population. Physicians and toxicologists will be expected to deal with these cases, yet information is not readily at their disposal because of the rapid emergence of new products on the market, rapid changes in the patterns of drug use and abuse, and inadequate scientific data about rare toxicologic phenomena. To aid in dealing more effectively with the problem, many communities have established Poison Control Centers, which are coordinated through a *National Clearinghouse for Poison Control Centers* in the U.S. Department of Health, Education, and Welfare.[4] These centers can serve the whole population on a 24 hr basis. They maintain files on the toxic ingredients of household and commercial products, they supply information and advice to physicians on the treatment of poisonings, and some of them also provide treatment facilities. Statistical summaries are published periodically by the *National Clearinghouse*. Departments of public health in the various states have divisions concerned with accidental poisonings and occupational toxicology. Every physician and pharmacist should be familiar with these consultative facilities, and he should also have at his instant disposal a concise reference manual on the general and specific treatment of poisonings.[11,12,16,16a]

ENVIRONMENTAL TOXICITY

A wholly new toxicologic phenomenon of modern times is the occurrence of mass poisoning through contamination of food, water, or air. There are three main reasons why the problem has become so much more serious than in the past. *First*, very toxic chemicals are being introduced in large numbers, as noted already, which were never before present in the biosphere. *Second*, the growth of industrial civilization has reached the point where for the first time its products can significantly contaminate the biosphere in a particular geographic region or even over the whole planet. *Third*, systems of mass distribution now ensure that any incident of toxicity will probably involve large numbers of people spread over a wide area.

The best historic analogy to our modern mass poisonings is probably the periodic epidemics of ergotism known since the Middle Ages in Europe.[17] Ergot comes from a fungus that grows on rye, containing alkaloids affecting blood vessels and brain. Thus, eating bread made from contaminated flour leads to arteriolar spasm, gangrene, and hallucinations or other psychotic behavior. As recently as 1951, such an outbreak occurred, with a large part of the population of a French village experiencing transient psychosis.[18] But as long as food production remained essentially decentralized, such episodes affected only the immediate locality. Today, in contrast, a single lot of canned foods contaminated, for example, by botulinus toxin can kill people scattered over the entire world. In Morocco, in 1959, the adulteration of olive oil with petroleum oil containing triorthocresyl phosphate caused some degree of demyelination paralysis in 10,000 people.[19]

Intelligent decisions about how to deal with the problems of environmental toxicity require an understanding of the pharmacologic principles governing uptake of substances by different routes,[20] accumulation and steady-state levels, acute and chronic organ damage by chemicals, and genetic, carcinogenic, and teratogenic effects.

Pesticides

We shall consider the two main groups of insecticides in recent use—the chlorinated hydrocarbons, such as DDT (dichlorodiphenyltrichloroethane) and the organic phosphates, such as parathion.[21–23]

DDT was introduced in 1945 for the control of malaria mosquitoes, with astounding success. It is a highly potent contact poison of the nervous system in insects. It is very stable, so it persists for a long time, offering continuous protection for many months after a single application. In typical use to reduce mosquito infestation, it is painted on interior walls. Very likely the main cause of the sharp reduction in malaria incidence after World War II was the widespread use of DDT.

The compound is surprisingly nontoxic to man. A median toxic dose for acute exposure is estimated to be about 10 mg kg^{-1}, or 700 mg for the average man. A single 1500 mg dose in a volunteer produced some neurologic disturbances (paresthesias, tremors), which disappeared within 24 hr. At the 6th and 12th hour after administration of the compound, lice that were fed on the subject died. Volunteers have taken 0.5 mg kg^{-1}, or 35 mg daily, for over a year without any demonstrable adverse effects, and without abnormality of nervous or hepatic function. When very large doses taken accidentally have produced serious poisoning, tremors, hyperexcitability, and convulsions were seen.[24] Thus, DDT is toxic to the nervous system in man and other vertebrates, as in insects, but it is many orders of magnitude more potent in insects, for reasons as yet unknown. Table 5-1 illustrates some typical actions of DDT on various species at different concentrations, in relation to actual levels of exposure.

The problems associated with DDT and other chlorinated hydrocarbon insecticides arise from their widespread use in agriculture. Their persistence, which is advantageous in the control of malaria mosquitoes, creates problems when they are sprayed over fields, forests, orchards, swamps, and lakes. The greater the use, the greater the contamination of waterways by runoff from the soil. The organic hydrocarbons are not, of course, absolutely stable; they are metabolized by various organisms (cf. Chapter 3) and they are degraded by photochemical reactions. These processes of elimination, however, are too slow to have prevented a steady increase in DDT concentration in the soil and water over the past quarter century of use.

TABLE 5-1. Some critical concentrations of DDT.
(Data from Pesticide Commission Report, 1969.[21])

Concentration or amount	Comment
0.05 μg/L[a]	Found in Lake Michigan.
0.1 μg/L	Kills some mollusc larvae.
0.3μg/L	Inhibits photosynthesis and causes damage in Chlorella.
5.0 μg/L	Kills crab larvae.
42.0 μg/L	Permissible level in drinking water, U.N. standard.
5000.0 μg/L	Kills trout eggs.
10 μg day^{-1}	Intake by inhalation at highest air level ever observed (1560 ng m^{-3}).
72–200 μg day^{-1}	Intake in average diet.
35,000 μg day^{-1}	Daily intake for 12–18 months in volunteers, without toxicity.

[a] Concentrations are often given in parts per billion. 1 ppb. = 1 μg/L.

Of greater concern than their mere chemical stability is the accumulation of the chlorinated hydrocarbons in the food chain.[25] This is a direct consequence of their very high lipid/water partition. The principles governing accumulation of DDT in the lipid stores and membranes of an organism are very similar to those already discussed in Chapter 4, in connection with the lipid-soluble volatile anesthetics. Here the concentrating process begins with the lowest forms, such as algae, and proceeds, with successive steps of magnification at successively higher levels in the food chain. For example, a fish may be unharmed by a low ambient concentration of DDT in the lake water, for the daily intake at the gills and by ingestion is not sufficiently great to establish a toxic steady state plateau in the tissue water. However, if the same fish feeds on crustaceans that in turn have fed on algae, the daily intake of DDT may be many times greater. As the storage depots of the food organisms are digested, their DDT is released and distributed in the body fluids and storage depots of the predator species. For example, typical concentrations of DDT in California species of plankton, bass, and grebes are 5.3, 4 to 138, and up to 1600 parts per million respectively. In Wisconsin, DDT residues in crustacea, chub, and gull were 0.41, 4.52 and 20.8 ppm respectively.[25] The net result is that although the waters may contain what seems a negligible and surely nontoxic concentration of DDT (cf. Table 5-1), the species high on the food chain may be exposed to a toxic level. It appears that serious damage has already been done to trout fisheries in certain areas, and to certain bird species through toxic effects on the reproductive process (especially the laying down of egg shells). Ironically, while many insect species have become resistant to DDT (cf. Chapter 8), natural fish and bird predators on these same species may have been reduced in number or even eliminated.

As would be expected, at a given daily dose of DDT, a steady-state is eventually established, at which the excretion (primarily in urine) equals the intake. At the same time, there is a plateau level in the body water, in equilibrium with that stored in body fat at a high lipid-water ratio (typically about 300:1) so that the fat contains most of the DDT in the body. Figure 5-1 shows the relationship between DDT in fat and the daily intake in volunteer human subjects. This relationship permits fat

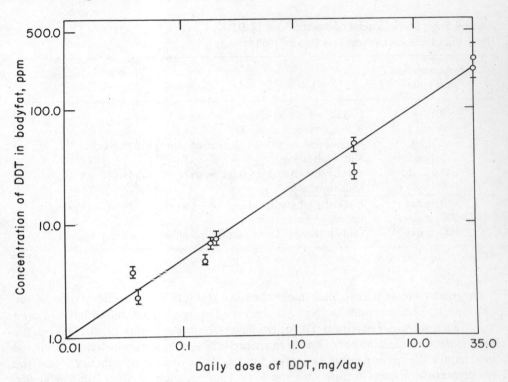

FIGURE 5-1. Relationship between equilibrium concentration in body fat and daily dose of DDT. *Points show means and standard errors. Daily dose of DDT is shown on a logarithmic scale. Measurements were made on fat samples after a constant level had been attained. (From HEW Report on Pesticides, Figure 4.[21])*

analyses (e.g., in autopsy material) to be used for monitoring environmental exposure to DDT.[26,27] Data from such studies point to an average intake of about 100 μg day^{-1} for the general population, a figure that closely matches independent estimates from analyses of various foods on the consumer market.

Figure 5-2 depicts the rate of attainment of the plateau level in fat at constant daily intake of DDT. This is analogous to the establishment of a plateau by intravenous infusion, where the biologic half-life can be estimated from the half-time of approach to the plateau (p. 314). Here we estimate a biologic half-life of about 6 months in the fat depots, a figure that agrees with the measured rate of decline in fat levels after discontinuing DDT intake.

A common point of confusion concerns the levels in fat. DDT in fat, as far as we know, is not harmful. It is only as an indicator of the aqueous concentration in contact with the vital organs that we are concerned about it. As analytic methods become more and more sensitive, we shall be able to detect in human tissues and excreta trace amounts of more and more substances present in the environment. Obviously, the mere presence of a foreign compound is not necessarily hazardous, even if that compound is known to be toxic at much higher concentrations. For example, the acute toxicities of the various chlorinated hydrocarbons vary over a 1000-fold range, whereas the assay sensitivities are approximately the same for all of them.[28] Tolerance limits will have to be established for each substance.

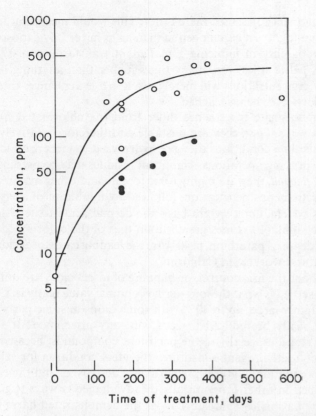

FIGURE 5-2. Accumulation of DDT in body fat. *Concentration of DDT in small samples of body fat is shown as a function of time, with constant intake of DDT by mouth at two dosage levels. Open circles: 35 mg day^{-1}; solid circles: 3.5 mg day^{-1}. Concentration is given in parts per million. From HEW Report on Pesticides, Figure 9.[21]*)

Although there is no persuasive evidence that DDT has caused or threatens to cause any toxic damage in man, evidence has developed implicating it as a carcinogen in mice.[29] This will be discussed more fully in Chapter 11. It suffices to point out here that carcinogenic properties require a different analysis from ordinary toxicity. In principle, continuous exposure to a toxic agent at a low enough concentration will cause no harm. Suppose, for example, that a toxic effect is due to enzyme inhibition or to occupancy of a transport protein in competition with an endogenous ligand. A significant biochemical effect will necessarily require a significant fractional occupancy of the sites. If the concentration is so low that only a few percent of the sites are occupied, there will be no toxic effect, regardless of how long—even for a lifetime— the agent is present. In other words, there should be a threshold of toxicity, below which the agent is safe. This threshold will, of course, vary somewhat from individual to individual, and the slope of the LDR curve for the toxic effect may be different for different agents. But there is bound to be some low concentration that is safe for virtually everyone. Carcinogenesis, mutagenesis, and teratogenesis are governed by different principles; this is why separate chapters are devoted to them in this book. The point here is that we do not know whether or not there is a threshold, and therefore it is safest for the moment to assume there is not. This would mean that for a carcinogen like DDT (assuming it is a carcinogen in man as in mice), any exposure at all carries some finite probability of inducing a malignant transformation. Even though the concentrations fed to mice were many times higher than anything to which man is exposed, lower concentrations will merely result in a lower cancer rate, but without a perfectly safe level ever being reached.

The organophosphate insecticides differ from the chlorinated hydrocarbons in two important ways. *First*, they are unstable and therefore relatively nonpersistent. Especially in alkaline conditions they are hydrolyzed to inert products. However, in the field, after spraying operations, significant residues may be present for many days or even weeks. *Second*, they are highly toxic to man and other mammals, by virtue of their rapid percutaneous penetration, followed by inhibition of acetylcholinesterase in the nervous system. On a weight basis the dermal acute toxicity in this group is, on the average, about 100 times greater than that of the chlorinated hydrocarbons. These insecticides (e.g., parathion, p. 407) are the leading cause of accidental poisoning among agricultural workers in California.

Decisions about the use, control, or banning of insecticides are difficult. The main question to be settled is what the long-term economic value really is. Crop losses from insects are certainly large, up to 30% with some crops in some parts of the world.[21] But can these really be reduced to zero with any insecticide? It seems doubtful. Resistance develops, especially to the persistent compounds, because long exposure to low levels of a lethal agent constitutes the ideal condition for selecting resistant mutants in a population. Natural predators are destroyed, and the ecologic balance may be disturbed in other economically disadvantageous ways (e.g., destruction of honey bees, or of a shellfish industry). Does the demonstrated harm to reproductive function in certain birds foretell a similar effect in the human species, which has not yet come to light? And how many people (if any) will develop cancer because of exposure to a present or future environmental level of DDT? How shall we balance economic gain and increased food supply against harm to some number of humans and the extinction of peregrine falcons?

The chlorinated hydrocarbons will certainly be used sparingly and selectively in the future or they will be abandoned entirely because so many insect pests have become resistant to them, and because of the possible carcinogenic hazard. But it must be recognized that the present alternative, a greatly increased use of the organophosphates, will cause problems of another kind. These insecticides, although they are relatively nonpersistent, are also extremely toxic, posing a very serious hazard to agricultural workers.

Air Pollution

Atmospheric pollution by combustion products ("smog") can produce toxicity on a mass scale. The Donora Pennsylvania, catastrophe of 1948 resulted in 5910 cases of illness (43% of the exposed population) and 20 fatalities.[30-38] Follow-up studies of the afflicted individuals revealed distinctly higher morbidity and mortality rates in the ensuing years.[38] A similar episode in the greater London area, December 5-9, 1952, apparently claimed several thousand lives. Very large numbers of people became ill with signs of respiratory distress. A retrospective analysis of the death

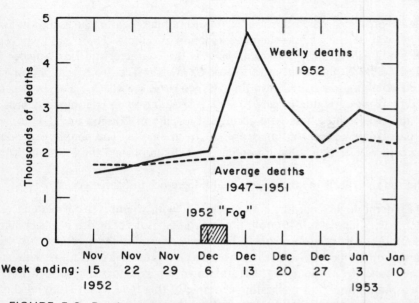

FIGURE 5-3. Deaths associated with the London "fog" of December 1952. *Solid curve shows weekly number of deaths in Greater London before and after the "fog." The dates of the "fog" (December 5–9) are shown by hatched area. Broken curve shows weekly average number of deaths for the preceding 5 years. (From Goldsmith, Figure 1.[39])*

records (Fig. 5-3) showed that about 4000 more deaths occurred at the time of the "fog" than would have been expected on the basis of data for the previous 5 years.[39–42]

Although acute episodes of severe air pollution like those cited above command attention because they are so dramatic, it has become obvious that many urban environments are continuously polluted to an alarming extent. Table 5-2 records some typical data for two urban areas. For some pollutants, it will be observed, the maximum 24 hr values are as much as ten times greater than the annual mean, and well into the range of manifest toxicity, as will be shown below. The chief components

TABLE 5-2. Typical components of smog.
Data are ppm for average Chicago air, for 24 hr maximums in Chicago (parentheses), and for typical photochemical-oxidant smog in California. (Adapted from Ayres and Buehler, Table I,[32] and Cadle and Allen, Table 1.[48])

Compound	Chicago		California
SO_2	0.08	(1.14)	0.20
$NO + NO_2$	0.16	(1.0)	0.20
CO	13.0	(66.0)	40.0
Total oxidants (as O_3)	0.02	(0.23)	0.5
Hydrocarbons	2.8	(14.9)	4.4
Suspended particulates	0.14	(0.24)	—

of smog are products of combustion from automobiles, heating fuels, and industrial plants, as well as their photochemical reaction products. There are two general types of smog. *Photochemical-oxidant smog* is the characteristic Los Angeles type, characterized by a high concentration of ozone, derived from the photolysis of NO_2 and combination of the resulting oxygen atoms with O_2. The brown color of this type of smog is due largely to NO_2. *Reducing smog* is composed primarily of SO_2 and particulates; this type occurred typically in London and Tokyo, where a high particulate concentration is present from smoke. The simple expedient of banning coal with a high sulphur content virtually abolished the awesome London smogs.

Studies on the effects of smog upon health have been of three types:

(a) Epidemiologic recording of sickness,[43-47] with attempts to correlate increased incidence with increases in air pollution, or comparisons of health status in different communities (e.g., urban vs. rural). These investigations show consistently higher incidence of pulmonary and cardiovascular disease in association with smog, but they suffer from the defect that unknown other factors may also distinguish the two populations. An interesting example of this type was a study of the performance of a high school athletic team through several seasons.[49] A striking linear relationship was found between the oxidant level in the air and decrements of performance, with the smallest effects demonstrable at 0.1 ppm. The maximum hourly oxidant level in Los Angeles reaches about 0.6 ppm, and the mean level exceeds 0.1 ppm.

(b) Exposure of animals or human volunteers to known levels of a particular pollutant. This procedure has produced clear enough adverse effects, particularly upon pulmonary airway resistance, but in general seems to underestimate the toxicity. The reason probably is that several of the components of smog have additive or synergistic effects. Thus, SO_2 alone is not nearly so damaging as in the presence of particulates, when H_2SO_4 is formed; and hydrocarbons alone (derived from automobile exhausts) are much more innocuous than when they react with ozone to form free radicals, aldehydes, and peroxy derivatives.

(c) Exposure of animals or humans to ambient air and to filtered air in the course of a severe smog.[50] Such experiments have shown no difference among normal subjects, but a significant relief of symptoms and of physiologic abnormalities of pulmonary function among patients with emphysema when they breathed filtered air. In addition, asthmatic attacks in some patients were correlated with days of high oxidant level.

Oxides of nitrogen (NO and NO_2) are derived not only from automobile exhausts but also from fuels used in heating. Animals exposed to concentrations between 5 and 10 ppm have markedly reduced resistance to respiratory infections.[51] In man, respiratory symptoms develop in the same concentration range, which is about ten times that found in ordinary photochemical smogs. Air quality standards for nitrogen oxides in California have been established at 0.25 ppm but present levels in Los Angeles average about 0.7 ppm.

Oxides of sulfur (SO_2, SO_3) are generated from fuel oil and petroleum refining processes. In numerous reports, increased incidence of respiratory illness has been associated with levels exceeding 0.05 ppm and increased mortality is found above 0.2 ppm.[52] Plant life is also affected adversely at these levels.

The particulates in smog may contain significant quantities of asbestos fibers, known to produce lung cancer in those exposed occupationally,[53,54] but no evidence has yet linked lung cancer convincingly to any kind of air pollution.[55,56] Cigarette smoking, at any rate, presents the major environmental hazard of this kind. Lead, derived principally from the combustion of leaded gasolines, is causing increasing concern; it will be considered later.

Carbon monoxide illustrates the difficulties in assessing the possible toxic effects of chronic environmental exposure to a known toxic agent at low levels.[57] The acute toxic action of CO is fairly specific; it combines with hemoglobin, forming a complex 200 times tighter than that between hemoglobin and O_2. One consequence is to reduce the oxygen-carrying capacity of the blood to an extent related directly to the percent saturation with CO–Hb. A second, and more important, consequence is to change the shape of the O_2–Hb dissociation curve, so that the positive cooperativity (Hill effect) is largely abolished, and the unloading of oxygen at the tissues thereby disturbed (p. 54). One would expect significant tissue anoxia to be produced only at fairly high saturation of Hb with CO, and this is the case; significant changes in pulse rate, cardiac output, and blood pressure occur at about 30% saturation or above. This blood level is in equilibrium with 75 ppm of air, a level rarely if ever attained in the general urban atmosphere. Atmospheric CO is produced primarily by automobiles and the levels fluctuate with conditions conducive to air pollution in general. Ambient levels have rarely exceeded 50 ppm, but are frequently in the 10 ppm range. As must obviously be true, persons exposed for several days to environmental levels of CO mirror these levels in their blood. Thus exposure in the 10–20 ppm range leads to levels of 4–8% saturation. Since CO acts like a gas of high solubility in blood (because of its uptake by Hb), the establishment of equilibrium with the ambient air is a slow process, taking 4–6 hr, as explained for other high-solubility gases in Chapter 4.

Cigarette smoking adds very considerably to the CO level, heavy smokers attaining a level of 7% saturation. It has been found, therefore, that all studies on environmental exposure to CO are overshadowed by the exposure due to smoking. When smokers and nonsmokers are examined separately, it is readily shown that groups especially exposed to CO, such as automobile drivers and traffic policemen, have demonstrably elevated CO–Hb levels. The question, however, is whether any adverse effects are associated with these low levels. To date, no conclusive evidence has been forthcoming. Decrement in performance on a task requiring accurate estimation of a time interval of approximately 1 sec was demonstrated down to 50 ppm; this finding could be interpreted as showing negligible decrement at a concentration rarely exceeded in ambient air. It required 1.5 hr of continuous exposure, and then the hemoglobin was only 2% saturated.

An attempt has been made to relate CO levels in the Los Angeles basin with case fatality rates for patients with myocardial infarction. There was certainly a positive correlation, but since CO levels vary concurrently with many other components of smog, and since meteorologic conditions are related directly to air pollution, there is no way to tell certainly from these data whether CO itself played any role.

The CO problem raises important cost-benefit questions. Reduction of environmental CO levels would require very substantial changes in the style of urban industrial life in all countries. Thus far, there are no real indications of toxicity from chronic exposure to even the highest levels that occur in a bad smog. It seems clear, therefore, that carbon monoxide is not among the most serious air pollution problems. Moreover, cigarette smoking far outweighs any contribution from the ambient atmosphere in raising blood CO–Hb levels. How much toxicity would have to be demonstrated, to warrant the curbing of private automobiles or the banning of internal combustion engines? This is the kind of difficult question we have to face increasingly with agents that have some demonstrable toxicity, as already discussed in relation to the chlorinated hydrocarbon pesticides.

Lead

Lead poisoning was once considered to be solely an occupational disease of painters and industrial workers.[58–60] Then, about 50 years ago, the large-scale poisoning of urban children was brought to light.[61] Slum dwellings in the Eastern and Midwestern cities of the United States contained leaded paints and plaster (up to 50% Pb by weight). As such housing fell into disrepair, crumbling plaster and flaking paint found their way into the respiratory and gastrointestinal tracts of the infants and young children growing up there. By the 1960's, this had become a national scandal, for lead had become a prime cause of poisoning among children, especially in the lower socioeconomic, minority ethnic groups.[62–63b] Mortality rates in lead poisoning are high, and permanent sequelae are extremely frequent. The most common effects in adults are anemia, with hemolysis of mature red cells and impaired synthesis of hemoglobin,[64–65] gastrointestinal disturbances (colic), and peripheral neuropathy. The most serious effect, seen especially in children, is encephalopathy, with mental retardation, recurrent seizures, and motor disturbances (cerebral palsy) as lifelong consequences.[66] The nervous system is more susceptible to permanent damage, the younger it is, and this principle can be extrapolated back into the period of fetal life. Moreover, any single acute episode of toxicity involving the nervous system may cause permanent derangements, even though the toxic agent is removed immediately; this applies to chlorinated hydrocarbon pesticides[67] as well as to lead, mercury, and other metals.[68] One may wonder, therefore, how many cases of mental retardation and other neurologic problems of unknown etiology in these socioeconomic groups might have been caused by childhood lead poisoning.

Dramatic epidemics of mass poisoning are certain to come to public attention and thus initiate measures to identify and counteract the offending agents. In contrast, poisoning that goes on, year after year, especially if its victims belong to an ethnic or socioeconomic minority, tends to escape notice. This is partly because the connection between the noxious agent and the illness it causes may not be apparent, and partly because the same underprivileged groups do not find adequate medical care. Lead poisoning, however, lends itself to an aggressive case-finding approach, because simple tests reveal and quantitate the presence of the metal in body fluids and tissues. Since lead is deposited in bone and teeth, evidence of past exposure can be sought by x rays, by analysis of deciduous teeth in children, or by the bluish-grey "lead line" in the gums of heavily exposed individuals in the presence of poor dental hygiene.[69] Blood and urine, however, are analyzed more readily in mass surveys; they reflect the daily intake of lead quite accurately.

Overt signs and symptoms of lead poisoning do not usually occur at blood lead levels lower than 0.4 μg ml^{-1}; clinical toxicity is observed frequently at 0.8 μg ml^{-1} and above, with encephalopathy associated with levels in excess of 1–2 μg ml^{-1}.

However, in a very important recent study,[70] interference with a step in hemoglobin synthesis was demonstrated at blood lead levels previously considered to be harmless. The enzyme Δ-amino levulinic acid (ALA) dehydrase catalyzes the conversion of ALA to porphobilinogen in the pathway of heme synthesis. Figure 5-4 shows the correlation between blood lead levels and the activity of this enzyme in erythrocytes

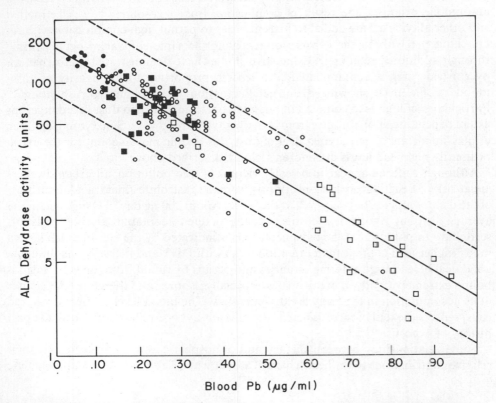

FIGURE 5-4. Relationship of ALA dehydrase activity to blood lead. *Measurements were made in 158 Swedish workers and students with different degrees of exposure to Pb. Ordinates are values of erythrocyte amino levulinic acid dehydrase activity (note logarithmic scale); abscissas are values of blood Pb. Different symbols represent various occupational groups. (From Hernberg et al., Figure 1.[70])*

for a large number of Swedish workers and students with various degrees of occupational exposure to lead. Some decreases in the average enzyme activity of exposed workers as compared with medical students can be observed even below 0.20 μg ml^{-1}. At 0.4 μg ml^{-1}, where ALA excretion is known to increase sharply, and mild clinical toxicity may be seen, the enzyme activity is more than 50 % inhibited (note logarithmic scale of ordinates). Pb also appears to cause some interference with Na$^+$-K$^+$ ATPase activity in red cells, though not at quite such low concentrations [71]

In view of the demonstrated damage to human health at blood levels above 0.4 μg ml^{-1} it is remarkable that large-scale testing programs in New York and Chicago in 1970,[72,73] showed that 10 % of all children in these cities had lead in excess of 0.6 μg ml^{-1} in their blood. Moreover, a surprisingly large fraction of these children lived in good housing, suggesting that in some manner the entire urban environment (not only delapidated slum dwellings) had become contaminated to a dangerous extent. Similar indications of a widespread incidence of high blood lead levels among children were obtained in a study of small cities in Illinois.[74]

What has happened seems fairly clear now. In the past several decades lead has been polluting the air of urban centers all over the world, more than 98 % of it derived from automobile exhausts, the result of combusting leaded gasoline.[75,76,77] Tetraethyl and other alkyl leads are added to fuels in order to permit high compression without knocking, yet without the expense of achieving the same equivalent octane rating through additional refining.[75] Exhaustive studies have demonstrated that urban air over a wide area is contaminated with lead in proportion to the density of auto-mobile traffic, even showing a diurnal fluctuation with commuter rush hours.[78] Particulates of high lead content fall out and contaminate urban dust to a dangerous extent depending upon distance from heavily traveled roadways. Since young children at play inhale and ingest a great deal of dust, this finding may account for the extra-ordinarily high lead levels in children's blood, described above.

Although children appear to be early victims of lead pollution, all urban dwellers are at risk.[79] Lead is absorbed only poorly from the gastrointestinal tract (about 10 % of the dietary intake), but very well at the lungs. About 300 μg day^{-1} is ingested in the average diet, but a good deal of this probably is due to contamination of foodstuffs secondary to pollution of the biosphere. This is indicated by the fact that fish have a much higher lead content than other foods (as with DDT and mercury), as though a good deal of lead were entering estuaries and oceans by runoff from the land. Lead is bound extremely tightly in many tissues, especially in bone; and therefore (cf. Chapter 4) its accumulation in the body is extremely slow. The blood level (principally in red cells) reflects the daily intake, whereas the amount in bone reflects primarily the past history of exposure.[60]

Some relationships between dietary and atmospheric sources of lead and their relative contributions to the health hazard are shown in Table 5-3. At low atmospheric

TABLE 5-3. Atmospheric lead pollution.
(Compiled and adapted from Environmental Prevention Agency, Table 7.[76])

Air (μg m^{-3})	Absorbed (μg day^{-1})			Expected blood level (μg g^{-1})
	Air	Diet	Total	
0.0005	Clean natural air.			
2	14	30	44	0.21
2–5	Approximate range in general urban air.			
10	69	30	99	0.40
	Significant increase in ALA excretion starts here.			
24–38	Measured in downtown Los Angeles and near freeways during commuter rush hours.			
50	345	30	375	0.72
	Frank clinical toxicity starts in this range.			

lead levels, the principal source of the absorbed lead is dietary, with about 30 μg daily absorption, sufficient to inhibit ALA dehydrase, as shown already in Figure 5-4. At ambient lead levels in the range now found frequently in urban air, about 14 $\mu g\, day^{-1}$ is absorbed by the inhalation route. The measured concentrations of atmospheric Pb in our major cities, averaged on a year-round basis, produce blood levels around 0.2 $\mu g\, ml^{-1}$—so called "normal" levels—at which erythrocyte ALA dehydrase is nearly 50% inhibited. Much higher levels occur regularly near busy automobile routes and occasionally over a wide area during a smog condition. If people were exposed constantly to air lead concentrations in the range that have been measured on freeways during commuter rush hours, serious lead poisoning would certainly ensue.

It must be concluded that the contamination of the urban atmosphere with lead presents a clear and present danger to health. Traffic policemen, garage workers and others whose occupations involve continued exposure to motor vehicle exhaust are most seriously affected.[79a] The poisoning of children in the micro-environment of slum dwellings a few decades ago forecast what would happen on a wider scale as lead pollution increased. Infants and children remain at high risk because of the dangerously high Pb concentrations in urban dust and soil, where they play, particularly near heavily traveled automobile routes. The general population is already exposed, on a continuous basis, to a Pb concentration that interferes with an essential step in heme synthesis. It is not known if this moderate inhibition of ALA dehydrase of red blood cells is in itself harmful. However, much higher air Pb concentrations occur from time to time—concentrations that we know would cause clinical toxicity if sustained.

In summary, the pollution of city air by a number of different substances presents an immediate and real hazard to health. Matters are already out of control, in that millions of city dwellers daily breathe several pollutants at concentrations high enough to cause and aggravate pulmonary diseases like bronchitis, emphysema, and asthma. The average levels of some of those, derived largely from automobile exhausts but also to some extent from industrial sources, have reached the threshold of toxicity for man. Thus, sudden intensification of the smog in a local area, due to temperature inversion or development of water-vapor fog, can and does precipitate severe acute toxicity, with definite increase in morbidity and mortality. Those at greatest risk for this type of injury, due to SO_2, NO_2, O_3, and other noxious gases, are patients with preexisting pulmonary or cardiovascular disease; but it may be surmised that there are also significant long-term effects on the health of normal people. Pollution by mercury and lead is more insidious. These metals cumulate in the body over weeks, months, and years, so the cause-effect relationship between them and their toxicity is obscured. Moreover, since some of the known toxic actions are on the brain, subclinical toxicity could well take the form of subtle changes in brain functions such as behavior and learning ability. The lead pollution problem brings into very sharp focus serious questions regarding society's ability to make rational and timely decisions in areas where there is a clash of economic interests and public health interests.

Enough toxicological data are in hand to warrant the immediate implementation of plans to phase out the production of leaded gasoline, which is virtually the sole source of the pollution, and which is not even a necessity of modern life. The petroleum industry itself has estimated that complete removal of lead from gasoline, and substitutions of other types of processing to yield equivalent grades of fuel, would add only one or two cents per gallon to the cost.[75]

Mercury

The history of mercury poisoning is much like that of lead poisoning, in that what used to be a rare occupational hazard has today become a serious problem for whole populations.[80] The general principle is further illustrated, that the wholesale pollution of the biosphere by numerous products and by products of our technology has placed vastly greater numbers of people at risk, who may have no occupational relationship at all to these poisons.

As an occupational hazard, mercury poisoning affected chiefly miners and those in the hat-felt industry. Metallic mercury vapor was responsible, and the effects were primarily on the kidneys and nervous system ("mad as a hatter"), presumably following oxidation to mercuric ion in the body. Mass poisoning appeared with the introduction of alkyl mercury compounds in certain industrial processes and as fungicides. As with the chlorinated hydrocarbon pesticides, the magnification of organic mercurial concentrations through the food chain was responsible. The process is exemplified by the remarkable story of Minamata Disease.[81,82] In 1956 a new factory on the shores of Minamata Bay (Japan) began producing vinyl chloride and acetaldehyde. Wastes containing methyl mercury were disposed of by dumping them into a nearby creek. Within a year, a strange illness appeared in families of fishermen along the bay. Neurological symptoms predominated, beginning with memory loss, paresthesias, ataxia, and narrowing of visual field, and progressing to severe emotional instability and loss of muscle coordination (athetoid movements). Small children and newborns were affected most severely. By 1960 there had been 85 adult cases, 22 fetal and childhood cases, and 41 deaths.

The astute observation that cats in the affected households suffered from the same symptoms eventually led to discovery of the cause, and the whole chain of causation, from the factory to man, was worked out. High concentrations of methyl mercury entered the bay, were taken up and stored by lower organisms, which were eaten by shellfish, and eventually by people and cats. Since metallo-organic compounds pass the blood-brain barrier much more readily than free metal ions, methyl mercury salts are more toxic than mercuric salts to the nervous system, relative to their renal toxicity.

As soon as the factory waste was diverted from Minamata Bay, the epidemic subsided. But although the danger of organic mercurials had been so well publicized, poisonings continued elsewhere.[83,84,84a] As late as 1969 there was a miniature epidemic of mercury poisoning in a New Mexico farm family.[85] Grain intended for seed purposes and treated with a fungicide (cyanomethyl mercury guanidine), and containing significant mercury residues, was fed to hogs. The meat of these animals was eaten over a period of 3 months. Of 10 children thus exposed, three experienced ataxia, agitation, visual impairments, and severe behavioral abnormalities. The mother was pregnant at the time and remained grossly healthy, but her infant, who had been exposed in utero, suffered brain damage. Interestingly, the urine Hg level was 15 times higher in the newborn infant than in the mother. By 6 weeks of age, no more Hg was detectable in the infant's urine, but electroencephalographic abnormalities and myoclonic jerks developed subsequently. Evidently the damage done to the nervous system became manifest only slowly. Poisoning from ingestion of Hg-treated seed grain occurred on a mass scale in Iraq in 1972; 500 deaths resulted.[86]

Episodes like those cited above direct attention to the general question: To what extent is mercury pollution of the air, water, and food supply a serious hazard? The data are not reassuring. As with the chlorinated hydrocarbon pesticides, mercury is persistent in the environment. Alkyl mercury compounds, the most toxic form of the element, are used in very large quantities for preventing mildew in grain. Inorganic mercury salts are converted to methyl mercury by bacterial action.[87]

The biologic half-life of mercury (as methyl mercury) in man has been measured to be about 70 days (k_e approximately 1 % per day). Mercury is stored in many tissues, especially in liver and brain. Severe toxic effects on the central nervous system have been found with brain content of 12 mg, and distribution studies with radioactive ^{203}Hg have shown that at the steady-state, 10–20 % of the total Hg in the body is in the brain.[88] Then a total body burden of about 100 mg would be toxic. Since the daily elimination is 1 % of that present, the corresponding daily intake at the steady-state would be 1 mg. By applying an arbitrary safety factor of 1/10, an "Allowable Daily Intake" of 0.1 mg day^{-1} was obtained.[89] This would correspond to the ingestion of 200 g daily of fish containing 0.5 ppm. But fish in Lake Michigan, in Swedish coastal waters, and elsewhere have been found to contain more than this amount of mercury, sometimes as much as ten times more, or well into the known toxic range for long-term exposure.[80,90] High Hg content was found, not only in Swedish fish, but also (as might be expected) in fish-eating birds and seed-eating rodents. Analysis of Hg content of feathers from museum specimen birds permitted a chronologic analysis of the course of environmental pollution with this element, as shown in Figure 5-5. The specimens contained increasing amounts of mercury the more recently they had been acquired, with a very sharp increase corresponding to the introduction of mercury into new industrial and agricultural uses following World War II.

The justified alarm over mercury contamination of fish has led to some control measures, such as prohibiting the dumping of mercury-containing wastes into sewage effluents, and phasing out mercurial fungicides. Dealing with the increasing threat of atmospheric pollution by mercury will be more difficult. It is known from experience with the inhalation of mercury fumes in industry that a concentration of about 100 μg m^{-3} causes symptoms, even when inhaled for a short time. For continuous exposure, and to allow for the much greater toxicity of organic than of inorganic mercury, a "safe" air standard would seem to be approximately 1 μg m^{-3}, as established in Germany. In clean open air, (e.g., over the ocean), the mercury level is 0.001 μg m^{-3} or below, but open air urban levels are up to 100 times higher. At San Francisco, for example, the breeze from the ocean carried 0.002 μg m^{-3}, but when the breeze shifted, to bring air from surrounding industrial regions, the level rose above 0.02.[80] None of these data suggest that we are yet approaching the acutely toxic level of Hg in the air we breathe, but they show clearly that the atmosphere is being polluted to a significant extent, principally from burning of industrial fuel.

Special hazards are associated with the evaporation of Hg vapor into confined spaces where people live or work.[91] For example, in offices recently painted with latex-based paints containing Hg compounds as mold retardants, remarkably high Hg levels were found in the air. A similar danger is present wherever metallic mercury is used, as in dentists' offices. At 24° the concentration of Hg vapor in equilibrium with Hg metal is 20 μg m^{-3}, far in excess of the "safe" range. If 1 ml of Hg is spilled in an

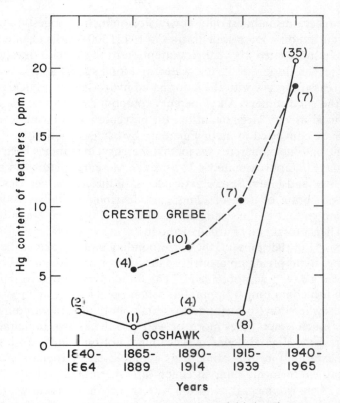

FIGURE 5-5. Mercury levels in two species of birds. *The mercury content of feathers is given in museum specimens of Swedish birds over more than a century. The number of samples is indicated in parentheses. (From Wallace et al., Figure 4.*[80]*)*

average sized room of 30 m³, this hazardous air concentration would be constantly present until all had evaporated—a process that would require 20,000 complete changes of the room air.

The allowable concentrations of Hg in food, water, and air are derived, as explained above, by applying an arbitrary safety factor to the levels known to cause acute or chronic toxicity. This may be risky, since other kinds of biologic damage may occur at even lower concentrations. Organic mercurials are more potent mutagens (chromosome breakage) even than colchicine, which has been regarded as very potent in this respect. And although the possibility of carcinogenesis has not yet been studied adequately, there is reason to worry that any potent mutagen may be a carcinogen (cf. Chapter 11). The alkyl mercury compounds are also teratogens at concentrations lower than cause illness in the mother. Thus, it may well prove necessary to reduce the environmental burden of Hg still further, if truly safe levels are to be achieved.

Food Additives

About 3000 different substances are added intentionally to foods during their manufacture, processing, or packaging.[92] Each person in the United States ingests over 1 kg of additives every year, on the average. A food additive is a substance or a mixture of substances, other than a basic foodstuff, which is present in food as a result of any aspect of production, processing, storage, or packaging. Additives are used for many purposes, such as to aid preservation and thus extend shelf life, to enhance flavor or color, to improve texture, or to increase yields in the production process.[93]

Some of the same problems discussed already in connection with pesticides and various forms of environmental pollution are seen also with food additives. Obviously, substances that are clearly toxic will not be knowingly added to foods, although occasionally they occur accidentally, as with aflatoxins in moldy peanuts (cf. Chapter 11). All chemicals intentionally added to foods must be subjected to rigorous testing to establish their safety, unless they are "generally regarded as safe" (abbreviated GRAS). The GRAS list compiled by the Food and Drug Administration contains about 600 items. No doubt most of these are reasonably safe as used, but evidence of hazard turns up from time to time, even among compounds that have long been on the list. The artificial sweetening agents known as cyclamates are an example; after being on the GRAS list for years, they were found to cause bladder cancer in rats. Another example is the food dye, Red 2, which was used for many years before it was found to interfere with reproduction in animals.

Another example of long delay in discovering adverse effects is seen in the story of monosodium glutamate, used as a flavor enhancer. This commonplace amino acid is responsible for the flavor-enhancing quality of seaweed, as used in Oriental cooking. It must obviously be fairly safe, since it is a major component of all dietary proteins. Indeed, human subjects have ingested over 100 g of it daily for several weeks, without significant toxic effects.[93a] Yet some people were discovered to have an unusual reaction—severe headache ("Chinese restaurant syndrome"). Moreover, very young animals (mice and monkeys) were found to develop hypothalamic lesions from excessive intake of monosodium glutamate; its use has therefore been banned in foods prepared for infants.

Occasionally, a new and untested additive leads to an epidemic of toxicity. In the autumn and winter of 1965–1966, 48 patients were admitted to various Quebec hospitals with an unusual kind of cardiomyopathy. All were heavy drinkers of a local brand of beer. Investigation brought to light the fact that cobalt sulfate was being added to draft beer made by one brewery, in order to counteract the antifoaming properties of traces of detergents in tavern glassware. Evidently, cobalt is cardiotoxic even at the low concentrations used here (approximately 0.7 mg liter^{-1}) when combined with alcohol, or in alcoholics. The precise role of cobalt was never worked out, but shortly after its removal, the epidemic ceased.[93b]

The history of diethylstilbestrol (DES) as a poultry and beef additive illustrates the difficulty of establishing limits for residues in foods.[93c] This synthetic estrogen was introduced into cattle feed, to increase the rate of weight gain and the ratio of protein to fat. Thus, the compound offered strong economic advantages. The Food and Drug Administration (FDA) approved the use of DES with the condition that it be withdrawn from feed 48 hr prior to slaughter, so that none would remain in the meat. The definition of "none" depends, of course, upon the sensitivity of existing methods of assay. In 1965, the available methods permitted detection only as low as 10 parts per billion, yet mice fed DES at a level of 6.5 ppb developed tumors. The 1958 revision of the United States Food and Drug laws included a provision (the Delaney amendment) setting a zero requirement for residues of any substance capable of causing cancer in any species. In the next 7 years, especially with better detection methods, increasing numbers of slaughtered animals were found to contain DES in their livers.

Eventually, in 1972, this use of DES was banned. One interesting aspect of the DES story was the demonstration of harm in a test species at a dietary level too low to be detected. The major question about permissible levels of carcinogens—is there a dose low enough to be safe?—will be discussed in Chapter 11.

In summary, toxicity on a large scale, due to numerous chemical agents, as well as to drugs, has become a major worldwide social and ecological problem.[94] From the standpoint of the individual, it matters little whether a potentially harmful agent gains access to his body through deliberate administration by a physician or through his own intake of food, air, or water. For all the chemical hazards, including drugs, toxicity data have to be obtained, a method has to be devised for quantitatively evaluating the danger, and acceptable limits of exposure have to be worked out. In the next section we shall turn our attention to these matters.

THE EVALUATION OF DRUG TOXICITY IN LOWER ANIMALS AND IN MAN

Broadly speaking, any adverse drug effect may be thought of as a manifestation of drug toxicity. It will be useful, however, to consider separately and in considerable detail, in later chapters, the following special categories of adverse drug effect: idiosyncrasy, drug allergy, tolerance and physical dependence, mutagenesis, teratogenesis, and carcinogenesis. In the present chapter, we shall consider adverse effects that are dose related, and experienced by most or all of the exposed population, usually at drug levels (or doses) in excess of those associated with a therapeutic action.

Sometimes a toxic effect is simply an extension of the therapeutic effect at a higher dose level. Coumarin anticoagulants, for example, prolong the clotting time of the blood. Overdosage leads to a bleeding tendency from excessive prolongation of the clotting time. Often, on the other hand, toxicity takes the form of a *side effect* more or less unrelated to the primary drug action. Examples are the nausea and vomiting seen frequently with the cardiac glycosides, and the gastrointestinal distress that often accompanies the ingestion of ferrous sulfate.

If quantitative estimates of efficacy and toxicity could be carried out routinely in humans, the decision whether a new drug should be adopted for clinical use would be a fairly straightforward task. We would begin at a low dosage, and increase the dose cautiously, watching carefully for toxic effects. If the desired therapeutic effect could be obtained with little or no toxicity in a large number of patients, we would accept the drug as efficacious and safe. In order to determine the margin of safety, we might increase the dosage well beyond the therapeutically effective range, with the aim of seeing by how much the therapeutic dose could be exceeded before toxicity ensued. Consider the following hypothetical illustration:

	Effective daily dose	Daily dose causing a toxic effect
Drug A	1 mg	2 mg
Drug B	100 mg	500 mg

We assume that A and B, at their effective doses, have equally useful therapeutic actions. In the usual situation, the two drugs being compared would be congeners with the same mechanism of action but different potencies. Here, A is 100 times more potent than B, yet it is relatively more toxic. Drug A produces toxicity at only twice its therapeutic dose, whereas B can be given safely up to five times its therapeutic dose.

Obviously, such deliberate exploration of toxic doses in humans is out of the question. Therefore the initial evaluations have to be based upon experiments with lower animals, and these have to explore the qualitative as well as the quantitative aspects of toxicity. It is important at this stage to find out what kinds of harmful effect may be expected, and at what dosages they may be manifested. Because species differences are considerable, several animal species have to be used. A convenient measure of potency is the *median effective dose* (ED50), that dose which would produce the specified effect in 50% of all subjects. If the effect being measured is death, the corresponding measure is the *median lethal dose* (LD50), and if the effect is a toxic one, the expression *median toxic dose* (TD50) is appropriate. Because of biologic variation it is meaningless to speak of "minimum lethal dose," "minimum toxic dose," or "maximum tolerated dose," as was customary at one time.

Drug potency may be of great interest to the medicinal chemist or pharmacologist who wishes to investigate the relationship between chemical structure and biologic activity, but usually it is of no great importance to the clinician. Thus, it would ordinarily matter little whether the dose of a drug is 10 μg or 10 mg. But there is an important exception to this generalization. If a drug is to be placed in a depot, for slow absorption over a long time, the greater the potency the better, for then the total amount employed can be reasonably small. Potency may also be an advantage with oral medication, if the material is a gastric irritant (usually because of some property unrelated to the therapeutic action), for then the less that can be administered the better.

The essential attribute we seek in a drug is efficacy at a safe dose. Ideally, this means that there should be a wide range of dosage between the effective and the toxic dose. The ratio TD50/ED50 (or often, in animals, LD50/ED50) is called the *therapeutic ratio* (also "therapeutic index"). A low ED50 characterizes a potent drug; but if the TD50 is also low, the margin of safety may be wholly inadequate. The therapeutic ratio is an initial crude indication of how safe a drug is likely to be. It is especially useful in a congeneric series, where molecular modifications are likely to alter both potency and toxicity but not necessarily to the same extent.

One problem in applying the therapeutic ratio concept is that few drugs are without some toxic side effect even at ordinary therapeutic dosage. The seriousness of the disease, the benefit likely to be derived from using the drug, and the degree of damage likely to be sustained as a result of drug toxicity all have to be weighed. A "minimum loss approach" has been proposed, which would give appropriate weight to these factors.[95] Curiously, some of our most useful drugs are also among the most toxic; neither digitalis glycosides nor the opiate analgesics have favorable therapeutic ratios.

A simple procedure for a preliminary assessment of the toxicity of a drug is the determination of lethal dosage in mice. The method will be described in some detail because it is applicable to any estimation of a quantal drug effect. *Quantal effects* (in contrast to graded effects, cf. chapter 1) are all-or-none responses. Each individual is categorized as responding or not responding, according to whatever criterion of response has been adopted. In studies of lethal toxicity each animal is classified as dead or alive at a specified time after drug administration. For any toxic agent there will be some low dose that kills no animals, some high dose that is uniformly lethal, and an intermediate dosage range in which a varying fraction of a population will be killed.

Some animals in a population will be sensitive to a drug, some will be resistant. As a rule, the sensitivity of animals to different doses of a drug is distributed normally with respect to the logarithm of the dose. If log dose is plotted on the horizontal axis and the relative frequency of animals sensitive to the various doses is plotted on the vertical axis, a gaussian (normal) distribution is usually approximated. This is illustrated in Figure 5-6 for three hypothetical drugs. The doses are expressed as

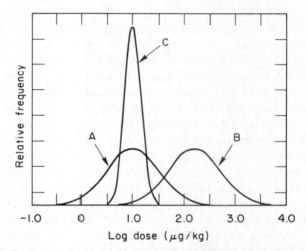

FIGURE 5-6. Theoretical distributions of sensitivities to the lethal effects of drugs in a population. *The mean (and median) sensitivity to drug A is 1.0 log unit, i.e., 10 μg kg^{-1}, and the standard deviation is ±0.5 log units. The mean sensitivity to drug B is 2.2 log units, i.e. 160 μg kg^{-1}, and the standard deviation is the same as for drug A. Drug C has the same median lethal dose as drug A, but the population is much more homogeneous with respect to the drug's lethal action; the standard deviation is only ±0.16 log units.*

μg kg^{-1} and the logarithms are plotted on the x axis. The y axis shows relative frequencies of animals dying at the different dose levels. The mean (also median) sensitivity is the dose at which one-half the animals die (the LD50), i.e., all animals sensitive to a lower dose are killed, whereas all animals sensitive to a higher dose survive. Curve A represents a drug that is lethal to one-half the animals at a dose of 10 μg kg^{-1} (log dose = 1). A small fraction of the population is killed even at doses below 1 μg kg^{-1} (log dose = 0). Another small fraction is not killed until the dose is raised above 100 μg kg^{-1} (log dose = 2.0). The standard deviation for this drug is ±0.5 log units; thus, two-thirds of the population of animals is killed at doses between 0.5 and 1.5 on the log scale, or between one-third and three times the LD50.

Curve B represents a drug for which the standard deviation of sensitivities is exactly the same as for drug A, but whose toxicity is much lower. The LD50 is at 2.2 log units, or 160 μg kg^{-1}, so this drug is only 1/16 as toxic as drug A.

Finally, curve C represents a drug that has the same toxicity as drug A, but to which the population responds in a much more homogeneous way. The standard deviation is only ± 0.16 log units. The antilog of 0.16 is 1.45; thus, two-thirds of the population are killed by this drug in the dosage range from 1/1.45 to 1.45 times the LD50 (between 69 and 145% of the LD50) or at doses between 6.9 and 14.5 μg kg^{-1}.

All quantal log dose-response (LDR) curves can be made identical by simply stretching or contracting the log dose scale. The convenient way to do this is to choose the standard deviation as the unit for this scale, and to designate the median lethal dose as zero. This is shown in Figure 5-7, curve 1. In reality, actual doses would be

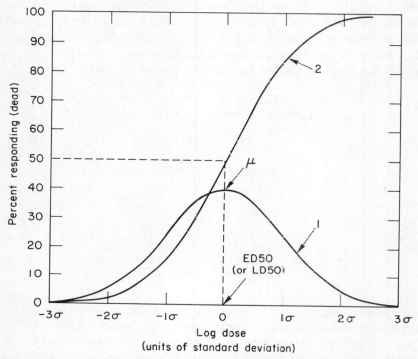

FIGURE 5-7. The quantal log dose-response curve. *The horizontal axis shows log dose in units of the actual deviation; the graph is therefore perfectly general. Curve 1 represents the normal distribution of sensitivities of individual animals to the drug; curve 2 is the cumulative normal distribution; μ represents the mean (also median) sensitivity, σ the standard deviation of sensitivities. For responses in general, the ED50 is the median effective dose; when death is the criterion of response, the median effective dose is called median lethal dose (LD50).*

indicated on the new generalized scale. Thus, curves A and B of Figure 5-6 would be drawn identically in the center of such a graph, except that the actual central value of log dose for curve A would be 1.0, whereas that for B would be 2.2. The central value for curve C would be 1.0, but the log dose values would be spread out to make the smaller standard deviation, 0.16, occupy the same linear distance as the standard deviation 0.5 of the other two curves.

In practice, what one determines is not the sensitivities of individual animals, but rather the cumulative number of animals that respond as the dosage is increased.

Therefore, a more useful form of graphic presentation is the cumulative (integral) form of the normal distribution (Figure 5-7, curve 2). This is the total area of the gaussian curve summed from left to right and expressed as percent of the total area. Thus, at any dose the cumulative curve gives the percent of animals responding to that dose and to all lower doses. These curves and their rationale are the same as those presented in chapter 1, Figure 1-84, where we discussed an interpretation of the LDR curve as a quantal distribution of receptor sensitivities.

In the normalized form shown here, the position, shape, and slope of the quantal LDR curve (curve 2) are fixed. At one standard deviation below the ED50, 16% respond; at one standard deviation above the ED50, 84% respond. At $-\sigma/2$, 31% respond; at $+\sigma/2$, 69% respond. These fixed relationships provide the basis for transforming quantal LDR curves to straight lines, which can be analyzed readily by statistical procedures. Instead of showing "percent responding" on the y axis, each percent response is converted to a *normal equivalent deviation* (N.E.D.), i.e., to the corresponding multiple of the standard deviation, as shown below:

Percent response	N.E.D.
2	-2.0
7	-1.5
16	-1.0
31	-0.5
50	0
69	$+0.5$
84	$+1.0$
93	$+1.5$
98	$+2.0$

This is the same procedure used to construct "probability graph paper"; the normal equivalent deviations are equally spaced on the y axis, but for convenience the "percent" scale is retained. On such paper a cumulative gaussian normal distribution assumes the form of a straight line throughout its entire range.

In order to circumvent the use of negative numbers, integer 5 is added to every N.E.D. The resulting new units are called *probits* (for "probability units") (Table 5-4). Thus, 50% response (N.E.D. = 0) corresponds to probit 5; 16% response (N.E.D. = -1.0) corresponds to probit 4; 93% response (N.E.D. = $+1.5$) corresponds to probit 6.5; and so on. From a practical standpoint one is rarely concerned with probit values smaller than 2 or greater than 8, since these represent percent responses well below 1% and above 99% respectively.

Figure 5-8 presents log dose-probit curves for three hypothetical drugs. In the theoretical normalized curve (Figure 5-7, curve 2) the log dose scale was in units of the standard deviation; the corresponding probit curve would be a straight line with slope 1.0. In Figure 5-8, we represent the logarithms of actual doses as abscissas, so that the position on the log dose axis reflects the potency of the drug. The customary measure of potency, the ED50, is the point on the log dose scale corresponding to probit 5. Drug A is evidently the most potent; its ED50 is antilog 1.3 = 20 mg. The slope of a log dose-probit line is determined by the biologic variation in sensitivity

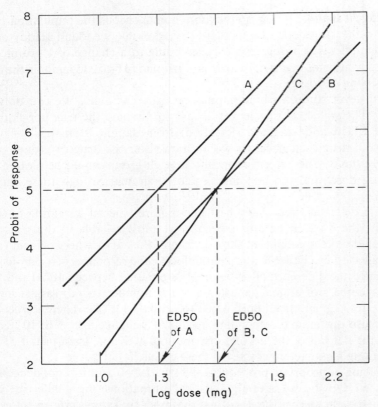

FIGURE 5-8. Log dose-probit curves for three hypothetical drugs.

TABLE 5-4. Conversion of percent to probit.
Each row of the table contains the probits corresponding to a decade of percents. To find, for example, the probit corresponding to 23%, enter the row labeled 20; under column headed 3 find probit 4.26. (Adapted from Finney,[97] Table I, originally Fisher and Yates,[98] Table IX. By permission of Cambridge University Press and Oliver and Boyd.)

%	0	1	2	3	4	5	6	7	8	9
0	—	2.67	2.95	3.12	3.25	3.36	3.45	3.52	3.59	3.66
10	3.72	3.77	3.82	3.87	3.92	3.96	4.01	4.05	4.07	4.12
20	4.16	4.19	4.23	4.26	4.29	4.33	4.36	4.39	4.42	4.45
30	4.48	4.50	4.53	4.56	4.59	4.61	4.64	4.67	4.69	4.72
40	4.75	4.77	4.80	4.82	4.85	4.87	4.90	4.92	4.95	4.97
50	5.00	5.03	5.05	5.08	5.10	5.13	5.15	5.18	5.20	5.23
60	5.25	5.28	5.31	5.33	5.36	5.39	5.41	5.44	5.47	5.50
70	5.52	5.55	5.58	5.61	5.64	5.67	5.71	5.74	5.77	5.81
80	5.84	5.88	5.92	5.95	5.99	6.04	6.08	6.13	6.18	6.23
90	6.28	6.34	6.41	6.48	6.55	6.64	6.75	6.88	7.05	7.33

to the drug; it is equal to $1/\sigma$, so the more homogeneous the population the steeper will be the line. In general, the standard deviation may be found readily on a probit plot as the difference in log dose corresponding to a change of 1 probit. Thus, the standard deviation of sensitivities to drug A is found to be 0.3 log unit on the dose scale, i.e., a doubling of dosage.

We can never study a whole population experimentally. We can only examine a sample. The statistical problem is always to estimate the true population values (e.g., the LD50 and standard deviation) from sample statistics.[96] To estimate the LD50 of drug A in mice, we would administer the drug to groups of animals at different doses. The percent mortality in each group would be plotted as probit against log dose, and the best line would be drawn through these experimental points.

Accurate determination of the best line requires special weighting of the points. Obviously, the data on percent response are most reliable in the region of 50% response and quite unreliable at the extremes of the curve, where percent response is strongly affected by chance factors that influence the responses of a very few animals. For example, the difference of one animal responding between 10/20 and 11/20 (the ratios of numbers of animals affected to total number tested) results in a change from 50% to 55% and from probit 5.00 to probit 5.13. The difference between 1/20 and 2/20, also one animal responding, results in a change from 5 to 10%, and, since this is in the flat tail of the normal distribution, a change from probit 3.36 to 3.72. The weighting factors compensate for these effects.[96,99,100]

By applying appropriate procedures the true LD50 and its confidence limits can be estimated. Obviously, as in all statistical estimations, the smaller the variability of the data (i.e., the steeper the slope) and the larger the sample size, the more accurate will be the estimate of the LD50, and the smaller will be its confidence range. The whole technique of statistical analysis of quantal LDR data is known as *probit analysis*. For a full working knowledge of this technique the reader is referred elsewhere.[97,99] Especially popular is a short-cut method employing nomograms in place of rather elaborate computations.[100] In the remainder of this discussion we shall examine some illustrative applications of the method to toxicity and efficacy evaluations.

Table 5-5 and Figure 5-9 present the results of a series of determinations on the lethal toxicity of an organophosphate cholinesterase inhibitor, guthion, in mice. The drug was given intraperitoneally to groups of eight or ten animals. At sufficient dosage the mice died from convulsions and other manifestations of central and peripheral acetylcholine accumulation. The entire experiment was replicated five times. The data illustrate the greater variability encountered in small groups, and the "smoothing" effect of pooling all the data into a single large sample. In these graphs the dose scale is logarithmic, but actual doses (rather than their logarithms) are indicated; this is often convenient where log probability (or probit) paper is readily available. From the probit plot for the pooled data we see that the LD50 is estimated to be 7.0 mg kg^{-1}. At probit 4.0, the corresponding dosage is 5.4 mg kg^{-1}. Now the ratio of these doses, corresponding to a difference of one probit, is $7.0/5.4 = 1.30$, and $\log 1.30 = 0.114$; this is our estimate of σ. This standard deviation is remarkably small. The entire range from 2% mortality (probit 3) to 98% mortality (probit 7), 4 probits in all, is spanned by less than a threefold range of dosage ($4 \times 0.114 = 0.456$; antilog $0.456 = 2.86$). Consequently, with this drug, even small groups of mice

TABLE 5-5. Toxicity of guthion in mice.
The drug was administered intraperitoneally, dissolved in 50% dimethyl-sulfoxide, to female mice. The number dead were recorded after 90 min. Data are number dead/total. LD50 values and confidence limits computed according to Litchfield and Wilcoxon.[100] (Data from student laboratory exercise, Department of Pharmacology, Stanford University School of Medicine, 1966.)

Dose	Raw data					
	Experiment number					
(mg kg^{-1})	1	2	3	4	5	Totals
4	—	0/10	—	0/10	1/10	1/30
5	0/8	1/10	0/8	1/10	1/10	3/46
6	3/8	2/10	2/8	2/10	4/10	13/46
7	3/8	5/10	5/8	5/10	5/10	23/46
8	7/8	5/10	7/8	5/10	5/10	29/46
10	8/8	10/10	7/8	10/10	9/10	44/45

LD50 values and confidence limits

Experimental numbers	LD50 (mg/kg)	95% confidence limits	
		Lower	Upper
1	6.8	6.15	7.50
2	7.4	6.55	8.35
3	6.7	6.00	7.40
4	7.6	6.66	8.57
5	6.8	5.80	7.95
Pooled	7.0	6.59	7.43

yield acceptable confidence limits for the LD50, as shown in Table 5-5; and the confidence range for the pooled data is narrower still.

Let us now return to Figure 5-8. Curve B represents a drug that is less potent than A but has the same slope. One might wish, typically, to compare the toxicities of A and B quantitatively. From data obtained in groups of mice one will ask: "Is A really more toxic than B, or does the separation of sample lines on a log dose-probit plot arise by chance?" If there is a real difference, how much more toxic is A than B?" "What is the true potency ratio (or toxicity ratio) of the two drugs, and what confidence limits can be placed on such a ratio?" Illustrative examples of such comparative toxicity evaluations will be presented, but again the reader is referred elsewhere for details of the procedures for arriving at these estimates.

If two log dose-probit curves are not parallel, it makes no sense to compare their potencies. Consider B and C in Figure 5-8. Evidently the two drugs do not kill mice by the same mechanism, for the population responds more uniformly to C than to B. At probit 5 (LD50), both have the same potency. At probit 6 (84% lethality), C is

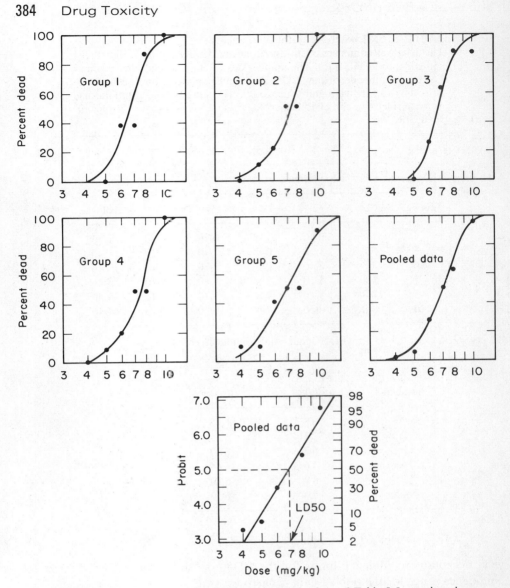

FIGURE 5-9. Toxicity of guthion in mice. *The data of Table 5-5 are plotted as log-dose percent mortality curves for each group of mice and for the pooled data. Horizontal scale is logarithmic, but actual doses are indicated. The log dose-probit curve for the pooled data is shown at bottom.*

more potent; at probit 4 (16% lethality), B is more potent. Any statement about comparative toxicity would have to be qualified by specifying what portion of the dose-mortality curve was under consideration.

    Initial toxicity tests are often carried out just as described above. Even while determining the mouse LD50 values, however, important clues may be obtained about mechanisms of toxicity. Do the animals convulse before death? Does respiration cease before the heart fails? Are there signs of gastrointestinal disturbance? Does muscular paralysis occur? Although species often differ from each other, a particular toxic effect may nevertheless occur universally, so that information gathered in any species should guide one's eventual testing of a drug in man.[101]

In order to arrive at an estimate of the therapeutic ratio, a method must be chosen for demonstrating the therapeutic effect in test animals, if that is possible. Here, the most appropriate species can be used, not necessarily the same as for the toxicity tests. It might be thought that a meaningful comparison of therapeutic and toxic doses would have to be carried out in one and the same species. However, even if lethal and therapeutic effects were both measured in mice, the therapeutic ratio thus arrived at could not be assumed to apply to man. The whole procedure should rather be regarded as an arbitrary one, primarily useful for comparing different drugs. Thus, two agents might be studied for their ability to reduce blood sugar levels in diabetic dogs. The dose required to bring about some specified effect, such as lowering the blood sugar concentration to some arbitrary value within a certain time, would be determined in a series of dogs, so that an ED50 value could be found for each drug. The LD50 values for the same two drugs would be obtained in mice, as already described. Then that drug with the greatest ratio [LD50 (mice)]/[ED50 (hypoglycemia, dogs)] would be considered the most promising in this particular evaluation.

It has been argued that to express the margin of safety as the therapeutic ratio LD50/ED50 is wholly unrealistic. Certainly in man the median lethal dose is of academic interest only. Even the median toxic dose would not be a useful measure because one is interested in obtaining therapeutic effects in nearly all patients, if possible, at a dosage that is toxic to practically none. The criterion we really want is a therapeutic ratio based on a dose that is toxic to perhaps 1% of patients, and a dose that is effective in 99% of patients. We might look for the ratio LD1/ED99 in animal tests. If all quantal LDR curves had the same slopes, then it would make no difference what ratio were chosen; the ratio LD1/ED99, for example, would always be a fixed fraction of the ratio LD50/ED50. But variation of slopes with different drugs and even different effects of the same drug complicates the situation.

Figure 5-10 illustrates theoretically how slopes influence the interpretation of a therapeutic ratio. Judged by the TD50/ED50 criterion, drug A appears safer; its therapeutic ratio is 2 dose units on the log scale, whereas the therapeutic ratio for B is only 1 dose unit. Because the slopes in A are rather flat, however, there is a larger overlap of efficacy and toxicity. The ED90 dose (probit 6.28), for example, corresponds to TD10 (probit 3.72); thus, at a dose effective in 90% of those treated, 10% of the animals would experience drug toxicity. In contrast, with drug B, despite the smaller margin of safety at probit 5, one can select a dose that is effective in 99% (probit 7.33) yet causes toxicity in only 1% (probit 2.67). Drug B seems preferable because the steep slopes of its log dose-effect and log dose-toxicity curves reduce the extent of overlap. But from a practical standpoint steep curves have serious disadvantages. Fluctuations in drug level are inevitable because of variation in drug absorption and elimination and because of periodicity of dosage schedules (cf. Chapter 4). The steeper the curve, the more readily can overshoot occur into the toxic range. Thus, inadvertent overdosage would be more hazardous with B than with A because a relatively smaller dose range lies between the TD1 and TD99. The situation becomes even more complex if, as frequently happens, the effect and toxicity curves are not even parallel.

Data of this kind on efficacy and toxicity in man are presented in Figure 5-11. Digitoxin was administered therapeutically to patients with atrial fibrillation. A reduction of 40–50% in heart rate was the criterion of therapeutic response, vomiting

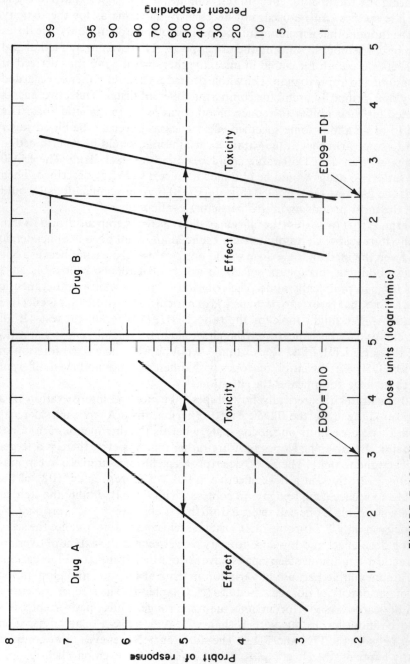

FIGURE 5-10. Effect of slope on the method of expressing the therapeutic ratio. *Log dose-probit curves for 2 hypothetical drugs, A and B, showing relationship between therapeutic effect and toxicity. These curves are steeper for drug B than for drug A. Scale of abscissas is in equal logarithmic increments of dosage. See text for analysis.*

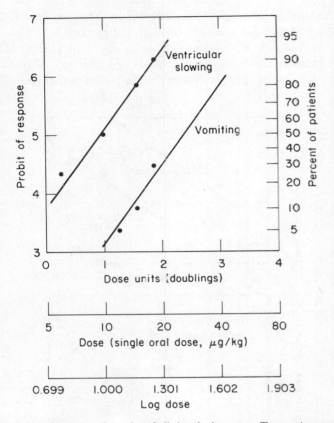

FIGURE 5.11. Therapeutic ratio of digitoxin in man. *Ten patients with atrial fibrillation were given a single oral dose of digitoxin at intervals of 1 week. The percent of patients showing a decrease of 40–50% in heart rate is shown in curve at left, the percent responding with nausea and vomiting is shown in curve at right. The dose scale on the x axis is shown in three ways. At top the unit dose is 5 µg kg^{-1}, and successive doublings of this dose are indicated by integers 1, 2, 3, 4. On middle line is scale of actual doses spaced logarithmically. On bottom scale are logarithms of doses. (Redrawn from Marsh, Figure 7.*[102] *By permission of Charles C. Thomas.)*

was the criterion of toxic response. The rather flat slopes indicate how variable human responses are likely to be. Here, the standard deviation is 0.21 on the log scale, corresponding to a dose factor of 1.6 (antilog 0.21 = 1.6). At a dose of 10 µg kg^{-1}, a therapeutic response would be obtained in only one-half of all patients. At 16 µg kg^{-1}, only 84% would respond; at 6.2 µg kg^{-1}, 16% would respond. The therapeutic ratio is not large. Measured at probit 5, TD50 = antilog 1.42, and ED50 = antilog 0.98; therefore TD50/ED50 = antilog (1.42 − 0.98) = 2.8. But the overlap of the curves is so great that a therapeutic ratio computed as TD1/ED99 would be much smaller than unity, i.e., at a dosage producing a therapeutic result in 99% of patients, vomiting would occur in much more than 1%. As a matter of fact, even at the ED50 three patients in every 100 would display this toxic symptom. Thus digitoxin has to be administered very cautiously, and the dosage has to be individualized. A cardiac glycoside with a larger therapeutic ratio would be a very useful drug, and pharmaceutical firms have spent much money and effort on the search. But, although many compounds with digitalis-like activity are known, none has yet been found to have a therapeutic ratio substantially greater than that of digitoxin.

A comparative study of two analgesic drugs in man is presented in Figure 5-12. These are not quantal LDR curves; responses are averages of measured graded effects in a large number of patients. Studies of pain relief in man are extraordinarily

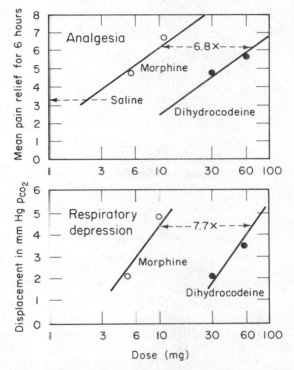

FIGURE 5-12. Comparison of analgesic and respiratory depressant effects of morphine and dihydrocodeine in man. *Patients with pathologic pain were used. Pain relief was scored on an arbitrary scale for 6 hr after drug administration. Average pain relief for 68 administrations of each drug at 2 doses is shown in upper curves. Respiratory depression was measured by the diminished sensitivity of alveolar ventilation to CO_2; results are shown in lower curves. (Adapted from Seed et al., Figures 2 and 4.[103])*

difficult to carry out properly. Subjects and drug sequences have to be randomized, double-blind technique is essential, and placebo reactions must be taken into account[104] (cf. chapter 14). Nevertheless, some clear-cut results have been obtained, as in these experiments. About 68 mg of dihydrocodeine was equivalent to 10 mg of morphine in analgesic potency, indicating that dihydrocodeine is the less potent drug by a factor of 7. However, it might well be superior for clinical use if it could be shown, at doses producing the same degree of analgesia, to be less potent in causing respiratory depression, a serious side effect of morphine. The figure shows clearly, however, that the relative potencies of the two drugs in producing respiratory depression were just about the same as for their analgesic effects. Moreover, both drugs produced some degree of respiratory depression even at the lowest analgesic doses.

As with nausea and vomiting in the case of the digitalis glycosides, so also here in the series of morphine-like analgesics it has not yet been possible to separate the major side effect from the desired therapeutic action.

Information about the metabolism of a drug is important in the evaluation of its toxicity. As pointed out in Chapter 3, drugs may be metabolized quite differently in different species; not only do rates vary, but the pathways may be dissimilar. No firm predictions can be made about this from one species to another; and although there is probably a general similarity between man and the other primates, even here no systematic proofs have been adduced. The mode of drug metabolism can affect the toxicity in several ways. Sometimes a metabolite is responsible for the principal toxic effects. Then if the preclinical testing is conducted in animals that do not form a toxic metabolite, whereas humans do, serious toxicity may be discovered unexpectedly during the clinical trials. Conversely, if the species used for testing does form such a metabolite, but man does not, a potentially safe and useful drug might be discarded. Another source of misleading information is species variation in rates of drug metabolism (p. 283). Yet another problem is raised by the development of drug tolerance when a drug induces an increase in the level of the microsomal drug-metabolizing enzymes, and the drug itself is a substrate, so that its rate of metabolism increases with continuing administration.

In addition to acute lethality determinations in mice, and animal tests of biologic effectiveness, new compounds that are candidates for clinical evaluation must undergo a rigorous series of acute and chronic toxicity tests. These tests, now largely prescribed by the Food and Drug Administration, are carried out in a variety of laboratory animals, the highest dose level being set sufficiently high to produce clear-cut toxicity. Hematologic studies and liver and kidney function tests are done routinely, and complete autopsy and histologic examinations are performed. Specially designed experiments seek carcinogenic activity or teratogenic effects in pregnant animals. Table 5-6 summarizes the usual procedures carried out in the stage of preclinical testing.

The usefulness of so much routine toxicologic testing has been questioned sharply,[101,106-107a] but it could also be argued from unfortunate experiences of recent years that extraordinary caution is justified before allowing new drugs to be introduced for widespread use in humans. The only relevant data that could help decide how much testing and what kinds of testing are useful would come from retrospective studies of drugs after their introduction into clinical use. Looking back through the results of animal testing at that stage, one could then get some index of predictability for human toxicity. Unfortunately, this has rarely been done. In one study of this kind[108] six unrelated drugs were considered: a glucocorticoid, a central depressant, an agent that blocks the oxidation of alcohol, a synthetic antibacterial drug, an antibiotic, and a tranquilizer. Each had been subjected to the usual routine acute and chronic toxicity tests, and each had been used in at least 500 patients. Some kinds of human toxicity could not possibly have been detected in certain species; vomiting, for example, does not occur in the rat. Some toxic effects were seen in the dog but not in man. Others occurred in man but not in other species; included here were the very important symptoms of toxicity on the central nervous system, such as headaches, depression, nightmares, tinnitus, giddiness, heartburn, etc., which cannot be detected in nonhuman species.

The study discussed above shows how characteristic differences in species responses to drugs can diminish the predictive value of animal testing. Even more

TABLE 5-6. Toxicologic procedures in animals.
(From Abrams et al.,[105] Table II. By permission of C. V. Mosby.)

I. ACUTE
  1. LD50 determination in rats or mice
  2. Pyramiding single-dose studies in dogs
  3. Local effects (topical or parenteral agents)

II. SUBACUTE
  1. Administration (6–13 weeks) to 40 rats (three dose levels)
  2. Administration (4–13 weeks) to 6 dogs (three dose levels)

III. CHRONIC
  1. Administration (1 year) to rats (three dose levels)
  2. Administration (six months) to dogs (three dose levels)
  3. Administration (six months) to a third species
  4. Reproduction experiments in rats and rabbits

IV. SPECIAL STUDIES
  1. Metabolism: absorption, blood, and tissue levels, transportation across membranes, excretion
  2. Effects on physiologic functions: blood pressure, cardiac output, respiration, renal function, central nervous system activity, hormonal effects, influences on appetite
  3. Histochemical studies when indicated

---

perplexing is the finding that the same toxic effect may occur in many species, but under different conditions and in response to different drugs. The evaluation of teratogenic action is plagued by this problem. As illustrated at length in Chapter 12, there seems to be no reliable way to predict for a new drug whether or not it is likely to cause fetal malformations in the human, even though it often turns out to be easy enough to demonstrate such an action in some animal under some condition, once the teratogenicity in the human has become evident. If salicylates, for example, were tested under certain conditions in the rat, they would be classed as teratogens, whereas in mice and humans they do not seem to be teratogenic. On the other hand, thalidomide, which is a potent teratogen in the human, does not produce fetal malformations in rats.[109] It is likely that in this important area testing in other primates may yield the most consistent correlations with the human.[110]

In summary, the whole subject of preclinical testing is in a state of flux. It would be foolish to require a lengthy set of routine tests that will have no predictive value. On the other hand, enough is known about the unpredictability of species differences to suggest that testing in the lower animals should include many species. Certainly in many cases a pattern of toxicity will emerge that can serve as a guide for what to expect in man. This is especially true of certain kinds of toxicity involving physiologic and biochemical processes that are equally important in all animal life. Examples are interference with protein and nucleic acid synthesis, steroid metabolism, neurotransmitter function, blood formation, renal tubular absorption and secretion, myocardial contractility, and so on. In general, the best approach would seem to be determined largely by the potential benefit of the new agent. Delay in the introduction of a new drug incident to exhaustive preclinical testing is of no great consequence for patients if effective drugs of the same type are already available. However, in the rare instance where a new agent promises great benefit or even life-saving properties in a disease for which no adequate remedy exists, more risk is obviously acceptable, and the preclinical testing phase should be shortened.

Once a drug has been subjected to adequate preclinical testing, and its animal toxicity is known, it can be evaluated for therapeutic effect in man. A dose is selected that is well below what has been found to have any effect at all in animals. The subjects are under the constant supervision of clinical investigators who are on their guard for signs of untoward reactions. Naturally, the number of subjects is small, and doses are carefully increased to the point where the desired therapeutic effect is obtained or signs of toxicity appear. It is later on, when tight control of the drug is relaxed, and it becomes more widely available for clinical use under less rigidly controlled conditions, that difficulties often arise.

Regulations of the Food and Drug Administration prescribe appropriate procedures to be followed and the kind of information that must be accumulated and submitted before approval is given for wider distribution of a drug. Nevertheless, it has been a recurring theme, documented amply in the medical literature, that a drug heralded as having little or no toxicity when first introduced turns out to have significant toxic effects. Several reasons may be suggested for this consistent underestimation of the toxicity of new agents.

The toxic reaction may be a rare event.   Suppose the incidence of toxicity is only 1 in 1000. It is very unlikely to be picked up in preliminary testing, but it will surely emerge after the drug has been used widely. Drug toxicity associated with idiosyncratic responses based on genetic abnormalities falls into this class. Examples are the prolonged apnea occasionally seen after succinylcholine administration (p. 444), the primaquine-induced hemolytic anemias (p. 455), and the porphyrias enhanced by drugs (p. 463). But many rare toxicities are not known to have a genetic basis. The antibiotic chloramphenicol was used extensively for 2 years before it was realized that at high dosage it could cause severe agranulocytosis and aplastic anemia, sometimes fatal; the incidence was only 1 out of 50,000 or 100,000 patients.[111,112] After chloramphenicol had been in use for 17 years it was discovered that its prolonged use could lead to visual impairment.[113,114] Of course, a useful drug should be retained in clinical use even when it is found to have rare toxic effects. On the other hand, such a drug should not be used for trivial purposes, and not at all if a safer compound will serve equally well.

Rare or sporadic toxicity may sometimes be caused by impurities irregularly associated with a drug, or to a drug metabolite, rather than by the drug itself. The volatile anesthetic halothane provides an instructive example. After about a decade of use it became evident that severe liver damage could occur rarely, probably at an incidence of about 1 in 10,000 administrations. An analysis of the commercially available halothane by gas chromatography revealed the presence of several contaminants. One of these, dichlorohexafluorobutene, was present to the extent of about

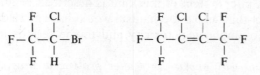

Halothane   Dichlorohexafluorobutene

0.02%.[115,116] This material could be shown to be hepatotoxic. The commercial synthesis of halothane was altered to eliminate this contaminant, but very rare cases of liver toxicity still occur.[117] There appears to be no way to decide, in view of the uncertainty of the incidence data, whether or not the situation has been improved. The halothane experience raises a general question: Might other drug toxicities also be due to impurities, by-products, isomers, and so on, not ordinarily removed by conventional procedures for drug synthesis or isolation? Obviously, the standards of purity that were acceptable 25 years ago have to be revised to conform to modern analytical and preparative techniques.

A major advance in understanding and dealing with rare toxicities is to determine the metabolic products of new drugs in man, when the first clinical tests are made. These drug metabolites are then subjected to toxicity and efficacy testing in animals.

A problem with rare toxicities is the difficulty of collecting adequate information. Suppose a physician observes that one of his patients develops a blood dyscrasia. Is it a manifestation of the existing disease? Is it a sign of a new disease process? Or is it caused by a drug; and if so, by which of several drugs the patient may have been taking? The blood disorder may even appear well after drug therapy has been terminated, and the history of previous medication may be uncertain. Unless the physician suspects a particular drug, the case is not likely to be reported at all. Occasionally, a physician will write a letter of inquiry to the pharmaceutical firm that markets the drug, asking if other physicians have had similar experiences. New regulations of the Food and Drug Administration require pharmaceutical firms to make their files of such letters available to inspectors.

Some organized attempts have been made to collect information on untoward drug effects. For example, the Registry of Blood Dyscrasias, under the auspices of the American Medical Association, solicited information for several years about blood disorders associated with drug administration and frequently published pooled data and interpretations. However, such an approach to the reporting problem does not secure information about the frequency of toxic reaction. The "denominator"— the total drug usage—is missing, and without that, no useful correlations can be deduced about the hazard or relative safety of a particular drug.

This data-collection and evaluation service of the AMA, under the new name of Registry of Adverse Drug Reactions,[118] has now been expanded to include all drugs. Other data-collection mechanisms have been established to assess teratogenic hazards (Perinatal Collaborative Study), the toxicity of halothane anesthesia (National Halothane Study), and so forth. Extensive tabulations of rare untoward drug reactions have been published.[119] What the public welfare really requires, in place of these ad hoc procedures, is a nationwide or worldwide data-collection system, feeding into a computerized monitoring program. Such a system, for which the technology is already at hand, would detect unusual associations between particular drugs and adverse effects. Whenever such an association occurred at a frequency greater than expected by chance, attention would be called quickly and automatically to the potential hazard. A pilot system of this kind is described beginning on p. 814. It is evident in retrospect that such a mechanism would have alerted us at least a year in advance to the chloramphenicol toxicity and to the serious teratogenic effects of thalidomide (p. 717).

The toxic reaction may appear only after prolonged drug administration. This presents a thorny problem because, if chronic toxicity studies in animals are carried on for a very long time (e.g. the lifetime of the animal), the introduction of useful new drugs will inevitably be delayed. Even after a drug fails to cause any harm to animals in a toxicity test of very long duration, it may nevertheless still produce damage on long-term administration to humans. With respect to any new drug that is to be used constantly, year in and year out, in patients, the argument could be made that safety on long-term administration remains unproved. At the time of their introduction into widespread use, this could have been said about vitamins, hormone preparations, antimalarials, food additives, steroid oral contraceptives, and even the chlorination or fluoridation of water supplies.

Possible carcinogenicity epitomizes the dilemma. The conservative point of view, now in effect, is that any compound, at any dose, that causes cancer in animals (usually mice) is liable to be prohibited for human use. It is not known, however, whether the human is more or less susceptible to carcinogenic agents than are mice. Nor is it known if an agent that causes a low incidence of tumors in mice poses any real threat to man, especially when given only infrequently, at lower relative dosage, to adults who may already have lived more than one-half their life span. A parenteral iron preparation (iron dextran injection) was withdrawn from the market because it was found to cause cancer under some conditions in mice. Subsequently, because it was considered to be of value therapeutically, its re-introduction was permitted. Nevertheless, as with chloramphenicol, the wise physician will keep the possible toxicity in mind and not use such a drug if safer ones can be used instead. Here the standard orally administered iron preparations are usually adequate; only in special circumstances is a parenteral iron preparation called for.

Chronic administration of streptomycin results in a high incidence of neurologic damage, manifested by hearing deficit and disorders of equilibrium. Yet the great potential benefit of this drug in certain cases of tuberculosis and other infections may outweigh even so serious a hazard.

At the other extreme we have instances in which toxic new drugs were introduced, and serious damage was caused without valid evidence of therapeutic efficacy. A notorious example was triparanol (MER-29), an agent that was shown to inhibit the reductive conversion of desmosterol (24-dehydrocholesterol) to cholesterol. Administration of this drug lowers blood cholesterol levels and accordingly raises blood desmosterol levels.[120] It might have been predicted, a priori, that an inhibitor of cholesterol biosynthesis would have widespread effects on the body, including a decrease in the production of corticosteroids. Nevertheless, the drug was introduced and vigorously promoted for the treatment of hypercholesterolemia, especially in atherosclerotic individuals. Only later did it become apparent that triparanol caused severe chronic toxicity, including cataracts, ichthyosis, alopecia, leukopenia, and diminished libido.[121,122] As a result, the drug was removed from the market. The therapeutic efficacy of this drug in atherosclerosis had never been established. Curiously, too, the manufacturer's reports on the preclinical tests gave little indication of chronic toxicity, yet animal experiments afterwards clearly demonstrated severe chronic toxicity in rats.[123] Subsequently it was charged in the courts that evidence of chronic toxicity had been concealed; the defendants pleaded no contest and were heavily fined.[124,125] It seems fair to point out that episodes like this, coupled with abuses in drug promotion and advertising, helped create the atmosphere in which legislation was passed (in 1962) giving stricter regulatory powers to the Food and Drug Administration.

The toxic effect may not have been detected in any of the animal species used for preclinical testing. The effect may even be unique to man, or to some particular period of human life. The failure of animal testing to reveal toxicity is characteristic of the nonlethal adverse effects that commonly limit the use of drugs in man. Examples of reactions not readily observable in experimental animals are headache, nausea, insomnia, and psychotic disturbances. Some toxic manifestations in humans may be utterly bizarre and unexpected. The thalidomide episode (p.717) is typical of this class of toxic reaction. The drug causes fetal malformations when taken by pregnant women. Prior to the epidemic of human toxicity, no laboratory tests for teratogenic effects had been developed. Many animal species are not affected.

Another example of wholly unexpected, bizarre toxicity is that caused by the monoamine oxidase inhibitor tranylcypromine in people who eat cheeses rich in tyramine or whose intake of sympathomimetic amines is otherwise enhanced (p. 272).

The newborn infant is peculiarly vulnerable to certain types of drug toxicity. He has a low level of drug-metabolizing enzymes, and his renal excretory system is not fully developed. Drug toxicities in the newborn, that once seemed inexplicable, are now better understood and can be avoided. These include chloramphenicol toxicity (p. 291), and kernicterus caused by vitamin K or sulfonamides displacing unconjugated bilirubin from plasma proteins (p. 821). Another interesting example of the vulnerability of the very young to otherwise innocuous agents is the often-fatal methemoglobinemia seen in infants less than six months old, whose feeding formulas are made with water (e.g., rural well water) containing inorganic nitrate. A nitrate concentration as low as 50 mg liter^{-1} may be toxic. Three factors are responsible. First, the low acidity of the stomach contents of infants permits invasion of the upper gastrointestinal tract by nitrate-reducing bacteria. The resulting nitrite is absorbed, and it is the direct cause of the methemoglobinemia.[126] Second, fetal hemoglobin is more easily converted to methemoglobin than is the adult form, and young infants still have considerable amounts of fetal hemoglobin in their blood. Third, infants are less able than older children to reduce methemoglobin back to the ferrous form, because they are deficient in the essential enzymes.[127] These last two factors also explain why the young infant is more prone to develop methemoglobinemia from other compounds like sulfonamides, ethylaminobenzoate, *p*-nitroaniline, and aniline dyes.[128]

TREATMENT OF TOXICITY

Principles of Nonspecific Therapy

Certain immediate measures are called for in every case of poisoning, regardless of the cause. First attention is given to maintaining respiration and circulation. Then it is important to find out what drug was taken, and how much of it, so that rational procedures can be followed. Further absorption of the toxic agent into the circulation should be stopped or retarded, but the appropriate steps depend upon the route of administration. If the drug was ingested and the patient remains conscious, vomiting should be induced. Various means may be employed, such as mechanical gagging, emetics (e.g., syrup of ipecac, mustard powder) by mouth, and injection of apomorphine. However, vomiting should not be induced if the toxic agent is corrosive (lye, kerosene, etc.), for it may cause hemorrhage or perforation of the esophagus or stomach. If the patient is unconscious, and a noncorrosive agent was ingested, then gastric lavage may be carried out, but only after insertion of an endotracheal tube, to avoid the possibility of asphyxiation by inhalation of vomitus. Activated charcoal or large amounts of protein may be given by mouth to adsorb toxic material and retard its further absorption from the gastrointestinal tract. Quantitative studies on the absorption of various substances have shown that plain activated charcoal is more effective than the so-called "universal antidote" containing magnesium oxide and tannic acid as well.[129,130] If the drug was given subcutaneously or intramuscularly, attempts may be made to delay its absorption by applying tourniquets proximal to the injection site, as in the first-aid treatment of snake bite. Obviously, if the toxic substance is being absorbed through the skin, thorough washing is indicated.

The most important reason for ascertaining exactly what agent is responsible for the toxic effects is that some poisons can be treated with specific antidotes. If a patient is found unconscious and no further information can be obtained, then general supportive therapy will be initiated, the principles of which are discussed below. But the prognosis may be improved greatly, indeed the victim's condition may even be changed for the better in a moment, if the poison is identified and the specific antidote is given. Unfortunately, in all too many cases it is hard to find out what poison was taken. It is not yet customary to label all prescription medications with the name of the drug. Frequently, a child or a person attempting suicide has emptied a container that bears no indication of the nature of the contents. Time has to be wasted in frantic telephone calls to relatives, pharmacists and physicians in the attempt to identify the medication. All medications should be labeled. This is accomplished very simply; the physician has only to request it on the prescription blank. Household and commercial products that are potentially toxic are now required to bear appropriate cautionary labels and to name the toxic ingredients. Poison control centers have useful files of information about toxic substances in household and commercial use.

Inasmuch as no specific antidotes are known for most drugs and poisons, the aims of treatment are to support the vital functions and hasten drug elimination. These essentials of nonspecific treatment are illustrated well by the management of poisoning due to barbiturates, the agents most frequently used in suicide attempts. Because here the life-threatening toxic effects are central respiratory depression and secondary circulatory collapse, primary attention is directed to maintaining a free airway and administering artificial respiration as required. Gastric lavage is never undertaken in an unconscious patient unless a cuffed endotracheal or tracheotomy tube is in place, to avoid any possibility of airway occlusion by vomitus. Even when the airway is protected, gastric lavage is limited to those occasions when the poison has been ingested very recently and is known not to be corrosive to the mucosa of the esophagus and stomach.

There has been much controversy over the use of analeptic drugs in poisonings by barbiturates or other central depressant drugs. These analeptics (pentylenetetrazol, picrotoxin, bemegride) are certainly capable of stimulating the respiration of experimental animals depressed by barbiturates; and when the depression is mild, they also show an awakening effect. However, their effectiveness is much diminished at deeper levels of barbiturate depression. In the 1940's in Denmark, a concerted attack on the problem of poisoning by central depressants was initiated.[131-133] Treatment was centralized in certain hospitals, where emergency teams stood ready day and night. Emphasis was placed upon restoring and maintaining the vital functions, and experts were trained in the important techniques. The mortality rate fell dramatically (Figure 5-13). When analeptics were completely abandoned (in 1949), the results continued to improve. Over a period of 15 years the mortality was reduced from 25 % to less than 1 %. It is difficult to attribute this impressive accomplishment to any single

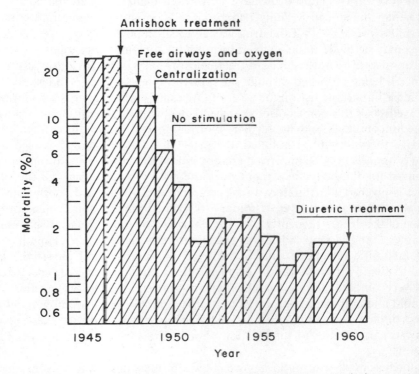

FIGURE 5-13. Mortality trend in poisonings due to central depressants upon improvement of nonspecific treatment methods in Copenhagen. *Barbiturates accounted for more than 75% of the poisonings. Scale of ordinates is logarithmic. The figures are from the official Danish medicostatistical bureau; only hospitalized patients were included. "Centralization" refers to the treatment of all cases of poisoning at a few designated centers. (From Myschetzky and Lassen, Figure 5.[132])*

factor; and it is also difficult to prove conclusively from data of this kind that analeptics make matters worse, as the Danish workers claim. It is fair to say that the only important result one could hope for in analeptic treatment would be restoration of respiratory function, and this can be achieved more reliably and with better quantitative control by mechanical means. The "awakening" effect is of no consequence, since the patient will awaken spontaneously when the barbiturate has been eliminated; and the danger of excessive analeptic action, namely convulsions, is a real one. Moreover, the proper use of analeptics, to ensure a sufficient effect yet avoid overstimulation, would require constant intravenous infusion of a short-acting compound (e.g., pentylenetetrazol), with constant monitoring and regulation, a task that should only be undertaken by an expert. The consensus today supports the Danish view that analeptics should never (or almost never) be used.

If adequate oxygenation is maintained by artificial respiration, the blood pressure can usually be supported by intravenous fluids. The use of pressor amines in hemorrhagic and traumatic shock has been abandoned in recent years[134,135] in favor of agents like isoproterenol, which strengthen myocardial contractility and cause peripheral vasodilation, and of α-adrenergic blocking agents like phenoxybenzamine, which relax arterioles and thereby promote better tissue perfusion. In hemorrhagic and traumatic shock the arterioles are constricted reflexly, the catecholamine content of the blood is very high, and blood volume is diminished; despite high peripheral resistance blood pressure is low, so that blood flow through the tissues is poor and venous return and cardiac output are low. It is still somewhat uncertain to what extent the same physiologic disturbances are present in barbiturate overdosage, and to what extent the hypotension may be caused by loss of sympathetic tone at the arterioles, resulting from depression of central vasomotor outflow. In barbiturate poisoning, if intravenous fluids alone will not restore an adequate blood pressure, it may be rational to use pressor amines. However, the increasing tendency is to avoid complicating a relatively simple problem of central depression by administering additional drugs, each with its own potential toxicity. Moreover, systolic blood pressures as low as 60 mm Hg are compatible with adequate perfusion of the vital organs. Attention is properly focused upon the central venous pressure (measured by a polyethylene catheter threaded up the antecubital vein to the vena cava) and the urine output (measured by an indwelling catheter), rather than upon blood pressure alone.[136,137]

Another significant advance of recent years has been the increasing use of hemodialysis, as simpler and cheaper units have become available. It is interesting to note that the original artificial kidney was designed by J. J. Abel (1857–1938), the first American pharmacologist, with a view to the treatment of drug poisoning.[138] The modern artificial kidney is used successfully to remove such drugs as salicylates, long-acting barbiturates, glutethimide, bromide, and methanol from the blood. Hemodialysis is primarily useful in hastening the elimination of drugs that would otherwise persist at dangerous levels for a very long time; thus, it is pointless in the typical case of poisoning by a short-acting barbiturate. Moreover, drugs that are largely bound to plasma protein at toxic concentrations cannot be removed efficiently by dialysis.

Peritoneal dialysis, which is less complicated but also less efficient than hemodialysis, is occasionally used, especially in infants. Here an isotonic fluid is introduced into the peritoneal cavity, then evacuated and replaced periodically.[139] The toxic drug diffuses across the peritoneal membranes in accordance with its concentration gradient. Efficiency is enhanced by application of the ion trapping principle (p. 144) through the use of buffered slightly alkaline solutions to remove weak acids like phenobarbital ($pK_a = 7.2$). Peritoneal dialysis, like hemodialysis, requires very careful attention to fluid and electrolyte balance.[140]

The beneficial effects of acidosis or alkalosis in promoting the redistribution of weak acids or bases in the various body compartments have already been considered in detail (p. 175). Administration of bicarbonate results in a transient plasma alkalosis, which promotes a shift of barbiturate out of the brain (and other tissues) into the plasma by the ion-trapping mechanism. This effect of altered plasma pH upon the distribution of a weak electrolyte between tissues and plasma was illustrated in Figure 2-22. Since the nonionized form of a drug is at the same concentration on both sides of biologic membranes, it follows that the magnitude of the inequality of *total* drug concentration will depend upon two factors, the pH gradient and the pK_a of the drug. The limits between which the plasma and urine pH values can be manipulated are narrow—a few tenths of a pH unit for the plasma, a few pH units for urine. The proportional rate of change of the nonionized form with respect to pH is given by the following equation,[141] obtained by differentiating the Henderson–Hasselbalch equation (cf. p. 19):

$$\frac{d(HA)/d(pH)}{(HA)} = -\ln 10 \left[\frac{10^{pH}}{10^{pH} + 10^{pK_a}} \right]$$

This expression gives the change of (HA) relative to the concentration already present. When the equation is solved for pH 7.4 and the proportional change in (HA) is plotted as a function of pK_a, the curve shown in Figure 5-14 is obtained. It can be

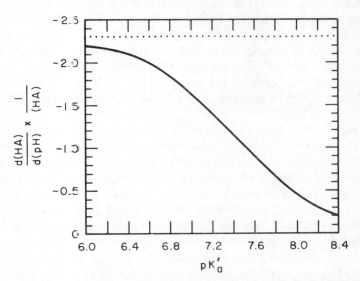

FIGURE 5-14. Proportional rate of change with pH of the nonionized form of a weak acid at pH 7.4. *The curve is plotted from the equation given above. Proportional rate of change of the nonionized form of the acid is given as ordinates, pK_a' as abscissas. The dotted line is the asymptote approached by the function as pK_a' decreases. (From Waddell and Butler, Figure 1.[141])*

seen that the maximal proportional rate of change is obtained with weak acids whose pK_a is about 6 or lower, and the minimal value is attained with drugs whose pK_a is about 8 or higher. This shows quantitatively how much more effective is alkalinization of plasma, urine, or peritoneal wash fluids for removing the more acidic drugs (like salicylates or even phenobarbital [$pK_a = 7.2$]) than acids that are weaker than phenobarbital. In the barbiturate class, it so happens that most of the short-acting compounds, like pentobarbital and secobarbital, have pK_a values in the range 7.6–8.0,[142] and are therefore more difficult to eliminate by ion-trapping mechanisms.

The shifting of acidic drugs from tissues into plasma by producing a transient metabolic alkalosis would be of no long-term benefit were it not for the accompanying effect on reabsorption from tubular urine; the excreted bicarbonate alkalinizes the urine, so that the back-diffusion of the drug is greatly retarded and the total drug output in the urine is increased. Quite apart from the influence of alkalinization, forced diuresis in itself significantly increases the renal clearance of any drug that is largely reabsorbed under conditions of low urine output.[143] This phenomenon is shown clearly in Figure 5-15. At both acid and alkaline urine pH, the renal clearance

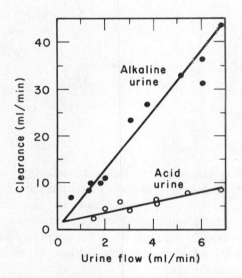

FIGURE 5-15. Renal clearance of phenobarbital as a function of urine flow in dogs. *Diuresis was induced by oral water, intravenous mercaptomerin, or intravenous sodium sulfate. In lower curve, urine pH was below 7.0; in the experiments shown in upper curve, sodium bicarconate was given intravenously so that urine pH was 7.8–8.0. Clearances were computed from the concentration of unbounded drug in plasma. (From Waddell and Butler, Figure 4.[141])*

of phenobarbital was found to be a linear function of the urine flow. The osmotic diuretics, urea or mannitol, are commonly used to promote a diuresis as great as 12 liters in 24 hr, alkalinization being achieved with bicarbonate or lactate. Such a regimen has been shown to reduce the period of barbiturate coma by two-thirds, compared with patients not so treated; the need for tracheotomy was reduced by one-half, and the overall mortality was further reduced compared with that achieved by respiratory management alone.[132,144] Of course, forced diuresis of any type is not employed in the presence of anuria or serious renal damage occasioned by the toxic material. Alkaline diuresis becomes distinctly less advantageous with increasing pK_a value of the drug.

The efficiency of various techniques of promoting the clearance of long-acting barbiturates is summarized in Table 5-7. Hemodialysis effects the greatest increase in clearance, but since it is used intermittently, the total amount of barbiturate removed per day is about the same as with alkaline diuresis.

TABLE 5-7. Efficiency of various types of active treatment of acute barbiturate intoxication.

Values shown below are approximate only, and are estimates from various studies with long-acting barbiturates. The values given for hemodialysis assume 8 hr of dialysis plus 16 hr of spontaneous clearance per 24 hr. (Data of Myschetzky[132] Table 6).

Treatment	Urine volume (liters 24 hr^{-1})	pH	Clearance (ml min^{-1})	Clearance (liters 24 hr^{-1})
Spontaneous	1.5	6	1	1.5
Diuretics				
mercurials, fluids	5	6	3.5	5
mannitol	9	6	6	9
osmotic diuretic plus alkalinization	12	7.5–8	17	24
Hemodialysis (8 hr only)			35	18

Principles of Antidotal Treatment

The limited number of specific antidotes that are available[145] are listed in Table 5-8. They will be discussed as examples of the various mechanisms of antidotal action. As more information becomes available about the biochemical mechanisms of toxicity, more such antidotes will undoubtedly be developed. Unlike the discovery of new drug actions, where chance has often been more important than foresight, rational selection and even deliberate synthesis have played important roles in the development of specific antidotes.

Mechanism 1. Antidote Complexes with Poison, Rendering It Inert

Heavy Metals. The treatment of poisoning due to heavy metals offers the simplest example of this mechanism. Chelating agents are used to form tightly bound nontoxic complexes with the metal ions. This reduces the concentration of free metal ions in the body fluids and thus promotes the dissociation of bound metal from tissue enzymes and other functional macromolecules. Typically the metal-chelate complexes are water soluble and can be excreted by the kidney. Thus the total body load of metal is reduced. The principles of chelation, with some examples, have already been presented in Chapter 1.

Poisoning by arsenic or mercury is specifically combatted by dimercaprol. This antidote was developed during World War II for protection against the arsenical gas lewisite; hence the original designation British anti-lewisite (BAL).[146] This compound holds the distinction of being the first antidotal agent synthesized on a rational basis. Arsenic was known to inhibit enzymes containing essential sulfhydryl groups, and small SH-containing molecules like cysteine and glutathione were found to offer some protection to experimental animals. The principle of chelation in stable 5-membered or 6-membered ring compounds (cf. Chapter 1) suggested that dithiols might complex arsenic more firmly than monothiols do. Out of many compounds tested, dimercaprol (dimercaptopropanol) proved most effective. The vicinal sulfhydryl

TABLE 5-8. Toxic agents, specific antidotes, and mechanisms of antidotal action.

Toxic agent	Specific antidote
Mechanism 1: Antidote complexes with poison, rendering it inert	
Arsenic, mercury	Dimercaprol (BAL)
Lead, plutonium, uranium	Dimercaprol; calcium disodium edetate (EDTA); diethylene-triamine pentaacetic acid (DTPA); penicillamine
Iron	Sodium ferrocyanide (by mouth); deferoxamine
Copper	Penicillamine; EDTA
Thallium	Dithizone (?)[a]
Formaldehyde	Ammonia (by mouth)
Heparin	Protamine
Botulinus toxin and other toxins	Botulinus antitoxin and other antitoxins
Various drugs	Specific antibodies (?)[a]
Digitalis glycosides	Steroid binding resins
Cholinesterase inhibitors	Pralidoxime
Cyanide	Methemoglobin (formed by nitrite administration)
Mechanism 2: Antidote accelerates metabolic conversion of poison to nontoxic product	
Cyanide	Thiosulfate
Mechanism 3: Antidote blocks metabolic formation of poison from less toxic precursor	
Methanol	Ethanol
Selenocystathionine	Cystine
Fluoroacetate	Acetate; monoacetin
Mechanism 4: Antidote specifically accelerates excretion of poison	
Bromide	Chloride
Strontium, radium	Calcium salts
Mechanism 5: Antidote competes with poison for essential receptors	
Carbon monoxide	Oxygen
Curare (tubocurarine)	Neostigmine; edrophonium
Coumarin anticoagulants	Vitamin K
Morphine, related narcotics	Naloxone; related antagonists
Thallium	Potassium salts
Amino acid analogs	Amino acids
Mechanism 6: Antidote blocks receptors that are responsible for toxic effect	
Cholinesterase inhibitors	Atropine
Mechanism 7: Antidote restores normal function by repairing or by-passing effect of poison	
Agents that produce methemoglobinemia	Methylene blue
Digitalis glycosides	Potassium salts; β-adrenergic blocking agents; procaine amide
Botulinus toxin	Guanidine
Methotrexate, other folic acid antagonists	Folinic acid; thymidine + purine + glycine
5-Fluorouracil	Thymidine
6-Mercaptopurine	Purines

[a] The symbol (?) indicates practical efficacy of antidote not well established, or doubtful.

groups form a stable mercaptide ring with appropriate metal ions, while the alcohol group serves to confer water solubility upon the whole complex. Dimercaprol

$$
\begin{array}{ll}
CH_2-SH & CH_2-S \\
| & | \quad \quad As-R \\
CH-SH & CH-S \\
| & | \\
CH_2OH & CH_2OH
\end{array}
$$

dimercaprol   arsenic mercaptide

finds use chiefly in arsenic, mercury, and lead poisonings, but it is also effective in the less common poisonings by gold, bismuth, and polonium. Scattered reports indicate its probable usefulness in antimony, chromium, and nickel poisonings. Unfortunately, like other thiols, it has considerable toxicity of its own, so that it has to be administered very cautiously. No exact dosage can be stated. Enough has to be given to complex stoichiometrically with all the toxic metal ions, but a large excess over this has to be avoided. The difficulty of choosing a correct dose is increased by the complicated time course to be expected; free metal ions in the body fluids will be complexed immediately, but the widthdrawal of bound metal from the tissues proceeds much more slowly.

A specific antidote to lead poisoning is calcium disodium edetate (EDTA), the structure and properties of which were presented earlier (p. 11). The very high stability constants of EDTA for lead, nickel, cobalt, and several other metals were shown in Table 1-3. The relatively nontoxic calcium disodium complex, rather than EDTA itself, is used clinically to avoid complexing the essential ionized calcium in the blood plasma. Thus, only metals with greater affinity than calcium will be bound, by displacing Ca^{2+} from the $CaNa_2$-EDTA complex. The stability constant for the complex with Pb^{2+} is 10^7 times greater than that for the Ca^{2+} complex. Dimercaprol and penicillamine (see below under Copper) also bind lead effectively.[146a,146b,146c]

Radioactive metals present special toxicity problems. The amounts in the body are likely to be small, but the long biologic and radioactive half-lives of these elements enhance their toxicity. Plutonium, which is extremely toxic, will be produced in very large amounts by fission-type nuclear reactors; it already poses a significant public health hazard. Plutonium is most effectively removed from the body by complexing it with diethylenetriaminepentaacetic acid (DTPA), a compound closely related to EDTA. Treatment is most successful when it is carried out shortly after exposure and before the plutonium is entirely sequestered in bone.[147,148] Uranium is complexed and removed effectively by calcium disodium edetate.[149] Alkalinization of the urine by administration of bicarbonate also promotes excretion of the uranyl ion, apparently as a nontoxic bicarbonate complex. Strontium and radium are difficult to remove by the known chelating agents, because their binding constants for EDTA and similar compounds are too close to that of calcium; a different principle, competitive displacement, is employed (p. 415).

Iron. Iron poisoning occurs frequently in young children who eat toxic amounts of ferrous sulfate tablets intended for the treatment of iron deficiency anemias in an adult member of the household. The high stability constants of the complexes between iron and EDTA or DTPA (Table 1-3) suggest that calcium disodium edetate ought to be the agent of choice in treating iron poisoning or diseases in which there is abnormal deposition of iron in the tissues. Experimental studies, confirmed by clinical experience, indicate that, although there may be some protective effect with early enough administration, reliable antidotal action cannot be achieved. The reason probably is that iron is bound even more firmly to naturally occurring chelating compounds in the body, such as transferrin, ferritin, and possibly other tissue components.

The absorption of iron from the gastrointestinal tract can be blocked, and its local deleterious actions prevented, by the oral administration of complexing agents. The most promising, in experimental studies, is sodium ferrocyanide ($Na_4Fe(CN)_6$).[150] The ferrocyanide ion is capable of associating with another iron atom (either Fe^{2+} or Fe^{3+}) to form a complex that is extremely insoluble throughout the pH range encountered in the gastrointestinal tract. The EDTA chelates, in contrast, tend to dissociate in an acid medium. Ferrocyanide itself appears to have a very low toxicity when administered by mouth. Clinical reports on the usefulness of this antidote have not yet appeared.

A newly introduced agent for the systemic treatment of iron poisoning is deferoxamine,[151–154] obtained by isolation of a siderochrome pigment from a streptomycete and removal of the bound iron by a chemical procedure. The structure of this compound is shown in Figure 5-16. It chelates iron in an octahedral complex, as shown,

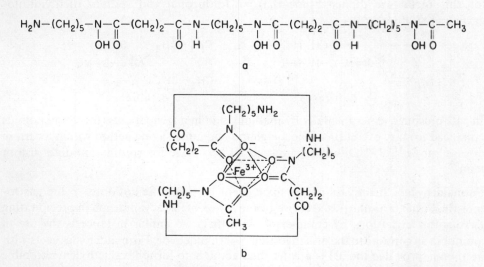

FIGURE 5-16. Deferoxamine and its complex with iron. (*From Moeschlin and Schnider, Figure 1.*[152])

and the stability constant of the complex is greater than 10^{30}. Deferoxamine will remove iron from transferrin and from ferritin, but not from hemoglobin or the cytochromes, to which the metal is bound even more tightly. Thus the chelate stability constant is just in the right range for the removal of excessive iron without disrupting the biologically indispensable iron compounds.

Copper.   Copper poisoning is unusual; when it occurs, calcium disodium edetate may be used. There is, however, a rare genetic disease (Wilson's disease) (cf. Chapter 6) characterized by deficiency of the copper-binding plasma protein, ceruloplasmin, and deposition of copper in the tissues (especially liver and brain). Here, once the disease is diagnosed, large amounts of copper have to be mobilized and excreted, and then the same therapy must be continued on a lifelong basis. An effective orally active drug for this purpose is penicillamine:[155,156]

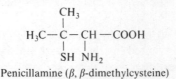

Penicillamine (β, β-dimethylcysteine)

Penicillamine chelates copper about as effectively as does its parent compound cysteine (p. 116). The methyl substituents on the β-carbon atom, however, render the agent more resistant to degradation by cysteine desulfhydrase or L-amino acid oxidase, thus prolonging its biologic half-life.[157] The major drawback to its use is that some patients become allergic to it.

Thallium. Thallium acetate and sulfate were used until recently as rodenticides and as poisons for ants and roaches. Thallium acetate has also been used in Europe as a depilatory agent, especially in children with ringworm. Thus, occasionally, accidental ingestion of thallium salts occurs. The only chelating agents shown to be effective for this metal are diphenylthiocarbazone (dithizone) and sodium diethyldithiocarbamate (dithiocarb):

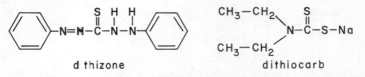

d thizone   dithiocarb

In rats poisoned experimentally by thallium, and in a few patients, these compounds enhanced urinary excretion of the metal and had a life-saving action within a certain dosage range.[158,159] Dithizone, however, is too toxic for routine antidotal use in man.

Formaldehyde. Inactivation of a toxic agent by a specific antidote, in the gastrointestinal tract, was illustrated above by the action of ferrocyanide ion in precipitating ferrous (or ferric) ions by complexing with them. A similar instance is the use of ammonia as antidote to the oral ingestion of formaldehyde. Formaldehyde reacts with ammonia, provided the pH is greater than about 8, to form hexamethylenetetramine (methenamine):

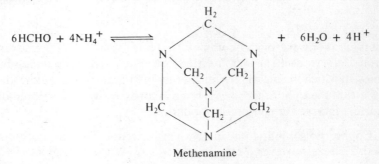

Methenamine

This reaction is more commonly employed in the use of methenamine as a urinary antiseptic. Here, the compound is administered by mouth and excreted into the urine, which must be kept acid in order to drive the reaction to the left, liberating formaldehyde, the presumed antibacterial agent. If a patient has swallowed formaldehyde, the administration of dilute ammonia or of ammonium salts in an alkaline buffered medium should eliminate the highly toxic free formaldehyde from the gastrointestinal tract by driving the same reaction to the right.[160] However, formaldehyde is so reactive that even a short delay would probably make the antidote useless.

Heparin.   Direct combination between an antidote and the toxic agent is also illustrated by the treatment of toxicity due to heparin. This and related polysulfonated polysaccharides interfere with blood coagulation directly, in vitro as well as in vivo. Heparin is believed to block the conversion of prothrombin to thrombin, and also the thrombin-mediated conversion of fibrinogen to fibrin. Because it blocks thrombin formation directly, it is used increasingly in the prophylactic treatment of people with recent myocardial infarction. Its toxicity, manifested as hemorrhages and the consequences of hemorrhages, is primarily an extension of the therapeutic action. Several polycations react directly with heparin in vivo or in vitro, forming nontoxic complexes that are pharmacologically inert. The low-molecular-weight, basic protein protamine, for example, terminates the effects of heparin rapidly when injected intravenously in approximately equimolar amounts.[161] The protamine-heparin complex is excreted by glomerular filtration. In open heart surgery, where heparin is used most commonly, it is desirable to terminate the anticoagulant effects promptly at the conclusion of the operative procedure.

Botulinus Toxin.   The specific antitoxins, although more often considered to lie within the realm of immunology than pharmacology, are certainly germane to this discussion of specific antidotes. The principle of neutralizing a toxin in vivo by an antitoxin represents the most specific example of the direct complexing mechanism whereby the poison is rendered inert. Botulinus toxin is chosen as prototype for consideration here because so much is understood about its mode of action. It is the most potent poison known, with lethal dose estimated to be 0.3 μg in man.[162] The toxin, now isolated as a crystalline protein, is absorbed from the gastrointestinal tract, and then acts throughout the nervous system to block the release of acetylcholine. This causes neuromuscular blockade and paralysis.

If a nerve-muscle preparation in vitro is exposed to a toxin-antitoxin mixture, no abnormality ensues. If the same preparation is exposed to toxin alone, there is a lag of about 30 min, after which the typical neuromuscular blockade develops. After the toxin has been in contact with the tissue, the blockade will develop inevitably, even in the presence of antitoxin. Thus, something that antitoxin cannot reverse happens rapidly, and results later in damage to the mechanism for release of stored acetylcholine.

Botulism is a rare but frequently fatal disease, acquired by eating preserved foods (often meat or fish) in which the causative organism (*Clostridium botulinum*) has grown because of faulty sterilization.[163] At least four antigenically different strains (A, B, E, F) are commonly involved. Antitoxin is prepared in horses by repeated challenge and eventual collection of blood serum. Multivalent antitoxin, effective against all four strains, is obviously indicated whenever doubt exists as to the antigenic type of the toxin.

There has been an element of fatalism about the treatment of this disease, conditioned largely by the difficulty of proving conclusively that the antitoxin is useful. The total number of cases seen annually in the whole world is very small, and certainly no one would deliberately conduct a placebo-controlled trial on desperately ill patients who might be saved by antitoxin. Moreover, the experimental indications that the toxin quickly produces irreversible effects have led to the opinion that once symptoms are manifested it is already too late to treat. Probably this pessimism is unfounded. Whatever the explanation may be, some dramatic recoveries have been seen after antitoxin treatment, even in patients who seemed to be running an inexorably lethal course.[164] There have been some indications that slow absorption of toxin from the intestinal tract might be responsible for the protracted downhill course of some patients. Thus, antitoxin, even late in the disease, could block further progression of symptoms by complexing free toxin as it entered the circulation.

Various Drugs and Specific Antibodies.   The principle of neutralizing a poison by a specific antibody is applied to other bacterial toxins, such as tetanus and diphtheria, as well as to snake venoms. The principle is also possibly applicable to the treatment of drug toxicity, since antibodies can be prepared against numerous drugs. The technique, described fully in Chapter 7, entails attaching the drug covalently to a protein, thereby forming an antigen. Various species (rabbits, goats, horses) respond to injections of such an antigen by making antibodies directed against the drug. Protection against digoxin toxicity in dogs by means of an antibody to digoxin has already been demonstrated.[165]

Digitalis.   Toxicity due to uncontrolled overdosage with these drugs is a serious and common medical problem, which is discussed at length later in this chapter. An interesting development has been the introduction of new steroid-binding resins (cholestyramine, colestipol) to complex and remove drugs of this class.[166] The principle is based on the known enterohepatic circulation of the steroids. They are excreted in the bile and reabsorbed in the intestine; their prolonged biologic half-lives are in part attributable to this process. The resin is administered by mouth in large quantities (e.g., 10 g). Since the digitalis glycosides are effective at very low doses, the total amounts in the body are not great even in the toxic range. Consequently, the binding capacity of the resin does not have to be very large; resins capable of binding only a few nanograms per milligram (i.e., a few ppm) had remarkable effects. In one study, the plasma half-life of digitoxin was reduced from about 5 days to 3 days, and that of digoxin from about $1\frac{1}{2}$ days to 16 hr. The resin, binding the glycoside, prevents its reabsorption, and carries it through the intestinal tract and into the feces.

Cholinesterase Inhibitors.   A somewhat more complex illustration of the direct action of an antidote upon a poison is found in the treatment of poisoning due to cholinesterase inhibitors. Here, a specific reagent, pralidoxime, was "tailor-made" to remove the inhibitors from the active site of the enzyme by a nucleophilic attack, and simultaneously to interact with them and form an inert complex.

The organic phosphate cholinesterase inhibitors were developed initially as insecticides and later were investigated as chemical warfare agents ("nerve gases"). Some of these compounds and their LD50 values are shown in Table 5-9. Accidental poisoning occurs frequently, especially among agricultural workers.[168]

TABLE 5-9. Some organic phosphate anticholinesterases
LD50 values were determined in mice, intraperitoneally or subcutaneously From Holmstedt,[167] Tables A–E.

LD50	Structure
Diisopropyl fluorophosphate (DFP) 4 mg kg^{-1} i.p.	H_3C–CH–O–P(=O)(F)–C–CH with CH_3 groups (diisopropyl fluorophosphate structure)
Tetraethyl pyrophosphate (TEPP) 0.7 mg kg^{-1} i.p.	$(C_2H_5O)_2P(=O)$–O–$P(=O)(OC_2H_5)_2$
Isopropyl methyl phosphonofluoridate (Sarin, GB) 0.42 mg kg^{-1} i.p.	H_3C–P(=O)(F)–O–CH(CH_3)$_2$
Methylfluorophosphorylcholine 0.1 mg kg^{-1} i.p.	$(CH_3)_3N^+$–CH_2–CH_2–O–P(F)(=O)–CH_3
Diethyl 4-nitrophenyl thionophosphate (parathion) 10–12 mg kg^{-1} s.c.	$(C_2H_5O)_2P(=S)$–O–C_6H_4–NO_2
Diethyl 4-nitrophenyl phosphate (paraoxon) 0.6–0.8 mg kg^{-1} s.c.	$(C_2H_5O)_2P(=O)$–O–C_6H_4–NO_2

The organic phosphates act by phosphorylating and thereby inactivating the "serine enzymes," as described in Chapter 1. Toxic manifestations are due to inactivation of acetylcholinesterase. Plasma cholinesterase is also inactivated; this seems to do no harm in itself, but the activity of the plasma enzyme provides a convenient assay by which to judge the extent of poisoning. Acetylcholinesterase is found in erythrocytes (where its function is unknown), at parasympathetically innervated effector organs (smooth muscles, glands), at the skeletal muscle end-plates, at autonomic ganglia, and in the central nervous system. At all these sites, the enzyme normally hydrolyzes and thus terminates the action of the neurotransmitter acetylcholine (AcCh). Symptoms of accumulation of AcCh appear if the acetylcholinesterase activity is reduced by about one-half, and death ensues if the enzyme activity falls below 10–20% of normal activity.[169] When death occurs, it is usually due to respiratory failure, caused in part by neuromuscular paralysis, in part by central depression.

The immediate treatment of poisoning due to cholinesterase inhibition relies upon the principle (to be discussed later) of blocking the receptors upon which the excessive AcCh acts, and the specific antidote employed for this purpose is atropine (p. 422). In severe poisoning, however, a real problem is that the spontaneous recovery of enzyme activity is very slow. The phosphoryl-enzyme bond (Figure 1-5) is hydrolyzed spontaneously at a negligible rate. The main contribution to spontaneous recovery appears to be the generation of new enzyme protein. The plasma cholinesterase, synthesized in the liver, recovers with a half-time of about 10 days, a rate comparable to that of the synthesis rates of several other liver proteins. The erythrocyte acetyl-cholinesterase activity recovers at a rate of about 1% per day, a time course typical of the formation of new red blood cells.

If a more powerful nucleophilic reagent than water could be employed, it might be possible to rupture the phosphoryl-enzyme bond and regenerate active enzyme. Hydroxylamine does this in vitro. When acetylcholinesterase was inhibited by tetra-ethyl pyrophosphate and allowed to recover its activity by spontaneous hydrolysis, less than 5% of the control activity returned in 7 days, only 50% in 28 days. Hydroxy-lamine caused a rapid regeneration of active enzyme (30 min) to a variable extent depending upon the concentration of hydroxylamine, with complete reactivation at 0.5 M.[170]

The sequence of reactions between the enzyme and a fluorophosphate inhibitor may be represented as follows, where —G: signifies the electron-rich group in the esteratic site of the protein:

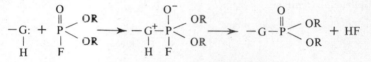

Formation of phosphorylated enzyme

Hydrolysis of phosphorylated enzyme (very slow)

Reactivation of phosphorylated enzyme by hydroxylamine (fast)

High concentrations of hydroxylamine are not tolerated in vivo, but it was reasoned[171] that if such a nucleophilic reagent could be combined with a molecular structure specific for the active site of the enzyme, a therapeutically useful reactivating agent might well be formed. Working from the knowledge that in acetylcholinesterase an anionic site is disposed at 5 A distance from the esteratic site (cf. Chapter 1), hydro-xylamine was incorporated into a molecular structure having a quaternary nitrogen atom at the appropriate distance. Similarly, an organic phosphate that included a quaternary nitrogen atom 5 A from the electronegative phosphorus atom should be very effective as an inhibitor. Thus, methylfluorophosphorylcholine (Table 5-9), an analog of AcCh, is one of the most potent anticholinesterases known.

Several such oximes have been synthesized. One of these, pralidoxime (N-methyl-pyridinium 2-aldoxime, formerly known as 2-PAM), is now widely used as an antidote to cholinesterase inhibitors. Under certain conditions pralidoxime is almost a million times more potent than hydroxylamine. Yet, as might be expected on theoretical grounds, it is not much better than hydroxylamine in reactivating other phosphorylated serine enzymes (e.g., chymotrypsin) whose substrate specificities imply an entirely different molecular architecture at their active sites. The structures of pralidoxime and some congeners are shown in Figure 5-17. The practical efficacy of pralidoxime combined with atropine is illustrated in Table 5-10. Atropine alone

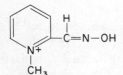

pralidoxime
(2-PAM, N-methylpyridinium
2-aldoxime)

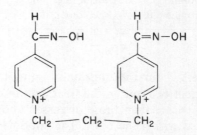

TMB-4
(1,1'-trimethylene bis(4-formylpyridinium)
dioxime)

CH₃—C—C=N—OH

monoisonitrosoacetone
(MINA)

CH₃—C—C=N—OH

diacetyl monoxime
(DAM)

FIGURE 5-17. Oximes used in anticholinesterase poisoning. *In upper row associated anions are not shown; 2-PAM is available as the iodide or chloride, TMB-4 as the chloride.*

increased the LD50 of sarin in rabbits. Combined treatment with pralidoxime and another oxime (TMB4), but without atropine, was ineffective. But the pralidoxime-atropine combination protected the animals against 90 LD50 doses of sarin.

The same principles apply to poisoning by the carbamate inhibitors of acetylcholinesterase (e.g., neostigmine, physostigmine), which are often used clinically, and also to those used as insecticides. These inhibitors form carbamylated enzymes analogous to the phosphorylated enzymes discussed above (cf. Figure 1-5), except that their rates of spontaneous hydrolysis are much faster.[173] Thus, although on theoretical grounds pralidoxime should be useful in the treatment of carbamate poisoning, it is found that atropine and supportive treatment suffice.

TABLE 5-10. Antagonism of the lethal effects of sarin by intravenous oximes and atropine.

Rabbits were injected i.v with graded doses of sarin, followed by various combinations of oximes and atropine 30 sec later, also i.v. (From O'Leary et al.,[172] Table 2.)

Antidotal treatment	Sarin LD50 (μg kg^{-1}) (95% confidence limits)	Multiples of untreated sarin LD50
None	14.7 (12.6–17.4)	1.0
Atropine, 2 mg kg^{-1}	38.0 (24.5–48.8)	2.6
2-PAM chloride, 7.5 mg kg^{-1} +		
TMB4 chloride, 7.5 mg kg^{-1}	18.4 (16.3–20.9)	1.3
Atropine plus 2-PAM chloride, 5 mg kg^{-1}	365 (342–400)	25
Atropine plus 2-PAM chloride, 10 mg kg^{-1}	1321 (985–1770)	90

Cyanide. A final illustration of antidotal action by complexing and removing the toxic agent is found in the treatment of cyanide poisoning. Here, the mechanism is more intricate than those discussed above because the actual complexing agent is produced within the body. The antidote is methemoglobin, produced in vivo from hemoglobin, by the action of sodium nitrite. Methemoglobin, in turn, complexes cyanide ion. Another but equally important part of the treatment makes use of a different principle—acceleration of the metabolic conversion of cyanide to a non-toxic product—and it will be discussed fully later (p. 411).

Cyanide combines with the ferric iron atom in heme proteins in the tissues, destroying their capacity to undergo oxidation and reduction in the normal electron transport process. Contrary to popular impression, cyanide is not a very potent poison in the quantitative sense, since the lethal dose is approximately 50–200 mg. But it can cause death extremely rapidly, primarily by inactivating cytochrome oxidase in tissues. Administration of oxygen, theoretically at least, should do no good, since the utilization of O_2 at the tissue level is impaired, not the oxygen supply; hemoglobin remains fully oxygenated in cyanide poisoning.

The first aim of treatment is to bind as much cyanide ion as possible in an inert form. This is accomplished by converting a portion of the blood hemoglobin to methemoglobin, thus making a large amount of ferric heme available for interaction with CN^-. The affinity of CN^- for cytochrome oxidase is actually greater than for methemoglobin;[174] nevertheless, a very large total amount of methemoglobin can withdraw enough cyanide from tissue cytochrome oxidase to be life saving. A normal adult has nearly 1000 g of blood hemoglobin, containing about 4 g of iron. Thus, if 50% of the hemoglobin is converted to methemoglobin, binding capacity is created for almost 1 g of cyanide ion, more than the fatal dose in man. Serious symptoms of anoxia due to methemoglobinemia are not seen until more than one-half of the total amount of hemoglobin has been oxidized.

The mechanism whereby nitrites oxidize hemoglobin to methemoglobin is still imperfectly understood There may be a coupled oxidation of NO_2^- to NO_3^-, and of oxyhemoglobin to methemoglobin hydroxide, with simultaneous reduction of water,[175] as follows:

$$Hb^{++} \cdot O_2 \longrightarrow Hb^{+++} + e^- + O_2$$

$$Hb^{++} \cdot O_2 \longrightarrow Hb^{+++} + e^- + [O] + [O]$$

$$NO_2^- + [O] \longrightarrow NO_3^-$$

$$H^+ + [O] + 2e^- \longrightarrow OH^-$$

$$OH^- = OH^-.$$

Although the exact mechanism is still not known, these steps yield the overall reaction

$$NO_2^- + 2Hb^{++} \cdot O_2 + H_2O \longrightarrow NO_3^- - 2Hb^{+++} \cdot OH^- + O_2$$

Because speed is essential, sodium nitrite is injected intravenously. There would be considerable advantage in a first-aid antidote that could be administered quickly by anyone. It has been suggested, therefore, that the vapor of amyl nitrite be inhaled; small ampoules of the volatile liquid are available. Although this is probably better than nothing, the rate of production of methemoglobin by this means is unavoidably slow, and the total amount that can be produced even in several minutes of amyl nitrite inhalation is but a fraction of the desirable amount.

Mechanism 2. Antidote Accelerates Metabolic Conversion of Poison to Nontoxic Product

Cyanide.   The second aim in the treatment of cyanide poisoning exemplifies this mechanism. The CN^- ion is normally converted in vivo to the innocuous thiocyanate (CNS^-) by the cyanide-thiosulfate sulfur transferase (p. 266). However, the rate of this reaction is ordinarily slow because the requisite sulfur donors (such as thiosulfate) are present in the body in limiting amounts. The reaction can be accelerated considerably by administering thiosulfate. Experiments with dogs have shown that the LD50 of cyanide can be increased 3-fold by sodium thiosulfate alone, 5-fold by sodium nitrite alone, and 18-fold by a combination of both antidotes.[176] Thus, two different mechanisms of antidotal action together form the basis of the treatment of cyanide toxicity: nitrite to form methemoglobin and complex the cyanide, thiosulfate to accelerate the metabolic conversion of cyanide to thiocyanate. In experimental animals, a further degree of protection was obtained by injecting the sulfur transferase enzyme together with thiosulfate;[177] but pure preparations of the enzyme are not available for clinical use.

In addition to the two antidotal mechanisms already described, a third approach appears to yield beneficial results in cyanide poisoning: administration of oxygen. As already noted, the hemoglobin is fully saturated in cyanide poisoning, so that oxygen would not be expected to be useful. Apparently, however, increasing the physically dissolved plasma O_2 tension bypasses some of the cyanide blockade of tissue O_2 utilization (see mechanism 7). Table 5-11 summarizes clear-cut experiments in mice.

Groups of 10 animals were used to determine the LD50 of potassium cyanide alone, and with various treatments. Eight different conditions were studied. The slopes of all the quantal LDR curves were substantially the same, as shown in the

TABLE 5-11. Antidotal effects in cyanide poisoning in mice.

Groups of ten Swiss–Webster male mice were used to determine the LD50 of KCN (administered subcutaneously) by the method of Litchfield and Wilcoxon.[100] $NaNO_2$ (100 mg kg^{-1}) was administered subcutaneously, $Na_2S_2O_3$ (1.0 g kg^{-1}) intraperitoneally; O_2 was given as a mixture of 95% O_2, 5% CO_2. The 95% confidence limits for slope and for LD50 are given in parentheses. (From Way et al.,[178] Table 1. By permission of American Association for the Advancement of Science.)

Experiment	Treatment before KCN	Slope function	LD50 (mg kg^{-1})
1	Control (air)	1.27 (1.03–1.56)	8.50 (7.73–9.44)
2	O_2	1.28 (1.02–1.70)	11.3 (10.3–12.4)[a]
3	$NaNO_2$	1.13 (1.06–1.21)	21.2 (19.9–22.6)
4	$NaNO_2 + O_2$	1.10 (1.02–1.20)	22.5 (21.4–23.6)[b]
5	$Na_2S_2O_3$	1.33 (0.98–1.70)	34.6 (30.2–39.1)
6	$Na_2S_2O_3 + O_2$	1.15 (1.06–1.24)	42.2 (40.0–44.5)[a]
7	$NaNO_2 - Na_2S_2O_3$	1.12 (1.03–1.26)	53.5 (51.2–55.6)
8	$NaNO_2 + Na_2S_2O_3 + O_2$	1.12 (0.96–1.31)	73.0 (69.8–76.8)[a]

[a] Significantly different from experiments 1, 5, and 7.
[b] Not significantly different from experiment 3.

third column. The LD50 values and their 95% confidence limits are given in the last column. The protective effects of nitrite and of thiosulfate individually and the increased protection afforded by both together are shown in experiments 1, 3, 5, and 7. The effect of furnishing 95% oxygen is indicated in experiments 2, 4, 6, and especially in experiment 8 as compared with experiment 7. Even though the exact mechanism is unknown, it is appropriate to furnish O_2, possibly even at increased pressure, as part of the treatment of severe cyanide poisoning.

Mechanism 3. Antidote Blocks Metabolic Formation of Poison from Less Toxic Precursor

Methanol. This mechanism is illustrated by the treatment of methanol poisoning with ethanol. Methanol poisoning is principally due to the consumption of alcoholic beverages that have been adulterated with methanol. Mass poisonings occur sporadically, as in Georgia in 1951, when 323 people were poisoned, of whom 41 died.[179] Methyl alcohol in large doses is a depressant of the central nervous system in all animals, a property it shares with other aliphatic alcohols. This general depressant action is rarely the cause of death in methanol poisoning. The two characteristic and serious toxic effects of methanol are due to metabolites—formaldehyde and formic acid. Formaldehyde selectively damages retinal cells, causing blindness; formic acid produces acidosis. Both of these toxic actions are seen only in man and other primates, so experimental investigations have been rather limited.[180]

Ethanol and methanol are oxidized by the same enzyme system; alcohol dehydrogenase converts alcohol to aldehyde (acetaldehyde, formaldehyde), then aldehyde dehydrogenase converts aldehyde to acid (acetic acid, formic acid). This provides the basis for the use of competitive substrate inhibition to block the conversion of methanol to the more toxic formaldehyde and formic acid.[181] The formaldehyde that is responsible for retinal damage may be formed in the retina itself rather than in the liver, since alcohol dehydrogenase is present in retinal cells, where it normally catalyzes the reversible oxidation of vitamin A, an alcohol, to the aldehyde retinene.[182] The rate of metabolism of methanol is independent of concentration over a wide range, just as with ethanol (cf. p. 305).[183] Methanol oxidation was studied in a purified system with alcohol dehydrogenase from monkey liver. Ethanol competitively inhibited the reaction, and its affinity for the enzyme was about 10-fold that of methanol.[184] In the body, methanol is oxidized very slowly, only about one-seventh as rapidly as ethanol, so the antidotal treatment with ethanol has to be prolonged for several days. Hemodialysis is also effective in removing methanol.

There is good evidence that another system, involving hydrogen peroxide and catalase, also pays a part in the oxidation of methanol to formaldehyde.[185,186] The purified catalase, like the alcohol dehydrogenase, is active with ethanol as substrate and is inhibited competitively by ethanol when methanol is the substrate.[185] Apparently, in vivo, methanol is metabolized slowly by both pathways. Ethanol, on the other hand, is primarily oxidized by alcohol dehydrogenase; but it has a greater affinity than methanol for both catalase and alcohol dehydrogenase. Consequently, ethanol can inhibit the oxidation of methanol, whereas methanol has but little effect upon ethanol oxidation.

Selenocystathionine. A more unusual instance of this antidotal mechanism is found in the treatment of poisoning due to selenocystathionine. Selenium analogs of the sulfur-containing amino acids occur in nature and cause poisoning in livestock and occasionally in man. These compounds occur in certain plants growing in seleniferous soils of the western United States[187] and in the nuts of *Lecythis ollaria*, a Venezuelan tree.[188] The compounds found in plants include selenomethionine, selenomethylcysteine, and selenocystathionine. The toxic syndrome of selenocystathionine poisoning in man is characterized by nausea, vomiting, dizziness, and fainting. In rats (and possibly in man) there is liver damage. Characteristically, a week or two after ingestion of selenocystathionine, there is generalized loss of hair. The livestock disease ("alkali disease," "blind staggers") is also characterized by hair loss and by deformation of keratinized structures like the hoof. In mammalian cells growing in vitro, cystine blocks the cytotoxic effect. Cystine is a competitive inhibitor of cystathionase, a pyridoxal enzyme that cleaves and deaminates cystathionine (or selenocystathionine) to cysteine (or selenocysteine) and α-ketobutyric acid.

$$\text{cleavage by} \atop \text{cystathionase}$$

$$\underset{\underset{\text{NH}_2}{|}}{\text{HOOC}-\text{CH}}-\text{CH}_2-\text{Se}-\text{CH}_2-\text{CH}_2-\underset{\underset{\text{NH}_2}{|}}{\text{CH}}-\text{COOH}$$

Selenocystathionine

Cells that lack this enzyme are not sensitive to selenocystathionine.[189] Thus, in poisoning by this substance, the actual toxic agent appears to be the cleavage product selenocysteine. By competing with selenocystathionine for the active site of cystathionase, cystine blocks conversion to the toxic product. Apparently, cystine also antagonizes the toxicity by supplying intracellular cysteine, which in turn competes with selenocysteine for incorporation into protein (mechanism 5). This competition, presumably, takes place at the active site of the cysteine-activating enzyme, which couples cysteine (or selenocysteine) to the appropriate transfer RNA molecule. Although the antidotal effects of cystine described here have been observed only in cell cultures, it seems likely that cystine will prove a useful antidote in poisoning by the selenium amino acid analogs in man and animals.

Fluoroacetate.   Another illustration of antidotal action by blocking the metabolic conversion of a precursor to a toxic product is seen in the treatment of fluoroacetate toxicity. This halogenated acetic acid derivative (CFH_2COOH) is found as a toxic constituent of *Dichapetalum cymosum*, a plant indigenous to South Africa, where it constitutes a hazard to livestock. The compound has been used as a rodenticide (under the designation "1080"), and thus several cases of accidental human poisoning have occurred. There is invariably a latent period after fluoroacetate administration. Then, after a delay of 1 or 2 hr, symptoms of myocardial and central nervous system malfunction appear. These include nausea, apprehension, convulsions, and defects of cardiac rhythm which can culminate in ventricular fibrillation. The metabolism of fluoroacetate has been studied thoroughly.[190] The compound enters the tricarboxylic acid cycle in competition with acetate, and is then metabolized to fluorocitrate. Fluorocitrate inhibits aconitase, the enzyme responsible for the conversion of citrate

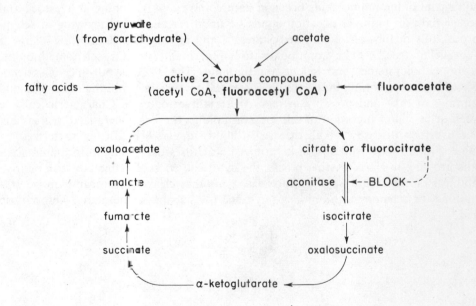

FIGURE 5-18. Metabolism and site of action of fluoroacetate. (*Adapted from Peters.*[191])

to isocitrate.[191] Thus, both citrate and fluorocitrate accumulate after fluoroacetate administration. These relationships are illustrated in Figure 5-18. The toxic effects seem to result from the disruption of energy supply consequent to the blockade in the tricarboxylic acid cycle.

Acetate, or acetate precursors (ethanol, acetamide), serve as antidotes by competing with fluoroacetate, as would be expected, and such compounds have had a limited but definite protective action in experimental fluoroacetate poisoning by diminishing the accumulation of citrate and of fluorocitrate.[192,193] Best results have been obtained with monoacetin, the monoacetate ester of glycerol.[194]

Mechanism 4. Antidote Specifically Accelerates Excretion of Poison

Bromide.   An example is the effect of chloride ions in accelerating the removal of bromide ions from the body. Accumulation of bromide in the extracellular fluids leads to a toxic syndrome characterized by disturbances of function in the central nervous system. Early symptoms are impaired mental processes, drowsiness, dizziness, irritability, and emotional instability. More severe effects include mania, delirium, delusions, hallucinations, and coma. Neurologic disorders are also typical (tremors, motor incoordination, slurred speech), as well as dermatitis, abnormal function of the exocrine glands, and gastrointestinal disturbances. The slow time course of the accumulation of bromide in the body, which accounts for the insidious development of bromism, has been discussed fully in Chapter 4. The specific antidotal administration of chloride was also described there. It depends upon the nearly identical handling of the chloride and bromide anions in the kidney. Increased chloride intake results in chloride diuresis. The excretion of bromide will be in nearly the same ratio to chloride as in the extracellular fluid.

As a specific illustration of the chloride-bromide relationship, assume the following: Cl^- concentration (extracellular fluid) = 100 meq liter^{-1} = 3.6 g liter^{-1}; total body Cl^- = 3.6 g × 12 liters extracellular fluid = 43 g; daily excretion of Cl^- in urine = daily Cl^- intake = 5 g, or 5/43 (about 10%) of the total body Cl^-; Br^- concentration, toxic level = 20 meq liter^{-1}, or 20% of the chloride concentration, on a molar basis.

If the chloride intake and output remained unchanged, then about 10% of the body bromide would be excreted daily, because this is the fraction of body chloride that is excreted daily. If an additional 5 g of chloride is administered each day, this excess will also be excreted, since the kidney functions to maintain a constant halide concentration in the extracellular fluid. Thus, as total halide excretion doubles, the excretion of bromide will be doubled, from 10 to 20% per day. It is not difficult to administer 5–10 g of sodium chloride or ammonium chloride daily, but very much larger amounts are impractical; thus the maximum effect that can be achieved is to increase the rate of bromide excretion several-fold. However, since bromide poisoning rarely presents itself as an acute emergency, slow elimination of the poison is usually not a serious handicap.

Strontium and Radium.   Another example of the same principle is the accelerated removal of strontium and radium by the administration of calcium. Both metals compete with calcium for the mechanisms that mediate absorption, binding to proteins, transport across membranes, deposition in bone, and renal excretion.[195]

Most investigations have concerned strontium, because radioactive ^{90}Sr is a product of nuclear explosions. It appears in fallout debris and thus may make its way into the human body by the oral and inhalation routes. The isotope is a beta emitter with a radioactive half-life of 28 years; its effective half-life after deposition in bone (taking account of both radioactive and biologic half-lives) is about 7 years. The corresponding figure for ^{226}Ra is 44 years. Neither of these metals can be removed from the body efficiently by chelating agents of the EDTA type because the binding constants are too close to those of calcium, which is always present in great excess over the traces of strontium or radium that would be of concern.

The absorption of strontium from the gastrointestinal tract is less efficient than that of calcium. Investigations in man, using ^{85}Sr (a gamma emitter, radioactive half-life 64 days) and ^{45}Ca showed that even on a low-calcium diet the molar absorption of calcium was two to three times that of strontium; and higher calcium intakes correspondingly reduced the absorption of strontium.[196] Milk is an important source of calcium in man; inasmuch as youngsters drink more milk than adults, they should be protected better. But because milk from cows exposed to fallout may be a prime source of ^{90}Sr intake, the situation is complex.[197]

Preferential transport of calcium relative to strontium occurs in the renal tubules as well as the gastrointestinal tract. Consequently, although both are almost completely reabsorbed, a smaller fraction of strontium than of calcium in tubular urine is reabsorbed. Experiments in man[198] showed that with low calcium intake the calcium clearance was low, and the clearance ratio of strontium to calcium was about 5:1. Raising the calcium intake by a factor of 10 caused a corresponding increase in the calcium clearance, since the tubular reabsorption mechanisms operate to maintain calcium homeostasis in the plasma. At the same time there was a 6-fold increase in strontium clearance. These effects are similar, in principle, to those of increased chloride intake upon bromide excretion, except that the renal clearance of strontium is considerably greater than that of calcium, whereas the bromide clearance is slightly less than that of chloride (p. 327). The excretion of strontium can also be increased by metabolic acidosis, causing demineralization of bone, and thereby promoting the mobilization of bone calcium and sequestered strontium. In man, the excretion of strontium is accelerated by calcium gluconate or by acidosis produced by ammonium chloride, and more so by administering both together.[199] Nonspecific ways of accelerating the excretion of a poison from the body are important in the treatment of toxicity when no specific antidotes are available, and they are also appropriate in conjunction with specific antidotes. These procedures (hemodialysis, peritoneal dialysis, ion trapping) were discussed at the beginning of this chapter.

Mechanism 5. Antidote Competes with Poison for Essential Receptors

Carbon Monoxide.   The treatment of carbon monoxide poisoning by administration of oxygen exemplifies this mechanism. Carbon monoxide is a product of incomplete combustion. It is found wherever the internal combustion engine is in use, is an industrial hazard, and it causes accidental poisoning in households where it is present in heating or cooking gas. Suicide by the use of automobile exhaust gas is common. About 5000 deaths annually in the United States are caused by carbon monoxide.

Carbon monoxide may be considered an antimetabolite of oxygen. It combines reversibly with hemoglobin to form carboxyhemoglobin. There are two consequences of importance. First, a certain number of binding sites for oxygen are occupied, so the oxygen-carrying capacity of the blood is decreased. Second, the binding of one or more molecules of CO to a molecule of hemoglobin with its four heme groups increases the affinity of the remaining sites for oxygen. The basis of this action is apparently the same as the well-known effect of one bound oxygen molecule upon the affinity of hemoglobin for the next one, namely, an induced allosteric modification of the protein (p. 52).[200] Thus, the ability of hemoglobin in the erythrocytes to give up oxygen to the tissues at low partial pressures of oxygen is seriously interfered with. This shifting of the oxyhemoglobin dissociation curve to the left (Figure 5-19) causes

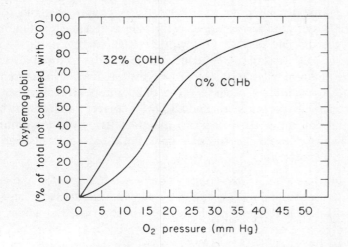

FIGURE 5-19. Effect of carbon monoxide on oxyhemoglobin dissociation. *Vertical axis shows oxyhemoglobin as percent of total hemoglobin not combined with CO,*

$$\left(\frac{oxyhemoglobin}{oxyhemoglobin + hemoglobin} \times 100 \right). \ Horizontal \ axis \ shows \ partial \ pressure \ of \ O_2$$

in mm Hg. Curve at right, in the absence of CO; that at left, in the presence of 32% *carboxyhemoglobin. (From Roughton and Darling, Figure 2.[201])*

a degree of tissue anoxia far greater than could be accounted for by the simple loss of oxygen-carrying capacity. Dogs were poisoned with CO until 75% of their hemoglobin was carboxyhemoglobin. The animals collapsed, and those that survived showed serious damage from tissue anoxia. In contrast, transfusion experiments showed that 75% of the blood could be replaced with CO-saturated blood without serious consequence.[202]

In man, little effect is seen with concentrations of carboxyhemoglobin up to about 35% of the total hemoglobin. As the concentration approaches 50%, headache, flushing, weakness, vomiting, and collapse occur. The color of the patient's skin may become cherry-red because of peripheral vasodilation and the bright-red color of carboxyhemoglobin itself. At still higher concentration, coma, intermittent convulsions, and respiratory failure are seen.

The affinity of CO for hemoglobin is about 250 times that of O_2. This means that the dangerous level of 50% carboxyhemoglobin (i.e., equal parts CO-hemoglobin and O_2-hemoglobin) will be reached when the concentration of CO in the inspired air is only 1/250 that of O_2, or 0.08%. The uptake of CO and the kinetics of its equilibration and elimination are governed by the same principles as those already discussed in connection with anesthetic gases (Chapter 4). Although the aqueous solubility of CO is low, its solubility in blood is very high because of its binding to hemoglobin; therefore its behavior is that of a typical high-solubility agent. Like the high-S anesthetic gases, it attains equilibrium slowly, and its uptake rate is very sensitive to changes in respiratory minute volume. Thus an active person, with a high respiratory exchange, will absorb CO faster (and be poisoned faster) than a person at rest.

The patient is removed from the contaminated environment and kept at rest, avoiding all stimulants, in order to reduce tissue oxygen demand to the lowest possible level. Respiration is maintained artificially, if necessary, with administration of pure O_2 or a mixture of 95% O_2, with 5% CO_2, to promote the competitive displacement of CO. Raising the O_2 concentration in the inspired air from 20% to 100% reduces the biologic half-life of carboxyhemoglobin in man from 250 min to about 40 min, as would be expected.[203] Use of a compression chamber at 2 atmospheres O_2 pressure works faster still and also helps correct tissue anoxia by supplying enough O_2 in solution in the plasma to maintain tissue oxygen requirements.[204] In severe poisoning, exchange transfusion is indicated to furnish an immediate supply of fresh hemoglobin.

Curare.   In curare poisoning, the competition between the poison and acetylcholine at receptors in the skeletal muscle end-plate provides the basis for antidotal action by a competitive displacement mechanism. Tubocurarine, the active principle of of curare, is used as a muscle relaxant in surgery. The major effect of overdosage is a prolonged flaccid paralysis of striated muscles, secondary to a stabilization of the membrane potential at the end-plate (cf. Chapter 1). In the presence of tubocurarine the usual amounts of AcCh released by motor nerve terminals no longer produce a sufficient local depolarization at the end-plate to trigger a propagated muscle action potential, so the muscle does not contract. It can be shown, with isolated nerve-muscle preparations, that higher concentrations of AcCh will provoke a response in the curarized end-plate, and the relationship between tubocurarine and AcCh appears to be competitive over a wide dose range (cf. Chapter 1). It is not practical to administer AcCh itself as an antidote. First, it is destroyed almost at once by the circulating plasma and erythrocyte cholinesterases. Second, its access from the circulation to the muscle end-plate is somewhat restricted by lipid membrane barriers. The antidotal procedure, therefore, is to administer a cholinesterase inhibitor. Neostigmine, physostigmine, and similar drugs, by retarding the destruction of AcCh liberated by nerve impulses, allow a higher steady-state level of AcCh to accumulate locally. Thus, for any given rate of arrival of nerve impulses at the motor nerve terminals, the local AcCh concentration will be higher in the presence of a cholinesterase inhibitor. The organic phosphate cholinesterase inhibitors would act in the same way, but their effects would long outlast the period of curare-induced paralysis. The most useful antidote in the class of cholinesterase inhibitors is neostigmine; its efficacy is attributed not only to cholinesterase inhibition, but also to a mild direct stimulatory action on the muscle end-plate.

Edrophonium is a structural analog of neostigmine; but it is not a carbamate ester, and it is a very poor inhibitor of cholinesterase:

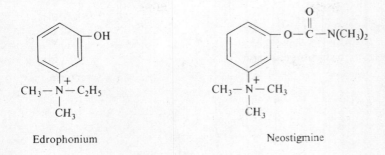

Edrophonium   Neostigmine

Edrophonium reverses the paralysis caused by tubocurarine even faster than does neostigmine. In contrast to neostigmine, which has a long duration of action, the effect of a single dose of edrophonium wears off very quickly. The exact mechanism of edrophonium action remains uncertain, but its direct stimulatory actions on the end-plate presumably play a role. Possibly edrophonium and neostigmine both displace tubocurarine from AcCh receptor sites in the muscle end-plate.[205]

Coumarin.   Another instance of this mechanism, the competitive reversal of toxic effect by the antidote, is the treatment of coumarin toxicity by vitamin K. The coumarins are anticoagulants; the most frequently used are bishydroxycoumarin, warfarin, and phenindione (Figure 5-20). They are employed therapeutically to depress the coagulability of blood in order to prevent venous thrombosis, and in certain other conditions.[206] Because they are also widely used as rodenticides, poisoning sometimes occurs in children. The coumarins act by depressing the synthesis of 4 plasma protein factors (the so-called prothrombin complex—factors II, VII, IX, and X) required in the normal process of blood coagulation. These proteins are synthesized in the liver, but only in the presence of adequate levels of vitamin K. The exact role of vitamin K is not known, but studies with perfused rat livers have shown that the vitamin K effect is not blocked by actinomycin D.[207] This suggests that the vitamin promotes some aspect of protein synthesis subsequent to transcription of the genetic message into specific messenger RNA, possibly the conversion of a precursor into active prothrombin.[207a]

The coumarins may be regarded as structural analogs of vitamin K, and their effects are like those of vitamin K depletion. It is not certain, however, whether they compete with the vitamin at a receptor site, or whether they interfere with the metabolism of the vitamin. It appears that vitamin K in the liver is normally in equilibrium with its epoxide, which is biologically inactive. After warfarin administration, the epoxide concentration in the liver rises, and the conversion of the epoxide to vitamin K is inhibited. In vitamin K deficiency, either the vitamin itself or the epoxide is active in promoting prothrombin synthesis. After warfarin administration, only vitamin K is effective, not the epoxide.[208]

The coumarin anticoagulants act slowly, as would be expected. They have no effect whatsoever upon blood clotting when added in vitro. Their actions take several days to develop, so acute toxicity is not usually a problem. Serious toxicity can develop with long-term use and inadequate control of the prothrombin time. A cause of

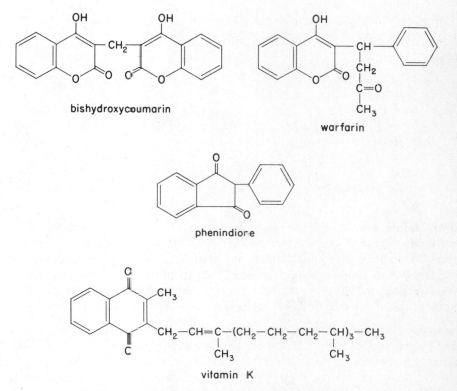

FIGURE 5-20. The coumarin anticoagulants and vitamin K.

toxic overdosage might be an unanticipated decrease in the rate of coumarin metabolism secondary to changes in the intake of other drugs, as described in Chapter 3.
Poisoning could be the result of ingesting coumarin rat poisons. The toxic manifestations are principally hemorrhagic episodes affecting various organs. Vitamin K
derivatives are specific antidotes, but one cannot expect an immediate response;
sufficient time must elapse for some new protein synthesis to occur. The lipid-soluble
vitamin K_1 is more effective than the water-soluble analogs,[209] and it acts within a
few hours.

Morphine and Morphine-Like Narcotics.   The mechanism of competition for a
receptor site also seems to explain the dramatic antidotal actions of narcotic antagonists like naloxone in poisoning by morphine and morphine-like narcotics.
The agents that stereospecifically antagonize the analgesic and narcotic effects of
morphine and related drugs were discussed in Chapter 1.

Morphine poisoning usually occurs as a result of self-administered overdosage.
The victim will be in a deep stupor or coma, with severely depressed respiration.
Naloxone can be life saving in these circumstances. It reverses all the narcotic effects
promptly, and marked stimulation of respiration is seen.

Formerly, nalorphine or levallorphan were used as narcotic antidotes, but these
compounds have mixed actions in man—some agonist effects of their own, as well as
the desirable antagonist effects.[210,211] At high doses they can even cause respiratory

depression. Naloxone, on the other hand, is a pure antagonist with no significant actions of its own. It is therefore the only appropriate antidote for narcotic overdoses. In a physically dependent addict, naloxone can precipitate a severe withdrawal syndrome. (cf. Chapter 9).

Numerous experiments with different species have shown the competitive nature of the antagonist : agonist relationship. In the presence of an antagonist, the LDR curve for a narcotic is shifted to the right (i.e., to higher doses) without change of slope or of maximum.[212] The extent of this shift on the log dose scale is the same for all agonists with a fixed dose of a given antagonist. The behavior is that to be expected of compounds competing for the same receptor sites, as discussed thoroughly in Chapter 1.

Figure 5-21 presents the results of an interesting experiment on two meperidine derivatives. The analgesic ED80 dose was first determined by subcutaneous administration in rats; criterion of response was failure to tail flick despite the application

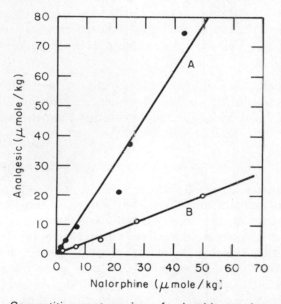

FIGURE 5-21. Competitive antagonism of nalorphine against two narcotic analgesics. *Rats were tested by the tail-flick method. The ED80 doses for two phenyl-piperidine derivatives were 1.16 μmole kg^{-1} for drug A, 0.31 μmole kg^{-1} for drug B; the ratio of potencies was 3.7. For each increment of the analgesic dose, an amount of nalorphine was found that would just antagonize the increased analgesia, and this dose of nalorphine (abscissa) was plotted against the total dose of the analgesic (ordinate). The ratios of the slopes of the two straight lines is 3.7. (From Grumbach and Chernov, Figure 3.*[213])

of heat for a period of 20 sec. The ED80 doses proved to be 1.16 μmole kg^{-1} for the less potent compound (A), 0.31 μmole kg^{-1} for the more potent one (B). The ratio of these doses is 3.7. Now the analgesic doses were increased, and in each instance the amount of nalorphine required to antagonize the increased analgesic effect was determined.

Each dose pair for constant effect was plotted as a single point, the nalorphine dosage on the horizontal axis, the analgesic dosage on the vertical axis. Straight lines that diverged from the origin resulted. Thus, for a given drug there was an invariable antagonistic ratio. For example, 1 μmole of nalorphine always antagonized 1.5 μmole of drug A, but only 0.4 μmole of the more potent drug B. Remarkably, the slopes of the two lines have the same ratio, 3.7, as the ED80 doses of the two drugs. These findings again imply a strictly competitive interaction between narcotic agent and narcotic antagonist, as though differences in affinities for the same receptor site were involved. Similar results were obtained when levallorphan was used as the antagonist.

Thallium.   Some ion antagonisms may represent competition at receptor sites on membranes or enzyme active centers. In thallium poisoning, for example, potassium ion has been found to counteract many of the toxic actions and also to promote the renal excretion of thallium. The protective effect of KCl administration in rats poisoned with Tl_2SO_4 has been reported, and in the same experiments NaCl was without effect.[158]

Although the mechanisms are still unknown, the chemical similarities between Tl^+ and K^+ lend plausibility to a hypothesis of competition for the same receptor sites.

Amino Acid Analogs.   Amino acid analogs (e.g., ethionine, fluorophenylalanine), which have been investigated as potential anticancer agents, are all toxic. The analogous natural amino acids are effective antidotes; they compete for incorporation into protein, as described for selenocysteine (p. 414).

Mechanism 6. Antidote Blocks Receptors that are Responsible for Toxic Effect

Cholinesterase Inhibitors.   A good example is the use of atropine to prevent the toxic effects of cholinesterase inhibitors. It interacts with AcCh receptors, rendering them insensitive to the large amounts of AcCh that accumulate in this type of poisoning. Atropine acts upon receptors at the parasympathetic effector organs and in the central nervous system; it has but slight action at autonomic ganglia and practically none at the neuromuscular junction. Atropine should be given liberally to counteract the effects of cholinesterase inhibitors, certainly in dosage sufficient to produce clear signs of atropinization, e.g., mydriasis, tachycardia, dry hands and mouth, and hot, flushed skin. From the competitive relationship between atropine and AcCh (Figure 1-81) it may be deduced that much more atropine will be required in anticholinesterase poisoning than is needed to atropinize a normal person. Atropine is especially helpful in antagonizing the life-threatening bronchiolar constriction and excessive bronchial secretions produced by AcCh accumulation.

Atropine alone can protect experimental animals against several LD50 doses of an organic phosphate cholinesterase inhibitor. However, since the neuromuscular junction is not responsive to atropine, the paralysis of the respiratory muscles produced by excessive AcCh will not be relieved. Prompt artificial respiration is therefore called for. As was shown in Table 5-10 atropine and the reactivating agent pralidoxime each have some protective effects, and the antidotal action is greatly enhanced when both agents are used together; combination therapy is now standard.

Mechanism 7. Antidote Restores Normal Function by Repairing or Bypassing Effect of Poison

Agents that Produce Methemoglobinemia. The use of methylene blue to combat methemoglobinemia illustrates the repair of a damaged receptor by an antidote. The oxidized, ferric form of hemoglobin is a chocolate-colored pigment called methemoglobin. Erythrocytes normally contain small amounts of methemoglobin, presumably a steady-state level resulting from spontaneous oxidation. They also contain two enzyme systems that reduce methemoglobin back to hemoglobin; these are methemoglobin diaphorase (diaphorase I), using NADH as coenzyme, and methemoglobin reductase (diaphorase II), using NADPH. A great many substances can produce methemoglobin,[214] for example, nitrites, chlorates, phenacetin, acetanilid, sulfanilamide, nitrobenzene, quinones, aniline, and aniline dyes. The production of methemoglobin by acetanilid and by aniline metabolites (p. 230), and the sensitivity of infants to nitrate in their drinking water and to aniline dyes (p. 394) have been discussed. Nitrites are probably the commonest cause of methemoglobinemia; the reader is referred to a fascinating account of medical detection in a mass poisoning caused by the substitution of sodium nitrite for table salt.[215]

Methemoglobin will not carry oxygen; therefore extensive methemoglobinemia is incompatible with life. When one or more of the four iron atoms in a hemoglobin molecule is oxidized to the ferric state, the affinity of O_2 for the other sites is increased. The oxyhemoglobin dissociation curve is shifted to the left, as with carboxyhemoglobin (but not so markedly) (Figure 5-19), so the delivery of O_2 to the tissues is impaired.[216] Patients with methemoglobinemia are therefore more anoxic than they would be if an equivalent loss of hemoglobin were sustained by hemorrhage. Early symptoms of anoxia are seen below 50% methemoglobin, but oxygenation becomes seriously inadequate only at higher levels; the lethal concentration is apparently above 70%.[217]

Methylene blue causes the reduction of methemoglobin to hemoglobin, and it is an effective antidote for methemoglobinemia, regardless of its cause. The dye acts as an intermediate electron acceptor between NADPH and methemoglobin; it undergoes a cyclic reduction to its colorless form, leucomethylene blue:

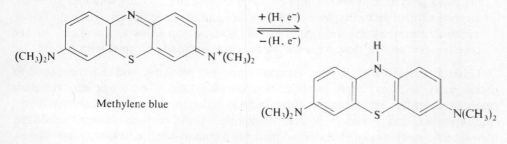

The direct reaction between NADPH and methemoglobin is catalyzed by methemoglobin reductase (diaphorase II), as already noted, and this reaction is accelerated by the intervention of methylene blue.[218] The electron transport sequence is as follows.[219]

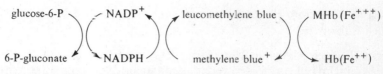

In the absence of methemoglobin, oxygen will serve as a terminal electron acceptor, oxidizing leucomethylene blue; thus, for example, methylene blue stimulates glucose oxidation by erythrocytes.

The effectiveness of intravenous methylene blue in treating severe methemoglobinemia has been demonstrated experimentally in dogs;[217] at methemoglobin concentrations in excess of 80%, only 1 dog out of 12 survived in a control series, but 8 out of 9 treated animals recovered rapidly and completely. The efficacy of methylene blue in man has also been shown.[220] Care should be exercised in the use of methylene blue, as higher doses paradoxically cause methemoglobinemia (by direct oxidation), as well as producing hemolysis and central nervous system depression.[221] Oxygen administration is also indicated, to increase the concentration of physically dissolved O_2 carried to the tissues in the plasma.

Digitalis.   Another example of an antidote repairing or bypassing the effect of a poison is seen in the treatment of digitalis toxicity. Were this poisoning not so common an occurrence, it might well be omitted here entirely because the antidotal mechanisms (and for that matter the mechanisms of the therapeutic or toxic actions of digitalis) are still so poorly understood. Nevertheless, there are clearly specific, effective antidotes, which will be discussed.

Digitalis toxicity occurs frequently and is difficult to avoid, for two reasons. First, as explained earlier, the drug has a very long biologic half-life, so it tends to accumulate, with an equally long half-time. Second, because the therapeutic ratio is very small, as shown earlier in this chapter, relatively small overshoots beyond the intended plateau, or unpredictable fluctuations of the drug level or of the patient's sensitivity to the drug can have serious consequences.

There are three major types of toxic manifestation.[222] These were well described in 1775 by Withering,[223] who introduced this drug into medicine:

> I found him [a Yorkshire tradesman] incessantly vomiting, his vision indistinct, his pulse forty in a minute. Upon enquiry, it came out that his wife had stewed a large handful of green foxglove leaves in a half pint of water and given him the liquor which he drank at one draught . . . this good woman knew the medicine of her country, but not the dose of it, for the husband narrowly escaped with his life.

Gastrointestinal disturbances, especially nausea, vomiting, and diarrhea, tend to occur early, and may serve as significant warning signs. Neurologic and ophthalmologic disorders are common; these include flickering sensations, colored vision, photophobia, and a variety of central manifestations such as vertigo, headache, drowsiness, restlessness irritability, weakness, convulsions, delusions, and stupor. The third class of toxic action comprises the cardiac effects proper, mainly depressed conduction and many kinds of cardiac arrhythmia.[224] The appearance of an irregularity of the pulse not previously present in a patient receiving a digitalis glycoside is very serious, because it has been shown in animal experiments that such effects do not occur until about 60% of the fatal dose has been given. The increased automaticity of the cardiac tissues may be expressed as paroxysmal or nonparoxysmal atrial tachycardia, premature ventricular beats, bigeminal pulse, nodal tachycardia, or ventricular tachycardia, with various degrees of associated heart block. Fatal ventricular fibrillation may supervene abruptly. It has been estimated that in as many as one-half of all cases one of these cardiac arrhythmias is the first sign of toxicity, without any premonitory gastrointestinal or neurologic symptoms.[225] The pattern of toxic effects is rather variable, not only between patients, but even in the same patient on different occasions. On the other hand, there is no evidence of any regular patterns of toxicity distinguishing one digitalis glycoside from another.[226]

It would seem elementary that signs of digitalis toxicity should call for immediate discontinuance of the drug. Surprisingly, this is not always done. Since many arrhythmias arise from the primary cardiac disease under treatment, the dose of digitalis may even be increased in the mistaken opinion that insufficient therapeutic effect has been obtained.[227] It is important, therefore, not only to recognize the toxic arrhythmias by electrocardiography, but also to monitor the plasma level of the drug by radioimmunoassay or similar rapid assay technique.

Discontinuing the administration of digitalis is essential and further absorption can be prevented with steroid-binding resins (p. 406), but these resins are unlikely to have any immediate effect because the drug is eliminated so very slowly (p. 323). The most important antidote is potassium ion. It is still unclear exactly what roles the monovalent and divalent cations play in cardiac contraction or impulse initiation and conduction. There is no doubt, however, that administration of digitalis in toxic doses leads to an abnormal efflux of potassium from the heart. Conversely, the sensitivity of the heart to the toxic effects of digitalis glycosides is increased by lowering the perfusing potassium concentration (in animal experiments), and diminished by raising the potassium level. These early observations led to clinical experimentation and controlled observation, which revealed similar actions in man.[227-230] A significant precipitating cause of digitalis toxicity may be the hypokalemia produced by the vigorous use of diuretics in cardiac patients. Arrhythmias caused by digitalis (particularly atrial tachycardias) can often be abolished by oral or slow intravenous administration of KCl or other potassium salts.[227,231] The amount required is about 50–100 meq (3–7 g of KCl). This increases the plasma K^+ to 1 or 2 meq liter^{-1} above its normal level of 3.5–5.0 meq liter^{-1}, and presumably restores potassium to the depleted heart. On theoretical grounds (cf. Chapter 2), better control can be maintained by continuous intravenous infusion of a dilute solution of a potassium salt than by oral administration; and fine control is important here because excessive potassium levels are dangerous.

Other methods are effective in combatting digitalis toxicity on the heart. It has long been known that epinephrine and related catecholamines can precipitate cardiac arrhythmias, especially in the digitalized heart, and that sympathetic denervation reduces the sensitivity of the heart to the toxic actions of digitalis. These findings have led to the introduction of beta-receptor blocking agents in the treatment of digitalis toxicity, apparently with some success.[232] Procaine amide, a derivative of the local anesthetic procaine, also has proved useful in reducing cardiac arrhythmias, especially ventricular ectopic beats, caused by digitalis.

Botulinus Toxin.   Guanidine hydrochloride appears to have some beneficial effect in the treatment of botulism,[233] a type of poisoning with an extremely poor prognosis. The basic defect caused by botulinus toxin is a blockade of acetylcholine release from cholinergic nerve terminals. The exact mechanism is not known. Guanidine overcomes various types of neuromuscular block. In curarized muscle, for example, it causes an increase in amplitude of the diminished end-plate potential. It does not alter the sensitivity of the end-plate to iontophoretically applied acetylcholine, nor does it inhibit acetylcholinesterase. Thus, it appears to act by facilitating the release of acetylcholine by action potentials arriving at the cholinergic terminals.[234] The effect, therefore, is to bypass or repair the functional damage caused by botulinus toxin. It is not known, however, if guanidine acts at the same biochemical step as botulinus toxin.

Folic Acid Antagonists.   The bypass mechanism of antidotal action is also well illustrated in the field of chemotherapy, where the toxic effects of antimetabolites can be antagonized by end-products of the inhibited reactions. Sulfonamides, for example, block the synthesis of folic acid in sensitive bacteria. This action is antagonized competitively by p-aminobenzoic acid (PABA),[235] but noncompetitively by folic acid.[236] In other words, in the presence of folic acid, the sulfonamide drug no longer had any effect, because folic acid is the sole essential product of the inhibited reaction. The same principle applies to any toxic agent. If all end-products of the pathways blocked by the agent are made available, then the toxicity is effectively bypassed.

In mammalian cells, several reduced derivatives of folic acid serve as cofactors in the transfer of single carbon atoms. These derivatives, such as 7,8-dihydrofolic acid (FAH_2), 5,6,7,8-tetrahydrofolic acid (FAH_4), N^5-formyl FAH_4 (folinic acid, leucovorin, citrovorum factor), and N^5,N^{10}-anhydroformyl FAH_4, are essential for the interconversion of glycine and serine, the synthesis of thymidylic acid from deoxyuridylic acid, and for two different steps in purine biosynthesis.[237]

The folic acid antagonists are the first drugs to have been used with some degree of success in cancer chemotherapy,[238] and they are still widely employed in the treatment of childhood leukemia. Because they interfere with essential functions in all cells, they have a high toxicity. Methotrexate (Figure 5-22), the drug of this class in common use today, combines reversibly but very tightly with folic acid reductase and inactivates it. The combination is practically stoichiometric, with a dissociation constant of only 3×10^{-11} M, representing an affinity 10^5 times greater than that of folic acid for the same enzyme.[239] The effect is primarily to block endogenous synthesis of glycine, thymidylate, and the purines.[240] These end products of single carbon transfer overcome the methotrexate toxicity completely and noncompetitively. This can be accomplished by a mixture of thymidine (which generates thymidylic acid in the cell), of a purine such as hypoxanthine or adenine, and of glycine; cells growing in vitro in such a mixture are indifferent to all concentrations of methotrexate.[241]

5-Fluorouracil and 5-Fluorodeoxyuridine.   5-Fluorouracil and 5-fluorodeoxyuridine (Figure 5-22) participate in normal intermediary metabolism, forming ribonucleosides and phosphorylated derivatives. The antitumor effect of these compounds can be attributed to inhibition of DNA synthesis secondary to a block of thymidylate synthesis. Both agents are converted to 5'-fluoro-2'-deoxyuridine 5'-monophosphate (FUdRP), which inhibits the enzyme thymidylate synthetase competitively.[242] Since thymidine is converted readily to thymidylic acid by a kinase, thymidine acts as a specific and effective antidote; in the presence of thymidine, the need for de novo thymidylate synthesis is obviated.

6-Mercaptopurine.   Another inhibitor of DNA synthesis is 6-mercaptopurine (Figure 5-22). The active compound is apparently the derivative 6-mercaptopurine

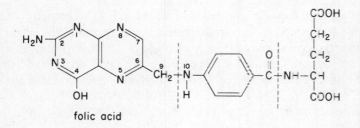

folic acid

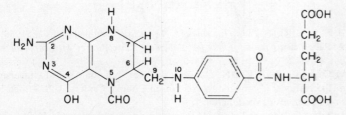

N⁵-formyltetrahydrofolic acid
(folinic acid, leucovorin, citrovorum factor)

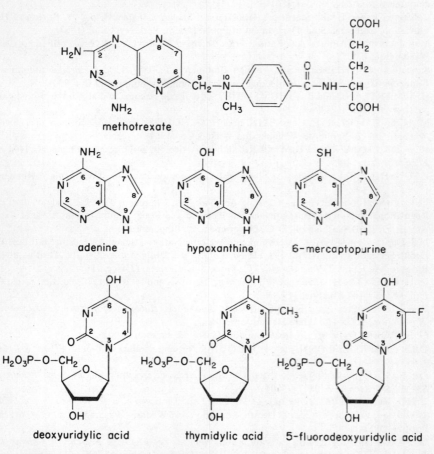

methotrexate

adenine   hypoxanthine   6-mercaptopurine

deoxyuridylic acid   thymidylic acid   5-fluorodeoxyuridylic acid

FIGURE 5-22. Some essential metabolites, and their antimetabolites used in cancer chemotherapy.

ribonucleoside 5'-phosphate, formed within the cell. The primary mechanism of action of this compound in cancer chemotherapy is its inhibition of the conversion of inosinic acid to adenine and guanine nucleotides.[243] Both hypoxanthine and adenine are effective antidotes. Guanine is less effective, probably because of its rapid degradation and limited capacity for conversion to adenine nucleotides in the cells.

REFERENCES

1. Cited in H. E. SIGERIST *The Great Doctors.* New York, Doubleday & Co. (1958).
2. C. BERNARD: *Lecons sur les Effets des Substances Toxiques et Médicamenteuses.* Paris, J.-B. Baillière et Fils (1857).
3. P. F. D'ARCY and J. P. GRIFFIN: *Iatrogenic Diseases.* London, Oxford University Press (1972).
4. Bulletin of the National Clearinghouse for Poison Control Centers, U.S. Public Health Service, September–October, 1970. Washington, D.C.
5. F. S. LISELLA: Morbidity and mortality: pesticides and other chemicals. In *Principles of Chemical Epidemiology.* U.S. Environmental Protection Agency, Chamblee, Georgia (1971) pp. 1–14.
6. R. G. SCHERZ: Prevention of childhood aspirin poisoning: clinical trials with three child-resistant containers. *New Eng. J. Med.* 285:1361 (1971).
7. California Public Health Statistical Report: *Vital Statistics*, Table 31, p. 209. Bureau of Health Education, California State Department of Public Health, Berkeley, Calif. (1967).
8. Manufacturing Chemists Association: *The Chemical Industry Facts Book*, 4th ed., 1960–61. Washington, D.C.
9. Subcommittee on Interstate and Foreign Commerce, Report 1158: *Hazardous Substances for Household Use.* U.S. Senate, 86th Congress, 2nd session. Washington, D.C. (1960).
10. H. S. MARTLAND and R. E. HUMPHRIES: Osteogenic sarcoma in dial painters using luminous paint. *Arch. Pathol.* 7:406 (1929).
11. M. N. GLEASON, R. E. GOSSELIN, and H. G. HODGE: *Clinical Toxicology of Commercial Products*, 3rd ed. Baltimore, Williams and Wilkins Co. (1969).
12. W. B. DEICHMANN and H. W. GERRARDE: Toxicology of Drugs and Chemicals. New York, Academic Press, 1969.
13. I. SUNSHINE, Ed.: *Handbook of Analytical Toxicology.* Cleveland, The Chemical Rubber Co., 1969.
14. Federal Hazardous Substances Labeling Act, Part 191, Chapter I, Title 21, Code of the Federal Regulations; and implementing regulations by Food and Drug Administration, Federal Register, August 12, 1961. Washington, D.C., Government Printing Office.
15. U.S. Department of Health, Education, and Welfare, National Center for Health Statistics: Public Health Service Publication No. 600, *The Facts of Life and Death*, Table 22, p. 20, "Deaths and Death Rates for Accidents." Washington, D.C., Government Printing Office, 1965.
16. R. H. DREISBACH: *Handbook of Poisoning*: diagnosis and treatment, 7th ed. Los Altos, Calif., Lange Medical Publications (1971).
16a. Report of the President's Science Advisory Committee, *Handling of Toxicological Information.* Washington, D.C., The White House, June 1966.
17. G. BARGER: *Ergot and Ergotism.* London, Gurney & Jackson (1931).
18. DRS. GABBAI, LISBONNE, and POURQUIER: Ergot poisoning at Pont St. Esprit. *Brit. Med. J.* 2:650 (1951).
19. DR. FARAJ: Intoxication collective par une huile à base de cresylphosphates. *Semaine Hôp. Paris*, *Suppl. Med. Monde* 36:2807 (1960).
20. J. PIOTROWSKI: *The Application of Metabolic and Excretion Kinetics to Problems of Industrial Toxicology*; U.S. Department of Health, Education and Welfare. Washington, D.C., Government Printing Office (1971).
21. U.S. Department of Health, Education and Welfare, *Report of the Secretary's Commission on Pesticides and Their Relationship to Environmental Health.* Washington, D.C., Government Printing Office (1969).

22. O. B. COPE: *Research in Pesticides*. New York, Academic Press (1965).
23. U.S. Environmental Protection Agency, *Principles of Chemical Epidemiology*. Chamblee, Georgia, (1971).
24. See ref. 5.
25. G. M. WOODWELL: Toxic substances and ecological cycles. *Sci. Am.* 216:24 (March, 1967).
26. W. S. HOFFMAN, H. ADLER, W. FISHBEIN, and F. C. BAUER: Relation of pesticide concentrations in fat to pathological changes in tissues. *Arch. Environ. Health* 15:758 (1967).
27. E. R. LAWS, JR., A. CURLEY, and F. J. BIROS: Men with intensive occupational exposure to DDT: a clinical and chemical study. *Arch. Environ. Health* 15:768 (1967).
28. C. G. HUNTER, J. ROBINSON, and M. ROBERTS. Pharmaco-dynamics of Dieldrin (HEOD). *Arch. Environ. Health* 18:12 (1969).
29. J. R. M. INNES, B. M. ULLAND, M. G. VALERIO, L. PETRUCELLI, L. FISHBEIN, E. R. HART, A. J. PALLOTA, R. R. BATES, H. L. FALK, J. J. GART, M. KLEIN, I. MITCHELL, and J. PETERS: Bioassay of pesticides and industrial chemicals for tumorigenicity in mice: a preliminary report. *J. Nat. Cancer Inst.* 42:1101 (1969).
30. G. B. MORGAN, G. OZOLINS, and E. C. TABOR: Air pollution surveillance systems. *Science* 170:289 (1970).
31. E. IGLAVER: A reporter at large: the ambient air. *The New Yorker Magazine* April 13, pp. 51–52 (1968).
32. S. M. AYRES and M. E. BUEHLER: The effects of urban air pollution on health. *Clin. Pharmacol. Ther.* 11:337 (1970).
33. R. A. PAPETTI and F. R. GILMORE: Air pollution. *Endeavour* 30:107 (1971).
34. A. C. STERN, Ed.: *Air Pollution*. New York, Academic Press (1968).
35. R. H. DREISBACH: *Handbook of the San Francisco Region*. Palo Alto, Ca., Environment Studies (1969).
36. B. ROUECHÉ: The fog. In *Eleven Blue Men*. New York, Berkeley Publishing Corp. (1953) pp. 171–189.
37. H. H. SCHRENK, H. HEIMANN, G. D. CLAYTON, W. M. GAFAFER, and H. WEXLER: Public Health Bull. No. 306, *Air Pollution in Donora, Pa*. Washington, D.C. (1949).
38. D. J. THOMPSON and A. CIOCCO: Sickness, change of residence, and death. I. General results of follow-up in two population groups. *Brit. J. Prevent. Social Med.* 12:172 (1958).
39. J. R. GOLDSMITH: Effect of air pollution on humans. In *Air Pollution*, vol. 1, chapt. 10, pp. 335–386, ed. by A. C. Stern. New York, Academic Press, (1962).
40. J. FRY: Effects of a severe fog on a general practice. *Lancet* 1:235 (1953).
41. Reports on Public Health and Medical Subjects, No. 95. London, Ministry of Health (1954).
42. S. M. FARBER and R. H. L. WILSON, eds.: *The Air We Breathe. A Study of Man and His Environment*. Springfield, Ill., Charles C. Thomas (1961), p. 414.
43. L. B. LAVE and E. P. SESKIN: Air pollution and human health. *Science* 169:723 (1970).
44. P. M. LAMBERT and D. D. REID: Smoking, air pollution and bronchitis in Britain. *Lancet* 1:853 (1970).
45. D. D. REID and C. M. FLETCHER: International studies in chronic respiratory disease. *Brit. Med. Bull.* 27:59 (1971).
46. E. GOLDSTEIN: Evaluation of the role of nitrogen dioxide in the development of respiratory diseases in man. *California Medicine* 115:21 (1971).
47. H. A. SULTZ, J. G. FELDMAN, E. R. SCHLESINGER, and W. E. MCSHER: An effect of continued exposure to air pollution on the incidence of chronic childhood allergic disease. *Amer. J. Pub. Health* 60:891 (1970).
48. R. D. CADLE and E. R. ALLEN: Atmospheric photochemistry. *Science* 167:243 (1970).
49. W. WAYNE, P. F. WEHRLE, and R. E. CARROLL: Oxidant air pollution and athletic performance. *J. Amer. Med. Assoc.* 199:151 (1967).
50. L. O. EMIK, R. L. PLATA, K. I. CAMPBELL, and G. L. CLARKE: Biological effects of urban air pollution. *Arch. Environ. Health* 23:335 (1971).
51. R. EHRLICH: Effect of nitrogen dioxide on resistance to respiratory infection. *Bacteriological Reviews* 30:604 (1966).
52. U.S. Department of Health, Education, and Welfare: *Air Quality Criteria for Sulfur Oxides: Summary and Conclusions*, Public Health Service Publication No. 5016. Washington, D.C., Government Printing Office (1969) pp. 344–844.

53. J. C. WAGNER, C. A. SLEGGS, and P. MARCHAND: Diffuse pleural mesothelioma and asbestos exposure in the North Western Cape Province. *Br. J. Industr. Med.* 17:260 (1960).
54. D. HUNTER: *The Diseases of Occupations*, 4th ed. Boston, Little Brown and Co. (1969).
55. A. BOUHUYS and J. M PETERS: Control of environmental lung disease. *New Eng. J. Med.* 283:573 (1970).
56. J. C. WAGNER, J. C. GILSON, G. BERRY, and V. TIMBRELL: Epidemiology of asbestos cancers. *Brit. Med. Bull.* 27:71 (1971).
57. National Academy of Sciences; National Academy of Engineering: *Effects of Chronic Exposure to Low Levels of Carbon Monoxide on Human Health, Behavior, and Performance*. Washington, D.C., National Research Council for the Environmental Studies Board (1969).
58. I. R. CAMPBELL and E. G. MERGARD: *Biological Aspects of Lead: An Annotated Bibliography (1950–1964)*. U.S. Environmental Protection Agency Publisher No. AP-104. Washington, D.C., U.S. Government Printing Office (1972).
59. Symposium on lead. *Arch. Environ. Health* 8:202 (1964).
60. R. A. GOYER: Lead toxicity: a problem of environmental pathology. *Am. J. Path.* 64:167 (1971).
61. R. C. GRIGGS, I. SUNSHINE, V. A. NEWHILL, B. W. NEWTON, S. BUCHANAN, and C. A. RASCH: Environmental factors in childhood lead poisoning. *J. Am. Med. Assoc.* 187:703 (1964).
62. H. WILLIAMS, E. KAPLAN, C. E. COUCHMAN, and R. R. SAYERS: Lead poisoning in young children. *Pub. Health Records* 67:230 (1952).
63. V. F. GUINEE: Lead poisoning in New York City. *Trans. N. Y. Acad. Sci.* 33:539 (1971).
63a. M. W. OBERLE: Lead poisoning: a preventable childhood disease of the slums. *Science* 165:991 (1969).
63b. J. J. CHISOLM, JR. and E. KAPLAN: Lead poisoning in childhood—comprehensive management and prevention. *J. Pediar* 73:942 (1968).
64. P. D. BERK, D. P. TSCHUDY, L. A. SHEPLEY, J. G. WAGGONER, and N. I. BERLIN: Hematologic and biochemical studies in a case of lead poisoning. *Am. J. Med.* 48:137 (1970).
65. H. A. WALDRON: The anaemia of lead poisoning: a review. *Br. J. Industr. Med.* 23:83 (1966).
66. M. A. PERLSTEIN and R. ATTALA: Neurologic sequelae of plumbism in children. *Clin. Pediatrics* 5:292 (1966).
67. C. R. ANGLE, M. S. McINTIRE, and R. L. MEILE: Neurologic sequelae of poisoning in children. *J. Pediat.* 73:531 (1968).
68. R. D. SNYDER: Congenital mercury poisoning. *New Eng. J. Med.* 284:1014 (1971).
69. H. L. NEEDLEMAN, C. C. TUNCAY, and I. M. SHAPIRO: Lead levels in deciduous teeth of urban and suburban American children. *Nature* 235:111 (1972).
70. S. HERNBERG, J. NIKKANEN, G. MELLIN, and H. LILIUS: δ-Aminolevulinic acid dehydrase as a measure of lead exposure. *Arch. Envir. Health* 21:140 (1970).
71. S. HERNBERG: Life span, potassium fluxes, and membrane ATPases of erythrocytes from subjects exposed to inorganic lead. *Work—Environment—Health*, Vol. 3, Supplement 1 (1967).
72. L. A. BLANKSMA, H. K SACHS, E. F. MURRAY, and M. J. O'CONNELL: Incidence of high blood lead levels in Chicago children. *Pedriatics* 44:661 (1969).
73. M. J. SPECTOR, V. F. GUINEE, and B. DAVIDOW: The unsuitability of random urinary delta aminolevulinic acid samples as a screening test for lead poisoning. *J. Ped.* 79:799 (1971).
74. P. R. FINE and R. H. SUHS: Pediatric lead poisoning in Illinois. In *Principles of Chemical Epidemiology*. Chamblee, Georgia, Environmental Protection Agency (1971) p. 119.
75. L. DANIELSON: *Gasoline Containing Lead*. Stockholm, Sweden, Swedish Natural Science Research Council, Bulletin No. 6 (1970).
76. Environmental Protection Agency: *Health Hazards of Lead*. United States Government, Working Paper, February 1972.
77. T. J. CHOW and J. L. EARL: Lead aerosols in the atmosphere: increasing concentrations. *Science* 169:577 (1970).
78. P. R. ATKINS: *The Natural Removal of Lead Pollutants from a Suburban Atmosphere*. Dissertation, Department of Civil Engineering, Stanford University (1968).
79. Department of Public Health, State of California, *Lead in the Environment and Its Effects on Humans*. Berkeley (1967).
79a. J. R. GOLDSMITH and A. C. HEXTER: Respiratory exposure to lead: epidemiological and experimental dose-response relationships. *Science* 158:132 (1967).
80. R. A. WALLACE, W. FULKERSON, W. D. SHULTS, and W. S. LYON: *Mercury in the Environment: The Human Element* ORNL-NSF Environmental Program, Oak Ridge National Laboratory, reprinted March 1971.

81. R. M. MILLER: Prenatal origins of mental retardation; epidemiological approach. *J. Pediat.* 71:455 (1967).

82. L. T. KURLAND, S. N. FARO, and H. SIEDLER: Minamata disease: the outbreak of a neurologic disorder in Minamata, Japan, and its relationship to the ingestion of seafood contaminated by mercuric compounds. *World Neurology* 1:370 (1960).

83. Environmental negligence: the mercury problem (editorial). *Am. J. Pub. Health* 61:1745 (1971).

84. Methyl mercury (editorial). *Science* 169:237 (1970).

84a. J. G. DATHAN and C. C. HARVEY: Pink disease—ten years after (the epilogue). *Brit. Med. J.* 1:1181 (1965).

85. A. CURLEY, V. A. SEDLAK, E. F. GIRLING, R. E. HAWK, W. F. BARTHEL, P. E. PIERCE, and W. H. LIKOSKY: Organic mercury identified as the cause of poisoning in humans and hogs. *Science* 172:65 (1971).

86. F. BAKIR *et al.*: Methylmercury poisoning in Iraq. *Science* 181:230 (1973).

87. J. M. WOOD, F. S. KENNEDY, and C. G. ROSEN: Synthesis of methyl–mercury compounds by extracts of a methanogenic bacterium. *Nature* 220:173 (1968).

88. B. ABERG, L. EKMAN, R. FALK, U. GREITZ, G. PERSSON, and J.-O. SNIHS: Metabolism of methyl mercury (^{203}Hg) compounds in man: excretion and distribution. *Arch. Env. Health* 19:478 (1969).

89. T. B. EYL: Current concepts: organic-mercury food poisoning. *New Eng. J. Med.* 284:706 (1971).

90. T. B. EYL, K. R. WILCOX, JR., and M. S. REIZEN: Mercury, fish and human health. *Mich. Med.* 69:873 (1970).

91. R. S. FOOTE: Mercury vapor concentrations inside buildings. *Science* 177:513 (1972).

92. H. J. SANDERS: Food additives; Part I. *Chemical and Engineering News*, Oct. 10, 1966, p. 100.

93. G. O. KERMODE: Food additives. *Sci. Am.* 226:15 (March, 1972).

93a. M. L. KAPLAN and P. G. KELLEHER: Monosodium glutamate: feeding of large amounts in man and gerbils. *Science* 169:1208 (1970).

93b. Y. L. MORIN, A. R. FOLEY, G. MARTINEAU, and J. ROUSSEL: Quebec beer-drinkers cardiomyopathy: forty-eight cases. *Can. Med. Ass. J.* 97:881 (1967).

93c. N. WADE: DES: A case study of regulatory abdication. *Science* 177:335 (1972).

94. R. CARSON: *Silent Spring*. Boston, Houghton Mifflin Co. (1962).

95. M. A. SCHNEIDERMAN, M. H. MYERS, Y. S. SATHE, and P. KOFFSKY: Toxicity, the therapeutic index, and the ranking of drugs. *Science* 144:1212 (1964).

96. J. W. TREVAN: The error of determination of toxicity. *Proc. Roy. Soc. B.* 101:483 (1927).

97. D. J. FINNEY: *Probit Analysis*, 2nd ed. London, Cambridge University Press (1952).

98. R. A. FISHER and F. YATES: *Statistical Tables for Biological, Agricultural and Medical Research.* London, Oliver and Boyd (1938).

99. A. GOLDSTEIN: *Biostatistics: An Introductory Text.* New York, Macmillan Co. (1964).

100. J. T. LITCHFIELD, JR. and F. WILCOXON: A simplified method of evaluating dose-effect experiments. *J. Pharmacol. Exper. Ther.* 96:99 (1949).

101. G. ZBINDEN: Experimental and Clinical Aspects of Drug Toxicity. *Adv. Pharmacol.* 2:1 (1963).

102. D. F. MARSH: *Outline of Fundamental Pharmacology.* Springfield, Ill., Charles C. Thomas (1951).

103. J. C. SEED, S. L. WALLENSTEIN, R. W. HOUDE, and J. W. BELLVILLE: A comparison of the analgesic and respiratory effects of dihydrocodeine and morphine in man. *Arch. Int. Pharmacodyn.* 116:293 (1958).

104. R. W. HOUDE, S. L. WALLENSTEIN, and W. T. BEAVER: Clinical measurement of pain. In *Analgetics*, ed. by G. deStevens. New York. Academic Press (1965).

105. W. B. ABRAMS, R. E. BAGDON, and G. ZBINDEN: Drug toxicity and its impact on drug evaluation in man. *Clin. Pharmacol. Ther.* 5:273 (1964).

106. J. M. BARNES and F. A. DENZ: Experimental methods used in determining chronic toxicity. *Pharmacol. Rev.* 6:191 (1954).

107. G. ZBINDEN: The problem of the toxicologic examination of drugs in animals and their safety in man. *Clin. Pharmacol. Therap.* 5:537 (1964).

107a. G. ZBINDEN: Animal toxicity studies: a critical evaluation *Appl. Ther.* 8:128 (1966).

108. J. T. LITCHFIELD, JR.: Evaluation of the safety of new drugs by means of tests in animals. *Clin. Pharmacol. Ther.* 3:665 (1962).

109. H. KALTER: Experimental investigation of teratogenic action. *Ann. N.Y. Acad. Sci.* 123:287 (1965).

110. C. S. DELAHUNT and L. J. LASSEN: Thalidomide syndrome in monkeys. *Science* 146:1300 (1964).

111. P. R. MC CURDY: Chloramphenicol bone marrow toxicity. *J. Am. Med. Ass.* 176:588 (1961).

112. A. A. SHARP: Chloramphenicol-induced blood dyscrasias: analysis of 40 cases. *Brit. Med. J.* 1:735 (1963).

113. J. G. COCKE, JR., R. E. BROWN, and L. J. GEPPERT: Optic neuritis with prolonged use of chloramphenicol. *J. Pediat.* 68:27 (1966).

114. N. N. HUANG, R. D. HARLEY, V. PROMADHATTAVEDI, and A. SPROUL: Visual disturbances in cystic fibrosis following chloramphenicol administration. *J. Pediat.* 68:32 (1966).

115. E. N. COHEN, H. W. BREWER, J. W. BELLVILLE, and R. SHER: The chemistry and toxicology of dichlorohexafluorobutene. *Anesthesiology* 26:140 (1965).

116. E. N. COHEN, J. W. BELLVILLE, H. BUDZIKIEWICZ, and D. H. WILLIAMS: Impurity in halothane anesthetic. *Science* 141:899 (1963).

117. Summary of the national halothane study. *J. Am. Med. Ass.* 197:775 (1966).

118. Council on Drugs, American Medical Association. Publications of the Registry on Adverse Reactions, Vol. 1. Chicago, 1964–1963.

119. P. S. NORMAN and L. E. CLUFF: Adverse drug reactions and alternative drugs of choice. In *Drugs of Choice*, 1968–1969, ed. by W. Modell, St. Louis, C. V. Mosby Co. (1967) Ch. 3, pp. 29–46.

120. J. AVIGAN, D. STEINBERG, H. E. VROMAN, M. J. THOMPSON, and E. MOSETTIG: Studies of cholesterol biosynthesis. I. The identification of desmosterol in serum and tissues of animals and man treated with MER-29. *J. Biol. Chem.* 235:3123 (1960).

121. R. W. P. ACHOR, R. K. WINKELMANN, and H. O. PERRY: Cutaneous side effects from use of triparanol (MER-29): preliminary data on ichthyosis and loss of hair. *Proc. Staff Meetings Mayo Clinic* 36:217 (1961).

122. R. C. LAUGHLIN and T. F. CAREY: Cataracts in patients treated with triparanol. *J. Am. Med. Ass.* 181:339 (1962).

123. L. VON SALLMAN, P. GRIMES, and E. COLLINS: Triparanol-induced cataracts in rats. *Arch. Ophthalmol.* 70:522 (1963).

124. New York Times, June 5, 1964, p. 11.

125. M. MINTZ: *The Therapeutic Nightmare.* Boston. Houghton Mifflin Co. (1965).

126. M. CORNBLATH and A. F. HARTMANN: Methemoglobinemia in young infants. *J. Pediat.* 33:421 (1948).

127. J. D. ROSS and J. F. DESFORGES: Reduction of methemoglobin by erythrocytes from cord blood: further evidence of deficient enzyme activity in the newborn period. *Pediatrics* 23:718 (1959).

128. F. RIEDERS: Noxious gases and vapors I: carbon monoxide, cyanides, methemoglobin, and sulfhemoglobin. In *Drill's Pharmacology in Medicine*, 4th ed., ed. by J. R. DiPalma. New York, McGraw–Hill (1971) Ch. 58.

129. R. E. GOSSELIN and R. P. SMITH: Trends in the therapy of acute poisonings. *Clin. Pharmacol. Therap.* 7:279 (1966).

130. A. L. PICCHIONI, L. CHIN, H. L. VERHULST, and B. DIETERLE: Activated charcoal universal vs. "universal antidote" as an antidote for poisons. *Toxicol. Appl. Pharmacol.* 8:447 (1966).

131. C. CLEMMESEN and E. NILSSON: Therapeutic trends in the treatment of barbiturate poisoning. The Scandinavian method. *Clin. Pharmacol. Ther.* 2:220 (1961).

132. A. MYSCHETZKY and N. A. LASSEN: Urea-induced, osmotic diuresis and alkalization of urine in acute barbiturate intoxication. *J. Am. Med. Ass.* 185:936 (1963).

133. C. CLEMMESEN: Treatment of narcotic intoxication. *Danish Med. Bull.* 10:97 (1963), and other papers in the same volume, pp. 100–144.

134. R. C. LILLEHEI, J. K. LONGERBEAM, J. H. BLOCH, and W. G. MANAX: The nature of irreversible shock: experimental and clinical observations. *Ann. Surgery* 160:682 (1964).

135. M. NICKERSON: Sympathetic blockade in the therapy of shock. *Amer. J. Cardiol.* 12:619 (1963).

136. H. SHUBIN and M. H. WEIL: The mechanism of shock following suicidal doses of barbiturates, narcotics and tranquilizer drugs, with observations on the effects of treatment. *Amer. J. Med.* 38:853 (1965).

137. L. WEINSTEIN and A. S. KLAINER: Management of emergencies. IV. Septic shock—pathogenesis and treatment. *New Eng. J. Med.* 274:950 (1966).

138. J. J. ABEL, L. G. ROWNTREE, and B. B. TURNER: On the removal of diffusible substances from the circulating blood of living animals by dialysis. *J. Pharmacol. Exper. Ther.* 5:275 (1914).

139. J. P. KNOCHEL, L. E. CLAYTON, W. L. SMITH, and K. G. BARRY: Intraperitoneal THAM: an effective method to enhance phenobarbital removal during peritoneal dialysis. *J. Lab. Clin. Med.* 64:257 (1964).

140. J. F. MAHER and G. E. SCHREINER: Hazards and complications of dialysis. *New Eng. J Med.* 273:370 (1965).

141. W. J. WADDELL and T. C. BUTLER: The distribution and excretion of phenobarbital. *J. Clin. Invest.* 36:1217 (1957).

142. M. E. KRAHL: The effect of variation in ionic strength and temperature on the apparent dissociation constants of thirty substituted barbituric acids. *J. Phys. Chem.* 44:449 (1940).

143. J. C. STRICKLER: Forced diuresis in the management of barbiturate intoxication. *Clin. Pharmacol. Ther.* 6:693 (1965).

144. N. A. LASSEN: Treatment of severe acute barbiturate poisoning by forced diuresis and alkalinisation of the urine. *Lancet* 2:338 (1960).

145. A. K. DONE: Pharmacological principles in the treatment of poisoning. *Pharmacol. Physicians* 3:1 (1969).

146. L. A. STOCKEN and R. H. S. THOMPSON: Reactions of British antilewisite with arsenic and other metals in living systems. *Physiol. Rev.* 29:168 (1949).

146a. R. A. KARK, D. C. POSKANZER, J. D. BULLOCK, and G. BOYLEN: Mercury poisoning and its treatment with N-acetyl-D,L-penicillamine. *New Eng. J. Med.* 285:10 (1971).

146b. S. SELANDER: Treatment of lead poisoning: a comparison between the effects of sodium calciumedetate and penicillamine administered orally and intravenously. *Br. J Indust. Med.* 24:272 (1967).

146c. J. J. CHISOLM, JR.: The use of chelating agents in the treatment of acute and chronic lead intoxication in childhood. *J. Pediat.* 73:1 (1968).

147. M. W. ROSENTHAL, J. F. MARKLEY, A. LINDENBAUM, and J. SCHUBERT: Influence of DTPA therapy on long-term effects of retained plutonium. *Health Phys.* 8:741 (1962).

148. W. D. NORWOOD: Therapeutic removal of plutonium in humans. *Health Phys.* 8:747 (1962).

149. R. DAGIRMANJIAN, E. A. MAYNARD, and H. C. HODGE: The effects of calcium disodium ethylenediamine tetraacetate on uranium poisoning in rats. *J. Pharmacol. Exper. Ther.* 117:20 (1956).

150. V. NIGROVIĆ and A. CATSCH: Tierexperimentelle Untersuchungen zur Behandlung der akuten Eisenvergiftung. *Arch. exper. Pathol. Pharmakol.* 251:225 (1965).

151. V. H. BICKEL, E. GÄUMANN, W. KELLER-SCHIERLEIN, V. PRELOG, E. VISCHER, A. WETTSTEIN, and H. ZÄHNER: Über eisenhaltige Wachstumsfaktoren, die Sideramine, und ihre Antagonisten, die eisenhaltigen Antibiotika Sideromycine. *Experientia* 16:129 (1960).

152. S. MOESCHLIN and U. SCHNIDER: Treatment of primary and secondary hemochromatosis and acute iron poisoning with a new, potent iron-eliminating agent (desferoxamine-B). *New Eng. J. Med.* 269:57 (1963).

153. J. JACOBS, H. GREENE, and B. R. GENDEL: Acute iron intoxication. *New Eng. J. Med.* 273:1124 (1965).

154. N. MOVASSAGHI, G. G. PURUGGANAN, and S. LEIKIN: Comparison of exchange transfusion and deferoxamine in the treatment of acute iron poisoning. *J. Pediat.* 75:604 (1969).

155. H. V. APOSHIAN: Penicillamine and analogous chelating agents. *Ann. N.Y. Acad. Sci.* 179:481 (1971).

156. I. STERNLIEB and I. H. SCHEINBERG: Penicillamine therapy for hepatolenticular degeneration. *J. Am. Med. Ass.* 189:748 (1964).

157. H. V. APOSHIAN: Biochemical and pharmacological properties of the metal-binding agent penicillamine. *Fed. Proc.* 20:185 (1961).

158. A. LUND: The effect of various substances on the excretion and the toxicity of thallium in the rat. *Acta Pharmacol. Toxicol.* 12:260 (1956).

159. F. W. SUNDERMAN: Diethyldithiocarbamate therapy of thallotoxicosis. *Amer. J. med. Sci.* 253:209 (1967).

160. A. LUND: Rational treatment of formaldehyde poisoning. *Acta Pharmacol. Toxicol.* 3:323 (1947).

161. T. W. PARKIN and W. F. KVALE: Neutralization of the anticoagulant effects of heparin with protamine (salmine). *Amer. Heart J.* 37:333 (1949).

162. C. LAMANNA: The most poisonous poison. *Science* 130:763 (1959).

163. C. S. PETTY: Botulism: The disease and the toxin. *Am. J. Med. Sci.* 249:345 (1965).

164. R. L. WHITTAKER, R. B. GILBERTSON, and A. S. GARRETT, JR.: Botulism, Type E. Report of eight simultaneous cases. *Ann. Int. Med.* 61:448 (1964).

165. D. H. SCHMIDT and V. P. BUTLER, JR.: Reversal of digoxin toxicity with specific antibodies. *J. Clin. Invest.* 50:1738 (1971).

166. G. BAZZANO and G. S. BAZZANO: Digitalis intoxication: treatment with a new steroid-binding resin. *J. Am. Med. Ass.* 220:828 (1972).

167. B. HOLMSTEDT: Pharmacology of organophosphorus cholinesterase inhibitors. *Pharmacol. Rev.* 11:567 (1959).

168. Occupation Disease in California Attributed to Pesticides and other Agricultural Chemicals (1963). Report prepared by G. D. Kleinman. State of California Department of Public Health, Bureau of Occupational Health, Berkeley, Calif.

169. D. GROB and J. C. HARVEY: Effects in man of the anticholinesterase compound sarin (isopropyl) methyl phosphonofluoricate). *J. Clin. Invest.* 37:350 (1958).

170. I. B. WILSON: Acetylcholinesterase. XIII. Reactivation of alkyl phosphate-inhibited enzyme. *J. Biol. Chem.* 199:113 (1952).

171. I. B. WILSON: Molecular complementarity and antidotes for alkylphosphate poisoning. *Fed. Proc.* 18:752 (1959).

172. J. F. O'LEARY, A. M. KUNKEL, and A. H. JONES: Efficacy and limitations of oxime-atropine treatment of organophosphorus anticholinesterase poisoning. *J. Pharmacol. Exper. Ther.* 132:50 (1961).

173. I. B. WILSON, M. A. HARRISON, and S. GINSBURG: Carbamyl derivatives of acetylcholinesterase. *J. Biol. Chem.* 236:1498 (1961).

174. H. G. ALBAUM, J. TEPPERMAN, and O. BODANSKY: A spectrophotometric study of competition of methemoglobin and cytochrome oxidase for cyanide in vitro. *J. Biol. Chem.* 163:641 (1946).

175. K. BETKE, I. GREINACHER, and O. TIETZE: Oxydation menschlicher und tierischer Oxyhämoglobine durch Natrumnitrit. *Arch. exper. Pathol. Pharmakol.* 229:220 (1956).

176. K. K. CHEN, C. L. ROSE, and G. H. A. CLOWES: Comparative values of several antidotes in cyanid poisoning. *Am. J. Med. Sci.* 188:767 (1934).

177. C.-J. CLEMEDSON, H. I. HULTMAN, and B. SORBO: The antidote effect of some sulfur compounds and rhodanese in experimental cyanide poisoning. *Acta Physiol. Scand.* 32:245 (1954).

178. J. L. WAY, S. L. GIBBON, and M. SHEEHY: Cyanide intoxication: protection with oxygen. *Science* 152:210 (1966).

179. M. N. COOPER, G. L. MITCHELL, JR., I. L. BENNETT, JR., and F. H. CARY: Methyl alcohol poisoning: an account of the 1951 Atlanta epidemic. *J. Med. Assoc. Georgia* 41:48 (1952).

180. J. R. COOPER and M. M. KINI: Biochemical aspects of methanol poisoning. *Biochem. Pharmacol.* 11:405 (1962).

181. O. RÖE: The roles of alkaline salts and ethyl alcohol in the treatment of methanol poisoning. *Quart. J. Stud. Alcohol.* 11:107 (1950).

182. M. M. KINI and J. R. COOPER: Biochemistry of methanol poisoning. 4. The effect of methanol and its metabolites on retinal metabolism. *Biochem. J.* 82:164 (1962).

183. G. R. BARTLETT: Combustion of C^{14} labeled methanol in intact rat and its isolated tissues. *Am. J. Physiol.* 163:614 (1950).

184. M. M. KINI and J. R. COOPER: Biochemistry of methanol poisoning. 3. The enzymic pathway for the conversion of methanol to formaldehyde. *Biochem. Pharmacol.* 1:207 (1961).

185. M. E. SMITH: Interrelations in ethanol and methanol metabolism. *J. Pharmacol. Exper. Ther.* 134:233 (1961).

186. T. R. TEPHLY, R. E. PARKS, JR., and G. J. MANNERING: Methanol metabolism in the rat. *J. Pharmacol. Exper. Ther.* 143:292 (1964).

187. I. ROSENFELD and O. A. BEATH: *Selenium: Geobotany, Biochemistry, Toxicity, and Nutrition.* New York, Academic Press (1964).

188. L. ARONOW and F. KERDEL-VEGAS: Cytotoxic and depilatory effects of extracts of *Lecythis ollaria. Nature* 205:1185 (1965).

189. L. ARONOW: Metabolism of seleno-cystathionine and effects on mammalian cells growing in vitro. *Fed. Proc.* 25:196 (1966).

190. R. A. PETERS: Mechanism of the toxicity of the active constituent of *Dichapetalum cymosum* and related compounds. *Adv. Enzymol.* 18:113 (1957).

191. R. A. PETERS: Biochemistry of some toxic agents. II. Some recent work in the field of fluoroacetate compounds. *Bull. Johns Hopkins Hosp.* 97:21 (1955).

192. R. A. PETERS and R. W WAKELIN: The synthesis of fluorocitric acid and its inhibition by acetate. *Biochem. J.* 67:280 (1957).

193. S. GITTER: The influence of acetamide on citrate accumulation after fluoroacetate poisoning. *Biochem. J.* 63:182 (1956).

194. M. B. CHENOWETH, A. KANDEL, L. B. JOHNSON, and D. R. BENNETT: Factors influencing fluoroacetate poisoning. Practical treatment with glycerol monoacetate. *J. Pharmacol. Exper. Ther.* 102:31 (1951).

195. A. ENGSTRÖM, R. BJÖRNERSTEDT, C. J. CLEMEDSON, and A. NELSON: *Bone and Radiostrontium.* New York, Wiley (1958).

196. H. SPENCER, M. LI, J. SAMACHSON, and D. LASZLO: Metabolism of strontium-85 and calcium-45 in man. *Metabolism* 9:916 (1960).

197. F. C. GRAN and R. NICOLAYSEN: A theoretical analysis of radio-strontium metabolism and deposition in humans. *Acta Physiol. Scand.* 61:Suppl. 223 (1964).

198. J. SAMACHSON and H. SPENCER–LASZLO: Urinary excretion of calcium and strontium 85 in man. *J. Appl. Physiol.* 17:525 (1962).

199. H. SPENCER and J. SAMACHSON: Removal of radiostrontium in man by orally administered ammonium chloride two weeks after exposure: the effect of low and high calcium intake. *Clin. Sci.* 20:333 (1961).

200. J. WYMAN, JR.: Linked functions and reciprocal effects in hemoglobin: a second look. *Adv. Prot. Chem.* 19:223 (1964).

201. F. J. W. ROUGHTON and R. C. DARLING: The effect of carbon monoxide on the oxyhemoglobin dissociation curve. *Amer. J. Physiol.* 141:17 (1944).

202. D. L. DRABKIN, F. H. LEWEY, S. BELLET, and W. H. EHRICH: The effect of replacement of normal blood by erythrocytes saturated with carbon monoxide. *Am. J. Med. Sci.* 205:755 (1943).

203. F. J. W. ROUGHTON and W. S. ROOT: The fate of CO in the body during recovery from mild carbon monoxide poisoning in man. *Amer. J. Physiol.* 145:239 (1945).

204. A. L. BARACH: Hyperbaric oxygen and current medical uses of oxygen. *N. Y. State J. Med.* 63:2775 (1963).

205. P. G. WASER: The cholinergic receptor. *J. Pharm. Pharmacol.* 12:577 (1960).

206. C. MERSKEY and A. DRABKIN: Anticoagulant therapy. *Blood* 25:567 (1965).

207. J. W. SUTTIE: Control of prothrombin and factor VII biosynthesis by vitamin K. *Arch. Biochem. Biophys.* 118:166 (1967).

207a. D. V. SHAH and J. W. SUTTIE: The effect of vitamin K and warfarin on rat liver prothrombin concentrations. *Arch. Biochem. Biophys.* 150:91 (1972).

208. R. G. BELL and J. T. MATSCHINER: Vitamin K activity of phylloquinone oxide. *Arch. Biochem. Biophys.* 141:473 (1970).

209. A. S. DOUGLAS and A. BROWN: Effect of vitamin-K preparations on hypoprothrombinaemia induced by dicoumarol and tromexan. *Brit. Med. J.* 1:412 (1952).

210. L. LASAGNA and H. K. BEECHER: The analgesic effectiveness of nalorphine and nalorphine-morphine combinations in man. *J. Pharmacol. Exper. Ther.* 112:356 (1954).

211. A. S. KEATS and J. TELFORD: Nalorphine, a potent analgesic in man. *J. Pharmacol. Exper. Ther.* 117:190 (1956).

212. B. M. COX and M. WEINSTOCK: Quantitative studies of the antagonism by nalorphine of some of the actions of morphine-like analgesic drugs. *Brit. J. Pharmacol.* 22:289 (1964).

213. L. GRUMBACH and H. I. CHERNOV: The analgesic effect of opiate-opiate antagonist combinations in the rat. *J. Pharmacol. Exper. Ther.* 149:385 (1965).

214. O. BODANSKY: Methemoglobinemia and methemoglobin-producing compounds. *Pharmacol. Rev.* 3:144 (1951).

215. B. ROUECHÉ: Eleven blue men. In *Eleven Blue Men.* New York, Berkeley Publishing Corp. (1953) pp. 78–89.

216. R. C. DARLING and F. J. W. ROUGHTON: The effect of methemoglobin on the equilibrium between oxygen and hemoglobin. *Am. J. Physiol.* 137:56 (1942).

217. O. BODANSKY and H. GUTMANN: Treatment of methemoglobinemia. *J. Pharmacol. Exper. Ther.* 90:46 (1947).

218. F. M. HUENNEKENS, R. W. CAFFREY, R. E. BASFORD, and B. W. GABRIO: Erythrocyte metabolism. IV. Isolation and properties of methemoglobin reductase. *J. Biol. Chem.* 227:261 (1957).

219. E. BEUTLER and M. C. BALUDA: Methemoglobin reduction. Studies of the interaction between cell populations and of the role of methylene blue. *Blood* 22:323 (1963).

220. A. F. MANGELSDORFF: Treatment of methemoglobinemia. *A.M.A. Arch. Ind. Health* 14:148 (1956).

221. N. GOLUBOFF and R. WHEATON: Methylene blue induced cyanosis and acute hemolytic anemia complicating the treatment of methemoglobinemia. *J. Pediat.* 58:86 (1961).
222. A. P. SOMLYO: The toxicology of digitalis. *Am. J. Cardiol.* 5:523 (1960).
223. W. WITHERING: An account of the foxglove, and some of its medical uses; with practical remarks on dropsy, and other diseases. Reproduced in its entirety in *Medical Classics* 2:305 (1937).
224. C. FISCH, K. GREENSPAN, S. B. KNOEBEL, and H. FEIGENBAUM: Effect of digitalis on conduction of the heart. *Progr. Cardiovasc. Dis.* 6:343 (1964).
225. P. L. RODENSKY and F. WASSERMAN: Observations on digitalis intoxication. *Arch. Int. Med.* 108:171 (1961).
226. G. CHURCH, L. SCHAMROTH, N. L. SCHWARTZ, and H. J. L. MARRIOTT: Deliberate digitalis intoxication. A comparison of the toxic effects of four glycoside preparations. *Ann. Int. Med.* 57:946 (1962).
227. B. LOWN and H. D. LEVINE: *Atrial Arrhythmias, Digitalis and Potassium.* New York, Landsberger Medical Books (1958).
228. J. SAMPSON and E. M. ANDERSON: The treatment of certain cardiac arrhythmias with potassium salts. *J. Am. Med. Ass.* 99:2257 (1932).
229. E. BRAUNWALD and F. J. KLOCKE: Digitalis. *Ann. Rev. Med.* 16:371 (1965).
230. J. J. SAMPSON, E. C. ALBERTON, and B. KONDO: The effect on man of potassium administration in relation to digitalis glycosides, with special reference to blood serum potassium, the electrocardiogram, and ectopic beats. *Amer. Heart J.* 26:164 (1943).
231. B. M. COHEN: Digitalis poisoning and its treatment. *New Eng. J. Med.* 246:225, 254 (1952).
232. J. P. P. STOCK and N. DALE: Beta-adrenergic receptor blockade in cardiac arrhythmias. *Brit. Med. J.* 2:1230 (1963).
233. M. CHERINGTON and D. W. RYAN: Treatment of botulism with guanidine. *New Eng. J. Med.* 282:195 (1970).
234. M. OTSUKA and M. ENDO: The effect of guanidine on neuromuscular transmission. *J. Pharmacol. Exp. Ther.* 128:273 (1960).
235. D. D. WOODS: The relation of *p*-aminobenzoic acid to the mechanism of the action of sulphanilamide. *Brit. J. Exper. Pathol.* 21:74 (1940).
236. D. D. WOODS: The biochemical mode of action of the sulphonamide drugs. *J. Gen. Microbiol.* 29:687 (1962).
237. J. L. STOKES: Substitutions of thymine for "folic acid" in the nutrition of lactic acid bacteria. *J. Bacteriol.* 48:201 (1944).
238. S. FARBER, L. K. DIAMOND, R. D. MERCER, R. F. SYLVESTER, JR., and J. A. WOLFF: Temporary remissions in acute leukemia in children produced by folic acid antagonist, 4-aminopteroyl-glutamic acid (Aminopterin). *New Eng. J. Med.* 238:787 (1948).
239. W. C. WERKHEISER: Specific binding of 4-amino folic acid analogs by folic acid reductase. *J. Biol. Chem.* 236:888 (1961).
240. W. C. WERKHEISER: The biochemical, cellular, and pharmacological action and effects of the folic acid antagonists. *Cancer Res.* 23:1277 (1963).
241. M. T. HAKALA and E. TAYLOR: The ability of purine and thymine derivatives and of glycine to support the growth of mammalian cells in culture. *J. Biol. Chem.* 234:126 (1959).
242. P. REYES and C. HEIDELBERGER: Fluorinated pyrimidines 26. Mammalian thymidylate synthetase: its mechanism of action and inhibition by fluorinated nucleotides. *Mol. Pharmacol.* 1:14 (1965).
243. J. S. SALSER and M. E. BALIS: The mechanism of action of 6-mercaptopurine. I. Biochemical effects. *Cancer Res.* 25:539 (1965).

CHAPTER 6
Pharmacogenetics and Drug Idiosyncrasy

INTRODUCTION

Pharmacogenetics concerns unusual drug responses that have a hereditary basis.[1-9] When such responses take the form of extremely high or low sensitivity to an ordinarily effective dose, or the responses are of a qualitatively different sort than normally seen, they may be called idiosyncratic. *Idiosyncrasy* is defined as "... a characteristic distinguishing an individual; characteristic susceptibility; eccentricity."[10] Although the word has long been used in pharmacology to describe peculiar drug reactions, a precise definition has been lacking. We define drug idiosyncrasy as a genetically determined abnormal reactivity to a drug. A complete understanding of an idiosyncratic reaction requires knowledge of the mechanism whereby the usual drug effect is altered in the genetically variant person, of the biochemical abnormality that constitutes the phenotypic expression of the genetic defect, and also of the pattern of inheritance of the genotype.

Idiosyncrasy should not be a catchall classification for unexpected reactions to drugs. Accidental overdosage, inadvertent injection into a vein, or excessively rapid intravenous administration may all provoke severe or even fatal reactions. Insoluble preparations of penicillin, for example, meant for depot use but introduced into a vein by accident, can cause massive pulmonary embolism. Too rapid intravenous injection of mercurial diuretics may cause ventricular fibrillation. A special kind of acute untoward reaction results from the rapid intravenous administration of drugs that are capable of releasing histamine from tissues. Sudden onset of intense generalized itching and burning sensations, lacrimation, erythema, blood pressure collapse, tachycardia, vomiting, and urticaria may present an alarming picture. In asthmatic patients, a severe asthmatic crisis may be precipitated. Allergic reactions to drugs present a special pattern of responses, discussed in the next chapter. Strange and surprising as all these kinds of adverse reactions may be, they have nothing to do with idiosyncrasy.

437

Mere sensitivity to a moderately low dose of a drug or resistance to a moderately high dose does not qualify as idiosyncrasy. Population heterogeneity is an obvious feature of all dose-response relationships, so that a wide dose range may separate the most sensitive from the least sensitive individuals. When guinea pigs were pretreated with an antihistamine drug and then exposed to a lethal dose of histamine, the dose required to protect 84% of the animals was 10 times greater than that which protected 16% of them.[11] The remarkably wide variation in human response to digitoxin was illustrated in Figure 5-11. It is likely that this commonly observed biologic variation in responsiveness to drugs has a genetic basis, a conclusion that is strengthened by the fact that variation is substantially less in inbred strains of animal than in cross-breeding wild strains. The characteristic feature in idiosyncratic sensitivity to low doses or resistance to high doses is a discontinuity from the ordinary distribution of dose sensitivities.

A few words of explanation are in order about the nomenclature used to describe the mode of inheritance of a drug idiosyncrasy.[12] The term *sex-linked* describes a trait carried on the X chromosome. If the male (whose sex chromosome pattern is XY) carries one allele for the trait, he has no normal allele; he is said to be *hemizygous*. The female (XX) carrying a sex-linked abnormality may be *heterozygous* or *homozygous* for the trait. The term *autosomal* refers to a trait carried on any of the 22 pairs of chromosomes (in man) other than X or Y; here the ordinary principles of heterozygosity or homozygosity apply to both sexes. With reference to the inheritance of a trait, the terms *dominant, codominant, recessive* are meaningful. If the trait is expressed in heterozygotes as well as in homozygotes, it is called dominant. If alternative expressions of the trait are possible, each independent of the others, it is called codominant; a classical example is blood group, in which alleles A and B are codominant over O, so that genotypes AO and BO belong to blood groups A and B, respectively (dominance), but genotype AB has both blood group antigens A and B (codominance). Finally, if the trait is only expressed in homozygotes, or (if sex-linked) in hemizygotes, it is called recessive.

Difficulties arise in applying the terminology of classical genetics to traits in which the underlying molecular abnormalities are understood. Let us consider a drug idiosyncrasy that depends upon the presence of an altered enzyme. And suppose, as is often true, that alleles for altered forms of the enzyme are independently expressed, i.e., that the allelic forms of the gene are *autonomous*, so that each gives rise to its corresponding gene product, the enzyme. At the molecular level, the abnormalities are inherited without dominance (autonomously); but if one looks at the drug idiosyncrasy, various results are possible. The heterozygote will contain normal enzyme and altered enzyme. If the normal enzyme suffices to protect against expression of the idiosyncrasy, then responses to the drug will be normal in heterozygotes and abnormal in homozygotes, and the trait will be described as recessive. On the other hand, if the presence of altered enzyme suffices to confer the idiosyncratic response, then heterozygotes and homozygotes will both display the trait, and it will be described as dominant. Finally, in the same example, if attention is focused upon the enzymes (as upon blood group substances in the earlier example), then the inheritance would be described as "without dominance," or codominant, since each allelic form of the gene is independently expressed. Whenever use of the older nomenclature would be confusing, we shall avoid terminologic ambiguities by stating in which genotypes each drug idiosyncrasy is expressed, and then describing separately how the gene products are determined, if known.

Twin studies have played an important part in distinguishing between environmental and hereditary components of biologic variation in general and of pharmacogenetic variation in particular. Drug responses are compared in pairs of identical (homozygous) and fraternal (heterozygous) twins. Ideally, the two members of a pair should live apart, so that environmental factors will be equally diverse for all subjects. The most illuminating studies have dealt with differences in rates of drug metabolism, since plasma half-lives of drugs can be measured with precision.[13] Twin zygosity was confirmed by means of typing for about 30 blood groups. The subjects were all adults who had not taken any drugs for at least one month. Almost all lived in different households, had different diets, and presumably were exposed to a variable extent to insecticides, chlorinated hydrocarbons, and other environmental chemicals that might influence the liver microsomal drug oxidizing system.

Table 6-1 gives illustrative data for bishydroxycoumarin, antipyrine, and phenylbutazone. The fraternal twins showed typical wide variations in plasma half-lives, as seen commonly in human populations, but the half-lives were remarkably similar within each pair of identical twins. The mean differences between members of a pair, for fraternal and identical twins, respectively, were 10.1 and 1.5 hr for bishydroxycoumarin, 5.3 and 0.2 hr for antipyrine, 1.0 and 0.1 days for phenylbutazone. Obviously, hereditary control of drug metabolism is predominant. The contribution of heredity to the large individual variations in plasma half-life can be estimated quantitatively, as a "heredity coefficient," from the formula:

$$\frac{(\text{Variance within pairs of fraternal twins}) - (\text{Variance within pairs of identical twins})}{(\text{Variance within pairs of fraternal twins})}$$

Values can range from zero, indicating a negligible hereditary contribution, to unity, indicating virtually complete hereditary influence. For the three drugs shown, and also for ethanol, the values exceeded 0.97. Halothane metabolism yielded a value of 0.88. In a study of nortriptyline metabolism by other investigators,[14] a value of 0.98 was obtained.

Rates of metabolism of certain drugs vary together. For bishydroxycoumarin and phenylbutazone, individuals who metabolize one slowly are likely to metabolize the other slowly; similar correlation has been found for desmethylimipramine, nortriptyline, and oxyphenylbutazone.[15] But this is not a general rule; a person may metabolize one drug unusually slowly and another at a normal rate or even unusually rapidly. Thus, it appears that the drug-specific as well as nonspecific components of the liver microsomal system are under independent genetic control.

Twin studies have also provided information about the genetic control of phenobarbital-induced increase in drug metabolism. The reduction in plasma half-life of antipyrine in response to phenobarbital yielded a heredity coefficient of 0.99. In this experiment, there were no important differences in phenobarbital blood levels. As shown in Figure 6-1, however, there was a direct relationship between the initial antipyrine half-life and the extent to which the half-life was shortened by phenobarbital. Thus, subjects who metabolized antipyrine slowly showed the greatest increase in metabolism due to phenobarbital.

TABLE 6-1. Plasma half-lives of three drugs in fraternal and identical twins.
(Modified from Vesell, Table 2.[13])

| Twin | Age, sex | Half-life | | |
		Bishydroxy-coumarin, hours	Antipyrine, hours	Phenyl-butazone, days
		Fraternal twins		
AM	21, F	45.0	15.1	7.3
SM	21, M	22.0	6.3	3.6
DL	36, F	46.5	7.2	2.3
DS	36, F	51.0	15.0	3.3
SA	33, F	34.5	5.1	2.1
FM	33, F	27.5	12.5	1.2
JaH	24, F	7.0	12.0	2.6
JeH	24, F	19.0	6.0	2.3
FD	48, M	24.5	14.7	2.8
PD	48, M	38.0	9.3	3.5
LD	21, F	67.0	8.2	2.9
LW	21, F	72.0	6.9	3.0
EK	31, F	40.5	7.7	1.9
RK	31, M	35.0	7.3	2.1
Mean differences		10.1	5.3	1.0
		Identical twins		
HoM	48, M	25.0	11.3	1.9
HoM	48, M	25.0	11.3	2.1
DT	43, F	55.5	10.3	2.8
VW	43, F	55.5	9.6	2.9
JG	22, M	36.0	11.5	2.8
PG	22, M	34.0	11.5	2.8
JaT	44, M	74.0	14.9	4.0
JaT	44, M	72.0	14.9	4.0
CJ	55, F	41.0	6.9	3.2
FJ	55, F	42.5	7.1	2.9
GeL	45, M	72.0	12.3	3.9
GuL	45, M	69.0	12.8	4.1
DH	26, F	46.0	11.0	2.6
DW	26, F	44.0	11.0	2.6
Mean differences		1.5	0.2	0.1

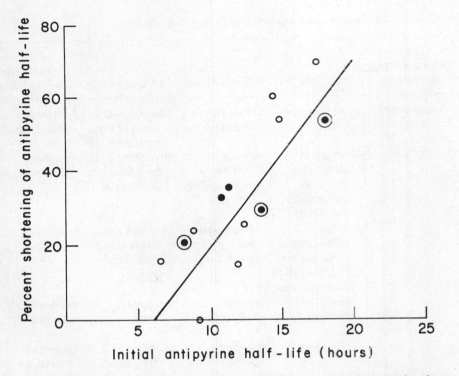

FIGURE 6-1. Effect of phenobarbital on plasma half-life of antipyrine in fraternal and identical twins. *Open circles are fraternal twins, solid circles are identical twins, concentric circles are identical twins with the same data. (From Vesell, Figure 10.[13])*

Gene mutations may abolish the synthesis of specific proteins or cause the production of altered proteins. Although the complete absence of a given protein need not necessarily be incompatible with life, it will often be so. Therefore, the mutations that can find phenotypic expression are only a selection of all possible mutations. Included are those protein deletions that are not lethal, as well as a wide variety of modified proteins usually altered by single amino acid substitutions, as in the hemoglobin variants. Isozymes fall into the same category. These are modified enzymes, still functional, but often displaying altered affinities for substrates and inhibitors, altered reaction velocities, changes in state of aggregation or allosteric interaction, or modified responses to temperature and ionic environment.

In view of the importance of proteins to all aspects of drug action, it is not surprising that an altered phenotype can be the basis of an idiosyncratic drug reaction. Indeed, the phenotypic abnormality is often first revealed by a person's abnormal response to a drug, so that drugs prove to be excellent tools for the discovery of hitherto unsuspected hereditary defects. We can devise, *a priori*, a classification of mechanisms of pharmacogenetic abnormality based upon the general principles relating drugs to proteins. Table 6-2 lists 6 mechanisms, with examples of each. The list includes all the drug idiosyncrasies whose mechanisms are understood. These will be discussed in the remainder of this chapter.

TABLE 6-2. Mechanisms and examples of drug idiosyncrasies.

Type of pharmacologic abnormality	Drug	Genetic basis	Disease or trait	Mode of hereditary transmission
1. Drug toxicity due to impaired drug metabolism	Succinylcholine	Altered plasma cholinesterase	Succinylcholine apnea of long duration	Autosomal autonomous
	Nitrites and other drugs that cause methemoglobinemia	Deficient NADH methemoglobin reductase	Hereditary methemoglobinemia	Autosomal recessive
	Isoniazid, certain other drugs that are metabolized by acetylation	Deficient liver acetyl transferase	Increased toxicity of isoniazid and related drugs	Autosomal recessive
	Diphenylhydantoin	Impaired hydroxylation	Increased toxicity	Autosomal dominant
	Acetophenetidin	Reduced O-dealkylation	Methemoglobinemia	Autosomal recessive
2. Increased sensitivity to drug effect	Nitrites and other drugs that cause methemoglobinemia	Abnormal hemoglobins (M and H)	Propensity to develop methemobinemia	Autosomal; hemoglobin M autonomous, not known if heterozygotes sensitive to methemoglobinemia-producing drugs; hemoglobin H recessive
3. Novel drug effect	Primaquine and other drugs	Deficient glucose-6-phosphate dehydrogenase in erythrocytes	Favism, drug-induced hemolytic anemia	Sex-linked autonomous
	Barbiturates and other drugs	Abnormal inducibility of δ-aminolevulinic acid synthetase	Hepatic porphyria	Autosomal dominant
	Anesthetic agents	?	Malignant hyperthermia	Autosomal dominant

TABLE 6-2. (*continued*)

Type of pharmacologic abnormality	Drug	Genetic basis	Disease or trait	Mode of hereditary transmission
4. Decreased responsiveness to drug	Coumarin anticoagulants	?	Warfarin resistance	Autosomal dominant
	Vitamin D (calcium?)	?	Vitamin D-resistant rickets	Sex-linked dominant
	Phenylthiourea (PTC)	Altered chemo-receptors?	Nontasters (association with thyroid disease?)	Autosomal recessive
	Vitamin B_{12}	Absence of intrinsic factor	Poor absorption of vitamin B_{12} = juvenile pernicious anemia	?
	Succinylcholine	Isozyme of plasma cholinesterase with high activity	Resistance to succinyl-choline paralysis	Autosomal autonomous
	Mydriatic agents	?	Racial differences in drug effectiveness	?
	Purine analogs (allopurinol, 6-MP)	Partial or complete loss of HG-PRTase	Gout	X-linked
5. Abnormal distribution of drug	Copper	Deficient ceruloplasmin	Wilson's disease	Autosomal recessive
	Iron	Increased tissue ferritin (hemosiderin)	Hemochroma-tosis	?
	Thyroxine	Increased or decreased thyroid-binding globulin	Elevated or depressed protein-bound iodine	Autosomal dominant
6. Differences in use of and response to psychotropic drugs (?)	Caffeine, nicotine, others	?	Differences in drug habituation and abuse (?)	?

DRUG TOXICITY DUE TO IMPAIRED DRUG METABOLISM

Succinylcholine Hydrolysis

This drug is a depolarizing type of neuromuscular blocking agent, widely used to produce muscular relaxation during surgical procedures (p. 31). The deserved popularity of succinylcholine rests upon its ability to cause skeletal muscle relaxation of short duration because of its very rapid metabolic degradation by the cholinesterase of plasma and liver (acylcholine acyl-hydrolase, sometimes called "pseudocholinesterase"). The drug level, established quickly by intravenous infusion and maintained readily, drops rapidly within a few minutes after the infusion is discontinued. The degradative reaction is a simple hydrolysis to the pharmacologically inert succinyl-monocholine:

$$(CH_3)_3\overset{+}{N}-CH_2CH_2-O-\overset{O}{\overset{\|}{C}}CH_2CH_2\overset{O}{\overset{\|}{C}}-O-CH_2CH_2-\overset{+}{N}(CH_3)_3$$

choline   succinylmonocholine

hydrolysis

succinylcholine (succinyldicholine)

Occasional patients manifest a bizarre response to succinylcholine; a prolonged muscular relaxation and apnea lasting as long as several hours after discontinuance of the infusion. Investigation revealed that many of these individuals have an atypical plasma cholinesterase.[1]

The atypical cholinesterase hydrolyzes various substrates at considerably reduced rates. This alone might suggest merely that the amount of enzyme is reduced. However, the entire pattern of affinities for substrates and inhibitors differs from the normal. Figure 6-2 illustrates this pattern for succinylcholine as a substrate (Figure 6-2a) and for succinylcholine as an inhibitor of the hydrolysis of benzoylcholine (Figure 6-2b). It can be seen that the affinity of the atypical enzyme for succinylcholine is more than 100-fold decreased compared with the normal. The concentrations of succinylcholine that are used clinically to produce neuromuscular paralysis during anesthesia are well below those required to saturate the enzyme. Consequently, the reduced affinity of the abnormal enzyme for succinylcholine is sufficient cause of the abnormally prolonged duration of action of the drug in patients with atypical cholinesterase.

It has proved convenient to use dibucaine, a local anesthetic that is completely stable in the presence of cholinesterase, to characterize the enzyme. The affinity of dibucaine as an inhibitor of the normal cholinesterase is about 20 times its affinity for the atypical enzyme. Under arbitrarily standardized conditions, with benzoylcholine as substrate and dibucaine at 10^{-5} M, the rate of hydrolysis of benzoylcholine by the normal enzyme is inhibited about 80%, but the atypical cholinesterase is little affected. The percent inhibition by dibucaine under these conditions is called the "dibucaine number." The results of testing a large number of randomly selected people are shown in Figure 6-3a. Most of the subjects clustered in a roughly normal distribution around dibucaine number 78, with a remarkably small coefficient of variation (about 4%). A small group had intermediate dibucaine numbers in the

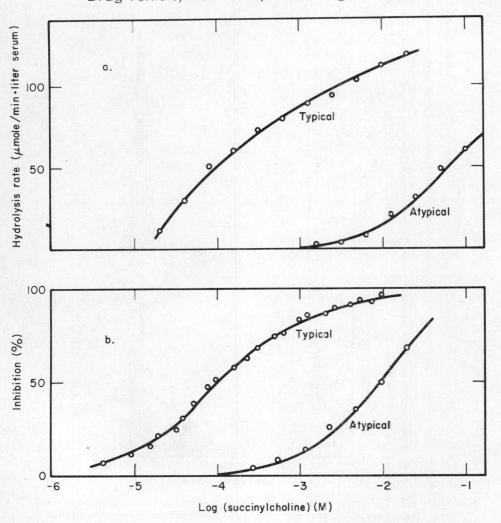

FIGURE 6-2. Interactions of succinylcholine with plasma cholinesterase. (*From Kalow, Figure 19 and 21.*[1])

range 40–70; there was no overlap with the normal range. Two subjects had very low dibucaine numbers (less than 20). In investigations on an even larger scale, it has been found that the incidence of very low dibucaine numbers is about 1 in 3000, and these people invariably respond to succinylcholine by prolonged paralysis.

Family studies leave little doubt that the presence of atypical cholinesterase is a genetically determined characteristic. Very low dibucaine numbers correspond to the homozygous condition. Intermediate values apparently arise from plasma containing a mixture of normal and atypical enzyme. This is indicated, for example, in Figure 6-4, where inhibition curves are shown for plasma with normal, intermediate, and low dibucaine numbers. The behavior of the "intermediate" plasma is what would be expected of a mixture; inhibition is first manifested at the very low inhibitor concentration to which the normal plasma responds, but complete inhibition is approached only at the very high concentrations required by the atypical enzyme.

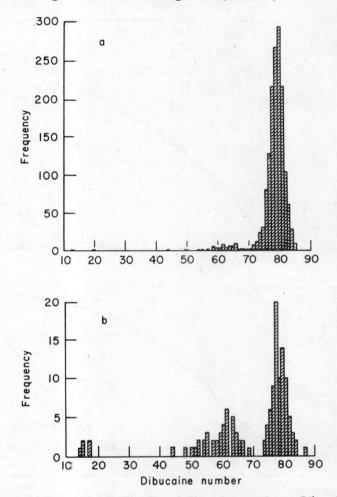

FIGURE 6-3. Frequency distribution of dibucaine numbers. *Dibucaine numbers represent percent inhibition of plasma cholinesterase activity by dibucaine at a fixed concentration in a standardized test, with benzoylcholine as substrate. (From Kalow, Figure 22.[1])*

Figure 6-3b shows the results of dibucaine studies of families of subjects with low or intermediate dibucaine numbers. The frequencies of low and intermediate dibucaine numbers are much greater than in the population as a whole. All the data are compatible with the existence of two allelic autosomal autonomous genes. Thus, the defect occurs in, and is transmitted by, both sexes. Homozygous normals produce a given quantity of the normal enzyme, individuals homozygous for the abnormal gene produce only atypical cholinesterase. Heterozygotes produce a mixture of the enzymes, much as carriers of sickle cell trait produce both hemoglobins A and S.[12]

The gene for atypical cholinesterase has a widespread distribution throughout the world. Application of the Hardy–Weinberg law (p. 453) to the frequencies of the phenotypes led to estimates of the gene frequency of about 2% in all the population groups studied, including British, Greek, Portuguese, North African, Jewish, and some Asiatic ethnic groups.[16] This uniformity is rather unusual and contrasts

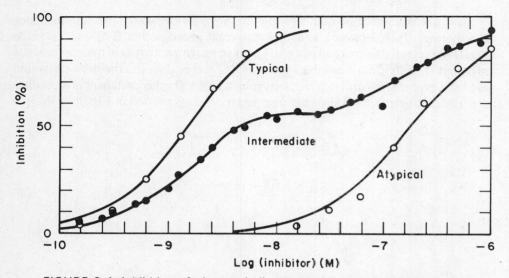

FIGURE 6-4. Inhibition of plasma cholinesterase by a neostigmine analog. *The inhibitor used was an analog of neostigmine known by the code name Ro2-0683. The substrate was benzoylcholine. The percent inhibition of enzyme activity is shown for 3 kinds of plasma. At left, typical plasma; at right, atypical plasma; middle curve, plasma with intermediate dibucaine number. (Modified from Kalow, Figure 25.[1])*

sharply with some of the drug idiosyncrasies to be discussed later. Subsequent studies, however, revealed significant differences. The allele appears to be absent in Japanese, Eskimos, and South American Indians, and it is very rare in Negroes, Australian aborigines, Filipinos, and Orientals other than Japanese.[17]

Other variants of the plasma cholinesterase have been discovered. The atypical cholinesterase already discussed is relatively insensitive to a number of inhibitors other than dibucaine: one of these is the fluoride ion. In family studies, it was found that some individuals had enzyme with normal or almost normal sensitivity to dibucaine inhibition but resistance to fluoride inhibition. The fluoride resistance was shown to be determined by a different allele of the same gene by demonstrating its segregation, as follows. In two families fluoride-resistant, dibucaine-resistant males mated to homozygous normal females had two kinds of children: fluoride-resistant but not dibucaine-resistant, or dibucaine-resistant but not fluoride-resistant; of 10 children of such matings, not one was of the same phenotype as either parent. Only the homozygote for fluoride resistance exhibits prolonged apnea when exposed to succinylcholine,[18,19] just as is true of the dibucaine-resistant atypical enzyme variant.

Another variant discovered through family studies is the so-called "silent" gene, thought at first to be an *amorphic* allele for this enzyme, i.e., one that determines no gene product at all or an enzyme protein so altered as to be completely inactive. Evidence for the presence of this allele is the existence of individuals who should be heterozygotes according to the presumed genotypes of their parents, yet who seem to be homozygotes. Figure 6-5a presents an illustration of this variant. The two females III-1 and III-2 (the *propositi*, i.e., the subjects who first came to the attention of the investigators) had abnormally low dibucaine numbers and extremely low enzyme activity; they appeared to be atypical homozygotes. Their father (II-2), their grandfather (I-2), and their paternal uncle (II-1) all were, as expected, heterozygotes for the

atypical enzyme (dibucaine numbers and enzyme activities were both intermediate).
Their mother (II-3), however, and their maternal grandmother (I-5) and maternal
aunt (II-4) presented an unusual pattern. They had enzyme activities in the intermediate
range, but their dibucaine numbers were normal rather than intermediate (as would
have been expected for ordinary heterozygotes). This and other instances of a peculiar
inheritance pattern[20] has led to the interpretation diagrammed in Figure 6-5b. It is

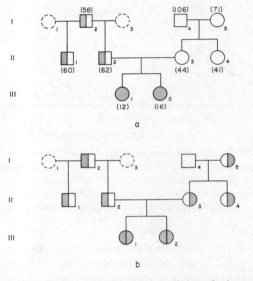

FIGURE 6-5. Inheritance of the amorphic allele of the plasma cholinesterase gene. (*From Lehmann and Liddell, Figures 12 and 13.*[16] *By permission of
Grune & Stratton.*)

assumed that the individuals with low cholinesterase activity but normal sensitivity
to dibucaine have one allele for normal cholinesterase and one amorphic ("silent")
allele. Then, as shown, the paradoxes are resolved; the two daughters carry one atypical
allele and one amorphic allele. The concept of a "silent" allele is supported strongly
by the discovery of a woman completely lacking in plasma cholinesterase activity,
presumably a homozygote for this allele. Married to a normal homozygote, this subject has given birth to two children, both with low plasma cholinesterase activity.

Later investigations on the "silent gene" variant revealed that what was "silent"
was not the gene but the gene product, i.e., that protein variants of the cholinesterase
were formed but were qualitatively so altered as to lack enzyme activity.[21] More
sensitive assay techniques revealed a complex heterogeneous mixture of defective
enzymes in these cases, some with very low but measurable enzyme activity, most with
abnormal immunologic properties.

Electrophoretic and molecular sieving techniques have revealed that plasma cholinesterase normally consists of a group of isozymes, probably in different states of
molecular aggregation, with a mean molecular weight of about 350,000.[22-24] Four
bands (designated C1–C4) are ordinarily found after electrophoresis. The kinetic
properties with respect to substrates and inhibitors (including dibucaine and fluoride)
are the same for all 4 components; genetically determined modification is expressed

in all four simultaneously. Thus, it has been suggested that these bands may differ principally in their states of molecular aggregation rather than in their primary structure. The data, however, do not require such an interpretation; analytic data on amino acid composition and sequence will eventually clarify this point.

Rarely, a plasma was found that yielded an additional band (C5) in electrophoresis. The cholinesterase activity in such cases was about 30% higher than normal; the sensitivity to inhibition by dibucaine or fluoride was not decreased. Since normal cholinesterase is present as well as an additional activity represented by the unusual electrophoretic band, it could not be expected that these individuals would show any unusual response to succinylcholine; an increase of this magnitude in the rate of destruction of succinylcholine would, in all likelihood, escape detection in view of its already rapid metabolism. Family studies indicated that the abnormality was transmitted as an autosomal autonomous characteristic. About 5% of healthy British subjects had this variant in their plasma.[25]

Finally, a variant was found to have greatly elevated enzyme activity, 2–3 times normal, associated with resistance to succinylcholine.[26,27] This variant is discussed later in the chapter (p. 474).

The role of various genotypes in determining the idiosyncratic response to succinylcholine is indicated in a study of 78 patients who displayed prolonged apnea after receiving the drug.[28] Enzyme activity was determined with acetylcholine as substrate; in this method the normal range is 72–166 units. Dibucaine and fluoride numbers were also determined. The genotypes were deduced from the results of these determinations and confirmed in family studies in about one-fourth of the cases. The frequencies of the various genotypes and the activities of plasma cholinesterase in each group are shown in Table 6-3. (Note that these genotype frequencies refer to the special patient

TABLE 6-3. Genotype frequencies and cholinesterase activity in patients with succinylcholine apnea.

Cholinesterase activity was determined with acetylcholine as substrate; normal range is 72–166 units. Mean ± standard devia-is shown. Genotypes were deduced from inhibition studies with dibucaine and fluoride. (From Thompson and Whittaker,[28] Table I.)

Genotype	Plasma cholinesterase activity	Percent of total
Normal-normal	86.1 ± 25.4	32.1
Normal-atypical	62.7 ± 19.6	12.8
Normal-fluoride resistant	88.0 ± 29.4	7.7
Atypical-fluoride resistant	64.7 ± 15.0	9.1
Atypical-atypical	40.5 ± 8.6	38.5

group, not to the population as a whole.) Atypical homozygotes comprised 38% of the patient group, whereas the frequency of this genotype in the population as a whole is about 1 in 3000. Curiously, one-third of all the patients who experienced prolonged apnea were of normal genotype with normal plasma cholinesterase activity.

The state of knowledge about plasma cholinesterase variants and their relationship to succinylcholine idosyncrasy is summarized in Table 6-4.

TABLE 6-4. The principal variants of plasma cholinesterase.
Enzyme activity was measured with benzoylcholine as substrate. Dibucaine and fluoride numbers are percent inhibition by these substances under standard conditions. (Data compiled from Lehmann and Liddell, Table 4[16] and Harris et al.[25] By permission of Grune & Stratton.)

Type of enzyme	Enzyme activity (units/ml)	Subject's response to succinylcholine	Dibucaine number	Fluoride number
Normal	60–125	Rapid hydrolysis	71–83	57–68
"Atypical"				
heterozygote	26–90	Rapid hydrolysis	52–69	42–55
homozygote	<35	Prolonged apnea	15–25	20–25
"Fluoride-resistant"				
heterozygote	Normal	Rapid hydrolysis	71–78	50–55
homozygote	Normal	Prolonged apnea	64, 67	34, 35
"Silent gene"				
heterozygote	Variably decreased	Rapid hydrolysis		
homozygote (1 case)	None	Prolonged apnea		
Electrophoretic variant (five bands instead of four)	About 30% higher than normal	Rapid hydrolysis	Normal	Normal
Elevated activity	2–3 × normal	Succinylcholine resistance (very rapid hydrolysis)	Normal	Normal

Hereditary Methemoglobinemia

A somewhat different example of how an abnormally prolonged drug effect can arise on the basis of a genetic defect is found in hereditary methemoglobinemia.[29–32] Here nitrites and other drugs that cause methemoglobinemia (e.g., aniline derivatives) have an unexpectedly long duration of action because one of the enzymes involved in the reduction of methemoglobin to hemoglobin in erythrocytes is absent. Ordinarily there is a small steady-state level of methemoglobin (about 1% of total hemoglobin), presumably arising by spontaneous oxidation of Fe^{2+} to Fe^{3+} in the hemoglobin molecules. The ferric iron is continuously reduced again by four different reductive mechanisms in the red cell.[33] Three of these mechanisms utilize ascorbic acid, gluta-thione, or NADPH as the reducing agents. The fourth and most important is NADH methemoglobin reductase. This enzyme is alternatively oxidized by methemoglobin and reduced by NADH, whereby methemoglobin is reduced to hemoglobin. In hereditary methemoglobinemia, the NADH methemoglobin reductase is absent.[34] The trait is due to an autosomal recessive allele, so the disease is manifested in homozygotes of either sex. It is ordinarily detected by the presence of cyanosis at birth.

Figure 6-6 illustrates the effect of a single dose of sodium nitrite in a person with hereditary methemoglobinemia and in a normal person. The amount of methemoglobin formed was about the same in both subjects, but whereas it had almost disappeared within 6 hr in the normal, there was no conversion whatsoever in the abnormal subject.

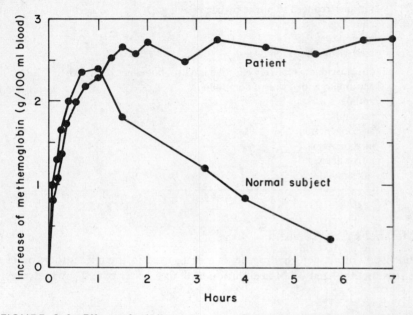

FIGURE 6-6. Effect of nitrite upon a patient with hereditary methemoglobinemia. *At zero time, 0.5 g sodium nitrite was injected intravenously in a normal subject and in a patient with this hereditary disease. Increase in blood methemoglobin content is shown on vertical axis. (From Eder et al., Figure 5.[35])*

Table 6-5 lists a number of drugs that may be responsible for causing methemoglobinemia; these should be avoided, if possible, in people with hereditary methemoglobinemia. The therapeutic management of methemoglobinemia, if it does develop, follows the principles outlined already (p. 423); methylene blue and oxygen are the agents of choice.

The indirect oxidants listed in Table 6-5 act only after metabolic transformation in vivo. Thus, genetic alterations of the pathways of drug metabolism can cause greater formation of products that directly cause methemoglobinemia. Acetophenetidin is a good example. This compound is normally metabolized by O-dealkylation in the liver to N-acetyl-p-aminophenol, which is further metabolized and conjugated (Figure 3-1). Two sisters developed severe methemoglobinemia after ordinary doses of acetophenetidin.[37] Investigation revealed very little O-dealkylation in these subjects; instead, there was N-deacetylation, producing a primary amine, followed by hydroxylation to yield an o-aminophenol derivative (2-hydroxyphenetidin) known to be potent in causing methemoglobinemia. The genetic deficiency in O-dealkylation could not be corrected by administering phenobarbital; on the contrary, the methemoglobinemia in response to acetophenetidin became worse, probably due to stimulation of the hydroxylation reaction.

TABLE 6-5. Drugs that can cause methemoglobinemia.
(Adapted from Prankerd,[36] tables pp. 139, 140. By permission of
Charles C. Thomas.)

Direct oxidants (effective in vitro and in vivo)
  nitrites
  nitrates (reduced to nitrite by bacteria in gut)
  chlorates
  quinones
  methylene blue (high doses)

Indirect oxidants (scarcely effective in vitro, but effective in vivo)
  arylamino and arylnitro compounds
  aniline
  acetanilid
  acetophenetidin
  nitrobenzenes
  nitrotoluenes
  sulfonamides

Slow Metabolism of Isoniazid

Isoniazid (isonicotinic acid hydrazide) is a drug used in the chemotherapy of tuberculosis. It is metabolized by N-acetylation and, to a lesser extent, by hydrolysis:[38]

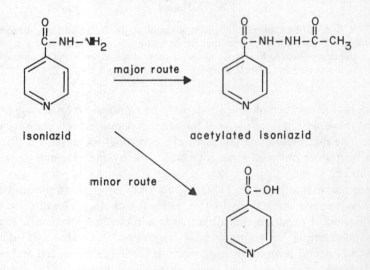

When blood concentrations of isoniazid were measured 6 hr after a standard dose
in a large number of subjects, a bimodal distribution was found. Some people
metabolized this drug very slowly, some rapidly. In a sample of 291 unrelated people,
52.2% metabolized the drug slowly. Age, sex, and race seemed to have no influence.
Preliminary familial data suggested that the trait, slow metabolism, was recessive.

In the following analysis, we shall designate the allelic genes controlling the metabolism rate as *slow* and *rapid*, the phenotypes as SLOW and RAPID. The hypothesis that a recessive allele was responsible for the slow metabolism of isoniazid could be tested by examining the offspring of a large number of matings. If a recessive trait is expressed phenotypically in fraction q of the population, then, according to the Hardy–Weinberg Law,[12] the frequency of the recessive allele is $\sqrt{q}$, since the phenotype arises only from matings of $q \times q$, which occur randomly with a probability of q^2. Thus, the allele frequencies here are $\sqrt{0.522} = 0.723$ for the recessive *slow*, and therefore 0.277 for the dominant *rapid*.

Matings of phenotypes SLOW × SLOW should give only SLOW offspring, since *slow-slow* is the only genotype represented.

Matings of phenotypes RAPID × RAPID are more complicated. We have first to know the frequencies of all three possible genotypes, *slow-slow*, *slow-rapid* (or *rapid-slow*), and *rapid-rapid*:

slow-slow	$(0.723)^2 = 0.522$	[phenotype SLOW]
slow-rapid	$2(0.723 \times 0.277) = 0.401$	[phenotype RAPID]
rapid-rapid	$(0.277)^2 = 0.077$	
	$\overline{1.000}$	

Now the sum of the genotype frequencies that make up the phenotype population RAPID is 0.478; therefore, the frequency of the genotype *slow-rapid* in this population is $0.401/0.478 = 0.839$. In mating of RAPID × RAPID, the phenotype SLOW (genotype *slow-slow*) can only arise by *slow-rapid* × *slow-rapid*, which will occur with probability $(0.839)^2$, and one-fourth of these matings will yield *slow-slow*:

$$slow\text{-}slow \ (0.839)^2/4 = 0.174$$

Thus, the phenotypic expectations for matings of the kind RAPID × RAPID are:

SLOW	17.4%
RAPID	82.6%

The expectations for matings of the kind RAPID × SLOW are readily computed in the same way.

Table 6-6 shows the results of such studies on parents and children. The data reveal a remarkably good agreement between observed and expected outcomes in each category, in confirmation of the hypothesis that slow metabolism of isoniazid is an autosomal recessive trait.

The enzyme responsible for the polymorphism of isoniazid inactivation has been shown, with human liver homogenates, to be an acetyl transferase, using coenzyme A. The reaction mechanism is discussed in Chapter 3. Sulfamethazine and hydralazine are acetylated by the same enzyme and are therefore subject to the same genetic variation. However, sulfanilamide and p-aminobenzoic acid, which appear in human urine in acetylated form, did not show polymorphism, nor were they acetylated by human liver homogenates.[38a] Presumably a different enzyme is responsible for the acetylation of these drugs.

Population studies have shown a remarkably wide range in the frequency of the *slow* gene.[40] The lowest values were found among Canadian Eskimos, Japanese, and Chinese (0.22, 0.31, and 0.39, respectively). The highest values were found among Egyptians, Scandinavians, Israelis, and Finns (0.91, 0.82, 0.87, 0.80). It is not known

TABLE 6-6. Rates of isoniazid metabolism in parents and children.
Numbers in the expected categories are computed on the basis of the hypothesis that slow metabolism of isoniazid is due to a recessive allele, as described in the text. (From Evans et al.,[39] Table X.)

Parental phenotypes	No. of matings	No. of children	No. of children of each phenotype			
			RAPID		SLOW	
			Expected	Observed	Expected	Observed
SLOW × SLOW	16	51	0	0	51	51
RAPID × SLOW	24	70	40.6	42	29.4	28
RAPID × RAPID	13	38	31.3	31	6.7	7
TOTALS	53	159		73		86

what selective advantage might be conferred by slow acetylation to account for its high frequency in certain racial groups or geographic settings.

Slow inactivators of isoniazid have less N-acetyltransferase in their livers than do rapid inactivators, but the properties of the purified enzymes obtained from both phenotypes appear to be identical. [41,42] It would seem, therefore, that slow inactivators synthesize the enzyme more slowly, or degrade it more rapidly, than normal.

When isoniazid is given to slow inactivators, it accumulates to toxic levels and can result in serious neuropathies.[43] Similar toxicity may be seen with phenelzine and hydralazine. In patients with both tuberculosis and epilepsy, who are treated simultaneously with isoniazid and diphenylhydantoin, an interesting drug interaction may occur.[44,45] Isoniazid is known to inhibit the metabolism of diphenylhydantoin by preventing hydroxylation.[46] In patients of SLOW phenotype, the accumulation of isoniazid can cause major inhibition of diphenylhydantoin metabolism, resulting in diphenylhydantoin toxicity. With appropriate doses of the two drugs, this complication is not seen in patients of RAPID phenotype.

Defective hydroxylation of diphenylhydantoin can also occur independent of any isoniazid effect.[47] This is an autosomal dominant trait. Affected individuals develop toxic signs such as nystagmus, ataxia, and mental confusion at quite ordinary doses of the anticonvulsant. Blood levels were shown to be extraordinarily high. Toxic effects subsided when dosage was lowered. This example illustrates that a very great range of drug metabolizing capacities in the population, with the extremes identifiable clearly as due to genetic factors is seen more and more frequently the more widely plasma drug levels are monitored.

INCREASED SENSITIVITY TO DRUG

Abnormal Hemoglobins

The genetically altered hemoglobins may confer abnormal sensitivity to nitrites and other drugs that cause methemoglobinemia, even though the reductive processes in the erythrocytes are normally operative. In sickle cell anemia, the replacement of glutamic acid by valine at position 6 in both β-chains results in a hemoglobin that appears to be normal when it is carrying oxygen, but forms molecular aggregates in the absence of oxygen.[48,48a] This change in the properties of hemoglobin causes a grossly visible "sickling" of the erythrocytes at low oxygen tension, and such erythrocytes agglutinate in the capillaries and are subject to lysis. Hemoglobin M, like hemoglobin S, differs from normal hemoglobin A by a single amino acid residue,[49] but the replacement may occur at several different positions. Histidine at position 58 on the α-chain or position 63 on the β-chain may be replaced by tyrosine; valine at position 67 on the β-chain may be replaced by glutamic acid; and there are other forms of this abnormal hemoglobin. At least two of the four iron atoms in hemoglobin M are very readily oxidized to the ferric state. Hemoglobin H consists of four β-chains instead of the usual two α- and two β-subunits. This abnormal hemoglobin is also unusually sensitive to oxidation. The life span of the affected erythrocytes is about 40 days instead of the usual 120 days. Methemoglobin accumulates in the older cells, and they become much more susceptible to lysis. In people with either of these hemoglobin anomales, the drugs listed in Table 6-5 can be dangerous; sulfonamides, for example, may cause hemolytic anemia.

NOVEL DRUG EFFECT

Primaquine Sensitivity

The antimalarial drug primaquine can ordinarily be administered at a dosage of 30 mg daily with only insignificant side effects. About 5–10% of Negro males given

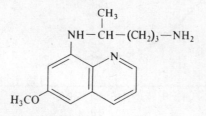

Primaquine

this normal dosage of primaquine develop a profound acute hemolytic anemia. The response is not merely an exaggerated sensitivity to an ordinary side effect of the drug; even at much higher doses no comparable hemolytic crises could be provoked in white patients of Northern European stock, nor in certain other ethnic groups, although very mild degrees of hemolysis could be detected by laboratory tests.

Radioactive chromic ion (^{51}Cr) is bound so tightly to erythrocytes that it can be used conveniently as a tag to follow the fate of infused red cells. With this technique for studying the defect in primaquine idiosyncrasy, it could be shown[50] that, when cells from reactors were transfused into normal individuals and primaquine was then administered, hemolysis of these labeled erythrocytes occurred. On the other hand, normal cells transfused into reactors were unaffected by the drug. Thus, the abnormality is localized to the erythrocyte.

Radioactive iron (^{59}Fe) can be used to label the newest erythrocytes differentially. With this technique, it was shown that in a primaquine reaction only erythrocytes older than about 55 days are hemolyzed. A single dose of ^{59}Fe was administered. A few days later, a challenging dose of primaquine caused hemolysis but no release of ^{59}Fe. Thus, only the older erythrocytes were lysed, not those that had been produced in the presence of the radioactive iron. By giving the primaquine challenge to different subjects at various times after the ^{59}Fe, it was found that radioactive cells were lysed after about 55 days. This explained the clinical observation that even massive hemolytic episodes were self-limiting; recovery occurs despite continued drug administration (Figure 6-7). After a long enough drug-free interval, however, primaquine is again capable of inducing a hemolytic crisis.

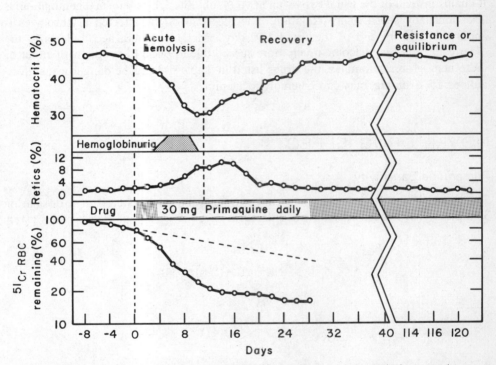

FIGURE 6-7. Clinical course of primaquine-induced hemolytic anemia. *Composite data from 3 Negro male reactors with similar degree of glucose-6-phosphate dehydrogenase (G6PD) deficiency. Primaquine was started at day zero. Eight days before, each subject had been injected with a sample of his own erythrocytes labeled with ^{51}Cr. Hematocrit is shown at top, reticulocytes at middle, red cell survival at bottom. Broken line represents normal course of erythrocyte destruction. Note hemoglobinuria at height of hemolytic crisis. (From Kellermeyer et al., Figure 1.[51] By permission of C. V. Mosby, originally from the Bulletin of the World Health Organization 22:625, 1960.)*

Reactors develop hemolytic anemia not only in response to primaquine, but also to acetanilid and other aniline derivatives including sulfanilamide, to naphthalene and its metabolites, and to nitrofurantoin, and some other nitro compounds. A compound present in fava beans also provokes a hemolytic crisis in sensitive individuals; hence the name *favism* is also given to this genetic anomaly. A list of some agents that can induce hemolytic anemia in this condition is given in Table 6-7.

TABLE 6-7. Agents reported to be capable of inducing hemolytic anemia in subjects with genetically determined idiosyncratic susceptibility. (Adapted from Marks and Banks,[52] Table 3.)

Primaquine	Quinine
Pamaquine	Quinidine
Pentaquine	p-Aminosalicylic acid
Quinocide	Antipyrine
Sulfanilamide	Probenecid
Sulfapyridine	Acetanilid
Sulfisoxazole	Phenylhydrazine
Sulfacetamide	Acetophenetidin
Sulfamethoxypyridazine	Pyramidone
Salicylazosulfapyridine	Chloroquine
Sulfones (sulfoxone)	Chloramphenicol
Naphthalene	Fava bean
Methylene blue	Viral respiratory infections
Vitamin K	Infectious hepatitis
Acetylsalicylic acid	Infectious mononucleosis
Nitrofurantoin	Bacterial pneumonias and septicemias (e.g., typhoid)
Furazoladone	Diabetic acidosis
	Uremia

Some of the active compounds cause hemolysis of reactor cells in vitro, but others evidently have to be metabolized first, since they are inactive in vitro. Naphthalene is in this latter category, whereas its oxidation products, α- and β-naphthol, are active both in vivo and in vitro. Primaquine itself is not very effective in vitro, presumably a metabolite is the active hemolytic agent. It has long been known that aniline and nitro compounds are capable of causing hemolytic anemia; therefore, it is of great practical importance to recognize that all these hemolytic reactions, as well as favism, can be manifestations of the same idiosyncrasy. However, some of the same drugs at very high doses can cause hemolysis of normal erythrocytes. Primaquine can produce some hemolysis in normal subjects at 120 mg daily, four times the usual dosage. Combined with high doses of acetanilid, it regularly causes a severe hemolytic reaction. Finally, phenylhydrazine in high dosage is well known to cause serious hemolytic crises in all exposed individuals; indeed, in animals it is used experimentally to destroy red cells and thereby provoke a massive synthesis of reticulocytes.

One of the most effective hemolytic agents, acetylphenylhydrazine,[53] can be used in vitro for identification of reactor erythrocytes. Under appropriate conditions, in the presence of oxygen and glucose, normal erythrocytes incubated with acetylphenylhydrazine maintain normal levels of reduced glutathione (GSH). Under the same conditions, GSH levels of reactor cells show a profound decline (Figure 6-8), presumably through conversion to oxidized glutathione (GSSG). Apparently, deficiency of sulfhydryl compounds, like GSH in the red cells, can cause hemolysis because agents that bind or oxidize −SH groups are hemolytic for both normal and reactor cells. The in vitro acetylphenylhydrazine test has proved extremely useful in predicting those who will react adversely to primaquine and related drugs, and in carrying out family studies to establish the genetic basis of the abnormality.

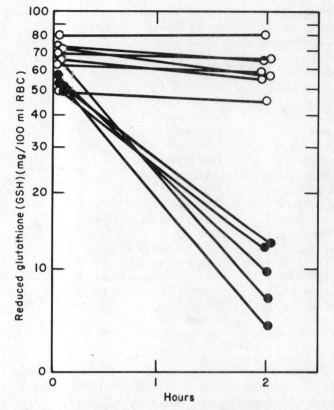

FIGURE 6-8. The acetylphenylhydrazine test for primaquine sensitivity of erythrocytes. *Glutathione content was measured initially and after 2 hr of incubation with acetylphenylhydrazine (5 mg/ml). Open circles are erythrocytes from normal subjects, solid circles are erythrocytes from primaquine-sensitive subjects. (From Beutler, Figure 4.*[50] *By permission of Grune and Stratton.)*

The basis of the curious GSH instability in response to hemolytic drugs remained obscure until it was discovered that reactor cells have a deficiency in the enzyme glucose-6-phosphate dehydrogenase (G6PD). No other enzyme activity thus far examined is depressed. Glutathione reductase and G6PD are coupled systems:

$$GSSG + NADPH + H^+ \xrightarrow[\text{reductase}]{\text{GSSG}} 2\,GSH + NADP^+$$

$$glucose\text{-}6\text{-}phosphate + NADP^+ \xrightarrow{\text{G6PD}} 6\text{-}phosphogluconic\ acid + NADPH$$

Figure 6-9 shows the amount of reduced glutathione formed in dialyzed homogenates of normal and primaquine-sensitive erythrocytes under three different conditions. In part a, NADPH was supplied, so that the activity of the glutathione reductase could be measured directly; the homogenates from the primaquine-sensitive cells behaved normally. In part b, glucose-6-phosphate and NADP were supplied, so that the reduction of NADP was prerequisite to the reduction of oxidized glutathione (as shown in the equation above). Since glucose-6-phosphate was the only other substrate in the system, its oxidation had to furnish the hydrogen for NADP reduction, and

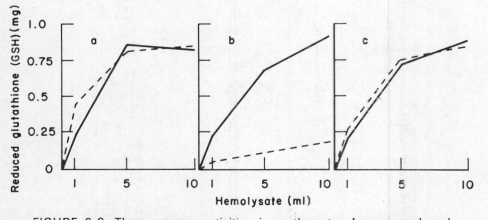

FIGURE 6-9. Three enzyme activities in erythrocytes from normal and primaquine-sensitive subjects. *The amount of reduced glutathione formed from a fixed amount of oxidized glutathione in a fixed time was measured, as a function of the amount of dialyzed hemolysate used. Solid curves are for normal subject, dashed curves are for primaquine-sensitive subject. a, NADPH was supplied and the activity of glutathione reductase was measured directly. b, Glucose-6-phosphate and NADP were supplied; therefore the reduction of GSSG to GSH was coupled to the activity of G6PD. c, 6-Phosphogluconate was supplied instead of glucose-6-phosphate, so the GSSG reduction depended on the activity of 6-phosphogluconic dehydrogenase. (From Carson et al., Figure 1.[54] By permission of the American Association for the Advancement of Science.)*

thus the whole reaction was made to depend upon the activity of the enzyme G6PD. The primaquine-sensitive erythrocytes were obviously deficient in this enzyme. Finally, in part c, 6-phosphogluconate was supplied; its oxidation now furnished NADPH, and again the homogenates from primaquine-sensitive cells behaved normally. In this way, the defect was localized to G6PD alone. Thus, the specific enzyme defect in reactor cells is known, and a reasonable connection has been established between the resulting inability to utilize glucose in the oxidative pathway to pentose and the inability to maintain GSH needed for the integrity of the erythrocyte.

Random testing of erythrocytes in vitro from Negro subjects has revealed a clear bimodality among males with respect to the residual GSH values at the end of the acetylphenylhydrazine test. Most of the population values clustered at about 60 mg per 100 ml of erythrocytes, with a spread from about 35–100; there were no values at all in the range 20–35, but about 15% of the males had GSH contents below 20. In females, the results were different. There was a much greater dispersion of data; only about 2% had very low values, and about 5% fell into an intermediate group distinct from the highs and the lows. Families of primaquine reactors were found to have a much higher incidence of low values among males and females, and a much higher incidence of intermediate values among females, than the population as a whole. Primaquine-sensitive fathers had normal sons, but passed the trait to all their daughters. A few color-blind primaquine-sensitive males passed both defective genes together to their daughters (color blindness is known to be carried on the X chromosome).

The pattern of inheritance of this trait is that of an autonomous sex-linked defect. Because males carry the defect on their single X chromosome (they are hemizygous),

TABLE 6-8. Properties of glucose-6-phosphate dehydrogenase (G6PD) in deficient subjects belonging to different population groups. Enzyme activity is expressed as percent of normal. Michaelis constants are indicated for reaction with substrate (G6P) and with coenzyme (NADP). Stability is the thermal stability of enzyme activity when whole hemolysates are incubated. Electrophoretic mobility was measured in starch gel. (Adapted from Marks and Banks,[52] Table 2.)

Ethnic or geographic group	Enzyme activity (% of normal)		Substrate affinities		Stability	Electrophoretic mobility
	Red cells	White cells	K_m G6P	K_m NADP		
Negro males	10–15	Normal or slightly decreased	Normal	Normal	Decreased	Normal fast component missing
Barbieri, males[a] (Northern Italian)	50	Normal	Slightly increased	Increased	Normal	Fast[b]
Sicilian	1–4	Decreased	Slightly increased	Increased	Decreased	
Sardinian	<1	Decreased	—	—	Decreased markedly	Fast[b]
Sephardic Jew	3–6	Decreased	Slightly decreased	Slightly decreased	Decreased	Normal

[a] An Italian family with a particular kind of G6PD deficiency.
[b] Normal fast and slow components missing; new very fast component present.

it is expressed phenotypically; these are the primaquine-sensitive group, with very low GSH values in the in vitro test. Female heterozygotes have intermediate values because the normal gene on one X chromosome and the defective allele on the other are both expressed. Obviously, heterozygous females will pass the defect to half their sons. Affected males have normal sons because they pass only their Y chromosome to them, and they have heterozygous daughters because they pass the defective X chromosome to all of them. If there were really complete phenotypic expression without dominance, then heterozygotes should fall into a well-defined intermediate group, and the frequency of the intermediates would be mathematically determined by the known gene frequency. This does not seem to occur. In the populations studied, more women were found with normal values in the GSH test than would be expected from the frequency of affected males (which, for a sex-linked trait, is the same as the gene frequency). This finding, and the wide dispersion of values, suggest that there is variable expression (variable penetrance), i.e., some other factors influence the degree to which the trait is expressed in identical genotypes.

Subsequent studies have shown that G6PD deficiency is not a simple absence of the enzyme but rather a heterogeneous trait. At least 80 distinct variants of the enzyme have been identified,[55] with different levels of activity, affinities for glucose-6-phosphate or NADP, pH optima, thermal stability, and electrophoretic mobility. A few examples from different ethnic groups are shown in Table 6-8. Severe deficiency of enzyme activity is correlated well with sensitivity to drug-induced hemolysis, provided in vitro measurements are made at the same concentrations of substrates and cofactors that would occur in vivo.[56,57]

The G6PD abnormality itself is usually without demonstrable adverse effect unless the erythrocytes are challenged by certain drugs; however, there is some evidence of decreased life expectancy among affected males.[58] From the point of view of genetic theory, high incidence of an abnormal gene in a given ethnic group implies some significant survival value for the heterozygous carrier females.[12] Analogous reasoning with respect to carriers of the sickling trait led to the discovery[59] that such heterozygotes are more resistant to serious forms of malaria than is the normal population. Prepubertal (especially infant) mortality from malaria is considerably lower in those individuals. Reactors to primaquine and fava beans are also found predominantly among groups which live in, or trace their ancestry to, malaria-hyperendemic areas (Table 6-9).[60,61] The postulated resistance to malaria infection of G6PD-deficient erythrocytes was shown in an interesting study. One of the X chromosomes in every cell of a female is known to be inactivated during its maturation, apparently on a random basis. Thus, females are mosaics with respect to traits controlled by the X chromosome. A female heterozygous for G6PD deficiency was shown to contain two kinds of erythrocytes. During acute *Plasmodium falciparum* infection, the normal erythrocytes were much more heavily infested with parasites than were the deficient ones.[62]

A curious by-product of the investigations on primaquine was the finding that all newborn infants are susceptible to drug-induced hemolytic anemia.[63] Among the eliciting drugs is menadione and other vitamin K analogs, which are naphtho-quinone derivatives; these drugs, given to prevent neonatal hemorrhage, can cause hemolysis. There is apparently no G6PD defect in the erythrocytes of normal infants, but low GSH levels are found. The abnormality persists for only a week or two.

TABLE 6-9. Incidence of glucose-6-phosphate dehydrogenase deficiency.
(From Marks and Banks,[52] Table 1.)

Group	Incidence (%)
ASHKENAZIC JEWS (males)	0.4
SEPHARDIC JEWS (males)	
Kurds	53
Iraq	24
Persia	15
Cochin	10
Yemen	5
North Africa	<1–4
ARABS	4
IRANIANS	8
SARDINIANS (males)	4–30
GREEKS (including Cyprus and Crete)	0.7–3
NEGROES	
American	13
Nigerians	10
Bantu	20
Leopoldville	18–23
Bashi	14
Pygmies	4
Watutsi	1–2
ASIATICS	
Chinese	2
Filipinos	13
Indians—Parsees	16
Javanese	3
Micronesians	0–1
AMERICAN INDIANS	
Oyana (males)	16
Carib (males)	2
Peruvian (males)	0
ESKIMOS	0

Malignant Hyperthermia

Rarely, after administration of a general anesthetic, a patient experiences rapidly
developing muscular rigidity and extreme hyperthermia, leading to death in over
60 % of cases.[64] The incidence has been estimated at only about 1 in 20,000. The familial
pattern is very clear; for example, one kindred has been described with 18 cases. The
trait is inherited as an autosomal dominant. The precipitating agent may apparently
be any general anesthetic, although most cases have been seen after halothane,
currently the most widely used anesthetic. Patients developing malignant hyperthermia have usually (though not always) also received the muscle relaxant succinylcholine. The molecular basis of the trait is still obscure.

Hepatic Porphyria

Another example of idiosyncrasy causing a novel response to a drug is the precipitation of acute attacks of porphyria by barbiturates and other drugs.[65,66] The porphyrias are abnormalities of the regulation of heme synthesis, in which large amounts of heme precursors such as δ-aminolevulinic acid (ALA) and porphobilinogen (PBG) are excreted. These are transformed to porphyrins with deep red color, so that the urine of patients with acute porphyria may turn red on standing, a useful diagnostic criterion. There are three known genetic forms of the disease: acute intermittent porphyria (Swedish type), variegate porphyria (South African type), and hereditary coproporphyria. Acute attacks are characterized by sudden increase in the plasma levels and urinary or fecal excretion of porphyrins or their precursors, and by various symptoms, such as abdominal pain, neuritis, and psychosis (in Swedish porphyria), or cutaneous photosensitivity and ulcerative lesions (in South African porphyria). All three forms of the disease are familial, with the trait transmitted as an autosomal dominant. The incidence of acute intermittent prophyria is about 1.5 per 100,000 in Sweden and Australia. Variegate porphyria, which can be traced to a single Dutch emigrant who settled in Capetown in 1686,[12] may affect as many as 1% of Afrikaners. In another type of porphyria, known as porphyria cutanea tarda, the role of heredity is uncertain. The effects are primarily in the skin, with ulcerative lesions, and the abdominal and neurologic symptoms are absent. This disease is seen chiefly among the Bantu peoples, in association with high alcohol intake and chronic liver disease.

Acute attacks of porphyria can be caused by otherwise innocuous drugs, and these attacks are sometimes fatal. Most frequently the barbiturates are involved,[67] but sulfonamides, aminopyrine, and phenylbutazone are among the numerous compounds that have been implicated.[68] Compounds containing an allyl group are especially prone to provoke acute attacks; allylbarbiturates (e.g., secobarbital) and allylisopropylacetamide (Sedormid) are prominent examples. Moreover, some of the compounds that are most dangerous to victims of hereditary porphyria are also capable of causing porphyria in normal people as well as in experimental animals or even hepatic cell cultures. Such toxic porphyrias have been well documented in human populations. A large-scale epidemic occurred in Turkey in 1955 after widespread consumption of wheat treated with the fungicide hexachlorobenzene. Another mass outbreak occurred in 1964 among workers in a factory producing the herbicide

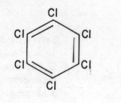

hexachlorobenzene

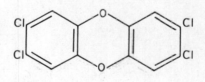

tetrachlorodibenzo-p-dioxin

2,4,5-T; the responsible agent was identified as a contaminant, tetrachlorodibenzo-p-dioxin.[69] It is possible that genetically affected individuals are merely more sensitive than normals to compounds that are intrinsically capable of disturbing heme synthesis.

The principal steps in heme biosynthesis are shown in Figure 6-10.[70] ALA synthetase condenses glycine and succinyl-CoA, yielding ALA. Then two molecules of ALA are condensed by ALA dehydrase to form PBG. Further enzymic transformations join

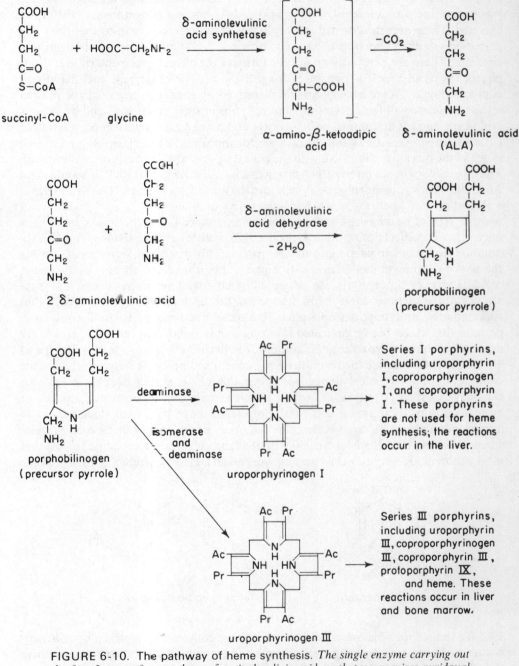

FIGURE 6-10. The pathway of heme synthesis. *The single enzyme carrying out the first 2 steps of the pathway, δ-aminolevulinic acid synthetase, requires pyridoxal phosphate. The precursor pyrrole, porphobilinogen, is polymerized into either the series I or series III porphyrins. Ac, acetic acid residue; Pr, propionic acid residue.*

four molecules of PBG to form a porphyrin skeleton. Side chain modifications yield the several uroporphyrinogens and corresponding uroporphyrins, and the coproporphyrinogens and corresponding coproporphyrins. Eventually, protoporphyrin IX combines with Fe^{2+} to form heme, a step catalyzed by the enzyme ferrochelatase. The first step, mediated by ALA synthetase, is rate-limiting for the whole pathway.

Several agents that produce acute porphyria in vivo have been shown to cause a large increase in the level of ALA synthetase in the liver of experimental animals and in embryonic chick liver cells in vitro.[71,72] Addition of various drugs led to the production of porphyrins detectable by fluorescence microscopy. Porphyrins were also readily formed if ALA was added. Actinomycin D, added to the cultures, blocked the drug-induced porphyrin formation, but not that caused by ALA. Since the effect of actinomycin is to prevent DNA-dependent RNA synthesis, it would appear that the direct effect of the drugs was to induce the synthesis of ALA synthetase, and thereby to cause an increase in porphyrin production.

Further studies strengthened this interpretation.[73,74] The induction of ALA synthetase was shown to occur only in liver cells and to be reversible on withdrawal of the inducing agents. During induction of this enzyme, there was no general increase in protein synthesis, i.e., the inducing effect was a specific one. Moreover, the inducing agents did not prevent the normal breakdown of ALA synthetase, the half-life of which was 4–6 hr in the presence or absence of inducers. Evidently, heme synthesis is normally controlled by a regulatory mechanism that represses the synthesis of ALA synthetase and thereby maintains a low rate of synthesis of heme. Heme itself is supposed to be the repressor, acting to shut down transcription of the operon coding for ALA synthetase.[75] Heme, therefore, should be able to overcome the effects of inducers; this has been demonstrated in vitro in the liver cell system.[73,74]

Drugs like allylisopropylacetamide and the allylbarbiturates are probably converted to metabolites that cause massive destruction of cytochrome P450 in the liver (cf. Chapter 3), depleting the pool of free heme and diverting heme from its repressor role so that increased production of ALA synthetase is triggered.[76–78] Ordinary inducers of the liver microsomal drug metabolizing system, on the other hand, like phenylbutazone or the non-allyl barbiturates, may also lower intracellular heme levels; in this case, the increased diversion of heme into cytochrome P450, which accumulates, may also result in decreased repression of ALA synthetase by heme. Such a mechanism might account for the porphyrogenic effects of such drugs in susceptible individuals.[78a]

Steroids may be involved too.[79] The onset of hereditary porphyria in the adolescent years suggests a role of the sex hormones; moreover, estrogens are known to precipitate attacks of porphyria cutanea tarda. Normally, steroid hormones like 11-β-hydroxy-Δ^4-androstenedione are metabolized by a liver enzyme, steroid-Δ^4-5α-reductase. The products are 5α derivatives. In patients with acute intermittent porphyria, however, decreased activity of this enzyme has been found. As a result, there is increased production of 5β-H (A : B cis) derivatives, in which the Δ^4 double bond remains unreduced. Such 5β metabolites are potent inducers of ALA synthetase.

What might the biochemical defect or defects be in hereditary porphyria? An abnormality of the mechanisms regulating heme synthesis could be responsible. There might, for example, be a change analogous to that seen in operator constitutive mutants in bacteria,[75] i.e., an insensitivity to an endogenous repressor (heme), resulting in increased transcriptions, i.e., increased ALA synthetase production despite normal heme levels. This hypothesis is consistent with the fact that the disease is caused by a dominant gene, which means that the normal allele does not confer protection as it usually would in a trait caused by absence or defective function of an enzyme.

On the other hand, it is difficult to account for the several types of porphyria on the basis of a single abnormality of regulation of heme synthesis, because different intermediates accumulate and are excreted (Figure 6-11).[80] In acute intermittent porphyria,

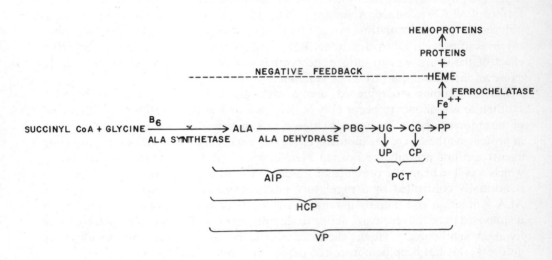

FIGURE 6-11. Biochemical defects in the hepatic porphyrias. *Heme biosynthesis is shown, as well as the intermediates excreted in excessive amounts in the several types of porphyria. ALA = δ-aminolevulinic acid; PBG = porphobilinogen; UG = uroporphyrinogen; UP = uroporphyrin; CG = coproporphyrinogen; CP = coproporphyrin; PP = protoporphyrin; AIP = acute intermittent porphyria; HCP = hereditary coproporphyria; VP = variegate porphyria; PCT = porphyria cutanea tarda. (Modified from Kaufman and Marver, Figure 1.[80])*

ALA and PBG are found as though there were a metabolic block to the further conversion of PBG to uroporphyrinogen. In hereditary coproporphyria, uroporphyrin and coproporphyrin are elevated in addition to ALA and PBG, a pattern that suggests a metabolic block between coproporphyrinogen and protoporphyrin. In variegate porphyria, all four of the above are excreted in increased amounts, as well as protoporphyrin, implicating a defective ferrochelatase step. Finally, in porphyria cutanea tarda, the chief excretory products are the uro- and coproporphyrins. Such primary defects anywhere along the pathway to heme would, of course, lead to compensatory increase in production of ALA synthetase. The postulated metabolic blocks must be partial rather than complete, since complete absence of heme would be incompatible with life. In this view of the disease, the increased ALA synthetase activity would represent a compensation for the primary metabolic defect, sufficient to maintain adequate heme synthesis despite the considerable loss of intermediates to the urine and feces.

DECREASED RESPONSIVENESS TO DRUG

Coumarin Resistance

The coumarin anticoagulants inhibit blood clotting by blocking the synthesis of four proteins essential to the clotting process: factors II (prothrombin), VII (proconvertin), IX (plasma thromboplastin component), and X (Stuart-Prower factor). Vitamin K is required for the synthesis of these specific proteins in the liver, and the coumarins antagonize vitamin K competitively. The structures of these compounds were presented in Figure 5-20, where the close chemical similarity between the coumarins and vitamin K is apparent.

The observation[81] that a patient required 20 times the average daily dose of warfarin to maintain the desired prolongation of prothrombin clotting time led to the discovery of a genetic trait that confers resistance to all the coumarins. Figure 6-12 shows a

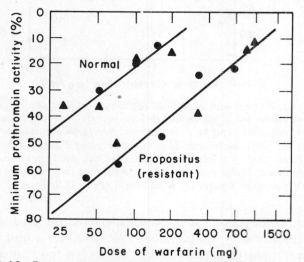

FIGURE 6-12. Dose-response relationship for warfarin in a normal and a resistant subject. *Response is expressed as the minimum level of prothrombin complex activity attained after a single dose, in terms of percent of normal activity. Circles are oral doses, triangles are intravenous doses. (From O'Reilly et al., Figure 2.[81])*

comparison of the responses to warfarin in this patient (the propositus) and a normal subject. The minimum level of prothrombin activity achieved after each dose is plotted against the log dose. The striking insensitivity of the propositus is apparent. Since oral and intravenous doses produced equivalent responses, both in the normal subject and in the propositus, it follows that defective absorption is not to blame for the warfarin resistance. Moreover, the rate of disappearance of warfarin, as judged by the return of prothrombin activity to normal levels after discontinuing the drug, was found to be exactly the same in the propositus and in the normal subject. Nor was the extent of protein binding of warfarin unusual in the propositus.

Figure 6-13 shows the effects of a fixed dose of warfarin in normal subjects and in the family of the propositus. Here the plasma concentration of warfarin and the reduction in prothrombin complex activity were measured 48 hr after a single dose of warfarin (1.5 mg kg^{-1}). The familial character of the warfarin resistance is obvious.

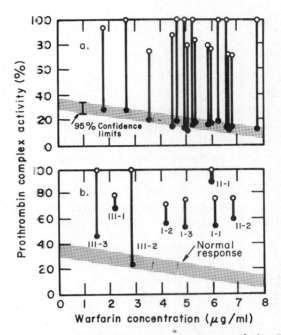

FIGURE 6-13. Normal and abnormal responses to warfarin. *Plasma concentrations of warfarin and prothrombin complex activity were measured 48 hr after single doses of warfarin (1.5 mg kg⁻¹) in 16 normal subjects (above), and in 8 members of the family of the warfarin-resistant subject (propositus) of Figure 6-12 (below). Open circles are initial levels of prothrombin complex activity, solid circles are levels after warfarin. Roman and Arabic numerals identify generation and individual respectively, in the coumarin-resistant kindred (cf. Figure 6-14). (From O'Reilly et al., Figure 5.[81])*

Figure 6-14 shows the pedigree of the same family. Individuals displaying warfarin resistance are represented by black symbols. We have here a trait that (1) appears in successive generations, (2) appears in both sexes, (3) is transmitted by both sexes, and (4) in matings between affected and normal individuals is sometimes transmitted and sometimes not. This trait is exceedingly rare. Many thousands of people have

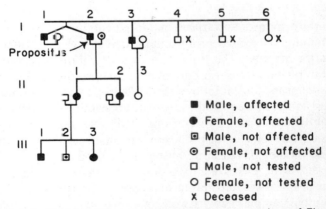

FIGURE 6-14. Kinship of the coumarin-resistant propositus of Figure 6-12. *(From O'Reilly et al., Figure 6.[81])*

been given coumarin anticoagulants, and most of them have been under rigorous laboratory control of their prothrombin clotting times. Yet there are only two known kindreds with coumarin resistance.[82] For a rare trait, the demonstrated pattern of inheritance can only mean that the trait is autosomal and dominant, for the following reason. If a trait is recessive, then the rarer it is, the lower the probability that the mate of an affected individual will also be carrying the abnormal allele; thus, the offspring would be heterozygotes and phenotypically normal. Therefore, a trait that is very rare and appears in successive generations (as in this family) is probably not recessive, and affected individuals are probably heterozygotes. This is a second example (cf. drug-induced porphyria) of an idiosyncratic reaction to drugs determined by a dominant gene.

Vitamin K appears to act in the synthesis of prothrombin at a translational or or post-translational level rather than upon the transcription of DNA into messenger RNA.[83] The vitamin may be required for the conversion of an inactive prothrombin precursor, which does not bind calcium, to active prothrombin, which does bind calcium.[84,85] Exactly how the coumarins interfere with this process is not clear. One theory is that coumarin anticoagulants alter the metabolism of vitamin K, promoting accumulation of the inactive vitamin K epoxide at the expense of vitamin K itself, perhaps by inhibiting the reduction of epoxide continuously formed in the liver.[86] The molecular basis of coumarin resistance is not yet known.

Warfarin has been in use as a rodenticide for a quarter of a century. Warfarin resistance has been observed in wild rats in Scotland,[87,88] Denmark,[89] and elsewhere.[90] The same principle applies here as with insect resistance to insecticides and bacterial resistance to antibiotics. If an agent is lethal to most of a population and if genes conferring resistance are present at all, the strong selective pressure will lead to replacement of the original sensitive population by a resistant one.

Vitamin D-Resistant Rickets

Another instance of decreased responsiveness to a drug is the special form of rickets that is resistant to vitamin D. Now that improved nutrition and vitamin supplementation have reduced the incidence of classical rickets, this form of the disease is recognized more readily. It is characterized by retarded growth and low plasma phosphate levels, with or without skeletal deformities.[91,92] The plasma calcium level is usually not abnormally low, but there is a profound renal loss of phosphate. These abnormalities do not respond to ordinary doses of vitamin D even when given parenterally; but huge doses of vitamin D, more than 1000 times the usual amount, are effective. Intravenous infusion of a calcium salt temporarily restores the renal tubular reabsorption of phosphate to normal, and massive oral doses of calcium have the same effect.

By measuring plasma phosphate levels in families of affected individuals, it was established that the disease is familial.[93,94] The trait was found in both men and women. Seven affected males had 10 sons, all of them normal, and 15 daughters, all with the disease. This shows conclusively that the disease is inherited as a sex-linked, dominant trait. A male carries the defective gene for this disease on his single X chromosome, which will be passed to his daughters but not to his sons. That the daughters, who must have been heterozygotes, were affected, shows that the trait is dominant.

The pathogenesis of vitamin D-resistant rickets remains controversial. Probably many of the manifest abnormalities are secondary to excessive parathyroid activity. Thus, for example, if poor calcium absorption from the intestine were the primary defect, lower plasma calcium levels would be expected. But feedback control mechanisms, including increased output of parathyroid hormone, would tend to raise plasma calcium by improving calcium absorption and promoting bone resorption.[95] The secondary hyperparathyroidism would also be responsible for the decreased renal tubular reabsorption of phosphate and the consequent hypophosphatemia. If a protein involved in calcium transport across the intestinal wall were synthesized under the influence of vitamin D,[96] then the abnormality could be analogous to that postulated for coumarin resistance; here the gene defect might yield a modified receptor with poor affinity for Vitamin D.

Inability to Taste Phenylthiourea

Receptors with a high degree of stereospecificity for chemical agents mediate the senses of taste and olfaction, acting somehow as transducers between the chemical stimuli and the specific sensory signals that are transmitted to the brain. It is not surprising, therefore, that genetic defects should cause altered responsiveness in these systems. Such hereditary abnormalities are known for both taste and smell. We shall discuss the one best understood by geneticists—the inability to taste phenyl-thiourea (phenylthiocarbamide, PTC):

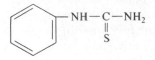

phenylthiourea (PTC)

PTC is perceived by most subjects as a very bitter substance at concentrations less than 0.15 mM, but a minority note no bitterness at all until much higher concentrations (sometimes 100 times higher) are reached. With a dilution series test, each concentration differing by a factor of 2 from the one before, a fairly reproducible taste threshold can be established for each subject. Figure 6-15 presents the frequency distributions obtained in one investigation with PTC (top) and with quinine (bottom) in the same subjects. The bimodality found with PTC but not with quinine shows that all bitter tastes do not activate the same chemoreceptors, and that people who are deficient in their ability to taste PTC may nevertheless taste quinine quite normally. For convenience, the subjects who taste PTC only at very high concentrations are categorized as "nontasters."

The question of whether the trait is dominant or recessive can be settled by means of mating analysis and application of the Hardy–Weinberg law, as was illustrated for isoniazid metabolism (p. 453). The reader is referred to that discussion for the detailed derivation. Here (Table 6-10) we see that matings between tasters yielded both tasters and nontasters in large numbers, whereas matings between nontasters yielded almost entirely nontaster offspring (the few exceptions in studies like this could be due to misclassification or illegitimacy). This finding indicates that the nontaster trait is recessive, the taster character dominant. Quantitative agreement with this hypothesis

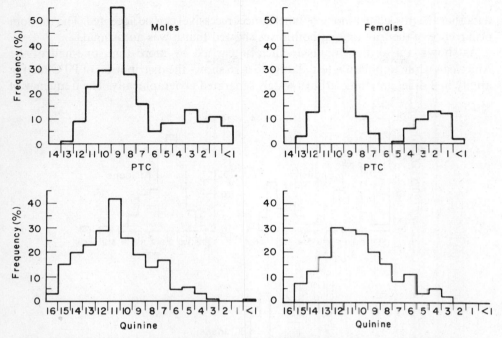

FIGURE 6-15. Distribution of taste thresholds for phenylthiourea (PTC) and quinine. *The most concentrated solutions are numbered 1 (0.13% PTC or 0.0187% quinine sulfate). The sets of increasing integers (toward left on the x-axes) represents serial 2-fold dilutions. Category labeled < 1 represents subjects unable to taste even the most concentrated solution. Tests were performed with a Belgian population of 225 males and 200 females.* (*From Leguebe, Figures 1–4.*[97])

is tested as outlined earlier, using the frequency of nontasters in the whole population (0.298, based on more than 3000 persons tested) to estimate the gene frequencies. Thus, $q^2 = 0.298$, $q = 0.545$, where q is the frequency of the nontaster allele. The computations for matings of tasters and nontasters, and for matings of tasters and tasters, yield, for the expected fraction of nontasters $q/(1 + q)$ and $[q/(1 + q)]^2$, respectively. The results shown in Table 6-10 agree so nearly perfectly with the observed

TABLE 6-10. Inheritance of the inability to taste phenylthiourea.
The expected fraction of nontasters was computed from the Hardy–Weinberg law on the assumption that it is a recessive trait, as described in the text. (From Stern,[12] Table 20; by permission of W. H. Freeman. Adapted from L. H. Snyder, *Ohio J. Sci* 32:436, 1937.)

Parents	No. of families	Offspring Tasters	Nontasters	Observed	Expected
Taster × taster	425	929	130	0.123	0.124
Taster × nontaster	289	483	278	0.366	0.354
Nontaster × nontaster	86	5	218	0.978	1.000

data that the postulated mode of inheritance (recessive) can be accepted. The random occurrence of the trait among both sexes showed that it was autosomal.

As shown above, the nontaster allele is carried by more than one-half of the American white population tested. Figure 6-16 shows the distribution of PTC-tasting ability in 3 different ethnic groups widely separated geographically. The frequency of

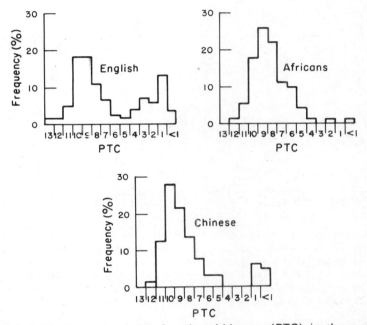

FIGURE 6-16. Taste thresholds for phenylthiourea (PTC) in three ethnic groups. *Thresholds were measured in 155 English males, 74 African Negroes, and 66 Chinese. Frequencies are plotted as percent of total in each group. The concentrations and serial dilutions were the same as in Figure 6-15. (From Barnicot, Figure 1.[98] By permission of Cambridge University Press.)*

tasters among American Indians (not shown in Figure 6-16) was found to be 98%, among Arabs only 63%. As with other drug idiosyncrasies, the implication of such differences is that some property directly or indirectly associated with the allele has been subject to long-term selective pressures of differing degree in the several geographic environments. The PTC nontaster trait is also found in primates other than man; 8 of 28 chimpanzees were judged to be nontasters.

An analog of PTC is a formerly widely used sweetening agent, ethoxyphenylurea:

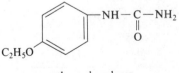

ethoxyphenylurea

When sulfur is substituted for oxygen in the urea moiety of this compound, the taste changes from sweet to bitter. It is concluded that the bitter taste of PTC is due to the grouping

$$-NH-\underset{\underset{S}{\|}}{C}-NH_2$$

The same grouping is found in the thiouracil family of drugs, which block the synthesis of thyroid hormones:

$$\begin{array}{c} O=C-CH=CH \\ \quad|\qquad\qquad| \\ NH-C-NH \\ \quad\underset{\underset{S}{\|}}{} \end{array}$$

thiouracil

This relationship suggested that a genetic abnormality involving an altered chemoreceptor for the thiouracil grouping might in some way also lead to defective thyroid function. Although the rationale seems far-fetched, surveys have shown that there is a significant increase over random expectation in the incidence of nodular goiter among male nontasters,[99] and also in the number of nontasters among a group of athyrotic cretins.[100]

Juvenile Pernicious Anemia

The juvenile form of this disease clearly has a genetic basis, whereas the role of heredity in adult pernicious anemia has not been worked out. The fundamental defect in pernicious anemia is inability to absorb vitamin B_{12} from the gastrointestinal tract. The absorption is dependent upon the presence of a mucoprotein synthesized in the gastric mucosa and secreted into the stomach. This protein, of molecular weight about 50,000, is called "intrinsic factor."[101] It binds to the mucosa of the ileum, and if it is carrying a molecule of B_{12}, the vitamin is transported across the mucosal cells and absorbed directly into the blood. In pernicious anemia, this specific protein is absent. The treatment of choice is vitamin B_{12} given parenterally, but intrinsic factor from a domestic animal (usually hog) may also be effective. Massive doses of B_{12} by mouth result in some degree of absorption even in the absence of intrinsic factor.

Juvenile pernicious anemia has an early onset, usually before two years of age, whereas the adult form is rarely seen before age 35. Megaloblastic anemia and neurologic disturbances are characteristic of both types of the disease, but gastric achlorhydria, present in the adult, does not occur in the majority of the juveniles. The genetic basis of the juvenile disease is indicated by the very high incidence among siblings—e.g., 5 pairs among 26 cases.[102] Several types of defect have been characterized in this disease. In one, there was a congenital absence of secretion of intrinsic factor, whereas the ileal phase of B_{12} absorption was normal. In another, there was normal intrinsic factor but defective ileal absorption. In yet another, the intrinsic factor was immunologically normal but was unable to promote B_{12} absorption in the ileum.[103] The frequent consanguinity of parents of affected children indicates autosomal recessive inheritance of the trait.

There are analogous diseases characterized by defective absorption of essential nutrients from the gastrointestinal tract. In cystic fibrosis, for example, there is known to be deficient production of enzymes, resulting in poor absorption of fats and the fat-soluble vitamins.

Resistance to Succinylcholine

Decreased responsiveness to succinylcholine has been reported,[104] in contrast to the prolonged effect of the drug in patients with atypical cholinesterase. The propositus, a 29-year-old male, was unaffected by a dose of succinylcholine that reduced grip strength (as measured by a hand dynamometer) of control subjects to about 10% of normal within a minute. At twice the test dose, there was only a transient 50% reduction in his grip strength. Analysis of his plasma cholinesterase by electrophoresis revealed a new component with mobility not normally observed. The enzyme activity was 3 times normal, a much greater increase than in the C5 variant described earlier (p. 449). The same plasma cholinesterase abnormalities were found in the mother, one sister, and one daughter, but not in three other siblings or a son. One brother and one daughter were not tested. The abnormal enzyme is evidently inherited as an autosomal autonomous characteristic. Inasmuch as one representation of the allele is sufficient to cause an excessively rapid destruction of succinylcholine, the succinyl-choline resistance behaves as a dominant trait. The allele that controls synthesis of the atypical cholinesterase, discussed earlier, has to be present on both homologous chromosomes for succinylcholine apnea to be manifested because any normal enzyme suffices to destroy the drug rapidly enough. Consequently, succinylcholine apnea appears to be a recessive trait. This illustrates well the semantic difficulties discussed on p. 438.

The unusual electrophoretic mobility of the genetically abnormal cholinesterase in succinylcholine-resistant subjects indicated that the high cholinesterase activity did not result simply from an increased amount of the normal enzyme. However, the specific activity (i.e., the catalytic efficiency of the active center) of the variant enzyme appeared to be normal, as indicated by immunoinactivation or titration with DFP. Moreover, measurement of the rate of return of enzyme activity after DFP treatment showed a rate of enzyme synthesis much higher than normal.[27]

Hypoxanthine-Guanine Phosphoribosyltransferase Deficiency

This enzyme (HG-PRTase) serves to reutilize oxypurines ingested in the diet or arising from the breakdown of nucleic acids by converting them to the corresponding mononucleotides. The mononucleotides of hypoxanthine (inosinic acid) and of guanine (guanylic acid) act as feedback inhibitors of the first enzyme in the de novo biosynthesis of purines, 5-phosphoribosyl-1-pyrophosphate amidotransferase (p. 272). A different enzyme, adenine-PRTase, performs the analogous "salvage" function for adenine.

A severe hereditary form of HG-PRTase deficiency is known as the Lesch–Nyhan syndrome. This is a sex-linked disease characterized by neurologic disorders, including choreoathetosis, spasticity, mental retardation, and compulsive self-mutilation; affected individuals usually do not survive beyond childhood. There is also an abnormally high blood level of uric acid and excessive uric acid excretion because the large amounts of hypoxanthine, guanine, and xanthine not salvaged are diverted into the oxidative pathway to uric acid. One form of gout is also associated with deficiency of HG-PRTase.[105,106]

In normal individuals and in patients suffering from gout who have normal HG-PRTase activity, allopurinol (p. 273), which inhibits xanthine oxidase, has two characteristic actions. First and most obvious, it decreases the formation of uric acid so that urate blood levels and urate excretion decrease. Increased levels of the oxypurine precursors lead, through normal HG-PRTase activity, to increased purine mononucleotides, which inhibit the de novo synthesis of purines. The net result is a decrease in the total purine excretion, as well as the excretion of uric acid, as shown in Figure 6-17. In patients with Lesch–Nyhan syndrome, however, or patients with gout accompanied by HG-PRTase deficiency, since the purines are not converted to

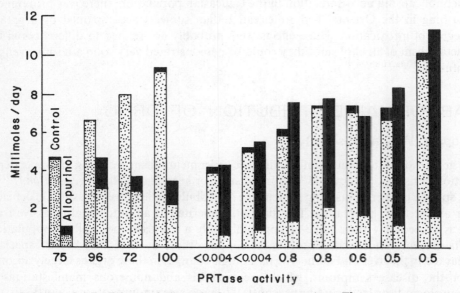

FIGURE 6-17. Effects of allopurinol on purine excretion. *The excretory patterns of uric acid (stippled) and other oxypurines (solid) are shown. In each patient, a pair of histograms show control result at left, result after allopurinol at right. HG-PRTase activity is given along the x axis as nmoles per mg protein per hour. The group of 4 individuals at left of figure had normal HG-PRTase activity. All the patients at right had absent or abnormally low activity. (From Kelley et al., Figure 24.*[106]*)*

mononucleotides, they are excreted into the urine. The result is a decrease in urate excretion accompanied by an equivalent increase in purine excretion. Thus, an abnormal response to allopurinol can be explained by the genetically determined deficiency of HG-PRTase. Such patients also react abnormally to purine analogs that have to be converted to nucleotides in order to act; examples are 6-mercaptopurine, 6-thioguanine, 8-azaguanine, and azathioprine.

Racial Differences in Drug Response

Finally, there are numerous racial differences in response to drugs in man, indicating that genetic influences play a role. Very few of these are well documented as yet. One clear example is the difference in response to *mydriatic agents.*[107] Whites of European stock display what we generally regard as a typical dilation of the pupil when ephedrine and similar agents are applied in the conjunctival sac. At the same drug concentration, Negroes show practically no response. A similar insensitivity of Negroes to the mydriatic effect of atropine was also reported.[108] Since ephedrine and atropine produce mydriasis by completely different mechanisms, it seems likely that the difference between the racial groups arises from some anatomic or physiologic peculiarity of the iris rather than from any drug-specific alteration of a receptor.

An interesting study revealed important differences in an autonomic response after administration of alcohol between Orientals and American Indians on the one hand and Americans of Caucasian stock on the other. Cutaneous flushing was quantitated by a spectrophotometric measurement on the ear lobe. At fixed small doses of alcohol causing no vasodilation in the Caucasian population, there was pronounced flushing in the Oriental and American Indian subjects accompanied by a greater degree of intoxication. These effects were probably not related to differences in the metabolism of alcohol since they could be demonstrated very soon after intravenous infusion.[108a,108b]

ABNORMAL DISTRIBUTION OF DRUG

Copper (Wilson's Disease)

A genetically determined abnormality of copper metabolism, resulting in copper deposition in tissues, is known as Wilson's disease or *hepatolenticular degeneration*.[109,110] A specific copper-containing protein, the α_2-globulin called ceruloplasmin, is deficient or absent from the plasma. The disease is inherited as an autosomal recessive trait. It is exceedingly rare; there are probably only a few cases per million population. The accumulation and deposition of copper occurs in all tissues but is especially marked in the liver and brain. The pathologic changes in these organs largely account for the disease symptoms, which are cirrhosis and numerous manifestations of neurologic disorder, including psychosis. The excessive amounts of copper in the tissues are largely bound to the various tissue proteins, which appear to be quite normal otherwise. Moreover, ceruloplasmin is evidently the only copper protein that is deficient in this disease, others, like tyrosinase and erythrocuprein, are present in normal amounts.

Ceruloplasmin normally contains about 98% of the plasma copper, not reversibly bound but incorporated into the protein structure at the time of synthesis. The daily intake of copper in the diet amounts to a few milligrams, more or less, depending upon what foods are eaten. Of this amount, approximately 1 mg is normally absorbed, and this corresponds roughly to the amount of copper incorporated daily into newly synthesized ceruloplasmin. Thus, the plasma water and tissues normally contain only negligible amounts of free copper. In the normal steady state, the same amount of ceruloplasmin that is synthesized each day is also destroyed and eliminated daily. It is presumably excreted into the intestine together with its associated copper.

When ceruloplasmin is absent, or present in insufficient amount, a decreased total amount of copper is found in the plasma, but a much greater than normal amount of free copper. Copper ions, therefore, escape from the circulation into the tissue water, where they become bound to various tissue components. Incidentally, more copper becomes available for renal excretion, so that more appears in the urine; but despite this increased urinary output, the patient with Wilson's disease is in positive copper balance. Figure 6-18 shows the characteristic abnormalities of copper content in plasma and urine. The daily retention of copper in Wilson's disease may be as little as 50 μg; this would account for the accumulation of nearly 200 mg in the tissues of a 10-year-old child affected by the disease. Because the process of accumulation is slow

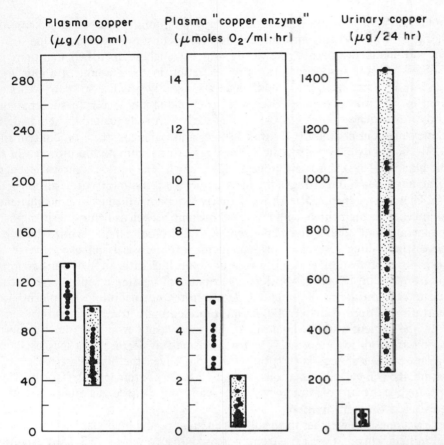

FIGURE 6-18. Plasma copper, plasma ceruloplasmin, and urinary copper in normal subjects and in patients with Wilson's disease. *At left, total plasma copper; middle, plasma ceruloplasmin, assayed by a method using a copper oxidase activity as the measure of ceruloplasmin; right, total urinary copper, daily output. Data from the individual subjects are represented by solid dots within vertical bars showing range. Open bars, normal subjects; stippled bars, patients with Wilson's disease. (Modified from Bearn, Figure 5.[113])*

and symptoms do not develop until considerable copper deposition has occurred, the clinical manifestations of this disease are rarely seen before the age of 6, and sometimes not until much later in life.

The specific drug for treatment or prevention is penicillamine,[111,112] which chelates copper and eliminates it from the body, as described already in Chapters 1 and 5. Because penicillamine is highly effective, it is all the more important to detect ceruloplasmin deficiency as early in life as possible. Routine screening of all infants might not be considered practical in view of the rarity of the condition, but certainly all relatives of patients in whom the diagnosis has been made should be investigated thoroughly and treated if evidence of the abnormality is found.

Iron (Primary Hemochromatosis)

Genetically determined abnormal distribution of iron characterizes the disease known as primary ("idiopathic") hemochromatosis.[114-116] Here there is a progressive accumulation of iron in the tissues. In the normal young adult, the body contains about 1 g of iron, and this amount remains fairly constant throughout life. In the patient with hemochromatosis, the steady state is somehow disturbed, and there is a daily excess of iron absorption over iron excretion in the amount of about 2 mg. The disease is rarely seen until middle age, presumably because so many years are required for the iron content of tissues to reach damaging levels. In such patients, the body iron reaches 20–40 g. Most of the excess iron is deposited as hemosiderin, a complex pigment containing ferritin. In liver and pancreas, the iron content may reach 50–100 times the normal, and lesser degrees of accumulation are seen in the thyroid gland and in skin spleen, kidney, and stomach. The pancreas shows degeneration of acinar tissue and scarring of the islets; diabetes is a common manifestation of the disease. There is usually portal cirrhosis of the liver, accompanied by liver insufficiency. The skin becomes pigmented, with increased melanin as well as hemosiderin deposits. The pancreatic and skin involvement account for the older name, "bronze diabetes."

One distinguishing feature of primary hemochromatosis is an elevation of the plasma iron concentration resulting in an abnormally high saturation of transferrin, the plasma iron-binding protein. Transferrin is capable of binding essentially all plasma iron up to concentrations of about 350 μg/ml. In the normal adult, the plasma iron concentration is approximately 120 μg/ml, representing a transferrin saturation of 35%. In the patient with hemochromatosis, the plasma iron and the transferrin saturation are both twice normal. The total plasma transferrin is not increased, and there is no evident change in its affinity for iron. Given the high plasma iron concentration, the clinical manifestations of the disease are not remarkable; iron overload after prolonged therapy of refractory anemia leads to the same syndrome of cirrhosis, diabetes, and skin pigmentation.

There is a question whether the positive iron balance and high plasma iron concentration in hemochromatosis arise from increased absorption or decreased excretion. What data are available indicate that the rate of elimination of iron is not diminished in this disease. The nature of the primary defect is not yet known, presumably it is an abnormality of the mechanism that prevents the net absorption from dietary sources of more iron than is required to meet the very small daily needs of the body. Therapy of hemochromatosis entails the removal of iron from the body. Hitherto this has been attempted by periodic bleeding, but recently trials have been initiated with iron-binding compounds like deferoxamine (p. 403).

The recognition of primary hemochromatosis as a genetically determined disease was delayed for several reasons. The late development of the clinical manifestations in patients means that members of antecedent generations of patients' families are often not available for study. The incidence of the disease is very low—less than 1 in 20,000 hospital admissions. Criteria for distinguishing the disease from other kinds of iron overload ("hemosiderosis" from multiple blood transfusions, dietary overload in Bantu tribesmen) had to be worked out. Now measurements of plasma iron and transferrin saturation permit identification of the trait even in young subjects many years before symptoms appear. Investigations by this method show a very high frequency of abnormality in families of patients with overt disease.

Hemochromatosis is much more common in males than in females, but in this instance, the sex difference may have no genetic connotation. Women lose iron through pregnancy, lactation, and menstruation. The loss attributed to menstruation, when prorated over the whole month, amounts to no less than 0.8 mg per day.[117]

which is nearly one-half the daily overload of 2 mg in hemochromatosis. Accordingly, the disease usually develops later in women than in men, so that the apparent incidence in a population containing both sexes and all ages would be higher among males.

One family study[118] spans four generations (Figure 6-19). The wife in the first generation (I-2) had developed diabetes at age 49 and died of cardiac failure (cardiac

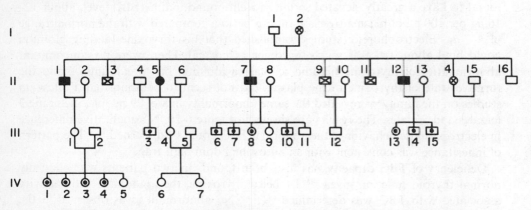

FIGURE 6-19. A family pedigree of primary hemochromatosis. *Squares are males, circles females. Open symbols, normal; solid symbols, "bronze diabetes," i.e., frank hemochromatosis with pigmentation; symbols containing X, subjects with 1–2 signs of hemochromatosis; symbols containing dot, subjects with elevated plasma iron level and no other demonstrable abnormality. (With modifications, from Boulin and Bamberger, chart p. 3158.[118])*

damage occurs frequently in hemochromatosis); she was also said to have developed pigmentation of the skin. There was no evidence of disease in her husband (I-1). Of 9 children, all but 1 showed some indication, more or less severe, of hemochromatosis. In the third generation, 8 of 15 subjects had elevated plasma iron levels, although none yet showed signs of disease. Finally, 4 of 7 children in the fourth generation also had elevated plasma iron levels. Throughout the kindred, the abnormal trait appeared in both males and females. The same arguments that applied to the analysis of the mode of inheritance of coumarin resistance (Figure 6-14) apply here. A trait that is very rare and that appears in successive generations is probably not recessive, and affected individuals are probably heterozygotes. In this case, primary hemochromatosis would be autosomal and dominant. Anomalies in the pedigree, illustrated in the figure, are difficult to interpret. Classification of II-16 as normal, for example, is a problem because his mother was affected, so illegitimacy cannot be invoked as an explanation. Another problem is the appearance of the trait in the fourth generation among children whose parents were apparently normal. The usual slow development of the disease, and a variable severity, may lead to a missed diagnosis in some affected individuals.

Increased or Decreased Thyroxine-Binding Globulin

Another genetic abnormality in the binding of a drug to a plasma protein concerns thyroxine. This hormone is carried in the plasma bound in roughly equal amounts to three kinds of plasma protein: (1) albumin, (2) a protein ("prealbumin") that migrates more rapidly toward the anode than does albumin, and (3) thyroxine-binding α-globulin (TBG).[119] TBG also binds triiodothyronine.[120] Its affinity is much greater for thyroxine than for triiodothyronine, and this probably explains why triiodothyronine is distributed so much more readily into the tissues. Less than 0.1% of total plasma thyroxine is present in the free form.[121]

During a routine health examination, a man with normal thyroid function was found to have a greatly elevated serum protein-bound iodine (PBI) level, about 12–16 μg per 100 ml of plasma over a 9-month period, compared with the normal range of 4–7 μg. Electrophoretic studies established that his thryoxine-binding globulin could bind about twice as much thyroxine as normal. There were no concomitant abnormalities of thyroxine binding to plasma albumin or "prealbumin," and the turnover rate of thyroxine in the plasma did not seem to be abnormal. Follow-up studies on the family[122] revealed the same abnormality in 8 of 29 people, including 3 females and 5 males. The results are shown in Figure 6-20. No qualitative difference in electrophoretic behavor of the abnormal TBG could be discerned.[123] The pattern of inheritance was consistent with an autosomal dominant trait.

Deficiency of TBG capacity has also been found. In two patients with clinically normal thyroid function given ^{131}I-labeled thyroxine, the amount of radioactivity associated with TBG was determined.[119,124] No abnormality was observed in the electrophoretic pattern of the plasma proteins, and there was no alteration of binding of the labeled thyroxine in the "prealbumin" and albumin regions. However, only a trace of radioactivity migrated with the electrophoretic mobility of TBG. Estrogen

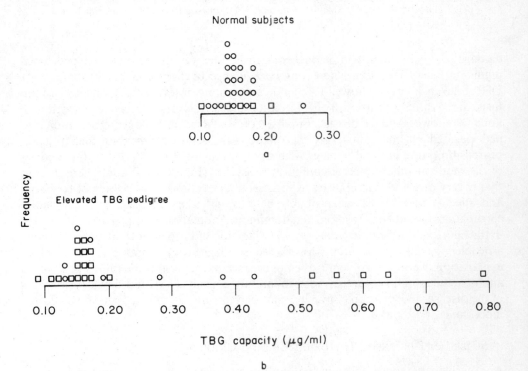

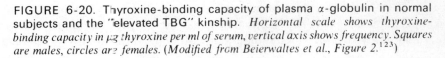

FIGURE 6-20. Thyroxine-binding capacity of plasma α-globulin in normal subjects and the "elevated TBG" kinship. *Horizontal scale shows thyroxine-binding capacity in μg thyroxine per ml of serum, vertical axis shows frequency. Squares are males, circles are females. (Modified from Beierwaltes et al., Figure 2.[123])*

treatment, which usually increases the thyroxine-binding capacity of TBG, had no effect. The apparent volume of distribution of thyroxine was only slightly increased over control values, but the plasma half-life of the ^{131}I-labeled hormone was shorter than normal by about 50%. Total daily excretion of thyroid hormones into the urine was within normal limits. Evidently, the rate of entry of labeled thyroxine into tissues (especially liver) was increased as a result of the TBG deficiency.[125] Since plasma binding would normally retard the passage of a substance from the blood plasma into the tissues, it seems reasonable that a decreased binding of thyroxine should lead to an increased rate of its passage into tissues.

Family studies indicate that the defect is genetically determined and sex-linked.[126,127] An interesting proof of the X-chromosome linkage of the trait was provided by the discovery of a female with Turner's syndrome (XO), who must have inherited the syndrome from her mother, since her father had normal TBG.[128,129]

DIFFERENCES IN USE OF AND RESPONSE TO PSYCHOTROPIC DRUGS

Most drug idiosyncrasies are discovered by chance when a drug is administered to a person who happens to carry a genetic trait determining the idiosyncratic response. Psychotropic drugs have the special property that they are sought out for self-administration by people who wish to experience a particular effect. The sought-after action may be euphoria, stimulation, tranquilization, or other modifications of mood or behavior. The multiplicity of genetic determinants of brain function, and the manifold actions of the psychotropic drugs, caution against oversimplified approaches. Suppose, however, that there were intrinsic differences in response to the psychotropic agents. Then one would also expect to find corresponding differences in the habitual use of these drugs, for if a person failed to obtain the desired effect, he would not continue to resort to that drug. It is well known, for example, that most people react with extreme displeasure to an initial dose of an opiate narcotic, both nausea and dysphoria being common responses. It was once supposed that administration of opiates in legitimate medical practice might "create" addicts. There is no valid evidence of this claim, although it is true that the incidence of addiction is high in the health professions, where there is easy access to addicting drugs.[130] It is quite obvious, however, that of the many millions of patients who receive morphine, an insignificantly small fraction ever seek to take the drug again. Likewise, in the population as a whole, very few of those who could obtain morphine or heroin illegally, if they wished, become addicts. It is noteworthy that although D-amphetamine has been used very widely to counteract fatigue and sleeplessness, only an occasional person who used it became habituated to it. And despite the nearly universal exposure of the population to the "legal" psychotropic drugs (alcohol, caffeine, and nicotine), some become habituated and some do not. Certainly socioenvironmental reasons can be found, ex post facto, to explain each case of addiction to heroin, the barbiturates, or alcohol, or of habituation to lysergic acid diethylamide, marijuana, nicotine, or amphetamine. But most people afflicted by the same adverse environmental circumstances do not seek escape through drug abuse. Despite the present paucity of evidence, therefore, the possibility should be entertained that the characteristic effects of psychotropic drugs upon mood, which underlie the development of drug abuse, may be at least in part genetically determined.

Investigation in this field has not yet transcended the difficulties of designing experiments free of self-selection or other kinds of bias, and of working out methods suitable for quantitation of subjective responses. It has been found, for example, that housewives who drink large amounts of coffee responded entirely differently to a test dose of caffeine in a placebo-controlled experiment than did housewives who never drink coffee.[131] The coffee drinkers felt more alert and had a sense of well-being after caffeine, as compared with placebo. The nondrinkers obtained significantly fewer effects of this kind; on the other hand, caffeine made them feel nervous and "jittery." But it is not known if the group habituated to coffee would have reacted in the same way at an earlier age, before their first exposure to caffeine. Large individual differences are observed in the sensitivity of people to the sleep-disturbing actions of caffeine,[132,133] but again it is not clear whether or not these are innate differences, independent of any prior exposure to caffeine. One investigation on the coffee-drinking and smoking habits of monozygotic and dizygotic twins suggests that these two kinds of drug-seeking behavior[134] are subject to genetic influences. Differences in sensitivity to alcohol among Orientals and American Indians as compared with Caucasians, already noted (p. 476), could possibly be related to drinking habits in these groups.[108a,108b]

REFERENCES

1. W. KALOW: *Pharmacogenetics: Heredity and the Response to Drugs*. Philadelphia, W. B. Saunders (1962).
2. J. B. STANBURY, J. B. WYNGAARDEN, and D. S. FREDRICKSON, eds.: *The Metabolic Basis of Inherited Disease*, 3rd ed. New York, McGraw-Hill (1972).
3. B. N. LA DU and W. KALOW, eds.: Pharmacogenetics. *Ann. N.Y. Acad. Sci.* 151:691 (1968).
4. Pharmacology Society Symposium: Pharmacogenetics. *Fed. Proc.* 31:1253 (1972).
5. B. N. LA DU: Genetic factors modifying drug metabolism and drug response. In *Fundamentals of Drug Metabolism and Drug Disposition*, B. N. La Du, H. G. Mandel, and E. L. Way, eds. Baltimore, Williams and Wilkins (971), pp. 308–377. Ch. 15.
6. E. S. VESSELL: Genetic aspects of drug metabolism in man. In *Drug Metabolism in Man. Ann. N.Y. Acad. Sci.* 179: 514–773 (1971).
7. E. S. VESELL: Drug therapy, pharmacogenetics. *New Eng. J. Med.* 287:904 (1972).
8. H. W. GOEDDE: Genetically determined variability in response to drugs. *Pharm. Weekbl.* 107:437 (1972).
9. B. N. LA DU: Pharmacogenetics: defective enzymes in relation to reactions to drugs. *Ann. Rev. Med.* 23:453 (1972).
10. Webster's *New International Dictionary of the English Language*, 3rd ed. Springfield, Mass., G. and C. Merriam Co (1968).
11. J. T. LITCHFIELD, Jr. and F. WILCOXON: A simplified method of evaluating dose-effect experiments. *J. Pharmacol. Exp. Therap.* 96:99 (1949).
12. C. STERN: *Principles of Human Genetics*, 2nd ed. San Francisco, W. H. Freeman, (1960).
13. E. S. VESELL: Genetic and environmental factors affecting drug response in man. *Fed. Proc.* 31:1253 (1972).
14. B. ALEXANDERSON, D. A. PRICE EVANS, and F. SJÖQVIST: Steady-state plasma levels of nortryptyline in twins: influence of genetic factors and drug therapy. *Brit. Med. J.* 4:764 (1969).
15. W. HAMMER, S. MARTENS, and F. SJÖQVIST: A comparative study of the metabolism of desmethylimipramine, nortriptyline, and oxyphenylbutazone in man. *Clin. Pharmacol. Therap.* 10:44 (1969).
16. H. LEHMANN and J. LIDDELL: Genetical variants of human serum pseudocholinesterase. *Progress in Medical Genetics*, 3:75 (1964).

17. A. H. LUBIN, P. J. GARRY, and G. M. OWEN: Sex and population differences in the incidence of a plasma cholinesterase variant. *Science* 173:161 (1971).

18. J. LIDDELL, H. LEHMANN, and D. DAVIES: Harris and Whittaker's pseudocholinesterase variant with increased resistance to fluoride. *Acta Genet. Statist. Med.* 13:95 (1963).

19. M. WHITTAKER: The pseudocholinesterase variants: esterase levels and increased resistance to fluoride. *Acta Genet. Statist. Med.* 14:281 (1964).

20. H. W. GOEDDE, D. GEHRING, and R. A. HOFMANN: Biochemische Untersuchungen zur Frage der Existenz eines "silent Gene" im Polymorphismus der Pseudocholinesterasen. *Humangenetik* 1:607 (1965).

21. K. ALTLAND and H. W. GOEDDE: Heterogeneity in the silent gene phenotype of pseudocholinesterase of human serum. *Biochem. Genetics* 4:321 (1970).

22. B. N. LA DU and B. DEWALD: Genetic regulation of plasma cholinesterase in man. In: *Advances in Enzyme Regulation*, ed. by G. Weber. New York and Oxford: Pergamon (1971). Vol. 9, p. 317.

23. H. HARRIS, D. A. HOPKINSON, and E. B. ROBSON: Two-dimensional electrophoresis of pseudocholinesterase components in normal human serum. *Nature* 196:1296 (1962).

24. H. HARRIS and E. B. ROBSON: Fractionation of human serum cholinesterase components by gel filtration. *Biochim. Biophys. Acta* 73:649 (1963).

25. H. HARRIS, D. A. HOPKINSON, E. B. ROBSON, and M. WHITTAKER: Genetical studies on a new variant of serum cholinesterase detected by electrophoresis. *Ann. Human Gen.* 26:359 (1963).

26. H. W. NEITLICH: Increased plasma cholinesterase activity and succinylcholine resistance: a genetic variant. *J. Clin. Invest.* 45:380 (1966).

27. A. YOSHIDA and A. G. MOTULSKY: A pseudocholinesterase variant (E Cynthiana) associated with elevated plasma enzyme activity. *Am. J. Human Gen.* 21:486 (1969).

28. J. C. THOMPSON and M. WHITTAKER: A study of the pseudocholinesterase in 78 cases of apnoea following suxamethonium. *Acta Gen. Statist. Med.* 16:209 (1966).

29. A. S. KEITT: Hereditary methemoglobinemia with deficiency of NADH-methemoglobin reductase. In *The Metabolic Basis of Inherited Disease*, 3rd ed., ed. by J. B. Stanbury, J. B. Wyngaarden, and D. S. Fredrickson. New York, McGraw-Hill (1972), pp. 1389–1397.

30. W. KALOW: Human hereditary defects with altered drug response. In *Pharmacogenetics: Heredity and the Response to Drugs*, Philadelphia, W. B. Saunders (1962) pp. 146–205.

31. R. F. SMITH, T. WHEELER, and A. GRAYBIEL: Hereditary methemoglobinemia: A family study with attention to the redox state of the myoglobin. *Johns Hopkins Med. Journal* 126:28 (1970).

32. G. E. BLOOM and H. S. ZARKOWSKY: Heterogeneity of the enzymatic defect in congenital methemoglobinemia. *New Eng. J. Med.* 281:919 (1969).

33. J. W. HARRIS: *The Red Cell*. Cambridge, Harvard University Press (1970).

34. E. M. SCOTT: The relation of diaphorase of human erythrocytes to inheritance of methemoglobinemia. *J. Clin. Invest.* 39:1176 (1960).

35. H. A. EDER, C. FINCH, and R. W. MC KEE: Congenital methemoglobinemia. A clinical and biochemical study of a case. *J. Clin. Invest.* 28:265 (1949).

36. T. A. J. PRANKERD: *The Red Cell*. Springfield, Mass., Charles C. Thomas (1961).

37. N. T. SHAHIDI: Acetophenetidin-induced methemoglobinemia. *Ann. N.Y. Acad. Sci.* 151:822 (1968).

38. J. W. JENNE: Partial purification and properties of the isoniazid transacetylase in human liver. Its relationship to the acetylation of p-aminosalicylic acid. *J. Clin. Invest.* 44:1992 (1965).

38a. D. A. P. EVANS and T. A. WHITE: Human acetylation polymorphism. *J. Lab. Clin. Med.* 63:394 (1964).

39. D. A. P. EVANS, K. A. MANLEY, and V. A. MC KUSICK: Genetic control of isoniazid metabolism in man. *Brit. Med. J.* 2:485 (1960).

40. B. N. LA DU: Isoniazid and pseudocholinesterase polymorphisms. *Fed. Proc.* 31:1276 (1972).

41. J. W. JENNE: Partial purification and properties of the isoniazid transacetylase in human liver. Its relationship to the acetylation of p-aminosalicylic acid. *J. Clin. Invest.* 44:1992 (1965).

42. W. W. WEBER, S. N. COHEN, and M. S. STEINBERG: Purification and properties of N-acetyltransferase from mammalian liver. *Ann. N.Y. Acad. Sci.* 151:734 (1968).

43. S. DEVADATTA, P. R. J. GANGADHARAM, R. H. ANDREWS, W. FOX, C. V. RAMAKRISHNAN, J. B. SELKON, and S. VELU: Peripheral neuritis due to isoniazid. *Bull. World Health Organ.* 23:587 (1960).

44. H. KUTT, K. VEREBELY, and F. MC DOWELL: Inhibition of diphenylhydantoin metabolism in rats and in rat liver microsomes by antitubercular drugs. *Neurology.* 18:706 (1968).

45. H. KUTT, R. BRENNAN, H. DEHEJIA, and K. VEREBELY: Diphenylhydantoin intoxication. *Am. Rev. Resp. Dis.* 101:377 (1970).

46. H. KUTT, W. WINTERS, and F. H. MC DOWELL: Depression of parahydroxylation of diphenylhydantoin by antituberculosis chemotherapy. *Neurology* 16:594 (1966).

47. H. KUTT, M. WOLK, R. SCHERMAN, and F. MC DOWELL: Insufficient parahydroxylation as a cause of diphenylhydantoin toxicity. *Neurology* 14:542 (1964).

48. M. MURAYAMA: Molecular mechanism of red cell 'sickling.' *Science* 153:145 (1966).

48a. G. J. BREWER, ed.: Hemoglobin and Red Cell Structure and Function. In *Advances in Exp. Med. Biol.* 28 (1972).

49. M. F. PERUTZ: *Proteins and Nucleic Acids.* Amsterdam, Elsevier Publishing Co. (1962).

50. E. BEUTLER: The hemolytic effect of primaquine and related compounds: a review. *Blood* 14:103 (1959).

51. R. W. KELLERMEYER, A. R. TARLOV, S. L. SCHRIER, P. E. CARSON, and A. S. ALVING: The hemolytic effect of primaquines. XIII. Gradient susceptibility to hemolysis of primaquine-sensitive erythrocyte. *J. Lab. Clin. Med.* 58:225 (1961).

52. P. A. MARKS and J. BANKS: Drug-induced hemolytic anemias associated with glucose-6-phosphate dehydrogenase deficiency: a genetically heterogeneous trait. *Ann. N.Y. Acad. Sci.* 123:198 (1965).

53. G. A. STUART: Observations on the mechanism of action of acetylphenylhydrazine in normal and glucose-6-phosphate dehydrogenase (G-6PD) deficient erythrocytes. *Br. J. Haemat.* 16:435 (1969).

54. P. E. CARSON, C. L. FLANAGAN, C. E. ICKES, and A. S. ALVING: Enzymatic deficiency in primaquine-sensitive erythrocytes. *Science* 124:484 (1956).

55. A. G. MOTULSKY, A. YOSHIDA, and G. STAMATOYANNOPOULOS: Glucose-6-phosphate dehydrogenase variants. *Ann. N.Y. Acad. Sci.* 179 636 (1971).

56. H. N. KIRKMAN: Glucose-6-phosphate dehydrogenase variants and drug-induced hemolysis. *Ann. N.Y. Acad. Sci.* 151:753 (1968).

57. A. YOSHIDA: Hemolytic anemia and G6PD deficiency. *Science* 179:532 (1973).

58. N. L. PETRAKIS, S. L. WIESENFELD, B. J. SAMS, M. F. COLLEN, J. L. CUTLER and A. B. SIEGELAUB: Prevalence of sickle-cell trait and glucose-6-phosphate dehydrogenase deficiency. Decline with age in the frequency of G-6-PD-deficient Negro males. *New Eng. J. Med.* 282:767 (1970).

59. A. C. ALLISON: Malaria n carriers of the sickle-cell trait and in newborn children. *Exper. Parasitol.* 6:418 (1957).

60. A. C. ALLISON: Glucose-6-phosphate dehydrogenase deficiency in red blood cells of East Africans. *Nature* 186:531 (1960).

61. A. R. TARLOV, G. J. BREWER, P. E. CARSON, and A. S. ALVING: Primaquine sensitivity. Glucose-6-phosphate dehydrogenase deficiency: an inborn error of metabolism of medical and biological significance. *Arch. Int. Med.* 109:209 (1962).

62. L. LUZZATTO, E. A. USANGA, and S. REDDY: Glucose-6-phosphate dehydrogenase deficient red cells: resistance to infection by malarial parasites. *Science* 164:839 (1969).

63. W. H. ZINKHAM and B CHILDS: Effect of vitamin K and naphthalene metabolites on glutathione metabolism of erythrocytes from normal newborns and patients with naphthalene hemolytic anemia. *Amer. J. Dis. Children* 94:420 (1957).

64. W. KALOW: Succinylcholine and malignant hyperthermia. *Fed. Proc.* 31:1270 (1972).

65. H. S. MARVER and R. SCHMID: "The porphyrias." In *The Metabolic Basis of Inherited Disease*, 3rd ed., edited by J. B. Stanbury, J. B. Wyngaarden, and D. S. Fredrickson. New York, McGraw-Hill (1972) pp. 1087–1140.

66. A. GOLDBERG and C. RIMINGTON: *Diseases of Porphyrin Metabolism.* Springfield, C. C. Thomas (1962).

67. L. EALES and G. C. LINDER: Porphyria—the acute attack. An analysis of 80 cases. *South African Med. J.* 36:284 (1962).

68. S. GRANICK: Hepatic porphyria and drug-induced or chemical porphyria. *Ann. N.Y. Acad. Sci.* 123:188 (1965).

69. A. POLAND and E. GLOVER: 2,3,7,8-Tetrachlorodibenzo-p-dioxin: a potent inducer of δ-aminolevulinic acid synthetase. *Science* 179:476 (1973).

70. S. GRANICK and S. SASSA: "δ-Aminolevulinic acid synthetase and the control of heme and chlorophyll synthesis." In *Metabolic Pathways*, Vol. 5. New York, Academic Press (1971).

71. S. GRANICK and G. URATA: Increase in activity of δ-aminolevulinic acid synthetase in liver mitochondria induced by feeding of 3,5-dicarbethoxy-1,4-dihydrocollidine. *J. Biol. Chem.* 238:821 (1963).

72. S. GRANICK: Induction of the synthesis of δ-aminolevulinic acid synthetase in liver parenchyma cells in culture by chemicals that induce acute porphyria. *J. Biol. Chem.* 238:PC2247 (1963).

73. S. GRANICK: The induction in vitro of the synthesis of δ-aminolevulinic acid synthetase in chemical porphyria: a response to certain drugs, sex hormones, and foreign chemicals. *J. Biol. Chem.* 241:1359 (1966).

74. L. J. STRAND, J. MANNING, and H. S. MARVER: The induction of δ-aminolevulinic acid synthetase in cultured liver cells. *J. Biol. Chem.* 247:2820 (1972).

75. F. JACOB and J. MONOD: Genetic regulatory mechanisms in the synthesis of proteins. *J. Mol. Biol.* 3:318 (1961).

76. G. ABBRITTI and F. DE MATTEIS: Decreased levels of cytochrome P-450 and catalase in hepatic porphyria caused by substituted acetamides and barbiturates. Importance of the allyl group in the molecule of the active drugs. *Chem-Biol. Interactions* 4:281 (1971/1972).

77. W. LEVIN, E. SERNATINGER, M. JACOBSON, and R. KUNTZMAN: Destruction of cytochrome P450 by secobarbital and other barbiturates containing allyl groups. *Science* 176:1341 (1972).

78. F. DE MATTEIS: Loss of haem in rat liver caused by the porphyrogenic agent 2-allyl-2-isopropylacetamide. *Biochem. J.* 124:767 (1971).

78a. F. DE MATTEIS: Mechanisms of induction of hepatic porphyria by drugs. *Proceedings Fifth Int. Congr. Pharmacol.*, San Francisco (1972), p. 198.

79. A. KAPPAS, H. L. BRADLOW, P. N. GILLETTE, R. D. LEVERE and T. F. GALLAGHER: A defect of steroid hormone metabolism in acute intermittent porphyria. *Fed. Proc.* 31:1293 (1972).

80. L. KAUFMAN and H. S. MARVER: Biochemical defects in two types of human hepatic porphyria. *New Eng. J. Med.* 283:954 (1970).

81. R. A. O'REILLY, P. M. AGGELER, M. S. HOAG, L. S. LEONG, and M. L. KROPATKIN: Hereditary transmission of exceptional resistance to coumarin anticoagulant drugs. The first reported kindred. *New Eng. J. Med.* 271:809 (1964).

82. R. A. O'REILLY: The second reported kindred with hereditary resistance to oral anticoagulant drugs. *New Eng. J. Med.* 282:1448 (1970).

83. H. F. DE LUCA and J. W. SUTTIE (eds.): *The Fat Soluble Vitamins*. Madison, University of Wisconsin Press (1970).

84. J. STENFLO and P. O. GANROT: Vitamin K and the biosynthesis of prothrombin. *J. Biol. Chem.* 247:8160 (1972).

85. G. L. NELSESTUEN and J. W. SUTTIE: The purification and properties of an abnormal prothrombin protein produced by dicumarol-treated cows. *J. Biol. Chem.* 247:8175 (1972).

86. R. G. BELL, J. A. SADOWSKI, and J. T. MATSCHINER: Mechanism of action of warfarin. Warfarin and metabolism of vitamin K. *Biochemistry* 11:1959 (1972).

87. C. M. BOYLE: Case of apparent resistance of *Rattus norvegicus* Berkenhout to anticoagulant poisons. *Nature* 188:517 (1960).

88. J. H. CUTHBERT: Further evidence of resistance to warfarin in rats. *Nature* 198:807 (1963).

89. M. LUND: Resistance to warfarin in the common rat. *Nature* 203:778 (1964).

90. W. B. JACKSON and D. KAUKEINEN: Resistance of wild Norway rats in North Carolina to warfarin rodenticide. *Science* 176:1343 (1972).

91. F. ALBRIGHT, A. M. BUTLER, and E. BLOOMBERG: Rickets resistant to vitamin D therapy. *Amer. J. Dis. Children* 54:529 (1937).

92. T. F. WILLIAMS and R. W. WINTERS: Familial (hereditary) vitamin D-resistant rickets with hypophosphatemia. In *The Metabolic Basis of Inherited Disease*, 3rd ed., ed. by J. B. Stanbury, J. B. Wyngaarden, and D. S. Fredrickson. New York, McGraw-Hill (1972). pp. 1465–1485.

93. R. W. WINTERS J. B. GRAHAM, T. F. WILLIAMS, V. W. MC FALLS, and C. H. BURNETT: A genetic study of familial hypophosphatemia and vitamin D resistant rickets. *Trans. Ass. Amer. Physicians* 70:234 (1957).

94. J. B. GRAHAM, V. W. MC FALLS, and R. W. WINTERS: Familial hypophosphatemia with vitamin D resistant rickets. II. Three additional kindreds of the sex-linked dominant type with a genetic analysis of four such families. *Amer. J. Human Genet.* 11:311 (1959).

95. F. W. LAFFERTY, C. H. HERNDON, and O. H. PEARSON: Pathogenesis of vitamin D-resistant rickets and the response to a high calcium intake. *J. Clin. Endocrinol.* 23:903 (1963).

96. R. H. WASSERMAN and A. N. TAYLOR: Vitamin D_3-induced calcium-binding protein in chick intestinal mucosa. *Science* 152:791 (1966).

97. A. LEGUEBE: Génétique et anthropologie de la sensibilité à la phenylthiocarbamide. I. Fréquence du gène dans la population belge. *Bull. Inst. Roy. Sci. Nat. Belgique* 36:article 27 (1960).

98. N. A. BARNICOT: Taste deficiency for phenylthiourea in African Negroes and Chinese. *Ann. Eugenics* 15:248 (1950–51).

99. F. D. KITCHIN, W. HOWEL-EVANS, C. A. CLARKE, R. B. MC CONNELL, and P. M. SHEPPARD: P.T.C. taste response and thyroid disease. *Brit. Med. J.* 1:1069 (1959).

100. G. R. FRASER: Cretinsm and taste sensitivity to phenylthiocarbamide. *Lancet* 1:964 (1961).

101. V. HERBERT and W. B. CASTLE: Intrinsic factor. *New Eng. J. Med.* 270:1181 (1964).

102. O. R. MC INTYRE, L. W. SULLIVAN, G. H. JEFFRIES, and R. H. SILVER: Pernicious anemia in childhood. *New Eng. J. Med.* 272:981 (1965).

103. M. KATZ, S. K. LEE, and B. A. COOPER: Vitamin B_{12} malabsorption due to a biologically inert intrinsic factor. *New Eng. J. Med.* 287:425 (1972).

104. H. W. NEITLICH: Increased plasma cholinesterase activity and succinylcholine resistance: a genetic variant. *J. Clin. Invest.* 45:380 (1966).

105. W. N. KELLEY, F. M. ROSENBLOOM, J. MILLER, and J. E. SEEGMILLER: An enzymatic basis for variation in response to allupurinol. Hypoxanthine-guanine phosphoribosyltransferase deficiency. *New Eng. J. Med.* 278:287 (1968).

106. W. N. KELLEY, M. L. GREENE, F. M. ROSENBLOOM, J. F. HENDERSON, and J. E. SEEGMILLER: Hypoxanthine-guanine phosphoribosyltransferase deficiency in gout. *Ann. Int. Med.* 70:155 (1969).

107. K. K. CHEN and E. J. POTH: Racial differences as illustrated by the mydriatic action of cocaine, euphthalmine and ephedrine. *J. Pharmacol. Exp. Therap.* 36:429 (1929).

108. T. G. SCOTT: The eye of the West African Negro. *Brit. J. Ophthalmol.* 29:12 (1945).

108a. P. H. WOLFF: Vasomotor sensitivity to alcohol in diverse Mongoloid population. *Am. J. Hum. Gen.* 25:193 (1973).

108b. P. H. WOLFF: Ethnic differences in alcohol sensitivity. *Science* 175:449 (1972).

109. I. H. SCHEINBERG and I. STERNLIEB: Wilson's disease. *Annu. Rev. Med.* 16:119 (1965).

110. A. G. BEARN: Wilson's disease. In *The Metabolic Basis of Inherited Disease,* 3rd ed., ed. by J. B. Stanbury, J. B. Wyngaarden and D. S. Fredrickson. New York, McGraw-Hill (1972), pp. 1033–1050, Ch. 43.

111. I. STERNLIEB and I. H. SCHEINBERG: Penicillamine therapy for hepatolenticular degeneration. *J. Am. Med. Ass.* 189:748 (1964).

112. I. STERNLIEB and I. H. SCHEINBERG: Prevention of Wilson's disease in asymptomatic patients. *New Eng. J. Med.* 278:352 (1968).

113. A. G. BEARN: Genetic and biochemical aspects of Wilson's disease. *Am. J. Med.* 15:442 (1953).

114. T. H. BOTHWELL and C. A. FINCH: *Iron Metabolism.* Boston, Little, Brown and Co. (1962).

115. J.-C. DREYFUS and G. SCHAPIRA: Iron overload. The metabolism of iron in hemochromotosis. *Iron Metabolism,* a CIBA Symposium, ed. by F. Gross. Berlin, Springer-Verlag (1964) pp. 296–325.

116. M. POLLYCOVE: Hemochromatosis. In *The Metabolic Basis of Inherited Disease,* 3rd ed., ed. by J. B. Stanbury, J. B. Wyngaarden, and D. S. Fredrickson. New York, McGraw-Hill (1972), pp. 1051–1084, Ch. 44.

117. J. MILLIS: The iron losses of healthy women during consecutive menstrual cycles. *Med. J. Australia* 2:874 (1951).

118. R. BOULIN and J. BAMBERGER: L'Hémochromatose familiale. *Sem. Hôp. Paris* 29:3153 (1953).

119. W. R. BEISEL, H. ZAINAL, S. HANE, V. C. DI RAIMONDO, and P. H. FORSHAM: Low thyroidal iodine uptake with euthyroidism associated with deficient thyroid-binding globulin but normal cortisol binding. *J. Clin. Endocrinol.* 22:1165 (1962).

120. A. H. GORDON, J. GROSS, D. O'CONNOR and R. PITT-RIVERS: Nature of the circulating thyroid hormone-plasma protein complex. *Nature* 169:19 (1952).

121. J. E. RALL, J. ROBBINS, and C. G. LEWALLEN: The Thyroid. *The Hormones*, Vol. 5, ed. by G. Pincus, K. V. Thimann, and E. B. Astwood, New York, Academic Press (1964) pp. 159–439.

122. W. H. BEIERWALTES and J. ROBBINS: Familial increase in the thyroxine-binding sites in serum alpha globulin. *J. Clin. Invest.* 38:1683 (1959).

123. W. H. BEIERWALTES, E. A. CARR, JR., and R. L. HUNTER: Hereditary increase in the thyroxine-binding sites in the serum alpha globulin. *Trans. Ass Am. Physicians* 74:170 (1961).

124. S. H. INGBAR: Clinical and physiological observations in a patient with an idiopathic decrease in the thyroxine-binding globulin of plasma. *J. Clin. Invest.* 40:2053 (1961).

125. R. R. CAVALIERI and G. L. SEARLE: The kinetics of distribution between plasma and liver of ^{131}I-labeled L-thyroxine in man: observations of subjects with normal and decreased serum thyroxine-binding globulin. *J. Clin. Invest.* 45:939 (1966).

126. J. S. MARSHALL, R. P. LEVY, and A. G. STEINBERG: Human thyroxine-binding globulin deficiency. A genetic study. *New Eng. J. Med.* 274:1469 (1966).

127. J. T. NICOLOFF, J. T. DOWLING, and D. D. PATTON: Inheritance of decreased thyroxine-binding by the thyroxine-binding globulin. *J. Clin. Endocrinol.* 24:294 (1964).

128. S. REFETOFF and H. A. SELENKOW: Familial thyroxine-binding globulin deficiency in a patient with Turner's syndrome (XO). Genetic study of a kindred. *New Eng. J. Med.* 278:1081 (1968).

129. ANONYMOUS: The thyroid and the Lyon. Editorial. *New Eng. J. Med.* 278:1119 (1968).

130. H. ISBELL: Methods and results of studying experimental human addiction to the newer synthetic analgesics. *Ann. N.Y. Acad. Sci.* 51:108 (1948).

131. A. GOLDSTEIN and S. KAISER: Psychotropic effects of caffeine in man. III. A questionnaire survey of coffee drinking and its effects in a group of housewives. *Clin. Pharmacol. Ther.* 10:477 (1969).

132. A. GOLDSTEIN, R. WARREN, and S. KAIZER: Psychotropic effects of caffeine in man. I. Individual differences in sensitivity to caffeine-induced wakefulness. *J. Pharmacol. Exp. Therap.* 149:156 (1965).

133. A. GOLDSTEIN, S. KAIZER, and R. WARREN: Psychotropic effects of caffeine in man. II. Alertness, psychomotor coordination, and mood. *J. Pharmacol. Exp. Therap.* 150:146 (1965).

134. F. CONTERIO and B. CHIARELLI: Study of the inheritance of some daily life habits. *Heredity* 17:347 (1962).

CHAPTER 7
Drug Allergy

INTRODUCTION

Drug allergy is an adverse reaction to a drug resulting from previous sensitization to that same drug or a closely related one. The term "hypersensitivity" has often been used to describe the allergic state. This word is inappropriate as applied to drug allergy because its literal meaning invites confusion with other kinds of adverse drug reaction. One could properly describe as "hypersensitive" the normal therapeutic responses of the people at the lower end of the frequency distribution in a quantal log dose-response curve, i.e., those individuals who are sensitive to a very low dose of a drug. One could also reasonably describe as "hypersensitivity" an idiosyncratic response at a low dosage level to the therapeutic or toxic effects of a drug in a genetically predisposed person. There has been a lack of precision in the diagnosis of drug allergies and often a failure to apply clear-cut criteria to their classification. Ambiguous terminology adds to the confusion. We shall avoid the term "hypersensitivity" and describe as drug allergy those drug reactions that have an obvious (or inferred) immunologic basis.[1-7]

In order for a drug to produce an allergic reaction, a prior *sensitizing* contact is required, either with the same drug or with one closely related chemically. A period of time is required—usually about 7–14 days—for the synthesis of significant amounts of drug-specific antibodies. Then exposure to the drug (the *eliciting* contact) results in an antigen-antibody interaction, which provokes the typical manifestations of allergy. However, there need be no drug-free interval between the sensitizing contact and the eliciting contact; thus, allergic sensitization could occur early and allergic response later during the same course of treatment. The manifestations of allergy are numerous. They involve various organ systems, and they range in severity from minor skin lesions to fatal anaphylactic shock. The pattern of allergic response differs in different species. In man, involvement of the skin is most common, whereas in the guinea pig, for example, bronchiolar constriction leading to asphyxia is typical. The pattern of response is somewhat conditioned by the route of sensitization and the route of subsequent administration and by the particular drug employed. A certain drug may preferentially elicit one or several responses from among the whole pattern of possible responses. Sulfonamide allergy, for example, is usually manifested by dermatitis, conjunctivitis, or fever; penicillin, on the other hand, most frequently elicits urticaria ("hives") and generalized itching. Unrelated drugs, once they have sensitized,

489

may also elicit the same allergic response, such as dermatitis, anaphylaxis, or angioedema. Thus, the allergic response is a consequence of the antigen-antibody interaction and has nothing directly to do with the chemical structure of the eliciting drug.

Drug allergy may be compared and contrasted with drug toxicity and drug idiosyncrasy, as follows:

1. *Occurrence.* This is not necessarily a distinguishing criterion, since all three kinds of adverse drug reactions may be common or rare, depending upon the drug. Most idiosyncrasies are rare because any given abnormal genotype is likely to be rare, but if a genetic polymorphism (e.g., PTC nontasters) is related to a drug idiosyncrasy, the frequency may be quite high. Although drug allergy, with most drugs, is seen in no more than a few percent of all who are exposed, some chemicals can cause allergic sensitization in nearly everyone exposed to them. Genetic predisposition to allergy probably plays a role;[8–10] affected individuals are evidently capable of being sensitized to many different allergens. In contrast, the genetic predisposition to drug idiosyncrasy takes the form of an unusual reaction to a particular drug or class of drugs.

2. *Dose relationship.* Toxic side effects are clearly dose related, as are idiosyncratic responses in susceptible individuals. In both cases, the usual dose-effect principles apply, since the responses are mediated directly by specific drug-receptor interactions. In contrast, allergic responses have an erratic relationship to dosage. Extremely small doses (e.g., traces of antibiotics in foodstuffs) suffice to sensitize in some cases. It is also clear that minute doses can elicit allergic responses in previously sensitized individuals, and the magnitude of the response has little to do with the size of the eliciting dose. Sometimes a mere trace of drug (e.g., a fraction of a microgram contaminating a syringe) elicits life-threatening manifestations of allergy; sometimes full therapeutic doses evoke only mild allergic effects. It appears that the magnitude of an allergic response is determined primarily by immunologic factors in the individual and that the drug (at whatever dose) may serve chiefly to "trigger" the reaction.

3. *Prior contact with drug.* Although prior exposure to a drug is not necessary for toxic side effects or idiosyncratic responses, it is essential for allergic reactions. However, sensitization may occur covertly by environmental or dietary exposure (e.g., penicillin in cow's milk or in moldy foods) so that allergic responses may occur without known prior exposure.

4. *Chemical specificity.* Toxic side effects and drug idiosyncrasies are directly and specifically determined by the chemical structure of the drug, and typical structure-activity relationships can be established. In drug allergy, the responses are determined by antigen-antibody reactions, and they are largely independent of which drug molecule elicits them. Here the structure-activity relationships concern the chemical structures of the sensitizing drugs and of the eliciting drugs. Some are more effective than others in sensitizing. If a particular drug does sensitize, then only this drug or closely related congeners will elicit the allergic response. Thus, the interactions leading to the allergic state as well as those producing allergic responses may show a high degree of specificity related to chemical structure, as discussed later in this chapter.

5. *Mechanisms.* In drug allergy, the immunologic basis can often be established by demonstrating circulating antibodies in serum or altered immunologic responses in tissues. The antibodies are specific for the sensitizing drug and closely related compounds, but as already indicated, the manifestations of drug allergy are unrelated to any particular drug. In contrast, the nature of a toxic or idiosyncratic reaction to a drug is determined by that drug. A corollary is that toxic or idiosyncratic reactions

are overcome or prevented by antagonists that are specific for the drug that precipitated the reaction. In drug allergy, on the other hand, specific drug antagonists are
useless, but antihistamines, epinephrine, and hydrocortisone, whose actions are
directed toward the general manifestations of the allergic response, may be effective.

IMMUNOLOGIC BASIS OF DRUG ALLERGY

The earliest observations on immunization concerned the reactions of the organism
to the introduction of foreign cells or foreign proteins. The formation of antibody
proteins directed rather specifically against the sensitizing antigens was soon demonstrated by a variety of methods. In some instances, the combination of antibody with
antigenic materials caused a precipitin reaction—the formation of an insoluble
antibody-antigen complex. In cellular reactions, such as the lysis of sensitized erythrocytes, the complement system of serum (see below) was shown to be required,
and the ability of antibody-antigen complexes to bind complement provided the
basis for an antibody assay. Antibodies fixed in skin or carried there by lymphocytes
could be demonstrated by local erythema and wheal formation elicited by application
of the appropriate antigen.

Immunoglobulins

We now understand that antibodies are a heterogeneous group of globulins, the
immunoglobulins of classes IgA, IgC, IgM, IgD, and IgE.[11-13] The elucidation of
the structure and function of these molecules is one of the outstanding achievements
of modern medical science.[80] The common features of the immunoglobulins are shown
in Figure 7-1. These comprise a symmetrical structure of heavy and light chains
each with a variable and a constant region. In the constant region of a given immunoglobulin class, the polypeptide chain is the same (or nearly the same) in its
amino acid sequence. This homology extends across species and is found even in
primitive organisms. In contrast, the variable region is composed of a variety of
different amino acid sequences, although the total number of amino acid residues
remains the same. Clearly it would be impossible to sequence any such protein,
which is only one of hundreds or thousands circulating in low concentration in the
plasma. The key to understanding the system came with the discovery that patients
with multiple myeloma had a neoplastic clone of cells producing large amounts of a
single immunoglobulin. This myeloma protein circulates in the plasma and is deposited in tissues, and a portion of the molecule (the Fab light chain region) appears
in the urine as Bence–Jones protein. No two myeloma patients produce exactly the
same immunoglobulin, but each patient produces enough of a single one to permit
the amino acid sequence to be worked out. In this way, the light and heavy chains
were sequenced, and the variable and constant regions were found.

The antigen binding sites are evidently composed of residues contributed by the
variable portions of a light and a heavy chain. It is generally accepted that lymphoid
cells differentiate in such a way that a given cell retains the capacity to produce only a
single immunoglobulin. All the lymphoid cells together, however, produce thousands
of different immunoglobulins. According to the clonal theory,[14] if a cell comes into
contact with an antigen, any part of which happens to "fit" its antigen binding site,
that cell is stimulated to divide and increase its production of that particular globulin.
Since each region of a given antigen may more or less fit a number of different antigen

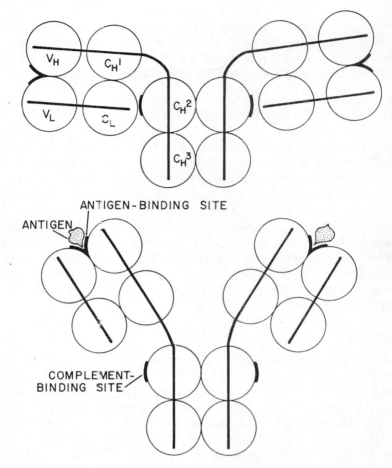

FIGURE 7-1. Structure of a typical immunoglobulin molecule. *The polypeptide chains are shown as solid lines; NH$_2$-terminal regions comprise the antigen binding site.* V$_H$ = *variable region, heavy chain;* C$_H$ = *constant regions, heavy chain;* V$_L$, C$_L$ = *variable and constant regions, light chain. Upper diagram depicts an immunoglobulin molecule free of antigen; lower diagram suggests conformation change upon antigen binding, exposing complement binding state. (From* The Structure and Function of Antibodies *by G. M. Edelman. Copyright © 1970 by Scientific American, Inc. All rights reserved.*[11]*)*

binding sites, a considerable array of different antibodies is likely to be produced directed toward the several antigenic determinants of the antigen molecule. Some types of antibody, such as IgG and IgM, are secreted into the plasma where they comprise the well-known soluble γ-globulins. Others, such as IgE, are found in serum only in very small amounts and are cytotropic—they are carried to cells in the skin and other tissues, where they become fixed to the cell surface.

Some of the immunoglobulins contain complement binding sites. Complement is a system of at least 11 serum proteins activated by an antigen-antibody complex of the IgG or IgM class. Formation of the antigen-antibody complex exposes a complement-binding site (Figure 7-1) A cascade of protein conversions is initiated, much as in the blood coagulation system. The resulting liberation of proteins with deleterious effects on cell surfaces may cause cell death or may lead to release of histamine from mast cells and platelets, enhanced phagocytosis by leukocytes, contraction of smooth muscle, and so on.[15]

Allergic responses are mediated by humoral or cytotropic antibodies or by lymphoid cells.[16] Those caused by humoral antibodies are usually of rapid onset, and have, therefore, been called *immediate* type reactions. Sensitization by a systemic route is common. Reactions mediated by lymphoid cells have been called *delayed* type reactions ("tuberculin type") because hours to days elapse after the administration of an eliciting dose of antigen to a sensitized person or animal. In this type, the skin is the major route of sensitization and the chief site of allergic reaction.

A more rational classification is based on mechanism rather than elapsed time.[17] Type I describes anaphylactic type reactions. These are caused by cytotropic (also called "reaginic") circulating antibodies (IgE), which become fixed to the surface of certain tissue cells. Then attachment of antigen to those cell-bound antibodies initiates an explosive release of pharmacologically active agents, including histamine, serotonin, heparin, and pharmacologically active polypeptides, to be described below. In Type II reactions, the antigen is localized on the surface of a target cell (usually an erythrocyte, leukocyte, or platelet), and the antibody is present in serum. Antibody-antigen complex causes agglutination or (in the presence of complement) lysis. Type III includes serum sickness, polyarthritis, and glomerulonephritis. Here antigens are present for long periods in the circulation. As they form, soluble antigen-antibody complexes localize in blood vessels, where they cause tissue damage in the presence of complement. Type IV reactions include the delayed type allergies in which tissue injury results from interaction of antigen with sensitized lymphocytes; this type is seen in most infections whether caused by viruses, bacteria, fungi, or larger parasites.

Covalently Bonded Drug-Protein Conjugates

Drugs that provoke allergic reactions are usually small molecules rather than proteins, so that special techniques had to be developed to investigate the immunologic basis of drug allergies. These techniques were worked out in the course of a remarkable series of experiments, largely in the laboratory of Karl Landsteiner (1892–1943) who summarized the methods and results in a classic treatise.[18] Prior to these experiments, it was assumed that antigen specificity resided entirely in the protein used as antigen. The basic discovery that upset this idea and opened the way to further progress was the finding that when proteins were acylated they would display altered specificity as antigens. Acylation was carried out with the anhydrides or chlorides of butyric, isobutyric, trichloroacetic, and anisic acids. These groups were coupled chiefly to ϵ-amino groups of lysine residues. Immune serum prepared against an acylated protein would react more strongly with the acylated protein than with the same protein that had not been acylated. Numerous compounds of low molecular weight could be linked to proteins by acylation or by diazo coupling reactions (to tyrosine, histidine, or lysine residues) to form "artificial conjugated antigens." The simple chemicals thus conjugated to proteins were called *haptens*.

The proof that immunologic specificity could be directed against a hapten was obtained by experiments in which the same hapten was used for immunizing and for testing but attached to proteins derived from different species—e g., hapten-horse serum for immunizing a rabbit, and hapten-chicken serum for testing the antibodies by a precipitin reaction. In these investigations, it was discovered that antibodies to a

TABLE 7-1. Specificity and cross-reactivity of immune sera to azoprotein antigens.

The compounds shown at top (A to D) were diazotized and coupled to horse serum proteins. These were used to immunize rabbits, and the rabbit antisera were used in the tests. The same four compounds and four others (A to H) were diazotized and coupled to chicken serum proteins; these were used as antigens in the tests. The testing procedure consisted of adding a few drops of an immune serum to a dilute solution of the hapten-protein antigen and recording the intensity of precipitation (0 to 4+). (Modified after Landsteiner and Lampl,[19] Table III. By permission of Springer.)

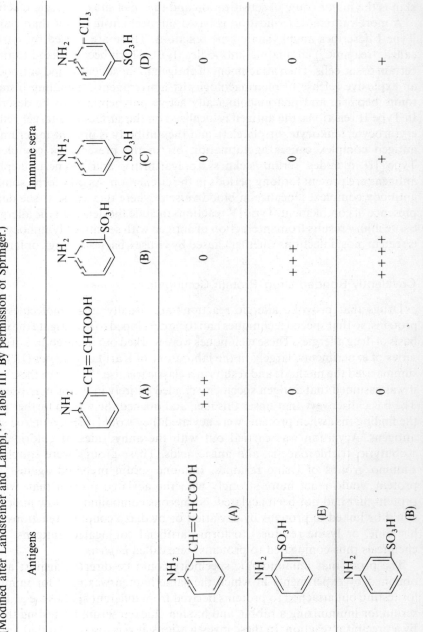

Antigens	Immune sera			
	(A)	(B)	(C)	(D)
(A)	+++	0	0	0
(E)	0	+++	0	0
(B)	0	++++	+	+

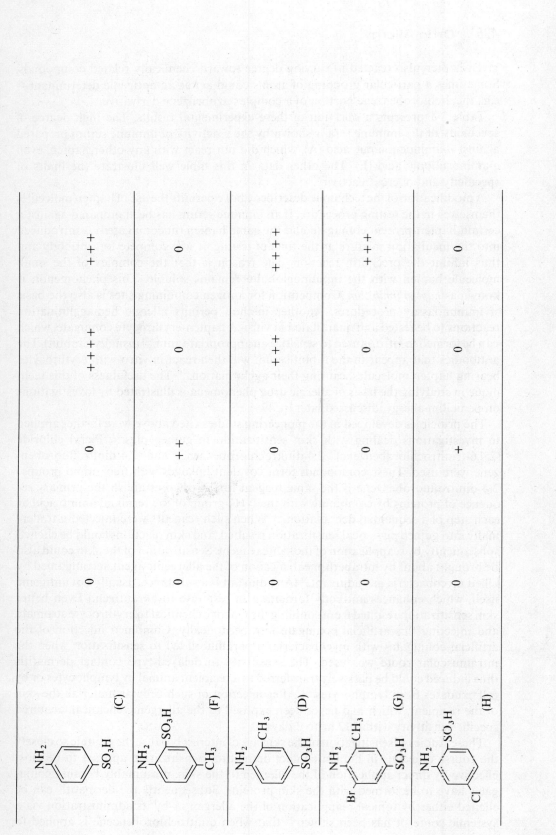

given hapten also reacted in varying degree toward chemically related compounds. Sometimes a particular grouping of atoms could act as an antigenic determinant— e.g., the 2-chlorobenzene portion of a complex azobenzene derivative.

Table 7-1 presents a selection of these experimental results. The high degree of specificity of the immune sera is shown by the reactivity of immune serum prepared against o-aminocinnamic acid (A), which did not react with any other hapten, even o-aminosulfonic acid (E). The other data in this table well illustrate the limits of specificity and of crossreactivity.

A modification of the technique described above permits the use of hapten molecules themselves in the testing procedure. If an immune serum has been prepared against a certain hapten-protein conjugate and the same hapten (unconjugated) is introduced into the incubation mixture at the time of testing, it will compete for antibody and thus inhibit the precipitin reaction. The reason is that the complex of the small molecule hapten with the immunoglobulin remains soluble. This phenomenon is known as *hapten inhibition*. Competition for antigen combining sites is also the basis of immunoassay procedures. Another method permits allergic hemagglutination reactions to be tested and quantitated in vitro. A hapten-erythrocyte conjugate, which can be formed in vitro, is used to sensitize an appropriate animal (usually a rabbit). The antibodies that appear in the rabbit serum will then react in vitro with erythrocytes bearing hapten molecules causing their agglutination.[20] The usefulness of this technique in studying the basis of allergic drug phenomena is illustrated by investigations on penicillin allergy, discussed later (p. 498).

The principles developed in the pioneering studies cited above were further applied in investigations dealing with skin sensitization in guinea pigs.[21] Picryl chloride (2,4,6-trinitrochlorobenzene), 2,4-dinitrochlorobenzene, and 2,4-dinitrofluorobenzene were used. These compounds form covalent linkages with free amino groups; 2-4-dinitrofluorobenzene is the same reagent first used to establish the primary sequence of proteins by combining with the NH_2-group of the terminal amino acid at each step of a sequential degradation.[22] When such reagents were injected intradermally into guinea pigs, local sensitization resulted, and skin reactions could be elicited subsequently by reapplication of the same reagent. Sensitization of the skin could also be brought about by intraperitoneal injection of the allergenic agent accompanied by killed mycobacteria as "adjuvant." (An adjuvant is a substance, usually not antigenic itself, which enhances antibody formation in response to an antigen.) Even better skin sensitization resulted from coupling the reactive chemical to erythrocyte stromata and injecting this artificial conjugate intraperitoneally. Combined injection of the artificial conjugates with mycobacteria in paraffin oil led to sensitization when the intramuscular route was used. The sensitivity to delayed-type contact dermatitis thus induced could be passively transferred to a recipient animal by lymphocytes or by cell exudates from lymphocytes.[23] After injection of such cellular material, the skin of the recipient, which had never been exposed to the allergenic chemical, acquired specific sensitivity within 12 hr to 2 days.

These studies of sensitization of the skin are of interest because they mimic so closely the course of events in human contact dermatitis. Sensitization appears to be most effective by direct application of the allergen to the skin, presumably because conjugates have to be formed with the skin proteins. Subsequently the dermatitis can be elicited either by topical reapplication of the allergen or by its administration via a systemic route. It has been shown[24] that when dinitrochlorobenzene is applied to guinea pig skin, nearly all of it that becomes fixed in the epidermis is bound to lysine groups in the proteins of the Malpighian layer at the junction of the epidermis and corium. This binding is thought to be essential for the development of the typical delayed-type skin allergy. Dinitrochlorobenzene conjugates with homologous (i.e., guinea pig) serum or with heterologous protein (egg albumin) caused sensitization of the immediate type, with circulating antibodies demonstrable but no skin allergy. On the other hand, conjugates of the same hapten with guinea pig skin protein injected into the foot pad of the guinea pig led to a typical delayed-type allergy of the contact dermatitis type; no circulating antibodies developed, but passive transfer could be achieved with lymphoid cells. Thus, it appears that the development of allergic contact dermatitis requires sensitization with a conjugate of hapten and skin protein.

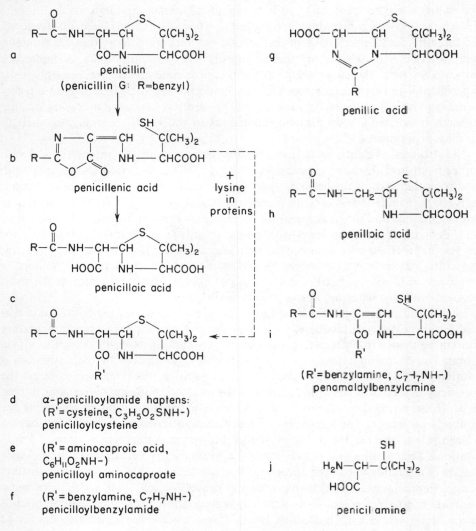

FIGURE 7-2. Structures of penicillin and derivatives. *Arrows indicate spontaneous transformations of the penicillin structure. The derivatives shown here are referred to in Figure 7-3. (Adapted from de Weck, Figure 1.[27])*

The success of these experimental approaches in producing suitable models of drug allergy raised the question whether a hapten must necessarily form a covalent linkage to a protein in order to act as an antigen. In one study,[25] a series of reactive chemicals was tested on rabbits to see if there was any correlation between antigenicity and the ability to combine with free amino groups of proteins. The highest antibody titers were found with those compounds that were capable of forming covalent bonds at body pH and at low temperature and were not readily metabolized. A similar and even more dramatic indication of the importance of covalent attachment came from experiments with 2,4-dinitrochlorobenzene.[18] This compound causes an allergic contact dermatitis in factory workers exposed to it, and as indicated above, guinea pigs can also be sensitized to it. There are approximately 90 chloro- and nitro-substituted benzenes. In experiments carried out with 17 of these, it was found that guinea pigs could be sensitized to 10. Not one of the 7 inert compounds would combine with the amino group of aniline in vitro, but all 10 that sensitized were able to do so. On the other hand, most drugs in therapeutic use, including many that are prone to cause allergic sensitization, are not chemically reactive compounds, certainly not comparable with the diazotizing, acylating, or amine-combining reagents used experimentally. This paradox has led to the concept that allergenic drugs are transformed in vivo to more reactive derivatives. These are the true immunogens forming covalent bonds with body proteins, analogous to the artificial conjugates used to produce experimental allergy.

The strongest evidence for covalent binding in hapten-protein interactions in vivo comes from investigations on penicillin allergy.[26-29] It has been shown that both in vitro and in vivo penicillin undergoes slow transformation to much more reactive derivatives. Figure 7-2 shows the initial molecular rearrangement of penicillin to penicillenic acid and the subsequent transformation of this intermediate to penicilloic acid. Penicillenic acid can react with amino groups (e.g., ϵ-amino groups of lysine residues in proteins) prior to molecular rearrangement, as shown by the broken arrow, to yield α-amide derivatives of the penicilloic acid structure. A number of lines of investigation have implicated these penicilloic acid-protein conjugates as the most frequent antigenic determinants in penicillin allergy.

Typical evidence is presented in Figure 7-3. The method of hemagglutination was used. Erythrocytes were incubated with penicillin and then added to a reaction mixture containing penicillin antiserum produced by repeated injection of penicillin into a rabbit. The penicillin-treated red blood cells were agglutinated by the antiserum at dilutions up to 1/64. The technique of hapten inhibition was then used to assess the specificity of the antibodies and antigens in the reaction. Addition of the same hapten to which the antibodies were formed inhibits the hemagglutination by saturating the antibody molecules. The hapten inhibition was quantitated by finding what hapten concentration was needed to inhibit the agglutination completely at various serum dilutions. The resulting curves in Figure 7-3 are remarkable because they show clearly that the compounds whose structures were illustrated in Figure 7-2 fall into three distinct classes. Penicillin itself, penicillenic acid, and penicilloic acid (a, b, and c) were by no means the most effective inhibitors of the hemagglutination, and four related compounds (g, h, i, and j) were entirely ineffective. But the three α-penicilloylamide haptens tested were about 100 times more effective than penicillin itself or its two breakdown products. These results imply very strongly that the penicillin antiserum was really directed against such a penicilloyl derivative and, thus, by inference, that a penicilloyl conjugate

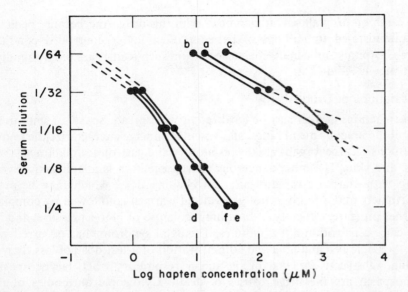

FIGURE 7-3. Inhibition of hemagglutination by haptens related to penicillin. *The designation of the various haptens refers to Figure 7-2. A suspension of erythrocytes was preincubated with benzylpenicillin (a, Figure 7-2), then added to rabbit benzylpenicillin antiserum. Hemagglutination resulted up to serum dilution 1/64. Addition of hapten to the reaction mixture could inhibit hemagglutination by combining with the serum antibody. Each experimental point here represents the hapten concentration needed to achieve complete inhibition of hemagglutination at the given serum dilution. With haptens g, h, i, and j (not shown), no inhibition resulted even at 10^{-3} M, the highest concentration tested. (Modified after de Weck, Figure 4.[27])*

was the actual sensitizing agent in vivo. Other investigations have led to the same conclusion, except that in man there are at least four other antigenic determinants besides the penicilloylamide conjugates.[26,28,29]

In summary, the argument that covalently bonded conjugates between a drug and a body protein are necessary for the development of drug allergy rests on two kinds of evidence. First, experimental allergy in animals has been produced readily with reagents capable of forming covalent bonds with proteins, whereas attempts to make animals allergic to drugs that are not particularly reactive have been unsuccessful. Second, the antigenic determinants in penicillin allergy, both in animals and in man, appear to be penicilloyl or related covalent conjugates with proteins (as described above) rather than the original penicillin molecule itself.

DRUG ALLERGY IN MAN

In this section, we shall consider (*1*) the various manifestations of drug allergy, (*2*) the frequency of allergic drug reactions in human populations and the factors that determine this frequency, (*3*) the methods of predicting allergic sensitivity in individual patients, (*4*) the methods of desensitizing, and (*5*) the management of allergic reactions. There is little doubt that penicillin is the leading cause of allergic drug reactions in general and also of serious systemic reactions.[30-32] Consequently, a great deal of the research on drug allergy in man deals with this drug. And because penicillin has been administered to millions of patients, often under controlled conditions in teaching hospitals and clinics, conclusions from such studies are often soundly based on statistically valid data.

Manifestations of Drug Allergy

Allergic reactions in man may be localized or widespread. Spasm of smooth muscle, edema of the mucous membranes, and vascular damage characterize the immediate-type response. Target organs are the respiratory and gastrointestinal tracts, the blood vessels, and skin. The most dangerous allergic reaction is anaphylaxis. Symptoms develop with alarming rapidity after an eliciting dose, which may be extremely small. Anxiety and a sensation of generalized warmth is followed by complaints of substernal pressure, difficulty in breathing, collapse of blood pressure, and anoxia. Death can occur within a few minutes. This fatal syndrome has occurred after the sting of a single bee and after the administration of a test dose of less than 1 μg of penicillin. Obstructive edema of the upper respiratory tract, laryngospasm, and bronchospasm are the usual causes of death. Cytotropic antibodies of the IgE type, known as *reagins*, are implicated in anaphylactic reactions.[7] IgE molecules have a high affinity for surface receptors on mast cells; attachment of allergen to the combining site of a fixed IgE molecule leads to massive release of histamine, serotonin, heparin, pharmacologically active peptides (kinins), and "slow reacting substance of anaphylaxis" (SRS-A, an acidic lipid). Circulating antibodies of the IgG and IgM types can combine with antigen before it reaches IgE antibodies fixed to tissues; these are known as *blocking antibodies*. They rarely cause a clinical syndrome and may prevent anaphylactic reactions.

Bronchial asthma alone may appear as an immediate allergic response unaccompanied by the more severe symptoms of anaphylaxis. There is experimental evidence that histamine is released during the allergic reaction. Human bronchial strips freshly obtained at autopsy were suspended in a tissue bath so that contractions of the smooth muscle could be recorded.[34] Bronchial strips from asthmatic subjects contracted in response to the same antigens (pollens, house dust) that had precipitated asthmatic attacks during life. At the same time, histamine was released into the bath. Control strips from nonallergic subjects did not contract, neither did they release histamine in response to the same allergens. But normal as well as allergic strips contracted when histamine was added to the bath. Antihistaminics completely blocked the response to added histamine but were ineffective against the contractions caused by allergens in sensitized strips. These experiments suggest that an antigen-antibody response in the previously sensitized tissue releases histamine, but they do not show that histamine is responsible for the muscle spasm. Probably some of the other pharmacologically active substances released contribute to the antigen-induced contraction. These findings essentially confirm in human tissues the principle underlying the classical Schultz–Dale phenomenon,[35] in which histamine release and muscle spasm are both elicited in guinea pig uterus in a tissue bath by specific antigens to which the animal had previously been sensitized. Consistent with the experimental in vitro results cited above, antihistamines are not effective in vivo in anaphylaxis or drug-induced asthma in man. Moreover, antihistamines themselves can cause bronchoconstriction in man, and they have been shown to cause contraction of isolated strips of guinea pig tracheal smooth muscle at concentrations in the usual therapeutic range.[36]

Other manifestations of the immediate type are conjunctivitis and rhinitis (as in hay fever), generalized urticaria, and angio-edema of various tissues. Angio-edema (also called angioneurotic edema) consists of swellings of the face, hands, feet, genitalia, and other regions. The syndrome is caused by dilation and altered permeability of small blood vessels chiefly in the subcutaneous tissues.

The "serum sickness syndrome" was first recognized as a response to antitoxin preparations containing horse serum. It is often elicited by foreign proteins as well as by drugs. The syndrome consists of fever, lymphadenopathy, and arthralgia, sometimes accompanied by urticaria. Polyarteritis nodosa and other collagen diseases may develop. Drug fever may often be seen alone, without the other reactions of the "serum sickness" group. The serum sickness syndrome is mediated by antigen, complement, and IgG antibody.

Dermatitis is a delayed response. The allergic reactions to systemic drug administration vary from trivial fixed eruptions to widespread and fatal exfoliative dermatitis, and the skin manifestations may assume a variety of forms. Fixed eruptions are remarkable; they occur in precisely the same cutaneous areas, sometimes no bigger than a fingertip, whenever the eliciting drug is administered. Contact dermatitis is the allergic response of skin to direct application of an eliciting drug. Lymphocytes infiltrate the cutis underlying the area of contact, and there is vascular dilation manifested by erythema. Vesicles form in the epidermis. Severe contact dermatitis may be accompanied by systemic allergic reactions, such as polyarteritis or other collagen diseases.[37] The role of histamine in allergic skin reactions is better established than in asthmatic and anaphylactic responses. Histamine is certainly released from skin as a consequence of the antigen-antibody reaction, and the blood level of histamine may be elevated.[38] Injection of histamine into the skin produces the "triple response" of erythema, wheal formation, and flare that also characterizes the delayed type of skin allergy.[18,39,40] Moreover, antihistaminic drugs are effective in antagonizing these phenomena when they occur as part of an allergic syndrome.

Many drugs have been held responsible for allergic disorders of the blood and the blood-forming tissues, such as hemolytic anemia, granulocytopenia (reduced number of circulating granulocytic leukocytes), and thrombocytopenia (reduced number of platelets).[41] Often there is a mere coincidence in time between administration of the drug and onset of the disease, without rigorous proof of an allergic basis. And frequently the disorder is actually an idiosyncratic one, as, for example, the hemolytic anemia due to primaquine. In some instances, however, it has been possible to demonstrate that drug allergy underlies the pathologic changes by demonstrating the presence of an antibody that reacts specifically with the suspected drug in a manner that can account for the destruction of blood cells. In some instances, this may come about through antigen attachment to the cells (as shown for penicilloyl derivatives in penicillin allergy) followed by antibody attachment and cell agglutination and the subsequent removal of affected cells in the reticuloendothelial system. Alternatively, an antibody-antigen complex may attach to cells and with the participation of complement may lead to cell lysis. A few examples will be cited.

A patient receiving the antischistosome drug stibophen (sodium antimony bispyrocatechol-2,4-disulfonate) developed an acute hemolytic anemia. Standard hematologic tests showed that the patient's serum in vitro could cause agglutination and hemolysis of his own or normal erythrocytes, but only in the presence of the drug. Serum from an unsensitized individual had no such effect.[42]

The antipyretic drug aminopyrine has been implicated in an allergic reaction leading to granulocytopenia.[43] The mechanism is an agglutination of leukocytes, which leads to their more rapid destruction. Three hours after a dose of aminopyrine, a patient developed pronounced leukopenia. At this time, 300 ml of the patient's whole blood was transfused into a normal recipient of the same blood group. The white blood cell count of the recipient fell precipitously (from 5000 to 1000 per cubic millimeter) soon after the transfusion. The decrease occurred mainly in neutrophils, eosinophils, monocytes, and, to a lesser degree, in lymphocytes. One week later, the recipient was given 300 ml of normal blood, and no decline in the white cell count occurred. Administration of aminopyrine itself to the recipient did not cause agranulocytosis. When a second recipient was tested with blood from the aminopyrine-sensitive donor, similar results were obtained; agglutination of the patient's own leukocytes or of normal leukocytes occurred when the patient's serum was added in vitro. Clearly, the sensitive individual had something in his blood after the aminopyrine injection that could agglutinate his own or others' leukocytes.

Blood platelets have been implicated as targets of allergic drug reactions.[44] This has been shown for allylisopropylacetylurea (Sedormid), a sedative formerly in very wide use in Europe. An antibody to the drug has been demonstrated in the serum of patients who, while taking this compound, developed thrombocytopenic purpura, a bleeding tendency caused by platelet deficiency. When a patient's serum, drug, platelets from either the patient or from a normal donor, and complement were incubated together, platelet lysis occurred. Without complement, the platelets agglutinated but did not lyse. Without drug, there was neither lysis nor agglutination. The factor in the patient's serum responsible for these immune reactions was an immunoglobulin. A very similar result was obtained with the antihistaminic drug 2-(N-phenyl-N-benzylaminomethyl)imidazoline (Antazoline), also capable of causing thrombocytopenic purpura. Other drugs, notably quinidine, have also been implicated in this disorder.

A controversy has raged for years about the rare aplastic anemia seen in patients treated with chloramphenicol. The infrequency of the reaction suggested to some that its basis was allergic, but rigorous criteria were never met. The reaction was known to occur most frequently in patients who had been undergoing prolonged therapy with the drug, a surprising finding for an allergic response, since previously sensitized patients would have been expected to react promptly. A careful clinical study showed[45] that the bone marrow toxicity is strictly dose related. A reversible depression of erythrocyte production could be produced in most patients at sufficient dosage. Inasmuch as chloramphenicol at high concentration does inhibit protein synthesis in mammalian cells in vitro, it seems likely that the aplastic anemia observed occasionally in patients is a direct toxic effect (or possibly in some patients an idiosyncratic sensitivity), but not an instance of drug allergy.

In some well-documented cases, the lymphoid system is the main target of drug allergy, and lymphadenopathy mimicking Hodgkin's disease may develop. In one case, a patient developed allergy to sulfisoxazole, diphenylhydantoin, primidone, and phenobarbital; circulating antibodies were demonstrated against all but the last of these.[46]

Involvement of the liver in an allergic drug reaction is very rare. A case of allergy to halothane in an anesthetist was clearly documented,[47] with recurrent attacks of hepatitis at every exposure to halothane but not to other anesthetic agents. The known metabolism of halothane in man is compatible with the format on of allergenic protein conjugates. Numerous drugs are known to cause the main types of liver injury: parenchymal cell damage and inflammation, or obstructive jaundice associated with inflammation of the bile canaliculi. Iproniazid has been associated with parenchymal damage and phenothiazines with injury of the obstructive-jaundice type. But evidence of allergic involvement has been only presumptive. Liver damage, for example, might not occur during an initial exposure to a drug but only on readministration, or there might be an associated dermatitis.

Frequency of Allergic Reactions to Drugs

The frequency of drug allergy in man is dependent upon the nature of the drug, the route of administration, the genetic predisposition of those who receive the drug, and the extent of prior exposure and of cross-reactivity to the same or related drugs.[48] There is really no way at present to arrive at a valid estimate of the frequency of allergic reactions to all drugs. There is not even universal agreement about the criteria for classification of a drug reaction as allergic. Consequently, many toxic or idiosyncratic reactions are considered allergic, while many allergic reactions are attributed to some other cause. Even were there no diagnostic difficulty, however, the pertinent statistical questions could not be answered. One would like to know what fraction of all patients treated with a given drug develop symptoms of allergy. One would like to know which of two drugs is less likely to cause allergy. Retrospective fact-gathering and haphazard reporting of reactions lead to distorted impressions. The only useful sort of investigation includes all patients who receive a drug, and all have to be followed to determine who has an allergic reaction and, equally important, who has not. As matters now stand, the mild allergic reactions, which are undoubtedly more common than the severe ones, are usually not even reported; they are treated by physicians everywhere, and the information is nowhere pooled or analyzed. Severe allergic reactions often result in hospitalization, hence are more likely to come to general attention. But knowing how many severe allergic reactions are attributable to a given drug does not help one assess the relative risk of using that drug unless one also knows how frequently the drug is administered. The number of allergic drug reactions, as an isolated statistic, is about as informative as the number of Fords, Chevrolets, and Alfa Romeos involved in automobile accidents in a year without knowledge of the number or kinds of cars on the highways or the miles driven per car. It now appears from large-scale surveillance studies (cf. Chapter 14) that relatively few drugs are allergenic, that the only drug of major concern is penicillin, and that allergic responses account for less than 10% of all adverse drug reactions.[50]

Drug allergy may be induced by any route of administration but not with equal efficiency. The oral route seems to be associated with a lower incidence of allergic sensitization than any other, whereas topical application of drugs to the skin is especially prone to sensitize. Industrial exposure to chemicals often results in the development of contact dermatitis among production workers. In one survey of more than 3000 cases of dermatitis due to occupational exposure, approximately one-sixth could be attributed to allergenic substances.[51] The number of compounds that are capable of causing contact dermatitis is extremely large and continually increases as new chemicals are synthesized. Contact dermatitis in workers engaged in the production of a new drug may serve as an omen of the probable development of drug allergy later in patients, after the drug is introduced for therapeutic use.

There are very great individual differences, as well as species differences, in the ability to become sensitized to drugs, and this "allergic predisposition" probably has a genetic basis.[8-10] Guinea pigs can be bred for high or low susceptibility to skin sensitization with 2,4-dinitrochlorobenzene.[52] Attempts were made to sensitize human subjects to contact dermatitis with p-nitrosodimethylaniline and 2,4-dinitro-chlorobenzene. Subjects were found to vary considerably in their susceptibility to sensitization by either compound; moreover, some became sensitized exclusively to one or the other, some to both, some to neither.[53]

We have already seen that prior exposure to a drug is essential for the sensitization that must precede an allergic response. But it should be borne in mind that mere absence of a recorded history of previous exposure by no means rules out the possibility of allergy, since histories of this kind are notoriously unreliable. Patients are commonly unaware of what medication they receive, multiple irrational drug mixtures abound, and memories tend to be much less persistent than antibody-forming capacity. Moreover, enough is known about cross-sensitization to make it apparent that the initial exposure may have been to a different but related drug or environmental chemical.

An investigation was conducted on the effect of prior exposure to sulfonamides upon the incidence of allergy.[54,55] The allergic responses considered were those characteristic of the sulfonamide compounds—drug fever, dermatitis, and conjunctivitis. Three sulfonamides were used: sulfathiazole, sulfapyridine, and sulfadiazine. Before starting a course of therapy, a careful history was taken to see if the patient had previously been exposed to any sulfonamide and, if so, to which one, and also to ascertain if the previous exposure had resulted in an allergic reaction. The results are summarized in Table 7-2. In a very large series of patients receiving a sulfonamide for the first time (control series), the incidence of allergic reactions developing during the course of therapy was 5.0%. In most of these, presumably, the drug was administered for weeks, long enough for sensitization and subsequent elicitation of the reaction to occur. Patients who had had previous treatment with a different drug and had not reacted to it were no more likely to develop an allergic reaction during their second

TABLE 7-2. Frequencies of several allergic responses to sulfonamides during first and second courses of drug treatment.
The allergic responses considered here were drug fever, dermatitis, and conjunctivitis. (From Dowling et al.,[55] Table III)

Reaction to first course	Sulfonamides administered during second course	Total no. of patients	Patients developing allergic reactions during second course	
			Number	Percent
No	Different drug	169	6	3.6
No	Same drug	144	16	11.1
Yes	Different drug	30	5	16.7
Yes	Same drug	48	33	68.8
	Control series of persons receiving one course only	737	37	5.0

course of treatment (incidence 3.6%) than if they were receiving the drug for the first time. But if the second course involved administration of the same drug as during the first course, even though there had been no reaction during the first course, the incidence of allergy was increased (to 11.1%). If there had been a reaction to the first course, then the incidence of reaction during the second course was still higher (16.7%), even when a different drug was used. Most significant, if the same drug that had caused an allergic reaction during the first course was administered again at a second course, the incidence of allergy jumped to 68.8%. The evidence is therefore clear that in the sulfonamide series there is both specificity and cross-reactivity. A patient sensitized to one drug is more likely to react to a second drug than if he had never been sensitized at all, but he is less likely to react to the second drug than to the one that sensitized him.

The extent of cross-reactivity after prior exposure in the penicillin group is less clearly worked out and more controversial. Several semi-synthetic derivatives have been made in recent years by adding various side groups to the 6-aminopenicillanic acid skeleton (Figure 7-4). Extravagant claims were made for some of these at the

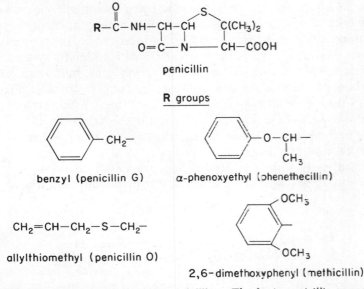

FIGURE 7-4. Structures of some penicillins. *The basic penicillin structure is shown above as 6-aminopenicillanic acid with an R substituent. Several R groups are shown below.*

time of their introduction, for example, that they could be given safely to patients who were allergic to penicillin G. In general, such claims have not been borne out, and cross-reactivity is the rule rather than the exception. Such cross-reaction has been demonstrated by actual allergic manifestations in patients and also by skin tests or red cell agglutination.[56,57] Conversely, patients who tolerate the new congeners usually show no positive skin test or hemagglutination with other types of penicillin, even though they might once have had an allergic reaction.[58] One of the methodologic difficulties here is that a patient who previously had an allergic reaction to penicillin might not necessarily react at the next challenge, even with the same drug. Thus, sound conclusions can only be obtained in large-scale well-controlled studies, of which there have been but few. Most careful investigations have revealed cross-reactivity in some patients, absence of cross-reactivity in others.[59,60]

This heterogeneity of allergic response is consistent with the experimental finding that there are several antigenic determinants, even with a single drug. One person may form antibodies directed toward a particular part of the drug molecule, another toward different chemical groups. If a patient happened to be allergically sensitized in a specific way toward benzylpenicillin, a derivative with a different R group might well fail to elicit the reaction. But another patient, in whom benzylpencillin was also the sensitizing drug, could have developed a less specific kind of allergic responsiveness and therefore react to any other penicillanic acid derivative. There is another consideration. A given individual may develop IgG and IgM antibodies, which will act as blocking antibodies, preventing cytotropic IgE interactions and tissue damage.[49] This is probably why some people who have positive scratch tests, i.e., have circulating IgE antibodies, will nevertheless not have an anaphylactic response to the therapeutic doses of penicillin. The practical consequence of all this is that one cannot predict with certainty how an individual patient will respond. It is often safest to avoid penicillin altogether if there is reason to fear a serious allergic reaction.

The incidence of allergic reaction to penicillin among all patients receiving it ranges from less than 1% to nearly 10% in various studies. In an extensive survey conducted in Australia,[51] 1.3% of nearly 7000 patients given systemic penicillin were reported to have an allergic reaction; probably some mild reactions were not reported. About one-tenth of the reported reactions could be considered life threatening, although there were no fatalities in this series. Table 7-3 shows that the reactions most commonly were of the delayed type, and Table 7-4 classifies all symptoms and signs, giving the frequency of each. The majority of all the reported reactions involved the skin (urticaria and erythema).

A controlled study with over 2000 college students[62] revealed an incidence of allergic reactions to penicillin of 3.3%. These were principally urticaria, angio-edema,

TABLE 7-3. Immediate and delayed reactions in penicillin allergy.
Survey of 6832 patients receiving penicillin. (From Research Committee of the New South Wales Faculty,[61] Table I.)

Reaction	Number of cases
IMMEDIATE	7
DELAYED	
less than 24 hr	24
1 to 7 days	33
8 to 14 days	14
over 14 days	3
period not specified	10
Total	91

TABLE 7-4. Symptoms and signs in penicillin allergy.
Survey of 6832 patients receiving penicillin. (From Research
Committee of the New South Wales Faculty,[61] Table III.)

Clinical features	Number of cases
FEVER	9
ARTHRALGIA	20
SKIN SIGNS	
bullae	4
erythema	46
purpuric spots	1
urticaria	64
subsequent desquamation	11
MOUTH SIGNS	
dryness	3
oral bullae	1
RESPIRATORY SIGNS	
laryngeal obstruction	2
bronchospasm	2
GENERAL COLLAPSE (coldness, sweating, etc.)	9
PARESTHESIAS	2

skin eruptions, and serum sickness. Of the 70 reactions, 27 were of the immediate type, the remainder were the delayed type.

Venereal disease clinics provide a good source of information about the frequency of allergic reactions to penicillin among the population as a whole, since groups attending these clinics (unlike those in a skin clinic, for example) are not likely to include an unusual number of individuals prone to allergic reactivity. Results of such surveys indicate a reaction rate of a few percent based upon very large numbers of people. Among more than 25,000 patients receiving penicillin in venereal disease clinics in 1959, 0.5% developed urticaria, and there were 8 instances of systemic anaphylaxis.[63] Very similar data on the overall incidence of allergic reaction to penicillin were obtained in a British study of nearly 900 patients treated for venereal disease.[64]

Prolonged treatment with penicillin may result in a high frequency of allergic reaction, and the allergy may develop unpredictably at any time during the course of therapy. For example, 32 adult patients were treated with benzathine penicillin G, a repository preparation, as part of a rheumatic fever prophylaxis program.[65] The drug was given intramuscularly once a month. Six patients developed some kind of allergic response, one at the first injection, others after several months. One patient who had displayed no previous sign of allergy died within a few minutes after her 20th injection, presumably from an anaphylactic reaction. The autopsy revealed no embolism in the lungs, such as would have resulted from inadvertent intravenous injection of the insoluble benzathine penicillin.

Penicillin is the major cause of anaphylaxis in man. A nationwide survey,[66] covering 29% of all general hospital beds in the country over a 3-year period, revealed 1070 cases of life-threatening drug reactions, of which 901 (84%) were caused by penicillin.

Of these 901 cases, 83 died, a fatality rate of nearly 10%. The frequency of severe reactions to penicillin showed no unusual distribution by age or sex. The route of administration emerged as a significant factor. There were 611 anaphylactoid reactions following intramuscular injection, of which 10% were fatal; after oral administration, there were only 49 reactions and none was fatal, presumably because of the slower entry of the drug into the circulation. Since the survey covered about one-third of all hospital beds in the country but included 3 years of data, it would appear that there were somewhat less than 100 fatalities per year in the country as a whole.

Tests for Predicting Drug Allergies

In view of the potential seriousness of drug allergies, it would obviously be valuable to have a reliable and safe method of testing for allergic sensitivity before administering a drug. For many years, skin and conjunctival tests were in vogue in which a very small amount of the drug solution was injected intradermally or dropped into the conjunctival sac. Local erythema or conjunctival inflammation was taken as sign of allergic sensitivity. These tests fell into disrepute for two reasons. First, they were unreliable in a capricious way. Patients with positive tests who were nevertheless given the drug therapeutically because of serious need often did not have allergic reactions, whereas patients with negative tests might have reactions of life-threatening severity. Second, the test itself could precipitate a full-blown anaphylactic response in some patients; indeed, deaths have been recorded as a result of skin testing, even though the amount used was only a minute fraction of the usual therapeutic dose. Recently, however, advances in identification of the true antigenic determinants for penicillin sensitization have led to the development of a more reliable skin test using penicilloyl-polylysine as the reagent.[67] The test consists of intradermal injection of the synthetic antigen followed by appraisal of the size of the wheal and erythema at the test site 20 min later. Some danger still persists, for example, 4 out of 16,239

TABLE 7-5. Relationship between skin test result and subsequent reaction to penicillin.

The skin test with penicilloyl-polylysine was scored according to size of wheal and erythema (− : negative reponse; ± : ambiguous response, wheal less than 12 mm in diameter; 2+ : positive, wheal 12–20 mm in diameter; 4+ : strongly positive, wheal more than 20 mm in diameter). Patients with 2+ or 4+ skin tests were given penicillin therapeutically only when it was felt that the need outweighed the risk. (Table constructed from data of Brown et al.,[67] text and Figure 3.)

Skin test response	No. of patients given penicillin therapeutically	Percent of patients reacting allergically to therapeutic course
−	13,530	0.5
±	782	1.3
2+	212	4.2
4+	206	10.2

patients tested developed generalized skin reactions after the test, and one had bronchospasm.

The predictive value of the penicilloyl-polylysine test can be assessed in the data presented in Table 7-5 and Figure 7-5. If history of prior contact with penicillin is ignored, then a strong correlation between skin test result and subsequent allergic

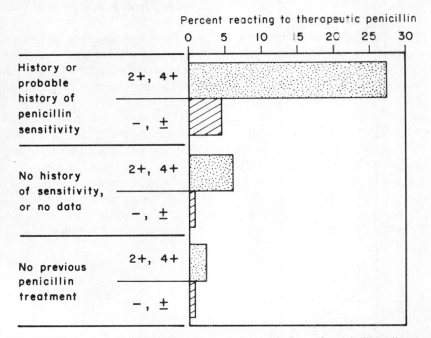

FIGURE 7-5. Relationship between previous history of penicillin allergy, skin test response, and subsequent allergic reaction to penicillin. *The percent of patients reacting to a therapeutic course of penicillin is shown as a function of previous history of allergic reaction to penicillin, and of reaction to the penicilloyl-polylysine skin test. These results are those of the patients analyzed in Table 7-7, and the meaning of skin test categories is the same as given there. (From Brown et al., Figure 4.[57])*

reaction is seen (Table 7-5). Among those with negative skin test, only 0.5% experienced any reaction. The percent experiencing an allergic reaction increased with increasing positivity of the skin test, to 10.2% among the group that had reacted most strongly. However, even in this strongly positive group, 9 out of 10 patients given penicillin therapeutically did not react adversely.

Figure 7-5 shows that the predictive value was even greater when previous history was taken into account. Of the patients with a history of penicillin sensitivity as well as a positive skin test, more than 1 in 4 experienced an allergic reaction; in the remaining categories, the response frequency was graded in an orderly manner. A meaningful way of summarizing these studies is to say that if a person without any history of penicillin allergy reacts positively to the skin test, the probability is increased greatly that he will experience an allergic reaction to therapeutically administered penicillin, as compared with one whose skin test is negative. In these experiments, "allergic reactions" included angio-edema, urticaria, generalized itching, erythematous skin eruptions, and anaphylaxis.

Skin testing with pen cilloyl-polylysine and a mixture of minor antigenic deter-minants has been used cuite extensively.[68,69] The procedure appears to be safe and of considerable predictive value. In one study,[70] 163 patients with no previous history of penicillin allergy were tested; there were 10 positive results. Of 66 patients with histories of penicillin allergy, 50 were found to be nonreactive in the test, and 37 of these received penicillin therapeutically without incident. Routine use of skin tests has significantly reduced the incidence of allergic reaction.[71,72]

An interesting test for allergic sensitivity is the *lymphocyte transformation test*. When circulating lymphocytes of allergic individuals are cultured in vitro in the presence of the specific ar tigen (but not otherwise), the cells undergo a transformation; they become larger, develop a basophilic cytoplasm, show increased RNA and DNA synthesis, and may even develop mitotic figures over a period of about four days. These blast cells are readily counted. When cells were cultured without antigen, or with an antigen unrelated to the allergenic drug to which patients were sensitized, fewer than 1% of the lymphocytes were transformed. Cells from patients allergic to penicillin, when cultured in the presence of penicillin, showed transformation in 4–45%. In patients who had received penicillin without allergic manifestations, the num-ber rarely (2 out of 33) exceeded 1%. Figure 7-6 shows similar results in aspirin allergy. The greatest advantage of the test is that it is conducted in vitro, with no possible risk to the patient. Its major disadvantage is that it requires four days to obtain the result.

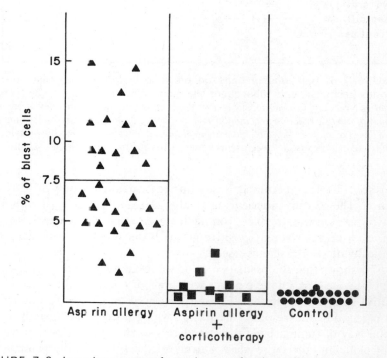

FIGURE 7-6. Lymphocyte transformation test for drug allergy. *Each point re-presents a result from cne test on one patient's lymphocytes. Patients known to be allergic to aspirin are shown at left, controls at extreme right. Center panel shows results in allergic patients treated with an antiinflammatory corticosteroid. (From Halpern, Figure 6.[17])*

Desensitization

If it is very important to give a drug to which a patient is known to be sensitive, and no alternative drug is available, then desensitization may be attempted. In at least some cases, this technique has been successful. Precautions against anaphylaxis must be taken; epinephrine, oxygen, and equipment for tracheostomy should be at hand. A very small amount of the drug (e.g., a few micrograms of penicillin) can be given intracutaneously. Every half hour the dose can be doubled, and eventually administration is switched to the subcutaneous route using a location that permits application of a tourniquet above the injection site. Finally, if therapeutic doses can be achieved without adverse reaction, the procedure may be considered successful.[73]

The scientific basis of desensitization is evidently complex. If a large amount of the allergen can be introduced without triggering the allergic reaction, the allergic state is inhibited. Hapten inhibition, blocking antibodies, and the ratio of antigen to antibodies may all play a role, as discussed earlier. In animals some striking examples have been demonstrated. When guinea pigs were fed 2,4-dinitrochlorobenzene for several weeks and then given a typical sensitizing course intracutaneously, there was a dramatic inhibition of the expected development of allergic sensitivity.[74] The protection was manifest even 6 months later. The protective effect of prefeeding was highly specific for the particular antigen; another hapten, o-chlorobenzoyl chloride, sensitized as usual even when it was given at the same time as the ineffective 2,4-dinitrochlorobenzene. Similar experiments with neoarsphenamine had been conducted many years before, with essentially the same result.[75] In all such cases, the protective feeding of hapten has to precede the attempted sensitization; the allergic responses cannot be modified once sensitization has occurred.

Another possible approach to desensitization is suggested by the experimental work on immunologic paralysis in skin homograft reactions. Tolerance to skin homografts can be induced in various species by prior injection of donor cells during fetal life of the recipient.[76] It would be of interest to ascertain whether prenatal exposure of the mother to certain allergenic drugs could reduce the incidence of allergic reactions to those same drugs later in the offspring.

Management of Drug Allergies

In the mild types of allergic reaction, the signs and symptoms subside when the drug is withdrawn. Antihistamines are helpful in relieving urticaria and itching. Anti-inflammatory steroids are effective in suppressing annoying skin reactions and are probably useful also when collagen is involved.

Life-threatening allergic manifestations develop very quickly and require instantaneous action. The important measures are to delay further drug absorption, to ensure an adequate airway, and to administer epinephrine or isoproterenol for bronchodilation. Antihistamines are useless and possibly harmful in that they may cause bronchoconstriction. In penicillin anaphylaxis, the intravenous injection of penicillinase has been advocated, with the purpose of destroying the drug. This is irrational because (a) the patient's life is in jeopardy from an antigen-antibody reaction that has already occurred and cannot be reversed, (b) the probable antigenic determinant of the allergic response (e.g., a penicilloyl derivative) is not a substrate for penicillinase, and (c) penicillinase is a foreign protein, which could cause further allergic reactions.

A tragic aspect of so many anaphylactic deaths is that the administration of penicillin was wholly unnecessary. In one survey of 30 fatal anaphylactic reactions to penicillin,[77] the drug had been given for a nonspecific skin eruption, a sprained toe, a traumatic injury to the finger, dermatitis associated with venous stasis, and prophylactically after intranasal surgery. In 12 of these fatal cases, the penicillin had been administered for an upper respiratory infection without fever. Penicillin could have served no useful purpose in any of these instances. It is also appalling that in systemic anaphylaxis, tracheostomy is rarely performed, yet the cause of death is often laryngeal edema or laryngospasm, and establishing an airway would save a life.

Although subcutaneous administration of epinephrine is the best treatment for anaphylaxis, there is bound to be some delay. even when a physician is at hand; the procedure is altogether impractical in the absence of a physician. An excellent first-aid treatment is the inhalation of an epinephrine aerosol. A stable suspension of epinephrine microcrystals, of particle size 3–5 microns (cf. Chapter 2), is available in an automatic aerosol dispenser.[78] Each dose of the inhalation delivers 0.16 mg of epinephrine to the respiratory tract, where it can act on the laryngeal tissues to prevent edema and on the bronchial tree to prevent smooth-muscle constriction. At the same time, the systemic absorption of the epinephrine is rather limited; thus, even five or more inhalations may produce only slight cardiovascular effects. Such an epinephrine aerosol device should obviously be included in any emergency kit and should also be carried by people known to be prone to anaphylactic reactions from drugs, foods, and bee stings.[79]

REFERENCES

1. W. C. BOYD: *Fundamentals of Immunology*, 4th ed. New York, Interscience Publishers (1966).
2. E. A. CARR, JR.: Drug allergy. *Pharmacol. Rev.* 6:365 (1954).
3. M. SAMTER and H. L. ALEXANDER, eds.: *Immunological Diseases*, 2nd ed. Boston, Little, Brown and Co. (1971).
4. M. L. ROSENHEIM and R. MOULTON, eds.: *Sensitivity Reactions to Drugs*. Springfield, Ill., Charles C. Thomas (1958).
5. Progress in immunology. In *First International Congress of Immunology* ed. by B. Amos. New York and London, Academic Press (1971).
6. M. SMATER and C. W. PARKER eds.: *Hypersensitivity to Drugs*. In International Encyclopedia of Pharmacology and Therapeutics. Oxford and New York, Pergamon Press (1972). Vol. 1, Section 75.
7. Therapeutic Conferences. Drug allergy. *Brit. Med. J.* 2:37 (1971).
8. A. S. WIENER, I. ZIEVE, and J. H. FRIES: The inheritance of allergic disease. *Ann. Eugenics* 7:141 (1936).
9. P. F. DE GARA: The hereditary predisposition in man to develop hypersensitivity: A critical review. In *Mechanisms of Hypersensitivity*, International Symposium, Henry Ford Hospital, ed. by J. H. Shaffer, G. A. LoGrippo, and M. W. Chase. Boston, Little, Brown and Co. (1958). pp. 703–712.
10. J. H. SANG and W. R. SOBEY: The genetic control of response to antigenic stimuli. *J. Immunol.* 72:52 (1954).
11. G. M. EDELMAN: The structure and function of antibodies. *Sci. Am.* 223:34 (Aug.. 1970).
12. F. W. PUTNAM: From animal matter to antibody—a trail of research in cancer. *Persp. Bio. Med.* 15:356 (1972).
13. T. B. TOMASI: Human immunoglobulin A. *New Eng. J. Med.* 279:1327 (1968).
14. F. M. BURNET: *The Canal Selection Theory of Acquired Immunity*. Nashville, Tenn., Vanderbilt University Press (1959).

15. S. RUDDY, I. GIGLI, and K. F. AUSTEN: The complement system of man. *New Eng. J. Med.* 287:489, 545, 592, 642 (1972).

16. Symposium on Membranes in Growth, Differentiation and Neoplasia. *Fed. Proc.* 32:34 (1973).

17. B. N. HALPERN: Antibodies produced by drugs and methods for their detection. In International Encyclopedia of Pharmacology and Therapeutics, *Hypersensitivity to Drugs*. Oxford and New York, Pergamon Press (1972). Vol. 1, Sec. 75.

18. K. LANDSTEINER: *The Specificity of Serological Reactions*. Cambridge, Mass., Harvard University Press (1945).

19. K. LANDSTEINER and H. LAMPL: Über die Abhängigkeit der serologischen Spezifizität von der chemischen Struktur. (Darstellung von Antigenen mit bekannter chemischer Konstitution der spezifischen Gruppen). XII. Mitteilung über Antigene. *Biochem. Z.* 86:343 (1918).

20. W. E. BULLOCK and F. S. KANTOR: Hemagglutination reactions of human erythrocytes conjugated covalently with dinitrophenyl groups. *J. Immunol.* 94:317 (1955).

21. M. W. CHASE: Experimental sensitization with particular reference to picryl chloride. *Int. Arch. Allergy Appl. Immunol.* 5:163 (1954).

22. F. SANGER and H. TUPPY: The amino-acid sequence in the phenylalanyl chain of insulin. 1. The identification of lower peptides from partial hydrolysates. *Biochem. J* 49:463 (1951).

23. M. W. CHASE, W. DAMESHEK, S. HABERMAN, M. SAMTER, and T. L. SQUIER: A symposium on the role of the formed elements of the blood in allergy and hypersensitivity. *J. Allergy* 26:219 (1955).

24. S. B. SALVIN: Contact hypersensitivity, circulating antibody, and immunologic unresponsiveness. *Fed. Proc.* 24:40 (1965).

25. P. G. H. GELL, C. R. HARRINGTON, and R. P. RIVERS: The antigenic function of simple chemical compounds: production of precipitins in rabbits. *Brit. J. Exper. Pathol.* 27:267 (1946).

26. C. W. PARKER: Immunochemical mechanisms in penicillin allergy. *Fed. Proc.* 24:51 (1965).

27. A. L. DE WECK: Studies on penicillin hypersensitivity. I. The specificity of rabbit "anti-penicillin" antibodies. *Int. Arch. Allergy Appl. Immunol.* 21:20 (1962).

28. A. L. DE WECK: Studies on penicillin hypersensitivity. II. The role of the side chain in penicillin antigenicity. *Int. Arch. Allergy Appl. Immunol.* 21:38 (1962).

29. B. B. LEVINE: Immunochemical mechanisms involved in penicillin hypersensitivity in experimental animals and in human beings. *Fed. Proc.* 24:45 (1965).

30. R. A. KERN and N. A. WIMBERLEY, JR.: Penicillin reactions: their nature, growing importance, recognition, management, and prevention. *Am. J. Med. Sci.* 226 357 (1953).

31. C. D. CALNAN: Cutaneous reactions to penicillin. *Postgrad. Med. 40: Supplement 152* (1964).

32. S. M. FEINBERG and A. R. FEINBERG: Allergy to penicillin. *J. Amer. Med. Ass.* 160:778 (1956).

33. L. P. JAMES, JR. and K. F. AUSTEN: Fatal systemic anaphylaxis in man. *New Eng. J. Med.* 270:597 (1964).

34. H. O. SCHILD, D. F. HAWKINS, J. L. MONGAR, and H. HERXHEIMER: Reactions of isolated human asthmatic lung and bronchial tissue to a specific antigen. Histamine release and muscular contraction. *Lancet* 2:376 (1951).

35. H. H. DALE: The anaphylactic reaction of plain muscle in the guinea-pig. *J. Pharmacol. Exp. Therap.* 4:167 (1913).

36. D. F. HAWKINS: Bronchoconstrictor and bronchodilator actions of antihistamine drugs. *Brit. J. Pharmacol.* 10:230 (1955).

37. D. M. PILLSBURY, W. B. SHELLEY, and A. M. KLIGMAN: Drug allergy and contact dermatitis of the allergic type. In *Dermatology*. Philadelphia, W. B. Saunders (1956). Ch. 17 and 18.

38. M. W. CHASE: Antibodies to drugs. In *Sensitivity Reactions to Drugs*, ed. by M. L. Rosenheim and R. Moulton. Springfield, Ill. Charles C. Thomas (1958) pp. 125–134.

39. H. H. DALE and P. P. LAIDLAW: The physiological action of β-iminazolylethylamine. *J. Physiol.* 41:318 (1910).

40. T. LEWIS: *The Blood Vessels of the Human Skin and Their Responses*. London, Shaw and Sons (1927).

41. E. A. CARR, JR. and G. A. ASTE: Recent laboratory studies and clinical observations on hypersensitivity to drugs and use of drugs in allergy. *Annu. Rev. Pharmacol.* 1:105 (1961)

42. J. W. HARRIS: Studies on the mechanism of a drug-induced hemolytic anemia. *J. Lab. Clin. Med.* 47:760 (1956).

43. S. MOESCHLIN and K. WAGNER: Agranulocytosis due to the occurrence of leukocyte-agglutinins (pyramidon and cold agglutinins). *Acta Haematol.* 8:29 (1952).
44. J. F. ACKROYD: The pathogenesis of purpura. In *Lectures on Haematology*, ed. by F. G. J. Hayhoe. London, Cambridge University Press (1959). p. 217.
45. J. L. SCOTT, S. M. FINEGOLD, G. A. BELKIN, and J. S. LAWRENCE: A controlled double-blind study of the hematologic toxicity of chloramphenicol. *New Eng. J. Med.* 272:1137 (1965).
46. D. S. ROBINSON, M. G. MAC DONALD, and F. P. HOBIN: Sodium diphenylhydantoin reaction with evidence of circulating antibodies. *J. Amer. Med. Ass.* 192:171 (1965).
47. G. KLATSKIN and D. V. KIMBERG. Recurrent hepatitis attributable to halothane sensitization in an anesthetist. *New Eng. J. Med.* 280: 515 (1970).
48. H. L. ALEXANDER: *Reactions with Drug Therapy*. Philadelphia, W. B. Saunders (1955).
49. G. T. STEWART: Penicillin allergy. *Clin. Pharm. Therap.* 11:307 (1970).
50. I. T. BORDA, D. SLONE, and H. JICK: Assessment of adverse reactions within a drug surveillance program. *J. Amer. Med. Ass.* 205:645 (1968).
51. J. V. KLAUDER: Actual causes of certain occupational dermatoses. *Arch. Dermatol.* 85:441 (1962).
52. M. W. CHASE: Inheritance in guinea pigs of the susceptibility to skin sensitization with simple chemical compounds. *J. Exper. Med.* 73:711 (1941).
53. K. LANDSTEINER, A. ROSTENBERG, JR., and M. B. SULZBERGER: Individual differences in susceptibility to eczematous sensitization with simple chemical substances. *J. Invest. Dermatol.* 2:25 (1939).
54. H. F. DOWLING and M H. LEPPER: "Drug fever" accompanying second courses of sulfathiazole, sulfadiazine and sulfapyridine. *J. Am. Med. Sci.* 207:349 (1944).
55. H. F. DOWLING, H. L. HIRSH, and M. H. LEPPER: Toxic reactions accompanying second courses of sulfonamides in patients developing toxic reactions during a previous course. *Ann. Int. Med.* 24:629 (1946).
56. R. H. SCHWARTZ and J. H. VAUGHAN: Immunologic responsiveness of man to penicillin. *J. Amer. Med. Ass.* 186: 151 (1963).
57. G. T. STEWART: Cross-allergenicity of penicillin G and related substances. *Lancet* 1:509 (1962).
58. P. P. VAN ARSDEL, JR.: Allergic reactions to penicillin. *J. Amer. Med. Ass.* 191:238 (1965).
59. E. F. LUTON: Methicillin tolerance after penicillin G anaphylaxis. *J. Amer. Med. Ass.* 190:39 (1964).
60. C. W. PARKER and J. A. THIEL: Studies in human penicillin allergy: a comparison of various penicilloyl-polylysines. *J. Lab. Clin. Med.* 62:482 (1963).
61. Research Committee of the New South Wales Faculty of the Australian College of General Practitioners: Report on a survey of allergic reactions to penicillin. *Med. J. Australia* 1:827 (1959).
62. K. P. MATHEWS, F. M HEMPHILL, R. G. LOVELL, W. E. FORSYTHE, and J. M. SHELDON: A controlled study on the use of parenteral and oral antihistamines in preventing penicillin reactions. *J. Allergy* 27:1 (1956).
63. W. J. BROWN, W. G. SIMPSON, and E. V. PRICE: Reevaluation of reactions to penicillin in venereal disease clinic patients. *Public Health Rep.* 76:189 (1961).
64. R. R. WILLCOX and G R. FRYERS: Sensitivity to repository penicillins. *Brit. J. Venereal Dis.* 33:209 (1957).
65. I. HSU and J. M. EVANS: Untoward reactions to benzathine penicillin G in a study of rheumatic-fever prophylaxis in adults. *New Eng. J. Med.* 259:581 (1958).
66. H. WELCH, C. N. LEWIS, H. I. WEINSTEIN, and B. B. BOECKMAN: Severe reactions to antibiotics. A nationwide survey. *Antibiot. Med.* 4:800 (1957).
67. B. C. BROWN, E. V. PRICE, and M. B. MOORE, JR.: Penicilloyl-polylysine as an intradermal test of penicillin sensitivity. *J. Amer. Med. Ass.* 189:599 (1964).
68. G. T. STEWART: Allergenic residues in penicillins. *Lancet* 1:1177 (1967).
69. F. R. BATCHELOR, J M. DEWDNEY, J. G. FEINBERG, and R. D. WESTON: A penicilloylated protein impurity as a source of allergy to benzyl-penicillin and 6-aminopenicillanic acid. *Lancet* 1:1175 (1967).
70. N. F. ADKINSON, JR., W. L. THOMPSON, W. C. MADDREY, and L. M. LICHTENSTEIN: Routine use of penicillin skin testing on an inpatient service. *New Eng. J. Med.* 285:22 (1971).
71. B. B. LEVINE and D. M. ZOLOV: Prediction of penicillin allergy by immunological tests. *J. Allergy* 43:231 (1969).

72. J. W. LENTZ and L. NICHOLAS: Penicilloyl-polylysine intradermal testing for penicillin hyper-sensitivity. *Brit. J. Vener. Dis.* 46:457 (1970).

73. Anon.: Penicillin allergy. *Medical Letter* 6:77 (1964).

74. M. W. CHASE: Inhibition of experimental drug allergy by prior feeding of the sensitizing agent. *Proc. Soc. Exp. Biol. Med.* 61:257 (1946).

75. M. B. SULZBERGER: Hypersensitiveness to arsphenamine in guinea-pigs. I. Experiments in prevention and in desensitization. *Arch. Dermatol.* 20:669 (1929).

76. N. A. MITCHISON: Immunological tolerance and immunological paralysis. *Brit. Med. Bull.* 17:102 (1961).

77. A. ROSENTHAL: Follow-up study of fatal penicillin reactions. *J. Amer. Med. Ass.* 167:1118 (1958).

78. A. SELTZER: A useful device for treating acute allergic drug reactions—the Medihaler-Epi. *Med. Ann. Dist. Columbia* 27:131 (1958).

79. J. H. SHAFFER: Stinging insects—a threat to life. *J. Amer. Med. Ass.* 177:473 (1961).

80. G. M. EDELMAN: Antibody structure and molecular immunology. *Science* 180:830 (1973).

CHAPTER 8
Drug Resistance

ORIGIN OF ACQUIRED DRUG RESISTANCE

Drug resistance is a state of insensitivity or of decreased sensitivity to drugs that ordinarily cause growth inhibition or cell death. The term is customarily used in reference to microorganisms or to cell populations (notably neoplasms) undergoing continuous growth in higher organisms. We are concerned here with *acquired* resistance, i.e., with populations initially sensitive that undergo a change in the direction of insensitivity.[1-3]

The Mutation-Selection Mechanism

The typical course of events in the development of drug resistance is that a strain of bacteria exposed to a growth-inhibitory or lethal drug responds normally at first. The growth rate is reduced or the population size is diminished. Eventually, however, although the drug is still present, growth resumes. The organisms that display this renewed growth are no longer susceptible to the same drug concentration. If the organism is a pathogen and the resistance has developed in a patient under treatment, the patient relapses and the infection becomes refractory to the old drug regimen. This phenomenon has been recognized since the latter part of the 19th century in microorganisms, and more recently in mammalian cells in vitro and some kinds of cancer cells in vivo. Acquired drug resistance is an important limitation to the use of antibiotics and many other antimicrobial and anticancer agents.

For a long time, it was assumed that the drug played some directive role in causing a biochemical adaptation in the cells. It has become clear, however, in most cases that have been studied adequately, that this view is incorrect. Instead, spontaneous mutants, which differ genetically from the original population in that they are already resistant to the drug action, survive and give rise to a wholly new, drug-resistant population. The drug provides a strong selective pressure in favor of the resistant cell by preventing growth of all the nonmutant wild-type sensitive cells. Thus, in acquired resistance, the bulk of the initial cell population usually does not become resistant. It responds to drug in the expected way, and it is then replaced by cells of a different kind, which are less sensitive to the drug action.[4,5] Occasionally, a growth-inhibitory drug may have mutagenic properties and thus nonspecifically increase the

517

probabilities of many kinds of mutation ; no example is known of a drug that selectively increases the mutation rate at the particular gene locus concerned with sensitivity and resistance to itself.

Evidence for the Mutational Origins of Drug Resistance

The question whether or not exposure to a drug is instrumental in causing development of resistance to that drug remained controversial for a long time. The difficulty arose from the fact that the drug necessarily had to be present in order to demonstrate resistance. How, then, could one tell if it had played a part in causing the altered cell response? Was drug resistance an adaptation to the drug, or a spontaneous change having survival value? The first solution to this problem was reached by means of an ingenious statistical approach known as a *fluctuation test*.[6] In its original form, this test was used to prove that acquired resistance of bacteria to bacteriophage arose spontaneously, before contact with the phage. Later, the same procedure was applied to determine the origin of bacterial resistance to a number of antibacterial drugs.

The design of the fluctuation test is illustrated in Figure 8-1. It was applied as follows to streptomycin resistance.[7] A drug-sensitive culture was diluted so that very

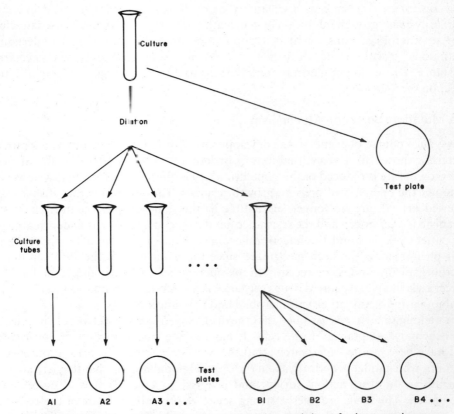

FIGURE 8-1. Fluctuation test to determine origin of drug resistance. *Small numbers of bacteria are inoculated into culture tubes. After growing out, they are plated onto test plates Only the test plates contain drug. The numbers of drug-resistant colonies on the plates of series A are compared with those of series B. (After Luria and Delbrück.[6])*

small inocula (50–300 cells) could be placed in each of a series of culture tubes. By plating an appropriate portion of the original culture on an agar test plate containing a lethal concentration of streptomycin, the frequency of drug-resistant cells in the original culture was estimated; each resistant cell would give rise to a resistant colony on the test plate, whereas no other cells would grow. It could then be asserted with confidence that none of the small inocula contained any cells already resistant to streptomycin; for example, if the frequency of resistant cells was 10^{-5}, then there would be only one chance in 1000 that a given inoculum of 100 cells contained a resistant cell. The culture tubes were incubated to permit multiplication of the small inocula to full-grown cultures (10^8 to 10^9 cells). Then came the critical step in the test. A sample from each culture tube was plated on a single test plate containing drug; about 20 culture tubes were thus plated (series A). From the 21st tube, identical platings were made onto 15 more test plates containing drug (series B). Now the plates of both series were incubated, and the numbers of resistant colonies were counted.

Let us suppose that drug resistance arises only after contact of bacteria with drug. Then in this experimental design, drug resistance would arise on the test plates. Since all test plates received equal inocula, the numbers of resistant colonies should be approximately the same on them all. On the other hand, if the drug resistance arose prior to contact with drug (i.e., in the culture tubes), then there might well be differences in the numbers of drug-resistant cells in the different tubes. If a spontaneous event leading to drug resistance occurred early in the growth of a culture, then by the time of plating onto the test plates, a sizeable clone of resistant cells would have developed. If the spontaneous event occurred late, then only a few resistant cells would be present in that tube when it was plated. The variation between plates in series B affords a measure of the random fluctuations to be expected from the experimental technique itself, when all platings are made from the same culture.

The question, then, is whether the variation in series A is substantially greater than the variation in series B. The answer was unambiguous. The mean number of resistant colonies was very similar in both series; however, the variation was much greater in series A. In series A, the mean was 106 colonies per plate, the variance was 2914, and the range was 48–291. In series B, the mean was 131, but the variance was only 151, and the range was 110–155. When numbers of items or events are counted, the random variation in repeated counts is expected to be such that the variance will be equal to the mean. This was approximately true in series B, but the variance in series A was much greater than could reasonably have come about by chance ($P < 0.001$). In other words, events in the tubes, but not in the plates, determined the numbers of drug-resistant cells obtained. Thus, it was concluded that phage resistance, streptomycin resistance, and so on, owed their origins to spontaneous random events occurring during growth of a culture of microorganisms. Several variants of the fluctuation test, some much simpler to perform, all led to the same conclusions.[8] An interesting application of the same concept to mice with transplantable leukemia yielded a similar indication about the origin of drug resistance of the leukemic cells to a cancer chemotherapeutic agent.[9]

A more direct and perhaps more convincing way of showing that resistant variants are present prior to contact with a drug is by means of the *replica plate technique*.[10] A culture of bacteria is spread uniformly over the surface of an ordinary nutrient agar plate and incubated until confluent heavy growth is present. This master plate is then pressed onto a sterile velvet surface, so that many cells from every part of the plate are transferred to the pile of the fabric. Fresh agar plates are then pressed, in succession, onto the same velvet surface; a few cells from every part of the velvet are thus transferred onto the surface of each "replica" plate. The replica plates (but not the master plate) contain the growth-inhibitory drug or antibacterial agent, so that only resistant cells will be able to grow. Figure 8-2 shows the outcome of such an experiment in

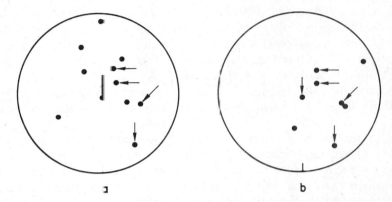

FIGURE 8-2. Replica plate demonstration of origin of resistance. *Plates* a *and* b *were spread with phage. By means of velvet, as described in the text, a master plate with confluent growth of a phage-sensitive bacterial population was replicated onto plates* a *and* b. *All phage-resistant colonies are shown; arrows indicate those in congruent positions on both plates. (From Lederberg, Figure 2.[10])*

which the antibacterial agent was phage. Eleven resistant colonies grew on one replica plate, eight on the other. Of these colonies, five pairs occupied identical locations on the two plates. Obviously, in these same positions on the master plate (which contained no phage) small clones of resistant cells must have been already present. It was concluded, therefore, that phage resistance arose spontaneously prior to contact with the selective antibacterial agent. Similar results have been obtained with streptomycin, penicillin, and other antibacterial drugs.

An extension of the replica plate procedure permitted the isolation of a pure strain of streptomycin-resistant *Escherichia coli* that had never been exposed to streptomycin at any stage of the procedure. Replica plating was used to locate a position on the master plate corresponding to that of a resistant colony on a replica plate. A bacteriologic loop was used to transfer cells from this position into a culture tube containing broth. After incubation, this culture was used to prepare a fresh master plate, and the entire procedure of replica plating was repeated. A large number of resistant colonies was now obtained on the replica plates. Again, cells were taken from a position on the new master plate corresponding to a resistant colony on the replica plate, and the whole procedure was repeated. Eventually, a pure culture of a streptomycin-resistant strain was obtained in this way, despite the fact that the cells had never been in contact with streptomycin. The drug was contained only in the replica plates; the cultures, progressively enriched for resistant cells, were grown only on master plates and in broth tubes containing no drug.

Drug resistance, like other genetic properties, can be transferred in the laboratory between cells of the same or closely related species by mechanisms that mediate the intercellular transfer of DNA.[11] Thus, specific drug resistance "markers" have been used in transformation experiments in which DNA of the resistant strain is used to transform the genotype of some cells of a sensitive strain. Drug resistance has also been transduced by means of a phage, which carries over a portion of the genome of the resistant cell; this is then integrated into the genetic apparatus of the recipient, drug-sensitive cell. Drug resistance has also been transferred by mating techniques in which DNA of a donor cell is introduced into a recipient cell by direct contact of the two.

A remarkable mechanism mediates the simultaneous transfer of resistance to several entirely unrelated antibacterial agents, whereas resistance arising through spontaneous de novo mutation characteristically is specific for one particular class of agents. Known as *transmissible multiple drug resistance*, it is found principally in the enteric bacteria.[12,13] In the early 1960's, it was found that patients with bacillary dysentery harbored strains of *Shigella* that were resistant to several antibacterial agents. When these strains were cultured in vitro with drug sensitive strains of *Shigella* or even with other Gram-negative bacteria (*E. coli*, *Klebsiella*, *Proteus*), the genes for multiple drug resistance were transferred to the sensitive strains without simultaneous transfer of any other genetic markers from the donor strain. Cell contact was required for this transfer. The resistance (R) factors were identified as extrachromosomal (episomal) closed circular rings of DNA. R^+ strains of bacteria have been found not only in hospital populations but also in domestic livestock, especially when antibiotics were routinely present in the feed.[13a] They have also been found in the enteric bacteria of a human population never exposed to antibiotics for therapeutic purposes.[13b] Thus, the transfer factors evidently occur widely; the extensive use of antibiotics merely favoring their proliferation by a selection mechanism. They constitute a significant problem in hospital patients, as evidenced by a study in which stool cultures from 100 apparently normal hospitalized infants revealed multiple drug resistant bacteria in 81 of them.[14,15]

Two independent elements are required for the resistance transfer phenomenon, a resistance transfer factor (RTF) and one of many possible R factors, which determine the pattern of drug resistance. At least 10 antibiotics may be involved in different combinations, including ampicillin, chloramphenicol, kanamycin, neomycin, streptomycin, and others. Some R factors carry genes for resistance to only a few of these, some to as many as seven. Resistance to phage, heavy metals (Hg, Ni, Co), and ultraviolet irradiation may also be transferred by episomes. No transfer can occur without the RTF gene, which controls the process operating during conjugation. Thus, a strain that harbors only RTF is drug sensitive; a drug resistant strain lacking RTF cannot transfer its resistance. The biochemical processes controlled by R factors and directly responsible for drug resistance are varied. They may, for example, cause malfunction of a process that normally concentrates an antibiotic intracellularly (tetracycline resistance, p. 526), or they may lead to production of an enzyme that inactivates the antibiotic (penicillin, chloramphenicol, aminoglucoside resistance, p. 529).

Patterns of Emergence and Spread of Drug Resistance

In the mutational development of the usual, chromosomal type of drug resistance, two distinct patterns are seen: the multiple-step ("penicillin type") and the facultative large-step ("streptomycin type") patterns. In the multiple-step pattern,[16] each isolation of resistant organisms in the laboratory leads only to a small increase in the degree of resistance. If a culture is placed in contact with a very high concentration of drug, all cells are affected and none will grow. At a suitable low concentration, while most of the population is held in check, a few resistant mutants will grow. These mutants are still sensitive to the drug at a somewhat higher concentration. Evidently no possible mutation can confer a high degree of resistance. On the other hand, if the population of mutants having a low level of resistance is grown in the presence of a somewhat higher drug concentration, one can select for another mutation superimposed on the first, which will confer a higher degree of resistance. In this way, step by step, quite high levels of resistance can be achieved. It was formerly thought that this pattern necessarily implied a multigenic determination of resistance (i.e., that each mutation affected one gene and many such genes were concerned in the action of the drug) so that the effects of successive mutations would be more or less additive. Our present understanding of mutation mechanisms makes an alternative view likely—that a single gene could well be involved but that mutations at different sites within this gene can lead to corresponding alterations at different positions on the gene product (presumably protein). Consider an enzyme the target of the drug action. The configuration of the combining site will be subject to modification by amino acid substitutions throughout the protein, and the configurational change might be expected to show additive effects when several substitutions are introduced. Each small change could reduce the affinity for the drug by a small amount, and these affinity decrements could be additive. That this reasoning has concrete applicability to drug-sensitive enzymes in microorganisms will be shown later (p. 542).

The *facultative large-step pattern* in mutational development of drug resistance is seen typically with streptomycin. If a sensitive culture is plated on a low concentration of the antibiotic, resistant colonies of different kinds can be obtained. Some are resistant to a low concentration of drug, others to a higher concentration; a few are completely insensitive to streptomycin at any concentration. It has been shown by recombination techniques that the various kinds of resistant genotypes represent alleles of the same gene locus. Evidently mutational substitution at certain sites leads to much greater change in drug sensitivity than at others. The biochemical basis of streptomycin resistance will be discussed in detail later.

The large-step pattern is a far more serious threat to successful chemotherapy than is the multiple-step pattern; for where it applies, an infectious disease may escape from drug control abruptly and completely at any time. For this reason, combined chemotherapy is especially indicated with drugs and organisms showing this pattern. The treatment of tuberculosis illustrates the point. The basis of combined chemotherapy is the complete independence of the mutational events leading to resistance to different drugs provided that the drugs are not simply congeners acting by the same mechanism. Suppose two drugs, X and Y, which inhibit growth of a pathogen, and a spontaneous mutation rate 10^{-6} for resistance to each of these. If 10^6 cells divide once, there will arise, on the average, one resistant to X and one mutant resistant to Y. But because the mutational events are independant, the probability is vanishingly small (10^{-12}) that a cell resistant to both drugs will arise. Thus, X-resistant mutants will be killed by Y, Y-resistant mutants will be killed by X, and the disease will be kept under control. This is the rationale for the combined treatment of tuberculosis with streptomycin plus isoniazid, streptomycin plus p-aminosalicylic acid, or isoniazid plus p-aminosalicylic acid.

It would appear that the logic of combined chemotherapy applies to all infections. But where control is readily accomplished with a single drug and large-step resistance is not a problem, a second drug does not usually offer sufficient advantage to outweigh its additional risks. This was thought to be the case with gonorrhea, since the *Neisseria* were highly sensitive to penicillin. Even here, however, resistance has become a major problem over the years. The appropriate procedure will always be to use high enough doses to discourage the emergence of multiple-step mutants and to employ in vitro sensitivity tests in order to choose the most effective drug. The problem of infectious episome-mediated multiple drug resistance further complicates rational therapy; if organisms become resistant simultaneously to several drugs, combined chemotherapy with those same drugs would obviously offer no advantage.

Important factors determining the ease with which drug resistance makes its appearance and then spreads in a human or animal population are: (*1*) the intensity of endemic or epidemic infection in that population, and (*2*) the extent of drug usage. If the total number of parasites harbored in the host population is high and the drug is widely used, opportunity is provided for the occurrence of mutations conferring resistance as well as for selection of the resistant genotype so that it becomes dominant. This principle frequently operates in shifts from sensitivity to resistance among numerous pathogenic microorganisms.

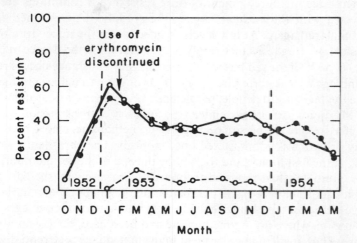

FIGURE 8-3. Erythromycin resistance among strains of *Staphylococcus* in a hospital population. *Nose and throat culture data were collected periodically at a hospital for contagious diseases. Resistance of staphylococci to high concentration of erythromycin (100 μg ml⁻¹) was determined. (Sensitive strains responded to 1 μg ml⁻¹.) Erythromycin was introduced at the end of September 1952 and discontinued in February 1953. Vertical axis shows percent of all strains isolated that were resistant to the drug; horizontal axis shows month and year. Solid curve, hospital personnel; upper broken curve, patients at time of discharge from hospital; lower broken curve, patients on admission to hospital. (From Dowling et al., Figure 1.[16a])*

An example studied particularly carefully[16a,17] is summarized in Figure 8-3. In preparation for the introduction of the then new antibiotic erythromycin at a contagious disease hospital in Chicago, nose and throat cultures were obtained from all patients and from all personnel concerned with patient care. Whenever staphylococci were found, their sensitivity to erythromycin was determined in vitro. On September 28, 1952, the use of erythromycin was begun. Nose and throat cultures were made periodically. In February, the use of erythromycin was discontinued. The figure shows that at the outset, the incidence of erythromycin resistance was negligible. It rose quickly, so that by January 60% of the staphylococci cultured from hospital personnel were resistant. The incidence among patients on discharge exactly paralleled this trend. For the first several months, no resistant organisms were harbored by patients at the time of their admission to the hospital. By March 1953, however, this was no longer true, presumably because of the widespread use of the antibiotic in the community by that time. The data show clearly that the resistant strains were being transmitted from hospital personnel to the patients, and that the bacterial flora in the carriers became resistant to erythromycin coincident with its introduction into use in the hospital. The conclusions about transmission of the resistant strains were confirmed by detailed analyses of the serologic types of the organisms. Following discontinuance of erythromycin, there was a gradual decline in the frequency of resistant strains. Similar observations on the rise and decline of bacterial resistance associated with intensity of therapeutic use have been made with penicillin, tetracyclines, and other antibiotics.

The prophylaxis of malaria provides another illustration of how mass use of a drug can encourage the development of drug resistance if conditions are favorable. In mice infected with *Plasmodium berghei*, the antifolic drug pyrimethamine is an effective antimalarial agent. At low levels of infection in the mice, drug treatment is very successful and drug resistance rarely occurs. But when the degree of parasitemia is high (e.g., 40–50% of the red blood cells parasitized), resistance occurs readily.[18,19]

Similar findings were reported from field trials on human malaria in East Africa.[20] In an isolated village of 130 people, parasitemia (*P. falciparum*) was demonstrated in 84 of them. Mosquito carriers abounded; the intensity of transmission was estimated at about 1 infective bite per person per night. Pyrimethamine, whose biologic half-life is only a day or two, was administered once monthly. The parasitemia rate fell from 64% to 23% in the first month and to 21% by the end of the second month. But then it started to climb and had returned to pretreatment levels by the end of the sixth month despite continuation of the pyrimethamine regimen. The malarial infections in this village were now unresponsive to the drug. But in two other villages in the same geographic region, where no pyrimethamine had been used, the plasmodia were still drug sensitive. Thus, inadequate treatment in the first village preferentially eliminated the drug-sensitive plasmodia, leaving a reservoir of infectious organisms in which mutants resistant to pyrimethamine could survive and multiply. An effective chemotherapeutic attack on any disease that infects a large part of the population requires sufficiently vigorous and continuous treatment to reduce the number of infectious organisms to a very low level. This principle was epitomized by Ehrlich in the early days of chemotherapy by the injunction, "Frapper fort et frapper vite!"[21] It is also essential to take simultaneous measures (such as mosquito eradication in malaria) to block the transmission of the disease to prevent the spread of drug-resistant organisms.

It would be useful to have reliable means for suppressing the emergence of drug resistance during chemotherapeutic treatment of infections or of cancer. The measures already discussed are: (1) the use of a combination of drugs, and (2) the attempt to treat intensively so as to eradicate the infectious organisms quickly. Another possible approach might be the use of antimutagenic agents, which would suppress the spontaneous mutation rate and thereby decrease the frequency of emergence of drug-resistant mutants.[22] It has also been found that bacteria harboring R factors can sometimes be "cured" by treatment with intercalating agents like ethidium bromide and acridines, which apparently prevent replication of the episomes.[23]

BIOCHEMICAL MECHANISMS OF DRUG RESISTANCE

That individual cells can become drug resistant by mutation implies that deletion or modification of an enzyme, or alteration of the properties of some other cell component whose synthesis is under gene control, can be responsible for the altered response to drug.[24–26] A number of possible general mechanisms have been suggested,[27] which are used as a basis for the following classification of mechanisms.

Mechanism 1. Decreased Intracellular Drug Level

D-serine. The decrease of drug concentration inside cells could come about by altered permeability of the cells, so that the rate of drug entry by diffusion is reduced. Or if the drug is actively transported into the cell, a defect in an enzyme (permease) or protein carrier that participates in this process could reduce the intracellular drug concentration. D-serine resistance in *E. coli* exemplifies this mechanism.[24] This amino acid isomer inhibits growth of sensitive cells. Resistant cells no longer take it up, nor can they concentrate glycine from the medium, as do the wild-type cells. Evidently a glycine permease is responsible for the entry of both glycine and D-serine into the sensitive cell, and this activity is lost in the resistant cells. Since the endogenous pathway of glycine synthesis in this organism remains intact, the permease is dispensable and the D-serine-resistant cells are able to grow.

Sulfonamides, Methotrexate, and 6-Mercaptopurine. An investigation into sulfonamide resistance in *E. coli* revealed two kinds of resistance.[28] In one kind, an enzyme with altered affinity for sulfonamide was isolated from the cells (cf. p. 544). In the other kind, although the cells were resistant to sulfonamides, the cell-free extracts (including sulfonamide-sensitive enzyme) displayed no differences from the wild type. It was concluded that the explanation of resistance must be the failure of the sulfonamide to enter the cells; however, no direct proof was offered.

Permeability changes have been implicated more directly in the acquired resistance of mouse leukemia cells to methotrexate (amethopterin), a potent inhibitor of dihydrofolate reductase.[29,30] Moreover, in studies of patients with various types of lymphatic cell neoplasm there was a good correlation between uptake of methotrexate in vitro in the various cells types and subsequent clinical response to the chemotherapy. The leukocytes of patients with chronic lymphocytic leukemia, which is known to be unresponsive to methotrexate, took up very little of the drug.[31] Decreased uptake has also been postulated to explain resistance to 6-mercaptopurine in a certain subline of ascitic carcinoma in mice. Cell-free extracts were able to form 6-mercaptopurine ribonucleotide, the actual toxic agent. Yet whole cells failed to achieve levels of the active compound as high as those observed in sensitive cell strains.[32] It should be noted, however, that this kind of evidence is not proof of a permeability or uptake defect. Frequently drug resistance is due to the appearance of a drug-inactivating enzyme; preparation of a cell lysate might well dilute or remove this enzyme or an essential cofactor.

Tetracycline, Chloramphenicol.   Tetracycline resistance carried by R factors has been shown to be due to defective drug uptake.[33] R⁻ strains actively accumulate tetracycline intracellularly, where the drug inhibits ribosomal function. R⁺ strains are inducible for the property of inhibiting the uptake process. This means that R⁺ strains are constitutively of low resistance; but in the presence of tetracycline, they become efficient in excluding the drug and consequently are resistant. An R factor has also been found that carries a mutant constitutive gene conferring immediate resistance by excluding tetracycline without the necessity of prior exposure.[34] A mutant of *E. coli*, resistant to chloramphenicol, has also been shown to contain a defective uptake and binding system.[35] This drug blocks protein synthesis by binding to the 50S ribosomal subunit of the 70S bacterial ribosome.[35a] Organisms that are not sensitive to chloramphenicol (yeast, mammalian cells) have a different kind of ribosome which is incapable of binding the drug. *E. coli* cells that have become resistant by mutation have a much lower intracellular chloramphenicol concentration than sensitive cells, although isolated ribosomes of the resistant strain bound chloramphenicol just as well as those from the sensitive wild type. Resistance therefore has been attributed to an altered permeability, but inactivation of the drug at or near the plasma membrane has not been rigorously excluded. The most common mode of resistance to chloramphenicol is due to a drug-inactivating enzyme, discussed later.

Chloroquine.   Investigations into the mechanism of resistance of malaria parasites to chloroquine implicate impeded uptake of drug by organisms.[36,37] Chloroquine complexes with DNA and thus inhibits reactions that require the participation of DNA. Inhibition of DNA replication is thought to be the primary drug effect. The DNA-dependent RNA polymerase reaction (i.e., genetic transcription) is also inhibited in vitro, regardless of whether the cell-free system is derived from chloroquine-sensitive or chloroquine-resistant organisms. In whole bacterial cells, it has been shown that a chloroquine-sensitive strain, *Bacillus megaterium*, takes up about 10 times more of the drug than a chloroquine-insensitive strain, *Bacillus cereus*. Direct evidence relating uptake of drug to acquired resistance comes from experiments in mice using *Plasmodium berghei*. A drug-resistant strain was developed by serial passage in mice for 17 months in the presence of increasing concentrations of chloroquine. Uptake studies were carried out with ¹⁴C-chloroquine labeled in the quinoline ring. Figure 8-4 shows the relationship between the dose of drug and its concentration in red blood cells after 4 hr when the maximum was attained. Since the uptake by normal unparasitized erythrocytes was negligibly small, it is assumed that the content of drug in parasitized cells reflects its uptake by the plasmodia. The greatly diminished concentration in the resistant plasmodia as compared with sensitive plasmodia is evident. The highest level that could be attained in the resistant organisms, with a 40-mg kg⁻¹ dose of chloroquine, was the same as would be achieved at one-tenth the dose in sensitive plasmodia. The uptake curve for liver shows that the drug concentration in this organ increased linearly with dose. The selective toxicity and satisfactory therapeutic ratio of chloroquine acting upon sensitive plasmodia may well be related to the steep uptake curve for parasitized red cells at drug dosages so low that very little drug is taken up by vital organs of the host.

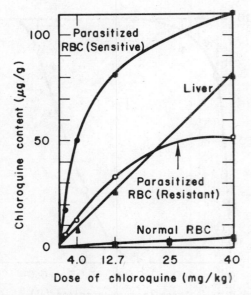

FIGURE 8-4. Uptake of chloroquine by sensitive and resistant plasmodia.
14C-chloroquine was given intraperitoneally to uninfected mice and to mice infected with a sensitive or resistant strain of Plasmodium berghei. *The data for infected mice refer only to parasitized red cells, the parasitized fraction having been determined by microscopic observation. The cells infected with resistant plasmodia contained 1.6 times more parasites per cell than the cells infected with sensitive parasites; thus, the drug content per parasite differs, between resistant and sensitive parasites, even more than shown. Chloroquine concentration in liver increased linearly with dose. (From Mccomber et al., Figure 3.*[37] *By permission of the American Association for the Advancement of Science.)*

Arsenite. A somewhat surprising but well-documented example of drug resistance attributable to decreased intracellular concentration of drug concerns growth inhibition of bacteria by arsenite.[38,39] This heavy metal anion strongly inhibits essential sulfhydryl enzymes like pyruvate (or α-ketoglutarate) dehydrogenase. A sample of soil was plated on a medium containing 10^{-2} M arsenite. One of the organisms that grew (a *Pseudomonas*) was studied to see how it was affected by arsenite. It was found that if this organism was grown in the absence of arsenite and then inoculated into a medium containing arsenite, there was always a lag before growth began. The growth rate, however, was the same up to very high concentrations of arsenite ($> 10^{-2}$ M). When the cells that had grown in the presence of arsenite were inoculated into fresh medium containing arsenite at the same concentration, growth began without any lag. It was then apparent that the organisms as isolated from the soil had the genetic endowment to adapt to the presence of arsenite. In this respect, they were analogous to strains of *Micrococcus* capable of becoming resistant to penicillin by producing penicillinase when exposed to penicillin.

The inhibition of dehydrogenase activities by arsenite was examined in *Pseudomonas* cells grown in the presence of arsenite and in cells grown in its absence. Figure 8-5 shows this comparison for the oxidation of L-ketoglutarate. The large difference observed here was seen also when pyruvate, succinate, or malate was the substrate. However, when these same dehydrogenase activities were tested in cell-free extracts, the difference between the two kinds of cells disappeared, i.e., the arsenite

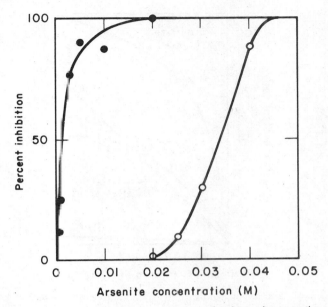

FIGURE 8-5. Effect of arsenite on oxidation of α-ketoglutarate in sensitive and resistant pseudomonas cells. *Solid circles, cells grown in ordinary medium; open circles, cells grown in presence of 10^{-2} M arsenite. (From Arima and Beppu, Figure 4.*[38])

resistance was abolished by cell lysis. These findings seemed to implicate some kind of exclusion mechanism at the cell membrane as the cause of arsenite resistance. Direct measurements confirmed this. Cells that had been grown in the presence or absence of arsenite (10^{-2} M) were equilibrated with several different concentrations of radioactive arsenite, and the uptake of radioactivity was measured. Results are shown in Figure 8-6 on a double-reciprocal plot. At any given arsenite concentration, the uptake by the population of resistant cells was smaller than that by sensitive cells. But the intercept on the y axis, representing the maximum uptake at "infinite" arsenite concentration, was the same for both kinds of cell. As in the use of this type of graph to analyze enzyme inhibition (p. 84), the identical y axis intercepts (analogous to V_{max}) signify the presence of a saturable process. Here, despite the exclusion of arsenite from resistant cells at low external arsenite concentrations, at very high concentrations the exclusion mechanism is, in effect, overwhelmed. The findings would be consistent with the presence of an inducible transport "pump" for extruding arsenite from the cells. The resistance develops within a period of only one or two cell generations, and it is lost quickly in the absence of arsenite. In this instance, therefore, the acquired drug resistance must be attributed to a phenotypic modification, and it is present in all cells of the resistant strain after exposure to arsenite.

Acquired resistance of trypanosomes to organic arsenicals has also been shown to depend upon decreased penetration by the drugs.[40] Of particular interest was the finding that the diminished uptake of arsenic by the cells occurred only with those arsenosobenzene compounds containing an amide substituent to which the resistance had developed, but not to other organic arsenicals to which there was no cross-resistance.

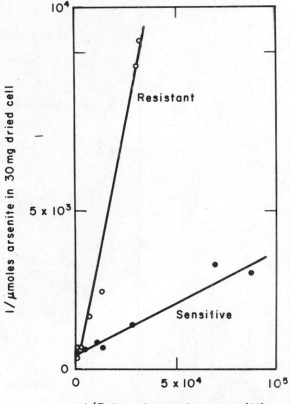

FIGURE 8-6. Uptake of arsenite by sensitive and resistant pseudomonas cells. *Solid circles, taken from ordinary medium; open circles, cells that had been grown in presence of 10^{-2} M arsenite. For the measurement of uptake radioactive arsenite was used and 20 min was allowed for equilibration. In the double-reciprocal plot shown here, the intercept on the y axis represents the maximum uptake at "infinite" external arsenite concentration. (From Beppu and Arima, Figure 3.[39])*

Mechanism 2. Increased Destruction of Drug

Penicillin.   A common type of resistance to penicillins, especially in *Micrococcus* (*Staphylococcus aureus*), is due to the production of enzymes that hydrolyze the drug to an inactive product.[41] The commonest type of penicillinase is a β-lactamase, yielding penicilloic acid; amidases also exist, producing 6-aminopenicillanic acid. Various penicillinases have been described, both of chromosomal and episomal origin.[42] Some are bound to the plasma membrane and must be converted from a hydrophobic to a hydrophilic form for secretion into the external medium: the usual product of a chromosomal gene is of this type. Others are located in the periplasmic region (between the plasma membrane and the cell wall) and are readily secreted into the medium; those produced by R factors are of this type.[43]

There are also many differences between the various penicillinases with respect to substrate specificity, sensitivity to inhibition by –SH reagents, and electrophoretic mobility. One class of β-lactamase does not hydrolyze ampicillin or carbenicillin

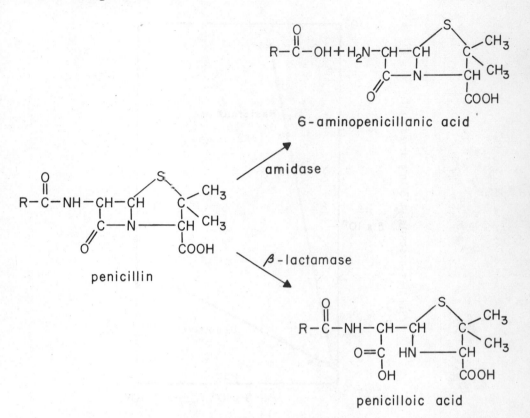

(synthetic penicillin derivatives) at all, while others hydrolyze them better than the naturally occurring benzylpencillin.

Strains with the chromosomal gene for a β-lactamase usually have very low basal levels of the enzyme but produce it upon contact with an appropriate penicillin, i.e., the enzyme is inducible. Mutation can render the enzyme constitutive, so that the level is high even in the absence of penicillin. Finally, R^+ strains transfer the capacity to produce a β-lactamase constitutively. The localization of the enzyme in close proximity to the site of action of the penicillins, which block the assembly of cell wall from peptidoglycan building blocks,[44] undoubtedly contributes to the drug resistance associated with penicillinase production. Moreover, a whole population of penicillinase-containing cells can act cooperatively to reduce the ambient penicillin concentration below effective levels. Many modified forms of penicillin have been introduced in an attempt to circumvent the resistance problem with considerable success. But the continual emergence of penicillinases with altered substrate specificities has tended to limit their effectiveness (cf. Chapter 13).

Aminoglycoside Antibiotics and Chloramphenicol. The aminoglycoside antibiotics include the streptomycins, gentamicins, kanamycins, neomycins, paromomycin, and spectomycin.[3] Spontaneous high-level chromosomal resistance to these antibiotics results from specific alteration at the receptor site on a ribosomal protein (cf. p. 555). Such resistance is usually specific for a single drug, and it has not been a major clinical problem. In contrast, resistance conferred by R factors is due to the presence of an enzyme that inactivates the drug, and cross-resistance among related drugs is the rule; this type of resistance is of great clinical significance.[45] Five different inactivating enzymes are known; all transfer a group (phosphate, adenylate, or acetate) to a sugar hydroxyl or amino group and thereby usually abolish antibiotic activity.[13] As illustrated in Figure 8-7, streptomycin phosphotransferase catalyzes the transfer of

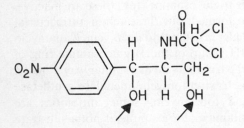

chloramphenicol

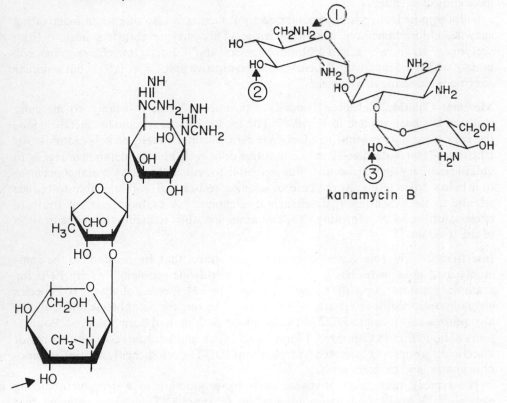

kanamycin B

streptomycin

FIGURE 8-7. Sites of inactivation of aminoglycoside antibiotics and chloramphenicol by enzymes under control of R factors. *Streptomycin phosphotransferase and adenylate synthetase inactivate at the hydroxyl group indicated by the arrow. The kanamycins are inactivated by acetylation at the amino group designated 1 and at the hydroxyl group designated 2. Gentamicin, which has a related structure, is inactivated by an adenylate synthetase at the hydroxyl group designated 3. Neomycin B has the same D-glucosamine as shown for kanamycin B. Chloramphenicol is acetylated at the hydroxyl groups indicated by the arrows. (Modified from Davies and Rownd, Figures 4, 5, and 7.[13])*

the terminal phosphate of ATP to the 3-OH of L-glucosamine, the third of the 3 sugar residues in the antibiotic. Streptomycin adenylate synthetase mediates the transfer of AMP (derived from ATP) to form a diester at the same —OH group of L-glucosamine: this enzyme can also inactivate kanamycin. Kanamycin acetyltransferase forms N-acetyl derivatives at the amino group of the D-glucosamine ring; these are inactive. N-acetyl derivatives of neomycin B are also formed, but these retain antibacterial activity, and therefore the enzyme does not confer resistance to neomycin. Kanamycin phosphotransferase phosphorylates the 3-OH group of the D-glucosamine ring of kanamycin and also inactivates neomycin and paromomycin in a similar way. Finally, gentamicin adenylate synthetase is analogous to streptomycin adenylate synthetase but inactivates gentamicin, kanamycin, and tobramycin. Some antibiotics are inhibitors of these inactivating enzymes. Gentamicin, for example, is not a substrate for kanamycin phosphotransferase but inhibits its activity. Such inhibitors might have clinical usefulness.

Chloramphenicol resistance conferred by R factors is also due to an inactivating enzyme, chloramphenicol acetyltransferase. This enzyme transfers acetate from acetyl-coA to form 3-acetoxychloramphenicol and 1,3-diacetoxychloramphenicol, both of which are inactive. This enzyme is constitutive in R$^+$ E. coli,[46,47] but a similar enzyme is inducible in S. aureus.

Mercuric Chloride, Selenite, Cyanide.   Episome-mediated resistance to mercuric chloride has been studied in E. coli.[48] The resistance was specific for mercuric ion; the cells were not resistant to phenylmercuric acetate, cobalt, nickel, cadmium, or zinc ions. The resistant cells, unlike sensitive cells, were able to metabolize $HgCl_2$ to volatile mercury derivatives and thus were able to reduce the heavy metal concentration below toxic levels. In the case of selenite, resistant E. coli was able to reduce selenite to the much less toxic elemental selenium.[49] A cyanide resistant strain of bacteria utilized CN^-, forming CO_2 and ammonia, thus reducing the concentration of the toxic ion.[50]

Insecticides.   The emergence of mutant insect strains that are resistant to the commonly used insecticides has become a major worldwide problem.[51,52] By 1970, for example, resistant populations had developed in 224 species, of which 105 species were of public health or veterinary importance. Among the Anopheline and Culicine mosquitoes, resistance to DDT, dieldrin, and malathion had been observed. Populations of houseflies in California, Florida, and Japan had become resistant to 4 major insecticide groups—chlorinated hydrocarbons (DDT), cyclodienes (dieldrin), organophosphates, and carbamates.

The typical mechanism of resistance is by production of a drug-metabolizing enzyme.[53,54] An example was presented in Chapter 3 (Table 3-1), showing that houseflies resistant to DDT demonstrated a greatly enhanced capacity to inactivate the toxic compound by dehydrochlorination. Houseflies resistant to carbamate insecticides have been shown to degrade these compounds more rapidly than do the sensitive strains.[55] The most extensive studies in insects have dealt with resistance to organophosphate cholinesterase inhibitors like malathion. As in the case of parathion (p. 249), malathion becomes an active inhibitor only upon its conversion to an oxygen analog known as malaoxon. Both malathion and malaoxon can be degraded by a phosphatase and by a carboxyesterase, as indicated in the structural formula that follows.

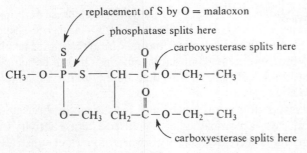

malathion

During the widespread use of malathion as a larvicide against mosquitoes, a resistant strain emerged.[56] Larvae of this strain were found to contain greatly increased activity of a mitochondrial carboxyesterase that degraded malathion to the monoester and the succinic acid derivative. Thus, less malathion remained available for conversion to malaoxon. The degradation of malaoxon was also increased in this strain compared with the sensitive strain. The enhanced esterase activity was thought to be due to an increased amount of the normal enzyme, since no alterations in affinity for malathion were found. However, affinities for other substrates were not studied, nor were pH optima or thermal stability.

Mating experiments showed that the increased carboxyesterase activity was inseparable from the malathion resistance. The data are shown in Table 8-1. The

TABLE 8-1. Carboxyesterase activity and malathion resistance in mosquito larvae. Larvae of *Culex tarsalis* were tested for sensitivity to malathion by determining the LC50 (concentration, in parts per million, killing 50% of the larvae). Carboxyesterase and phosphatase products were measured by an in vitro assay using radioactive malathion and identifying products by a chloroform extraction procedure; the data are percent of total radioactivity found in products in 30 min at 23°. (From Matsumura and Brown,[56] Table 12.)

Larvae	Malathion LC50 (ppm)	Carboxyesterase products (%)	Phosphatase products (%)
Resistant	1.8	4.4 ± 0.6	4.3 ± 0.8
Sensitive	0.043	0.8 ± 0.3	3.2 ± 0.9
F_1 hybrid	0.80	4.5 ± 1.0	
B_1 back-cross	0.75	4.2 ± 0.4	
B_2 back-cross	0.80	5.4 ± 0.6	

resistant larvae required 42 times higher malathion concentration for 50% kill than did the sensitive strain; under the conditions of the assay, the carboxyesterase activity was 5.5 times higher. There was no difference in phosphatase activity between the 2 strains. The first-generation hybrid (F_1) showed a resistance level somewhat lower than the resistant strain and a higher carboxyesterase activity. Selection for malathion resistance was carried out among the F_1 hybrids. Survivors of exposure to malathion (1 part per million) were crossed back to the sensitive line to obtain strain B_1. The same procedure was repeated with B_1, survivors being mated with the sensitive strain to obtain B_2. The table shows that the high carboxyesterase activity was retained in B_1 and B_2 strains, despite their genomes being 3/4 and 7/8, respectively, derived from the sensitive stock. Thus, selection for malathion resistance resulted in associated high activity of this particular degradative enzyme. It was concluded that the gene conferring malathion resistance is an allele of the wild-type gene that determines carboxyesterase activity

A similar investigation[57] of malathion resistance in houseflies showed that, although resistance was accompanied by increased esterase activity toward malathion or malaoxon, there was decreased activity toward other ester substrates (e.g., methoxy-butyrate). In mating experiments, this decreased activity was inseparable from the increased activity toward malathion or the resistance to malathion. Thus, it seems likely that the enhanced ability to degrade the insecticide resulted from a qualitatively altered enzyme rather than a simple increase in amount of a normal enzyme. The increase in esterase activity toward malathion and the concomitant decrease in activity toward methoxybutyrate suggested that the resistant strain might prove to be sensitive to a methyl ester analog of malathion; this was demonstrated to be true.[58] Thus, resistance to one particular insecticide does not necessarily confer cross-resistance, even to closely related congeners.

Most insecticides are oxidatively metabolized, apparently by a microsomal mixed-function oxidase system involving NADPH and a cytochrome P450 like that found in mammalian liver.[59] Induction of microsomal enzyme activity by insecticides is not usually observed; however, resistance emerges through selection of resistant mutants. Certain compounds, known as synergists, act as inhibitors (actually competitive substrates) of the mixed-function oxidase system, thereby protecting an active insecticide against destruction. An example shown below is piperonyl butoxide, which can saturate the microsomal system, thus enhancing the potency of another compound against resistant strains.[60]

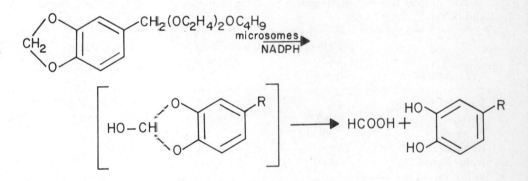

Mechanism 3. Decreased Conversion of Drug to a More Active Compound

_p_-Fluorophenylalanine.   An interesting example of this mechanism in bacteria is the acquired resistance to _p_-fluorophenylalanine (cf. p. 119). The active form of this drug is its complex with the phenylalanine transfer-RNA, a complex that is formed because the phenylalanine-activating enzyme accepts the fluoro analog. Once attached to transfer-RNA, the drug is incorporated into proteins instead of the natural amino acid, with deleterious consequences for the bacteria, presumably because the analog-containing proteins cannot function normally. Phenylalanine-activating enzyme was purified from wild-type cells and from resistant mutants.[61] The purified wild-type enzyme functioned with either phenylalanine or fluorophenylalanine as substrate. The enzyme from the resistant organism was completely inactive toward fluorophenylalanine when tested in a cell-free system containing phenylalanine transfer-RNA, ATP, and Mg^{2+}. The K_m values for phenylalanine, however, and for ATP were the same as for the normal enzyme. In addition to its inactivity toward fluorophenylalanine, the mutant enzyme had a much greater thermal stability than did the wild-type enzyme. It is supposed, therefore, that a mutation in the structural gene controlling the amino acid sequence of the activating enzyme was responsible for the acquired resistance to the drug. Presumably, a configurational change resulting from the amino acid replacement rendered the fluoro derivative incapable of combining, whereas the enzyme was still able to activate the natural amino acid.

Purine and Pyrimidine Analogs. Purine and pyrimidine analogs, when they act by incorporation into nucleic acids, have to be converted to nucleotides first; fluorouridylic acid, for example, is the active form of 5-fluorouracil. Changes in the enzymes mediating such conversions may be responsible for drug resistance. For example, ascites tumors in mice are inhibited by 5-fluorouracil. Several resistant sublines of ascites cell were studied to ascertain the mechanism of drug resistance.[62] The activity of the enzyme uridine kinase was found to be drastically decreased in resistant cells. This enzyme catalyzes the phosphorylation of uridine to uridylic acid and of fluorouridine to fluorouridylic acid, with ATP as phosphate donor; therefore, its deficiency would decrease the conversion of 5-fluorouracil to its active form. Uridine kinase was isolated and purified from wild-type and resistant cells. The enzyme from resistant cells precipitated at a lower concentration of ammonium sulfate than that from wild-type cells, it was more difficult to elute from an anion exchange column at pH 7.4, and it was more readily inactivated by heat. Thus, the presumptive basis of the decreased enzyme activity is a mutational alteration in enzyme structure.

A similar illustration is provided by resistance to the adenine analog, 2,6-diaminopurine by a *Salmonella* species.[63] The drug is a growth inhibitor in this organism, and resistant mutants can be obtained in its presence. The enzymes that convert purine bases to the corresponding nucleotides catalyze the transfer of a ribose phosphate moiety from phosphoribosyl pyrophosphate (PRPP), splitting out pyrophosphate; they are therefore called purine phosphoribosyl transferases (PRTases). These enzymes were purified and eluted from a DEAE-cellulose anion exchange column, the enzyme activity of each fraction being tested for activity with adenine, 2,6-diaminopurine, and hypoxanthine. The results are shown in Figure 8-8. The extract from wild-type *Salmonella* cells (top) yielded 2 distinct peaks of enzyme activity —one for adenine, forming adenosine monophosphate (AMP), the other for hypoxanthine, forming inosine monophosphate (IMP). The adenine PRTase also converted diaminopurine to its nucleotide. The extract from resistant cells (middle) showed two alterations: (1) the adenylate enzyme was eluted sooner from the column, whereas the IMP enzyme behaved normally in this respect, and (2) all trace of activity toward diaminopurine had disappeared. An equal mixture of the two extracts (bottom) illustrates the expected additive effects, showing that the resistant extract did not contain any inhibitor that would interfere with detection of activity toward diaminopurine, if it were present. Thus, it is reasonable to conclude that the acquired resistance to diaminopurine is due to a mutational modification of the adenine PRTase. The effect of the genetic change is to alter its ionic properties somewhat and to abolish its ability to interact with 2,6-diaminopurine as a substrate without altering its activity toward adenine.

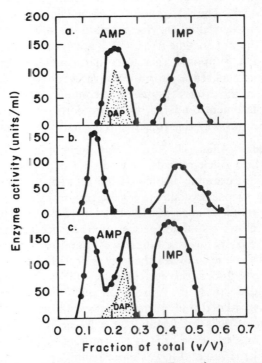

FIGURE 8-8. Elution of salmonella purine PRTases from an anion exchange column. *DEAE-cellulose column elution by linear NaCl gradient from 0 to 0.5 M in pH 7.6 buffer. Horizontal axis shows fraction of the total 400-ml volume run through the column; vertical axis shows enzyme activities. Each fraction was assayed for purine PRTase activity with PRPP as donor and adenine, 2,6-diaminopurine, and hypoxanthine individually as acceptors; thus, AMP, diaminopurine nucleotide (DAP), and IMP were formed. a, wild-type extract; b, diaminopurine-resistant extract; c, mixture of a and b. (From Kalle and Gots, Figure 1.[63] By permission of the American Association for the Advancement of Science.)*

An analogous example of this mechanism is of some importance in cancer chemotherapy. The purine analog 6-mercaptopurine (6-MP) is converted to the corresponding nucleotide by the "salvage pathway" in mammalian cells, involving the same reaction with PRPP just described for bacteria. In numerous instances in transplantable murine tumors and in other mammalian cells growing in vitro, acquired resistance to 6-MP entails loss of the purine PRTase.[64] Here the relevant enzyme is hypoxanthine-guanine PRTase, which is active with hypoxanthine, guanine, 6-MP, thioguanine, and azaguanine as substrates. As with 2,6-diaminopurine resistance in bacteria, the adenine PRTase activity is usually not affected. Drug failures with 6-MP in clinical cancer chemotherapy are seldom if ever due to acquired resistance of this kind.[65]

A model has been proposed for the possible exploitation, in cancer chemotherapy, of the property causing drug resistance.[66] A line of mouse fibroblasts resistant to 6-MP was developed in vitro, and the cause of the resistance was shown to be deficient conversion of 6-MP to the nucleotide. Such resistant cells should be unable to utilize exogenous purines like hypoxanthine and be completely dependent upon their de novo pathway of purine biosynthesis which forms purines from simpler precursors such as glutamine and phosphoribosylamine.

The de novo pathway can be blocked by antifolic drugs, which block single-carbon transfers, since single-carbon transfers are essential in biosynthesis of the purine ring. If cells are exposed to one of these antifolic drugs, methotrexate, and at the same time glycine, thymidine, and a purine are supplied, wild-type cells will be able to grow (cf. p. 426). The methotrexate inhibition will be overcome because all the end-products of the single-carbon transfer reactions are furnished. and the purine can be utilized by means of the "salvage pathway." The cells resistant to 6-MP. on the other hand, should be unable to grow in a hypoxanthine-supplemented medium because they cannot utilize this exogenous purine, and their endogenous synthesis of purines is shut off by methotrexate. The experiment is shown in Figure 8-9. The outcome was as

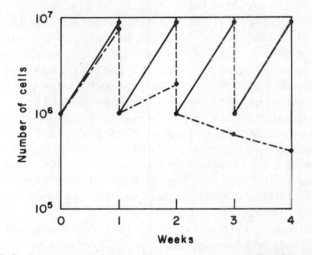

FIGURE 8-9. Selective inhibition of growth of mouse fibroblasts resistant to 6-mercaptopurine. *Weekly multiplication of cells in vitro, subcultured each week. Horizontal axis is number of weeks; vertical axis is number of cells, plotted on a logarithmic scale. The medium contained methotrexate (10^{-6} M), hypoxanthine and thymidine (3×10^{-5} M), and glycine (10^{-4} M). Solid line, normal cells; broken line, cell line resistant to 6-mercaptopurine. Cells were diluted and subcultured weekly as indicated by vertical broken lines. When adenine was substituted for hypoxanthine, both cell lines grew well (not shown). (From Tomizawa and Aronow, data of Table 4.[66])*

expected; the resistant cell line eventually failed to grow in a medium containing methotrexate, hypoxanthine, thymidine, and glycine, whereas the normal cell line continued to multiply under these conditions. When adenine was substituted for hypoxanthine, however, the resistant cells grew perfectly well.

Mechanism 4. Increased Concentration of Metabolite Antagonizing the Drug Action

One of the earliest investigations of sulfonamide resistance disclosed a striking example of this mechanism.[67] When the amount of p-aminobenzoic acid in resistant mutants of *Staphylococcus* was compared with that in the sensitive parent strains, an increase on the order of 100-fold was found in the resistant cells. This increase was sufficient to account for the observed degree of resistance by competitive antagonism of the sulfonamide inhibition. Few other examples of this mechanism have come to light, and even for sulfonamide resistance it is not the most frequent mechanism. Overproduction of a metabolite implies that there has been a mutational loss of control in a pathway that is subject to regulation by end-product ("feedback") inhibition or by end-product repression of enzymes. Several illustrations will be given on p. 546 of drug resistance due to mutational modification of enzymes subject to end-product inhibition. In these instances, the resulting increased metabolite levels seem to be incidental to the drug resistance rather than to be its cause.

Mechanism 5. Altered Amount of Target Enzyme

Enzyme levels in cells are regulated to meet the needs of the organism by controls exerted upon the processes of transcription (messenger-RNA synthesis) and translation (assembly of nascent protein)[68] Enzyme induction by a substrate or substrate analog illustrates the expansion of enzyme capacity by specific *derepression* of the gene, resulting in an increased rate of enzyme synthesis. The *repressor* is a protein, which interacts with a particular operator gene and thereby prevents (partially or completely) the transcription of the corresponding structural gene. Combination of an *inducer* with this protein releases the repression. Mutational alterations of several kinds can affect these control mechanisms. Complete release of repression, as by mutation in the regulatory gene that controls synthesis of the repressor, results in *constitutive formation* of an enzyme that is normally inducible; a great increase in its rate of synthesis results, and therefore its steady-state level in the cell becomes greatly elevated. Mutational modification of repressor conformation is also possible, resulting in altered affinities for inducers.

Mutational alterations in regulatory systems can lead to acquired drug resistance. If the drug happens to be a reversible inhibitor of a given enzyme and if the amount of that enzyme per cell increases, then the same drug concentration, producing the same percent inhibition, will no longer prevent growth. The actual enzyme activity in the presence of the drug will be greater than in the wild type, and the products of the enzyme reaction will be formed at a rate more than sufficient to meet the needs of the cell. If the drug happens to be an irreversible inhibitor, then a stoichiometric equivalent of drug will be required to produce any given inhibition; this will obviously require more drug when more enzyme is present.

Antifolic Drugs. This mechanism (increased amount of target enzyme) has been identified as a cause of acquired resistance to antifolic drugs in bacteria, in mammalian cells in culture, and in transplanted leukemic cells in vivo.[69] However, it is still uncertain whether treatment failure of human leukemia with antifolic agents is to be attributed to this cause.[70] The target of action of the antifolic drug is the enzyme dihydrofolate reductase, which catalyzes the reduction of dihydrofolate to the active tetrahydrofolate (p. 426). In one experiment, sarcoma-180 cells were grown in vitro and sublines resistant to methotrexate were isolated.[71] The activity of the enzyme was measured in cell extracts from sensitive and resistant cells. The activity of dihydrofolate reductase was much higher in the resistant than in the sensitive cell lines. A comparison was made between the degree of resistance and the extent of increase in enzyme activity. A cell line 67 times more resistant to methotrexate than the wild type had a 65-fold increase in enzyme activity. Another line, which was 174 times more resistant than the wild type, had 155 times more enzyme activity. Moreover, the extent of increase in enzyme activity in the two resistant strains was exactly paralleled by the degree of increase in binding capacity of the extracts for methotrexate. At the same time, it was shown that the K_m for folic acid and the rate of conversion of substrate per drug-binding site (i.e., per active center) were the same for the resistant and wild-type enzyme. Sublines of mouse sarcoma have been developed with much greater degrees of methotrexate resistance than those discussed above. One cell line was resistant to 3000 times the usually effective concentration of methotrexate, and it contained 300 to 400 times the normal amount of dihydrofolate reductase.[72] In cells like these, 5% of the total protein may be represented by this one enzyme.[73]

A very thorough study of the properties of dihydrofolate reductase from methotrexate-resistant bacteria (*Diplococcus pneumoniae*) revealed two distinct types of resistance.[74] In one type, the properties of the enzyme were altered; this will be discussed later. In the other type, two different mutations mapped genetically to about the same region of the genome led to very large increases in the amount of enzyme, but there was no detectable change in its properties. The level of drug resistance was measured by determining the amount of drug required to give the same degree of growth inhibition with wild-type and resistant cells and expressing this as a ratio. The two strains were 15 and 20 times more resistant, respectively, than the wild type. The K_m values for dihydrofolate and for NADPH were the same for the enzyme from the two resistant strains as for the wild-type enzyme; the pH optimum was also the same, 7.3. The enzyme activity per milligram of cell protein (expressed as moles of dihydrofolate reduced per minute) of the two strains was 14 and 18 times greater, respectively, than that of the wild-type enzyme. Finally, because methotrexate is bound very tightly to the enzyme, the number of drug-binding sites can be measured directly by determining the maximum amount of drug that can be bound per milligram of protein in the extract. This estimate agreed remarkably well with that based upon enzyme activity; the increase was 16-fold and 22-fold, respectively, over the wild-type enzyme. It seems justifiable to conclude, therefore, in these two cases that the observed degree of resistance to methotrexate was accounted for by a comparable increase in the amount of the target enzyme per cell, without significant change in the properties of the enzyme.

Neostigmine.   An unusual example of this mechanism is the acquired resistance of a strain of *Pseudomonas* to neostigmine.[74a] This organism contains a cholinesterase. It can utilize simple sources of carbon and nitrogen (e.g., glucose and ammonia) for growth, but its growth can be made to depend upon the cholinesterase by furnishing a choline ester as sole source of carbon or nitrogen. Thus, if acetylcholine has to be utilized, the cholinesterase activity becomes rate limiting for growth. Under these conditions, neostigmine, a cholinesterase inhibitor, acted as a growth inhibitor; when choline and acetate were furnished instead of acetylcholine, neostigmine had no growth-inhibitory effect whatsoever. Mutants resistant to neostigmine were obtained. These proved to contain a greatly increased amount of cholinesterase. All the properties of the enzyme that were measured proved to be identical with those of the wild-type cholinesterase. Thus, the acquired drug resistance could be attributed to an increased amount of the target enzyme.

Steroids.   Decrease in amount of a drug receptor protein can also result in drug resistance. Glucocorticoid hormones are used in the treatment of certain tumors of lymphatic origin. In vitro, they inhibit the growth of lymphosarcoma cells and of mouse fibroblasts. Specific glucocorticoid binding proteins, present in the cytoplasm and nuclei of steroid sensitive cells, are much reduced in amount in resistant cell lines.[75] The small amount that remains appears to have normal affinities for various glucocorticoids. Similar observations have been made in steroid sensitive and resistant lymphoma cells[76] and in lymphosarcomas maintained by serial passage in mice.[77] The steroid receptor protein evidently plays no essential role in the cell economy under these conditions, since the resistant lines grow well in its virtual absence. Obviously, in the intact animal, presence of the receptor confers the property of responsiveness to the steroid hormone.

Mechanism 6. Decreased Requirement for Product of Drug-Sensitive Enzyme (Hypothetical)

This mechanism is included for the sake of completeness, since it is logically plausible, although no examples have been discovered. Consider the reaction $X \rightarrow Y$, catalyzed by an enzyme that is subject to inhibition by a drug. A certain rate of production of Y is essential to the needs of the cell; thus the drug, by inhibiting the reaction, inhibits cell growth in the wild type. One can imagine the following way for this mechanism of resistance to operate. Suppose that in the wild-type cell, Y is being degraded (or drawn off into nonessential reactions) so that its steady-state level is kept low. In other words, the rate of reaction $X \rightarrow Y$ is assumed to be considerably greater than the rate at which Y has to be synthesized to meet growth needs. Under these conditions, mutational loss of an enzyme responsible for the degradation (or diversion) of Y could result in drug resistance. For then, even when it was largely inhibited by the drug, the reaction $X \rightarrow Y$ would produce Y fast enough to satisfy growth requirements. A similar argument would apply if a mechanism developed for the more efficient utilization of Y for the growth needs of the cell. On the other hand, there is no basis for supposing that Y could become nonessential to the cell. One might argue that by mutation, the drug-sensitive enzyme could be deleted, and the cell would then use an exogenous supply of Y. But if the wild-type cell was capable of deriving Y from an exogenous source, it would not have been inhibited by the drug. The mutation, then, would have to have opened a pathway not previously operative for utilizing an exogenous metabolite. The implausibility of an "alternative metabolic pathway" as a mechanism of acquired drug resistance is discussed below (mechanism 7).

Mechanism 7. Enhanced Biochemical Mechanisms for Bypassing or Repairing the Drug-Sensitive Reaction

Because the idea of bypassing a drug-sensitive step is simple and attractive, this mechanism used to be cited as the most likely explanation for acquired drug resistance. In this elementary formulation, however, it remains hypothetical; no examples have yet come to light. In order to explain acquired drug resistance on this basis, we would have to postulate some rather special conditions. Certainly, the bypass pathway could not have been present in wild-type cells because if it were, the organism would have been drug-resistant in the first place. And if the genetic specifications for the supposed alternative pathway were not present before, they could hardly be expected to spring up, fully formed, as the result of a single mutational step. It would have to be imagined, then, that the wild type contained inactive DNA corresponding to the enzymes for the alternative pathway. Possibly the genes were present in a form that could be activated by mutation. Possibly the pathway was repressed and could be derepressed by mutation in a regulatory gene.

On the other hand, enhanced ability to repair lethal damage caused by a drug has been well established as a mechanism of acquired resistance. An example is the ability of certain bacterial strains to repair damaged DNA resulting from exposure to alkylating agents or X-irradiation. The β-chloroethylamine alkylating agents (e.g.

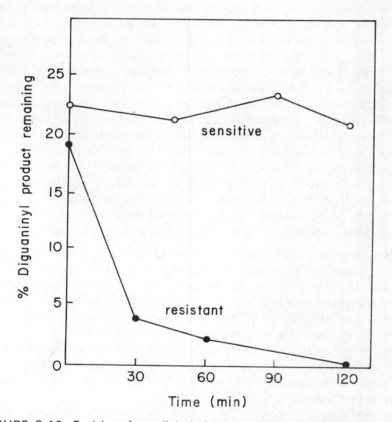

FIGURE 8-10. Excision of crosslinks in DNA treated with an alkylating agent. *Cultures of a sensitive and resistant strain of E. coli were treated briefly with ^{35}S mustard gas, a potent bifunctional akylating agent. The cultures were diluted and aerated to remove the toxic gas, then sampled at various times. DNA was extracted and hydrolyzed to remove purine residues. Diguanyl and guanine residues were separated and their radioactivity determined. The graph shows the bifunctionally alkylated guanine as a percent of total alkylated guanine, representing the degree of crosslinking of the DNA in vivo. Top curve: sensitive strain. Bottom curve: Resistant strain. (From Venitt, Figure 1.[67a])*

mechlorethamine) react with N-7 of guanine residues in DNA (p. 2). The bifunctional alkylating agents crosslink DNA sister strands, forming diguanin-7-yl derivatives joined by a $-CH_2CH_2-N(CH_3)-CH_2CH_2-$ bridge. With a sulfur mustard, the bridge contains S instead of N. Such crosslinked DNA is incapable of normal replication and strand separation. Mutant strains of *E. coli* resistant to the lethal effects of sulfur mustard were isolated. In these cells, the alkylation reactions proceeded as in sensitive strains, but repair processes were capable of excising the diguanyl residues, replacing the missing purines, and thus restoring functional DNA to the cell.[67a] This excision and repair process is a normal mechanism present in all cells; presumably it is concerned with monitoring the fidelity of DNA replication (cf. Chapter 10). The repair activity is greatly enhanced in resistant organisms as illustrated in Figure 8-10.

Mechanism 8. Decreased Affinity of Receptor for Drug

Our present understanding of the dependence of protein conformation upon amino acid sequence, and the recognition of induced allosteric modifications of protein structure, make this mechanism seem a plausible one. Random mutations in the structural gene controlling the target enzyme or other drug receptor protein result in many kinds of alteration. Some mutations may be "nonsense," interrupting the translation of the message because the altered codon corresponds to no amino acid. Other mutations may lead to gross changes in amino acid composition and sequence, as by the "frame shift" mechanism, so that no functional protein is formed. And some single amino-acid replacements are probably incompatible with the folding of the polypeptide chain into an active conformation. But a great many different amino acid substitutions will yield functional but altered proteins. From among the cells containing these altered proteins, the drug will select in favor of those with decreased affinity for the drug. That mutation in a structural gene can really result in decreased affinity for an enzyme inhibitor is well established. An example already discussed in Chapter 6 is the cholinesterase variant that is resistant to dibucaine.

***p*-Nitrobenzoic Acid.**   The first demonstration of this mechanism was accomplished years ago in whole cells by means of an elegant experiment.[27] A design was conceived that could rule out all plausible alternatives to the implication that resistance must be due to a target enzyme with altered affinity for the drug. The growth of *E. coli* is inhibited by *p*-nitrobenzoic acid (PNB), and this agent was found to compete with the utilization of two chemically similar metabolites, *p*-aminobenzoic acid (PAB) and *p*-hydroxybenzoic acid (POB). These metabolites have quite different functions in the cell, and both are required to reverse the inhibition caused by PNB. Thus, PNB evidently interacts with two distinct enzymes, a PAB enzyme and a POB enzyme. These relationships are represented in Figure 8-10.

In the experiment, wild-type cells were plated on inhibitory concentrations of PNB under two different conditions: (*1*) in the presence of PAB, and (*2*) in the presence of POB. Since both metabolites are required to overcome the action of PNB, growth was inhibited under both conditions. However, a few colonies resistant to the drug action appeared on both kinds of plate. The resistant cells isolated in the presence of PAB were still inhibited by PNB in the presence of POB, and, likewise, the cells isolated in the presence of POB were still sensitive to PNB in the presence of PAB. In other words, resistance developed independently to the two different actions—anti-PAB and anti-POB—of one and the same drug, PNB. This finding ruled out any mechanism of resistance (mechanisms 1 to 3) that depends upon decreased penetration, increased destruction, or decreased conversion of the drug, since all of the drug actions would then have been altered equally.

Sulfathiazole was known to inhibit *E. coli* growth by acting as a competitive antagonist to PAB. The corresponding hydroxy compound, phenosulfazole, was found to inhibit growth by competing with POB (see Figure 8-11). Mutants selected

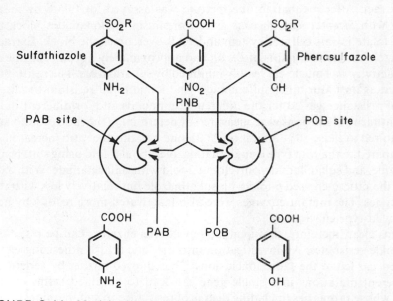

FIGURE 8-11. Model showing independent enzymes for utilization of *p*-aminobenzoic acid (PAB) and *p*-hydroxybenzoic acid (POB) in *Escherichia coli. Both enzymes are shown inhibited by p-nitrobenzoic acid (PNB), each is inhibited independently by the sulfonamides corresponding to PAB and POB, respectively. (R represents the substituted amide groupings of sulfathiazole and phenosulfazole.) (Modified from Davis and Maas, Figure 1.[27])*

for resistance to each of these compounds displayed the following behavior: The mutants resistant to sulfathiazole were not resistant to phenosulfazole. They were also not resistant to PNB even when POB was present, i.e., they were still sensitive to the anti-PAB action of PNB, despite their resistance to the anti-PAB action of sulfathiazole. The mutants resistant to phenosulfazole showed analogous properties. They were not resistant to sulfathiazole or PNB in the presence of PAB. Moreover, the mutants originally isolated on PNB also failed to show cross-resistance; neither the organism resistant to the anti-PAB action of PNB nor the one resistant to the anti-POB action of PNB was resistant to sulfathiazole or phenosulfazole. Thus, resistance at a single site can be specific for one inhibitor of that site. This finding rules out mechanisms 4 to 7. If, for example, the resistance were due to an increased concentration of the metabolite antagonizing the drug (mechanism 4), then resistance at the PAB site (or the POB site) would mean resistance to all competitive inhibitors at that same site. A similar argument applies to the other postulated mechanisms. Only mechanism 8, an altered target enzyme, is compatible with these experimental observations, for the loss of affinity resulting from a change in enzyme conformation could be specific for the chemical structure of one or another inhibitor.

Sulfonamides. The isolation of the target enzyme for sulfonamide action[78] made it possible to examine directly the question of altered enzymes in sulfonamide resistance. The synthesis of compounds with biologic activity characteristic of folic acid was studied in cell-free extracts by furnishing PAB, 2-amino-4-hydroxy-6-hydroxymethyl-dihydropteridine (the pteridine portion of the folic acid structure), ATP, Mg^{2+}, and a cell extract. After incubation, the mixture was assayed for folate by means of a bioassay with *Streptococcus faecalis* as test organism. Sulfonamides block the synthesis of folate in this cell-free system and PAB overcomes the block. Extracts from sulfathiazole-resistant mutants of *E. coli* had approximately normal enzyme activity, but this activity was much less readily inhibited by sulfathiazole. The resistant extract was tested against four other sulfonamides and found to be resistant to all, but the degree of resistance varied for the different compounds and for different mutants.[28] The quantitative alterations were measured by determining the ratio of sulfonamide to PAB required to cause 50% inhibition. With one mutant, the ratio increased some 3-fold compared to the wild type using sulfathiazole, about 5-fold using sulfabenzamide, sulfadiazine, and sulfanilamide, only about 2-fold with sulfacetamide. With a different mutant, the ratio increased 6-fold with sulfathiazole but relatively less with the other sulfonamides. The mutant enzymes were also inactivated more readily by heat than was the wild-type enzyme.

It seems clear, therefore, that qualitatively altered enzymes can be responsible for sulfonamide resistance. An investigation into the folic acid-synthesizing enzymes of *Pneumococcus* led to the same conclusions[79] but showed further by genetic analysis that different mutations in a single gene can lead to modified forms of the same enzyme, whose properties (including degree of resistance to sulfonamides) are altered in individually distinctive ways.

Antifolic Drugs. In the study of methotrexate resistance in bacteria in which increased amounts of dihydrofolate reductase were found (p. 539), some of the mutant strains were shown to have qualitatively different enzyme.[74] Strain R5 is a good example. This mutant had a resistance level 40 times greater than the wild type. The activity of dihydrofolate reductase in extracts was almost identical with that of the wild type, and the K_m values for dihydrofolate and for NADPH were nearly the same as those of the wild-type enzyme. However, the affinity of this enzyme for methotrexate was drastically reduced; indeed, the apparent mode of inhibition was changed from noncompetitive to competitive. This is illustrated in Figure 8-12. The velocity of the dihydrofolate reduction was measured at various substrate concentrations in the absence and presence of methotrexate, and the results were plotted by the double-reciprocal method (p. 85). The wild-type enzyme and the resistant mutant R6 both yielded straight lines intersecting on the x axis, typical of noncompetitive inhibition. The result for R5 was quite different. The methotrexate concentration had to be increased more than 10-fold in order to inhibit the reaction sufficiently; then the lines intersected on the y axis, as is typical of competitive inhibition. Further investigation of this enzyme revealed that the pH optimum was 0.6 units lower than that of the wild-type enzyme. The heat stability of this enzyme was indistinguishable from that of the wild type, but another resistant mutant yielded enzyme with reduced affinity for

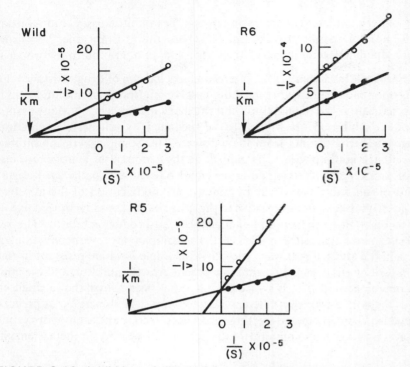

FIGURE 8-12. Inhibition of dihydrofolate reductase activity in extracts of wild-type and methotrexate-resistant cells. *Several mutant strains of Diplococcus pneumoniae were studied. Double-reciprocal plots are shown in the customary way, reciprocal substrate concentration (dihydrofolate) on the x axis, reciprocal velocity (moles dihydrofolate reduced per minute) on the y axis. At upper left, wild-type extract; upper right, extract from resistant mutant R6; at bottom, extract from resistant mutant R5. Solid circles, reaction in the absence of methotrexate; open circles, with methotrexate, 3.2 × 10⁻¹⁰ M for wild and R5, 6.45 × 10⁻⁹ M for R5. (Adapted from Sirotnak et al., Figures 1 and 2.*[74])

drug, shift to competitive inhibition, altered pH optimum, and markedly increased rate of heat inactivation at 45°.

Species differences in the properties of dihydrofolate reductase afford the basis for the chemotherapeutic efficacy of pyrimethamine, an important antimalarial. The enzyme from plasmodia does not differ greatly from that of mammalian tissues with respect to affinity for methotrexate, but the plasmodial enzyme is hundreds of times more sensitive to inhibition by pyrimethamine than are the mammalian enzymes.[80] Variants of *Plasmodium berghei* (mouse malaria), which were resistant to pyrimethamine, were isolated. Dihydrofolate reductase from this source was found to be increased in activity for the normal substrate and decreased in affinity for pyrimethamine. The increased activity could have been due either to more enzyme or to a higher turnover of substrate at each catalytic site. This question was resolved by titrating with methotrexate, which is bound so tightly that it can be used to estimate the number of sites. It was shown that the number of sites was increased in the resistant enzyme to exactly the same extent as the total activity, i.e., that the turnover number was the same as in the wild-type enzyme. There were also marked differences in the binding of pyrimethamine by the two enzymes. The inhibitor dissociation constant was about 0.3 nM for the sensitive strain, 14 nM for the resistant one.[81] Resistance is, therefore, due both to an increase in enzyme and an alteration in its properties.

"False Feedback Inhibitors." An interesting mechanism of drug resistance that also depends upon modified enzyme structure involves end-product inhibition, an important mechanism in the regulation of intermediary metabolism.[24] Many instances of end-product inhibition are known to be mediated by allosteric interactions, the allosteric site being distinct from the substrate site. Some growth inhibitors act as "false feedback inhibitors," i.e., by mimicking the action of the endogenous feedback inhibitor and thereby shutting off an essential biosynthetic pathway. Resistance to this kind of inhibition can occur by mutational modification of the allosteric site. Thus, the enzyme becomes insensitive to the drug; but at the same time, it may lose its ability to respond to the normal endogenous end-product inhibitor. The result is drug resistance if the cell can survive the accompanying overproduction of end-products in the affected pathway. The classic example is valine resistant in *E. coli*.[82] In strain K12 of this organism, valine is a potent growth inhibitor, and the inhibition is overcome noncompetitively by isoleucine. It has been shown that a single enzyme catalyzes the synthesis of two different α-acetohydroxy acids serving as precursors to valine and isoleucine, respectively; these are α-acetolactate and acetohydroxybutyrate. Valine acts as a feedback inhibitor of the acetohydroxy acid synthetase enzyme:

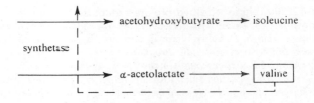

The enzyme has been isolated from valine-resistant mutants and shown to be resistant to valine inhibition, although in the absence of valine the rate of formation of product was the same as in the wild type. In general, mutational modification of an allosteric site can occur without any change in the substrate site; indeed, these sites are often on physically distinct subunits of an oligomeric enzyme molecule.

Tryptophan acts as a feedback inhibitor of its own synthesis by blocking a step in the conversion of shikimic acid 5-phosphate to anthranilic acid,[83] as illustrated in Figure 8-13. The amino acid analog 5-methyltryptophan (also shown in the figure) mimics the feedback inhibition caused by tryptophan and thus shuts off tryptophan synthesis. Since the analog cannot be utilized for protein synthesis, it is a growth-inhibitory drug. Mutants of *E. coli* were selected for resistance to the growth inhibition caused by 5-methyltryptophan. Extracts of these mutants were compared with wild-type extracts in a cell-free system for the conversion of shikimic acid phosphate to anthranilic acid in the presence of glutamine (as amino group donor), Mg^{2+}, and NAD. Results are shown in Figure 8-14. The concentration-dependent inhibition of anthranilic acid synthesis by both tryptophan and 5-methyltryptophan is apparent in the wild-type extract. The resistant extract shows a greatly diminished sensitivity not only to inhibition by 5-methyltryptophan but also to inhibition by tryptophan.

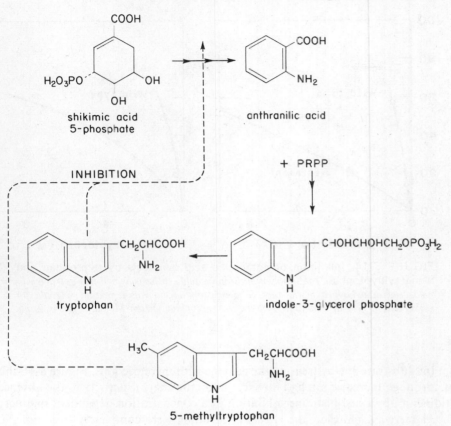

FIGURE 8-13. Feedback inhibition by tryptophan and 5-methyltryptophan. *The pathway of tryptophan biosynthesis is shown, from shikimic acid. Shikimic acid is a branch point, serving also as precursor to other aromatic metabolites. Compound arrows indicate intermediary reactions not shown. The site of feedback inhibition is one of the steps in the conversion of shikimic acid phosphate to anthranilic acid. (After Meister.[84])*

A by-product of the acquired resistance to the 5-methyl analog was, therefore, loss of regulatory control by tryptophan and a consequent overproduction of that amino acid and its excretion into the medium.

A similar example of acquired resistance to a feedback inhibitor concerns 2-thiazolealanine, an analog of histidine.[85] In a manner similar to that described for tryptophan, histidine regulates its own synthesis by inhibiting an early reaction, in this case the coupling of adenosine triphosphate (ATP) with ribose phosphate derived from 5-phosphoribosyl-1-pyrophosphate (PRPP). This feedback inhibition is illustrated in Figure 8-15. The phosphoribosyltransferase that catalyzes this reaction is specifically inhibited by histidine and also by 2-thiazolealanine. Growth inhibition is the consequence of the resulting histidine deficiency. The inhibition of histidine synthesis, either by histidine itself or by its analog, is noncompetitive with respect to the substrates (ATP, PRPP), and the inhibitory site can be distinguished clearly

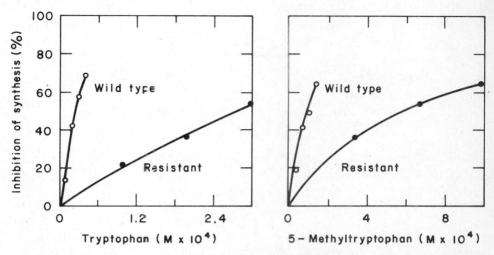

FIGURE 8-14. Inhibition of anthranilic acid synthesis by tryptophan and 5-methyltryptophan. *Inhibition of anthranilic acid synthesis by cell-free extracts was measured as described in the text. The resistant strain was a mutant selected for resistance to growth inhibition by 5-methyltryptophan. (From Moyed, Figures 2 and 3.[83])*

from the substrate site by treating the enzyme with mercuric ions. Figure 8-16 shows that, although mercuric ion had no effect upon the enzyme activity in the absence of histidine, it abolished histidine inhibition in a concentration-dependent manner; at 10^{-5} M mercuric chloride, the effects of histidine were completely overcome. This could not have been due to a complexing of histidine by mercuric ion inasmuch as there was a 100-fold excess of histidine. Thorough removal of mercuric ions by means of a sulfhydryl compound was found to restore the sensitivity of the enzyme to inhibition by histidine. Thus, the feedback inhibition is evidently brought about by combination of histidine (or 2-thiazolealanine) at an allosteric site.

A resistant mutant of *Escherichia coli* was isolated by the usual selection procedures. The phosphoribosyltransferase of these cells was found no longer to be sensitive to inhibition, either by 2-thiazolealanine or by histidine. Presumably, a mutation had altered the allosteric site or had affected the mode of interaction of the enzyme subunits so that allosteric inhibition was no longer possible. The mutant, therefore, not only grows despite the presence of the inhibitor but also overproduces histidine and excretes it into the culture medium.

In addition to this genetic mechanism of resistance to 2-thiazolealanine, an interesting phenotypic resistance has been demonstrated.[85] Histidine biosynthesis

FIGURE 8-15. Feedback inhibition by histidine and 2-thiazolealanine. *The pathway of histidine biosynthesis is shown. Compound arrows indicate intermediate steps not shown. The site of feedback inhibition by histidine or by its analog, 2-thiazolealanine, is the adenosine triphosphate phosphoribosyltransferase, which catalyzes addition of the phosphoribosyl moiety to ATP. Carbon atoms of ribose, nitrogen and carbon atoms from adenine, and nitrogen from glutamine form the imidazole ring. (After Smith and Ames.[86])*

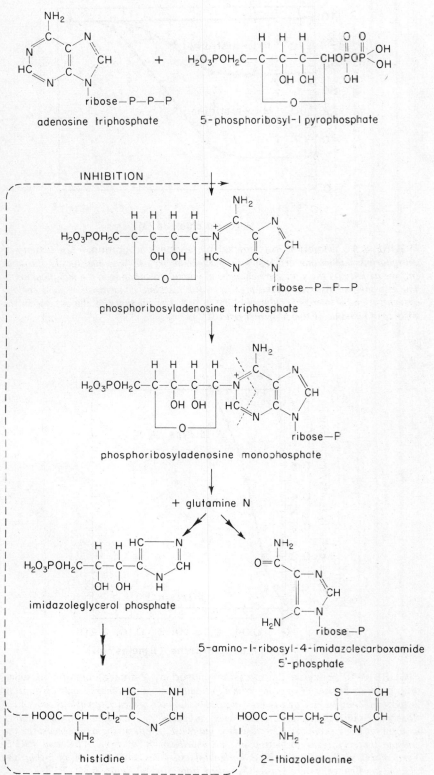

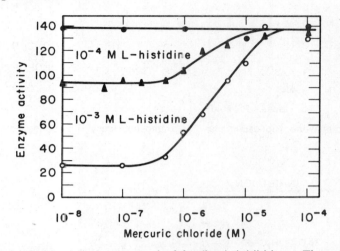

FIGURE 8-16. Mercuric ion reversal of feedback inhibition. *The activity of phosphoribosyladenosine triphosphate pyrophosphorylase was measured; units of enzyme activity on the y axis are changes in optical absorbancy in a 4 min incubation. The enzyme was assayed in the presence of 2 histidine concentrations and various concentrations of mercuric chloride. Line at top shows activity of the enzyme in the absence of histidine. (From Martin, Figure 9.[87])*

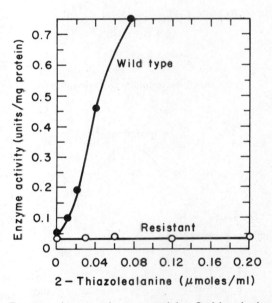

FIGURE 8-17. Enzyme derepression caused by 2-thiazolealanine in wild-type cells of *Escherichia coli*. *Wild-type cells and a mutant strain resistant to 2-thiazolealanine were grown to the same cell mass in the presence of various concentrations of 2-thiazolealanine. Extracts were prepared and assayed for their ability to form an early product in the histidine pathway. In effect, the assay measures the enzyme that catalyzes formation of phosphoribosyl-ATP from ATP and PRPP. Vertical axis gives enzyme activity; horizontal axis gives concentrations of 2-thiazolealanine in which cells were grown. (Modified from Moyed, Figure 6.[85])*

is regulated not only by feedback inhibition but also by end-product repression of some of the biosynthetic enzymes in the pathway. Under certain conditions, especially at low concentrations of 2-thiazolealanine, wild-type cells undergo the following adaptation. The histidine deficiency caused by the "false feedback inhibition" releases the enzymes from repression and an increased rate of enzyme synthesis ensues. Thus, the target enzyme upon which the inhibitor acts is greatly increased in amount. Despite the continued presence of the inhibitor, conversion of substrate to product now proceeds at a rate sufficient to meet the histidine needs of the cell and growth is resumed. Figure 8-17 illustrates the considerable increase in enzyme level in the wild type in the presence of 2-thiazolealanine. No such effect is to be expected in the genetically resistant strain and none occurs.

Rifampicin.   This antibiotic is one of several rifamycins derived from *Streptomyces*, which inhibit synthesis of bacterial RNA. They bind to bacterial RNA polymerase but not to the mammalian enzyme. RNA polymerase is a complex enzyme, composed of several subunits. It catalyzes the polymerization of nucleoside triphosphates into RNA, utilizing DNA as template. Rifampicin blocks the initiation of RNA synthesis, but not its continuation, through an interaction with the β subunit of the polymerase.[87a] Rifampicin resistant strains of *E. coli* contain RNA polymerase with altered physical properties, which neither binds rifampicin nor is inhibited by it.[88,88a] That the β subunit and not the σ factor of RNA polymerase is altered in rifampicin resistance was shown in a crossover in vitro experiment summarized in Table 8-2. The β subunit

TABLE 8-2. Sensitivity of RNA polymerase components to rifampicin. The assay mixture contained DNA from T4 phage or calf thymus (CT), unlabelled GTP, CTP, and UTP, Mg^{2+}, and an ATP generating system, radioactive AMP, and the β and/or σ components of RNA polymerase derived from rifampicin sensitive (s) or resistant (r) *E. coli*. Incubations were carried out for 10 min at 30°, following which the radioactivity incorporated into RNA was measured. (Modified from Di Mauro et al., Table 1.[88])

Polymerase component	DNA	CPM incorporated	
		without rifampicin	with rifampicin
β_s	T4	18	
	CT	770	5
β_r	T4	80	
	CT	1370	520
σ_s	T4	2	
σ_r	T4	9	
$\sigma_s + \beta_s$	T4	1480	13
$\sigma_s + \beta_r$	T4	1840	780
$\sigma_r + \beta_s$	T4	1220	14
$\sigma_r + \beta_r$	T4	2190	1026

(core enzyme) alone is inactive with T4 phage DNA but functions well with calf thymus DNA. Synthesis by β from rifampicin sensitive strains is inhibited by the antibiotic, whereas β from resistant strains is resistant in vitro. The σ component was inactive alone, whether derived from sensitive or resistant strains. With T4 DNA, a combination of σ and β components yielded good synthesis. Complete inhibition by rifampicin occurred only when β from sensitive cells was present; with β from resistant cells, the polymerase activity was resistant to inhibition. Thus, rifampicin resistance can be attributed to a mutant, altered form of the β subunit of RNA polymerase.

ANTIBACTERIAL AGENTS THAT INHIBIT PROTEIN SYNTHESIS

Several antibacterial agents act by altering the function of ribosomes in protein synthesis.[89,90] Mutant modifications in the protein synthesis system provide the basis for resistance to erythromycin, spectinomycin, streptomycin, and the tetracyclines.

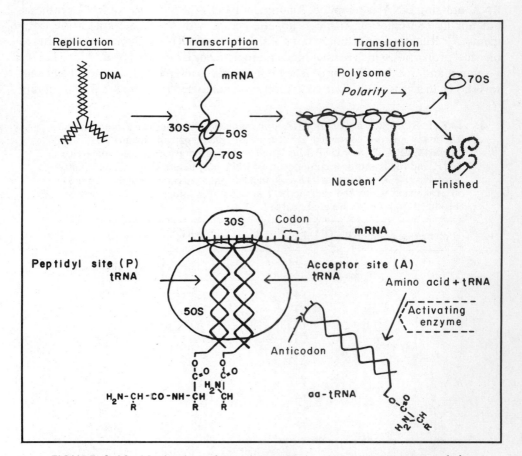

FIGURE 8-18. Mechanism of protein synthesis. *At top, transcriptions of the genetic message, and attachment of ribosomes to messenger-RNA. These may attach and begin translation of the message before transcription is completed. Nascent proteins are shown as hanging free from the ribosomes. At bottom, a magnified view of events on the single ribosome. The configuration of transfer-RNA is, in reality, more complex than represented here. (From Das et al., Figure 12.[92])*

The first stage of protein synthesis in prokaryotic cells is the formation of an initiation complex. The initial (N-terminal) amino acid is formylmethionine (fMet), which is activated by a synthetase enzyme to form an aminoacyl-transfer RNA, using the specific tRNA for fMet. The fMet-tRNA then combines with a 30S ribosomal subunit attached to a messenger RNA (mRNA) strand. The initiation codon, AUG, on the mRNA is matched by the complementary anticodon on the tRNA. At the initiation stage, fMet-tRNA is probably held in the peptidyl binding site (P) of the ribosome. Subsequently, incoming aminoacyl-tRNA molecules bind at another site, the acceptor site (A). The process is shown in Figure 8-18.

Three protein initiation factors (IF-1, IF-2, IF-3) and GTP are required in the formation of the completed initiation complex. IF-1 and IF-2 seem to be involved in the initial binding to the 30S ribosomal subunit, while IF-3 may be required for the association of the 50S subunit to form a complete 70S ribosome. Thus the initiation complex consists of the 70S ribosome, fMet-tRNA, and mRNA.

Chain elongation begins with entry of a second aminoacyl-tRNA into the A site. Which amino acid this will be is determined by the anticodon portion of its tRNA, which recognizes the base triplet of mRNA that is positioned at the A site, as determined by the genetic code (Table 8-3).[91] Insertion of aminoacyl-tRNA into the A

TABLE 8-3. The genetic code.
Each triplet codon is shown with its 5'-terminal nucleotide to the left, 3'-terminal to the right. The codons are translated from left to right. (Modified from H. A. Sober.[99])

UUU } Phe UUC	UCU UCC } Ser UCA UCG	UAU } Tyr UAC	UGU } Cys UGC
UUA } Lue UUG		UAA } stop UAG	UGA stop UGG Trp
CUU CUC } Leu CUA CUG	CCU CCC } Pro CCA CCG	CAU } His CAC CAA } Gln CAG	CGU CGC } Arg CGA CGG
AUU AUC } Ile AUA AUG Met, fMet	ACU ACC } Thr ACA ACG	AAU } Asn AAC AAA } Lys AAG	AGU } Ser AGC AGA } Arg AGG
GUU GUC } Val GUA GUG	GCU GCC } Ala GCA GCG	GAU } Asp GAC GAA } Glu GAG	GGU GGC } Gly GGA GGG

site (the codon recognition reaction) is mediated by another protein factor (elongation factor EF-Tu), and GTP is again required. A second elongation factor (EF-Ts) is required to regenerate EF-Tu. The first 2 amino acids are now adjacent to each other on the surface of the 50S portion of the ribosome, the anticodons of their respective tRNA molecules opposite their codons on the mRNA. A peptidyl transferase (one of the 20 or more proteins of the 50S ribosomal subunit) then forms a peptide bond between the free $-NH_2$ group of the amino acid in the A site and the $-COOH$ group of the amino acid in the P site, simultaneously cleaving the ester linkage to the terminal adenosine 3'-hydroxyl of the tRNA. A third elongation factor (EF-G) and

GTP are required in the next steps. The deacylated tRNA is released from the P site, and the newly formed peptidyl-tRNA moves from the A site to the P site, freeing the A site for the next aminoacyl-tRNA. At the same time, the ribosome moves an amount equal to 3 bases (about 10A) relative to the mRNA, bringing the next codon into position for recognition. This translocation of the ribosome and its nascent protein chain is in the direction defined by the polarity of the mRNA; phosphodiester bonds link the 5'-hydroxyl group of each ribose residue to the 3'-hydroxyl group of the adjacent ribose residue. Thus, at one end of the polynucleotide chain is a free 5'-hydroxyl, at the other end a free 3'-hydroxyl. The ribosomes move in the direction 5' → 3' as they translate the genetic message[93] and the nascent protein elongates at its —COOH end.[94]

Elongation continues until a termination codon (UAA, UAG, or UGA) is reached on the mRNA. Three release factors are known. A terminating tRNA, with an appropriate anticodon for one of the terminating codons, enters the A site. The completed protein is released from the ribosome, and the mRNA is detached at the same time. A new round of protein synthesis can begin if a 30S ribosomal subunit complexes with the mRNA. The same message is translated by a number of ribosomes in tandem (polysomes), as shown in Figure 8-18.

Complete primary base sequences of many tRNA molecules have been worked out, and considerable information is available about the higher order structures.[95,96] Figure 8-19 shows the elementary structure of alanine tRNA from yeast.[97,98] The occurrence at a central position of these and other tRNA molecules of a base triplet complementary to the known codon for the appropriate amino acid makes the anticodon hypothesis inescapable. Thus, for example, a codon assignment for alanine had been known to be GCC. The expected anticodon (written in the direction 3' → 5') would therefore be CGG, and the sequence CGI actually appears at the middle loop of alanine tRNA. The base-pairing properties of I (hypoxanthine) are similar to those of G (guanine). Similarly, UAC is a codon for tyrosine, and the complementary sequence AΨG is found in the same position in the middle loop of tyrosine tRNA. Ψ (pseudouracil) has the same base-pairing properties as U (uracil). The tRNA's are particularly rich in unusual bases, which are formed by modification of the four normal bases after polymerization. They may function to protect the small tRNA's from attack by endogenous nuclease enzymes.

Erythromycin. This macrolide antibiotic binds to the 50S ribosomal subunit from bacteria. Although it is structurally unrelated to chloramphenicol, it interferes with the binding of chloramphenicol to this subunit. The 50S subunits from an erythromycin resistant strain of *E. coli* did not bind the antibiotic. The proteins from 30S and 50S subunits were studied by prelabeling them through growth of the cells in medium containing a radioactive amino acid. Sensitive cells were grown in ³H-lysine medium, resistant cells in ¹⁴C-lysine. Samples of the ribosomal proteins from each strain were mixed and chromatographed on a carboxymethyl cellulose column. All the proteins from 30S ribosomes had the same ratio ¹⁴C to ³H. But of the 21 proteins from the 50S subunit, one from the resistant strain appeared in a different position in the elution diagram. Presumably, this was the protein that had undergone a mutational change responsible for the inability to bind erythromycin, thus conferring erythromycin resistance.[101] Another type of erythromycin resistance is apparently due to modification of the 28S RNA component of the 50S ribosomal

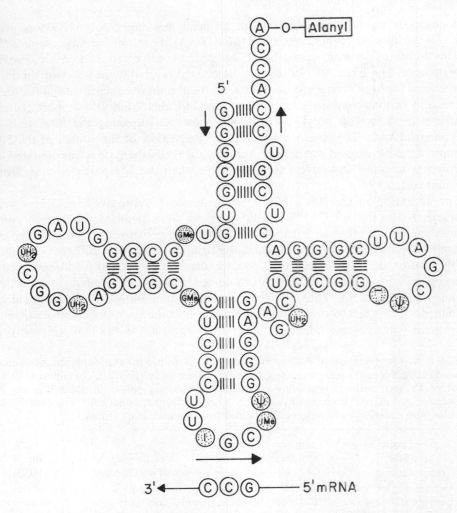

FIGURE 8-19. Nucleotide sequence of alanine transfer RNA. *The typical loop structure of tRNA molecules is shown. Amino acid attaches to terminal adenosine 3'-OH through an ester linkage. Anticodon loop is shown at bottom, aligned with an Ala codon of mRNA. Unusual bases are shown shaded.* ψ = *pseudouridine; I* = *inosine; UH$_2$* = *dihydrouridine; T* = *ribothymidine; GMe* = *methyl guanosine; GMe$_2$* = *dimethyl guanosine; IMe* = *methyl inosine. (From Watson, Figure 12-2.*[00])

subunit by formation of N6-dimethyladenine, not present in 28S RNA from sensitive strains.[101a]

Streptomycin. The antibiotic belongs to the group of aminoglycosides that includes spectinomycin, neomycin, kanamycin, gentamicin, and paromomycin. Chromosomal resistance in this group has been traced to alterations of a single protein in the 30S ribosomal subunit.

A major effect of streptomycin is to inhibit bacterial protein synthesis at the initiation stage by preventing elongation of the initiation complex (fMet + tRNA + 70S ribosome).[102] In vitro, protein synthesis directed by artificial polynucleotide messengers is partially inhibited; when artificial messenger polyAUG was used (AUG is the initiation codon, specifying fMet-tRNA), the inhibition was complete.[103]

The binding of streptomycin to the 30S subunit has been demonstrated in crossover experiments. The bacterial ribosome is dissociated reversibly into its two subunits by reducing the Mg^{2+} concentration. Mixtures of subunits from sensitive and resistant bacteria in various combinations could be tested for their ability to support protein synthesis in vitro with polyU as artificial messenger, directing the formation of polyphenylalanine. The results were clearcut. Regardless of the source of the 50S subunit, if the 30S subunit was derived from sensitive cells, the system was inhibited by streptomycin; but streptomycin was ineffective when the 30S particles came from resistant cells.[104]

The alteration in the 30S subunit responsible for streptomycin resistance was characterized as follows:[105,106] The 30S particles were dissociated into their component proteins (more than 20) and a 16S RNA. The proteins were fractionated on phosphocellulose. One of these, designated P10, appeared at very different positions on the elution diagram, depending upon whether it was derived from sensitive or resistant cells. Functional 30S particles could be reconstituted by mixing the purified proteins and 16S RNA. Thus, the role of each protein and of the RNA could be examined with respect to streptomycin binding, ribosome assembly in vitro, capacity for protein synthesis, and fidelity of translation. Table 8-4 shows that streptomycin

TABLE 8-4. Identification of P10 as the protein responsible for streptomycin resistance. Amino acid incorporation into protein was studied in two in vitro systems, one containing f2 RNA (in which Val incorporation was followed), the other containing polyU (in which Phe was incorporated). s = derived from sensitive cells; r = derived from resistant cells. The control 30S particles were undissociated ribosomes. (Modified from Nomura *et al.*, Table 3.[105])

Origin of proteins used for reconstitution		Inhibition of amino acid incorporation by Sm (%)		Relative degree of misreading of poly U message (%)	Binding of ^{3}H-DHSm (Relative values)
All except P10	P10	f2 RNA ^{14}C-valine	poly U- ^{14}C-phenylalanine		
s	s	74	35	(100)	(100)
s	r	10	7	8	5
r	r	3	4	3	5
r	s	78	35	(100)	(100)
Control 30 S (s)		69	45	(100)	(100)
Control 30 S (r)		10	2	7	4

sensitivity and the ability to bind streptomycin are uniquely associated with the P10 protein. The first column gives the source of all proteins other than P10 (sensitive, s, or resistant, r); the second column gives the source of P10. When P10 was derived from sensitive cells, the in vitro incorporation directed by f2 RNA (containing initiation codon AUG) was markedly inhibited by streptomycin; polyU-directed phenylalanine incorporation was also inhibited but not as strongly. When P10 was derived from resistant cells, there was little inhibition in either system. Misreading (see p. 557) was also associated with sensitive P10. Finally, the binding of ^{3}H-dihydrostreptomycin was greatly reduced in the presence of resistant P10. It was also shown that, in the complete absence of P10, initiation (as judged by f2 RNA-directed Val or fMet incorporation) was very poor, polyU-directed phenylalanine incorporation was only moderately decreased, and streptomycin neither inhibited protein synthesis nor induced misreading.

Very similar results were obtained with *tetracycline* and with *spectinomycin*, which also interact with 30S ribosomal subunits.[107,108,108a] An experiment with spectinomycin is shown in Figure 8-20. Here resistance was shown to be due to mutational change in a different 30S ribosomal protein, P4. A spectinomycin-sensitive strain of *E. coli* was grown in ^{3}H-lysine and a resistant strain in ^{14}C-lysine. The proteins extracted from the 30S particles were fractionated on a carboxymethyl cellulose column. The modified mutant form of P4 is evident at the left of the elution diagram.

The correct assembly of every protein in the cell according to the specifications of the genetic code (the translation of the genetic message) depends upon a high degree of fidelity in the matching of anticodon to codon. The structure of the 30S ribosome, which provides a matrix for this matching process, plays an important role in assuring this fidelity. As already indicated, the P10 ribosomal protein, which is concerned in the binding of streptomycin, is essential in this process. In the presence of streptomycin, ribosomes from streptomycin-sensitive cells bind the drug in such a way that the specific codon-anticodon interactions are distorted.[109-111] Thus, the "wrong" tRNA is permitted, at a fairly high frequency, to enter site A, and consequently the "wrong" amino acid is incorporated into the nascent protein. This misreading effect, in a cell-free system, is illustrated in Table 8-5. Under the experimental conditions

TABLE 8-5. Misreading of codons caused by streptomycin.

The cell-free system contained an extract of streptomycin-sensitive *Escherichia coli* supplemented with excess transfer-RNA. Reaction mixture contained: $12.5\,mM$ Mg^{2+}; polyuridylic acid (polyU), $10\,\mu g$ per $0.25\,ml$; polycytidylic acid (polyC), $15\,\mu g$ to $20\,\mu g$ per $0.25\,ml$. Incorporation into acid-insoluble material (protein) was measured. The control incorporation of *Phe* (set equal to 100) was 500 pmoles, that of *Pro* was 200 pmoles. (Data of Davies et al.[109] Tables 2 and 3.)

	Control	Streptomycin (4 μg/ml)
polyU		
Phe	100	60
Leu	5	10
Ile	8	30
Ser	4	20
Tyr	26	38
polyC		
Pro	100	230
His	1	12
Thr	17	41
Leu	1	3
Ala	1	4
Ser		55

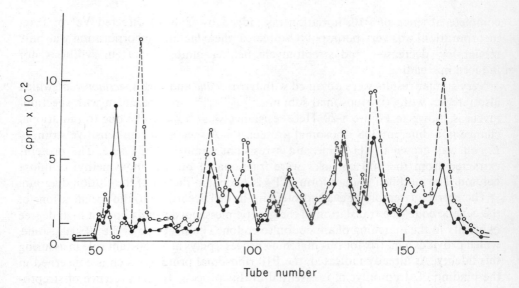

FIGURE 8-20. Altered form of ribosomal protein P4 in spectinomycin resistance. *Sensitive E coli were grown in ^{3}H-lysine, resistant mutant in ^{14}C-lysine. Proteins from 30S ribosomal subunits were extracted, mixed, and chromatographed on carboxymethylcellulose. Broken line = ^{3}H radioactivity; solid line = ^{14}C radioactivity. (From Bollen et al., Figure 5.[107])*

employed, phenylalanine was principally incorporated when polyU was used as messenger (UUU is the codon for *Phe*); there was also significant incorporation of tyrosine, very little of leucine, isoleucine, or serine. Addition of streptomycin reduced the incorporation of *Phe* as already shown, but it greatly increased the incorporation of *Leu*, *Ile*, and *Ser*. When polyC was used as messenger (CCC is the codon for *Pro*), streptomycin caused an increase in the incorporation of proline rather than an inhibition; but there was a dramatic and disproportionate increase in the incorporation of serine and histidine. The pattern that emerges from these misreadings of the genetic code appears in most cases to be a disturbance in the reading of the base in the 5'-position in the codon, but sometimes the base in the middle position is affected. The experimental observations in Table 8-5 are understandable by reference to the genetic code (Table 8-3) on the premise that the binding of streptomycin to the 30S ribosome subunit distorts the fit between tRNA and mRNA so that normal hydrogen bonding distances are altered. Thus, we might have UUU (*Phe*) read as though it were AUU (*Ile*), CUU (*Leu*), or UCU (*Ser*); or CCC (*Pro*) read as though it were UCC (*Ser*), CAC (*His*), and so on. Numerous misreadings in vivo would lead to the insertion of many wrong amino acids or even to the premature termination of nascent protein chains (e.g., by misreading of an amino acid codon as a terminating triplet UAG, UGA, or UAA). Clearly, normal protein synthesis would be completely disrupted and cell death would probably result.

A rare kind of acquired drug resistance is that known as *drug dependence*. Here the cells not only tolerate a growth-inhibitory drug but specifically require that drug for their growth. The phenomenon has been described for chloramphenicol and for isoniazid; the best-known and best-understood instance is streptomycin dependence.

Streptomycin-dependent strains of bacteria can be isolated on medium containing the drug by the usual procedures for selecting resistant mutants. On subculture, these organisms will grow only in the presence of streptomycin or very closely related congeners. The specificity of the requirement for streptomycin suggested that the drug must have played some directive role in the development of the dependent state, for it was hard to imagine that a specific requirement for a foreign substance could develop spontaneously. Nevertheless, it was shown conclusively by the replica plating technique[112] that streptomycin dependence arises by spontaneous mutation. Despite the superficial similarity to physical dependence in higher organisms (Chapter 9), this phenomenon has essentially the same genetic basis as the more usual kind of acquired drug resistance. Streptomycin sensitivity, various degrees of resistance, and dependence are determined by alleles of a single genetic locus.[113] A widespread misconception persists that dependence is an extreme form of resistance, that a cell becomes "more and more resistant and eventually becomes dependent." This is not correct. A sensitive cell may become resistant or dependent by a single mutational step.

Evidence that the misreading of the genetic message induced by streptomycin underlies the phenomenon of streptomycin dependence comes from experiments on phenotypic suppression.[114,115] Among certain strains of streptomycin-resistant bacteria, it has been possible to select for mutations that are suppressible by streptomycin. A concrete example will illustrate. An arginine-requiring mutant was isolated from a strain of *E. coli* with moderate resistance to streptomycin. The mutant was completely lacking in active ornithine transcarbamylase, the enzyme converting ornithine to citrulline in the biosynthetic pathway leading to arginine. Naturally, the organism was able to grown when arginine was supplied. However, it was also able to grow when streptomycin was furnished in appropriate concentration, regardless of whether arginine was present or not. When grown on streptomycin, the cells produced active ornithine transcarbamylase, i.e., the effects of the mutation were suppressed. Mating experiments showed that the site of the suppressible mutation was indeed in the ornithine transcarbamylase structural gene. Phenotypic suppression could also be demonstrated in streptomycin-sensitive organisms, provided very low concentrations of the drug were employed.

The interpretation of phenotypic suppression by streptomycin is as follows: The mutation in the structural gene had resulted in an altered codon specifying an amino acid replacement at a particular position in the sequence, which was not compatible with a functional state of the protein. Alternatively, the altered codon might specify termination ("nonsense"). By inducing misreading, streptomycin then caused the defective codon to be read in a tolerable way (i.e., as an amino acid compatible with enzyme function) with a certain frequency, and so a partial repair of the defective protein was effected. A hypothetical example, based upon the information in Table 8-3 and Table 8-5, may be cited. Suppose a triplet UCC, coding for serine in the wild-type enzyme, had mutated to CCC by a U → C transition (cf. p. 624). Then, in the mutant organism, proline is inserted at that position instead of serine, producing (let us assume) a protein that is unable to fold into the correct tertiary configuration and is therefore inactive. Streptomycin induces the misreading of CCC as serine with a high frequency (Table 8-5), and thus the correct amino acid will be inserted sometimes in the mutant organism. Some functional enzyme molecules will be formed, and some growth will occur in the presence of streptomycin. The misreading effect, of course, is rather general, so the partial restoration of activity of the mutated enzyme is accompanied by reduced activity of other enzymes.[116,117]

Mutants of the kind described above are classified as "conditionally streptomycin dependent" because a metabolite can substitute for streptomycin in supporting growth.[118] Streptomycin seems to act in its usual way (inducing misreading) when it remedies the phenotypic defect caused by the mutation. It is assumed that in the classical type of streptomycin dependence, where only the drug itself is effective, the P10 ribosomal protein has been altered in such a way that misreading occurs in the absence of drug, to an extent that disrupts protein synthesis completely. Then binding of streptomycin to the defective 30S particle would restore a more normal configuration, permit a higher frequency of correct codon-anticodon interactions, and thereby permit cell growth to occur.

SELECTION OF DRUG-RESISTANT CELLS IN ANIMALS AND MAN

To what extent might selection of resistant cells play a role in the development of drug tolerance in animals and man? Such a mechanism would presumably be operative only in tissues characterized by a high rate of cell renewal, in which a drug-resistant or drug-dependent variant could generate a clone sufficiently large to replace an original drug-sensitive cell population. Such tissues are principally the blood-forming elements of bone marrow, the gastrointestinal epithelium, male germinal cells, embryonic tissues, and neoplasms.[119]

Tolerance to massive acute hemolysis produced by primaquine after the initial occurrence could be thought of as resulting from a selection mechanism, although no resistant mutants are involved. In individuals who are genetically prone to react in this way (p. 455), the older erythrocites are sensitive, the younger cells are resistant. The first dose of primaquine therefore wipes out the older cell population, and the individual is then tolerant to further doses. If a regular dosage schedule is maintained, a certain small fraction of the total erythrocyte population will be lysed every day as new cells come of age; but massive acute hemolysis will not be manifested again unless primaquine is first discontinued for long enough to permit re-establishment of the normal age distribution of the erythrocyte population.

According to the clonal selection theory of immunologic tolerance,[120] mutation and selection underlie the development of a person's immunologic reactivity and his ability to recognize and not reject his own proteins. Lymphoid cells of the embryo become specialized, through mutation, for the production of a variety of immunoglobulins; each cell synthesizes one such antibody protein. Exposure to endogenous antigens during fetal development is postulated to cause the elimination of all those cells whose antibodies would interact with these antigens. As a reult of this selection process, the cells that remain resistant (in a sense) to endogenous proteins stand ready to be stimulated by foreign antigens during postfetal life.[121] When this occurs, they proliferate and thus greatly increase the production of particular antibodies. As suggested already in connection with the discussion of drug allergy (Chapter 7), it may be possible that exposure to a drug during fetal life confers protection in later life against that drug's producing an allergic response.

Neoplasmas that have a rapid growth rate might be expected to provide good examples of the mutation-selection process in the origin of drug resistance.[122] This is true of transplantable leukemia and ascitic carcinoma of mice; instances of acquired resistance to antifolic compounds, purine analogs, and glucocorticoids have been presented earlier in this chapter. But acquired resistance of leukemia or of a solid malignant neoplasm to drug therapy may have complex causes. Sometimes, although the disease becomes refractory, the cancer cells themselves may show little or no evidence of drug resistance. In one experiment,[123] mice were inoculated with leukemia cells and then treated with methotrexate. These animals survived about twice as long as untreated controls, but they died despite continuous drug therapy. Leukemia cells obtained from such animals at death and reinjected into fresh mice were found to be sensitive to methotrexate. Thus, the cause of death was certainly not the emergence of a drug-resistant mutant line of leukemia cells. Only after repeated animal passage in the presence of methotrexate was it possible to obtain a population of drug-resistant cells that would be indifferent to methotrexate when innoculated into fresh animals.

Figure 8-21 shows an experiment[124] in which ascites tumor cells were counted regularly by washing out the peritoneal cavities of the mice. Methotrexate administration on alternate days caused regular sharp declines in the cell number. Nevertheless, the treated groups died 12 days after injection of the tumor cells, with cell count about 30 million in the ascitic fluid. The untreated groups succumbed within 6 days, with

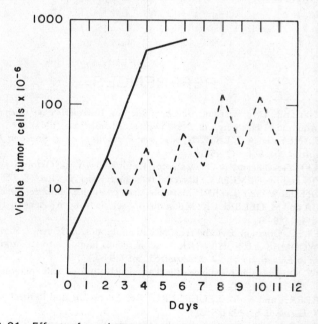

FIGURE 8-21. Effect of methotrexate on growth of tumor cells in mice. *An ascitic form of mouse leukemia was used. Mice were injected initially with about 3 million methotrexate-sensitive cells. Solid line shows cell counts from the abdominal cavity in untreated controls, which died by 6 days after injection. Broken line shows cell counts in mice treated with methotrexate (3 mg/kg) on days 2, 4, 6, 8, and 10. The treated animals were all dead by the 12th day. (From Welch, Chart 1.[124])*

cell count around 80 million. Cells recovered from the treated mice at death were not drug resistant, as proved by reinoculation into fresh animals. The most probable explanation for the death of the treated mice in this experiment is that the neoplastic cells had spread from the abdominal cavity to vital organs elsewhere in the body, where they were inaccessible to the drug.

Drugs like methotrexate, 6-mercaptopurine, and glucocorticoids can produce striking amelioration of the condition of patients with certain kinds of cancer. But the neoplastic process eventually becomes refractory to the drug therapy. It has often been assumed that drug failure under these conditions must be due to selection of genetically altered tumor cell lines, much as described earlier for microorganisms and transplantable murine tumors. Extensive data on "drug-resistant" human cancers have not yet been obtained, but it is interesting that thus far, at least, not a single convincing instance of drug resistance due to mutation and selection has come to light. Clearly, many other factors can account for therapeutic failure.[65,70,125] The drugs used in cancer chemotherapy, for example, have very poor therapeutic ratios. Therefore, they have to be used at maximum tolerated dosage, so that any increase of dose is likely to produce serious toxicity. Under these conditions, any change in the patient's circulation that reduces the efficiency of delivery of the drug to the tumor site may result in drug failure. Or a part of the tumor itself may be poorly vascularized and consequently receive too little drug. Invasion of the central nervous system by tumor cells can protect them from drugs unable to pass the drug-brain barrier readily. Alterations in metabolism or excretion of the drug may also contribute to the drug-refractory state.

REFERENCES

1. R. J. SCHNITZER: Drug Resistance in Chemotherapy. In *Experimental Chemotherapy*, Volume I, R. J. Schnitzer and F. Hawking, eds. New York, Academic Press (1963).
2. E. L. DULANEY and A. I. LASKIN, eds.: *The Problems of Drug-Resistant Pathogenic Bacteria. Ann. N. Y. Acad. Sci.* Vol. 182 (1971).
3. W. B. PRATT: *Fundamentals of Chemotherapy*. Oxford, New York, Oxford University Press (1973).
4. V. BRYSON and M. DEMEREC: Bacterial resistance. *Amer. J. Med.* 18:723 (1955).
5. V. BRYSON and W. SZYBALSKI: Microbial drug resistance. *Advance. Genet.* 7:1 (1955).
6. S. E. LURIA and M. DELBRÜCK: Mutations of bacteria from virus sensitivity to virus resistance. *Genetics* 28:491 (1943)
7. M. DEMEREC: Origin of bacterial resistance to antibiotics. *J. Bacteriol.* 56:63 (1948).
8. H. B. NEWCOMBE and R. HAWIRKO: Spontaneous mutation to streptomycin resistance and dependence in *Escherichia coli. J. Bacteriol.* 57:565 (1949).
9. L. W. LAW: Origin of the resistance of leukaemic cells to folic acid antagonists. *Nature* 169:628 (1952).
10. J. LEDERBERG and E. M. LEDERBERG: Replica plating and indirect selection of bacterial mutants. *J. Bacteriol.* 63:399 (1952).
11. W. BRAUN: *Bacteria. Genetics*, 2nd ed. Philadelphia, W. B. Saunders (1965).
12. T. WATANABE: Infective heredity of multiple drug resistance in bacteria. *Bacteriol. Rev.* 27:87 (1963).
13. J. E. DAVIES and R. ROWND: Transmissable multiple drug resistance in Enterobacteriaceae. *Science* 176:758 (1972).
13a. H. W. SMITH: Transfer of antibiotic resistance from animal and human strains of escherichia coli to resident E. coli in the alimentary tract of man. *Lancet* 1:1174 (1969).

13b. C. E. DAVIS and J. ANANDAN: The evolution of R factor. *New. Eng. J. Med.* 282:117 (1970).

14. D. S. FEINGOLD: Hospital-acquired infections. *New Eng. J. Med.* 233:1384 (1970).

15. E. C. MOORHOUSE: Transferable drug resistance in enterobacteria isolated from urban infants. *Brit. Med. J.* 2:405 (1969).

16. H. EAGLE: The multiple mechanisms of penicillin resistance. *J. Bacteriol.* 68:510 (1954).

16a. H. F. DOWLING, M. H. LEPPER, and G. G. JACKSON: Clinical significance of antibiotic-resistance bacteria. *J. Amer. Med. Ass.* 157:327 (1955).

17. M. H. LEPPER, B. MOULTON, H. F. DOWLING, G. G. JACKSON, and S. KOFMAN: Epidemiology of Erythromycin-Resistant Staphylococci in a Hospital Population—Effect on Therapeutic Activity of Erythromycin. In *Antibiotics Annual* 1953–54 (1953), p. 308.

18. I. M. ROLLO: "Daraprim' resistance in experimental malarial infections. *Nature* 170:415 (1952).

19. G. H. HITCHINGS: Pyrimethamine. The use of an antimetabolite in the chemotherapy of malaria and other infections. *Clin. Pharmacol. Therap.* 1:570 (1960).

20. D. CLYDE and G. T. SHUTE: Resistance of East African varieties of *Plasmodium falciparum* to pyrimethamine. *Trans. Roy. Soc. Trop. Med. Hyg.* 48:495 (1954).

21. P. EHRLICH: Chemotherapeutics: scientific principles, methods, and results. *Lancet* 2:445 (1913).

22. A. NOVICK: Mutagens and antimutagens. *Brookhaven Symp.* 8:201 (1956).

23. D. H. BOUANCHAUD and Y. A. CHABBERT. Practical effectiveness of agents curing R factors and plasmids. *Ann. N. Y. Acad. Sci.* 182:305 (1971).

24. H. S. MOYED: Biochemical mechanisms of drug resistance. *Annu. Rev. Microbiol.* 18:347 (1964).

25. R. J. SCHNITZER and E. GRUNBERG: *Drug Resistance of Microorganisms.* New York, Academic Press (1957).

26. G. E. W. WOLSTENHOLME and C. M. O'CONNOR, eds.: *Drug Resistance in Microorganisms.* Ciba Foundation Symposium. Boston, Little, Brown and Co. (1957).

27. B. D. DAVIS and W. K. MAAS: Analysis of the biochemical mechanism of drug resistance in certain bacterial mutants. *Proc. Nat. Acad. Sci. U.S.A.* 38:775 (1952).

28. M. L. PATO and G. M. BROWN: Mechanisms of resistance of *Escherichia coli* to sulfonamides. *Arch. Biochem. Biophys.* 103:443 (1963).

29. G. A. FISCHER: Defective transport of amethopterin (methotrexate) as a mechanism of resistance to the antimetabolite in L5178Y leukemic cells. *Biochem. Pharmacol.* 11:1233 (1962).

30. D. KESSEL. A comparison of 4-amino-4-deoxy-N^{10}-methylpteroic acid and methotrexate transport by mouse leukemic cells. *Mol. Pharm.* 5:21 (1969).

31. D. KESSEL, T. C. HALL, and D. ROBERTS: Modes of uptake of methotrexate by normal and leukemic human leukocytes in vitro and their relation to drug response. *Cancer Res.* 28:564 (1968).

32. A. R. P. PATERSON: Resistance to 6-mercaptopurine. II. The synthesis of thioinosinate in a 6-mercaptopurine-resistant subline of Ehrlich ascites carcinoma. *Canad. J. Biochem. Physiol.* 40:195 (1962).

33. T. J. FRANKLIN: Resistance of *Escherichia coli* to tetracyclines. *Biochem. J.* 105:371 (1967).

34. T. J. FRANKLIN and J. M. COOK: R factor with a mutation in the tetracycline resistance marker. *Nature* 229:273 (1971).

35. D. VAZQUEZ: Uptake and binding of chloramphenicol by sensitive and resistant organisms. *Nature* 203:257 (1964).

35a. B. WEISBLUM and J. E. DAVIES: Antibiotic inhibitors of the bacterial ribosome. *Bact. Rev.* 32:493 (1968).

36. J. CIAK and F. E. HAHN: Chloroquine: mode of action. *Science* 151:347 (1966).

37. P. B. MACOMBER, R. L. O'BRIEN, and F. E. HAHN: Chloroquine: physiological basis of drug resistance in *Plasmodium berghei*. *Science* 152:1374 (1966).

38. K. ARIMA and M. BEPPU: Induction and mechanisms of arsenite resistance in *Pseudomonas pseudomallei*. *J. Bacteriol.* 88:143 (1964).

39. M. BEPPU and K. ARIMA: Decreased permeability as the mechanism of arsenite resistance in *Pseudomonas pseudomallei*. *J. Bacteriol.* 88:151 (1964).

40. H. EAGLE and H. J. MAGNUSON: The spontaneous development of arsenic-resistance in *Trypanosoma equiperdum*, and its mechanism. *J. Pharmacol. Exp. Therap.* 82:137 (1944).

41. M. H. RICHMOND, G. W. JACK, and R. B. SYKES: The β-lactamases of gram-negative bacteria including pseudomonads. *Ann. N. Y. Acad. Sci.* 182:243 (1971).

42. M. G. SARGENT and J. O. LAMPEN: A mechanism for penicillinase secretion in *Bacillus licheniformis*. *Proc. Nat. Acad. Sci. U.S.A.* 65:962 (1970).

43. H. C. NEW: The surface localization of penicillinases in *Escherichia coli* and *Salmonella typhimurium*. *Biochem. Biophys. Res. Comm.* 32:258 (1968).

44. J. L. STROMINGER, K. ISAKI, M. MATSUHASHI, and D. J. TIPPER: Peptidoglycan transpeptidase and D-alanine carboxypeptidase: penicillin-sensitive enzymatic reactions. *Fed. Proc.* 26:9 (1967).

45. J. E. DAVIES, M. BRZEZINSKA, and R. BENVENISTE: R factors: biochemical mechanisms of resistance to aminoglycoside antibiotics. *Ann. N. Y. Acad. Sci.* 182:226 (1971).

46. Y. SUZUKI and S. OKAMOTO: The enzymatic acetylation of chloramphenicol by the multiple drug-resistant *Escherichia coli* carrying R factor. *J. Biol. Chem.* 242:4722 (1967).

47. W. V. SHAW and R. F. BRODSKY: Characterization of chloramphenicol acetyltransferase from chloramphenicol-resistant *Staphylococcus aureus*. *J. Bacteriol.* 95:28 (1968).

48. I. KOMURA and K. IZAKI: Mechanism of mercuric chloride resistance in microorganisms. *J. Biochem.* 70:885 (1971).

49. G. S. AHLUWALLA, Y. R. SAXENA and H. H. WILLIAMS: Quantitative studies on selenite metabolism in *Escherichia coli*. *Arch. Biochem. Biophys.* 124:79 (1968).

50. B. SKOWRONSKI and G. A. STROBEL: Cyanide resistance and cyanide utilization by a strain of *Bacillus pumilis*. *Can. J. Microbiol.* 15:93 (1969)

51. Insecticide resistance—the problem and its solution. *WHO Chronicle* 25:214 (1971).

52. A. W. A. BROWN and R. PAL: Insecticide resistance in arthropods. *WHO Monograph Series* #38, 2nd ed., Geneva (1971).

53. F. J. OPPENOORTH: Resistance in insects: the role of metabolism and the possible use of synergists. *Bull. WHO* 44:195 (1971).

54. R. D. O'BRIEN and I. YAMAMOTO, ed.: *Biochemical Toxicology of Insecticides*. New York and London, Academic Press (1970).

55. G. P. GEORGHIOU and R. L. METCALF: The absorption and metabolism of 3-isopropylphenyl *N*-methylcarbamate by susceptible and carbamate-selected strains of house flies. *J. Econ. Entomol.* 54:231 (1961).

56. F. MATSUMURA and A. W. A. BROWN: Biochemistry of malathion resistance in *Culex tarsalis*. *J. Econ. Entomol.* 54:1176 (1961).

57. F. J. OPPENOORTH and K. VAN ASPEREN: Allelic genes in the housefly producing modified enzymes that cause organophosphate resistance. *Science* 132:298 (1960).

58. W. C. DAUTERMAN and F. MATSUMURA: Effect of malathion analogs upon resistant and susceptible *Culex tarsalis* mosquitoes. *Science* 138:694 (1962).

59. J. E. CASIDA: "Insect Microsomes and Insecticide Chemical Oxidations" in *Microsomes and Drug Oxidations*, ed. by J. R. Gillette, A. H. Conney, G. J. Cosmides, R. W. Estabrook, J. R. Fouts, and G. J. Mannering. Academic Press, New York and London (1969), p. 517.

60. J. E. CASIDA: Mixed-function oxidase involvement in the biochemistry of insecticide synergists. *J. Agr. Food Chem.* 18:753 (1970).

61. W. L. FANGMAN and F. C. NEIDHARDT: Demonstration of an altered aminoacyl ribonucleic acid synthetase in a mutant of *Escherichia coli*. *J. Biol. Chem.* 239:1839 (1964).

62. O. SKÖLD: Studies on resistance against 5-fluorouracil. IV. Evidence for an altered uridine kinase in resistant cells. *Biochim. Biophys. Acta* 76:160 (1963).

63. G. P. KALLE and J. S. GOTS: Genetic alteration of adenylic pyrophosphorylase in *Salmonella*. *Science* 142:680 (1963).

64. W. BROCKMAN: Resistance to purine antagonists in experimental leukemia systems. *Cancer Res.* 25:1596 (1965).

65. J. D. DAVIDSON: Formal discussion on resistance to purine antagonists in experimental leukemia systems. *Cancer Res.* 25:1606 (1965).

66. S. TOMIZAWA and L. ARONOW: Studies on drug resistance in mammalian cells. II. 6-Mercaptopurine resistance in mouse fibroblasts. *J. Pharmacol. Exp. Therap.* 128:107 (1960).

67. M. LANDY, N. W. LARKUM, E. J. OSWALD, and F. STREIGHTOFF: Increased synthesis of *p*-aminobenzoic acid associated with the development of sulfonamide resistance in *Staphylococcus aureus*. *Science* 97:265 (1943).

67a. S. VENITT: Interstrand cross-links in the DNA of *Escherichia coli* B/r and B$_{s-1}$ and their removal by the resistant strain. *Biochem. Biophys. Res. Comm.* 31:355 (1968).

68. J. D. WATSON: Molecular Biology of the Gene. 2nd ed., New York, W. A. Benjamin (1970).

69. G. A. FISCHER: Increased levels of folic acid reductase as a mechanism of resistance to amethopterin in leukemic cells. *Biochem. Pharmacol.* 7:75 (1961).

70. J. R. BERTINO: Current studies of the folate antagonists in patients with acute leukemia. *Cancer. Res.* 25:1614 (1965).

71. M. T. HAKALA, S. F. ZAKRZEWSKI, and C. A. NICHOL: Relation of folic acid reductase to amethopterin resistance in cultured mammalian cells. *J. Biol. Chem.* 236:952 (1961).

72. M. T. HAKALA and T. ISHIHARA: Chromosomal constitution and amethopterin resistance in cultured mouse cells. *Cancer. Res.* 22:987 (1962).

73. M. T. HAKALA and E. M. SUOLINNA: Specific protection of folate reductase against chemical ·and proteolytic inactivation. *Mol. Pharmacol.* 2:465 (1966).

74. F. M. SIROTNAK, G. J. DONATI, and D. J. HUTCHISON: Genetic modification of the structure and amount of dihydrofolate reductase in amethopterin-resistant *Diplococcus pneumoniae*. *J. Biol. Chem.* 239:4298 (1964).

74a. B. W. SEARLE and A. GOLDSTEIN: Mutation to neostigmine resistance in a cholinesterase-containing *Pseudomonas*. *J. Bacteriol.* 83:789 (1962).

75. J. F. HACKNEY, S. R. GROSS, L. ARONOW, and W. B. PRATT: Specific glucocorticoid-binding macromolecules from mouse fibroblasts growing in vitro. *Molecular Pharm.* 6:500 (1970).

76. J. D. BAXTER, A. W. HARRIS, G. M. TOMKINS, and M. COHN: Glucocorticoid receptors in lymphoma cells in culture: relationship to glucocorticoid killing activity. *Science* 171:189 (1971).

77. A. F. KIRKPATRICK: Stereospecific glucocorticoid binding to subcellular fractions of the sensitive and resistant lymphosarcoma P1798. *Nature New Bio.* 232:216 (1971).

78. G. M. BROWN: The biosynthesis of folic acid. II. Inhibition by sulfonamides. *J. Biol. Chem.* 237:536 (1962).

79. B. WOLF and D. HOTCHKISS: Genetically modified folic acid synthesizing enzymes of Pneumococcus. *Biochemistry* 2:145 (1963).

80. R. FERONE, J. J. BUSCHALL, and G. H. HITCHINGS: *Plasmodium berghei* dihydrofolate reductase; isolation, properties, and inhibition by antifolates. *Mol. Pharmacol.* 5:49 (1969).

81. R. FERONE: Dihydrofolate reductase from pyrimethamine-resistant *Plasmodium berghei*. *J. Biol. Chem.* 245:850 (1970).

82. R. I. LEAVITT and H. E. UMBARGER: Isoleucine and valine metabolism in *Escherichia coli*. XI. Valine inhibition of the growth of *Escherichia coli* strain K-12. *J. Bacteriol.* 83:624 (1962).

83. H. S. MOYED: False feedback inhibition: inhibition of tryptophan biosynthesis by 5-methyl-tryptophan. *J. Biol. Chem.* 235:1098 (1960).

84. A. MEISTER: *Biochemistry of the Amino Acids*, 2nd ed. New York, Academic Press (1965).

85. H. S. MOYED: Interference with the feed-back control of histidine biosynthesis. *J. Biol. Chem.* 236:2261 (1961).

86. D. W. E. SMITH and B. N. AMES: Phosphoribosyladenosine monophosphate, an intermediate in histidine biosynthesis. *J. Biol. Chem.* 240:3056 (1965).

87. R. G. MARTIN: The first enzyme in histidine biosynthesis: the nature of feedback inhibition by histidine. *J. Biol. Chem.* 238:257 (1963).

87a. W. ZILLIG, K. ZECHEL, D. RABUSSAY, M. SCHACHNER, V. S. SETHI, P. PALM, A. HEIL, and W. SEIFERT: On the role of different subunits of DNA-dependent RNA polymerase from *E. coli* in the transcription process. *Cold Spring Harbor Symposia on Quant. Biol.* 35:47 (1970).

88. D. DI MAURO, L. SNYDER, P. MARINO, A. LAMBERTI, A. COPPO, and G. P. TOCCHINI-VALENTINI: Rifampicin sensitivity of the components of DNA-dependent RNA polymerase. *Nature* 222:533 (1969).

88a. D. RABUSSAY and W. ZILLIG: A rifampicin resistant RNA-polymerase from *E. coli* altered in the β-subunit. *FEBS Letters* 5:104 (1969).

89. T. CASKEY, P. LEDER, K. MOLDAVE, and D. SCHLESSINGER: Translation: its mechanism and control. *Science* 176:195 (1972).

90. A. L. LEHNINGER: Ribosomes and Protein Synthesis. In *Biochemistry*. Worth Publishers, New York (1970) Ch. 30.

91. Cold Spring Harbor Symposia on Quantitative Biology: *The Genetic Code*. Cold Spring Harbor, New York, Biological Laboratory (1966). Vol. 31.

92. H. K. DAS, A. GOLDSTEIN, and L. C. KANNER: Inhibition by chloramphenicol of the growth of nascent protein chains in *Escherichia coli*. *Mol. Pharmacol.* 2:158 (1966).

93. A. GOLDSTEIN, J. B. KIRSCHBAUM, and A. ROMAN: Direction of synthesis of messenger RNA in cells of *Escherichia coli*. *Proc. Nat. Acad. Sci. U.S.A.* 54:1669 (1965).

94. A. GOLDSTEIN, D. B. GOLDSTEIN, and L. I. LOWNEY: Protein synthesis at 0°C in *Escherichia coli*. *J. Mol. Biol.* 9:213 (1964).

95. S. H. KIM, G. J. QUIGLEY, F. L. SUDDATH, A. MC PHERSON, D. SNEDEN, J. J. KIM, J. WEINZIERL, and A RICH: Three-dimensional structure of yeast phenylalanine transfer RNA: folding of the polynucleotide chain. *Science* 179:285 (1973).

96. M. LEVITT: Detailed molecular model for transfer ribonucleic acid. *Nature* 224:759 (1969).

97. R. W. HOLLEY, J. APGAR, G. A. EVERETT, J. T. MADISON, M. MARQUISEE, S. H. MERRILL, J. R. PENSWICK, and A. ZAMIR: Structure of a ribonucleic acid. *Science* 147:1462 (1965).

98. J. T. MADISON, G. A EVERETT, and H. KUNG: Nucleotide sequence of a yeast tyrosine transfer RNA. *Science* 153:531 (1966).

99. H. A. SOBER, ed.: *Handbook of Biochemistry* 2nd ed. Cleveland, Ohio, Chemical Rubber Co. (1970), p. I-118.

100. J. D. WATSON: *Molecular Biology of the Gene*, 2nd ed. New York, W. A. Benjamin (1970).

101. K. TANAKA, H. TERAOKA, M. TAMAKI, E. OTAKA, and S. OSAWA: Erythromycin-resistant mutant of *Escherichia coli* with altered ribosomal protein component. *Science* 162:576 (1968).

101a. C. J. LAI and V. WEISBLUM: Altered methylation of ribosomal RNA in an erythromycin-resistant strain of *Staphylococcus aureus*. *Proc. Nat. Acad. Sci. U.S.A.* 68:856 (1971).

102. B. WEISBLUM and J. DAVIES: Antibiotic inhibitors of the bacterial ribosome. *Bact. Rev.* 32:493 (1968).

103. L. LUZZATTO, D. AFRION, and D. SCHLESSINGER: Mechanism of action of streptomycin in *E. coli*; interruption of the ribosome cycle at the initiation of protein synthesis. *Proc. Nat. Acad. Sci. U.S.A.* 60:873 (1968).

104. J. E. DAVIES: Studies on the robosomes of streptomycin-sensitive and resistant strains of *Escherichia coli*. *Proc. Nat. Acad. Sci. U.S.A.* 51:659 (1964).

105. M. NOMURA, S. MIZUSHIMA, M. OZAKI. P. TRAUB, and C. V. LOWRY: Structure and function of ribosomes and their molecular components. *Cold Spring Harbor Symposia on Quantitative Biology* 34:49 (1969).

106. M. OZAKI, S. MIZUSHIMA and M. NOMURA: Identification and functional characterization of the protein controlled by the streptomycin-resistant locus in *E. coli*. *Nature* 222:333 (1969).

107. A. BOLLEN, T. HELSER, T. YAMADA, and J. DAVIES: Altered ribosomes in antibiotic-resistant mutants of *E. coli*. *Cold Spring Harbor Symposia on Quantitative Biology* 34:95 (1969).

108. J. E. DAVIES, P. ANDERSON, and B. S. DAVIS: Inhibition of protein synthesis by spectinomycin. *Science* 149:1096 (1965).

108a. G. R. CRAVIN, R. GAVIN, and T. FANNING: The transfer RNA binding site of the 30S ribosome and the site of tetracycline inhibition. *Cold Spring Harbor Symposia on Quantitative Biol.* 34:129 (1969).

109. J. DAVIES, L. GORINI, and B. D. DAVIS: Misreading of RNA codewords induced by aminoglycoside antibiotics. *Mol. Pharmacol.* 1:93 (1965).

110. J. DAVIES, D. S. JONES, and H. G. KHORANA: A further study of misreading of codons induced by streptomycin and neomycin using ribopolynucleotides containing two nucleotides in alternating sequence as templates. *J. Mol. Biol.* 18:48 (1966).

111. R. MISKIN and A. ZAMIR: Effect of streptomycin on ribosome interconversion, a possible basis for the action of the antibiotic. *Nature* 238:78 (1972).

112. A. GOLDSTEIN: The origin of streptomycin-dependent variants of Escherichia coli. *J. Pharmacol. Exp. Therap.* 112:326 (1954).

113. D. A. MITCHISON: Microbial genetics and chemotherapy. *Brit. Med. Bull.* 18:74 (1962).

114. J. DAVIES, W. GILBERT, and L. GORINI: Streptomycin, suppression, and the code. *Proc. Nat. Acad. Sci. U.S.A.* 51:883 (1964).

115. L. GORINI and E. KATAJA: Phenotypic repair by streptomycin of defective genotypes in *E. coli*. *Proc. Nat. Acad. Sci. U.S.A.* 51:487 (1964).

116. L. GORINI: Streptomycin and the ambiguity of the genetic code. *New Scientist* 24:776 (1964).

117. W. F. ANDERSON, L. GORINI, and L. BRECKENRIDGE: Role of ribosomes in streptomycin-activated suppression. *Proc. Nat. Acad. Sci. U.S.A.* 54:1076 (1965).

118. L. GORINI: Induction of code ambiguity by aminoglycoside antibiotics. *Fed. Proc.* 26:5 (1967).

119. C. P. LEBLOND and B. E. WALKER: Renewal of cell populations. *Physiol. Rev.* 36:255 (1956).

120. F. M. BURNET: Immunological recognition of self. *Science* 133:307 (1961).

121. P. B. MEDAWAR: Immunological tolerance. *Science* 133:303 (1961).

122. R. W. BROCKMAN and E. P. ANDERSON: Biochemistry of cancer (metabolic aspects). *Ann. Rev. Biochem.* 32:463 (1963).

123. L. W. LAW: Differences between cancers in terms of evolution of drug resistance. *Cancer. Res.* 16:698 (1956).

124. A. D. WELCH: The problem of drug resistance in cancer chemotherapy. *Cancer Res.* 19:359 (1959).

125. Symposium: Conference on obstacles to the control of acute leukemia. *Cancer Res.* 25:1469–1679 (1965).

CHAPTER 9
Drug Tolerance and Physical Dependence

Drug tolerance is a state of decreased responsiveness to the pharmacologic effect of a drug resulting from a prior exposure to that drug or to a related drug. When exposure to drug A produces tolerance to it and also to drug B, the organism is said to be *crosstolerant* to drug B. The degree of tolerance, in general, may vary within very wide limits. Usually in the tolerant organism, although the ordinarily effective drug dose is less effective than it had been or even entirely ineffective, an increased dosage will again elicit the typical drug response. Thus, as a rule, tolerance is a quantitative change in sensitivity to a drug. Sometimes, however, the drug effect cannot be obtained at any dosage in the tolerant organism.

Physical dependence is a state sometimes associated with drug tolerance, especially in the nervous system, in which, as a consequence of exposure to a drug, the presence of that drug is required for normal function. If the dependent state is produced by exposure to drug A, as a result of which dependence also develops to drug B, the organism is said to be *cross-dependent* on drug B. The state of physical dependence can only be revealed by withdrawing the drug that is responsible. This elicits various pathophysiologic disturbances known collectively as a *withdrawal syndrome* (also "abstinence syndrome"). All manifestations of the withdrawal syndrome can be terminated abruptly and dramatically by readministering the drug.

TOLERANCE BY INDIRECT MECHANISMS

There are two mechanisms whereby an animal becomes tolerant to a drug even though the sensitivity at the cellular (or subcellular) sites of drug action does not change. *First*, the concentration of free drug in contact with the receptors may remain within normal limits even though the total drug dosage to the animal increases. This could occur by a reduction in the efficiency of drug absorption into the body, an increase in the rate of drug elimination, a diminution in the passage of drug across biologic membranes that separate the sites of action from the plasma water, or an increased amount of binding of the drug in an inert complex. *Second*, the biologic effect of the drug may be increasingly antagonized through homeostatic mechanisms, even though the drug continues to manifest its usual action upon its cellular receptors. Examples of both types of mechanism will be presented.

Reduction of the Ambient Drug Concentration (Metabolic Tolerance)

In the only well-documented instances of this mechanism, tolerance results from an increased rate of drug metabolism. Progressively diminished absorption from the gastrointestinal tract has been cited as the cause of tolerance in arsenic eaters, but the data are fragmentary and inconclusive.[1-3] About a century ago, this peculiar form of drug abuse was prevalent among the peasants of the province of Styria and elsewhere in Austria. Solid arsenic trioxide was eaten, usually in powdered form, in gradually increasing dosage. It was supposed to produce a ruddier complexion and an appearance of healthy well-being and to increase the endurance in mountain climbing.

The phenomenon of tolerance has some features in common with immune processes. Successive challenges produce diminishing effects, as though something were synthesized in the body that antagonizes the drug action or combines directly with the drug and inactivates it. However, the time course of tolerance development, e.g., hours to days with morphine, is shorter than that usually required for the synthesis of antibodies. Early claims that the serum of morphine-tolerant animals conferred protection against the lethal effects of morphine in normal animals[4] have been refuted.[5,6] The idea has been revived, however, by the proposal that drugs may induce the synthesis of "silent receptors" in the tissues, i.e., macromolecules that interact with the drug and inactivate it but do not produce any biologic effect.[7] Some experimental evidence has also been obtained, suggesting that some of the tolerance produced by repeated morphine injections may persist for a very long time, up to a year in rats. It has been claimed that even a single injection of morphine can produce some long-lasting decrease in sensitivity to subsequent morphine injections.[8] There are also indications that polypeptide hormones like parathyroid hormone and insulin may in some instances lead to antibody production and thus to a state of partial tolerance.

There is no doubt that metabolic tolerance develops toward any drug that induces synthesis of enzymes responsible for its own degradation, as described fully in Chapter 3. This kind of tolerance has a unique characteristic—its magnitude is strongly dependent upon the route of drug administration and upon the criteria of drug effect. Suppose such a drug is given intravenously to a normal animal and to one that has been pretreated with the drug for a long time. The maximum intensity of drug effect should be the same in both animals, but the effect should be terminated more quickly in the pretreated animal. This should be so because the dose distributes into the same volume of distribution and produces the same drug level in the body fluids of both animals. But the increased rate of metabolism in the pretreated animal will cause the level to fall faster. If lethality were the measure of drug action, we should probably not find any difference in LD50 between pretreated and normal animals. But if the total area under an effect-duration curve were the criterion (as for analgesia, p. 388), then the animal that degrades the drug faster will seem to have become tolerant. The situation is different when the drug is given by a route of slow absorption, for then the peak level attained after a single dose is cetermined by the balance between absorption rate and elimination rate. As the rate of drug metabolism increases, therefore, the peak intensity of drug effect will be reduced and ever larger doses will be required to attain the same peak effect.

Tolerance to barbiturates and to ethyl alcohol arises in part from cellular adaptations, to be discussed later (p. 591), and in part from an increased rate of drug metabolism, as already illustrated for pentobarbital in Table 3-2. In the experiment summarized there, the biologic half-life of the drug in rats was about 79 min after the first dose, only 26 min after the fourth dose. There was a corresponding reduction in sleeping time, but the plasma barbiturate level at the time of awakening was essentially the same in the normal and tolerant animals. The data are consistent with the finding[9] that tolerance to the sedative-hypnotic effects of barbiturates is not necessarily accompanied by an increase in the LD50. The rate of development of this kind of tolerance depends, as might be expected, upon the particular barbiturate and the species. It appears that a sufficiently high blood level has to be maintained for a certain length of time in order to cause an increased rate of synthesis of the liver microsomal enzymes. Rats and rabbits, for example, which metabolize hexobarbital very rapidly, had to be given that drug twice daily for several days in order to develop tolerance; dogs, which metabolize hexobarbital much more slowly, developed tolerance after a single dose.[10]

An increased rate of metabolism of ethyl alcohol associated with the tolerant state is illustrated in Figure 9-1. Six male subjects addicted to alcohol were studied under carefully controlled conditions on a hospital ward.[11] Their nutrition was adequate during the course of the experiment, and they received vitamin supplements daily.

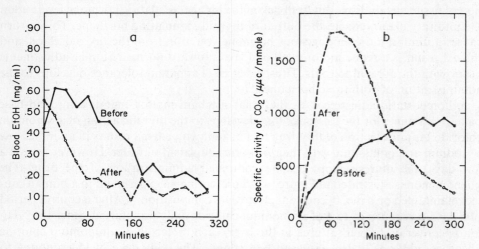

FIGURE 9-1. Increased metabolism of ethanol during tolerance. *Data from one subject, before and after a 7-day period of alcohol ingestion, during which the subject received 3.2 g of ethanol per kg per day in divided doses. A test dose of ethanol was given by mouth, and 1/2 hr later 10 μc of ethanol-1-^{14}C was given intravenously. At 20 min intervals, blood samples were removed for ethanol determination, and samples of expired air were collected for CO_2 assay and radioactivity determination. a, blood ethanol concentrations; b, specific radioactivity of CO_2. Solid lines, test before the 7-day period of drinking; broken lines, test after 7-day period of drinking. (Modified from Mendelson et al., Figures 3 and 7.[11] By permission of Grune & Stratton.)*

After a 4-day predrinking period, they were given a small test dose of ethyl alcohol by mouth and 30 min later, an intravenous injection of 10 μc of ethanol-1-^{14}C. Blood ethanol levels were followed, and carbon dioxide in the expired air was measured and its radioactivity determined. The specific radioactivity of the CO_2 served as a measure of the rate of oxidation of ethanol. The subjects were then given alcohol in large amounts regularly for 7 days. At the end of that time, another test dose was given. The data for one subject are summarized in the figure. At the left (a), it can be seen that the blood level established by the test dose declined much faster after the 7-day period of drinking than before. At the right (b), the specific radioactivity of carbon dioxide in the first 2 hr after the test dose is seen to be much higher after the drinking period than before. Evidently, as has also been shown in rats,[12] the administration of ethanol induces a large increase in activity of liver alcohol dehydrogenase, the rate-limiting enzyme in the oxidative pathway for ethanol.

Metabolic crosstolerance is a very common cause of "drug interaction," an effect of one drug on the therapeutic effect or toxicity of another administered simultaneously. Drug A (e.g., phenobarbital) might induce increased activity of the microsomal drug oxidizing system so that drug B (e.g., diphenylhydantoin) is metabolized more rapidly than before. The usual dose of diphenylhydantoin would no longer establish an effective blood level. Drug interactions are discussed in Chapter 14.

Homeostatic Adjustments Antagonizing the Drug Action

Tolerance to exogenous hormones frequently develops as a consequence of the operation of homeostatic adjustments. Two examples may be cited. Administration of thyroid hormone to a normal individual leads initially to the characteristic stimulation of tissue metabolism. But feedback of the higher circulating hormone levels upon the pituitary gland reduces the output of thyroid-stimulating hormone. This in turn causes a diminution of endogenous hormone secretion from the thyroid gland, and the net result is a reduction of the blood levels toward normal. Similar adjustments occur with the adrenal steroids. Thus, a degree of apparent tolerance develops to the administration of both these hormones.[13]

A homeostatic adjustment in the renal mechanisms for maintaining acid-base balance accounts for the tolerance that develops to the diuretic action of ammonium chloride. Administration of this drug to a patient with edema results in an initial loss of sodium and potassium, with their osmotic equivalent of water. However, within a few days, the diuresis stops despite continued administration of the drug. The phenomenon is illustrated in Figure 9-2, representing an experiment in a human subject maintained on a diet of constant electrolyte composition.[14] After a control period of 5 days, a regimen of 15 g of ammonium chloride daily was started. Since the NH_4^+ ion is converted to neutral urea in the liver, each molecule of ammonium chloride absorbed adds one hydrogen ion to body fluids. The daily dose of 15 g amounts to 280 milliequivalents of protons and chloride ions. The acidosis is compensated by the bicarbonate buffer system of the extracellular fluids, resulting in decreased plasma bicarbonate and increased plasma chloride. The increased chloride load presented to the renal tubules in the glomerular filtrate results in increased chloride excretion and an accompanying increased excretion of Na^+. Potassium excretion (from intracellular fluid) tends to rise after a day or two. By the second day of drug administration, the urinary ammonia excretion starts to increase; as it does, the sodium and potassium

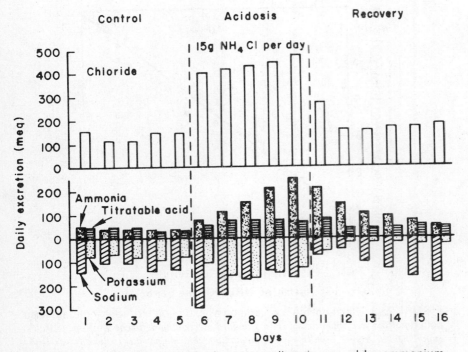

FIGURE 9-2. Development of tolerance to diuresis caused by ammonium chloride. *The subject of this experiment was maintained on a diet of constant composition throughout the experiment. Daily excretion of chloride is shown on top line, excretion of ammonia, titratable acid, sodium, and potassium at bottom. For convenience the scale for cation excretion is inverted. Units are milliequivalents. (From Pitts, Figure 26.[14] By permission of Charles C. Thomas.)*

excretions return to control levels. Thus, by the fifth day of ammonium chloride administration, the additional chloride excretion is being accompanied by a nearly stoichiometric equivalent of ammonia and hydrogen ions. The body is then in a state of compensated metabolic acidosis. The urine is acid (not shown in Figure 9-2), and the daily ammonium chloride intake is balanced by an equal ammonium chloride excretion. Complete tolerance has developed to the diuretic action of ammonium chloride. The reversibility of the various compensatory mechanisms is shown in the excretion pattern during the 6-day recovery period after cessation of drug administration.

The biochemical basis of the development of tolerance to ammonium chloride diuresis was demonstrated in rats.[15] Groups of animals were maintained on standard diets supplemented with various amounts of ammonium chloride. Measurements were made of urinary ammonia excretion and also of the activity of a renal enzyme, glutaminase (since urinary ammonia is derived from glutamine). The glutaminase activity increased in a few days to a new plateau that was proportional to the intake of ammonium chloride. This is shown in Figure 9-3, where the ammonia excretion is plotted against the glutaminase activity of kidney homogenates, and each point represents one rat. The cluster of points at low enzyme activity and low ammonia excretion represents untreated control rats; other points are data from rats on the ammonium chloride regimen. A perfectly linear relationship was found. The higher

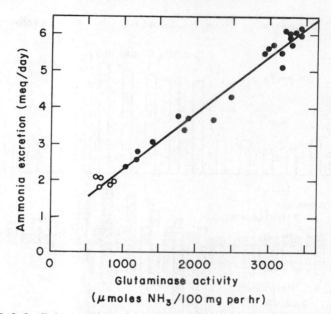

FIGURE 9-3. Relationship of ammonia excretion to renal glutaminase activity. *Rats were maintained on a standard electrolyte-deficient diet (open circles) supplemented from 2–5 millimoles of ammonium chloride per day (solid circles). Daily ammonia excretion was measured (ordinates), and renal glutaminase activity was determined (abscissas) and expressed as micromoles of ammonia produced per hour by 100 mg dry weight of tissue. (From Rector et al., Figure 2.[15])*

the daily dose of ammonium chloride, the higher the new steady-state level of renal glutaminase, and the higher the ammonia excretion. Evidently, the key to the development of tolerance to ammonium chloride diuresis is an increased rate of synthesis (or decreased rate of degradation) of this kidney enzyme in response to acidosis.

TOLERANCE AT THE CELLULAR SITES OF DRUG ACTION

Tolerance at the cellular sites of drug action could, in principle, result from a mutation-selection mechanism as described in Chapter 8 for development of drug resistance in parasitic microorganisms and neoplastic mammalian cells. A selection mechanism can often be ruled out, however, on the basis that too little time has elapsed relative to the rate of cell renewal at the sites of drug action. Thus, acute tolerance (*tachyphylaxis*) to some drugs may develop within a few minutes. Tolerance can sometimes be produced in isolated tissues in an organ bath, where no cell divisions occur and where all mechanisms involving the whole animal can be excluded. In the most striking instances of drug tolerance, the site of drug action is in the brain, where no cell renewal occurs, so that the cells becoming tolerant are necessarily the same ones that were formerly drug sensitive.

When drug tolerance is accompanied by physical dependence, all simple explanations, such as the mere exclusion of drug from the sites of action, or the inactivation or destruction of the drug, become inadequate. The mere absence of drug from the sites of action could not account for the functional changes that must underlie the dependent state. And the disturbances that ensue if the drug is withdrawn attest to its having been present and active at cellular sites of action during the period of drug tolerance.

Finally, the presence of cellular tolerance may be established unequivocally by direct measurement of drug concentrations in the appropriate body fluids. It may be demonstrated that sufficient drug is in contact with the target cells, yet no pharmacologic effect results. And it may be shown further that a typical response to the drug can be elicited if the ambient drug concentration is raised to a level much higher than is required in the nontolerant animal.

Acute Tolerance (Tachyphylaxis)

Sympathomimetic Amines.   It has been known for many years that repeated intravenous doses of certain sympathomimetic amines elicit smaller and smaller cardiovascular responses. Figure 9-4 shows a classical experiment with ephedrine.[16] A dog

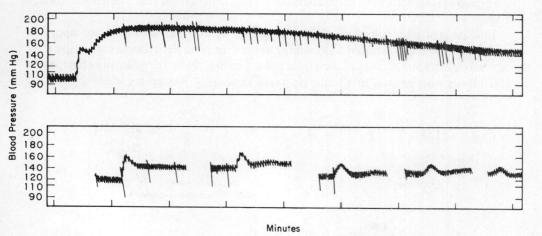

FIGURE 9-4. Ephedrine tachyphylaxis in the dog. *A 5-kg male dog was given barbiturate anesthesia and atropinized. The record, obtained on a kymograph drum, reads from left to right. Mean blood pressure is shown on the vertical axis, time (marks are 1 min apart) on the horizontal axis. The long upper tracing is the response to the first injection of ephedrine sulfate (3 mg kg^{-1} intravenously). The second injection of ephedrine (lower tracing) was given 25 min after the first; subsequent injections were made at 10-min intervals. (From Chen and Meek, Figure 1.[16])*

was anesthetized with a barbiturate and atropinized to block vagal effects, then given ephedrine sulfate, 3 mg kg^{-1} intravenously. There was a very large increase in the mean blood pressure due principally to arteriolar constriction and partly to increased cardiac output. Twenty-five minutes later the same dose was repeated, with much diminished effect; both the intensity of the response and its duration were reduced. Further repetition of the injection at 10-min intervals led quickly to a state of nearly complete tolerance to the drug. Similar effects have been demonstrated in many sympathetically innervated tissues outside the cardiovascular system, such as uterus, intestine, bronchioles, and nasal mucous membranes.[17]

In experiments like that depicted in Figure 9-4, it has been found that even after the establishment of tachyphylaxis to ephedrine, other agents (e.g., epinephrine) continued to manifest their usual pressor actions. The tolerance, therefore, could not be attributed to any general exhaustion of the contractile capacity of the arteriolar smooth muscle. The only alternative explanation seemed to be that there were receptors specific for each kind of sympathomimetic agent, and that these different classes of receptors became "saturated" more or less easily. Somehow, it was supposed, the occupancy of ephedrine receptors by ephedrine made them unresponsive to further ephedrine administration, while other receptors (e.g., those responsive to epinephrine) continued functioning.[17]

The concept of independent receptors appeared more and more dubious as the number of known sympathomimetic agents increased, for each one appeared to have its own pattern of tachyphylaxis. Among the phenylethylamines, for example, those with α-methyl groups (ephedrine, amphetamine) produced tachyphylaxis more readily than unsubstituted compounds like tyramine; the catecholamines themselves (epinephrine, norepinephrine) were found to produce little or no tachyphylaxis.[18] The chemical structures of these compounds and others to be discussed are shown in Figure 9-5.

Our current understanding of the mechanism of tachyphylaxis is based upon the discovery that many sympathomimetic amines of the phenylethylamine structure have no vasoconstrictor actions of their own but act indirectly by releasing norepinephrine (NE) from storage sites in adrenergic nerve endings.[19] Reserpine, which blocks the

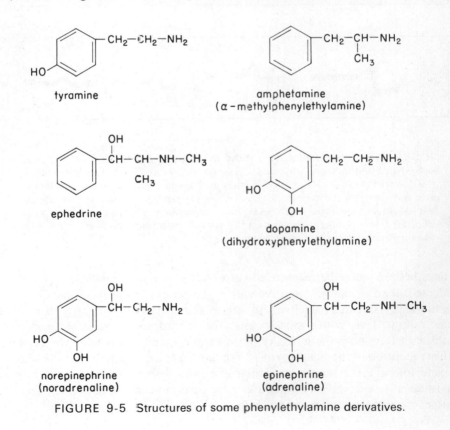

FIGURE 9-5 Structures of some phenylethylamine derivatives.

uptake of biogenic amines into vesicles at the nerve endings and thereby depletes the
neuronal stores of NE almost completely, was used as a tool to classify the various
sympathomimetic agents according to their modes of action [20] In reserpinized
animals, some of these compounds, like NE, retained full potency, i.e., they acted
directly upon the NE receptors on the postjunctional effector cells. Some had diminished effects, indicating a mixed action, partly dependent upon the presence of
NE stores in the nerve ending. Some agents, like tyramine, were devoid of their usual
cardiovascular effects in reserpinized animals, i.e., their whole action seemed to be
due to their ability to release NE from the storage vesicles.

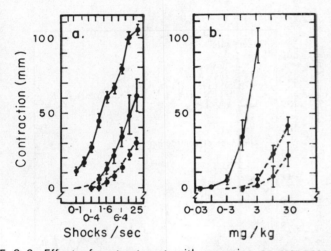

FIGURE 9-6. Effect of pretreatment with reserpine on response to nerve
stimulation and tyramine. *Spinal cats were pretreated with reserpine, 3 mg kg^{-1} 48
and 24 hr before testing (bottom curves), or 0.1 mg kg^{-1} 24 hr before testing (middle
curves). Controls were not reserpinized (upper curves). Vertical axis, contraction of
nictitating membrane, mm deflection on drum record. Horizontal axis (a) = stimulus
frequency to preganglionic sympathetic chain, shocks/sec; (b) = tyramine dose,
mg kg^{-1}. Vertical ranges are ± standard error. (From Trendelenburg, Figure 1.[21])*

Figure 9-6 illustrates the approximately parallel effects of NE depletion upon nerve
stimulation and upon the actions of tyramine. The experiment was done in cats whose
spinal cords had been transected in the cervical region in order to eliminate tonic
sympathetic activity.[21] The effects of supramaximal preganglionic stimulation at
various frequencies were compared with those of tyramine at increasing dosage, using
the contraction of the nictitating membrane as criterion of response. The control
animals received no reserpine; a group was given reserpine (0.1 mg kg^{-1}) 24 hr prior
to the testing; another group was given a higher dose of reserpine (3 mg kg^{-1}) 48 and
24 hr prior to the testing. The results show the systematic reduction of response to a
given stimulus frequency or a given dose of tyramine by the increasing doses of
reserpine. In other words, both nerve stimulation and tyramine work by releasing
NE. Prior depletion of NE by reserpine diminishes the amount of NE that can be
released effectively by either means. And increasing stimulus frequency or increasing
tyramine dosage partly overcomes the deficit caused by reserpine. In the same experiments, the blood pressure and heart rate responses to tyramine (not shown) were

similarly reduced by the reserpine pretreatment and partially restored by increasing doses of tyramine.

The observations cited above illustrate a mechanism whereby treatment with one drug (reserpine) produces tolerance to another (tyramine). Can tachyphylaxis to tyramine itself be explained in the same way, i.e., that tyramine depletes all the NE and therefore becomes ineffective? There is no doubt that tyramine releases NE and that the development of tachyphylaxis is associated with diminished NE release. Figure 9-7 illustrates this with the perfused isolated rat heart.[22] The experiment makes use of the fact that sympathetic nerve endings take up exogenous NE. This uptake and binding mechanism normally plays an important role in terminating the action of NE released

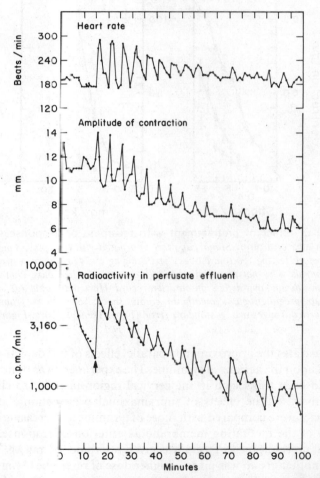

FIGURE 9-7. Tyramine tachyphylaxis and the rate of release of ^{3}H-norepine-phrine from perfused rat heart. *Rat hearts were perfused in vitro and the amplitude and rate of contraction were measured. At the outset, ^{3}H-norepinephrine was infused for 2–4 min. Then at 15 min (arrow) and every 5 min thereafter, an injection of tyramine (10 µg) was made into the perfusion cannula. The perfusate effluent was collected in 1-min fractions and radioactivity was determined; about 85% of this effluent radioactivity was identified as catecholamine. Note logarithmic scale of radioactivity. (Modified from Axelrod et al., Figure 1.[22] By permission of the British Medical Association.)*

into the region of the nerve-effector junction by a nerve stimulus. The stores of NE that are capable of being released by nerve stimuli can be labeled with radioactive NE taken up from the circulation. In the experiment, ^{3}H-NE was given by way of the perfusion fluid for a few minutes, following which 1-minute samples of the perfusate effluent were collected for determination of radioactivity. At the same time, the heart rate and amplitude of contraction were measured. During the initial period, the heart rate and contraction amplitude were fairly stable, and there was a rapid outflow of the recently infused ^{3}H-NE. An injection of tyramine at 15 min caused a sharp rise in heart rate and contraction amplitude and simultaneously a considerable additional outflow of ^{3}H-NE. Repeated injections of tyramine at 5-minute intervals resulted (after the second or third injection) in ever smaller responses of the heart. Although each injection continued to cause a measurable release of ^{3}H-NE, the actual amounts released became smaller at the same time that tolerance was developing to the biologic effects. In this connection, it is important to note that the scale of radioactivity in the figure is logarithmic, so that equal vertical distances represent smaller amounts of radioactivity near the bottom of the chart than near the top. Thus, whereas the initial tyramine injection at 15 min released about 4000 cpm additional radioactivity into the perfusion effluent, the injection at 20 min released only 1600 cpm, and the injection at 85 min released only 600 cpm.

The experiment described above might seem to support the simple view that tolerance to tyramine results from complete depletion of the neuronal NE. When residual NE was actually measured, however, by a chemical procedure, a considerable amount was found even after tyramine had become ineffective. Some of this residual NE was releasable by nerve stimulation: biologic responses to such stimulation were obtainable during tyramine tachyphylaxis, although their magnitudes were reduced (especially at low stimulus frequencies). The NE that was easily releasable by tyramine could be distinguished from the remainder of the neuronal stores by varying the conditions of administration of radioactive NE. Figure 9-8 shows such an experiment.[23] Rats were given ^{3}H-NE intravenously and killed 1 hr later; their hearts were assayed for catecholamine content by means of a fluorometric procedure, and catecholamine radioactivity was determined. Other animals were treated in the same way but were given a dose of tyramine 30 min after the ^{3}H-NE injection. The left panels (a) show that tyramine caused a depletion of about 40% in the catecholamine content and a decrease of about the same extent in the radioactivity, compared with control hearts. On the other hand, if the radioactive NE was given 48 hr prior to the tyramine injection and the animals were killed as before 30 min after tyramine (right panels, b), there was relatively less loss of radioactivity. In other words, the exogenous NE was readily releasable by tyramine soon after it was taken up, but there were also stores of NE, more slowly labeled in this experiment, which were resistant to release by tyramine.[24,25]

Tachyphylaxis to tyramine and related agents, as well as the tolerance to tyramine that is produced by reserpine, can be overcome by infusion of NE.[22] The administered catecholamine is taken up by sympathetic neurons and stored (as already discussed) in a "labile pool," whence it is easily released by tyramine. However, as might be expected, tachyphylaxis reappears very quickly under these circumstances for the newly bound NE is rapidly depleted.[26]

How do agents like tyramine release NE from the neuronal stores? It has been shown that tyramine itself is taken up and bound at the catecholamine storage sites,

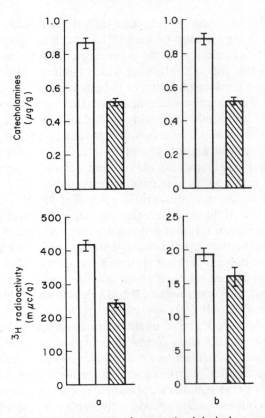

FIGURE 9-8. Differential release of recently labeled norepinephrine by tyramine. *Rats were given 10 μc of ³H-norepinephrine per 100 g body weight intravenously. Either 30 min later (a) or 48 hr later (b), some of the rats received tyramine (10 mg kg⁻¹) intravenously, and 30 min afterwards they were sacrificed. Heart catecholamine and radioactive catecholamine were determined; these data are given per gram of heart tissue ± standard errors. Open histograms, controls; hatched histograms, tyramine-injected rats (From data of Potter et al., Table 1.²³)*

displacing NE in the process.²² This bound tyramine is then releasable, either by nerve stimulation or by subsequent doses of tyramine. The releasable tyramine acts as a "false neurotransmitter." Since tyramine does not stimulate the catecholamine receptors in postjunctional effector cells, the diminished response in the tachyphylactic state is understandable; what is released as tachyphylaxis develops is a mixture containing tyramine and a decreasing amount of NE.²⁷

The enzymes of catecholamine metabolism can influence the development and duration of tachyphylaxis.²⁸ Present concepts are illustrated in Figure 9-9, and the biochemical pathways of synthesis and degradation of the catecholamines are shown in Figure 9-10. Extraneuronal metabolism of the catecholamines is mediated by catechol-O-methyl transferase (COMT); the major portion of exogenously administered catecholamines as well as the NE released by nerve stimulation or by tyramine are converted to O-methyl derivatives. Catecholamines within the neurons are metabolized principally by monoamine oxidase (MAO) located in the mitochondria. The NE that is liberated after reserpine treatment is oxidized by this enzyme, and

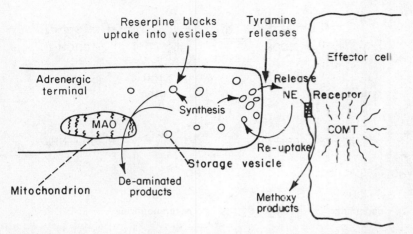

FIGURE 9-9. Schematic diagram of catecholamine transformations in the adrenergic neuron. *Synthesis of norepinephrine (NE) and its incorporation into storage vesicles takes place in the adrenergic neuron. Intraneuronal oxidation to deaminated products is catalyzed by monoamine oxidase (MAO) in mitochondria. Metabolism of released NE is catalyzed by catechol-O-methyl transferase (COMT) located in the postjunctional tissue. Reserpine prevents NE storage intraneuronally, tyramine releases it from the neuron.*

very little of it escapes to exert a pharmacologic action upon the effector cells. But in the presence of MAO inhibitors, the NE escapes and reserpine seems to acquire sympathomimetic stimulant properties. Tyramine is also metabolized by MAO. Thus, MAO inhibitors not only intensify the sympathomimetic effects of tyramine (p. 272) but also at the same time accelerate the development of tachyphylaxis to it by permitting a greater accumulation of tyramine (or its β-hydroxy metabolite, octopamine) in the catecholamine vesicles. The α-methyl derivatives of phenyl-ethylamines are not substrates of MAO, and consequently, tachyphylaxis develops much more readily to them than to tyramine.

Another complexity is revealed by studies on the dependence of tachyphylaxis upon dose and time. As might be expected, low doses of tyramine, widely spaced in time, produce no tachyphylaxis; presumably the accumulation of tyramine in the storage granules is limited under these conditions by its constant metabolic removal by MAO. Tolerance to high doses given at short intervals develops rapidly and persists. At intermediate doses, however, a peculiar effect has been described.[29] Tachyphylaxis develops after several doses, but this is followed by an "escape," i.e., a return of responsiveness to tyramine. The phenomenon is illustrated in Figure 9-11. The upper panel shows pressor responses in a spinal cat after the third and ninth injection of tyramine at 15-minute intervals and the return of a pressor effect at the 16th injection. The lower panel shows that the cardiac catecholamine content continued to decline throughout the injection series. These results are thought to be explained by the fact that tyramine depletion of NE pools can stimulate the synthesis of NE. Continued administration of tyramine could, therefore, furnish easily releasable NE in amounts sufficient to restore pressor action, without significantly replenishing the total NE store. This hypothesis gains some support from the finding that the escape from tachyphylaxis can be prevented by agents (e.g., disulfiram, p. 263) that block the

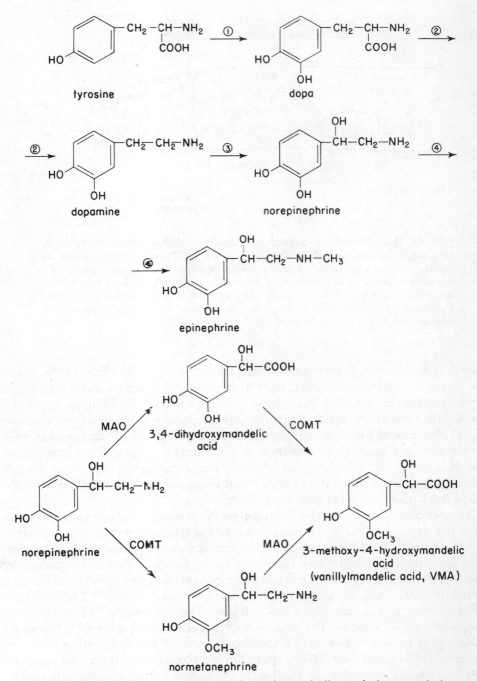

FIGURE 9-10. Pathways of synthesis and metabolism of the catechol-amines. *The synthetic pathway from tyrosine is shown above; enzyme 1 (tyrosine hydroxylase) appears to be the rate-limiting enzyme. The alternative degradative pathways for norepinephrine are shown below. Epinephrine is handled in analogous fashion. Several minor metabolites and conjugates, not shown here, are also found in the urine. Enzymes: 1, tyrosine hydroxylase; 2, dopa decarboxylase; 3, dopamine β-hydroxylase; 4, phenylethanolamine-N-methyl transferase; MAO, monoamine oxidase; COMT, catechol-O-methyl transferase.*

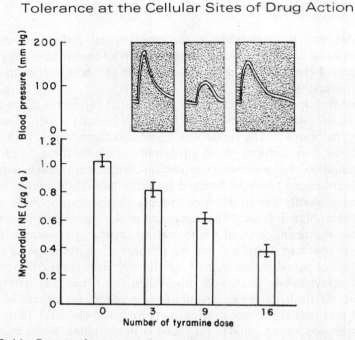

FIGURE 9-11. Escape from tyramine tachyphylaxis in the spinal cat. *Tyramine (800 μg kg⁻¹) was injected intravenously into spinal cats at 15-min intervals and blood pressure was recorded. Groups of cats were sacrificed at different times and the cardiac catecholamine contents were determined. Typical blood pressure tracings after the 3rd, 9th, and 16th tyramine dose are shown in upper panel. Mean catecholamine content ± standard error is shown in lower panel. (From Bhagat et al., Figures 1 and 2.[29])*

β-hydroxylation of dopamine, an essential step in the pathway of NE synthesis (Figure 9-10).[30]

Other Drugs That Provoke Acute Tolerance.

Stimulants of neuroeffector systems.   Drugs like acetylcholine and nicotine, which act by depolarizing a membrane to trigger an action potential, may cause a response initially and then block their own actions.[31,32] This effect is readily demonstrable by the local application of nicotine to a sympathetic ganglion. If the superior cervical ganglion of the cat is exposed and the contractions of the nictitating membrane are recorded, the application of a high concentration of nicotine to the ganglion will cause a maximum sustained contraction, which will spontaneously subside. The ganglion is then blocked, and application of nicotine or of carbachol will not elicit a further contraction of the nictitating membrane. A similar demonstration can be made with acetylcholine on smooth or striated muscle that is responsive to it. A rat uterus is suspended in a tissue bath under slight tension, in a special low-calcium medium that will inhibit spontaneous contractility. Small doses of acetylcholine now will produce brief contractions; a very large dose of acetylcholine causes a maximum sustained contraction, which (like that of the nictitating membrane) spontaneously subsides. Thereafter, the uterus will be completely unresponsive to acetylcholine. Repeated washing of the tissue gradually restores the sensitivity. Since this type of acute tolerance is commonly seen with depolarizing agents, it was at first attributed to persistent depolarization in the presence of the drug. A new response would be impossible until the membrane at the ganglion cell, muscle end-plate, or smooth muscle cell can repolarize. Direct measurements of transmembrane potentials, however, showed that after membrane repolarization occurred, yet the membrane remained refractory.[33]

Studies with morphine in electrically stimulated guinea pig ileum (p. 602) showed that acute tolerance could develop, although the primary action of morphine on this tissue is inhibitory.[34] The tissue was suspended in an organ bath and stimulated coaxially (i.e., by electrodes placed inside and outside the lumen) with shocks of sufficient strength to elicit maximum contractions, which were recorded on a kymograph. These contractions could be blocked by atropine or potentiated by neostigmine; they were evidently due to direct or indirect electrical stimulation of acetylcholine release. Morphine depressed the amplitude of the contractions. In the presence of morphine, the ileum retained its normal sensitivity to exogenously added acetylcholine. It appeared, therefore, that the primary effect of morphine was to diminish the output of acetylcholine caused by the electrical stimulation; direct assay of released acetylcholine confirmed this. When the tissue was left in contact with morphine, or fresh morphine solutions were added, the effects of the drug soon wore off, and even high concentrations were then without effect. In this tolerant state, the contractions were normal in the presence of morphine; when morphine was now washed out, the contraction amplitude decreased. The contractility in response to electrical stimulation could then be restored by morphine, as though some sort of physical dependence had developed. Neither acute tolerance nor "dependence" could be produced with atropine, an unrelated drug that also depresses contraction amplitude; but all the morphine congeners tested had the same effects as morphine itself. The relationship, if any, between these acute changes in sensitivity to morphine and the morphine tolerance that develops in vivo (cf. p. 599) is not clear.

Histamine.   Acute and chronic tolerance to histamine has been the subject of periodic study in the past, but the mechanisms have not been elucidated. In a typical experiment on an anesthetized cat, the administration of 10 μg of histamine intravenously produced a moderate fall of blood pressure. Repeated injections of histamine, in increasing larger doses, elicited diminishing hypotensive responses, so that within hours the dosage could be increased more than 100-fold.[35]

In another investigation[36] in guinea pigs, single daily histamine doses of 0.5 mg kg^{-1} were given subcutaneously. After a week, the daily dosage was increased by 0.5 mg kg^{-1}, and then a further increase of the same magnitude was made each subsequent week for 8 weeks. Two effects of histamine were chosen for study—bronchiolar constriction and stimulation of gastric acid secretion. Initially, and at the end of the 8-week period, the animals were tested for their sensivity to the pulmonary effect of histamine by placing them in an aerosol chamber and noting how much time was required for them to cough and become dyspneic. An increase in this time represents a decrease in sensitivity to the drug, but since no information is available about the rate of increase of the local histamine concentration in the bronchioles, no conclusions can be drawn about the quantitative aspects of tolerance. In control animals, the average time was 1 to 1.5 min and this was not significantly different in untreated animals retested after 8 weeks. In contrast, the animals that had received daily injections of histamine for 8 weeks showed a significant increase in time to more than 3 min. Free gastric acidity in untreated animals at the end of the experiment was 21.5 meq per liter (standard error ± 4.1) after a test dose of histamine; but in the histamine-treated animals, it was only 2.6 meq per liter (standard error ± 1.8). Thus, a striking degree of tolerance developed to this histamine action. An antihistamine drug given before each histamine injection did not prevent the development of tolerance in these guinea pigs.

Histamine releasers (e.g., tubocurarine, morphine) may at first produce hypotension and other effects attributable to histamine, but the effects diminish on repeated administration.[37] Many years ago, for example, it was shown that dogs became tolerant to the peripheral vasodilation caused by morphine.[38,39] Small doses repeated for many weeks led to little tolerance, but large doses caused tolerance rapidly. The vascular bed of a denervated leg in the tolerant animal was shown to be tolerant to morphine infusions. Thus, a large part of the acute vascular tolerance to morphine is really tolerance to histamine release or to histamine itself,[40] and the phenomenon is probably unrelated to narcotic tolerance in the brain. Presumably, the tolerance results in part from histamine depletion from storage sites in the skin and elsewhere and in part reflects the onset of tolerance to histamine itself. After tachyphylaxis has developed fully, there is no further release of histamine, although the histamine stores in tissues are by no means depleted.[41]

Nitrites.   It has long been common knowledge that workers engaged in nitroglycerin production or in the handling of dynamite (which contains nitroglycerin) experience throbbing headache, nausea, and other unpleasant symptoms upon first exposure but become readily "accustomed" to the compound.[42,43] The tolerance wears off in a few days, so that the term "Monday disease" has been used[44] to describe the renewed symptoms after a weekend off the job; and workers are said to avert this "disease" by carrying a small amount of nitroglycerin home with them in order to maintain their state of tolerance. Tolerance to this and other nitrite esters was studied in human volunteers.[45] Erythritol tetranitrate was given by mouth, glyceryl trinitrate (nitroglycerin) and ethylene glycol dinitrate by rubbing onto the skin, and methyl nitrate and amyl nitrate by inhalation. A "headache dose" was determined, which would just produce a moderately uncomfortable headache. When repetition of the dose failed to elicit headache, the dose was increased. In this way, tolerance was produced to all these esters, although the degree of tolerance could not be ascertained accurately. The investigators asserted that complete tolerance to one or two "headache doses" could be produced. Cross-tolerance was the rule for all the nitrites and nitrates mentioned above, but not for the hypotensive actions of unrelated drugs like histamine. In dogs in which tolerance to the nitrate esters was established,[46] it was found that the red blood cells had lost much of their ability to hydrolyze the esters. Since it is thought that the nitrate esters act pharmacologically as free nitrite, this decreased hydrolytic capacity could explain the tolerance. It would not, however, explain cross-tolerance to sodium nitrite, which was regularly observed.[45,47]

Urethane.   Acute tolerance to urethane has been demonstrated in isolated tissue.[48] A piece of rabbit ileum was suspended in an organ bath and its movements recorded by means of a lever and kymograph. When urethane (3 to 5 mg ml^{-1}) was added to the Ringer solution in the bath, the characteristic spontaneous pendular movements stopped immediately. Within 15 min, however, the movements began again and had returned to control levels an hour later. At this time, fresh urethane solution was without effect. However, replacement of the urethane solution with fresh Ringer solution caused a considerable increase in the amplitude of the contractions, as though some compensatory mechanism operating in the presence of the drug was unmasked by its removal.

Atropine.   Atropine tolerance has been demonstrated in dogs with isolated loops of intestine (Thiery-Vella loops) in which peristaltic activity was measured by pressure changes in small balloons within the gut lumen.[49] When atropine was first administered, the typical depression of motility was observed; but after 3 or 4 doses at 30-min intervals, the drug became wholly ineffectual. The peristaltic activity was then also resistant ("cross-tachyphylaxis") to atropine congeners but not to unrelated drugs like cocaine, nitrites, and ganglionic blocking agents, which still produced their usual inhibitory effects. Moreover, the tachyphylaxis to atropine developed even when the inhibitory effects of atropine were antagonized by simultaneous administration of methacholine and also when atropine was given repeatedly in doses too small to produce any inhibitory effects on the intestinal motility. The investigators proposed that atropine induced tolerance by occupying receptors persistently "in the face of a compensatory change" in the tissue, but no direct evidence has been adduced.

Tolerance and Physical Dependence in the Central Nervous System

From prehistoric times and in all ethnic groups, people have sought out drugs that would furnish pleasure and satisfaction, allay anxiety, or influence the psyche in other ways considered desirable. Among these agents are a great many to which tolerance may develop and also some upon which the user becomes physically dependent. Because of the confusion of legal, popular, and scientific meanings of "habituation" and "addiction," the Expert Committee of the World Health Organization considering nomenclature decided to abandon these older terms and to substitute a single more inclusive term, namely *drug dependence*.[50]

Drug dependence includes three distinct and independent components: tolerance, physical dependence, and compulsive abuse (psychic craving). Different drugs show these features to various degrees.[51] Marijuana (Cannabis) is subject to compulsive abuse, but tolerance and physical dependence do not occur.[52] A low degree of tolerance to cocaine, nicotine, and caffeine develops, also mild physical dependence.[53] The psychic craving for these stimulants may be very intense, as in habitual cigarette smokers who try to "break the habit." Similar craving, withdrawal headache, and behavioral changes such as irritability and restlessness are seen when a prolonged high intake of caffeine is suddenly stopped.[54,55] D-amphetamine (dextroamphetamine, D-amphetamine, D(+)-amphetamine) and D-lysergic acid diethylamide (LSD) are both subject to compulsive abuse, and tolerance develops to both;[56,57] but no very striking withdrawal syndrome occurs, although the severe depression after cessation of amphetamine abuse may represent a withdrawal effect. An example of tolerance and physical dependence without compulsive abuse is provided by the morphine congener and antagonist nalorphine. This drug has been given experimentally to human subjects, but although the dosage was raised progressively and a withdrawal syndrome ensued when administration was stopped, no psychic craving developed; moreover, nalorphine is not sought after by addicts.[58] Alcohol, barbiturates, and the narcotics display all three components of drug dependence to such a degree as to create major problems for the individual and for society. We shall later discuss these drugs in detail, since they have been investigated intensively with respect to tolerance and physical dependence.

The social evils of drug addiction are compounded when addiction is treated as a crime rather than a disease. Compulsive abuse originates in the strong pleasurable (euphoriant) actions of a drug that reinforce drug-seeking behavior in certain individuals.[59,60] The development of a high degree of tolerance forces the addict to much higher dosages in order to obtain the desired effects. Eventually, even though he no longer obtains any pleasurable result because of tolerance, physical dependence leads him to continue taking the drug at all costs to ward off the withdrawal syndrome. If the drug is illegal, its price in the black market is exorbitant; to sustain his needs, the victim of drug dependence is often forced into a life of criminality.[61-64]

Experimentation on tolerance and physical dependence requires that a clearly recognizable drug effect be studied, preferably one that can be measured quantitatively. In animals, one tries to choose a drug effect that can be localized to a particular region of the brain and that produces an objectively measurable change in a body function. Among the many such actions drugs can cause are: vomiting, respiratory depression or stimulation, convulsive seizures, stimulation or depression of coordinated motor activity, alteration of temperature control, sleep, and analgesia. The drug must then be administered on a regular schedule over a long period of time in order to establish whether or not tolerance develops with respect to the chosen criterion.

Modern quantitative methods of investigating animal behavior, especially operant conditioning and conditioned avoidance techniques, have been useful in studying tolerance and physical dependence because they are often quite sensitive to disruption by centrally acting drugs.[65-71] The return to normal patterns of behavior despite continued drug administration becomes an indicator of tolerance; further disturbance of the behavior pattern on withdrawal may be viewed as the equivalent of a withdrawal syndrome. Behavioral phenomena, however, are subject to adaptive modification by numerous influences, such as the repetition of a testing procedure or uncontrolled variations in external stimuli; these changes must be clearly distinguished, by means of adequate controls, from pharmacologic tolerance.[72] For example, if the response of the organism to the drug is capable of being attenuated by a learning process, the result may be misinterpreted as pharmacologic tolerance. Suppose that a behavioral task is chosen for study, e.g., the ability of trained rats to run through a maze to a food reward. A psychotropic drug may disrupt the task performance initially, but repeated administrations may have less and less effect. The apparent tolerance, however, could be due to the learning of a new skill, namely, the ability to run the maze in the drugged state. This "state-dependent learning" is now recognized as an important factor to be taken into account in all such experiments. It has also been shown that tasks learned in the presence of a psychotropic drug may subsequently be performed better in the drugged state. This can be confused with pharmacologic drug dependence, since the animal performs the task better with the drug than without it. To distinguish between such learning effects and true pharmacologic tolerance and dependence, it is necessary to use multiple criteria of drug action, including some that are unlikely to be modifiable by learning.[73]

An important advance has been the development of self-administration procedures, in which animals inject themselves intravenously by pressing a bar or lever. In this type of operant conditioning, the reinforcing (rewarding) properties of drugs can be examined directly. An animal is fitted with an indwelling polyethylene cannula in the jugular vein. A lever in the cage controls the administration of a drug solution, so that a fixed dose of drug is injected at each lever press or after a certain number of lever presses. In early experiments of this type with morphine in rats,[74] it was thought necessary first to make the animals passively tolerant and dependent by means of injections administered by the investigator. Then the lever pressing behavior was introduced as a means of relieving the discomfort of the withdrawal syndrome. Subsequently, the animal would maintain lever pressing behavior at a fairly constant rate, thus obtaining morphine injections on a continuing schedule. The rats tended to maintain a constant daily dose of morphine, increasing the rate of lever pressing if the drug concentration in the infusing solution was decreased, and decreasing the rate if the concentration was increased. When saline solution was substituted for morphine, the rate of lever pressing rose sharply. Then, with continued lack of reinforcement, the lever pressing behavior was extinguished. The greatly increased rate of lever pressing when drug was withdrawn could perhaps be analogized to the frantic "hustling" behavior of addicts in the early part of a withdrawal syndrome. It is interesting that, in these experiments, the rats did not continually increase their drug intake to higher and higher levels when they had every opportunity to do so, but rather established a constant daily intake well below what could have been obtained. Perhaps a maximum degree of tolerance had been reached.

Similar experiments with monkeys[75] revealed that drugs of the addicting type can serve as primary reinforcers. This means that the drug injection itself, in an animal that has never before received the drug, is reinforcing, tending to perpetuate the operant behavior (lever pressing) that immediately preceded the injection. All monkeys, under the appropriate experimental conditions, will addict themselves to just the

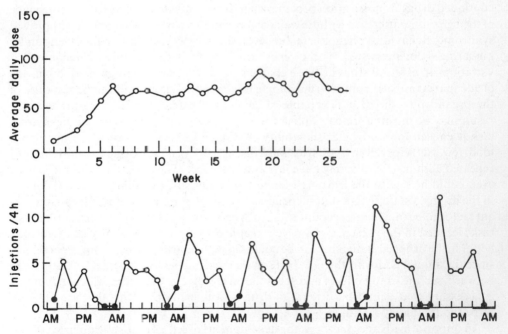

FIGURE 9-12. Morphine self-administration in the monkey. *Typical records for a male Rhesus monkey self-injecting morphine, 2.5 mg kg^{-1} per injection. Upper record: Average daily dose for 26-week period. Lower record: Diurnal pattern of drug intake during the fifth week, by 4-hr periods. The low point in each cycle is at 4:00 a.m.; the high point is at noon. (Adapted from Deneau et al., Figure 4.[75])*

same drugs that have abuse potential in man—especially the opiates, alcohol, barbiturates, cocaine, and amphetamines. Figure 9-12 shows a typical record of such self-administration behavior with morphine. Typically, as shown here, the animal increases its daily dose as tolerance develops, often reaching a very high daily intake and establishing a high degree of physical dependence. Eventually, as shown in the upper part of the figure, the daily intake stabilizes; however, as shown below, there is a marked diurnal cycle. Animals in this self-induced "addicted" state largely ignore other reinforcing activities such as satisfying hunger, thirst, or sexual drive in favor of exclusive preoccupation with self-administration of the drug. In this respect, self-addicted monkeys behave very much like human addicts.[76]

Animals on self-injection schedules, like human addicts, illustrate two kinds of conditioning that can lead to perpetuation of drug-seeking and drug-using behavior. Initially there is only the primary reinforcement, the "rewarding" quality of the drug's action on the brain. The mechanism is probably related to that of the well-known electrical self-stimulation phenomenon.[77] When electrodes are implanted in certain specific areas (e.g., medial forebrain bundle) stimulation has positively reinforcing properties, perhaps through excitation of neuronal "reward" pathways, such as must presumably exist to mediate the reinforcement of biologically useful behavior patterns (eating, drinking, sexual activity). It seems likely that drugs with positively reinforcing properties may also act upon such pathways, possibly by altering neurotransmitter synthesis, release, reuptake, metabolism, or postsynaptic action. The power of primary reinforcement is shown by the fact that monkeys will self-administer a drug like cocaine to the point of exhaustion, convulsions, and even death, although it does not produce physical dependence.[75]

If a drug produces physical dependence, there is an additional reinforcement—the relief of abstinence symptoms by administration of the drug. This secondary reinforcement plays an important part in shaping addict behavior, even after the development of tolerance has largely diminished the direct pleasurable aspects of drug injection. Each time mild or severe withdrawal discomfort grows, builds to a peak, and then is suddenly and completely eliminated by the next drug dose, the drug-seeking ("hustling") and drug-using behaviors are reinforced.[78]

Many of the characteristic subjective effects of centrally acting drugs can only be studied in humans because, if they occur in other species, we have no way to detect or measure them. Only in recent years have the techniques of the controlled clinical trial (cf. Chapter 14) been applied to the study of drug tolerance and physical dependence. A great deal of out present understanding in this field is derived from investigations on human volunteers carried out over a number of years at the U.S. Public Health Service hospital for addicts at Lexington, Kentucky. A very important advantage of this locale is that the patient-prisoners who volunteer to be subjects are under restraint, the wards can be locked, and external sources of drugs can be effectively cut off. Without these safeguards, one might well wonder if experimental conditions could actually be observed faithfully. Many examples in the remainder of this chapter will be drawn from this extraordinary series of clinical-pharmacologic experiments.

As a prototype of this kind of study, let us examine in detail an experiment carried out to see if tolerance could develop to LSD or to D-amphetamine in man.[57] A second question concerned the mechanism of action of these stimulant drugs. If they acted in the same way upon the same receptors, then tolerance to one would presumably confer tolerance to the other. The experiment was designed so that cross-tolerance could be tested as well as direct tolerance to the drug that had been administered chronically. The subjects were 10 former opiate addicts who had received no narcotic drugs for at least 6 months. The drugs, including a placebo control, were given "blind," i.e., without the subjects being aware of their nature. The subjects were divided into two groups. First, over a period of a few weeks, test doses of placebo, D-amphetamine, and LSD were given to both groups. Various measurements were made at hourly intervals, twice before the test dose and eight times thereafter; these included body temperature, pulse rate, blood pressure, pupillary diameter, and kneejerk. In addition, the subject was asked to respond to a series of questions about his mood, feelings, and sensations. Two doses of LSD (0.5 μg kg^{-1} and 1.5 μg kg^{-1}) and a single dose of D-amphetamine (0.6 mg kg^{-1}) were used. At the higher dose of LSD, as compared with placebo, there was a significant rise in temperature, pulse rate, blood pressure, and pupillary diameter, and a significant reduction of the threshold stimulus required to elicit the kneejerk. Moreover, there were significantly more positive answers to the questions about mood (e.g., "Do you have a weird feeling?") after the higher dose of LSD than after placebo. "Clinical grades" assigned by physician observers, based on the subjects' general behavior, were also significantly increased relative to placebo. With D-amphetamine, the significant changes were a rise in blood pressure, an increase in the number of positive answers on the questionnaire (e.g., "Does your memory seem sharper to you than usual?"), and increased "clinical grades."

One group of subjects was then given LSD, another group D-amphetamine, on a regular schedule, beginning with smaller doses and building up to 1.5 μg kg^{-1} of LSD and 0.6 mg kg^{-1} of D-amphetamine (the same as the test doses) daily for 13 days. The tests were then repeated on two successive days, using both drugs for each group of subjects. Thus, the group that had been receiving D-amphetamine chronically was tested for direct tolerance to D-amphetamine, and also for crosstolerance to LSD. The group that had received LSD chronically was tested for direct tolerance to LSD and crosstolerance to D-amphetamine. A rest period of two weeks was allowed to permit the tolerance to wane. Now the entire experiment was repeated with the same subjects, including a repeat of the initial testing, the period of chronic administration, and the final testing, except that the drugs were crossed over. The subjects that had been made tolerant to D-amphetamine in the first stage were now made tolerant to LSD, and vice versa.

The results of this experiment were extraordinarily clear-cut. After chronic administration of LSD, the effect of the test dose of LSD was diminished on all the variables measured, especially the pupillary dilation. The subjective actions of LSD also decreased greatly. The effects of a test dose of D-amphetamine, however, remained essentially unchanged. After chronic administration of D-amphetamine, on the other hand, direct tolerance developed with respect to the blood pressure elevation and the subjective effects, and there was no crosstolerance to LSD. The striking results obtained for the questionnaire responses in one part of this experiment are presented in Figure 9-13. The results with D-amphetamine during control periods are shown as the number of positive answers in the questionnaire as a function of time after administration of the test dose, in the curves labeled *Control*. The curve labeled *Test*, on the left, represents the responses to the test dose of D-amphetamine after the period of chronic administration of D-amphetamine; direct tolerance is essentially

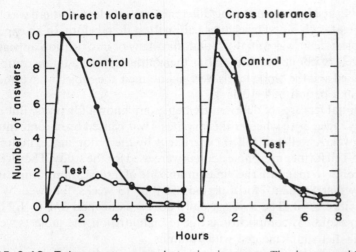

FIGURE 9-13. Tolerance to D-amphetamine in man. *The data are subjective positive responses to a questionnaire about the effects of D-amphetamine on mood. Time after administration of 0.6 mg kg⁻¹ D-amphetamine is shown on x axis. Direct tolerance (left) is shown by diminution of response after chronic administration of D-amphetamine for 13 days as compared with initial control. Absence of cross tolerance (right) is shown by nearly identical response to the control after chronic administration of LSD for 13 days. Both parts of the experiment were carried out at different times in the same subjects in a crossover design. (From Rosenberg et al., Figure 3.⁵⁷ By permission of Springer.)*

complete. On the right is seen the action of D-amphetamine in the same subjects after they had been made tolerant to LSD. There was no crosstolerance to D-amphetamine whatsoever. When similar curves were plotted (not shown) for the effects of test doses of LSD in LSD-tolerant and D-amphetamine-tolerant subjects, they looked very much like these. The clear conclusion is that although D-amphetamine and LSD have some similarities as stimulant drugs, their mechanisms of action are quite different. In contrast, crosstolerance does develop between LSD and two other hallucinogens, mescaline and psilocybin.

Alcohol, Barbiturates, and Related Depressants.   These central depressants produce effects, including tolerance and physical dependence, that are more dangerous to the addict and to society than occur with the opiate narcotics.[73-81] The desired effects with these agents are often obtained at the expense of motor incoordination, boisterous and aggressive behavior, and loss of judgment. The antisocial aspects of alcoholism are nowhere more evident than in the high mortality and injury rates associated with drunken driving. Yet our society imposes no penalties upon the use of alcohol. At the same time, it classes addicts to morphine or heroin as criminals, although no demonstrable antisocial behavior is associated with the pharmacologic actions of these drugs.

It was shown many years ago that tolerance to alcohol has a cellular basis, for both in animals and in man repeated administration leads to diminishing effects at given levels of alcohol in the blood. Dogs, for example, were given as much alcohol as they would tolerate for a period of 55 weeks.[82] Alcohol concentrations in the blood and cerebrospinal fluid were measured periodically. Throughout the range of blood levels, established by administering different doses of alcohol, there was less manifest intoxication at each blood level after habituation than before. In an experiment with human subjects,[83] it was initially found that signs of intoxication appeared at blood alcohol levels of about 2 mg ml^{-1}. But then, although the administration of alcohol was continued and the blood levels were maintained, the subjects nevertheless became sober within a period of 4–10 hr.

The essential features of delirium tremens were known for years. But considerable controversy raged as to whether this psychosis was caused by chronic intoxication or by withdrawal. A well-controlled experiment by the group at Lexington settled the question.[84] Ten former morphine addicts were used for the study. They were furnished enough alcohol to maintain the "maximum state of intoxication compatible with safe ambulatory management" for a period of up to 13 weeks, followed by abrupt and complete withdrawal. The average daily dose was around 1/4 to 1/2 liter of 95% ethanol. To avoid any complications due to malnutrition, the subjects were kept on a high-calorie diet supplemented with vitamins.

The "degree of intoxication" was evaluated by trained observers using an arbitrary scale from 0–4. There was fairly good agreement between blood levels and the estimated degree of intoxication. Initially, as the daily intake was being increased very cautiously, there was no evidence of intoxication. Then, as the blood concentration rose past 1 mg ml^{-1} the subjects became boisterous, noisy, and silly. During the third week, a curious fall in the blood alcohol concentrations occurred without any change in the daily intake. Its cause was not investigated, but it might reflect the appearance of increased activity of the liver enzymes that metabolize ethanol. As the blood alcohol level declined at this time, sobriety returned. When the daily dose was then increased, the blood level rose again, and the state of intoxication returned. Subsequently, the blood level continued to rise as the daily intake was adjusted upward, but the degree of intoxication lagged behind. Tolerance was demonstrable on electroencephalograph records as well as by these gross evaluations. An increase of slow-wave activity occurred initially at the higher blood levels, but this effect became less marked as the experiment proceeded, despite the rising blood levels in the final weeks.

During their state of chronic intoxication, none of the subjects developed any hallucinatory or convulsive behavior. The onset of withdrawal symptoms upon discontinuance of alcohol administration was quite rapid. About 8 hr after their last drink, the subjects became nervous, apprehensive, and very weak. Some suffered retching and vomiting. All six of the patients who had been drinking for 48 days or more manifested tremor, weakness, perspiration, nausea, vomiting, diarrhea, elevated blood pressure, and insomnia. Delirium and hallucinations occurred in four of the subjects. Convulsions of the grand mal type developed in two; one of these became so seriously ill he had to be treated with barbiturates. All the symptoms waned after a number of days, and 3 months later the subjects appeared to be quite normal in all respects. Three subjects who withdrew from the experiment within the first month developed only slight tremor and anorexia.

It is clear from this and similar experiments[85] that delirium tremens is a typical withdrawal syndrome manifested after prolonged intake of ethyl alcohol, that a severe degree of physical dependence may occur, and that the intensity of the withdrawal syndrome depends upon the duration of exposure to alcohol and the dosage schedule.

The experiments cited above clarified an aspect of alcoholism about which there had been much confusion. The natural history of the disease in humans runs a very long course, usually several decades, with gradual increase in the frequency and amount of alcohol intake. It had been thought, therefore, that the development of alcohol dependence must be very slow. It is apparent now, however, that the pharmacologic aspects of alcohol dependence can develop extremely rapidly, given continuous exposure to a high alcohol concentration for a relatively short time. In the development of alcoholism, it is the pattern of alcohol intake that changes slowly, over a period of many years. When the intake of alcohol becomes sufficient to sustain high blood and brain levels continuously for a period of days or weeks, alcohol dependence develops, and delirium tremens may then occur on withdrawal, as at the end of a typical drinking spree.

Animal models for the study of alcohol dependence were not available until recently. Most experimental animals will not drink voluntarily to the point of intoxication, so special techniques are required. In one such procedure known as "schedule-induced polydipsia," rats are fed with small food pellets dispensed only during fixed feeding periods scheduled evenly around the clock.[86] This leads to a considerably increased water intake (schedule-induced polydipsia). If the only source of water is an alcohol solution, the rats drink up to about 13 grams of ethanol per kilogram of body weight; this would correspond to a daily alcohol intake of more than a liter for a person of average weight. The animals consume nearly half their calories as ethanol. They are moderately intoxicated throughout most of each day at first, but the signs of intoxication gradually lessen, although blood levels remain in the usually intoxicating range (above 1 mg ml^{-1}) most of the time. After 3 or 4 weeks of this regimen, in one experiment, the ethanol administration was stopped. Within a few hours the rats became hyperactive, and convulsions could be induced by stimuli (e.g., jangling sounds) that had no effects in normal rats. Several of the animals died in the course of the convulsions.

What is the relationship between drug dose (and duration of exposure) and the degree of physical dependence, as measured by the intensity of the withdrawal syndrome? To answer this fundamental question, quantitative methods were required. First, the brain level of alcohol had to be held constant so that different levels and different durations of exposure could be studied. Second, some system of grading the withdrawal syndrome was necessary. Mice were housed in a vapor chamber containing a fixed concentration of ethanol.[87] By administering daily injections of pyrazole, the liver alcohol dehydrogenase could be inhibited. With alcohol metabolism thus largely blocked, a near-equilibrium could be established across the alveoli so that the ethanol level in blood was linearly related to its concentration in the inspired air, as described for volatile anesthetics in Chapter 4. During their stay in the vapor chamber, the mice were more or less intoxicated, depending upon the ethanol concentration. On removing the mice from the vapor chamber, various characteristic withdrawal signs were observed (including convulsions and death), and these could be scored according to their severity. As Figure 9-14A shows, the withdrawal reaction reached its peak at about 10 hr, then subsided completely in about 30 hr. The degree of dependence (intensity of withdrawal reaction) proved to be related linearly to the total exposure to alcohol, i.e., the blood level times the duration, as shown in Figure 9-15. It was found that even a single injection of alcohol produced a very slight but measurable degree of dependence.

This technique proved useful for studying the effects of various drugs on the course of the withdrawal reaction. Injections of ethanol abolished all the withdrawal signs

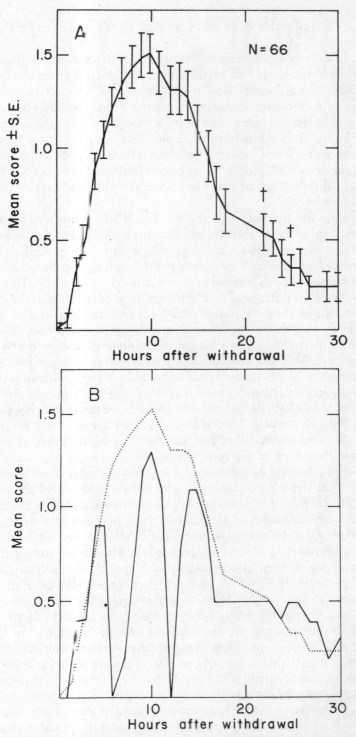

FIGURE 9-14. Withdrawal reaction of mice removed from vapor chamber.
A: Course of the withdrawal reaction in mice exposed for 3 days to a blood alcohol level of 1.8–2.3 mg ml^{-1}, then removed from the vapor chamber and left untreated. B: Modification of withdrawal syndrome by pentobarbital injections, 60 mg kg^{-1} at arrows. Dotted curve is that for the untreated mice, as above. (From Goldstein, Figures 1 and 4.[88])

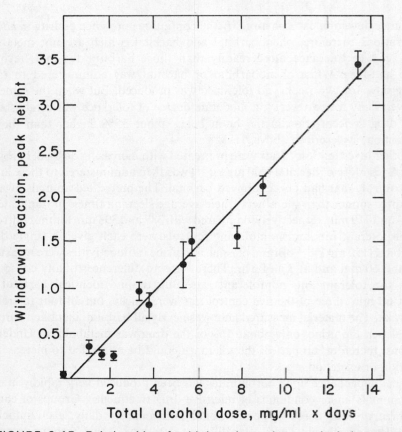

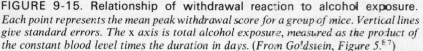

FIGURE 9-15. Relationship of withdrawal reaction to alcohol exposure. *Each point represents the mean peak withdrawal score for a group of mice. Vertical lines give standard errors. The x axis is total alcohol exposure, measured as the product of the constant blood level times the duration in days. (From Goldstein, Figure 5.[87])*

immediately, but they returned as the ethanol was eliminated. Pentobarbital had the same effect (Figure 9-14B), as was expected from the known cross-dependence of barbiturates and alcohol. Chlorpromazine, on the other hand, which is not useful clinically in alcohol withdrawal, made the withdrawal reaction worse.

Tolerance to the barbiturates and related drugs and physical dependence on them present a picture rather similar to what is seen with alcohol.[39,90] In both cases, experiments in animals have shown that, although a contribution to tolerance is made by increased drug metabolism due to induction of enzymes, the main feature of tolerance is an adaptation of the brain to higher drug levels. Neither with the barbiturates nor with alcohol does one see the impressive degree of tolerance that can develop with the narcotics; nevertheless, the tolerance is readily demonstrable. For example, rats were given barbital in daily doses of 200 mg kg^{-1} subcutaneously, a sufficient dose to produce anesthesia.[91] At the instant of awakening, each rat was sacrificed and the drug concentration was determined in its brain. In a group of animals thus killed after the second daily dose, the mean brain concentration was 184 mg kg^{-1}. After the fifth injection, the concentration at awakening was 248 mg kg^{-1}. a statistically significant increase ($P < 0.01$).

Tolerance development is favored by the continuous presence of drug in adequate concentration; therefore, phenobarbital and barbital, which are not metabolized rapidly, lead to tolerance more readily than those barbiturates that have short biologic half-lifes. When phenobarbital or barbital was administered to rats on alternate days for two weeks, no tolerance was produced. But when the same doses were given daily for two weeks, a moderate degree of tolerance was established, the waking drug concentration in the brain being about 35% higher than the initial concentration, as described above.[91]

In another investigation,[92] rats were pretreated with increasing doses of barbital for 13 days. A test dose of barbital (200 mg kg^{-1}) was then administered to these animals and to controls that had never received barbital. The pretreated animals awakened significantly sooner than the others; their average sleeping times, in duplicate runs, were 284 and 319 min, respectively, compared with 387 and 393 min for the control rats. Then the tolerant rats and nontolerant controls were each given a single dose of ^{14}C-barbital (150 mg kg^{-1}). Brain, plasma, and urine radioactivities were measured at 10, 30, and 60 min and at 3 and 6 hr. There were no differences of any consequence between the tolerant and nontolerant rats. But, despite identical barbital brain levels at 60 min, three of the five control rats were asleep, but all four tolerant rats were awake. The material measured here was nearly all barbital, identified chromatographically in the urine; only about 5% of the drug was metabolized. Under these conditions, therefore, no part of the tolerance could be attributed to increased drug destruction or excretion.

Physical dependence upon barbiturates has been produced very rapidly in experimental animals under conditions of intensive drug treatment.[93] Groups of cats were given three or four doses of pentobarbital intravenously daily, each sufficient to produce deep anesthesia. Then, after different durations of this barbiturate pretreatment, groups of the cats were tested to determine their thresholds for the induction of convulsive seizures with pentylenetetrazol. The periods of pentobarbital administration studied were from one day to three weeks. As the experiment continued, tolerance was manifested by a shortening of the duration of anesthesia, and it became necessary to increase the dosage to establish the same degree of anesthesia. On abrupt termination of the barbiturate injections, except in the group intoxicated for only one day, typical withdrawal syndromes developed. The cats showed increased hyperexcitability, tremors, startle responses, myoclonic jerks, and in at least one animal a spontaneous grand mal seizure. The pentylenetetrazol seizure thresholds were determined by infusing this convulsant drug intravenously at a slow constant rate and measuring the amount required to produce the onset of the tonic phase of muscular movements. The results are given in Table 9-1. They show that even after intoxication with pentobarbital for only 26 hr, although no spontaneous signs of withdrawal could be detected, the seisure threshold was already lowered, compared with initial thresholds determined in the same cats. After longer periods of intoxication, the lowering of seizure threshold during the withdrawal period was very marked, and it persisted for several days.

In man, tolerance to barbiturates is well known. A false impression long prevailed that physical dependence upon these agents did not develop, until experiments with human subjects,[94-95] very much like those on alcohol, showed otherwise. The experiments demonstrated that abrupt withdrawal from barbiturates precipitates a particularly violent withdrawal syndrome, characterized by weakness, tremor,

TABLE 9-1. Lowering of seizure threshold during barbiturate withdrawal in cats. Cats were given pentobarbital intravenously 3–4 times daily, in doses sufficient to cause deep anesthesia. Prior to the injections, seizure threshold was determined in each cat by infusing pentylenetetrazol intravenously and measuring how much was required to produce tonic muscular contractions. Then, after various durations of barbiturate intoxication, seizure threshold was again determined 20 and 90 hr after pentobarbital was discontinued. The data are average thresholds, as percents of initial threshold for each animal group. All the depressed thresholds differ significantly (P < 0.05) from the pretreatment value. (Data from Jaffe and Sharpless,[93] Table 1.)

No. of animals	Duration of barbiturate treatment	Threshold for pentylenetetrazol-induced seizures (% of pretreatment threshold)	
		20 hr after terminating barbiturate	90 hr after terminating barbiturate
8	26 hr	82	101
7	56 hr	72	107
7	5 days	46	103
4	3 weeks	31	59

insomnia, anxiety, vomiting, loss of weight, increased pulse and respiratory rates, increased blood pressure, convulsions of the grand mal type, and a psychosis closely resembling alcoholic delirium tremens. Because the withdrawal syndrome is so severe, abrupt withdrawal of barbiturates from an addicted patient must never be undertaken; the dosage has to be reduced very gradually over a long period of time.

New centrally acting drugs are too often introduced and used widely before the hazards of tolerance and physical dependence are fully realized. This was true of the mild tranquilizing agent meprobamate. Eventually, in a well-designed clinical trial, the withdrawal syndrome was demonstrated unequivocally.[96] Groups of about 25 patients each were given placebo or meprobamate (3.2 or 4.6 g) daily for 40 days. The design of the experiment was "double blind," i.e., neither the patients nor the observers knew the assignment of medications. Severe sedative effects were observed at both dosages of meprobamate; 35 out of the 47 patients receiving the drug had a staggering gait or could not stand unsupported. Over a period of about a week, however, despite continued dosage, tolerance developed, and these effects wore off. After 40 days, placebo was substituted for drug in identical capsules, so patients were unaware that medications were being changed. A variety of withdrawal symptoms ensued, of varying degrees of severity, involving 44 of the 47 patients. Insomnia and tremors were the most common; others included vomiting, severe anxiety, loss of appetite, hallucinations, and delusions resembling those seen after alcohol withdrawal. Three patients had grand mal convulsive seizures. Patients who had been receiving placebo for the first 40 days experienced no "withdrawal" effects, whereas the severity of the syndrome in the patients from whom meprobamate was withdrawn bore a direct relationship to the dosage previously administered.

The lesson of meprobamate—that tranquilizers very often turn out to be addicting —seems to be learned only slowly. In subsequent decades, other depressants with tranquilizing properties were introduced, each alleged to have low addiction liability and each in turn being abused on a large scale and causing physical dependence. Various drugs are preferred at different times and places; preferences wax and wane. Short-acting barbiturates like secobarbital and pentobarbital ("reds" and "yellows") remain, together with alcohol, the most favored and cheapest of the depressants. Serious drug abuse problems, with accompanying dependence, have been encountered with the benzodiazepines (chlordiazepoxide, diazepam).

Physical dependence upon alcohol, barbiturates, meprobamate, or other depressants of this class, entails no cross-dependence upon the opiate narcotics, but there seems to be complete cross-dependence within this group. Paraldehyde, for example, has been used traditionally in alcoholic delirium tremens, and barbiturates are also effective in this condition. To a large extent, the success of such agents may be due not so much to their own sedative properties as to their specific relief of the withdrawal syndrome by substituting for alcohol, and then permitting a more gradual withdrawal to be accomplished.[84]

Narcotics.

Pharmacologic effects of the narcotics.   This group of compounds comprises the natural opium alkaloids, of which morphine is the prototype, and related synthetic and semisynthetic drugs. Sometimes these are called, as a group, opiates (or opioid narcotics); we shall refer to them simply as narcotics. The compounds that have been studied most intensively are morphine, heroin (diacetylmorphine), and the synthetic congeners levorphanol, meperidine, and methadone. The structure-activity relationships among these drugs were discussed in Chapter 1, where their chemical formulas and conformations are also given (p. 34 ff.).

The narcotics have complex pharmacologic effects.[97–99] They are exceedingly valuable clinically for allaying severe pain and alleviating anxiety. The aspect of their psychotropic action that accounts for their abuse by addicts is described as *euphoria*. This is a peculiar state of wellbeing, which seems to defy exact description.[60,100] After intravenous administration of morphine or heroin, the addict experiences an immediate sensation of physical pleasure akin to sexual orgasm.[101] A feeling of relaxation follows, which may be accompanied by increased loquaciousness, increased motor activity, or facilitation of social interaction. With higher doses, sedation is the prominent effect, with indulgence in daydreams and fantasies. Libido and aggressiveness are decreased as the subject becomes increasingly withdrawn and unresponsive to his surroundings, often drifting into sleep. It seems very likely that the analgesia produced by these drugs is intimately connected with the euphoriant effect as a whole, and that what is primarily altered is the emotional reaction and anxiety engendered by painful stimuli. Indeed, patients with intractable pain commonly report, after receiving a narcotic analgesic, that the pain is still perceived but "no longer bothers" them. Many years of research have been devoted to the quest for an analgesic drug that would be free of addiction liability. In general, it has been found that these properties go together. In recent years, however, there has been some interest in the mixed agonist–antagonists (e.g., nalorphine, cyclazocine), which do have analgesic effects without apparent addiction liability.

Although, to some extent, the narcotics produce similar actions in all animal species, the euphoriant actions can be observed directly only in man. Moreover, man is much more sensitive to these drugs than are other species; the effective analgesic dose of morphine in man, for example, is about 0.2 mg kg^{-1}, whereas in the dog, it is at least 10 times higher. As in man, the predominant effects in monkeys, dogs, rabbits, and rats are sedative. In horses, cats, and mice, the predominant effects are excitatory. But these do not seem to be fundamental differences. In any species (including man), the narcotics produce a mixture of excitatory and depressant effects upon gross motor behavior, clearly excitatory effects like emesis, and specific actions such as analgesia and hypothermia that are not readily characterized as excitatory or depressant. Respiratory depression is produced in all animals. It is the cause of death from over-dosage in man and most other species. Even in mice, where motor activity is greatly stimulated by the narcotics, death is caused by respiratory depression, which appears to be superimposed on the excitation caused at lower doses.

Tolerance to the narcotics. Most investigations of tolerance or physical dependence in animals have used analgesia (antinociceptive action) as the criterion of drug effect. This has often been successful, but the results have to be interpreted with caution. In such investigations, animals are subjected to some standard procedure for inflicting a noxious stimulus, and their reaction is recorded. Often, the measure of analgesia is the latency of reaction to the stimulus. Analgesia is then defined as the drug-induced toleration of the noxious stimulus, and tolerance is defined as re-establishment of the reaction pattern despite the presence of the drug. Increasing the drug dosage should then once more produce analgesia, and the degree of tolerance can be defined in terms of the increase in drug dosage required to produce the same degree of analgesia as a standard dose did initially. However, the criteria of analgesia are somewhat uncertain, since the mere failure of an animal to lift its paw or flick its tail when heat or pressure is applied might signify interference with a simple spinal reflex rather than an analgesic action upon the brain. Moreover, in this type of experiment, whenever any influence causes the animal to become more responsive to noxious stimuli in the presence of drug, it will appear that pharmacologic tolerance has developed. At best, analgesia is an indirect measure of drug action in animals, and its interpretation remains somewhat uncertain. Experiments in which a narcotic drug directly produces a biologic response would seem better suited to the study of tolerance.

The duration of action of a single dose of a narcotic is determined by the route of administration and by the rate of elimination of the particular drug. If repeated doses are given at appropriate intervals, the intensity of response diminishes; then, in order to obtain the same response as formerly, the dose has to be increased. Thus, in the course of days or weeks, the tolerance, in human subjects or other species, may build up to a remarkable degree, until many times the lethal dose can eventually be tolerated. In man, for example, an initial dose of 100–200 mg of morphine would be sufficient to cause profound sedation, respiratory depression, anoxia, and death; but tolerant subjects have been known to take as much as 4 g without adverse effect.[102] Once tolerance has been established to one of the narcotics, the subject is found to be crosstolerant to all narcotics but not to drugs of a different series. Morphine-tolerant individuals are also tolerant to heroin, methadone, meperidine, and so on but not to alcohol or barbiturates. In other words, tolerance to narcotics is highly specific for the chemical structure of these compounds; it is not a physiologic adaptation to depressant agents in general.[103]

The usual course of addiction is for the addict to increase successive doses of narcotic just as much as is required to obtain the sought-for euphoric effect. The ability of addicts to "feel" this drug action and estimate its intensity has been used to establish the time course of the progression of tolerance in a remarkable experiment.[104] Postaddicts, who had not received any narcotic drugs for several months, were given heroin or morphine intravenously 4 times daily. The dosage was started at 18 mg, in divided doses, on the first day, and was increased stepwise to 180 mg on the 19th day of the experiment. After each injection, the addicts were asked simply to judge the intensity of effect on an arbitrary scale. A dose-response curve for these estimates was established by administering various doses to other groups of postaddicts and considering only their responses to the first dose administered. A "tolerance index" could then be constructed as follows. Any given subjective judgment of intensity could be converted to a standard dose that would have been required to produce that same estimated intensity in nontolerant subjects. The tolerance index was defined as the ratio of this equieffective standard dose to the actual dose administered. Initially, at the first dose the tolerance index would be 1.0 because the administered dose produces the same effect as the standard dose. As tolerance develops, the index becomes smaller, and it approaches zero as larger doses produce even smaller effects. The result of this experiment is shown in Figure 9-16. It indicates that tolerance to

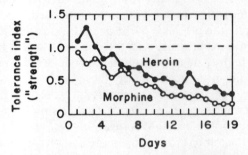

FIGURE 9-16. Course of development of tolerance to heroin and morphine. *Eight addicts were studied. Heroin or morphine was administered intravenously 4 times daily. Morphine dose was increased gradually from 18 mg on the first day to 180 mg on the 19th day. Heroin dose was increased from 7.2 mg to 76 mg. Subjects were asked to estimate the "strength" of the drug, and these estimates were converted to a "tolerance index" as described in the text. The tolerance index is the ratio of dose that would be required in a nontolerant subject to dose actually administered to achieve the same estimated effect in the tolerant subject. An index of zero would represent complete tolerance. (From Martin and Fraser, Figure 6.[104])*

morphine begins to develop without any lag, apparently at the very first dose administered. After 2–3 weeks, a 10 times higher dosage was required to yield the same effects. Eventually (not shown), doses up to about 20 times higher or more were tolerated, at which time the desired effects were no longer obtained at all. The course of development of tolerance to heroin is characterized by a short lag, but then it parallels the morphine course.

Similar experiments can be carried out with animals, using various objective responses as criteria. It had been suggested[105] that tolerance only develops to depressant effects of the narcotics. In man, however, tolerance involves all the typical psychotropic actions, some of which are depressant, some excitatory. In mice, the most obvious effect of the narcotics is to stimulate motor activity of a special kind, described as a stereotyped "running fit." Tolerance does develop to this excitatory action,[106] and, therefore, running activity has proved a useful tool for studying the time course and reversibility of tolerance. Home cages are fitted with light beams and photocells, with each interruption of a beam activating a counter. After the initial exploratory behavior subsides, the animals spend most of the time huddled together in a corner of the cage, so that background activity is very low. Removal from the cage, injection with saline solution, and replacement in the cage produced very little increase in the recorded activity. In contrast, an opiate induced a great increase in running, which continued at a constant rate for about 2 hr, then gradually diminished. When the same dose was injected at regular intervals (e.g., every 8 hr), less running activity was produced after each successive dose. At any time during this process, substantially increasing the opiate dose could reinstate nearly the full running activity seen after the initial injection. Thus, the capacity of mice to perform the motor act was not impaired; only the sensitivity to opiate had decreased.

In order to carry out quantitative experiments on the tolerance process, it was necessary to vary either the dose or the interval, holding the other constant. With a given narcotic, the dose-response relationship dictates the dose that will be required to produce a maximal response at the outset. Using this constant dose, one can vary the injection interval at will. Such experiments were carried out using levorphanol at the fixed dose of 20 mg kg^{-1}, which causes maximal running activity in the mouse receiving its first injection. As shown in Figure 9-17, each interval schedule led to a

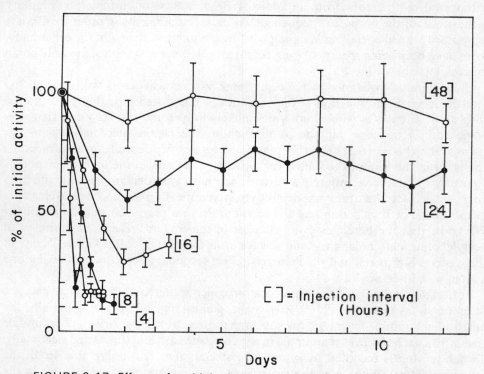

FIGURE 9-17. Effects of multiple doses of a narcotic on tolerance in mice. *Levorphanol (20 mg kg^{-1}) was injected i.p. on various interval schedules. Running activity was measured initially and after each injection. Points represent running activity as percent of initial running activity for each group of mice. Numbers in brackets represent the injection interval for each curve, 4, 8, 16, 24, and 48 hr. (From Goldstein and Sheehan, Figure 6.[106a])*

different rate of development of tolerance and also a different eventual degree of tolerance. The 4 hr interval was not much different from the 8 hr interval, suggesting that an intrinsic process limited the rate at which tolerance could possibly develop. At the 48 hr interval, no tolerance developed, i.e., whatever process was initiated by the single injection had worn off completely 48 hr later.

The best interpretation of these findings is that a single effective dose of a narcotic initiates a certain biochemical change, with its own intrinsic time course of onset and decay, which is responsible for tolerance (and dependence, see below). If the next dose is given before the increment induced by the previous dose has decayed, tolerance will build up, just as in the process of cumulative toxicity (cf. Chapter 4). The curves of Figure 9-17 are like those to be expected from such a model in which the plateau level of tolerance represents a steady state, at which the amount of new tolerance induced by each dose is just sufficient to last through the interval until the next dose is due. The model is that of a completely reversible process, which is complete at 24–48 hr. If the same thing applies to human addicts, it implies that there is some "safe" interval for morphine or heroin injections, at which tolerance and dependence would not build up; anecdotal evidence from addicts suggests that this interval may be a few days or so but that daily use leads to tolerance and dependence. The principles here seem to be very similar to those emerging in the study of alcohol dependence, as discussed earlier. As expected of a reversible process, tolerance disappears after withdrawal of a narcotic from an addict. Indeed, addicts often undergo voluntary withdrawal for the purpose of reducing their daily requirements in order to alleviate temporarily the financial hardship imposed by the tolerant state. On the other hand, there have been some reports of long persistent tolerance in animals, possibly on an immunologic basis.[8]

Understanding tolerance in molecular and biochemical terms will require first that the mechanism of action of the narcotics be elucidated. For that goal, studies with whole animals or whole brains are unlikely to be sufficient. We know that sites of narcotic action are widespread throughout the central nervous system—for example, blockade of reflexes in the spinal cord, respiratory depression in the medulla, analgesia in the wall of the fourth ventricle, hypothermia in the anterior hypothalamus.[107,108] But localization of a narcotic action to a particular anatomic site does not reveal if it acts there presynaptically or postsynaptically or on non-neural elements of the tissue, or if its action has any relationship to a particular neurotransmitter. We know that the narcotics cause changes in the content, release, or turnover of acetylcholine, catecholamines, and serotonin in the brain.[109] But which, if any, of these effects is primary, and which merely reflect secondary consequences of narcotic action, we still do not know.

Fortunately, an isolated tissue preparation which seems to contain typical narcotic receptors is available.[34,110,111] This is the guinea pig ileum, and especially the longitudinal muscle-myenteric plexus preparation from this organ. The muscle strip with attached plexus is mounted in a small tissue bath and stimulated electrically. Twitch tension is recorded by means of a strain gauge and polygraph. In all the following essentials, the muscle strip behaves like narcotic sensitive systems in the brain: (1) the required concentrations are very low, in the same range as pharmacologically effective concentrations in the whole animal; (2) the rank order of potencies for a great many narcotics corresponds extremely well with the order for analgesia or other typical narcotic effects; (3) the specific narcotic antagonists block or reverse the narcotic actions; (4) the narcotic effects are stereospecific for the D(−) isomers; (5) muscle strips prepared from animals made tolerant to narcotics are also tolerant to narcotics.

The myenteric plexus is by no means a simple neural network, but it is obviously a great deal simpler than the brain. Electrical stimulation acts upon the plexus, leading eventually to release of acetylcholine at the muscle; atropine, accordingly, abolishes the electrically stimulated twitch. It is known that morphine acts by decreasing the release of acetylcholine, but it is uncertain if this is an effect on the cholinergic terminals or on some other neural element of the plexus. Morphine tolerant muscle strips were found to be tolerant as well to the addition of catecholamines to the bath; these substances ordinarily have inhibitory actions like those of morphine.[112] The sensitivity to added acetylcholine, which provokes contraction of unstimulated muscle, was not changed. As Figure 9-18 shows, there was a pronounced supersensitivity to serotonin, which also causes muscle contraction. Serotonin supersensitivity in the central nervous system could be a primary mechanism of narcotic tolerance (cf. p. 612). It is likely that fundamental progress in understanding tolerance and dependence will be made in this (or a similar) isolated tissue in which the affected

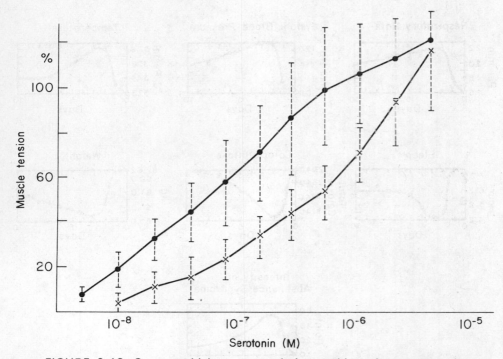

FIGURE 9-18. Supersensitivity to serotonin in morphine tolerant myenteric plexus-longitudinal muscle preparation. *Horizontal axis gives serotonin concentration; vertical axis gives muscle tension as percent of the maximal electrically stimulated tension in the same muscle strips. (×) = results for strips from nontolerant guinea pigs; (●) = results for strips from morphine tolerant guinea pigs. Standard errors are shown by broken vertical lines. Tension developed by serotonin addition to the bath was measured after electrical stimulation was turned off. (From Schulz and Goldstein, Figure 1.*[112a])

neurons and synapses are amenable to direct observation and experimentation, free of the complicating influences of the nervous system as a whole.

Physical dependence on the narcotics. Tolerance to the narcotics is invariably accompanied by physical dependence. The tolerant addict or experimental animal evidently functions well provided he continues to receive the drug. When a high degree of tolerance has been attained, even very large doses of narcotic may no longer produce any euphoriant effect; drug intake has to be continued in order to avoid withdrawal symptoms. If drug administration is stopped, profound derangements ensue. At first, there is restlessness and intense craving for the drug. Yawning, running nose, lacrimation, and perspiration follow, with chills, fever, vomiting, panting respiration, loss of appetite, insomnia, hypertension, aches and pains, and loss of weight. The pupils become dilated and there are associated signs of hyperactivity of the sympathetic nervous system. Pilomotor stimulation (gooseflesh) accounts for the vernacular description of withdrawal as "cold turkey." In animals, severe disturbances of body function and behavior may also occur during the withdrawal period.[53,113,114]

The invention of a procedure for quantitating the intensity of the withdrawal syndrome in man[115] has contributed much to understanding its nature and to the

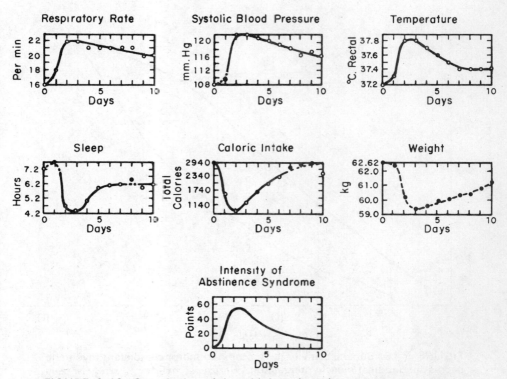

FIGURE 9-19. Quantitation of the withdrawal syndrome. *Sixty-five addicts were stabilized on a dosage of 240 to 340 mg of morphine daily, then withdrawn abruptly at day zero. Careful observations and measurements were made for 10 days. A representative sampling is shown in the upper 2 rows. The summation of scores (see text) for all the signs of withdrawal yielded the curve at bottom. (Adapted from Kolb and Himmelsbach, Figure 1.[116])*

study of addiction potential among new narcotics. Addicts or postaddicts are stabilized on a dosage of 240–340 mg of morphine daily. Careful measurements are then made on a regular schedule of respiratory rate, blood pressure, body temperature, hours of sleep, caloric intake, and body weight. At the same time, the presence or absence of certain signs (not subject to measurement) is noted, such as yawning, lacrimation, vomiting. For each manifestation, an arbitrary number of points is assigned, with a maximum limit set upon some, so that the total score will, to a degree, represent a balanced assessment of the intensity of the whole withdrawal syndrome. The evaluations and measurements are usually carried out once daily, but alternatively they can be carried out on an hourly schedule.

Figure 9-19 shows one of the earliest results of applying this technique. Sixty-five addicts were studied.[116] The various curves show the course of the physiologic variables that were measured quantitatively after withdrawal of morphine. The bottom curve is the total point score computed on a daily basis, including all the items listed above. The peak intensity at two days is evident, followed by a slow decline over a period of more than a week. The total intensity of the withdrawal syndrome is sometimes expressed as the area under such a curve.

The method has proved extremely useful for comparing different drugs. The course of withdrawal is almost the same for morphine and heroin; but it is very different for methadone, and this has had some practical application in the clinical management of withdrawal. Figure 9-20 shows an experiment in which subjects were stabilized on methadone and then withdrawn.[117] Although methadone fully satisfied the addict's requirement while it was being administered, the subsequent withdrawal effects developed more slowly and did not reach as great an intensity as after morphine withdrawal. However, the total duration of the withdrawal period was longer with methadone. The intensity of withdrawal effects after morphine is nearly unbearable

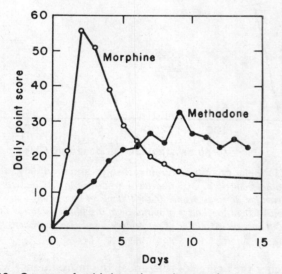

FIGURE 9-20. Course of withdrawal syndrome after morphine and after methadone. *Morphine and methadone were withdrawn (on day zero) after several months of administration. Intensity of the withdrawal syndrome was scored daily thereafter, as described in the text. Morphine data are average point scores of 65 subjects; methadone data are for 5 subjects. (From Isbell, Figure 5.[117])*

and may even be life threatening, whereas the maximum intensity of the methadone withdrawal is tolerable. Therefore, the standard procedure adopted for withdrawing addicts from morphine or heroin is to substitute methadone for whatever drug was being taken and then later to withdraw methadone.

The relationship between dosage administered during the period of addiction and the intensity of the subsequent withdrawal syndrome was studied in a large number of addicts who had been stabilized on various dosages of morphine from 40–400 mg daily.[118] For each group of subjects, the total score for intensity of the withdrawal syndrome was summed over 7 days. Figure 9-21 gives the result. Clearly, the higher the

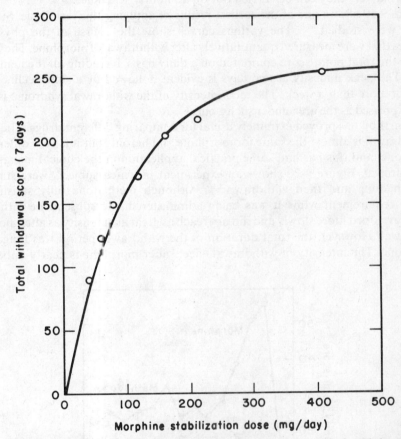

FIGURE 9-21. Relationship between dosage and intensity of withdrawal syndrome. *Data for intensity of withdrawal syndrome in 127 addicts who had been stabilized on various dosages from 40 to 400 mg of morphine daily before abrupt withdrawal. Total scores for 7 days of withdrawal are plotted against the stabilization dose prior to withdrawal. (Modified from Andrews and Himmelsbach, Figure 2.[118])*

dosage (i.e., the higher the degree of tolerance), the more intense was the subsequent withdrawal syndrome. The shape of the curve is interesting because it suggests that a maximum degree of physical dependence is reached at dosages of about 400 mg day^{-1}. This flattening of the curve, however, may be artificially exaggerated by the fact that certain scores cannot exceed arbitrary maximum values.

Many attempts have been made to modify the withdrawal syndrome, especially by drug treatment of one sort or another.[119] Tranquilizers and hypnotics, especially the benzodiazepines, afford symptomatic relief. Dramatic termination of the withdrawal syndrome is seen only with other narcotics. Moreover, one narcotic can be substituted for another at any time during the period of physical dependence and tolerance without precipitating signs of withdrawal. This crossdependence is the basis not only of the methadone withdrawal procedure described earlier, but also of methadone maintenance in which addicts are stabilized on an ambulatory basis by substituting oral methadone for their intravenous heroin, while allowing them to engage in productive occupations.[120] The effectiveness of methadone by the oral route contributes to the practicality of this procedure.

Narcotic antagonists, which block the primary effects of the narcotics,[121] also prevent the development of tolerance[122] and dependence. An example is shown in Figure 9-22. Monkeys were given morphine every 4 hr for 35 days at the fixed dose

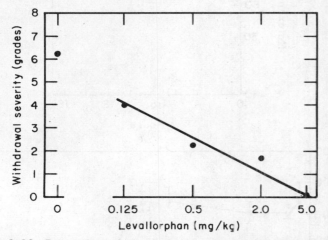

FIGURE 9-22. Prevention of physical dependence on morphine by levallorphan. *Levallorphan at various doses was administered simultaneously with morphine sulfate (5 mg kg^{-1}) every 4 hr, subcutaneously, to monkeys (Macaca mulatta). After 35 days the drugs were stopped and the intensity of withdrawal symptoms was assessed on an arbitrary grading scale. Note logarithmic dose scale. (From Seevers and Deneau, Figure 1.[123])*

of 5 mg kg^{-1}. The antagonist levallorphan was given with each morphine injection, a different dose being administered to each animal. After 35 days, the injections were stopped and the intensity of withdrawal symptoms was noted. Levallorphan blocked the establishment of physical dependence in a dose-related fashion; complete antagonism occurred at an approximately equimolar ratio. If tolerance and dependence are adaptations to the disturbances of homeostasis caused by narcotics, it is not surprising that agents which prevent the acute effects should also block the development of tolerance and dependence.

Antagonists can precipitate an immediate and severe withdrawal syndrome if administered to a physically dependent person or experimental animal. This phenomenon has been refined into an excellent tool for quantitating the intensity of physical dependence in mice.[124] A prominent feature of withdrawal in this species is a remarkable "jumping syndrome." In contrast to normal mice, which never spontaneously jump out of a jar or off a platform, mice that have been treated chronically with a narcotic and then given a single injection of an antagonist (e.g., naloxone) jump repetitively. Antagonists do not cause jumping in untreated animals up to the convulsant-lethal dose. As treatment with a narcotic becomes more intensive (high dose,

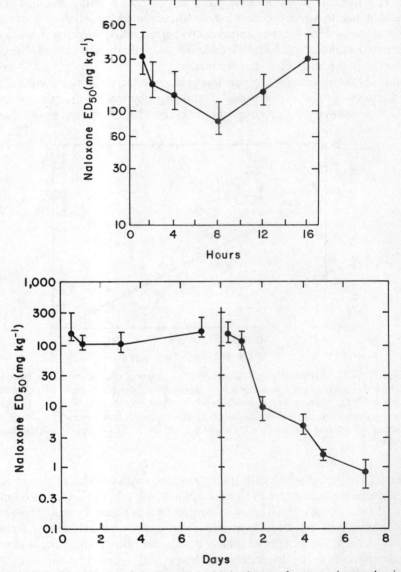

FIGURE 9-23. Effects of single and multiple doses of a narcotic on physical dependence in mice. *Levorphanol (20 mg kg^{-1}) was injected i.p. Withdrawal was precipitated in groups of mice by naloxone. Points represent naloxone ED50 with standard errors. In untreated animals, no dose of naloxone produces jumping. Top: Effect of a single dose of levorphanol given at time zero. Bottom: Effect of levorphanol on the steady state degree of dependence when given at 12 hr interval (left) or at 4 hr interval (right). (From Cheney and Goldstein, Figures 2 and 3.[125])*

shorter interval, longer duration), and simultaneously with the development of a higher and high degree of tolerance, the jumping can be elicited with lower and lower doses of naloxone. By measuring the naloxone ED50 in groups of mice, one can estimate the degree of dependence, although it is understood that there is no assurance of a quantitative linear correspondence between the severity of the disturbance underlying physical dependence and the naloxone ED50. Experiments employing this technique revealed a process much like that demonstrated for the development of tolerance in mice. Figure 9-23 shows that even a single injection of a moderate dose of narcotic produced some physical dependence, which reached a peak at about 8 hr, then waned and was gone after a day or so. This time course was unrelated to that of the narcotic in plasma, which had a measured half-life of less than 1 hr; however, persistent tightly bound narcotic at sites in the central nervous system cannot be ruled out.

The time course of onset and disappearance of physical dependence after one dose of levorphanol led to a prediction: that repeated injection of the same dose at 4 hr intervals would cause a cumulative effect, leading to intense physical dependence (very low naloxone ED50), whereas injections at a 16 hr interval, when the underlying process had largely waned, would lead to a measurable but low degree of dependence at the steady state. These predictions were borne out experimentally, as shown in Figure 9-23. Precipitated withdrawal effects after a very short exposure to a narcotic have also been observed in dogs[126] and in humans.[127] The possible mechanism underlying precipitated withdrawal will be discussed later in this chapter.

The methods and findings described here have been applied to the practical problem of assessing the addiction liability of new narcotic drugs. Addicts and former addicts are used as subjects for these testing procedures, which are carried out under "blind" conditions. For example, a narcotic drug is given on a certain injection schedule, and then saline injections are substituted without the subject's knowledge. Under these conditions, the ability of a new drug to induce physical dependence can be tested by administering it for a long enough period of time and then observing the intensity of the withdrawal syndrome (if any) when the drug is stopped. An alternative test is to substitute the new drug for morphine to see if it will prevent the onset of a morphine withdrawal syndrome. Curiously, the most reliable way of finding out if a new drug is addictive is to give it to addicts under controlled "blind" conditions and ask them if they like it! Addicts were able to identify morphine, heroin, and other narcotics and to distinguish them from barbiturates, amphetamine, and placebos with remarkable accuracy. "If one were to select, on the basis of single doses, the most important single subjective response identifying a drug as being subject to morphine-like abuse, probably this measure would be whether the former opiate addict identifies the drug as an opiate ('dope')."[128] If a new drug met with the approval of addicts, it was concluded that that drug would probably have a high addiction liability.

Theories of Tolerance and Physical Dependence.   The mechanism of the development of tolerance and physical dependence is still unknown, but there has been no dearth of theoretical speculation. Inasmuch as tolerance develops to intravenous injections of drugs, all explanations involving diminished absorption can be discounted. Moreover, in agreement with the earlier-cited results of experiments with alcohol and barbiturates, it has been shown by means of radioactive morphine in dogs that this drug is not excluded from the brain of the tolerant animal.[129] Dogs were made tolerant by injecting morphine at 8 hr intervals in increasing doses over a period of 5 weeks. The dose was stabilized at 2 mg kg^{-1} at each injection during the fifth week. Then, these dogs and others that had never received morphine were given a single subcutaneous dose of 2 mg kg^{-1} of radioactive morphine labeled in the N-methyl group. Periodically thereafter, dogs of both groups were sacrificed, and an exhaustive set of determinations was made on the tissues of various parts of the central nervous system. Plasma and cerebrospinal fluid levels were also determined. A method was used that determined only unconjugated morphine. The radioactive material after extraction was shown to be essentially all morphine (rather than any metabolite) by chromatography.

There were no remarkable differences in any part of the brain between nontolerant and tolerant dogs. In this same experiment, the plasma half-life of the injected morphine was the same in both groups of animals (about 1 hr). The radioactivity in cerebrospinal fluid of the tolerant dogs was somewhat higher than in the nontolerant dogs at comparable times. The plasma of tolerant animals contained less conjugated morphine than that of nontolerant animals, as would be expected from the demonstration (in rats) that liver glucuronide transferase activity decreases during the development of tolerance.[130] In summary, all the differences between tolerant and nontolerant animals seemed to be inconsequential and certainly not of sufficient magnitude to explain the tolerance.

Similar results have been obtained in rats[131] and in mice. In tolerant mice, the concentration of ultrafiltrable narcotic in the brain water was shown to be sufficiently high, yet virtually no pharmacologic effect was produced.[132] This demonstrated that the tolerance was not due to an inactivation of the narcotic molecules by binding to tissue components or to soluble macromolecules, as in an immunologic mechanism. Using various doses of radioactive narcotic in nontolerant and tolerant mice, curves could be established relating a pharmacologic effect (running activity) to the actual brain concentration (rather than the total dose) of the drug.[133] In the tolerant animals, the same brain concentrations produced much less effect than in controls.

Thus, it is clear in all species—even in those where metabolic tolerance plays some role—that, when tolerant animals receive large doses of a narcotic drug and display a largely reduced pharmacologic effect, the drug concentrations in their brains are sufficiently high. For narcotics, therefore, as also for alcohol and barbiturates, the principal mechanisms of tolerance and physical dependence have to be sought within the neural elements of the central nervous system.

A satisfactory theory should offer a unitary explanation of the fact that tolerance and dependence apparently develop, persist, and disappear together, as though they were reflections of the same underlying biologic change.[124] To explain the phenomena adequately, the theory should also account for the different time courses of the acute and chronic drug effects. Drug action is immediate, as soon as the drug can enter the nervous system and reach the receptors. Development of the tolerant-dependent state is slow, on the order of hours or days, so the mechanism that is responsible for tolerance and dependence must take effect comparably slowly. Presumably more is involved than merely activating existing neural circuits to oppose the drug action, for such effects would be expected to occur very quickly in the central nervous system. The actual time course suggests, instead, that what changes is the level of an enzyme, the storage and release of a neurotransmitter, the production and release of a hormone, the pattern of synaptic contacts, or some other process involving biosynthesis and macromolecular turnover.

Support for the view that the time course of the development of tolerance and dependence reflects a process of macromolecular synthesis comes from experiments with inhibitors of RNA and protein synthesis. Actinomycin D, puromycin, and cycloheximide have all been reported to block tolerance and dependence when given during the period of administration of the narcotic.[134,135,136] Such evidence must be examined very critically to see exactly what is meant operationally by "blocking the development of tolerance." For example, in an analgesia test, the normal animal makes a motor response (e.g., lifting paw or flicking tail) to a noxious stimulus. Morphine blocks this response. As tolerance develops, the motor response returns despite the administration of morphine. To block this means that the motor response does not occur, for whatever reason; certainly a generalized toxicity due to the inhibitor of RNA or protein synthesis would produce the same result. Experiments of this kind would be more convincing, therefore, if the criterion of drug effect were a motor phenomenon (e.g., running activity in mice), so that when tolerance was prevented, the animal would emit the motor behavior. In at least one or two of the reported experiments, adequate precautions were taken to exclude toxic effects due to the treatment.

Several theories have been advanced; these are not necessarily mutually exclusive but may merely deal with the phenomena in different terms. There are basically two kinds of theory. One kind postulates a continuous and unchanged interaction between the drug and its receptors, the effects of which are antagonized or compensated by changes elsewhere in other biochemical pathways or in other neuronal systems. The other attributes tolerance to a change in the drug receptors themselves—either a change in their number or a change in their properties—making them less sensitive to the drug.

The first kind of theory can be formulated in a very general way.[105,137,138] The drug action is seen as disturbing homeostasis. The primary drug effects are compensated for by the activation of pathways that produce opposite effects, thus restoring homeostasis in the presence of the drug. By analogy to the way the body deals with other disturbances of homeostasis, it is supposed that neural or hormonal mechanisms which counteract the drug effects may be involved. Then a higher drug dose would be required to produce the original effect again. The system would also be dependent, since removing the drug would permit the counteracting mechanism to upset homeostasis in the opposite direction. This immediate response to removal of the drug would correspond to the withdrawal syndrome, which would then wane as homeostasis was gradually restored in the absence of drug.

Assuming a centrally acting drug acted by increasing neurotransmitter levels at certain synapses, tolerance to the drug would develop if the brain became tolerant to high levels of the neurotransmitter. It is interesting to note, therefore, that rats can become tolerant to abnormally high levels of acetylcholine in the brain caused by prolonged exposure to a cholinesterase inhibitor.[139] The inhibitor, an organic phosphate compound, was injected at about one-half the LD50. It produced tremors, convulsions, and a variety of severe parasympathomimetic effects. When the same dose was repeated daily for 60 days, the effects diminished greatly; the animals, which had lost weight, began gaining again and the convulsions, tremors, and autonomic disturbances all but disappeared. Acetylcholinesterase and free acetylcholine levels in the rat brains were investigated. The course of enzyme inhibition and the conse-quent marked increase in acetylcholine following injection of the inhibitor were almost the same on the 50th day as on the 3rd day; if there was any real difference at all, the acetylcholine level was slightly higher on the 60th day, when the effects were minimal. Apparently, therefore, the brains of the tolerant animals had become refractory to high concentrations of acetylcholine. This was confirmed by measuring the LD50 of carbachol, an acetylcholine congener that is neither a substrate nor an inhibitor of acetylcholinesterase. The LD50 in the nontolerant rats was 2.0 mg kg^{-1} (95% confidence limits 1.5 to 2.7); in the tolerant rats it had nearly doubled to 3.9 mg kg^{-1} (2.9 to 5.2).

A more concrete version of a theory of the first kind postulates that postsynaptic receptors for an endogenous neurotransmitter become supersensitive [140, 140a] as in the well-known phenomenon of denervation supersensitivity.[93] It is known that, after denervation of sympathetically innervated effectors in the peripheral autonomic system, these effectors become supersensitive to norepinephrine. The principal cause is the loss of the uptake and storage capacity for norepinephrine that is ordinarily associated with adrenergic nerve endings which plays an important role in terminating the actions of norepinephrine. It is postulated that a long period of depression of the brain by narcotics, barbiturates, or alcohol could cause a kind of functional denerva-tion of central pathways which sensitizes them so that they over-react when the drug is withdrawn. Increased activity of the sensitized pathway would antagonize the drug effect. The mechanism could merely increase the number of receptors, leading to a higher probability of combination with neurotransmitter in the synaptic cleft; or a qualitative change could result in a greater intrinsic sensitivity of the receptors. Thus, despite continued drug effect at the site of drug action, biologic function would remain normal. Withdrawal of drug, as in the theory discussed earlier, would yield abnormal effects opposite to those caused by the drug in the first place.

A theory of the second kind is the "enzyme expansion" theory which applies specific concepts of biochemical regulation to the drug receptors.[141-143] These receptors, which could be enzymes or other functional macromolecules, are postulated to increase in amount as a consequence of occupancy by the drug, and this increase accounts for both tolerance and dependence. Suppose, for example, that the drug inhibits an enzyme responsible for synaptic transmission or other neuronal function and that the enzyme is subject to product repression. This common biochemical arrangement would account for all the main facts about tolerance and dependence. Let C be a product of the enzyme, E, which is inhibited by the drug; assume that the

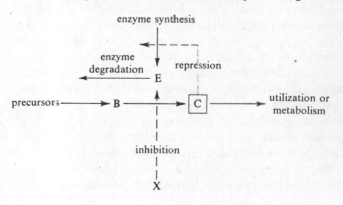

function of C is excitatory at the particular synapses where it is released. Then the normal steady-state level of E and the normal utilization of C determine the level of C and the normal state of excitation. The steady-state level of E is determined by its rates of synthesis and degradation, according to the plateau principle (Chapter 4).

This model predicts two kinds of results, of different time courses. The inhibition of E by the drug X will cause an *immediate* decline in the concentration or availability of C; if C was mediating an excitatory function, the effect will be depressant on that function. The decrease in C will increase the synthesis of E, and the enzyme level will rise. This will be a *delayed* effect, with time course of hours or days commensurate with the rate of protein turnover. The increased level of E will now produce C from B at the normal rate despite its partial inhibition by X, and the concentration of X will have to be raised in order to reduce the concentration of C again in the face of the higher enzyme level. Thus, tolerance will develop. When a high degree of tolerance has been produced, the following situation will be obtained. The level of total enzyme and the drug concentration are both very high. Most of the enzyme is inhibited. The level of free enzyme is about what it was normally; therefore the availability of C is normal; and neuronal function is normal in the presence of drug.

Withdrawal of drug will cause two effects. The *immediate* effect, as soon as drug concentration declines sufficiently, is to disinhibit the large excess of enzyme that is present. A great overproduction of C results, with effects (in this instance excitatory) opposite to those of the primary drug effect. This is the withdrawal syndrome. The *delayed* effect, requiring perhaps days, will be a restoration of the original state of affairs. The excess of C represses the new synthesis of E; as the level of E declines, the concentration of C also falls. Thus, physical dependence and tolerance develop together and disappear together. The most attractive feature of this theory is its consonance with modern biochemical concepts and its ability to explain both tolerance and physical dependence in a unitary manner, without special ad hoc assumptions.

An even simpler form of this theory[144] requires no end-product repression of the enzyme. It is assumed that the enzyme is undergoing continual synthesis and degradation and that the inhibitory interaction of drug with enzyme stabilizes the enzyme. As a consequence, the total amount of enzyme would increase (cf. Chapter 4), and tolerance would develop as above. No change in the rate of enzyme synthesis would be required.

Nothing in this drug-receptor expansion theory requires that the drug receptor be an enzyme, as originally postulated. The same principles would apply if the drug receptor were a component of a transport system, a macromolecule essential to neurotransmitter release, or a postsynaptic receptor for a neurotransmitter. The essential point is based directly upon the mass law, namely, that according to Michaelis–Menten kinetics (i.e., in Zone A, p. 92) the fractional occupancy is only a function of the free ligand concentration, not of the number of binding sites. Suppose there is a normal pool of drug receptors, all of them in the free state, and that occupancy of half the receptor pool by drug molecules produces the acute drug effect. The biochemical regulatory mechanism will now expand the receptor pool until normal function is again established, i.e., until the number of free receptors is normal. At the same ambient drug concentration, this will require that the total receptor pool be exactly doubled, since 50% occupancy by drug will then yield the same free receptor pool as initially. In order to replicate the original drug action, it will now be necessary for drug molecules to occupy half of the free receptors, in addition to those already occupied. In other words, the drug concentration will have to be increased sufficiently to cause 75% occupancy. Removal of drug would expose the 2-fold excess of receptor, producing abnormalities of physiologic function opposite to those initially caused by the drug. Finally, the regulatory mechanisms would gradually restore the receptor pool to normal.

In seeking to identify biochemical mechanisms, it is important to distinguish between biochemical correlates of acute drug effects and biochemical correlates of the tolerant-dependent state. Measurements have been made on a variety of substrates, enzymes, neurotransmitters, and other components of brain tissue in an effort to discover something that changes when drug is administered. There has been no dearth of positive findings. If a biochemical effect is consistently observed with active drugs of a given family but not with inactive congeners, if potencies for a biochemical effect and the pharmacologic effect are well correlated, if specific antagonists of pharmacologic action also block the biochemical effect, and if the biochemical effect diminishes as tolerance develops to the pharmacologic action, then the biochemical effect qualifies as an authentic *biochemical correlate* of the drug action. Let us consider a few examples.

It has been known for years that morphine stimulates adrenal medullary secretion. Direct studies with mice have shown increased synthesis of norepinephrine from radio-labeled tyrosine at the peak of drug effect, implying an increased stimulation of adrenergic pathways in the brain.[145] Other investigations have shown increased dopamine turnover; and abolition of certain narcotic effects when catecholamines are depleted by reserpine, α-methyltyrosine, or 6-hydroxydopamine treatment.[146-150] Increased catecholamine turnover (implying increased catecholamine release) certainly qualifies as a specific biochemical correlate of acute narcotic action. But, as with all other biochemical correlates, we face alternative interpretations: Is it an essential step in mediating the pharmacologic effect (drug → catecholamine release → pharmacologic effect): Is it a consequence of a pharmacologic effect (drug → pharmacologic effect → catecholamine release)? Or is it simply another and unrelated action of the drug (drug → pharmacologic effect; drug → catecholamine release)?

When slices of rat brain cortex are incubated in a manometric apparatus for measuring oxygen uptake, the respiration is found to be increased about 80% in 5 mM KCl, compared with the rate in a low-potassium medium. Morphine at a concentration of 1 mM was found to inhibit this stimulated oxygen uptake almost completely. Rats were given morphine daily to produce tolerance, and control animals were given saline injections instead. Groups of animals were sacrificed daily, and in vitro measurements of oxygen uptake were carried out in the presence and absence of morphine. As tolerance developed, the inhibitory effect of morphine was lost. After the injections were stopped on the seventh day, the sensitivity to inhibition by morphine gradually returned. Again, there is no way to decide if the phenomenon observed here is in the direct chain of causation between the drug-receptor interaction and the ultimate pharmacologic effect of the drug.

Finally, opiate narcotics diminish acetylcholine release in the guinea pig ileum, as in the brain. In brain, the diminished release is accompanied by a modest accumulation of this neurotransmitter in the cholinergic nerve terminals.[151-153] This phenomenon is clearly associated in some manner with the acute actions of narcotics, inasmuch as they meet the various criteria (including stereospecificity) for a specific biochemical correlate, but once more the causal relationship is unproved.

There is a basic difference in criteria for relating a biochemical effect to acute drug action, as described above, and to tolerance and dependence. It has been pointed out, on purely logical grounds, that any biochemical mechanism responsible for tolerance must act continuously while the animal is tolerant.[154] Its time course should coincide with that of the development of the tolerant-dependent state; it should be waxing while the biochemical correlates of acute drug action are waning.

Although the biochemical changes underlying the tolerant-dependent state are not yet known, a few examples will illustrate the kinds of change that meet the logical requirement outlined above. Morphine undergoes N-demethylation in rat liver microsome preparations. In tolerant animals, the N-demethylating capacity is greatly reduced.[155] If the N-demethylation of morphine were an essential step in its action and brain contained a system analogous to that in liver, tolerance could be accounted for by a decrease in N-demethylating capacity; however, physical dependence would not be explained. The turnover of dopamine in brain is persistently elevated during the tolerant-dependent state;[156,157] activation of dopaminergic pathways could, therefore, possibly play a causal role in establishing and maintaining tolerance and dependence, perhaps by opposing certain central actions of morphine. Finally, the supersensitivity to serotonin in the myenteric plexus of the morphine tolerant guinea pig (p. 603) could be responsible for tolerance by opposing the pharmacologic effect of morphine in this tissue.

REFERENCES

1. J. J. VON TSCHUDI: Uber die Giftesser. *Wiener Med. Wochenschr.* 1:453 (1851); 3:8 (1853).
2. W. HAUSMANN: Uber die Arsenikesser in Steiermark. *Arch. Int. Pharmacodyn.* 11:483 (1903).
3. H. E. ROSCOE: On the Alleged Practice of Arsenic-Eating in Styria. In *Memoirs of the Literary and Philosophical Society of Manchester*, 3rd Series. London, H. Bailliere (1862). Vol. 1, p. 208.
4. C. GIOFFREDI: L'immunizzazione per gli alcaloidi vegetali tentativi di sieroterapia negli avvelenamenti ricerche sperimentali. *Giorn. Int. Sci. Med.* 19:829 (1897).
5. E. J. PELLINI and A. D. GREENFIELD: Narcotic drug addition. II. The presence of toxic substances in the blood serum in morphine habituation. *Arch. Int. Med.* 33:547 (1924).
6. A. G. DU MEZ and L. KOLB: Absence of transferable immunizing substances in the blood of morphine and heroin addicts. *Public Health Rep.* 40:548 (1925).
7. H. O. J. COLLIER: A general theory of the genesis of drug dependence by induction of receptors. *Nature* 205:181 (1965).
8. J. COCHIN: Possible mechanisms in development of tolerance. *Fed. Proc.* 29:19 (1970).
9. C. M. GRUBER and G. F. KEYSER: A study on the development of tolerance and cross tolerance to barbiturates in experimental animals. *J. Pharmacol. Exp. Therap.* 86:186 (1946).
10. H. REMMER: Gewöhnung an Hexobarbital durch beschleunigten Abbau. *Arch. Int. Pharmacodyn.* 152:346 (1964).
11. J. H. MENDELSON, S. STEIN, and N. K. MELLO: Effects of experimentally induced intoxication on metabolism of ethanol-1-C^{14} in alcoholic subjects. *Metabolism* 14:1255 (1965).
12. R. M. DAJANI, J. DANIELSKI, and J. M. ORTEN: The utilization of ethanol. II. The alcohol-acetaldehyde dehydrogenase systems in the livers of alcohol-treated rats. *J. Nutrition* 80:196 (1963).
13. H. CLEGG, ed.: *Drugs in the Treatment of Disease.* London, British Medical Association (1961). pp. 276, 289.
14. R. F. PITTS: *The Physiological Basis of Diuretic Therapy.* Springfield, Ill., Charles C. Thomas (1959).

15. F. C. RECTOR, JR., D. W. SELDIN, and J. H. COPENHAVER: The mechanism of ammonia excretion during ammonium chloride acidosis. *J. Clin. Invest.* 34:20 (1955).

16. K. K. CHEN and W. J. MEEK: Further studies of the effect of ephedrine on the circulation. *J. Pharmacol. Exp. Therap.* 28:31 (1926).

17. C. V. WINDER, M. M. ANDERSON, and H. C. PARKE: Comparative properties of six phenethylamines with observations on the nature of tachyphylaxis. *J. Pharmacol. Exp. Therap.* 93:63 (1948).

18. M. D. DAY and M. J. RAND: Tachyphylaxis to some sympathomimetic amines in relation to monoamine oxidase. *Brit. J. Pharmacol.* 21:84 (1963).

19. J. H. BURN and M. J. RAND: The action of sympathomimetic amines in animals treated with reserpine. *J. Physiol.* 144:314 (1958).

20. U. TRENDELENBURG. A. MUSKUS, W. W. FLEMING, and B. GOMEZ ALONSO DE LA SIERRA: Modification by reserpine of the action of sympathomimetic amines in spinal cats; a classification of sympathomimetic amines. *J. Pharmacol. Exp. Therap.* 138:170 (1962).

21. U. TRENDELENBURG. Modification of the effect of tyramine by various agents and procedures. *J. Pharmacol. Exp. Therap.* 134:8 (1961).

22. J. AXELROD, E. GORDON, G. HERTTING, I. J. KOPIN, and L. T. POTTER: On the mechanism of tachyphylaxis to tyramine in the isolated rat heart. *Brit. J. Pharmacol.* 19:56 (1962).

23. L. T. POTTER, J. AXELROD, and I. J. KOPIN: Differential binding and release of norepinephrine and tachyphylaxis. *Biochem. Pharmacol.* 11:254 (1962).

24. L. T. POTTER and J. AXELROD: Studies on the storage of norepinephrine and the effect of drugs. *J. Pharmacol. Exp. Therap.* 140:199 (1963).

25. R. KUNTZMAN and M. M. JACOBSON: On the mechanism of heart norepinephrine depletion by tyramine, guanethidine and reserpine. *J. Pharmacol. Exp. Therap.* 144:399 (1964).

26. J. R. CROUT, A. J. MUSKUS, and U. TRENDELENBURG: Effect of tyramine on isolated guinea-pig atria in relation to their noradrenaline stores. *Brit. J. Pharmacol.* 18:600 (1962).

27. J. M. MUSACCHIO, I. J. KOPIN, and V. K. WEISE: Subcellular distribution of some sympathomimetic amines and their β-hydroxylated derivatives in the rat heart. *J. Pharmacol. Exp. Therap.* 148:22 (1965).

28. I. J. KOPIN: Storage and metabolism of catecholamines: the role of monoamine oxidase. *Pharmacol. Rev.* 16:179 (1964).

29. B. BHAGAT, E. K. GORDON, and I. J. KOPIN: Norepinephrine synthesis and the pressor responses to tyramine in the spinal cat. *J. Pharmacol. Exp. Therap.* 147:319 (1965).

30. J. M. MUSACCHIO, M. GOLDSTEIN, B. ANAGNOSTE, G. POCH, and I. J. KOPIN: Inhibition of dopamine-β-hydroxylase by disulfiram *in vivo*. *J. Pharmacol. Exp. Therap.* 152:56 (1966).

31. W. D. M. PATON and E. J. ZAIMIS: The methonium compounds. *Pharmacol. Rev.* 4:219 (1952).

32. W. D. M. PATON: Transmission and block in autonomic ganglia. *Pharmacol. Rev.* 6:59 (1954).

33. G. B. KOELLE: Neuromuscular blocking agents. In *The Pharmacological Basis of Therapeutics*, L. S. Goodman and A. Gilman, eds. Toronto, The Macmillan Company (1970).

34. W. D. M. PATON: The action of morphine and related substances on contraction and on acetylcholine output of coaxially stimulated guinea-pig ileum. *Brit. J. Pharmacol.* 12:119 (1957).

35. ST. KARÁDY: Über experimentelle Tieruntersuchungen zur Frage der Histamintachyphylaxie und Histaminresistenz. *Arch. Exp. Pathol. Pharmakol.* 180:283 (1936).

36. J. L. AMBRUS, C. M. AMBRUS, and J. W. E. HARRISSON: Effect of histamine desensitization on histamine induced gastric secretion of guinea pigs. *Gastroenterology* 18:249 (1951).

37. W. D. M. PATON: Compound 48/80: a potent histamine liberator. *Br. J. Pharmacol.* 6:499 (1951).

38. C. F. SCHMIDT and A. E. LIVINGSTON: The action of morphine on the mammalian circulation. *J. Pharmacol. Exp. Therap.* 47:411 (1933).

39. C. F. SCHMIDT and A. E. LIVINGSTON: The relation of dosage to the development of tolerance to morphine in dogs. *J. Pharmacol. Exp. Therap.* 47:443 (1933).

40. J. E. ECKENHOFF and S. R. OECH: The effects of narcotics and antagonists upon respiration and circulation in man. A review. *Clin. Pharmacol. Therap.* 1:483 (1960).

41. J. L. MONGAR and H. O. SCHILD: A comparison of the effects of anaphylactic shock and of chemical histamine releasers. *J. Physiol.* 118:461 (1952).

42. G. E. EBRIGHT: The effects of nitroglycerin on those engaged in its manufacture. *J. Amer. Med. Ass.* 62:201 (1914).

43. A. M. SCHWARTZ: The cause, relief and prevention of headaches arising from contact with dynamite. *New Eng. J. Med.* 235:541 (1946).

44. J. C. MUNCH, B. FRIEDLAND, and M. SHEPARD: Glyceryl trinitrate. II. Chronic toxicity. *Industr. Med. Surg.* 34:940 (1965).
45. L. A. CRANDALL, JR., C. D. LEAKE, A. S. LOEVENHART, and C. W. MUEHLBERGER: Acquired tolerance to and cross tolerance between the nitrous and nitric acid esters and sodium nitrite in man. *J. Pharmacol. Exp. Therap.* 41:103 (1931).
46. L. A. CRANDALL, JR.: The fate of glyceryl trinitrate in the tolerant and nontolerant animal. *J. Pharmacol. Exp. Therap.* 48:127 (1933).
47. H. B. MYERS and V. T. AUSTIN: Nitrite toleration. *J. Pharmacol. Exp. Therap.* 36:227 (1929).
48. K. HECHT: Untersuchungen über Giftgewöhnung. *Arch. Exp. Pathol. Pharmakol.* 113:338 (1926).
49. G. W. GRAY and M. H. SEEVERS: In vivo observations on the nature of atropine tachyphylaxis exhibited by intestinal smooth muscle. *J. Pharmacol. Exp. Therap.* 113:319 (1955).
50. WORLD HEALTH ORGANIZATION, Expert Committee on Drugs Liable to Produce Addiction: Report on the Thirteenth Session. WHO Tech. Rep. Ser. 273, Geneva (1964). p. 9.
51. Evaluation of Dependence-Producing Drugs. Report of a WHO Scientific Group. WHO Tech. Rep. Ser. 287, Geneva (1964).
52. G. E. W. WOLSTENHOLME and J. KNIGHT, eds.: *Hashish: Its Chemistry and Pharmacology.* Ciba Foundation Study Group No. 21. Boston, Little, Brown and Co. (1965).
53. G. A. DENEAU and M. H. SEEVERS: Pharmacological aspects of drug dependence. *Advance. Pharmacol.* 3:267 (1964).
54. R. H. DREISBACH and C. PFEIFFER: Caffeine-withdrawal headache. *J. Lab Clin. Med.* 28:1212 (1943).
55. A. GOLDSTEIN, S. KAISER, and O. WHITBY: Psychotropic effects of caffeine in man. IV. Quantitative and qualitative differences associated with habituation to coffee. *Clin. Pharmacol. Ther.* 10:489 (1969).
56. C. D. LEAKE: *The Amphetamines.* Springfield, Ill., Charles C. Thomas (1958).
57. D. E. ROSENBERG, A. B. WOLBACH, JR., E. J. MINER, and H. ISBELL: Observations on direct and cross tolerance with LSD and D-amphetamine in man. *Psychopharmacologia* 5:1 (1963).
58. W. R. MARTIN and C. W. GORODETZKY: Demonstration of tolerance to and physical dependence on N-allylnormorphine (nalorphine). *J. Pharmacol. Exp. Therap.* 150:437 (1965).
59. L. KOLB: Types and characteristics of drug addicts. *Mental Hygiene* 9:300 (1925).
60. A. WIKLER and R. W. RASOR: Psychiatric aspects of drug addiction. *Amer. J. Med.* 14:566 (1953).
61. J. A. O'DONNELL and J. C. BALL, eds.: *Narcotic Addiction.* New York, Harper & Row, 1966.
62. E. M. BRECHER: *Licit and Illicit Drugs.* Boston, Little, Brown and Co. (1972).
63. Reports of American Bar Association and American Medical Association Joint Committee on Narcotic Drugs, *Drug Addiction: Crime or Disease?* Bloomington, Indiana University Press (1969).
64. R. H. BLUM: *Society and Drugs.* San Francisco, Jossey-Bass Inc., (1969). Vol. 1–3.
65. P. B. DEWS and W. H. MORSE: Behavioral pharmacology. *Ann. Rev. Pharmacol.* 1:145 (1961).
66. H. STEINBERG, A. V. S. DE REUCK, and J. KNIGHT, eds.: *Animal Behavior and Drug Action.* Ciba Foundation Symposium. Boston, Little, Brown and Co. (1964).
67. M. RICHELLE: A note on behavioral tolerance to meprobamate. *J. Exper. Anal. Behavior* 8:45 (1965).
68. C. R. SCHUSTER and J. ZIMMERMAN: Timing behavior during prolonged treatment with *dl*-amphetamine. *J. Exper. Anal. Behavior* 4:327 (1961).
69. D. X. FREEDMAN, J. B. APPEL, F. R. HARTMAN, and M. E. MOLLIVER: Tolerance to behavioral effects of LSD-25 in rat. *J. Pharmacol. Exp. Therap.* 143:309 (1964).
70. D. X. FREEDMAN, G. K. AGHAJANIAN, E. M. ORNITZ, and B. S. ROSNER: Patterns of tolerance to lysergic acid diethylamide and mescaline in rats. *Science* 127:1173 (1958).
71. H. MOSKOWITZ and M. WAPNER: Studies on the acquisition of behavioral tolerance to alcohol. *Quart. J. Stud. Alc.* 25:619 (1964).
72. S. IRWIN: Influence of external factors and arousal mechanisms on the rate of drug tolerance development. *Arch. Int. Pharmacodyn.* 142:152 (1963).
73. D. A. OVERTON: Dissociated learning in drug states (state-dependent learning). In D. H. Elfron et al. (eds.), Psychopharmacology. A Review of Progress, PHS Publ. No. 1936, Washington, US Govt. Print. Office (1968). p. 918.

74. J. R. WEEKS: Experimental morphine addiction: method for automatic intravenous injections in unrestrained rats. *Science* 138:143 (1962).

75. G. DENEAU, T. YANAGITA, and M. H. SEEVERS: Self-administration of psychoactive substances by the monkey. *Psychopharmacologia* 16:30 (1969).

76. C. R. SCHUSTER and T. THOMPSON: Self-administration of and behavior dependence on drugs. *Ann. Rev. Pharmacol.* 9:483 (1969).

77. J. OLDS: Hypothalamic substrates of reward. *Physiol. Rev.* 42:554 (1962).

78. A. WIKLER: Some implications of conditioning theory for problems of drug abuse. *Behav. Sci.* 16:92 (1971).

79. H. ISBELL and H. F. FRASER: Addiction to analgesics and barbiturates. *Pharmacol. Rev.* 2:355 (1950).

80. M. VICTOR and R. D. ADAMS: The effect of alcohol on the nervous system. *Res. Publ. Ass. Res. Nerv. Ment. Dis.* 32:526 (1953).

81. E. M. JELLINEK: Phases of alcohol addiction. *Quart. J. Stud. Alc.* 13:673 (1952).

82. H. W. NEWMAN: Acquired tolerance to ethyl alcohol. *Quart. J. Stud. Alc.* 2:453 (1941).

83. I. A. MIRSKY, P. PIKER, M. ROSENBAUM, and H. LEDERER: "Adaptation" of the central nervous system to varying concentrations of alcohol in the blood. *Quart. J. Stud. Alc.* 2:35 (1941).

84. H. ISBELL, H. F. FRASER, A. WIKLER, R. E. BELLEVILLE, and A. J. EISENMAN: An experimental study of the etiology of "rum fits" and delirium tremens. *Quart. J. Stud. Alc.* 16:1 (1955).

85. J. H. MENDELSON, special ed.: Experimentally induced chronic intoxication and withdrawal in alcoholics. *Quart. J. Stud. Alc.* 25:Suppl. 2, 1964.

86. J. L. FALK, H. H. SAMSON, and G. WINGER: Behavioral maintenance of high concentrations of blood ethanol and physical dependence in the rat. *Science* 177:811 (1972).

87. D. B. GOLDSTEIN: Relationship of alcohol dose to intensity of withdrawal signs in mice. *J. Pharmacol. Exp. Therap.* 180:203 (1972).

88. D. B. GOLDSTEIN: An animal model for testing effects of drugs on alcohol withdrawal reactions. *J. Pharmacol. Exp. Therap.* 183:14 (1972).

89. M. H. WULFF: *The Barbiturate Withdrawal Syndrome.* Suppl. No. 14, EEG and Clinical Neurophysiology. Copenhagen, Munksgaard (1959).

90. H. ISBELL: Addiction to barbiturates and the barbiturate abstinence syndrome. *Ann. Intern. Med.* 33:108 (1950).

91. H. REMMER, M. SIEGERT, H. R. NITZE, and I. KIRSTEN: Die Gewöhnung an langwirkende Barbiturate. *Arch. Exp Pathol. Pharmakol.* 243:468 (1962).

92. A. G. EBERT, G. K. W. YIM, and T. S. MIYA: Distribution and metabolism of barbital-^{14}C in tolerant and nontolerant rats. *Biochem. Pharmacol.* 13:1267 (1964).

93. J. H. JAFFE and S. K. SHARPLESS: The rapid development of physical dependence on barbiturates. *J. Pharmacol. Exp. Therap.* 150:140 (1965).

94. H. ISBELL, S. ALTSCHUL, C. H. KORNETSKY, A. J. EISENMAN, H. G. FLANARY, and H. F. FRASER: Chronic barbiturate intoxication: an experimental study. *Arch. Neurol. Psychiatr.* 64:1 (1950).

95. H. F. FRASER, H. ISBELL, A. J. EISENMAN, A. WIKLER, and F. T. PESCOR: Chronic barbiturate intoxication: further studies. *Arch. Intern. Med.* 94:34 (1954).

96. T. M. HAIZLIP and J. A. EWING: Meprobamate habituation. A controlled clinical study. *New Eng. J. Med.* 258:1181 (1958).

97. F. F. FOLDES, M. SWERDLOW, and E. S. SIKER: *Narcotics and Narcotic Antagonists.* Springfield, Ill., Charles C. Thomas (1964). pp. 88–112.

98. N. B. EDDY, H. HALBACH, and O. J. BRAENDEN: Synthetic substances with morphine-like effect. Relationship between analgesic action and addiction liability, with a discussion of the chemical structure of addition-producing substances. *Bull. World Health Organ.* 14:353 (1956).

99. H. KRUEGER, N. B. EDDY, and M. SUMWALT: The pharmacology of the opium alkaloids. Part I. *Public Health Rep.* 56:Suppl. 165, 1941.

100. H. ISBELL and W. M. WHITE: Clinical characteristics of addictions. *Amer. J. Med.* 14:558 (1953).

101. R. D. CHESSICK: The "pharmacogenic orgasm" in the drug addict. *Arch. Gen. Psychiatr.* 3:545 (1960).

102. E. G. WILLIAMS and F. W. OBERST: A cycle of morphine addiction. Biological and psychological studies. I. Biological investigations. *Public Health Rep.* 61:1 (1946).

103. N. B. EDDY: "The Phenomena of Tolerance," in *Origins of Resistance to Toxic Agents*, ed. by M. G. Sevag, R. D. Reid, and O. E. Reynolds. New York, Academic Press, 1955.

104. W. R. MARTIN and H. F. FRASER: A comparative study of physiological and subjective effects of heroin and morphine administered intravenously in postaddicts. *J. Pharmacol. Exp. Therap.* 133:388 (1961).

105. M. H. SEEVERS and G. A. DENEAU: Physiological Aspects of Tolerance and Physical Dependence. In *Physiological Pharmacology: A Comprehensive Treatise*, ed. by W. S. Root and F. G. Hofmann. New York, Academic Press (1963). Vol. 1, part A, p. 565.

106. L. SHUSTER, R. V. HANNAM, and W. E. BOYLE, JR.: A simple method for producing tolerance to dihydromorphinone in mice. *J. Pharmacol. Exp. Therap.* 140 149 (1963).

106a. A. GOLDSTEIN and P. SHEEHAN: Tolerance to opioid narcotics. I. Tolerance to the "running fit" caused by levorphanol in the mouse. *J. Pharmacol. Exp. Therap.* 169:175 (1969).

107. V. J. LOTTI, P. LOMAX, and R. GEORGE: Temperature responses in the rat following intracerebral microinjection of morphine. *J. Pharmacol. Exper. Therap.* 150:135 (1965).

108. V. J. LOTTI, P. LOMAX, and R. GEORGE: N-Allylnormorphine antagonism of the hypothermic effect of morphine in the rat following intracerebral and systemic administration. *J. Pharmacol. Exp. Therap.* 150:420 (1965).

109. D. H. CLOUET, ed.: *Narcotic Drugs: Biochemical Pharmacology*. New York, Plenum Press (1971).

110. E. A. GYANG and H. W. KOSTERLITZ: Agonist and antagonist actions of morphine-like drugs on the guinea-pig isolated ileum. *Brit. J. Pharm.* 27:514 (1966).

111. B. M. COX and M. WEINSTOCK: The effect of analgesic drugs on the release of acetylcholine from electrically stimulated guinea-pig ileum. *Brit. J. Pharm.* 27:81 (1966).

112. A. GOLDSTEIN and R. SCHULZ: Morphine tolerant longitudinal muscle strip from guinea pig ileum. *Brit. J. Pharmacol.* 48:655 (1973).

112a. R. SCHULZ and A. GOLDSTEIN: Morphine tolerance and supersensitivity to serotonin in the myenteric plexus of the guinea pig. *Nature* 244:168 (1973).

113. T. THOMPSON and C. R. SCHUSTER: Morphine self-administration, food-reinforced, and avoidance behaviors in Rhesus monkeys. *Psychopharmacologia* 5:87 (1964).

114. F. HUIDOBRO and C. MAGGIOLO: Studies on morphine. IX. On the intensity of the abstinence syndrome to morphine induced by daily injections of nalorphine in white mice *Arch. Int. Pharmacodyn.* 158:97 (1965).

115. C. K. HIMMELSBACH: Studies of certain addiction characteristics of (a) dihydromorphine ("Paramorphan"), (b) dihydrodesoxymorphine-D ("Desomorphine"), (c) dihydrodesoxycodeine-D ("Desocodeine"), and (d) methyldihydromorphinone ("Metopon"). *J. Pharmacol. Exp. Therap.* 67:239 (1939).

116. L. KOLB and C. K. HIMMELSBACH: Clinical studies of drug addiction. III. A critical review of the withdrawal treatments with method of evaluating abstinence syndromes. *Amer. J. Psychiatr.* 94:759 (1938).

117. H. ISBELL: Methods and results of studying experimental human addiction to the newer synthetic analgesics. *Ann. N.Y. Acad. Sci.* 51:108 (1948).

118. H. L. ANDREWS and C. K. HIMMELSBACH: Relation of the intensity of the morphine abstinence syndrome to dosage. *J. Pharmacol. Exp. Therap.* 81:288 (1944).

119. C. K. HIMMELSBACH and H. L. ANDREWS: Studies on modification of the morphine abstinence syndrome by drugs. *J. Pharmacol. Exp. Therap.* 77:17 (1943).

120. V. P. DOLE and M. NYSWANDER: A medical treatment for diacetylmorphine (heroin) addiction. *J. Amer. Med. Ass.* 193:646 (1965).

121. L. A. WOODS: The pharmacology of nalorphine (N-allylnormorphine). *Pharmacol. Rev.* 8:175 (1956).

122. P. D. ORAHOVATS, C. A. WINTER, and E. G. LEHMAN: The effect of N-allylnomorphine upon the development of tolerance to morphine in the albino rat. *J. Pharmacol. Exp. Therap.* 109:413 (1953).

123. M. H. SEEVERS and G. A. DENEAU: A critique of the "dual action" hypothesis of morphine physical dependence. *Arch. Int. Pharmacodyn.* 140:514 (1962).

124. E. L. WAY, H. H. LOH, and F.-H. SHEN: Simultaneous quantitative assessment of morphine tolerance and physical dependence. *J. Pharmacol. Exp. Therap.* 167:1 (1969).

125. D. L. CHENEY and A. GOLDSTEIN: Tolerance to opioid narcotics, III. Time course and reversibility of physical dependence in mice. *Nature* 232:477 (1971).

126. W. R. MARTIN and C. G. EADES: A comparison between acute and chronic physical dependence in the chronic spinal dog. *J. Pharmacol. Exp. Therap.* 146:385 (1964).

127. A. WIKLER, H. F. FRASER, and H. ISBELL: N-allylnormorphine: effects of single doses and precipitation of acute "abstinence syndromes" during addition to morphine, methadone or heroin in man (post-addicts). *J. Pharmacol. Exp. Therap.* 109:8 (1953).

128. H. F. FRASER, G. D VAN HORN, W. R. MARTIN, A. B. WOLBACH, and H. ISBELL: Methods for evaluating addiction liability. (A) "Attitude" of opiate addicts toward opiate-like drugs, (B) a short-term "direct" addiction test. *J. Pharmacol. Exp. Therap.* 133:371 (1961).

129. S. J. MULÉ and L. A. WOODS: Distribution of N-C^{14}-methyl labeled morphine. I. In central nervous system of nontolerant and tolerant dogs *J. Pharmacol. Exp. Therap.* 136:232 (1962).

130. A. E. TAKEMORI: Enzymic studies on morphine glucuronide synthesis in acutely and chronically morphinized rats. *J. Pharmacol. Exp. Therap.* 130:370 (1960).

131. T. JOHANNESSON and L. A. WOODS: Analgesic action and brain and plasma levels of morphine and codeine in morphine tolerant, codeine tolerant and non-tolerant rats. *Acta Pharmacol. Toxicol.* 21:381 (1964).

132. J. A. RICHTER and A. GOLDSTEIN. Tolerance to opioid narcotics. II. Cellular tolerance to levorphanol in mouse brain. *Proc. Nat. Acad. Sci. U.S.A.* 66:944 (1970).

133. A. GOLDSTEIN, B. A. JUDSON and P. SHEEHAN: Cellular and metabolic tolerance to an opioid narcotic. *Brit. J. Pharmacol.* 47:138 (1973).

134. B. M. COX, M. GINSBERG, and O. H. OSMAN: Acute tolerance to narcotic analgesic drugs in rats. *Brit. J. Pharmacol.* 33:245 (1968).

135. E. L. WAY, H. H. LOH, and F.-H. SHEN: Morphine tolerance, physical dependence, and synthesis of brain 5-hydroxytryptamine. *Science* 162:1290 (1968).

136. M. COHEN, A. S. KEATS, W. KRIVOY, and G. UNGAR: Effect of actinomycin D on morphine tolerance. *Proc. Soc. Exp. Biol. Med.* 119:381 (1965).

137. C. K. HIMMELSBACH: Symposium: can the euphoric, analgetic and physical dependence effects of drugs be separated? IV. With reference to physical dependence. *Fed. Proc.* 2:201 (1943).

138. W. R. MARTIN and A. J. EISENMAN: Interactions between nalorphine and morphine in the decerebrate cat. *J. Pharmacol Exp. Therap.* 138:113 (1962).

139. J. BRODEUR and K. P. DUBOIS: Studies on the mechanism of acquired tolerance by rats to O,O-diethyl S-2-(ethylthio)ethyl phosphorodithioate (Di-Syston). *Arch. Int. Pharmacodyn.* 149:560 (1964).

140. H. O. COLLIER: Tolerance, physical dependence and receptors. *Advan. Drug. Res.* 3:171 (1966).

140a. H. O. COLLIER: Humoral transmitters, supersensitivity, receptors and dependence. In *Scientific Basis of Drug Dependence*, H. Steinberg, ed., London, Churchill (1969).

141. L. SHUSTER: Repression and de-repression of enzyme synthesis as a possible explanation of some aspects of drug action. *Nature* 189:314 (1961).

142. D. B. GOLDSTEIN and A. GOLDSTEIN: Possible role of enzyme inhibition and repression in drug tolerance and addiction. *Biochem. Pharmacol.* 8:48 (1961).

143. D. B. GOLDSTEIN: Effects of barbital on amino acid metabolism in *Escherichia coli*. *Mol. Pharmacol.* 1:31 (1965).

144. A. GOLDSTEIN and D. B. GOLDSTEIN: Enzyme expansion theory of drug tolerance and physical dependence. *Res. Publ. Ass. Res. Nerv. Ment. Dis.* 46:265 (1968).

145. C. B. SMITH and M. I. SHELDON: Effects of narcotic analgesic drugs on brain noradrenergic mechanisms. In *Agonist and Antagonist Actions of Narcotic Analgesic Drugs*, H. W. Kosterlitz, H. O. J. Collier, and J E. Villarreal, eds. London, Macmillan Co. (1972).

146. L.-M. GUNNE: Catecholamines and 5-hydroxytryptamine in morphine tolerance and withdrawal. *Acta Physiol. Scand.* 58, Suppl. 204:5 (1963).

147. H. WEIL-MALHERBE, E. R. B. SMITH, A. J. EISENMAN, and H. F. FRASER: Plasma catecholamine levels and urinary excretion of catecholamines and metabolites in two human subjects during a cycle of morphine addiction and withdrawal. *Biochem. Pharmacol.* 14:1621 (1965).

148. J. A. SCHNEIDER: Reserpine antagonism of morphine analgesia in mice. *Proc. Soc. Exp. Biol. Med.* 87:614 (1954).

149. M. MEDAKOVIĆ and B. BANIĆ: The action of reserpine and α-methyl-*m*-tyrosine on the analgesic effect of morphine in rats and mice. *J. Pharm. Pharmacol.* 16:198 (1964).

150. G. FRIEDLER, H. N. BHARGAVA, R. QUOCK, and E. L. WAY: The effect of 6-hydroxydopamine on morphine tolerance and physical dependence. *J. Pharmacol. Exp. Therap.* 183:49 (1972).

151. J. A. RICHTER and A. GOLDSTEIN: Effects of morphine and levorphanol on brain acetylcholine content in mice. *J. Pharmacol. Exp. Therap.* 175:685 (1970).

152. J. CROSSLAND and P. SLATER: The effect of some drugs on the "free" and "bound" acetylcholine content of rat brain. *Brit. J. Pharmacol.* 33:42 (1968).

153. K. HANO, H. KANETO, T. KAKUNAGA, and N. MORIBAYASHI: Pharmacological studies of analgesics. VI. The administration of morphine and changes in acetylcholine metabolism in mouse brain. *Biochem. Pharmacol.* 13:441 (1964).

154. H. O. J. COLLIER: Pharmacological mechanisms of drug dependence. *Proc. 5th Internat. Congr. Pharmacol.*, p. 141, San Francisco (1972).

155. J. COCHIN and J. AXELROD: Biochemical and pharmacological changes in the rat following chronic administration of morphine, nalorphine and normorphine. *J. Pharmacol. Exp. Therap.* 125:105 (1959).

156. D. H. CLOUET and M. RATNER: Catecholamine biosynthesis in brains of rats treated with morphine. *Science* 168:854 (1970).

157. S. J. ROSENMAN and C. B. SMITH: ^{14}C-Catecholamine synthesis in mouse brain during morphine withdrawal. *Nature* 240:153 (1972).

CHAPTER 10
Chemical Mutagenesis

If a drug produces permanent heritable change in a germ cell, the outcome will be an altered hereditary constitution (genotype) of the individual who will be the product of the union of that germ cell with another. A persisting change is thus introduced into the germ line of the species, unless the alteration is incompatible with survival. Permanent changes in the genotype (*mutations*) are produced by radiation and by chemical agents (*mutagens*). Mutations also occur spontaneously by unknown mechanisms. In the strict sense of the word, a mutation is a very sharply localized change in the genetic material (also called "point mutation"), as distinguished from deletions and other alterations of chromosome structure or number. In this discussion of chemical mutagenesis, we shall adopt the original broader meaning and consider all chemically induced modifications of the genotype.[1-5]

MOLECULAR BASIS OF MUTATION

The sum total of the genetic information that specifies the structure, function, and development of each individual of a species is encoded in the DNA.[6,7] The zygote of sexually reproducing organisms contains two copies of this information, one from the sperm, the other from the ovum. All the information contained in all the genes is in the form of a linear code of 3-letter words, the letters of which are the nucleotide bases, adenine (A), guanine (G), cytosine (C), and thymine (T). Thus, the "word" CGG specifies one piece of information, CAG another, and so forth. The mechanism whereby such information is translated into amino acid residues of proteins was discussed in Chapter 8. Now we are concerned with the replication of the genetic information and its passage from one generation to the next. The orderly replication of the genetic information is ensured by the mechanism of base-pairing by hydrogen bond formation in the double-stranded DNA helix. Since a given base on one strand uniquely specifies its partner on the complementary strand, the letters of the coding alphabet are really the four possible base pairs, A:T, T:A, G:C, and C:G. The obligatory pairing of purine against pyrimidine is ensured by the distance between the phosphate-deoxyribose backbones of the two helices; pyrimidine against pyrimidine would leave a gap between, and purine against purine would not fit the available space. The hydrogen bonding relationships are optimal for the matching of adenine to thymine and guanine to cytosine (Figure 1-11). The process whereby the double helix unwinds during replication, each strand acting as template for the synthesis of a new complementary strand—the semiconservative replication mechanism—guarantees that all of the genetic information will be partitioned equally to daughter cells at every cell division and thus be transmitted accurately from generation to generation.[8-11]

The following kinds of mutation are recognized:

1. *Base pair transformation.* A given base pair may be replaced in three ways. In one of these, the original purine is replaced by another purine, the original pyrimidine by another pyrimidine; this kind of change is called a *transition.* In the other possible changes, a purine is replaced by a pyrimidine or a pyrimidine by a purine; this is called a *transversion.*

2. *Addition or deletion* of a base pair. This kind of change is known as a *frame shift mutation* because the ordered translation of the codons, triplet by triplet, will be profoundly disturbed. All the bases distal to the point of insertion or deletion will be out of register. As can be imagined, the consequences are usually much more drastic than those of a single base pair transformation.

3. *Large deletions and rearrangements.* Deletions of the genetic material occur in all sizes. The basic mutational process here appears to be *breakage* followed by *reconstitution* of fragments. This occurs in single DNA molecules and also at the gross level of the chromosomes. Segments may be inverted, exchanges may occur between chromatids (the paired subunits of the chromosome), and material may be translocated from one chromosome to another.

4. *Unequal partition of chromosomes* between daughter cells. This is known as *nondisjunction.* It may occur at meiosis or mitosis and is frequently caused by chemical agents that disturb the formation and function of the system of spindle fibers.

A fundamental distinction has to be made between two modes of action of mutagens. Agents of one class act directly upon the existing genetic material and therefore can be effective at any time in the cell cycle. Agents of the second class are only able to modify the course of a dynamic process such as DNA replication or chromosome movement; such mutagens may be effective only at a particular time in the cell cycle.

A type of chemical mutagenesis that does not fall readily into either of the above categories is that due to the incorporation of radioactivity into DNA. The mutations occur in three ways: (*1*) The energy of a disintegration may rupture an internucleotide bond by a recoil effect. (*2*) Localized β or γ emission may be mutagenic by virtue of secondary bombardment of nearby purine or pyrimidine bases. (*3*) Transmutation of a radioactive atom may lead to altered chemical properties and thus affect the fidelity of subsequent replications. It is well known that ^{32}P incorporated into DNA of bacteria and viruses causes both lethality and point mutations, probably by the first two mechanisms. Both ^3H and ^{14}C are thought to be especially hazardous because they can be incorporated so readily into the nucleic acid bases and deoxyribose and thus into DNA. The special hazard of ^3H is that it is so difficult to monitor routinely; its decay energy is so low and the mean path length of its β particles so short that Geiger counters are ineffective for detecting contamination. The special hazard of ^{14}C is its exceedingly long radioactive half-life (more than 5000 years); incorporation in the human germ line could cause mutational effects over a period of millennia.[12]

The fidelity of the normal DNA replication process is remarkable. Spontaneous mutations, which are errors in this process, are rarely observed at a frequency greater than 1 per 10^5 replications. An interesting experiment[13] demonstrated this high degree of fidelity in vitro. The alternating copolymer of deoxyadenylic acid and thymidylic acid (dAT copolymer), in which each single strand has the base sequence ... ATATAT ..., was allowed to act as primer for the synthesis of new DNA catalyzed by DNA polymerase in the presence of all four deoxyribonucleoside triphosphates. As every A specifies a complementary T and vice versa, no G or C whatsoever should be incorporated; and the newly-synthesized material should also have a strictly alternating ... TATATA ... sequence. Both of these expectations were confirmed. Less than one residue of G per 28,000 A and T residues was found.

The molecular basis of this fidelity of replication is far from clear. Certainly the simple difference in bond energies between "correct" (A:T, G:C) and "incorrect" (A:C, G:T) purine-pyrimidine pairs could not alone account for it. Additional mechanisms must exclude or reject the wrong bases. An example of such a recognition mechanism is the system for enzymic repair of DNA.[14-16] The repair enzymes excise segments containing erroneous bases (e.g., thymine dimers formed by ultraviolet irradiation) in one strand of the DNA, and permit their replacement by the alignment and linking of correct bases properly paired against those of the other (normal) strand. Thus, defective regions of either strand are "patched." The existence of repair mechanisms greatly complicates the interpretation of data on mutagenesis, since the mutations we eventually see are only a small fraction of those originally produced, the remainder having been repaired. Direct evidence of this has been obtained in special mutant bacterial strains that lack the excision repair system. Such strains yield 10–100 times as many mutants when treated with a chemical mutagen as do wild-type strains. This property makes them useful as tester strains for mutagenesis screening.[4]

The sequence of base pairs in the DNA determines the corresponding sequence of bases in RNA. Only one strand of the DNA (the "sense" strand) is transcribed, serving as template for the synthesis of single-stranded RNA. The same base pairing mechanism operates as in replication, except that RNA contains uracil (U) instead of thymine so that we have the base pair A:U instead of A:T. A small fraction of the DNA specifies the structures of the two classes of ribosomal RNA and the modest number (64 or fewer) of transfer-RNA (tRNA) molecules. Most of the rest of the genome encodes the information for the sequence of amino acids in all the cell proteins and for regulatory processes involving operator genes and derepressor RNA. This information is first transcribed into messenger-RNA (mRNA), which serves as template for the assembly of proteins, as described in Chapter 8.

The fidelity of replication and transcription underlies the persistence of mutations, for any change that cannot be recognized as incorrect will remain encoded permanently in the genome. It is important to understand what is meant here by "incorrect." By the very nature of the genetic code, any of the four normal base pairs is correct. Suppose, for example, that a particular sequence of 450 base pairs specifies a corresponding sequence of 150 amino acids in an enzyme. If one of these base pairs is changed to any of the other normal pairs, the codon containing the new base pair may specify a different amino acid. Likewise, if one or more normal base pairs are added or deleted, or if a portion of the sequence is rearranged, the mutant DNA will be replicated in the usual way, and it will be perpetuated as long as its protein (or

RNA) products are compatible with survival. Indeed, this principle underlies all of evolution, for unless mutant DNA could function normally in replication and transcription, natural selection could not act upon the resulting phenotypes. It is only at a certain stage in the genesis of a mutation that an intrinsically abnormal base pair may be present. For instance, if an erroneous base pairing occurs during replication so that A on an existing strand pairs with C (instead of T) on the new complementary strand, there will be a transient abnormal pair A:C. This may be recognized and repaired by excision of a segment of the new strand that includes C and its restitution by a new segment. If there is no repair, normal base pairing will occur at the next replication in both daughter duplexes, and one of these will become a permanent mutant. The reason is simply that, by the usual rules of base pairing, A will pair with T, thus reconstituting the original base pair; but C will pair with G, yielding a G:C pair instead of the original A:T at this site.

Much of the fundamental work that led to our present understanding of the molecular basis of mutagenesis was done with mutants of bacteriophage T4 of *Escherichia coli*, known as rII mutants.[17,18] These are characterized by an abnormal plaque morphology (large plaques with very sharp edges, caused by unusually rapid lysis) and by their inability to grow on bacterial strain K, although they grow well on strain B. Thus, mutants are readily recognized by eye from among thousands of wild-type plaques, and wild-type revertants are efficiently selected by growth on bacteria of strain K. The rII mutants arise by a genetic change occurring anywhere within a particular region of the phage genome, designated the rII gene. The rII gene directs the synthesis of two proteins. The term *cistron*, in general use to describe the portion of a gene that codes for a single protein, originated in these investigations with rII mutants. It was found that certain pairs of mutants would grow on *E. coli* K if inoculated together but not separately. This phenomenon of complementation obviously depended upon each strain producing a normal gene product that could be used by the other. The test for this property was called a *cis-trans* test, whence the term *cistron*.

The exact location of a given mutation within the gene can be established by the method of recombination. Phage recombination results from breakage and reunion of DNA in two different phage particles. Two mutant strains of phage are inoculated together into a culture of *E. coli* B. The progeny, after lysis of the bacteria, are tested by spreading on strain K. Some wild-type plaques result, and their frequency is determined. If the experiment is done with two mutant strains thought to be different but in fact identical, then very few wild-type plaques are found, representing spontaneous back mutations.

As illustrated in Figure 10-1, a wild-type recombinant can arise only if the damaged portions of the genomes do not overlap. If the probability of breakage is constant throughout a gene, the frequency of recombination between two mutant sites is a measure of the linear distance between them. Since the selection of wild-type recombinants on *E. coli* strain K is very efficient, extremely low frequencies of recombination can be detected. Two mutants are presumed to have been altered at the same site if wild-type recombinants cannot be obtained. The resolving power of the method is on the order of a single base pair, i.e. mutants could probably be distinguished if they were mutated at adjacent base pairs. Deletions are recognized by their inability to yield recombinants with a series of mutants already mapped at different sites; deletions of a wide range of sizes have been thus identified.

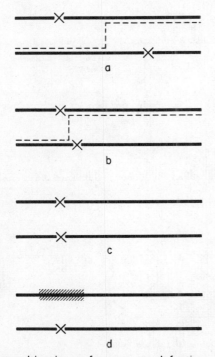

FIGURE 10-1. Recombination of mutants defective at different sites. *Each diagram represents phage DNA from 2 strains. Mutant sites are indicated by X. Broken line represents replication or breakage and reunion. Hatched segment is a deletion. a: Wild-type recombinant is possible because mutations are at different sites. b: Wild-type recombinant is possible, but will occur less frequently than in a. c and d: Wild-type recombinants impossible because mutations or deletions are at identical sites.*

As detected by this technique, spontaneous mutations and those caused by chemical mutagens were plotted on a map of the rII gene. The sites of a large number of spontaneous mutations are shown in Figure 10-2. They are scattered over the entire gene, but the distribution is far from random. At certain *hot spots* the mutability is many times greater than elsewhere. There are two prominent hot spots for spontaneous mutation, one near the terminus of the A cistron, the other in the middle of the B cistron. The spectrum of mutation sites in the terminal portion of the B cistron, after treatment by different chemical mutagens, is shown in Figure 10-3. The spontaneous sites for this region are the same as already depicted in Figure 10-2. These results indicate that the phenomenon of hot spots is not peculiar to spontaneous mutation but is seen with all the mutagens tested. It is also evident that hot spots are mutagen-specific. One of the spontaneous hot spots, for example, has no counterpart in any of the mutagen patterns. The largest hot spot in the 5-bromouracil pattern is not represented even once in the spontaneous pattern. The 2-aminopurine hot spot in segment 8 is represented by only an occasional mutant in any of the other patterns.

Hot spots were once taken at face value as representing sites of unusually high mutability. If this were true, a hot spot would have to be imbedded in a special and rather rare sequence of base pairs. The reason for this deduction is simply that the

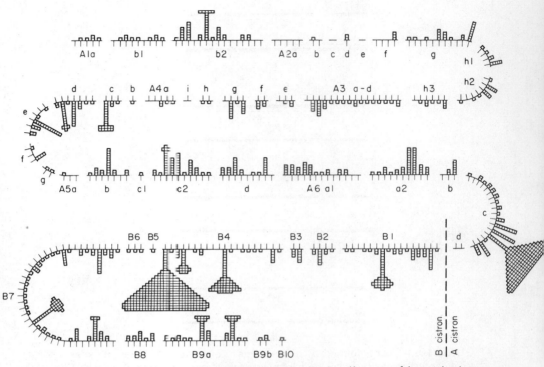

FIGURE 10-2. Spontaneous mutation sites in the rII gene of bacteriophage T4 of E. coli. *The various segments of the A and B cistron are designated by arbitrary numbers and letters. Each small square denotes one independent occurrence of a spontaneous mutation. (From Benzer, Figure 6.[17])*

normal base pairs could account, at most, for only four different degrees of mutability; and these would necessarily be associated with numerous sites throughout the gene. To account for exceptionally high mutability at one site, we would have to invoke some influence of neighboring base pairs. Suppose there is one extraordinary hot spot out of 1000 base pairs. Then a special sequence of at least 5 pairs will be required, since 5 is the smallest specified sequence that would occur randomly only once in 1000 base pairs (actual probability $4^{-5} = 1/1024$). But advances in our understanding of the genetic code and the way it functions render such an explanation unlikely.

First, the very nature of the code makes certain sites more mutable than others. As Table 8-3 indicates, each of the 20 amino acids is coded in mRNA by more than a single codon, some by as many as six different codons. It is clear from the table that most of the degeneracy of the code is attributable to the base in the third (3′) position. Every codon has at least one degenerate partner that differs in the third position but represents the same amino acid. One-half of the codons have three such degenerate partners. Obviously, a transition mutation in the DNA that results in a corresponding change in the third position in the RNA codon (purine for purine, or pyrimidine for pyrimidine) will have no effect whatsoever; the "mutation" will be undetectable. And for one-half of the codons even a transversion in the third position would be undetectable. Certain changes in the first position will also have no effect (e.g., AGA → CGA = *Arg*; CUG → UUG = *Leu*).

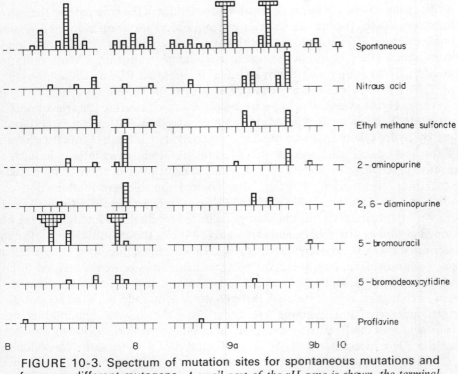

FIGURE 10-3. Spectrum of mutation sites for spontaneous mutations and for seven different mutagens. *A small part of the rII gene is shown, the terminal portion of the B cistron shown at bottom of Figure 10-2. Each small square denotes one independent occurrence of a mutation. The mutagens are listed next to each row, at the right. Mutation sites are indicated by symbols at bottom. (Modified from Benzer, Figure 8.[17])*

Second, the apparent mutability of a given site will be determined by the position and nature of the corresponding amino acid in the protein. It is now clear that functional proteins tolerate amino acid replacement at some positions but not at others. At certain critical locations, any alteration may produce a nonfunctional protein. But often the substitution of chemically similar amino acids (e.g., *Glu → Asp, Gln → Asn, Lys → Arg, Leu → Ile*) has but little effect on the protein function. From this point of view, a hot spot could be a site at which the base pair alteration results in a codon specifying an amino acid that is incompatible with protein function when it occupies that particular position in the amino acid sequence. In general, mutations that have large effects upon a phenotypic function will be detected; but mutations at other sites, which lead to tolerated modifications of protein structure, will be overlooked.

Third, the identification of a special role in polypeptide chain termination for the codons UAA and UAG[7,19,20] offers yet another explanation of hot spots. These codons, as well as UGA, specify no amino acid (i.e., "nonsense"). Therefore, codons that can be transformed into these by alteration of a single base pair will seem to be more mutable than codons that cannot because premature chain termination will nearly always produce a complete deficiency of the protein function. Thus, for example, a *Gln* position coded by CAA or CAG could readily be converted to "nonsense" by the single transition C → U, causing chain termination.

A surprising amount cf information about the nature of the base pairs at the various mutant sites in the rII gene can be deduced from observations on induced reversions. A single example will illustrate the method and the argument.[8,21-23] The base analog 5-bromouracil (BU) is known to cause pyrimidine transitions. Most mutations induced by BU are also revertible by BU. This implies that BU can cause both transitions, C → T and T → C, thereby transforming G:C (or C:G) to A:T (or T:A), and the reverse. Hydroxylamine acts preferentially upon C, causing the transition C:G (or G:C) to T:A (or A:T).[24-27] Most mutants caused by BU cannot be induced to revert by hydroxylamine. From this, it is inferred that most BU mutants have an A:T (or T:A) pair at the mutant site, i.e., that BU itself preferentially induces the transition G:C → A:T (or C:G → T:A). This conclusion is further strengthened by the fact that, even under conditions that favored the selective modification of G residues, most BU mutants could not be made to revert by treatment with an alkylating agent.[28,29] Explicit data about the changes induced by chemical mutagens have been obtained in studies with tobacco mosaic virus (TMV)[30]; these confirm the earlier conclusions in most respects. Here the virus RNA can be treated directly with a mutagenic agent, then inoculated into the plant host; and the virus protein obtained in large yield. Since the entire amino acid sequence of TMV protein has been determined, the observed changes can be correlated, through the genetic code, with the actions of the various mutagens. For example, treatment with the known deaminating agent nitrous acid resulted frequently in replacement of a threonine residue by isoleucine. Since the *Thr* codons are ACA, ACG, ACC, and ACU, whereas the *Ile* codons are AUC, AUA, and AUU, it is obvious that nitrous acid deaminated C to U in the second position of an ACC, ACA, or ACU codon. Similar detailed descriptions of mutagenesis are derived from other systems in which the gene product has been completely characterized.[31-33]

BASE PAIR TRANSFORMATIONS

The smallest unit of mutation is the single base pair. Base pair transformations can be brought about in two ways. A mutagen may react directly with a base in DNA and modify it chemically. At the next replication, the modified base may pair with a new partner. The subsequent replication will see the completion of the mutation process, for the new partner will pair correctly and thus an entirely different base pair will be substituted for the original one. Figure 10-4 illustrates these steps for the hypothetical case of an adenine residue being deaminated to hypoxanthine. Hypoxanthine, from the standpoint of base pairing, is rather like guanine, for it has an oxygen atom at the 6-position. The first replication may then yield a normal duplex containing A:T and an abnormal one containing H:C. In the next replication, H:C will yield G:C as one of its products. Whether the other product is H:T or H:C is relatively unimportant; a mutant allele of the original A:T pair has already been formed and can now maintain itself permanently in subsequent replications.

Certain experimental findings have suggested a different scheme. It is proposed[34] that when one base of a pair is altered by a mutagenic agent, its partner is excised and replaced before replication occurs, so that all the progeny are mutant. Alternatively, it is suggested[35] that at replication one strand acts as master strand, the base on that

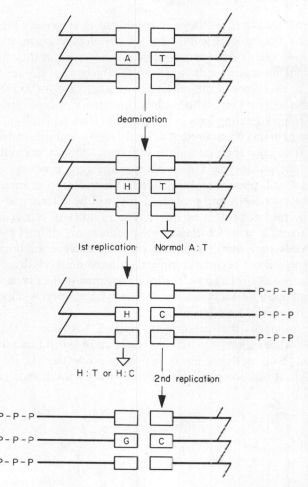

FIGURE 10-4. Mechanism of a mutagenic transformation by deamination.
*Adenine is deaminated to hypoxanthine, which pairs like guanine. The result is a
mutagenic transition, $A:T \rightarrow G:C$.*

strand determining both incoming bases; again, if the base on the master strand is
altered, all the progeny will be mutant.

The second way a mutagen can cause a base pair alteration is by affecting the
fidelity of replication. The mutagen itself may be incorporated into DNA and then
pair incorrectly at a subsequent replication. Or the mutagen may cause erroneous
base pairing in some less direct way, for example, by drastically altering the proportions
of the four bases available for the replication process.

Mutagens of the first kind, which modify bases of an already-formed DNA duplex,
are important experimental tools because they can be used in vitro. They have been
employed to modify bacterial and plant viruses, transforming-DNA and synthetic
deoxyribonucleotide polymers.[23,36] After treatment, the DNA can be introduced
into living cells to observe the results of the induced mutations; the treated synthetic
polymer can be studied in the DNA polymerase reaction to see how the synthesis
of a replica strand is modified.[37] Used experimentally, these direct-acting mutagens

are very efficient, inasmuch as they are employed at extremely high concentrations and often under nonbiologic conditions of pH, temperature, ionic environment, and so on. In vivo their efficiency would be much lower but they might nevertheless have a significant mutagenic action. Those mutagens that do act in vivo are likely to be effective at all stages of the cell cycle, whether or not the DNA is replicating. Mutagens of the second kind, which affect the fidelity of replication, will obviously be active only in proliferating cells at the time of DNA replication.

Once a base pair has been altered, several factors will determine the phenotypic delay, i.e., the time until the mutation is expressed. At first, the cell of mutant genotype has wild-type phenotype. This is because the gene products—messenger-RNA and protein—are still present and functional. Their disappearance and replacement by mutant messenger-RNA and protein (if any) will be determined by the messenger half-life and the rate of protein turnover. The rapidity of cell growth and division will influence the rate at which these gene products are diluted by simple partition into daughter cells. In multinucleate cells, only one nucleus will in general be mutant, so the phenotype will not become completely altered until cell divisions segregate the mutant nucleus into a cell of its own. In diploid organisms, the expression of the mutant trait will depend upon its dominance or recessivity, i.e., upon whether it is manifest in heterozygotes or only in homozygotes.

Among the mutagens that act directly upon DNA, one of the most specific is hydroxylamine, which appears to act selectively upon C residues under weakly acidic conditions. The resulting oxime has base pairing properties like those of T. In alkali, an entirely different reaction proceeds, whereby the pyrimidine or purine ring of T or

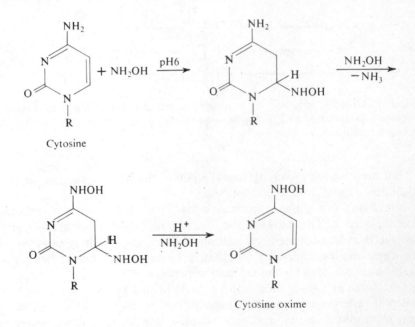

G is split, but this evidently leads to lethality rather than to a point mutation. The mutagenic effect of hydroxylamine, therefore, is almost exclusively to produce transitions in the direction $G:C \rightarrow A:T$.[24,25] It should be understood that the bacterial viruses that have been studied contain hydroxymethylcytosine rather than cytosine itself, but the base-pairing properties are identical to those of C, and no further distinction will be made here.

Nitrous acid is a nonspecific deaminating agent. It attacks all the bases except thymine, which has no amino group. As shown in Figure 10-5, it transforms adenine to hypoxanthine, whose base pairing properties are like those of guanine; the end

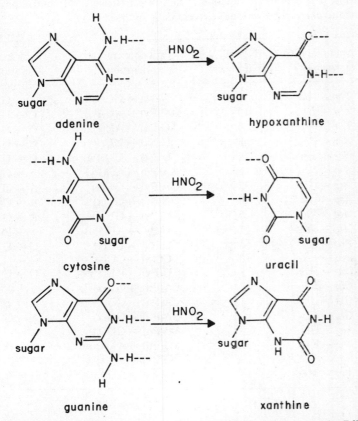

FIGURE 10-5. Deamination of nucleic acid bases by nitrous acid. *Effect of nitrous acid upon the 3 bases subject to deamination. Dashed lines represent hydrogen bonds in the DNA helix. (From Kotaka and Baldwin, Figure 1.[37])*

result is, therefore, a transition of the A:T → G:C type. Nitrous acid deaminates cytosine to uracil, which behaves like thymine; so the result is a transition of the reverse kind, G:C → A:T. Finally, it deaminates guanine to xanthine; but xanthine apparently acts like guanine in base pairing, so no mutation results.[11] In phage, a prominent effect of nitrous acid is to induce extensive deletions.[38]

That the mutagenic action of nitrous acid is due almost entirely to the postulated transitions, C → T and A → G, is indicated by extensive studies with tobacco mosaic virus,[30] summarized in Table 10-1. Nineteen different amino acid replacements were observed in the TMV protein after mutagenic treatment with HNO_2. Many of these occurred repeatedly, so that altogether 63 occurrences were identified. The table shows that when the codons (from Table 8-5) for the original amino acid and the

TABLE 10-1. Mutagenic action of nitrous acid on tobacco mosaic virus RNA.

The observed amino acid replacements in TMV protein are interpreted in terms of the most probable single-base alterations, from the genetic code as given in Table 8-5. The triplet codons are read from 5′ at left to 3′ at right. Degeneracy in the 3′ position is indicated by (x) = any base, (Pu) = either purine, (Py) = either pyrimidine. (From Siegel, Table I,[30] modified and updated to correspond with more recent data on the code.)

Amino acid replacement	No. of occurrences	Probable codon alteration	Base alteration
Thr → Ala	2	AC(x) → GC(x)	A → G
Thr → Ile	10	AC(Py) → AU(Py)	C → U
Thr → Met	3	AC(Pu) → AU(Pu)	C → U
Ser → Phe	8	UC(x) → UU(Py)	C → U
Ser → Leu	2	UC(x) → UU(Pu)	C → U
Asn → Ser	6	AA(Py) → AG(Py)	A → G
Asp → Gly	2	GA(Py) → GG(x)	A → G
Asp → Ala	4	GA(Py) → GC(x)	A → C
Ile → Val	5	AU(Py) → GU(x)	A → G
Ile → Met	1	AU(Py) → AU(Pu)	Py → Pu
Pro → Ser	3	CC(x) → UC(x)	C → U
Pro → Leu	6	CC(x) → CU(x)	C → U
Leu → Phe	1	CU(Py) → UU(Py)	C → U
Gln → Val	2	CA(Pu) → GU(x)	?
Gln → Arg	1	CA(Pu) → CG(x)	A → G
Glu → Gly	2	GA(Pu) → GG(x)	A → G
Arg → Gly	3	AG(Pu) → GG(x)	A → G
Arg → Lys	1	AG(Pu) → AA(x) or	G → A or
		CG(x) → AA(x)	?
Val → Met	1	GU(x) → AU(Pu)	G → A

replacement amino acids are considered, all but a few of the observations are accounted for by C→U or A→G transition. In only three instances, representing only one or two occurrences each, was it impossible to account for the result by the postulated transitions; and those may well have been spontaneous rather than mutagen-induced events. Significantly, there was not a single instance suggesting the modification of a U residue, in agreement with the chemical impossibility of deaminating U.

The data for proline and phenylalanine, shown in Table 10-1, provide an interesting proof that the viral RNA strand itself, and not a complementary strand, acts as template for the synthesis of TMV protein. The codon for *Pro* (CC(x)) cannot be derived from a codon representing another amino acid by deamination, and the codon for *Phe* (UU(Py)) cannot be transformed to any other codon by deamination. If a complementary strand were the template for protein synthesis, then *Phe* should be replaced readily but should not be a replacement, whereas *Pro* should be a replacement but should never be replaced. The reason is that the *Phe* codon UU(Py) on the complementary strand would be represented by AA(Pu) on the viral RNA strand; and this should be subject to deamination, but could never arise by deamination. Similarly, the *Pro* codon CC(x) on the complementary strand would be represented by GG(x) on the viral RNA; this should not be subject to mutagenic transformation by nitrous acid. In fact, as the table shows, the findings were exactly contrary; *Pro* was replaced nine times but was never a replacement, whereas *Phe* was a replacement nine times but was never replaced.

An extremely potent mutagen, which somewhat resembles nitrous acid in its action on DNA, is N-methyl-N'-nitro-N-nitrosoguanidine.[39,40] At first, it was thought that this agent might act indirectly by liberating nitrous acid or diazomethane, but now it is considered likely that it acts directly. Adenine is deaminated to hypoxanthine, and a nitroguanidinium addition product may also be formed. The reaction with cytosine also appears to be an addition to the amino group. This mutagen is principally remarkable because it produces a variety of mutations within living cells

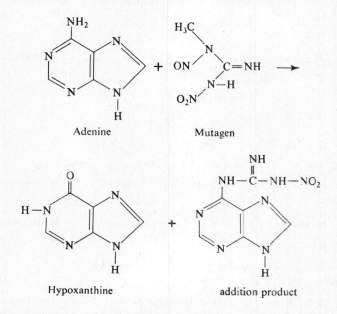

Adenine   Mutagen

Hypoxanthine   addition product

at a concentration (about 100 μg ml^{-1}) that is not lethal. This behavior contrasts sharply with that of many mutagens, which act readily upon isolated DNA but are effective in vivo only at concentrations that cause much killing. Extensive lethality at mutagenic dosage is also the rule for irradiation mutagenesis.

Alkylating agents such as ethyl methanesulfonate (EMS), ethyl ethanesulfonate (EES), and the nitrogen mustards can carry out an electrophilic attack upon various functional groups (amino, carboxyl, sulfhydryl, phosphate) in proteins and nucleic

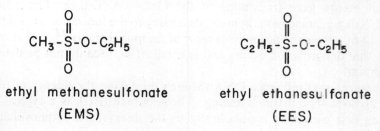

ethyl methanesulfonate   ethyl ethanesulfonate
(EMS)   (EES)

acids. The mutagenicity of these compounds is largely attributable to alkylation of position 7 of guanine, as shown in Figure 10-6. The effect of quaternizing the nitrogen atom is two-fold: to weaken the bond between N-9 and the deoxyribose moiety and to promote ionization at N-1 as shown.[42] It was first supposed that the bond-weakening effect at N-9 was the primary cause of the mutagenicity of alkylating agents. Depurination was postulated, followed presumably by the entry of any base opposite

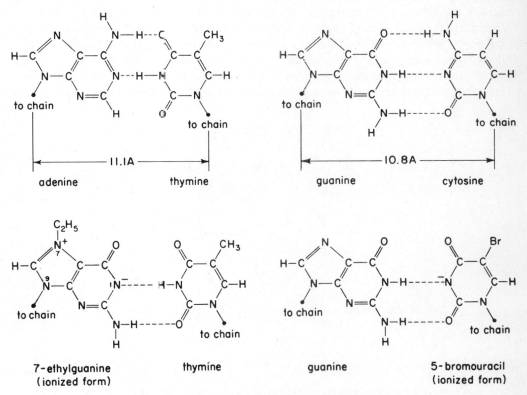

FIGURE 10-6. Normal and abnormal base pairing. *The 2 normal base pairs are shown on top line. Alkylation of guanine at position 7 permits ionized form to pair with thymine (lower left). Ionization of 5-bromouracil permits pairing with guanine (lower right). All hydrogen bond distances are 2.8 to 3.0 A. (Modified from Strauss, Figure 3.[41] By permission of Grune & Stratton.)*

the resulting gap at the next replication. Thus, it was predicted that G → A transitions and both kinds of transversion (G → C, G → T) would be produced. However, careful study of the effects of EMS upon phage T4 indicated that by far the most common mutational events were transitions of the G:C → A:T type. Thus, anomalous pairing of 7-alkylguanine with thymine, secondary to the ionization at N-1 (as shown in Figure 10-6), appears to account for most of the mutagenicity.[28,29,43] It is possible, of course, that depurination occurs and is lethal; if so, it could not be detected in a study of mutations.

The mutagens that influence DNA through modifying the fidelity of replication are base analogs. The thymine analog, 5-bromouracil (BU), is a typical example. After being first converted metabolically to the deoxyribose triphosphate, BU is incorporated extensively into DNA in place of T by entering the nascent DNA strand opposite A on the old strand. The extent of this replacement in some experiments has been quite remarkable, up to about one-half the total number of T residues. Obviously, the presence of BU instead of T does not seriously affect DNA function —either replication or transcription—since the organisms are viable and continue to grow and divide, either in normal medium or in the continued presence of BU. Thus, the A:BU pair functions like the A:T pair. At replication, BU specifies an incoming A on the nascent strand; at transcriptions, BU specifies A on the nascent messenger-RNA.

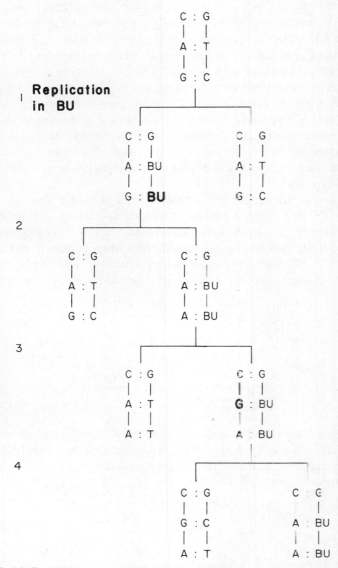

FIGURE 10-7. Mutagenesis by 5-bromouracil (BU). *The commonest mechanism is shown at replication I; BU enters opposite G, and the end result is a G:C → A:T transition. If BU that has already been incorporated pairs with an incoming G (as at replication 3), an A:T → G:C transition results.*

Errors of incorporation or of replication are probably attributable to the ionized form of BU, which undergoes base pairing as though it were C (Figure 10-6). This results from loss of a proton at N-1, so that a hydrogen bond can be formed with the H atom at N-1 of guanine. When it is being incorporated, BU may occasionally undergo this erroneous base pairing and thus enter opposite G, as illustrated in the first replication in Figure 10-7. At subsequent replications, this BU might behave "normally," as though it were T, and thus the end result would be a $G:C \rightarrow A:T$ transition. Since it has been shown that BU is more likely to be ionized when it is free (as the deoxynucleoside triphosphate) than after its polymerization into DNA, errors of incorporation (rather than of replication) are probably the principal mechanism of BU mutagenesis.[23] Alternatively, as shown at the third replication in Figure 10-7, a BU molecule, incorporated "correctly" in place of T, might behave as as though it were C, pairing with an incoming G. Then the transition $A:T \rightarrow G:C$ will be the end result. As already noted, the patterns of mutation induction and reversion observed in phage conformed to these expectations; transitions of the $G:C \rightarrow A:T$ type were most frequent, but $A:T \rightarrow G:C$ transitions also occurred.[44] As long as the strand containing BU persists, occasional mutations would be expected to occur at any subsequent replication, i.e., whenever an incoming G is paired against BU. This phenomenon has been observed in phage as a peculiar "mottling" of the plaques caused by new mutations arising after plaque formation has been initiated by phenotypically wild-type phage.[45]

The mechanisms are apparently similar for all the base analogs that can be incorporated. Purines replace purines, pyrimidines replace pyrimidines, so that transitions always result. The essential requirement is a certain ambiguity of structure with respect to those features that distinguish the normal purines or pyrimidines from each other. Thus, for example, 2-aminopurine resembles guanine at the 2-position but lacks the keto group at the 6-position. It seems to induce transitions in both directions.[8]

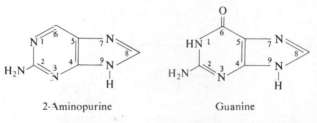

2-Aminopurine   Guanine

An interesting base-analog mutagen that may be of some significance in man is caffeine.[46,47] This is a fully methylated purine. Because it is substituted in the 7-position, it cannot form a stable bond to deoxyribose at the 9-position and is therefore not incorporated into DNA.

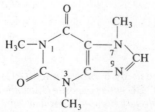

Caffeine (1,3,7-trimethylxanthine)

Because it is known to inhibit some enzymes of purine metabolism,[48] it has been proposed that it alters the normal base ratios in the DNA precursor pool, thereby causing errors of base pairing. It is also possible that it may intercalate between base pairs[49] in the manner of the acridines (p. 642) and thus cause frame shift mutations. Finally, there is evidence that caffeine greatly enhances the rate of ultraviolet-induced mutation by impairing the operation of the normal repair mechanisms for excising and replacing radiation-damaged segments of DNA.[50]

Many drugs of the base analog type have been employed in cancer chemotherapy in order to produce lethal damage in cells engaged in rapid DNA synthesis. Some also act as radiation sensitizers, increasing the killing effect of any given x-ray dose.[51] The lethal effect of x-irradiation is dependent upon the G:C content of the DNA. This is in contrast to ultraviolet irradiation, which is most effective upon DNA with high A:T content and which acts by dimerization of adjacent T residues. Alkylating agents, which act preferentially upon G:C pairs, have long been recognized to be "radio-mimetic" in their actions. Bromouracil and other halogenated uracil compounds that are incorporated into DNA are good x-ray sensitizers. Incorporation is not a necessary condition, however. Certain purine analogs, like 6-mercaptopurine, sensitize but are not incorporated. Nor is growth inhibition essential; 6-chloropurine sensitizes without any effect upon cell growth.

FRAME SHIFT MUTATIONS

These changes are point mutations of an entirely different type from the alterations of single base pairs discussed above. They result from the addition or deletion of a base. This mechanism of mutagenesis was discovered during investigations with acridine dyes such as proflavine and acridine yellow. When bacteria infected with

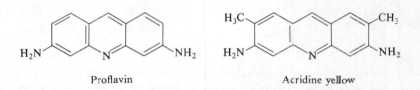

Proflavin   Acridine yellow

phage T4 were treated with an acridine, rII mutants were obtained that differed sharply from those already described, in that they could not be reverted by base analogs or by any of the other mutagens that cause transitions. Nor would acridines induce any reversion of transition mutants. On the other hand, many spontaneous mutants that were not revertible by the other mutagens could be reverted by treatment with acridines, and acridine mutants often reverted spontaneously. The elucidation of the mechanism of acridine mutagenesis was accomplished in a series of brilliant experiments that also established several fundamental principles of the coding and translation of genetic information.[52]

When the standard methods of recombination analysis were applied to acridine mutants, as described earlier, the mutations could all be mapped at single sites throughout the rII gene. These mutants were found to revert spontaneously (or by acridine treatment) in an interesting way. The revertants did not display truly wild-type behavior but differed in some discernible way (e.g., plaque morphology, growth rate) from the wild type. The behavior was designated "pseudowild."

Figure 10-8 illustrates the procedures that were used to unravel the mechanism of acridine mutagenesis. A proflavin-induced rII mutant was chosen as starting material. It was arbitrarily designated (+) for reasons that will shortly become clear. This

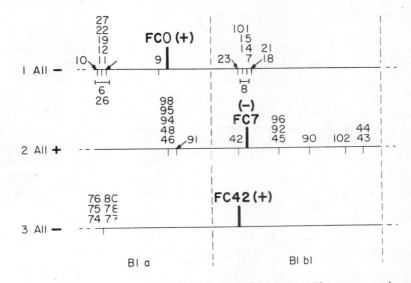

FIGURE 10-8. Reading-frame mutations in T4 phage. *This is a rough map, only approximately to scale, of the left end of the B cistron of the rII gene. The original mutant, FCO, was produced with an acridine dye. Line 1 shows the mapping of suppressors of FCO. Line 2 shows suppressors of FC7, one of the suppressors of FCO mapped on line 1. Line 3 shows, in turn, suppressors of FC42, seen on line 2 as a suppressor of FC7. For meanings of (+) and (−) see text. (Extracted from Crick et al., Figure 2.[52] This map is now known to contain minor errors. An accurate map is given in Barnett et al.[53])*

mutant strain (FC0, line 1 of Figure 10-8) was grown on *E. coli* B, and pseudowild revertants were isolated by plating on strain K. It will be recalled that the wild-type phage grows on strain B or strain K, but that rII mutants fail to grow on strain K. Recombination analysis showed that the spontaneous pseudowild revertants were in reality double mutants. The new mutation, in every case but one, fell into a cluster on either side of the original FC0 mutant site. Thus, the second mutation is an intragenic suppressor of the original mutation. The suppressors of FC0 are identified by number and are given the arbitrary designation (−). When, by recombination with wild type, the (−) suppressors were obtained free of the FC0 mutation, they all proved to be typical rII mutants. In other words, two rII mutations were somehow able to suppress each other when both were present in the same genome. One of these suppressors (FC7) was chosen for further study, as shown on line 2 of Figure 10-8. Again spontaneous pseudowild revertants were selected, as indicated, and again each of these proved to be a typical rII mutant. Since they were capable of suppressing the FC7 (−) mutation, they were designated (+). The process was repeated again; line 3 shows the analysis of FC42 (+) and its suppressors, designated (−).

These results were interpreted by supposing that acridines caused the insertion or deletion of a base. As a consequence, the "reading frame" (i.e., the ordered sequence of triplets) would be shifted, so that all codons distal to the mutation site would be changed. Clearly, no functional gene product could be synthesized under these circumstances. However, a shift of the reading frame in the opposite direction would restore correct reading, except in the region between the two mutation sites. This is illustrated schematically in Figure 10-9. Each normal codon is represented by a

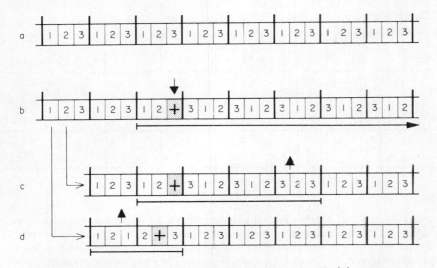

FIGURE 10-9. Mechanism of frame shift mutagenesis. *Each box represents a base pair. The base pairs in a codon are numbered 1, 2, and 3 in the reading direction from left to right (i.e., 5′ → 3′ on the messenger-RNA). Original configuration is shown in line a. Addition of a base produces configuration shown on line b, where all codons to right of addition are now missense. On line c, deletion of a base restores proper reading frame to right, leaves a few missense codons between the sites of addition and deletion. On line d, the deletion has been made to left of original addition, with a similar restorative result.*

sequence of bases numbered 1-2-3 (line a). The insertion of an extra base (line b) throws all codons to the right out of register (3-1-2 instead of 1-2-3). Finally (line c), deletion of a base restores the reading frame to the right of the deletion, leaving only the region between the two sites out of register. Presumably, if the original mutation and its suppressor are not too far apart, and if they occur in a region of the gene corresponding to a portion of the protein product that will tolerate some amino acid replacements, a partially functional protein can result, and pseudowild behavior is seen. Line d of Figure 10-9 shows a similar result when the deletion is to the left of the insertion.

By recombination and appropriate selection procedures, it was possible to construct artificial genomes containing any desired combination of (+) or (−) mutations. When two (+) or (−) mutations were combined in the same genome, the result was a typical rII mutant; the gene was nonfunctional. But remarkably, when three (+) or (−) mutations were combined, pseudowild behavior resulted. This constituted strong evidence that the genetic code was indeed a triplet code; for if each codon contained three bases, addition or deletion of that number should restore the reading frame and produce a wild-type protein containing one extra (or one missing) amino acid.

Direct confirmation of the insertion-deletion theory of acridine (and spontaneous) mutagenesis could not be obtained in the rII phage mutants because the gene product was unknown. It was predicted, however, that if pseudowild double mutants of the (+) and (−) types could be studied in a system in which the protein product of the

Wild

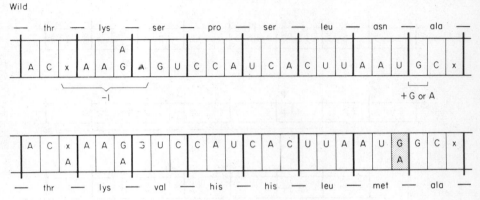

Pseudowild

FIGURE 10-10. Frame shift mutation in phage T4 lysozyme. *Portions of the amino acid sequences for the wild-type protein and for the lysozyme isolated from a pseudowild strain are presented. The pseudowild strain carries two frame shift mutations of opposite sign, i.e., an addition and a deletion. The codons corresponding to each amino acid are shown, as given in Table 8-3. The symbol x represents any one of the four bases. The polypeptide sequence is written with NH_2-terminus to left, polynucleotide sequence with 5'-terminus to left. (From Streisinger et al., Table 1.[33])*

gene was available, "a string of amino-acids would be altered, covering the region of the polypeptide chain corresponding to the region on the gene between the two mutants."[52] This proof was accomplished with the enzyme lysozyme of phage T4, by amino acid sequence determinations.[33,54] The frame shift predicted by the theory really occurs. An illustration is presented in Figure 10-10. The lysozyme from a pseudowild (+ and −) double mutant was found to differ from the wild-type enzyme with respect to five contiguous amino acids. The codons for all the amino acids in this region are shown. It is clear that the deletion of one base from the –thr–lys–ser– codons at the left and the insertion of a guanine or adenine residue in the –asn–ala– codons at the right would precisely account for the observed amino acid replacements. Because the polarity of each codon is known and it is also known that proteins are assembled from NH_2-terminus to COOH-terminus, this experiment shows conclusively that the genetic message is translated in the direction $5' \rightarrow 3'$ on the mRNA. The reason is that if the mRNA were translated in the direction $3' \rightarrow 5'$, every codon shown in Figure 10-10 would have to be reversed, left to right. If this were so, no set of codons corresponding to the wild-type sequence of amino acids could be converted to the pseudowild sequence by any simple transformation.

Acridine dyes cause the addition or deletion of bases at replication by becoming intercalated between the adjacent base pairs of the DNA.[55] These dyes (and similar compounds) are planar molecules of dimensions similar to those of normal base pairs (Figure 10-11). Physical measurements of several kinds have given convincing evidence that they do indeed interact with DNA in a manner consistent with intercalation. They cause a local spreading of the distance between adjacent base pairs and a localized unwinding of the helix to accommodate this distortion. An elegant proof employed supercoiled circular DNA.[56] Here the local unwinding at the point of intercalation forces a change in the degree of supercoiling, which is readily detectable as an alteration of buoyant density of the DNA. The use of this technique to demonstrate the intercalation of actinomycin D was described in Chapter 1.

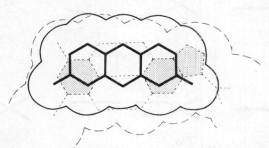

FIGURE 10-11. Relative sizes of an acridine (proflavin) and a base pair. *The purine-pyrimidine base pair is shown shaded, its three hydrogen bonds are represented by dotted lines. The acridine is superimposed in bold outline. (From Lerman, Figure 2.[55])*

If spreading apart adjacent base pairs by acridine intercalation permits the insertion of an extra base during replication, how does the same process account for base pair deletions? The similarity of acridine-induced and spontaneous mutations offers a clue. Reciprocal additions and deletions of bases may occur as a result of unequal crossover between homologous chromosomes of diploid organisms at meiosis, or during recombination due to DNA breakage and reunion in bacteria and phage.[9,55,57-59] Unequal crossover produces spontaneous mutation of the frameshift type, and acridines evidently increase the frequency of this event, very likely by interfering with the excision and repair processes.[60,61]

Mutations of the spontaneous and acridine type may well arise, as indicated above, through an unequal crossover. Crossover, the exchange of homologous segments between chromatids, occurs normally in meiosis, where it serves to assort genetic characters into new genomes. It also occurs between homologous chromatids at mitosis. Crossing over requires either actual breakage and reunion of chromatids or a reciprocal switching of the replication mechanism from one chromatid to another ("copy choice").[62] These possibilities are diagrammed in Figure 10-12. At the top of the figure are shown two homologous chromosomes in synaptic alignment at meiosis. The result, after centromere division, is the emergence of two new chromosomes, the reciprocal recombinants, in addition to the original pair.

Broken ends of chromatids are known to be "sticky," in the sense that they tend to heal together, a process in which the DNA ligases play an important part. An important consequence of this property is that once breakage is produced or repair of broken ends is inhibited, bizarre alterations of chromosome structure are possible.[63] An illustration of how gene duplications, inversions, and deletions can occur through

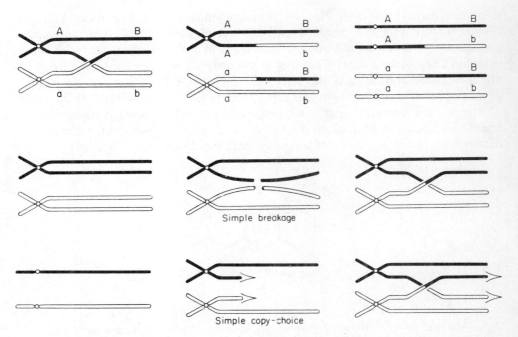

FIGURE 10-12. Crossover at meiosis. *In upper line, two homologous chromosomes are shown aligned, each comprised of two chromatids. Centromere is small circle at left. A and B are genes of one chromosome; a and b are the corresponding alleles on the other. Recombination yields two new genomes. Middle and bottom diagrams show alternative theories to account for crossover and recombination. (From Srb et al., Figures 6-2 and 6-15.[1])*

operation of a cycle of breakage, fusion, and bridge formation is shown in Figure 10-13. At the top of the figure, a chromosome from which a terminal segment has been broken is depicted. Such terminal fragments become lost because they are detached from the portion of the chromosome bearing the centromere, and therefore cannot move properly at mitosis or meiosis. If such a terminal deletion is compatible with continued life of the cell, the mutant will be defective in those characters controlled by the missing genes. After replication of the chromatid, the "sticky" broken ends join to form a dicentric chromatid. At the next anaphase, the centromeres will be pulled in opposite directions, forming an anaphase bridge, which eventually breaks. The new break heals after replication, and the cycle is repeated. A sequence of genes, A, B, and C, is shown to undergo several possible changes in the course of these events. Sometimes broken ends reunite to form ring chromosomes. Sometimes a whole segment may be transposed elsewhere on the same chromosome or even onto a different chromosome. A microphotograph showing anaphase bridges, detached terminal fragments, and extensive chromosome breakage is presented in Figure 10-14. Here an alkylating agent was administered to mice bearing a transplantable carcinoma, and the tumor cells were examined 48 hr later.

The precise morphologic classification of the individual chromosomes of a diploid set (the *karyotype*) makes it easy to recognize the kinds of gross chromosome alterations described above. Agreement between deductions from genetic evidence and observed aberrant morphology has been remarkable. Especially in the giant salivary gland chromosomes of *Drosophila* have structural alterations been discernible that

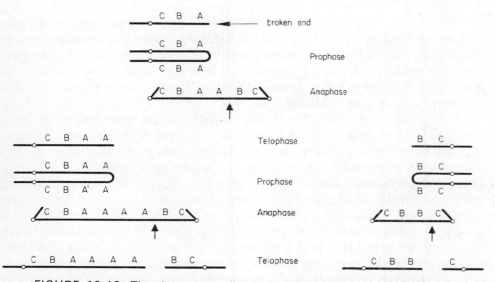

FIGURE 10-13. The chromosome breakage-fusion-bridge cycle. *A chromosome with a broken end is pictured at top. Open circle represents centromere. A, B, C are genes. Fusion of broken ends of the 2 chromatids is shown, yielding a dicentric chromosome. An anaphase bridge results in breakage (shown by arrow), followed by repetition of the cycle. Gene duplications and deletions result, as illustrated. (From McClintock, Figure 1.*[64])

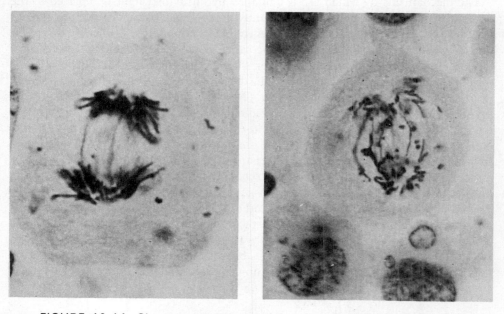

FIGURE 10-14. Chromosome abnormalities induced by mechlorethamine. *Mice bearing Walker carcinoma 256 were given the nitrogen mustard mechlorethamine, a single dose of 1 mg kg*[-1] *intraperitoneally. Microphotograph at left shows a cell at mitosis 48 hr later. Chromosome bridges (chiasmata) and fragments are evident. Photograph at right shows bridges and more severe fragmentation in a cell at mitosis 56 hr after drug treatment. ×2500. (From Koller, Figure 6.*[65] *By courtesy of the author.)*

were predicted from genetic evidence. In all such cases, the modified chromosomes replicate and undergo mitosis normally, provided the mutant phenotype is viable. In this way, even major chromosome abnormalities can become established in the germ line of the species. And since hereditary defects have been associated with such visible abnormalities, it follows that agents capable of breaking chromosomes are also capable of causing genetic damage.

Alkylating agents are very effective chromosome breakers, mimicking the action of x-irradiation. Chromosome breakage by x rays requires oxygen, however, whereas that caused by alkylating agents does not. Another difference is that delayed effects are much more commonly encountered with alkylating agents than with x rays. Crosslinking is evidently not the only mechanism underlying chromosome breakage, since monofunctional alkylating agents are effective, as are many of the chemical mutagens that induce base-pair transformations. Bromouracil, for example, is a good chromosome breaker in mammalian cells in vitro.[66,67] Hydroxylamine causes chromatid breaks and also inhibits the repair of breaks caused by x rays.[68] It seems likely, therefore, that chromosome breakage is related in some fundamental way to other mechanisms of mutagenesis.[69,70] Since breakage and reunion of the genetic material occur normally as part of the cell cycle, inhibition of repair mechanisms may play a central role in the action of chromosome breakers. Since it is now generally accepted that DNA forms the continuous skeletal backbone of a chromatid, the close relationship between chromosome breakage and induced aberrations in DNA replication (excision, incomplete repair) can be rationalized.

The mechanisms by which DNA damaged by ultraviolet light is repaired in the dark provide a basis for understanding how interference with repair could lead to chromosome breakage.[70a] The primary effect of ultraviolet light is to cause dimerization of adjacent thymine residues on the same strand of DNA. Such DNA cannot replicate normally because the daughter strand contains gaps, instead of adenine residues, opposite the thymine dimers. The dark repair process is complex, consisting of five steps: (1) recognition of damage; (2) chain incision above and below each thymine dimer; (3) excision of the damaged region; (4) repair replication, substituting a duplicate oligonucleotide segment for the excised segment, but with thymine monomers; (5) end-to-end ligation to restore the linear continuity of the DNA strand. In addition to this "cut-and-patch" mechanism, damaged DNA can be repaired by a recombination process, sister-strand exchange.[70b] Here interrupted replication of both strands of the duplex occurs, with gaps, as before, opposite thymine dimers. Then undamaged segments of original and replicate strands are ligated to form one new functional duplex. The reciprocal recombinant, of course, is nonfunctional. The two processes are illustrated in Figure 10-15.

Caffeine derivatives and related purines break chromosomes, despite the fact that they are not incorporated, but they are known to inhibit dark repair of DNA.[63,71,72]

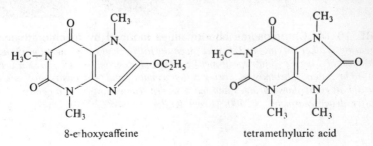

8-ethoxycaffeine   tetramethyluric acid

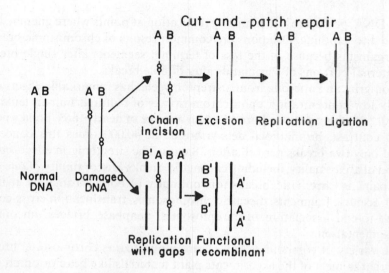

FIGURE 10-15. Two mechanisms of repair of DNA damaged by ultraviolet light. *For illustration, one thymine dimer is shown on each strand of a duplex but at different positions. Thick lines represent newly synthesized portion of the DNA.*

One of the best chromosome breakers is 8-ethoxycaffeine, which causes a variety of chromosome aberrations in bean root-tip cells during a stage in the mitotic cycle when DNA is not being synthesized.[73] Shortly after treatment, the chromosomes begin to appear "sticky"; after this stage, there is the usual progression to abnormal mitoses and fragmentation. The closely related tetramethyluric acid behaves differently in that it only affects cells that are in mitosis during treatment. Thus, after the initial "stickiness" and consequent breakage in some of the cells, no further aberrations are seen for about 24 hr. Then a new wave of chromosome abnormalities appears as the cells damaged originally come once more into mitosis. It has been suggested that tetramethyluric acid, which is less lipid soluble than 8-ethoxycaffeine, cannot penetrate the nuclear membrane and thus acts only at mitosis, when that membrane has disintegrated.[72] With both these agents, as with most chromosome breakers, the frequencies of aberrations per cell and of cells containing aberrations are dose related.

Deletions occur in all sizes, both spontaneously and consequent to treatment with a mutagen. In bacteriophage T4, deletions were recognized by the fact that they could not be caused to revert to the wild type and that they would not yield wild-type recombinants when crossed with certain point mutants.[18] The extent and position of each deletion was found by crossing it with point mutants whose positions had been mapped; every point mutant with which no wild-type recombinants were obtained must lie within the region of the deletion. The results of such studies led to a simple conclusion. Deletions can occur spontaneously anywhere along the rII gene. Their lengths range from a few base pairs to most of the gene. They can cross the boundary between two adjacent cistrons;[74] when this happens, the region of separation between the two protein products is deleted, and a continuous protein is synthesized, with a certain number of amino acids missing where one protein should end and the next should begin. Nitrous acid, it has already been pointed out, causes major deletions in phage DNA, perhaps by interrupting replication at points where guanine has been deaminated to xanthine. Deletions are common results of chromosome breakage in higher organisms because of the loss of terminal segments after single breaks and loss of internal portions of chromatids after double breaks.

Streptonigrin, an antibiotic from a streptomycete, has remarkable effects at extraordinarily low concentration upon chromosomes of cultured human leukocytes.[75] At 2×10^{-9} M, this compound produced an average of nearly three breaks per cell in 12 hr; in contrast, bromouracil deoxyriboside at 40,000 times this concentration produced only two breaks per cell after 28 days. The streptonigrin effects comprised every kind of abnormality, including chromatid breaks (discontinuity of one chromatid in a pair), isochromatid breaks (discontinuity of both chromatids at the same position), acentric fragments, dicentric chromosomes, translocation cross-configurations, end-to-end association of chromosomes, anaphase bridges, uncoiling, and severe fragmentation.

A wide variety of compounds have been implicated as chromosome breakers.[69] It is true that in most of the experiments plant materials like bean or onion root tips were used; but whenever human cells have been exposed in vitro to the same mutagens, similar effects were seen. In most investigations, fairly high concentrations of the agents were used in order to produce a large enough number of chromosome abnormalities for ready visualization. It is difficult to say what hazard may be presented by exposure of human cells in vivo to these same agents (some of which are drugs in common use) at ordinary doses. This problem is discussed in a wider context in a later section of this chapter.

METAPHASE POISONING (SPINDLE INACTIVATION)

The function of mitosis is to ensure the equipartition of the entire chromosome complement into two daughter cells at division. The function of meiosis is to partition the two representations of each chromosome into two germ cells. The processes that ensure the orderly preparation and execution of the anaphase movement—of sister chromosomes in mitosis, of homologous chromosomes in meiosis—are extremely complex.[76,77] The essentials are: (1) proper duplication and polar positioning of the centrioles, to which the spindle apparatus will be attached; (2) correct alignment of the chromosome pairs on the equatorial plate at metaphase, each attached by its centromere to a spindle fiber; and (3) proper synthesis and functioning of the spindle fibers, mediating the poleward migration of the chromosomes at anaphase. Metaphase poisons disrupt this sequence of events and thereby produce arrested or grossly abnormal meiosis or mitosis.[78-82]

An essential part of the mitotic apparatus are the microtubules of the spindle.[83] The subunits of the microtubules are composed of a protein, tubulin, which is capable of reversible polymerization and depolymerization (gel-sol transformation). Tubulin has a molecular weight of about 120,000. It consists of two major, different subunits (α, β), each of molecular weight 52,000, and possibly a third, subunit. Assembly of microtubules from tubulin can be demonstrated in vitro; the reaction requires Mg^{2+} and is blocked by Ca^{2+}, bound GTP plays a role, and dephosphorylation of the protein may be an essential step.

The classic example of a specific spindle poison is colchicine.[80]

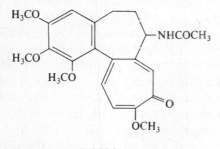

Colchicine

This curious molecule, with two seven-membered rings, is derived from the plant *Colchicum autumnale*, the meadow saffron. At very low concentrations (about 10^{-8} *M*), it disrupts spindle function by inhibiting the formation of fibrils; yet the specific protein of the mitotic apparatus can still be demonstrated. Each molecule of tubulin contains one colchicine binding site, with a binding constant of $2 \times 10^6 \; M^{-1}$. Colchicine does not disrupt intact microtubules, but rather prevents the polymerization reaction; since the microtubules are in a dynamic state, the net result is spindle dissolution. The effects of colchicine are highly specific; at concentrations sufficient to block mitosis, it does not inhibit DNA, RNA, or protein synthesis.[84] The cytologic picture of colchicine poisoning is so characteristic that it is called "colchicine mitosis" ("c-mitosis"). At low concentrations, unusual mitotic patterns develop, sometimes resulting in an incorrect distribution of chromosomes to the daughter cells. At higher concentrations, the drug produces complete metaphase arrest; this accounts for its usefulness as a tool for obtaining a great many cells in mitosis. Polyploidy is frequently the outcome of colchicine treatment because chromosomes in mitosis split but are unable to separate and thus, doubled in number, enter a new cycle of replication.

Another plant product with similar action is podophyllotoxin, a polycyclic lactone related to the coumarins, which are also metaphase poisons. Several medicinal plant

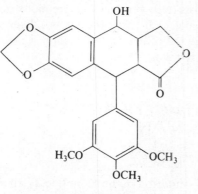

Podophyllotoxin

alkaloids, some carcinogens (e.g., methylcholanthrene), androgenic and estrogenic hormones, chloral hydrate, and ether are among the commonly used drugs that can act as spindle poisons. The efficacy of some anticancer agents (e.g., vinblastine) and some antifungal agents (e.g., griseofulvin) depends on their mitotic poisoning effect. Although the various spindle poisons produce similar abnormalities in the cytologic picture, their biochemical mechanisms of action are very different. Podophyllotoxin binds at the colchicine site on tubulin and presumably acts in the same way. The vinca alkaloids (vinblastine and vincristine), on the other hand, bind to tubulin at a different site. Two moles of GTP are also bound, at a site different from either the colchicine or vinblastine site. Griseofulvin does not compete with colchicine or vinblastine, and thus interacts at yet another site. The complexities of organization of tubulin into microtubules, of microtubules into a spindle apparatus, and of the energy-requiring mechanism whereby the spindle moves (or guides) the chromosomes to opposite poles indicate many distinct possibilities for specific interference by the various antimitotic drugs.

The complete arrest of mitosis is, of course, incompatible with survival. But partial metaphase inhibition can lead to a great variety of bizarre mitotic figures and unusual chromosome distributions in daughter cells. The only such effects that concern us here are those that do allow cell survival. One of the most serious, from the standpoint of genetic disease, is the unequal partition of chromosomes to daughter cells, an event known as *nondisjunction*. This occurs when both chromosomes of a pair move into the same cell because of faulty attachment of a spindle fiber to a centromere or some other defect in spindle function. Whether this occurs during mitosis in the gonadal germ cell line or during the meiotic divisions preceding the formation of spermatozoa and ova, abnormal gametes are produced. The gamete lacking a whole chromosome will usually not be capable of producing a viable zygote. But the gamete containing an extra chromosome can produce offspring. Down's syndrome ("mongolism"), characterized by mental deficiency as well as other abnormalities, is associated regularly with the presence of an additional copy of chromosome 21 ("21-trisomy").[85] People with this defect can be shown to have 47 chromosomes in all their body cells instead of the normal 46. Likewise, sexual abnormalities of several kinds have been traced to an unusual number of X or Y chromosomes.[86] The cause of "spontaneous" nondisjunction is unknown. The incidence of 21-trisomy increases significantly with increasing maternal age, but why older oocytes should be more prone to abnormal meiosis than younger ones remains obscure. The ability of exogenous compounds like colchicine to produce nondisjunction in some cells raises the possibility that drugs or other environmental agents may be contributing to the incidence of trisomy in man.

CHEMICAL MUTAGENESIS IN ANIMALS AND MAN

The Human Germ Line

Inherited defects arise by mutation in the germ line. Each person may be regarded as a differentiated clone of cells derived from the fusion of a paternal and maternal gamete to form a zygote. Mutations can be introduced into the human germ line only during the reproductive life of the individual, a period of about 30 years on the average. Therefore, the hazards of mutagenesis, chemical or otherwise, concern only the young population. These hazards are peculiar because genetic damage does not affect the exposed individual, but may remain concealed for generations until homozygosity makes it manifest.

Primordial germ cells are first distinguishable at about the sixth week of gestation. Development proceeds differently in the two sexes. In the female, all the primary oocytes (about 400,000) are produced from undifferentiated oogonia during fetal life. No further cell divisions occur until puberty, when the monthly maturation of single ova begins. The maturation process entails two meiotic divisions, followed by the degeneration of three of the four meiotic products as polar bodies.

In the male, a population of primary spermatogonia persists in the germinal layer of the seminiferous tubules of the testis. These *stem cells* undergo mitosis about once every 12 days, giving rise to nonequivalent daughter cells. One daughter cell retains the characteristics of a primary spermatogonium, the other migrates toward the lumen of the tubule and becomes a primary spermatocyte, the progenitor of four mature spermatozoa. In this way, stem cell renewal and sperm production continue throughout childhood and reproductive life; but before puberty, the sperms degenerate.[87]

The continuity of the male germ line through one human generation is shown schematically in Figure 10-16. Period 1 contains all the mitotic cycles (about 50 on the

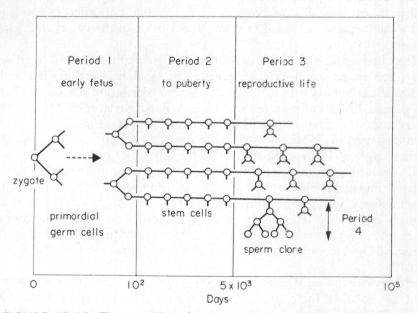

FIGURE 10-16. The germ line of man. *A schematic diagram showing the 4 periods of possible sensitivity to mutagens in the human male. (In the female, periods 2 and 3 are effectively absent, and period 4 represents the 2 meiotic divisions at the time of fertilization of the ovum.) (From Goldstein, Figure 25.[88])*

average) between the zygote and the population of primordial germ cells; its duration is about 6 weeks. We are not speaking here of the total number of cell divisions, which would be one less than the total cell population at the end of the period under consideration. We are concerned with the number of times the chromosomes of any given cell in the final population have replicated. In the female, another 17 mitotic cycles serve to produce all the primary oocytes in both ovaries. Period 2 lasts until puberty, about 12 to 14 years; period 3 encompasses the remainder of reproductive life. If the average generation time is taken to be 30 years, then these periods of stem cell renewal (average cycle 12 days) contain about 900 mitotic cycles in the male. (Periods 2 and 3 are absent in the female.) Finally, period 4 comprises the two meiotic divisions by which the male and female gametes are formed. Thus, on the average, a zygote is formed by the union of a sperm whose chromosomes have replicated approximately 950 times since the previous generation, and an ovum whose chromosomes have replicated only about 70 times in the same period.

It will be evident from this account that the occurrence of new mutations might follow a different course in the two sexes. *In the female*, mutagens that act only on replicating DNA or on the mitotic process should have effects primarily during fetal life. Mutagens that act on nonreplicating DNA might act throughout the lifetime. Agents that disturb meiosis would act only at the time of conception, when the meiotic divisions occur. This is probably the time when most spontaneous mutations occur. *In the male*, on the other hand, the risk of mutation by agents that act on replicating DNA or on the mitotic process should span the whole reproductive life cycle. The male stem cell line passes through so many more mitotic cycles than does the female that such mutagens should cause the accumulation of many more mutations in sperm than in ova, other factors being equal. Agents that only affect meiosis should act, in the male, during a period of a few weeks prior to the coitus that leads to conception.

It follows that mutations arising in relation to DNA replication and cell division, whatever their cause, should produce genetic defects whose incidence is correlated with paternal age but not with maternal age. Such a correlation is actually observed for two genetic diseases of man, hemophilia and chondrodystrophy. Mongolism, on the other hand, is correlated exclusively with maternal age, the implication of which has been discussed. As it remains somewhat uncertain which mutagenic agents act upon what stages of DNA replication or of the mitotic or meiotic cycle, only one practical conclusion can be derived, apart from the general injunction to minimize exposure to mutagens. Since by far the greatest number of mitotic cycles in the female germ line occurs during the first two months of fetal life, it seems wise to avoid unnecessary exposure of pregnant women to any drugs or potentially mutagenic environmental agents from a time just prior to conception through the first trimester of pregnancy. This recommendation relates also to potentially teratogenic agents (cf. Chapter 12).

Large differences in mutagenicity, depending upon the time of treatment with a mutagen, as shown in Table 10-2, are fairly typical. The data reflect differences in sensitivity of the various stages of spermatogenesis. Since spermatogenia in the stem cell line, premeiotic (primary) spermatocytes, postmeiotic (secondary) spermatocytes, spermatids, and spermatozoa are all present simultaneously, they are all necessarily exposed to the mutagen. But if the treatment is brief and matings are conducted on successive days, one can distinguish which stages of germ cell maturation are most sensitive. If the litters conceived shortly after treatment are affected, then the agent must have caused mutations in the mature spermatozoa. The data show, on the contrary, that the most sensitive forms were those that required 10 to 13 days to mature after treatment; in mice, these would be the postmeiotic spermatids. In *Drosophila*, too, the spermatids are the germ cells most sensitive to alkylating agents and radiation. The quantitative differences between the stages, in oogenesis as well as in spermatogenesis, may be very great.[90,91]

TABLE 10-2. Partial sterility and translocations induced in mice by an alkylating agent.

Triethylenemelamine (0.2 mg kg^{-1}) was administered in a single intraperitoneal injection to male mice. These were mated daily to untreated females 1, 2, and 3 days after injection, and again after 10, 11, 12, and 13 days. F_1 males were tested for partial sterility and examined cytologically for translocations. (Data of Cattanach,[89] Tables 1 and 2. By permission of Springer.)

Litter size in matings with treated males	
Days after drug	Average litter size
1	6.3
2	5.3
3	7.3
10	1.7
11	2.0
12	1.6
13	3.6
Control	8.5

Sterility and translocations in F_1 males			
Days after drug on which F_1 males were conceived	Number tested	% sterile or semisterile	% showing translocations
1–3	111	4.5	7.2
10–13	74	14.9	28.4

Some Common Methods of Testing Mutagenicity in Animals

Since direct experiments with chemical mutagens are obviously out of the question in humans, our assessment of the mutagenic hazards associated with exposure to drugs and other agents necessarily rests upon genetic investigations in other animals. One naturally supposes that the sensitivity of the genetic apparatus to mutagens will be almost the same in closely related species. Although much of modern genetics rests upon experiments with *Drosophila*,[92] mice have been used increasingly as a practical mammalian model.[93] Because large-scale breeding is often required, especially to detect low mutation rates, larger mammals are excluded on practical grounds. Induced dominant mutations are readily observed, but detection of induced recessive mutations requires the use of specially bred stocks.[94] Since recessive mutations are expressed in the homozygous state, a good test of mutagenesis is to mate an animal treated with a mutagen to an animal that is already heterozygous for certain traits. If the treatment induces a mutation at a corresponding locus, then some of the offspring will be homozygous for the mutant trait. In devising such tests, advantage is often taken of the fact that the male is hemizygous for the X chromosome; thus, for example, one-half the male offspring of a treated female with an induced X-chromosome mutation will display the mutant trait.

A good example of the adroit use of sex linkage in a test for mutagenesis is the classical *ClB method* in *Drosophila*.[95] The procedure requires a stock of females heterozygous for two mutant traits carried on the same X chromosome—bar eye (a visible characteristic) and a recessive lethal trait. Males are treated with a mutagen and then mated to the special females. Female F_1 offspring with bar eye are selected for the next round of breeding. These animals will have the maternal X chromosome carrying the bar eye allele and also the recessive lethal gene carried with it. Their other X chromosome is inherited from the treated males. The question is whether any recessive lethal mutations were induced in that X chromosome during the mutagen treatment. We are concerned here with mutations that are not allelic with the recessive lethal already carried by the female. In the occasional instance of induced mutation at the same gene locus, no F_1 offspring would be obtained, since the zygote would be homozygous for the lethal trait. The answer is obtained very simply by breeding these females with ordinary males and examining the sex of F_2 offspring. If a recessive lethal mutation is present in the X chromosome derived from the treated males, there will be no viable male F_2 offspring whatsoever because both maternal X chromosomes would then carry recessive (but nonallelic) lethal mutations and all F_2 males would express one or the other lethal trait. Conversely, if any males are found, then no recessive lethals had been induced.

Dominant lethal mutations are detected by exposing males to a mutagenic treatment, mating them to normal females, and then simply observing the number of viable offspring. This test is frequently employed in mice. To ensure detection of nonviable embryos, the pregnant females are sacrificed just before term in order to count the number of live embryos, the number of dead embryos, and the number of corpora lutea (whence the number of preimplantation deaths can be estimated, since each corpus luteum represents one ovum).[96–98] Dominant lethals are often due to major chromosome abnormalities that are incompatible with development of the zygote.

Chromosome translocations have been observed microscopically in mice after the following selection procedure.[89] The F_1 male offspring of males originally treated with a mutagen were mated with normal females and their litter size was used as a preliminary screening criterion. Whenever the average litter size derived from a given F_1 male was smaller than normal, a direct cytologic examination of that animal's testis was carried out. If 19 instead of the normal 20 chromosomes were seen consistently in metaphase configurations, a translocation was assumed to be present. Table 10-2 presented data of a typical experiment with an alkylating agent, in which dominant lethals as well as translocations were induced. The size of litters derived from treated males was greatly reduced 10 to 13 days after treatment. The translocation test showed that the male offspring of these same treated males carried translocations and were partially sterile, and again the peak effect was seen in offspring of males mated 10 to 13 days after drug treatment.

Another method, which has yielded important information about radiation mutagenesis in mice, is the *specific locus method*.[99] It depends upon the expression of mutations when they are homozygous; the traits considered here are readily observable, visible abnormalities such as unusual coat color or peculiar shape of the ear. A special stock of mice was bred, heterozygous for seven such traits carried on seven different autosomal genes. Males or females are exposed to the mutagenic treatment and then mated to mice of the opposite sex belonging to the special stock. Then the F_1 offspring are examined. When a mutation has been induced in one of the seven loci in a treated mouse, its offspring will be homozygous for that particular visible trait.

The method can be illustrated by an experiment on radiation mutagenesis. Males were given 600 roentgens of whole-body x-irradiation. They were then allowed to recover from the postirradiation sterility, so that the spermatozoa available for the matings developed from irradiated spermatogonia. These treated males were mated with females of the special stock, and unirradiated control males were also mated. In the control group in which 37,868 offspring were examined, two mutant animals were found. In the irradiated group in which 48,007 offspring were examined, 53 mutants were found. The mean mutation rate induced by x-irradiation was therefore computed to be $2.5 \pm 0.4 \times 10^{-7}$ per roentgen per locus. The disadvantage of this method is evident from the data; enormous numbers of animals have to be bred and examined. And although a good quantitative estimation can be made when mutagenesis is strong, the accuracy of estimate for a weak mutagen (e.g., one that only doubled the spontaneous mutation rate) would be very poor because of the extremely small number of mutations observed. Another problem is that the seven chosen genes differ considerably among themselves in their sensitivities to mutagenic treatments, so that "mean mutation rate" may have no relevance to actual rates at the most sensitive gene loci in man.

Cytogenetic methods may give direct evidence of mutagenic effects. This is exemplified by in vivo studies that revealed the mutagenic action of cyclohexylamine, a major metabolite of cyclamate, the artificial sweetener.[100] Male rats were given intraperitoneal injections of cyclohexylamine at different daily doses for 5 days. A metaphase blocker, colcemid, was then given, and 5 hr later smears of bone marrow and spermatogonial cells from the seminiferous tubules were prepared. The per cent of cells containing one or more chromosome breaks was computed. Control values were 2–3%. In treated animals, there was a dose-related increase in both cell types, to as high as 20%. Single chromatid breaks predominated; these are considered most serious from the standpoint of mutagenic hazard, since multiple breaks will usually lead to cell death, as discussed earlier.

Cell culture has also proved useful in evaluating mutagens. Established mammalian cell lines are cultured in the presence of a suspected mutagen at various concentrations. For cytogenetic studies, a metaphase blocker is added, and chromosomes are examined for abnormalities. This method, using a kangaroo rat cell line, demonstrated the dose-related production of chromatid breaks and exchange figures by DDT and its metabolites (DDD and DDE).[101] Mutagenesis in cell culture has also been demonstrated through the use of cell lines containing specific markers.[101a] These may be morphologic, biochemical (e.g., enzyme deficiency, and selection for induced revertants), or serologic (variants of cell surface antigens).

The most practical screening for mutagenicity can obviously be obtained with simple in vitro systems using microorganisms. A serious shortcoming, however, is the absence of host metabolic processes that normally operate upon a potential mutagen. A chemical may have no mutagenic action whatsoever, yielding negative results in tests carried out in vitro, yet be converted in the mammalian organism to a potent mutagen. Conversely, a compound that is strongly mutagenic in vitro may be metabolized to inert derivatives in vivo and thus present no mutagenic hazard. These considerations led to the development of a *host-mediated assay* for mutagenicity.[102,103,104] A test organism is chosen for convenience, e.g., a histidine auxotroph of an enteric bacterium. The mutagenic effect to be measured is an increase in the frequency of reversion to histidine independence. Alternatively, *Neurospora conidia* have been used, since a forward mutation in the pathway of adenine biosynthesis in this organism leads to production of a purple pigment that makes mutant colonies readily visible. The organism is grown intraperitoneally in a mouse or other mammalian host, to which the suspected mutagen is also administered. A great many compounds that are not mutagenic in vitro also lack mutagenic action in the host-mediated assay, and certain mutagens (e.g., streptozotocin, N-methyl-N'-nitro-N-nitrosoguanidine, methylazoxymethanol) are active both in vitro and in vivo. Dimethylnitrosamine is a compound that is known to be oxidatively dealkylated to diazomethane, which is a potent mutagen: the parent amine was inactive in vitro but highly mutagenic in the host-mediated assay. A similar situation was found with cycasin, a glycoside, which was inactive in vitro and active in the host-mediated assay; its aglycone, methylazoxymethanol, is known to be a potent mutagen.

Evaluation of the Hazards of Chemical Mutagens in Man

The difficulties of arriving at quantitative estimates of mutagenicity for chemical agents in human populations are very great. Indeed, it has yet to be shown that any chemical agent has produced genetic defects in man. Even in the case of radiation mutagenesis, which is generally accepted as a fact, most of the evidence comes from animal experimentation. The human exposed to radiation or to a chemical mutagen is not expected to be affected himself except at doses large enough to cause sterility. Even the offspring of the exposed person may seem unaffected if the induced mutation is recessive or incompletely expressed. Thus, many induced mutations will only be manifested in future generations through the eventual union of gametes both of which are heterozygous for the same recessive alleles. It follows that much of the data bearing directly upon the human species will have to be epidemiologic rather than experimental. It also follows that a conservative position with respect to mutagenic hazards in humans will be based frequently on common-sense judgments rather than on iron-clad proofs. By assuming a conservative position we mean that we wish to err, when in doubt, in the direction of overestimating the potential mutagenic hazard.[88,105,106]

A growing number of genetic diseases are being identified in man. Most estimates show[2] that every sperm or ovum carries several mutant genes accumulated over the past history of the race, and that as many as one person in three carries a new mutation not present in either of his parents. These accumulated and newly altered mutant genes are attributed to past and present "spontaneous" mutation. It is quite clear from what is known about radiation mutagenesis that lifelong exposure to background radiation could not account for more than a small fraction of the total spontaneous mutation rate. Occasionally, a "mutator gene" renders an organism and its progeny subject to very high spontaneous mutation rates, probably by production of an endogenous mutagen.[32,107–109a] In addition, the human race is exposed to many chemicals that are known to be mutagenic to lower forms of life. Since no estimates of the "spontaneous" mutation rate in man have been made in the absence of such exposure, the possibility must be entertained that some part of the apparent spontaneous rate may be due to exogenous chemical mutagens.

In organisms in which chemical mutagenesis has been demonstrated, the concentrations usually employed have been very high compared with those to which humans might be exposed. If extrapolation from such data to man is to have any validity, a knowledge of the dose-response relationship is essential. This has been worked out for very few mutagens. Especially important is the question whether the probability of mutation is a simple product of dose (concentration) by duration of exposure. Is prolonged exposure of humans to very low doses equivalent in mutagenic efficiency to short exposures at high doses in laboratory experiments? For radiation mutagenesis, it is now known that chronic low-dosage exposure is several times less efficient than acute high-dosage exposure.

In the present state of our ignorance, it would serve no purpose to list all drugs employed therapeutically and all environmental agents that might possibly be mutagenic to man. Such compilations are available,[111] but they may serve to distract attention from the few agents that deserve serious attention, either because of demonstrated strong mutagenicity in other species or because of widespread human exposure coupled with evidence of weak mutagenicity in other species. Foremost among these are the alkylating agents and the analogs of nucleic acid bases, both used commonly in cancer chemotherapy. The inorganic nitrite ion, used as a food preservative, is certainly mutagenic (as nitrous acid) at the acid pH of the stomach, and perhaps at tissue pH.[110] Organic nitrites are used medicinally, but their mutagenicity in vivo is unknown. Ethyl alcohol and nicotine are clearly mutagenic in various organisms, and a large part of the human race is exposed to them over long periods of time. Certain fungicides have been discovered to be mutagenic after being in widespread use.[113]

We shall take caffeine as prototype of a drug to which there is widespread exposure and which is certainly mutagenic in lower organisms.[46,47,63,112] People who drink coffee several times daily establish and maintain a mean concentration equivalent to about 1 μg ml^{-1} throughout their body water.[88] This estimate is based on the total area under the time-concentration curve for subjects drinking three to four cups of coffee daily; the actual level fluctuates with each cup of coffee that is drunk. Caffeine permeates all cells and also crosses freely from the mother's blood into the fetus. Hence, there is no doubt that the human germ line is exposed to this drug. Attempts to estimate what mutagenic effect, if any, will be produced by such exposure are beset by uncertainties. The evidence is summarized below.

Caffeine mutagenicity in *E. coli* is illustrated in Figure 10-17. Here the cells were grown at a constant exponential rate in a chemostat. The steady-state population was maintained by continuous inflow of fresh medium containing a limiting concentration of tryptophan (required by this strain) and continuous outflow of the same volume of the culture. A small sample was removed periodically and plated on phage T5. Resistant mutants give rise to colonies, which can be counted. In this system, the T5-resistant mutants grow at the same rate as the wild type. Therefore, if no new mutants arose, the proportion of mutants would remain constant. The observed linear increase in the proportion of mutants reflects a constant rate of appearance of new mutants; it is a direct measure of the mutation rate. It can be seen that when caffeine was added to the medium there was a short lag, and then the mutation rate increased 9-fold. The concentration of caffeine was 150 μg ml^{-1}, about 150 times the average concentration to which the germ cells of habitual coffee drinkers are exposed on a long-term basis.

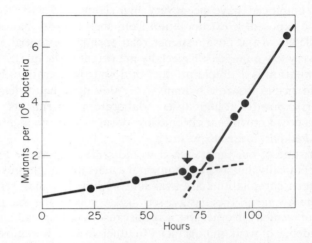

FIGURE 10-17. Mutagenic effects of caffeine on Escherichia coli. *The cells (strain B/1,t) were grown in a chemostat with limiting concentration of tryptophan in the input medium. Generation time = 5.5 hr. Samples were taken periodically and plated on phage T5. Ordinates are numbers of T5-resistant mutants per 10^6 cells. Caffeine (150 μg ml^{-1}) was added at arrow. (Modified from Novick, Figure 4.[114])*

If mutagenicity were a linear function of caffeine concentration without any threshold, and if all human genes were just as sensitive to caffeine as the gene controlling resistance to phage T5 in *E. coli*, then the following calculations might be in order: The concentration of caffeine that was employed produced an increment of the spontaneous mutation rate 8 times the spontaneous rate itself. Therefore, the concentration required to double the spontaneous rate of mutation of the T5 gene would be 150/8, or 19 μg ml^{-1}. The amount of radiation necessary to produce a doubling of the spontaneous mutation rate in man is estimated to be about 200 roentgens, if administered over a long period of time. Then chronic exposure of habitual coffee drinkers to 1 μg ml^{-1} of caffeine should be equivalent to approximately 200/19, or 10 roentgens of radiation.

There is no simple way to extrapolate from data on a single gene of *E. coli* the mutagenicity in the human. Uncertainties arise because of mutagen specificity even among genes of the same species; even in the same strain of *E. coli*, for example, caffeine was much less mutagenic on the gene controlling resistance to phage T6. Another problem is whether mutagenic action proceeds at a constant rate in time or at a constant rate per cell division cycle. Caffeine appears to act at a different time in the cell cycle in plants but in mammals, the data indicate it acts primarily at the time of DNA replication.[102] This was shown by labeling chromosomes with ^{3}H-thymidine and noting what fraction of abnormal chromosomes was labeled.[63] In onion root tips, all aberrations appeared in unlabeled chromosomes, and these were of the exchange type; in hamster cell cultures, only labeled chromosomes showed defects, and these were of the fragmentation type. The requisite concentration of caffeine was the same for both cell types, about 6 mg ml^{-1} or 6000 times that established in coffee drinkers.

Surveying caffeine mutagenicity in a number of different species is one way to test the generality of the bacteriophage data. Certainly, if the mutagenic action turns out to be very weak in all species and on all genes tested, one gains confidence about the safety of such a drug in man. In *Drosophila*, studies were carried out by feeding larvae on caffeine-containing medium (2.5 mg ml^{-1}) and also by injecting males with single doses (about 400 μg g^{-1}).[116] The method of sex-linked lethals (p. 654) was used. The spontaneous mutation rate in these experiments, despite the very high caffeine dosage, was increased only 5-fold, an effect equivalent to that obtained in *Drosophila* males with 150 roentgens of acute radiation. Even this weak effect could not be confirmed in another laboratory.[46]

The specific locus method was used to assess caffeine mutagenicity in mice.[117] Ordinary mice were given caffeine (1 mg ml^{-1}) in their drinking water and then mated: their offspring were also given caffeine until ready to be mated. Thus, the treated mice had been exposed constantly from conception to mating. About 32,000 offspring of treated males mated to special stock females were examined, and about the same number of offspring of the reciprocal matings were also examined. Only one specific locus mutant was found, corresponding to a mutation rate per locus per gamete of 0.01×10^{-5} to 2.5×10^{-5} (the wide range represents the 95% confidence limits). This mutation rate did not differ significantly from the spontaneous rate of 1.0×10^{-5}.

Another experiment assessed the frequency of dominant lethals and translocations induced by caffeine.[118] Male mice were given 3 mg ml^{-1} of caffeine in their drinking water. Male offspring of caffeine-treated males were studied at 6 weeks of age, first by determining litter sizes, then by examining testis preparations for translocations. Of 201 F_1 males examined in this way, only 13 produced small litters; none of these semi-sterile animals showed typical translocations. Moreover, no dominant visible effects were seen in either the F_1 or the F_2 generation.

The chromosome-breaking action of caffeine was studied in human (HeLa) cells in culture.[115] The cells were exposed to caffeine at various concentrations for 1 hr, then incubated for 24 hr; and chromosome analyses were carried out. As shown in Table 10-3, breaks and other abnormalities were produced, and the number of breaks was very nearly a linear function of caffeine concentration. The caffeine appeared to act only upon cells engaged in DNA replication. From the dose relationship, it can be estimated that a concentration of 1 μg ml^{-1} would produce a negligible increment in the spontaneous rate of chromosome breakage. In summary, the available data in bacteria, *Drosophila*, mice, and cells of human origin indicate that caffeine, at a concentration of 1 μg ml^{-1}, causes an increase of at most a few per cent in the spontaneous mutation rate. It seems probable, therefore, that caffeine is not a significant mutagen in man.

In the previous sections of this chapter, we have discussed the various systems that can be used to screen for mutagenicity. From the standpoint of predicting whether or not a drug or chemical agent is likely to be hazardous to the human germ line, it should be obvious that no one system is sufficient. Some have argued that, since the DNA of all organisms is similar in its fundamental structure and mechanism of replication, any convenient organism may be used. Certainly a compound that proves strongly mutagenic in any test system should be suspect, and compounds that are universally mutagenic in other species may be assumed to be mutagenic in man, too. Alkylating

660   Chemical Mutagenesis

TABLE 10-3. Chromosome breaks induced by caffeine in cells of human origin.
HeLa cells were cultured and treated for 1 hr with various concentrations of caffeine. Then the cells were washed with fresh growth medium and incubated another 24 hr. Chromosome analyses were performed, with the results tabulated below. Chromatid breaks (single chromatid) and isolocus breaks (both chromatids) were counted, and also translocations, dicentric chromosomes, and ring forms. (From Ostertag et al.,[115] Table 1.)

Caffeine (μg ml^{-1})	Number of Chromosomes	Chromatid or isolocus breaks	Trans-locations	Dicentrics	Rings
0	≈187	4			
500	2754	18		1	
1000	3693	47	*	2	
2000	4361	111	1		
3000	2663	106	1	2	
5000	5666	401	5	2	3
10,000	3456	763	11	3	

* 2 cells with 10 translocations.

agents, cyclohexylamine, nitrites and nitrosamines, base analogs, and streptonigrin are examples. On the other hand, a negative test in one organism cannot be taken as a guarantee of safety in man. Even a negative result in a host-mediated test system gives no real assurance, since species differ so greatly in the pattern of metabolites derived from a given parent compound.

These considerations have led to proposals for direct monitoring of mutagenesis in humans.[119,120,121,122] Of course, the approach can not be experimental, i.e., people can not be exposed deliberately to suspected mutagens. Rather, the aim would be to detect any sudden increase in mutation frequency in human populations; such early warning would then lead to intensive search for the cause. Any convenient mutant phenotypes could be chosen for continuous monitoring, and any indicator of a change in the genetic material would be regarded as a danger signal. Cytogenetic abnormalities of the translocation type would be suitable; aneuploidy, polyploidy, and chromosome breakage tend to be eliminated from the germ line through sterility or cell death, and are, therefore, probably not serious hazards to the germ line. Visible dominant mutations would be useful, provided their detection in newborns was unambiguous; several hundred of these are known already in man. Sex-linked recessive mutations could be used, but their expression is not very efficient; a newly arisen mutation on an X chromosome in the male or female germ cells has only a one-third chance of being expressed in the offspring. Autosomal recessives are obviously useless since they are only expressed, usually after many generations, in the homozygous state.

The sensitivity of a monitoring system presents a real problem, even if the mutant trait could be identified quickly in the newborn. The following computation indicates how difficult it would be to detect even a considerable increase in the spontaneous mutation rate.[119] Suppose a spontaneous rate of 10^{-5} per gamete. Then 3 million births—the total annual birth rate in the United States—would yield about 60 new mutants. An increase to 80 (i.e., an increase of one third) would be the smallest statistically significant change. Even then, with the warning evidence in hand, the formidable task would remain of identifying the presumed mutagenic agent through retrospective investigation of the 80 parental pairs.

An interesting suggestion has been advanced[119] to monitor, on a routine basis, the cytology of blood cells in newborns, or even in adults. The proposal rests upon the assumption that mutagenesis would affect somatic cells, not only the germ line—an assumption for which there is ample evidence in the results obtained with mutagens in cell culture systems. Moreover, whereas a mutant phenotype in a single newborn infant represents only a single mutational event, thousands of blood cells can be monitored in a single individual, thus amplifying greatly the sensitivity of detection. An alternative procedure would be to monitor the electrophoretic pattern of a number of different plasma proteins simultaneously in order to detect any mutant variant arising from a mutational event in the gamete or early stages of development of the zygote.

Another monitoring procedure that might prove valuable makes use of the sex ratio as an indicator of sex-linked lethal mutations.[123] The sex ratio is defined as the number of live-born boys per 100 live-born girls. If a man is exposed to a mutagen and a defect is induced on his X chromosome, then no male offspring will be affected (since sons inherit the paternal Y chromosome only), but female offspring may suffer partial or complete decrease of viability. Thus, the sex ratio at birth will increase to the extent that nonviable female zygotes or fetuses are present. Conversely, if females are exposed to a mutagen, one-half their male offspring will carry a mutant maternal X chromosome, and any recessive lethal alleles will be expressed. In this instance, the sex ratio will decrease. The method was used, with somewhat equivocal result, to ascertain whether or not genetic damage was produced among radiation-exposed survivors of the nuclear blast at Hiroshima.[124] There is also weak evidence suggesting that habitual smoking of cigarettes may be mutagenic; in several large statistical surveys, it was found that in matings between smoker men and nonsmoker women, the sex ratio of their offspring significantly exceeded that found among nonsmokers.[125] However, interpretation of this interesting finding is considerably beclouded by two facts: first, that the sex ratio in the entire white population of the United States is as high as 106 boys to 100 girls; and second, that even reciprocal matings (nonsmoker men with smoker women) yielded a high sex ratio, although mutation in the females should have lowered the sex ratio. Despite these difficulties, it may be that carefully constructed statistical studies in large populations containing both exposed and nonexposed people will be able to detect drug-induced mutations by their effects on the sex ratio.

REFERENCES

1. A. M. SRB, R. D. OWEN, and R. S. EDGAR: *General Genetics*, 2nd ed. San Francisco, W. H. Freeman (1965).
2. C. STERN: *Principles of Human Genetics*, 3rd ed. San Francisco, W. H. Freeman (1973).
3. R. M. HERRIOTT: Mutagenesis. *Cancer Res.* 26:1971 (1966).
4. A. HOLLAENDER, ed.: *Chemical Mutagens: Principles and Methods for Their Detection*. New York, Plenum Press (1971). Vol. 1–2.

4a. B. N. AMES: The detection of chemical mutagens with enteric bacteria. See p. 267 in ref. 4.
5. F. VOGEL and G. ROHRBORN, eds.: *Chemical Mutagenesis in Mammals and Man.* New York, Springer-Verlag (1970).
6. J. D. WATSON: *Molecular Biology of the Gene,* 2nd ed. New York, W. A. Benjamin (1970).
7. Cold Spring Habor Symposia on Quantitative Biology: *The Genetic Code.* Cold Spring Harbor, New York, Biological Laboratory (1966). Vol. 31.
8. E. FREESE: The difference between spontaneous and base-analog induced mutations of phage T4. *Proc. Nat. Acad. Sci. U.S.A.* 45:622 (1959).
9. J. W. DRAKE: The Molecular Basis of Mutation. San Francisco, Holden-Day (1970).
10. E. FREESE: Molecular mechanisms of mutations. See Ch. 1, p. 1 in ref. 4.
11. G. ROHRBORN: Biochemical mechanisms of mutation. See Ch. 1. p. 1 in ref. 5.
12. L. PAULING: Genetic and somatic effects of carbon-14. *Science* 128:1183 (1958).
13. T. A. TRAUTNER, M. N. SWARTZ, and A. KORNBERG: Enzymatic synthesis of deoxyribonucleic acid, X. Influence of bromouracil substitutions on replication. *Proc. Nat. Acad. Sci. U.S.A.* 48:449 (1962).
14. R. B. SETLOW: Physical changes and mutagenesis. *J. Cell. Comp. Physiol.* 64:suppl. 1, 51 (1964).
15. E. M. WITKIN: Radiation-induced mutations and their repair. *Science* 152:1345 (1966).
16. R. E. MOSES, J. L. CAMPBELL, R. A. FLEISCHMAN, G. D. FRENKEL, H. L. MULCAHY, H. SHIZUYA, and C. C. RICHARDSON: Enzymatic mechanisms of DNA replication in *Escherichia coli. Fed. Proc.* 31:1415 (1972).
17. S. BENZER: On the topography of the genetic fine structure. *Proc. Nat. Acad. Sci. U.S.A.* 47:403 (1961).
18. S. BENZER: On the topology of the genetic fine structure. *Proc. Nat. Acad. Sci. U.S.A.* 45:1607 (1959).
19. A. O. W. STRETTON and S. BRENNER: Molecular consequences of the amber mutation and its suppression. *J. Mol. Biol.* 12:456 (1965).
20. S. BRENNER and A. O. W. STRETTON: The *amber* mutation. *J. Cell. Comp. Physiol.* 64:suppl. 1, 43 (1964).
21. S. BENZER and E. FREESE: Induction of Specific Mutations with 5-Bromouracil. *Proc. Nat. Acad. Sci. U.S.A.* 44:112 (1958).
22. E. FREESE, E. BAUTZ-FREESE, and E. BAUTZ: Hydroxylamine as a mutagenic and inactivating agent. *J. Mol. Biol.* 3:133 (1961).
23. D. R. KRIEG: Specificity of chemical mutagenesis. *Progr. Nucleic Acid Res.* 2:125 (1963).
24. I. TESSMAN, R. K. PODDAR, and S. KUMAR: Identification of the altered bases in mutated single-stranded DNA. I. In vitro mutagenesis by hydroxylamine, ethyl methanesulfonate and nitrous acid. *J. Mol. Biol.* 9:352 (1964).
25. I. TESSMAN, H. ISHIWA, and S. KUMAR: Mutagenic effects of hydroxylamine in vivo. *Science* 148:507 (1965).
26. D. M. BROWN and J. H. PHILLIPS: Mechanism of the mutagenic action of hydroxylamine. *J. Mol. Biol.* 11:663 (1965).
27. E. FREESE, E. BAUTZ, and E. BAUTZ-FREESE: The chemical and mutagenic specificity of hydroxylamine. *Proc. Nat. Acad. Sci. U.S.A.* 47:845 (1961).
28. E. BAUTZ and E. FREESE: On the mutagenic effect of alkylating agents. *Proc. Nat. Acad. Sci. U.S.A.* 46:1585 (1960).
29. D. R. KRIEG: Ethyl methanesulfonate-induced reversion of bacteriophage T4rII mutants. *Genetics* 48:561 (1963).
30. A. SIEGEL: Artificial production of mutants of tobacco mosaic virus. *Adv. Virus Res.* 11:25 (1965).
31. C. YANOFSKY, B. C. CARLTON, J. R. GUEST, D. R. HELINSKI, and U. HENNING: On the colinearity of gene structure and protein structure. *Proc. Nat. Acad. Sci. U.S.A.* 51:266 (1964).
32. C. YANOFSKY, E. C. COX, and V. HORN: The unusual mutagenic specificity of an *E. coli* mutator gene. *Proc. Nat. Acad. Sci. U.S.A.* 55:274 (1966).
33. G. STREISINGER, Y. OKADA, J. EMRICH, J. NEWTON, A. TSUGITA, E. TERZAGHI, and M. INOUYE: Frameshift mutations and the genetic code. *Cold Spring Harbor Symp. Quant. Biol.* 31:77 (1966).
34. E. M. WITKIN and N. A. SICURELLA: Pure clones of lactose-negative mutants obtained in *Escherichia coli* after treatment with 5-bromouracil. *J. Mol. Biol.* 8:610 (1964).
35. H. E. KUBITSCHEK: Mutation without segregation. *Proc. Nat. Acad. Sci. U.S.A.* 52:1374 (1964).

36. F. LINGENS: Wirkungsmechanismus einiger chemischer Mutagene. *Arch. exper. Pathol. Pharmakol.* 253:116 (1966).

37. T. KOTAKA and R. L. BALDWIN: Effects of nitrous acid on the dAT copolymer as a template for DNA polymerase. *J. Mol. Biol.* 9:323 (1964).

38. I. TESSMAN: The induction of large deletions by nitrous acid. *J. Mol. Biol.* 5:442 (1962).

39. J. D. MANDELL and J. GREENBERG: A new chemical mutagen for bacteria, 1-methyl-3-nitro-1-nitrosoguanidine. *Biochem. Biophys. Res. Comm.* 3:575 (1960).

40. E. A. ADELBERG, M. MANDEL, and G. C. C. CHEN: Optimal conditions for mutagenesis by N-methyl-N'-nitro-N-nitrosoguanidine in *Escherichia coli* K12. *Biochem. Biophys. Res. Comm.* 18:788 (1965).

41. B. S. STRAUSS: Chemical mutagens and the genetic code. *Progr. Med. Geretics* 3:1 (1964).

42. P. BROOKES and P. D. LAWLEY: Reaction of some mutagenic and carcinogenic compounds with nucleic acids. *J. Cell. Comp. Physiol.* 64: suppl. 1, 111 (1964).

43. E. BAUTZ-FREESE: Transitions and transversions induced by depurinating agents. *Proc. Nat. Acad. Sci. U.S.A.* 47:540 (1961).

44. B. D. HOWARD and I. TESSMAN: Identification of the altered bases in mutated single-stranded DNA. II. In vivo mutagenesis by 5-bromodeoxyuridine and 2-aminopurine. *J. Mol. Biol.* 9:364 (1964).

45. D. PRATT and G. S. STENT: Mutational heterozygotes in bacteriophages. *Proc. Nat. Acad. Sci. U.S.A.* 45:1507 (1959).

46. I. D. ADLER: The problem of caffeine mutagenicity. See Ch. 24, p. 383 in ref. 5.

47. S. EPSTEIN: The failure of caffeine to induce mutagenic effects or to synergize the effects of known mutagens in mice. See Ch. 25, p. 404 in ref. 5.

48. A. L. KOCH: The mechanism of action of methyl xanthines in mutagenesis. In Symposium on *Information Theory in Biology*, ed. by H. P. Yockey, et al. New York, Pergamon Press (1958), p. 136.

49. P. O. P. TS'O, G. K. HELMKAMP, and C. SANDER: Interaction of nucleosides and related compounds with nucleic acids as indicated by the change of helix-coil transition temperature. *Proc. Nat. Acad. Sci. U.S.A.* 48:686 (1962).

50. M. LIEB: Dark repair of UV induction in K12 (λ). *Virology* 23:381 (1964).

51. H. S. KAPLAN, J. D. EARLE, and F. L. HOWSDEN: The role of purine and pyrimidine bases and their analogs in radiation sensitivity. *J. Cell. Comp. Physiol.* 64:suppl. 1, 69 (1964).

52. F. H. C. CRICK, L. BARNETT, S. BRENNER, and R. J. WATTS-TOBIN: General nature of the genetic code for proteins. *Nature* 192:1227 (1961).

53. L. BARNETT, S. BRENNER, F. H. C. CRICK, R. G. SHULMAN, and R. J. WATTS-TOBIN: Phase-shift and other mutants in the first part of the rII B cistron of bacteriophage T4. *Phil. Trans. B Roy. Soc.* 252:487 (1967).

54. E. TERZAGHI, Y. OKADA, G. STREISINGER, J. EMRICH, M. INOUYE, and A. TSUGITA: Change of a sequence of amino acids in phage T4 lysozyme by acridine-induced mutations. *Proc. Nat. Acad. Sci. U.S.A.* 56:500 (1966).

55. L. S. LERMAN: Acridine mutagens and DNA structure. *J. Cell. Comp. Physiol.* 64: suppl. 1, 1 (1964).

56. M. WARING: *Distortion of DNA Structure and Function by Intercalating Molecules.* Proc. Fourth Int. Cong. Pharmacol., Basel, Schwabe and Co. (1970), Vol. I, p. 308.

57. G. E. MAGNI: Origin and nature of spontaneous mutations in meiotic organisms. *J. Cell. Comp. Physiol.* 64: suppl. 1, 165 (1964).

58. G. E. MAGNI, R. C. VON BORSTEL, and S. SORA: Mutagenic action during meiosis and antimutagenic action during mitosis by 5-aminoacridine in yeast. *Mutation Res.* 1:227 (1964).

59. G. E. MAGNI: The origin of spontaneous mutations during meiosis. *Proc. Nat. Acad. Sci. U.S.A.* 50:975 (1963).

60. R. DULBECCO: Summary of 1964 biology research conference. *J. Cell. Comp. Physiol.* 64: suppl. 1, 181 (1964).

61. E. M. WITKIN: The effect of acriflavine on photoreversal of lethal and mutagenic damage produced in bacteria by ultraviolet light. *Proc. Nat. Acad. Sci. U.S.A.* 50:425 (1963).

62. J. H. TAYLOR: The Replication and Organization of DNA in Chromosomes. In *Molecular Genetics*, ed. by J. H. Taylor. New York, Academic Press (1963), Ch. 2

63. B. A. KIHLMAN: Root tips for studying the effects of chemicals on chromosomes. See Ch. 18, p. 489 in ref. 4.

64.   B. MC CLINTOCK: The stability of broken ends of chromosomes in *Zea mays*. *Genetics* 26:234 (1941).

65.   P. C. KOLLER: Comparative effects of alkylating agents on cellular morphology. *Ann. New York Acad. Sci.* 68:783 (1958).

66.   T. C. HSU and C. E. SOMERS: Effect of 5-bromodeoxyuridine on mammalian chromosomes. *Proc. Nat. Acad. Sci. U.S.A.* 47:396 (1961).

67.   E. H. Y. CHU: Effects of ultraviolet radiation on mammalian cells. I. Induction of chromosome aberrations. *Mutation Res.* 2:75 (1965).

68.   N. S. COHN: The effect of hydroxylamine on the rejoining of x-ray-induced chromatid breaks in *Vicia faba*. *Mutation Res.* 1:409 (1964).

69.   B. A. KIHLMAN: *Actions of Chemicals on Dividing Cells*. Englewood Cliffs, New Jersey, Prentice-Hall, Inc. (1966).

70.   B. A. KIHLMAN: Molecular mechanisms of chromosome breakage and rejoining. In *Advances in Cell and Molecular Biology*, ed. E. J. DuPraw. New York, Academic Press (1971).

70a.   P. HOWARD-FLANDERS, R. P. BOYCE, and L. THERIOT: DNA repair and genetic recombination: studies on mutants of *Escherichia coli* defective in these processes. *Rad. Res. Suppl.* 6:156 (1966).

70b.   W. D. RUPP and P. HOWARD-FLANDERS: Discontinuities in the DNA synthesized in an excision-defective strain of *Escherichia coli* following ultraviolet irradiation. *J. Mol. Biol.* 31:291 (1968).

71.   G. ODMARK and B. A. KIHLMAN: Effects of chromosome-breaking purine derivatives on nucleic acid synthesis and on the levels of adenosine 5'-triphosphate and deoxyadenosine 5'-triphosphate in bean root tips. *Mutation Res.* 2:274 (1965).

72.   B. A. KIHLMAN: Biochemical aspects of chromosome breakage. *Adv. Genet.* 10:1 (1961).

73.   D. SCOTT and H. J. EVANS: On the non-requirement for deoxyribonucleic acid synthesis in the production of chromosome aberrations by 8-ethoxycaffeine. *Mutation Res.* 1:146 (1964).

74.   S. BENZER and S. P. CHAMPE: A change from nonsense to sense in the genetic code. *Proc. Nat. Acad. Sci. U.S.A.* 48:1114 (1962).

75.   M. M. COHEN, M. W. SHAW, and A. P. CRAIG: The effects of streptonigrin on cultured human leukocytes. *Proc. Nat. Acad. Sci. U.S.A.* 50:16 (1963).

76.   D. MAZIA: Mitosis and the Physiology of Cell Division. In *The Cell, vol. III. Meiosis and Mitosis*, ed. by J. Brachet and A. E. Mirsky. New York, Academic Press (1961), Ch. 2.

77.   A. BAJER and J. MOLE-BAJER: Architecture and function of the mitotic spindle. See ref. 70.

78.   A. HUGHES: *The Mitotic Cycle*. New York, Academic Press (1952).

79.   H. STERN: The physiology of cell division. *Ann. Rev. Plant Physiol.* 7:91 (1956).

80.   P. DUSTIN, JR.: New aspects of the pharmacology of antimitotic agents. *Pharmacol. Rev.* 15:449 (1963).

81.   A. BARTHELMESS: Chemisch induzierte multipolare Mitosen. *Protoplasma* 48:546 (1957).

82.   A. BARTHELMESS and J. EINLECHNER: Chemisch induzierte multipolare Mitosen. II. *Protoplasma* 51:325 (1959).

83.   L. WILSON and J. BRYAN: Biochemical and pharmacological properties of microtubules. In *Advances in Cell and Molecular Biology*, Vol. 3, ed. E. J. DuPraw. New York, Academic Press (1974).

84.   E. W. TAYLOR: The mechanism of colchicine inhibition of mitosis. I. Kinetics of inhibition and the binding of H^3-colchicine. *J. Cell Biol.* 25: No. 1 (1965), p. 145.

85.   J. LEJEUNE: The 21 trisomy—current stage of chromosomal research. *Progr. Med. Genetics* 3:144 (1964).

86.   W. M. DAVIDSON and D. R. SMITH, eds.: *Proceedings of the Conference on Human Chromosomal Abnormalities*. London, Staples Press (1961).

87.   C. P. LEBLOND, E. STEINBERGER, and E. C. ROOSEN-RUNGE: Spermatogenesis. In *Mechanisms Concerned with Conception*, ed. by C. G. Hartman. New York, Macmillan Co. (1963), Ch. 1.

88.   A. GOLDSTEIN: Mutagens currently of potential significance to man and other species. In *Mutations. Second Macy Conference on Genetics*, ed. by W. J. Schull. Ann Arbor, University of Michigan Press (1962), p. 167.

89.   B. M. CATTANACH: The sensitivity of the mouse testis to the mutagenic action of triethylene-melamine. *Z. Vererbungs.* 90:1 (1959).

90.   T. ALDERSON and M. PELECANOS: The mutagenic activity of diethyl sulphate in *Drosophila melanogaster*. II. The sensitivity of the immature (larval) and the adult testis. *Mutation Res.* 1:182 (1964).

91. M. PELECANOS and T. ALDERSON: The mutagenic activity of diethyl sulphate in *Drosophila melanogaster*. III. The sensitivity of the immature (larval) and adult ovary. *Mutation Res.* 1:302 (1964).

92. S. ABRAHAMSON and E. B. LEWIS: The detection of mutations in *Drosophila melanogaster*. See Ch. 17, p. 461 in ref. 4.

93. D. GRAHN: Mammalian Radiation Genetics. In *Methodology in Mammalian Genetics*, ed. by W. J. Burdette. San Francisco, Holden-Day (1963), p. 127.

94. B. M. CATTANACH: Specific locus mutation in mice. See Ch. 20, p. 535 in ref. 4.

95. H. J. MULLER: The measurement of gene mutation rate in *Drosophila*, its high variability, and its dependence upon temperature. *Genetics* 13:279 (1928).

96. M. PARTINGTON and A. J. BATEMAN: Dominant lethal mutations induced in male mice by methyl methanesulphonate. *Heredity* 19:191 (1964).

97. A. J. BATEMAN and S. S. EPSTEIN: Dominant lethal mutations in mammals. See Ch. 21, p. 541 in ref. 4.

98. S. S. EPSTEIN and G. RÖHRBORN: Recommended procedures for testing genetic hazards from chemicals, based on the induction of dominant lethal mutations in mammals. *Nature* 230:459 (1971).

99. W. L. RUSSELL: X-ray-induced mutations in mice. *Cold Spring Harbor Symp. Quant. Biol.* 16:327 (1951).

100. M. S. LEGATOR, K. A. PALMER, S. GREEN, and K. W PETERSEN: Cytogenetic studies in rats of cyclohexylamine, a metabolite of cyclamate. *Science* 165 1139 (1969).

101. K. A. PALMER, S. GREEN, and M. S. LEGATOR: Cytogenetic effects of DDT and derivatives of DDT in a cultured mammalian cell line. *Tox. and Appl. Pharm.* 22:355 (1972).

101a. E. H. Y. CHU: Induction and analysis of gene mutations in mammalian cells in culture. See Ch. 15, p. 411 in ref. 4.

102. M. S. LEGATOR and H. V. MALLING: The host-mediated assay, a practical procedure for evaluating potential mutagenic agents in mammals. See Ch. 22, p. 569 in ref. 4

103. M. S. LEGATOR: The host-mediated assay, a practical procedure for evaluating potential mutagenic agents. See Ch. 15, p. 260 in ref. 5.

104. F. J. DE SERRES and H. V. MALLING: Measurement of recessive lethal damage over the entire genome and at two specific loci in the ad-3 region of a two-component heterokaryon of neurospora crassa. See Ch. 11, p. 311 in ref. 4.

105. H. V. MALLING: Chemical mutagens as a possible genetic hazard in human populations. *Am. Ind. Hyg. Ass. J.* 31:657 (1970).

106. M. HARRIS: Mutagenicity of chemicals and drugs. *Science* 171:51 (1971).

107. B. L. S. PIERCE: The effect of a bacterial mutator gene upon mutation rates in bacteriophage T4. *Genetics* 54:657 (1966).

108. A. GOLDSTEIN and J. S. SMOOT: A strain of *Escherichia coli* with an unusually high rate of auxotrophic mutation. *J. Bacteriol.* 70:588 (1955).

109. H. P. TREFFERS, V. SPINELLI, and N. O. BELSER: A factor (or mutator gene) influencing mutation rates in *Escherichia coli*. *Proc. Nat. Acad. Sci. U.S.A.* 40:1064 (1954).

109a. J. DRAKE, ed.: The genetic control of mutation. *Genetics* Vol. 73, supplement, April, 1973.

110. I. A. WOLFF and A. E. WASSERMAN: Nitrates, nitrites, and nitrosamines. *Science* 177:15 (1972).

111. A. BARTHELMESS: Mutagene Arzneimittel. *Arzneimittel-Forsch.* 6:157 (1956).

112. W. KUHLMANN, H.-G. FROMME, E.-M. HEEGE, and W. OSTERTAG: The mutagenic action of caffeine in higher organisms. *Cancer Res.* 28:2375 (1968).

113. M. S. LEGATOR, F. J. KELLY, S. GREEN, and E. J. OSWALD: Mutagenic effects of captan. *Ann. N.Y. Acad. Sci.* 160:344 (1969).

114. A. NOVICK: Mutagens and antimutagens. *Brookhaven Symp. Biol.* 8:201 (1956).

115. W. OSTERTAG, E. DUISBERG, and M. STÜRMANN: The mutagenic activity of caffeine in man. *Mutation Res.* 2:293 (1965).

116. L. E. ANDREW: The mutagenic activity of caffeine in *Drosophila*. *Amer. Naturalist* 93:135 (1959).

117. M. F. LYON, R. J. S. PHILLIPS, and A. G. SEARLE: A test for mutagenicity of caffeine in mice. *Z. Vererbungs.* 93:7 (1962).

118. B. M. CATTANACH: Genetical effects of caffeine in mice. *Z. Vererbungs.* 93:215 (1962).

119. J. F. CROW: Human population monitoring. See Ch. 23, p. 591 in ref. 4.

120. J. V. NEEL and A. D. BLOOM: The detection of environmental mutagens. *Med. Clin. of N. Am.* 53:1243 (1969).

121. E. B. HOOK: Monitoring human birth defects and mutations to detect environmental effects. *Science* 172:1363 (1971).
122. F. VOGEL: Monitoring of human populations. See Ch. 28, p. 453 in ref. 5.
123. F. VOGEL: Statistical examinations in human populations. See Ch. 27, p. 433 in ref. 5.
124. J. V. NEEL: *Changing Perspectives on the Genetic Effects of Radiation*. Springfield, Ill., Charles C. Thomas (1963).
125. A. DAMON, R. L. NUTTALL, E. J. SALBER, C. C. SELTZER, and B. MAC MAHON: Tobacco smoke as a possible genetic mutagen: parental smoking and sex of children. *Am. J. Epidemiol.* 83:530 (1966).

CHAPTER 11
Chemical Carcinogenesis

Cancer is the malignant unrestrained proliferation of somatic cells. It occurs spontaneously and can also be induced by ionizing radiation, viruses, and chemicals known as *carcinogens*. Chemical carcinogenesis was discovered in man long before it could be demonstrated experimentally in animals. In 1775, cancer of the scrotum was recognized as an occupational disease of chimneysweeps, and prolonged exposure to soot was presumed to be the cause.[1] In the following century, other instances of coal tar carcinogenesis in industrial workers came to light. But it was not until 1915 that cancer was produced experimentally by applying coal tar to an animal's skin.[2] The subsequent identification and isolation of the responsible polycyclic hydrocarbons, the systematic exploration of structure-activity relationships, the discovery of carcinogenic properties among other groups of compounds, and the elaboration of theories of chemical carcinogenesis are among the most interesting developments in modern pharmacology.[3-9]

MECHANISM OF ACTION OF CHEMICAL CARCINOGENS

Methods of Experimentation

Only the most potent agents produce cancer in every exposed animal. With less potent agents, the incidence is low and has to be compared with the frequency of spontaneous cancer; therefore, large numbers of animals may be required to demonstrate carcinogenicity. Exposure to a carcinogen usually has to be continued for a long time. But even when a brief exposure suffices, there is a long latent period before cancers start to appear. For these reasons, the experimental animals have to be maintained for a long time. Rodents (especially mice, rats, and hamsters) have proved most useful in laboratory studies.

Some carcinogens act primarily at the site of their application. If painted on the skin, they produce papillomatous epithelial growths that develop into squamous cell carcinomas. If injected subcutaneously, they produce sarcomas, i.e., malignant growths

667

of the fibroblasts in connective tissues. If given by mouth, they may produce tumors of the gastrointestinal tract. Other carcinogens are principally effective when incorporated into the diet; they act on the liver to produce malignant hepatomas or tumors of the bile ducts. Some carcinogens act at widely dispersed sites throughout the body, regardless of the route by which they are taken in. Cutaneous application of such a compound might lead not only to skin cancer at the point of application but also perhaps to cancer of the intestine, lungs, or kidneys. Illustrative of carcinogenesis at a remote site is the effect of the hydrocarbon 3-methylcholanthrene (Figure 11-6). When this substance was given to rats in the diet, it caused no hepatomas but produced cancer of the mammary glands in all the treated animals.[10] Similarly, administration of naphthylamine (p. 682) by any route leads to cancer of the bladder in susceptible species. The mammary cancers caused by 3-methylcholanthrene, the bladder tumors caused by naphthylamine, and indeed all cancers that develop in tissues remote from the site of carcinogen administration are not metastatic implants. They are primary tumors initiated by the carcinogen itself or by a product of carcinogen metabolism after absorption and distribution have taken place.

Species and strain differences bespeak the major role of genetic background in determining susceptibility to carcinogenesis. One source of variation is the known difference in activity of the drug-metabolizing enzymes among different species; this can account for differences of carcinogenic potency if the carcinogen has to be metabolized to an active product, or if an active carcinogen has to reach a remote site of action before it is transformed to an inert metabolite. A good example is 2-acetylaminofluorene (AAF), which is metabolized to an N-hydroxy derivative. This metabolite (or more likely an ester derived from it) is the active carcinogen (cf. p. 675). This conversion takes place in several species that develop cancer when AAF is administered. In the guinea pig, however, the N-hydroxylation reaction does not occur, and accordingly, AAF is not carcinogenic. Moreover, in species in which N-hydroxy AAF is formed, it is excreted in the urine as an inert conjugate with glucuronic acid. Thus, the liver glucuronyl transferase activity and the β-glucuronidase activity of the urine both profoundly influence the ability of systemically administered AAF to cause bladder cancer.

In addition to species differences in the metabolism of compounds to active carcinogens (also called *proximate carcinogens*), there may be intrinsic differences in sensitivity of tissues to the carcinogenic process. All animals are subject to chemical carcinogenesis, but the incidence of a given type of cancer may vary widely between species. The influence of genetic constitution is revealed in marked strain differences within a single species.[10a] Such differences are tissue specific, as is also true for differences with respect to spontaneous cancers. Mice have been bred selectively for a high incidence of spontaneous tumors at particular sites. For example, one strain may develop spontaneous mammary gland cancers at a rate of less than 1%, whereas the incidence in a specially bred strain may be as high as 90%. Sometimes a high susceptibility to spontaneous cancer of a particular tissue is associated with high sensitivity to induced chemical carcinogenesis at the same site, but this is not necessarily so. If a given carcinogen induces sarcomas at the site of subcutaneous injection and also lung carcinomas remote from the injection site, selective breeding may yield one strain in which the carcinogen produces only sarcomas, another in which only lung tumors develop. Azo dyes injected subcutaneously usually cause both sarcomas at the injection site and hepatomas, but some strains of mice develop few tumors of either kind in response to these agents. This pattern of genetic variation in susceptibility to cancer in general, susceptibility to cancer of particular tissues, and susceptibility to individual chemical carcinogens, may also apply in the human. It is well known that certain kinds of cancer tend to run in families, and there is also a high concordance rate for the occurrence of specific types of cancer in monozygous twins.

Sex differences in cancer incidence and in responses to carcinogens may be related to hormonal influences.[11,12] A strain of mice that developed mammary cancer at a high rate after administration of a hydrocarbon carcinogen was found to produce unusually large amounts of estrogen. Estrogen administration to other strains was found to increase the yield of mammary tumors caused by the same carcinogen.

Malignant growths of hormone-sensitive organs often remain responsive to the hormones that ordinarily stimulate these organs. For example, prostate cancer can be treated by castration, to remove the major source of testosterone, or by administering estrogenic hormones, which antagonize the effects of androgens. Thyroid tumors have been induced by pituitary thyroid-stimulating hormone or thiouracil (which causes increased output of the pituitary hormone). Pituitary hormones have also been used to produce tumors in the adrenal glands, ovaries, testes, and mammary glands. Insulin apparently plays some role in promoting tumor development, for the frequency of carcinogen-induced hepatomas and mammary carcinomas is much lower in alloxan-diabetic rats than in normal animals. It is not certain whether the hormones act as carcinogens in their own right or whether they alter the cellular environment in sensitive tissues in a way that makes them more susceptible to endogenous or exogenous carcinogens. Some phenanthrene derivatives having the same carbon ring skeleton as the naturally occurring steroids are potent carcinogens, even on tissues like skin which are not hormone-dependent. No such compounds have been found to arise by metabolism of steroid hormones, but they might possibly be produced from dietary steroids through metabolism by the intestinal flora.[13]

If species, strain, sex, hormonal status, diet, and route of administration are carefully controlled, then reliable dose-response relationships can be found and the relative potencies of carcinogens can be described quantitatively. Figure 11-1 shows log dose-response curves for three-hydrocarbon carcinogens administered to groups of mice by single subcutaneous injections. The eventual incidence of sarcomas at the injection sites was recorded. The curves are approximately parallel, suggesting a similar mechanism of action of the agents. Under these conditions, 3,4-benzpyrene was about one-fifth as potent as 1,2,5,6-dibenzanthracene or 3-methylcholanthrene. ED50 values and their confidence limits for carcinogenesis may be found in the same way as for any toxic drug action, as described in Chapter 5. At least a 10-fold increase of dose was required to span the range of response from an incidence of a few percent to an incidence of nearly 100%. This implies that laboratory experiments may tend to underestimate the likelihood that very small doses of a carcinogen will produce cancer in some animals. The reason is that with a small group of animals (e.g., less than 100) a dosage that causes no tumors at all will be judged ineffective, whereas the same dosage in a large population of the species would cause cancer in some animals. The same argument applies to estimating "safe" dosages of carcinogens in human populations on the basis of experimentation with a limited number of animals.

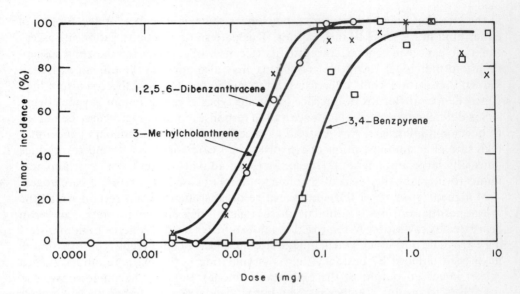

FIGURE 11-1. Dose-response relationship for carcinogens. *Three hydrocarbon carcinogens were administered subcutaneously, each to a group of 20 mice in a single dose. The incidence of sarcomas at the site of injection was noted. (From Bryan and Shimkin, Figure 5.[14])*

Initiation and Promotion

One of the most significant advances in understanding the mechanism of carcinogenesis was made about 20 years ago when it was discovered that the chemical induction of cancer involved two distinguishable processes, designated *initiation* and *promotion*.[15] Initiation is the production of an irreversible cellular change, which is a necessary but not sufficient condition for the development of cancer. Promotion is the process whereby a tumor is caused to develop in tissue in which initiation has already occurred.

The discovery of these independent processes arose from observations on the latent period. It had been found that after injecting a coal tar hydrocarbon subcutaneously (as in the experiments shown in Figure 11-1) there was a latent period of several weeks during which no tumors were observed. Then tumors began to appear in some mice, and during the subsequent months, if the dose of carcinogen was large enough, all the animals would develop cancer. Two variables were discerned—the total frequency of tumors eventually attained (the variable plotted in Figure 11-1) and the average latent period before the tumors appeared. As a rule, the more potent the carcinogen (as measured by the total tumor incidence), the shorter the average latent period was found to be; sometimes these variables seemed to be quite independent of each other. Such discrepancies led to the realization that the carcinogenic effect of the coal tar hydrocarbons was really a dual one. Other compounds were sought and found that had one or the other kind of action. Thus, two classes of substance could be identified—initiators of the carcinogenic process and promoters of the development of cancer.

An initiator could be painted once on an area of mouse skin. When this painted area was left untreated, no cancers appeared. But when the same area was treated repeatedly with a promoter, cancers developed with predictable frequency. The total tumor incidence varied with the initiator and its dose, but the latent period was determined only by the promoter and by its mode of application. If, after the single application of the initiator to the skin, the treatment with promoter was delayed, the latent period was correspondingly delayed; but the eventual incidence of cancer remained constant. Reversing the order of administration of initiator and promoter abolished the carcinogenic effect.

The essential features of initiation and promotion are summarized schematically in Figure 11-2. The diagram on the left depicts the tumor frequency as a function of time when different carcinogens were used for the single initial painting and the course

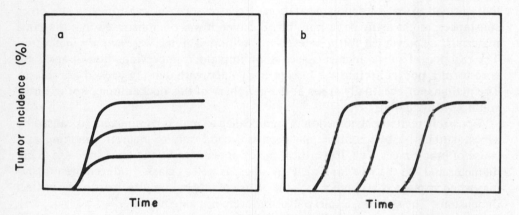

FIGURE 11-2. Initiation and promotion in carcinogenesis. (*From Berenblum and Shubik, Figures 2 and 3.*[15])

of treatment with the promoter was kept constant. The potencies of the several carcinogens are reflected in the different tumor frequencies attained, but the latent period was always the same. In the diagram on the right, a single carcinogen was used and the promoter treatment was delayed for different periods. Here the tumor frequency remained the same, but the latent period varied. The most striking separation of initiating action from promoting action was achieved in experiments in which an initiator (urethane) was given by mouth. No tumors developed anywhere except on areas of skin that were painted repeatedly with the promoter, croton oil; croton oil had no effect unless urethane had been administered previously. The conclusion drawn from all these experiments was that the initiator seems to cause an irreversible change in the cells of a certain number of mice after a single exposure, but that the altered cells are not able to develop into cancers except under the influence of a promoter.

Careful histopathologic studies of the early stages of carcinogenesis have revealed that promoting action is often associated with cell damage in the area where the malignancy will ultimately arise. Examples are the development of liver cancer following liver damage caused by carbon tetrachloride or other hepatotoxic agents, and development of skin cancers during the regenerative healing process after severe burn damage. Stimulation of cell growth seems to be an important component of the action of hormones in promoting carcinogenesis in target organs. Subcutaneous injection of hydrocarbon carcinogens with mixed initiating and promoting actions results in considerable local cell death, followed eventually by the appearance of malignant cells among survivors at the periphery of the affected area. And croton oil, a typical promoter in experimental carcinogenesis, contains a strongly irritant substance (a phorbol ester) that causes extensive cell damage. A possible mechanism of action of promoters is inhibition of DNA repair systems (cf. p. 646), a plausible explanation in view of the increasing evidence implicating somatic cell mutagenesis in the carcinogenic process.[16]

Remarkably, films of inert material implanted subcutaneously in rats cause a high incidence of sarcomas without administration of any accessory carcinogen.[17] Glass, plastic, and platinum foil were among the effective carcinogens. At first it was thought that a small extent of depolymerization of the plastics, or impurities in the other substances, might really be responsible. But then it was demonstrated that the same materials, in powdered form, or even as perforated films, were wholly ineffective. The reaction of subcutaneous tissues to an implanted impervious film of any kind is to form a pocket around the foreign body lined with densely packed fibroblasts. The malignancy eventually arises at the periphery of this pocket lining not in direct contact with the film.

A possibly related phenomenon of significance to man is carcinogenesis caused by asbestos fibers; asbestos fiber inhalation is second only to cigarette smoking as a cause of lung cancer.[18,19] The critical factor appears to be the fiber size—0.5–5 μm diameter and less than 80 μm long. Pure silica, as well as glass, produced mesotheliomas when implanted in contact with the pleura of rats but only as fibers of the critical dimensions. The same materials pulverized were not carcinogenic.[20]

The mechanism of carcinogenesis by implanted inert films and fibers is obscure.[21] Possibly the inert material, by modifying the cellular environment, acts like a promoter, favoring the development of tumors from spontaneously arising precancerous cells. One hypothesis implicates host immunologic defenses. According to this view, neoplastic cells arise from time to time under normal conditions, but the potentially cancerous cells are held in check or destroyed by immune processes. Thus, any interference with the immunologic mechanisms might allow a tumor to develop. It is known that patients receiving immunosuppressive drugs on a long-term basis (e.g., for maintenance of organ transplants) have a higher than normal incidence of cancer.[22]

Another hypothesis implicates latent oncogenic RNA viruses. The activation of such viruses (or viral "oncogenes" incorporated into the host genome), which has been proposed as a general mechanism for both chemical and radiation-induced carcinogenesis,[23] might also mediate the curious induction of cancer by inert films and fibers. Polycyclic hydrocarbon carcinogens have been shown to activate mouse leukemia virus[24] and adenovirus in cultured hamster cells.[25] Moreover, viral vaccines inhibited chemical carcinogenesis in mice.[26]

There are significant analogies between chemical and radiation (x-ray) carcinogenesis.[27] It has been proposed that radiation carcinogenesis may be mediated indirectly by carcinogens produced in the tissues as a consequence of ionizing radiation. These carcinogens could be free radicals or other reactive molecules, such as alkylating or arylating agents. That the tissue environment in the irradiated host plays an important role in radiation carcinogenesis was shown by means of transplantation experiments[28] in which thymus glands from nonirradiated mice, implanted into irradiated hosts, developed malignant tumors. Radiation seems to have both initiating and promoting actions.

The incidence of cancer in experimental animals is a function of the radiation dose, and the same relationship has been observed in human leukemia.[29,30] The dose relationship accords with the results obtained with chemical carcinogens that are pure initiators. On the other hand, exposure to x-rays results in tissue damage and tissue reaction as seen with croton oil and other promoters. Accordingly, regenerative hyperplasia of bone marrow regularly precedes the emergence of radiation-induced leukemia; and sensitivity to the induction of leukemia by x-rays is greatest at periods of rapid cell proliferation, as for example during fetal life.

Carcinogenesis and Mutagenesis

Cancer cells, once established, differ from their tissue of origin in that they have become independent of the control mechanisms that ordinarily limit cell growth and division in differentiated tissues. This is not merely a question of growth rate but of a balanced relationship between growth rate and the necessary rate of cell renewal. The normal mitotic rate in intestinal epithelium or in bone marrow is higher than in many cancers, but even these rapidly growing tissues are under strict regulation so that those cells that are shed into the intestinal lumen or destroyed in the circulation are exactly replaced. A vivid example of this kind of regulation is seen in the regeneration of excised tissue in a skin wound or after a partial hepatectomy. Cell proliferation is explosively rapid at first but ceases when the tissue mass has been restored. Most impressive of all is the regulation displayed during embryonic development, when differentiation of structure and function bring rapid cell proliferation to an abrupt end. In contrast, even a slowly growing cancer continues its cycles of mitotic activity and cell growth inexorably, disrupting the normal relationships between adjacent cells, invading into capillaries and lymph channels, implanting metastatically in remote parts of the body, and eventually killing the host.

Associated with the property of undisciplined growth and probably intimately related to it is the tendency of cancer cells to become undifferentiated, to lose the distinguishing morphologic and biochemical features of their tissue of origin. This is not, however, an all-or-none property but varies in degree from tumor to tumor and often progresses during the evolution of a particular tumor. Some cancers of endocrine organs may even continue to produce their usual hormones, and they may also respond to the appropriate tropic hormone. Thus, thyroid cancer may be stimulated by pituitary thyroid-stimulating hormone, prostate cancer by androgens, and breast cancer by estrogens.

Some mammary cancers in rats retain the hormone sensitivity of normal mammary tissue, and these regress after ovariectomy, whereas others continue to grow after such removal of the estrogen source. It has been shown that the estrogen sensitive tumors contain a specific cytoplasmic estradiol binding protein, which promotes the binding of the estrogen to chromatin in the nucleus. Cytoplasm from autonomous (estrogen-insensitive) tumors lacks this estrogen receptor protein, and no binding to chromatin could be demonstrated. Addition of cytoplasm from an estrogen-dependent tissue promoted binding of estradiol to chromatin from autonomous tumors, indicating that the lack of hormonal control was not due to any alteration of the chromatin.[31]

That the loss of responsiveness to growth controls is an intrinsic property of the cancer cells is further evidenced in a number of ways.[32] The very fact that cancer, whether spontaneous or carcinogen induced, can originate locally, in a particular tissue, rather than at multiple sites in the body, implicates a local cellular transformation as the essential prerequisite. When an area of mouse skin was painted once with an initiator and later transplanted to a different site, cancer developed only in the carcinogen-treated skin, regardless of how long transplantation was delayed. The same experiment was performed in a hybrid produced by mating a carcinogen-sensitive with a carcinogen-resistant strain of mice. This arrangement permitted transplantation of the carcinogen-treated skin of the hybrid to either of the parent strains. Cancer developed in the treated skin even after its transplantation to a resistant host in which the carcinogen would have been ineffective. Frequently, cancers that have achieved a sufficient degree of autonomy will grow malignantly after transplantation into hosts that would otherwise remain free of cancer.

A provocative development is the conversion of normal cells to cancer cells by carcinogens in vitro.[33-35] In one such experiment,[34] advantage was taken of a difference in chromosome number between two varieties of hamsters. Cells from lung tissue of the Chinese hamster (diploid number, $2n = 22$) were established in culture. They were grown for 12 days on agar containing a hydrocarbon carcinogen, while controls were grown on plain nutrient agar. All cells were then transferred to the ordinary agar. The carcinogen-treated cell cultures developed characteristic chromosome alterations, of the kind observed after chromosome breakage (e.g., terminal centromeres, cf. Chapter 10), but the cells not exposed to carcinogens rarely showed such changes. The altered cells, implanted in the cheek pouch of the Syrian hamster ($2n = 44$), produced sarcomas, whereas untreated cells did not. The chromosome complement of the tumors showed that they originated from the cells that had been maintained in culture, not from cells of the host animal. The tumors consistently showed abnormal chromosomes of the same kinds identified in the carcinogen-treated cell cultures. The chromosome abnormalities noted here are consistent with many observations on unusual numbers of chromosomes (aneuploidy) or bizarre anomalies of certain chromosomes in animal and human cancers.[36] There is, for example, an exceptionally high frequency of chronic myelogenous leukemia in mongoloid individuals who are trisomic for chromosome 21; a peculiar chromosome has also been observed in leukemia not associated with mongolism. In many cancers, however, the chromosomes appear to be normal in number and gross appearance. It could, of course, be argued that chromosome aberrations, when they occur, are the result rather than the cause of the cancer state.

It is abundantly clear that cancer cells differ genetically from their normal progenitors, and the phenotypic expression of this difference is the characteristic lack of response to growth-controlling mechanisms in the host. Since the initiation of the malignant change is abrupt, and since the change is apparently irreversible and heritable, it may be regarded as a somatic mutation. According to this view, initiation is tantamount to somatic mutagenesis. It is therefore supportive of this concept that ionizing radiation as well as alkylating agents and other mutagens also possess carcinogenic activity. Likewise, many substances originally discovered to be carcinogens have since proved to be mutagenic in microorganisms.[37] Spontaneous cancers might arise by spontaneous mutagenesis, perhaps initiated by unrecognized carcinogens.

The genotypic change alone may not suffice for the establishment of a cancer. The role of promoters could be to create a local environment favorable to the selection and propagation of the new mutants. One indispensible feature of this "favorable local environment" may simply be the opportunity for sufficient cell division to permit phenotypic expression of an altered genotype. It will be recalled that even in actively multiplying bacteria there is a lag between the induction of a mutation and its expression, during which the wild-type gene product has to be "diluted" in the cytoplasm of progeny cells. In most tissues of higher organisms the rate of cell renewal is very slow. One can imagine that promoters act by inducing proliferative tissue reactions during which the precancerous mutant cells are stimulated to multiply. The carcinogen-induced mutation would only be expressed after the loss of those wild-type gene products that were concerned in the cell's response to growth-controlling substances in the tissue environment. Once a clone of mutant cells had become sufficiently large, it would fully express the phenotypic characteristics of cancer cells, thus becoming autonomous and independent of the promoter.

Among the agents known to be carcinogenic in animals and also mutagenic (usually tested on bacteria) are nitrosamines, diazomethane, alkane sulfates and sulfonates, β-propiolactone, ethyleneimine, triethylene melamine, 1,2,3,4-diepoxy-butane, dimethylhydrazine, and the nitrogen and sulfur mustards. These highly reactive electrophilic compounds all interact covalently with DNA.[37,38] Other carcinogens, however, had proved not to be mutagenic, making it seem that there was no necessary relationship between carcinogenicity and mutagenicity. This apparent discrepancy was cleared up by the discovery of metabolic transformation to proximate carcinogens in the animal body. In other words, the compounds that had been tested for mutagenicity were those known to produce cancer when administered to animals, but they were not the metabolically derived carcinogens that actually initiated the neoplastic process in the tissues. Strong support for the somatic muta-genesis theory is now provided by the consistent finding that proximate carcinogens are also mutagens, even when the parent compounds are not. A good example is 2-acetylaminofluorene (AAF) (Figure 11-3). As shown, a number of derivatives are formed, of which only the ester metabolites, such as the N-acetoxy and N-sulfate esters, are proximate carcinogens; they give rise directly to reactive electrophilic derivatives. N-methyl-4-aminoazobenzene (MAB) (p. 685) is subject to an analogous set of metabolic conversions.

Figure 11-4 shows a typical experiment in which various agents were tested for their ability to inactivate transforming DNA in vitro. A tryptophan-requiring bacterial strain was used for the test; the transforming DNA contained the genes needed for tryptophan synthesis. Each transformed cell produced a clone that could grow on the tryptophan deficient agar. The figure shows that only the proximate carcinogens derived from N-methyl-4-aminoazobenzene or 2-acetylaminofluorene were capable of inactivating the transforming DNA, whereas the parent compounds were not. The N-hydroxy derivative of AAF was not active, but a variety of esters of this derivative were active. Results of this sort led to the suggestion that N-hydroxy-lation is required for metabolic activation, but it is not the proximate carcinogen. Rather, an endogenous ester such as the acetoxy or sulfate derivative is probably the proximate carcinogen. Other experiments showed that the same active compounds produced mutagenic alterations in the tryptophan operon of the transforming DNA.

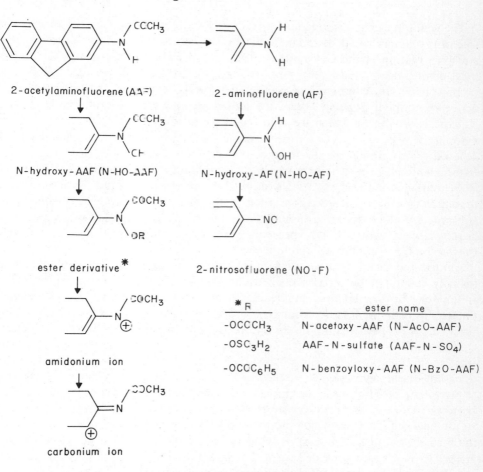

FIGURE 11-3. Metabolic conversion of 2-acetylaminofluorene to proximate carcinogens. *The various esters, represented by R, and listed at lower right, are converted readily to electrophilic reactant (carbonium compound) at lower left. Pathway for monomethylaminoazobenzene (MAB) (see p. 685) is analogous. (Modified from Miller and Miller, Figure 5.[39])*

Another study examined the mutagenic activity of a large number of carcinogens and chemically related noncarcinogenic chemicals on bacteriophage T4. Again, proximate carcinogens such as alkylating agents and N-acetoxy-AAF were potent mutagens, whereas mutagenic activity was much lower or absent in the noncarcinogenic compounds.[41] Mutagenic effects have also been demonstrated in mammalian cells treated with carcinogens. Here hamster cells growing in culture were exposed to various agents, and mutagenicity was assayed by testing for clones that had lost the ability to synthesize hypoxanthine-guanine phosphoribosyltransferase and thus had become resistant to 8-azaguanine (p. 475).[42] Both transition mutants (usually GC → AT) and frameshift mutants (cf. Chapter 10) have been identified.[41,43]

The considerable evidence suggesting a similarity between carcinogenesis and mutagenesis has led to the investigation of interactions between carcinogens and

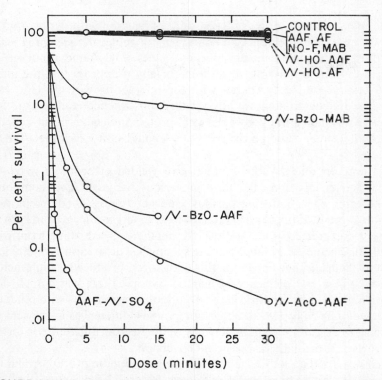

FIGURE 11-4. Inactivation of transforming DNA by proximate carcinogens in vitro. *Percent survival of functional DNA is shown as a function of time of exposure to various compounds in vitro. See text for description of method. All the agents were used at molar ratios between 7 and 20 per DNA nucleotide. For abbreviations, see Figure 11-3. (Modified from Maher et al., Figure 4.[40])*

DNA. Evidence of such interactions is indisputable, but the relationship to carcinogenesis is not clear. For one thing, noncarcinogenic congeners often also interact with DNA. Polycyclic hydrocarbons raise the "melting temperature" at which the strands of the double helix separate, i.e., they stabilize the hydrogen-bonded structure. DNA also solubilizes the normally water-insoluble hydrocarbons, as would be expected in any hydrophobic bonding to a polyanionic macromolecule. An intercalation mechanism is suggested by the size and planarity of the carcinogens: dibenzpyrene, for example, can be superimposed almost perfectly upon the adenine-thymine pair, much as was shown for a mutagenic acridine in Figure 10-11.[43a,44] One proposal envisions a perturbation by carcinogens of the statistical distribution of electrons over the whole DNA helix.[45]

It was known for many years that most alkylating agents are also carcinogenic. As already discussed, carcinogens that appear to be chemically inert are transformed metabolically to alkylating or arylating agents. A prominent action of monofunctional alkylating agents upon nucleic acids was noted in Chapter 10—an attachment to N at position 7 of guanine residues in DNA. Certain electrophilic reactants derived from carcinogens (e.g., AcO-AAF) also attach to guanine, but to C at position 8. Reactions of these types were observed after carcinogenic alkylating agents had acted upon mouse tissues in vivo.[46] The extent of reaction with tissue DNA seemed very low, with less than one molecule bound per 10^8 molecular weight (150,000 base pairs) of DNA. At the same time, one in 50 molecules of RNA and about one in every 1000 protein molecules were alkylated. Superficially it appears that the interaction with DNA was negligible compared with the interaction with protein. However, although it is difficult to suppose any serious consequence could ensue from the inactivation of so small a fraction of the total protein molecules in the cell, it is easy to imagine that a single "hit" on the cell's DNA could suffice to initiate the carcinogenic process.

Investigations on dimethylnitrosamine have yielded evidence of a relationship between carcinogenicity and alkylation in various tissues.[46] This compound is a very potent carcinogen, inducing various kinds of tumors in different tissues of experimental animals. It is converted to an active methylating agent in vivo (p. 686). When rats were treated with radioactive methyl-labeled dimethylnitrosamine, 7-methylguanine could be isolated from tissue nucleic acids, and N-methylhistidine from tissue proteins. In newborn rats, this carcinogen produced a high incidence of renal tumors and a low incidence of hepatic tumors; there was a high degree of methylation in the kidney but little in the liver. In this instance, as with other carcinogens that have to be converted to active compounds, differences in the sensitivity of various tissues to the carcinogenic action may well arise from differences in distribution of the enzymes that mediate the essential conversion.

More decisive are data on the correlation between binding to DNA and carcinogenic potency in a group of related carcinogens. Figure 11-5 presents graphically the

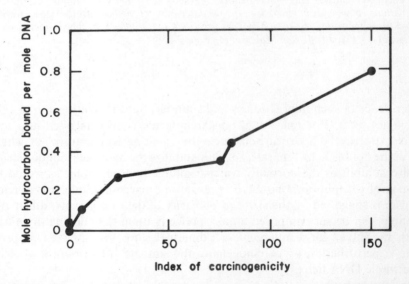

FIGURE 11-5. Relationship of carcinogenic potency to interaction with DNA. *The extent of binding certain carcinogenic hydrocarbons to mouse skin DNA is given on the y-axis, as moles of hydrocarbon bound per "mole" of DNA (estimated as containing 20,000 nucleotides, molecular weight 7×10^6). A measure of carcinogenic potency for application to mouse skin is given on the x-axis. Each solid circle represents a single hydrocarbon. The most potent carcinogen tested here was 7,12-dimethylbenzanthracene; the least potent were naphthalene and 1,2,5,6-dibenzanthracene. (From Brookes, Chart 5.[46])*

outcome of experiments in which seven different polycyclic hydrocarbons were painted on the skin of mice. In each case, the DNA was isolated and the bound hydrocarbon determined. It can be seen that although the total binding was small even for the compound bound in greatest amount, there was a good correlation between binding and carcinogenic potency. An important feature of this investigation was the fact that the binding was measured in the same tissue upon which the carcinogens acted directly. If an administered carcinogen had to be transformed metabolically to an active compound, which would then produce cancer at some tissue site, a correlation between DNA binding and potency would be expected only for the metabolic product, not for the administered substance itself.

The somatic mutation hypothesis has been criticized as too simplistic; doubt has been expressed, in view of the seemingly small extent of interaction between carcinogens and DNA, that "cancer mutations" could be regularly produced. But no special ability of carcinogens to cause these particular mutations need be supposed. It should be borne in mind that the animal body is a medium in which there is strong positive selection in favor of "cancer mutants." If a mutagen in contact with tissues induces a lethal mutation in some of the millions of cells present, those cells will simply die and be replaced, undetected by the investigator. Also undetected would be deletions of enzymes and other proteins resulting from viable mutations. But a single mutation leading to loss of responsiveness to growth regulation could give rise to a clone of cancer cells.

An interesting alternative to the somatic mutation hypothesis was developed around the finding that certain specific proteins, with which carcinogens react covalently, are no longer found in the corresponding cancer tissue.[47-51] It was pointed out that certain self-regulatory systems might exist in which the product of a structural gene, X, is an enzyme, which catalyzes the synthesis of an inducer, which acts at a regulatory site, promoting transcription of the very same structural gene, X. In such a hypothetical circuit, if a carcinogen destroyed the activity of the enzyme, the operon could remain shut permanently, giving rise to an apparently heritable defect. No convincing evidence in support of this ingenious theory has been adduced.

THE PRINCIPAL GROUPS OF CHEMICAL CARCINOGENS

Polycyclic Hydrocarbons

An intensive series of investigations during the period 1920–1940 sought to identify and isolate the active carcinogenic components of coal tar.[1] These studies led to the recognition of 3,4-benzpyrene (Figure 11-6) as the major coal tar carcinogen and also to the synthesis and biologic testing of many related compounds. Consequently, a rather detailed and quite satisfactory picture of structure-activity relationships in this group has emerged. In this chapter, the long established common terminology is retained. In the newer official terminology, the benzene rings of a reference compound, to which additional benzene rings are attached, are designated by letters; thus, 3,4-benzpyrene is benzo(a)-pyrene.[52] Figure 11-6 shows that all the carcinogenic hydrocarbons may be regarded as derivatives of phenanthrene. Phenanthrene itself, like the simpler anthracene, naphthalene, and benzene molecules, is completely

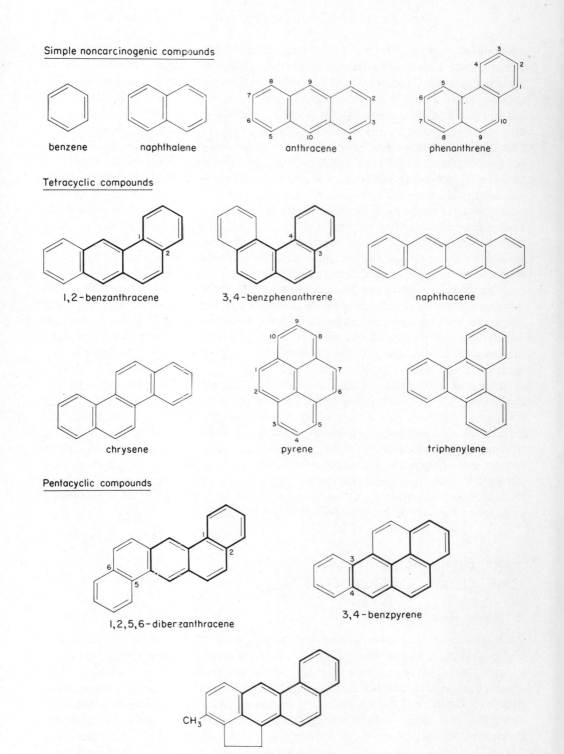

Simple noncarcinogenic compounds

benzene   naphthalene   anthracene   phenanthrene

Tetracyclic compounds

1,2-benzanthracene   3,4-benzphenanthrene   naphthacene

chrysene   pyrene   triphenylene

Pentacyclic compounds

1,2,5,6-dibenzanthracene   3,4-benzpyrene

3-methylcholanthrene

FIGURE 11-6. Structures of some polycyclic hydrocarbons. *The phenanthrene structure is emphasized in each of the carcinogenic compounds shown above. Phenanthrene itself is not carcinogenic, nor are pyrene, chrysene or triphenylene.*

devoid of carcinogenicity. Its tetramethyl derivative, 1,2,3,4-tetramethylphenanthrene (not shown) is weakly carcinogenic. Addition of a fourth benzene ring yields 1,2-benzanthracene or 3,4-benzphenanthrene, which are both carcinogenic. All other tetracyclic hydrocarbons are inert. Methyl substituents increase the carcinogenic potency of phenanthrene in a regular way; the 5,6-dimethyl derivative is nearly as potent as 1,2,5,6-dibenzanthracene. The related 3-methylcholanthrene is a very potent carcinogen, yet the homologous anthracene derivative (not shown), lacking the benzene ring at the 1,2-position (cf. 1,2-benzanthracene), is completely inactive. The potent carcinogen 3,4-benzpyrene is directly related to the 1,2-benzanthracene structure.

The principal necessary requirements for carcinogenicity may be summarized as follows: The entire polycyclic hydrocarbon must be coplanar. A phenanthrene nucleus must be present together with some substituents, preferably at least one additional benzene ring. The convex edge of the phenanthrene moiety must be free of substituents. In the series of tetracyclic hydrocarbons (Figure 11-6), most of the noncarcinogenic compounds fail to conform to the necessary specification. Naphthacene lacks the phenanthrene nucleus, chrysene and triphenylene contain substituents in forbidden positions. The noncarcinogenicity of pyrene is considered below. Potency of the carcinogenic hydrocarbons is usually enhanced by methyl substitutions at appropriate positions, and the cyclization of adjacent methyl groups (as in 3-methylcholanthrene) further increases potency.

The relationships described above were worked out on an empirical basis. Our understanding of them has been deepened by the development of an electronic theory.[53,54] The polycyclic hydrocarbons are by no means chemically inert but are characterized by a resonant system of π electrons, an orbital system extending over the entire molecule. Methods of quantum chemistry permit the calculation of electron densities associated with each part of the molecule. Such theoretical calculations led to the conclusion that a particular bond, represented by the 3,4-double bond of dibenzanthracene, was especially electron rich and therefore very reactive in the carcinogenic compounds. This bond was designated the "K region." For carcinogenic

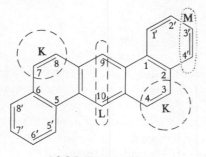

1,2,5,6-dibenzanthracene

activity, it appeared the electron density of the K region had to exceed a certain value, and at the same time the competing reactivity toward para substitution at the 9,10-positions ("L region") had to be less than a certain value. When these electronic indices were computed for a great many polycyclic hydrocarbons, the order with few exceptions corresponded to the order of carcinogenic potencies. The noncarcinogenic pyrene (Figure 11-6), for example, even though it contains a phenanthrene nucleus, has an insufficient reactivity at its K region. Thus, reactivity of the K region appeared to be the key to carcinogenicity among the polycyclic hydrocarbons.

The concept of K region reactivity received strong experimental support when complexes of hydrocarbon carcinogens with mouse skin proteins were isolated,[55] as already described. It was found that the carcinogenic hydrocarbons attached to tissue proteins through their K regions, whereas noncarcinogenic congeners did not. For example, the dicarboxylic acid derivative shown below was identified after the

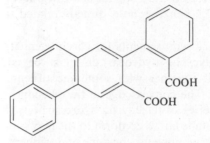

COOH
COOH

derivative of 1,2,5,6-dibenzanthracene

application of 1,2,5,6-dibenzanthracene to mouse skin. On the other hand, the dicarboxylic acid derivative itself did not bind to mouse skin proteins at all.

Further evidence indicated[43a,56,57] that formation of reactive epoxide intermediates and carbonium ions may precede the binding to cell constituents. An example would be the metabolic conversion of 1,2-benzanthracene to the corresponding epoxide. Aliphatic epoxides are alkylating agents, aromatic epoxides are arylating agents.

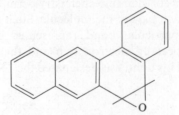

epoxide of 1,2-benzanthracene

Thus, it is likely that the mechanism of action of polycyclic hydrocarbons is basically the same as that of other carcinogens whose chemical reactivities are more obvious.

The main significance of the electronic theory was its ability to explain the empirical structure-activity findings in terms of a quantitative index of reactivity of a particular region of the carcinogen molecule. The theory directed attention toward chemical reactivity in a series of compounds that were generally regarded as inert, and thus set the stage for the discovery of covalent bonding between the polycyclic hydrocarbons and macromolecules in tissues.

Amines

Aromatic Amines.   Certain aromatic amines were first discovered to be carcinogenic in man as a result of industrial exposure. Naphthylamine, long used in the dye industry, was implicated in the causation of bladder cancer in exposed workers;

the latent period was estimated to be about 15 to 20 years.[58-60] Studies on the induction of bladder cancers by aromatic amines in experimental animals have shed light

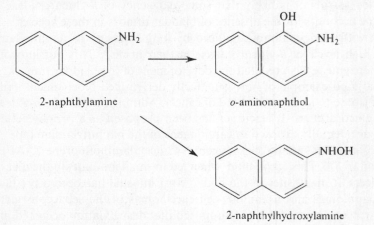

on how differences in metabolic pathways may affect carcinogenicity.[61-64] It seems abundantly clear now that the aromatic amines themselves are not carcinogenic but give rise to carcinogenic metabolites in vivo. Thus, 2-naphthylamine is transformed in the liver to two principal metabolites, the o-aminonaphthol and the hydroxylamine (N-hydroxy) derivative. When 2-naphthylamine itself was tested for carcinogenicity by direct implantation into the mouse bladder after incorporation into a wax pellet, no tumors were elicited. On the other hand, both the phenolic derivative and the hydroxylamine were potent carcinogens in this system.[61,65] It is doubtful, however, that o-aminonaphthol is a proximate carcinogen, since it is reabsorbed into the circulation after implantation in the bladder and can then be converted to the hydroxylamine and re-excreted into the urine.

The carcinogenic metabolites formed in the liver are rapidly conjugated there with glucuronic acid. In this manner, the tissues are usually protected from exposure to the carcinogens, for the glucuronides are inert. The glucuronides are excreted in the urine. In man and the dog, the urine is known to contain a soluble β-glucuronidase which, under acid conditions, releases free carcinogen in the ureters and bladder. This mechanism has been established in several ways.[61,65] It was shown that the carcinogenic activity responsible for producing bladder cancer is present in the urine rather than in the bladder circulation. Dogs were subjected to a surgical procedure whereby blind pouches of bladder were constructed; these pouches received their normal blood supply but were no longer in contact with urine. Naphthylamine administration produced no cancers in the pouches. If the ureters were transplanted to the sigmoid colon, tumors developed in them but not in the bladder. Finally, an inhibitor of β-glucuronidase (glucosaccharo-1,4-lactone) greatly reduced the incidence of bladder tumors in dogs when it was fed simultaneously with 2-naphthylamine.

It must be evident from the foregoing account that both the potency of an administered carcinogenic amine and the sites at which it will produce cancer depend upon the activity of drug-metabolizing enzymes. Conversion to N-hydroxy or other active products, formation of glucuronides (or sulfate esters), and enzymic hydrolysis at sites of excretion all influence the end result. It is found, for example, that in contrast to man and the dog, mice and rats are refractory to bladder carcinogenesis by aromatic amines. Since N-hydroxynaphthylamine is carcinogenic by implantation in the mouse bladder, and since 2-naphthylamine produces cancers at other tissue sites after it is fed to rats, it is likely that some deficiency of β-glucuronidase action in rodent urine accounts for the absence of bladder tumors in these species.

Patients with bladder tumors induced by long exposure to naphthylamine have unusually high levels of β-glucuronidase in their urine.[62] It is not known whether these high enzyme levels predated the development of the bladder tumors; if so, this would be a good example of how genetically determined biochemical individuality might predispose to a particular kind of cancer. Administration of a β-glucuronidase inhibitor (glucosaccharo-1,4-lactone) has been proposed as a prophylactic measure for people accidentally exposed to carcinogens of the naphthylamine type.

Another aromatic amine carcinogen is 2-acetylaminofluorene (AAF), already discussed on p. 675. This compound, when fed in small amounts in the diet of the rat, causes cancers at many sites in the body. Most unusual has been a predilection for inducing papillomas and squamous-cell carcinomas of the sebaceous gland in the external ear duct. Originally it was supposed that deacetylation occurred in the liver and that 2-aminofluorene was the active carcinogen. It became evident, however, that neither AAF nor 2-aminofluorene is directly carcinogenic. As already recounted for 2-naphthylamine, the analogous N-hydroxy derivative of AAF has been found to be a carcinogen.[66-68] AAF itself, for example, had no local carcinogenicity in rats after intraperitoneal injection, or in the intestinal tract after feeding. But the N-hydroxy derivative produced peritoneal sarcomas and gastric carcinomas upon direct contact, and esters of N-hydroxy-AAF were even more potent carcinogens.

The guinea pig provides a good further test of the hypothesis that metabolism to N-hydroxy-AAF is required for carcinogenesis, for this species does not carry out the N-hydroxylation reaction. Accordingly, AAF is not a carcinogen in this species. The guinea pig is not, however, intrinsically refractory; when N-hydroxy-AAF was fed or injected, intestinal, peritoneal, and subcutaneous cancers were readily obtained.

Another group of aromatic amines, important because of their widespread use in industry, includes 4-aminodiphenyl and 4-aminostilbene and their N-methyl derivatives.[58] In their carcinogenicity and metabolic conversion to N-hydroxy derivatives

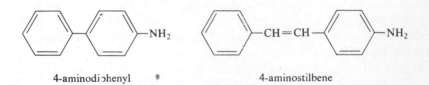

4-aminodiphenyl   4-aminostilbene

in vivo, these compounds closely resemble AAF and naphthylamine. They cause tumors in various tissues in the rat after feeding, especially in the acoustic sebaceous gland, intestine, liver, and kidneys. They also induce sarcomas at the sites of subcutaneous injection, but this does not rule out prior metabolic transformation to a proximate carcinogen, especially in view of the experimental finding that tumors can form at the site of injection of an inert substance after a carcinogen has been administered by mouth.

Finally, bladder cancers have been induced in mice by pellet implantation of saccharin, an aromatic amine that has been widely used as a noncaloric sweetening agent for human consumption.[69]

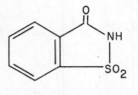

saccharin

Azo Dyes.   The azo dyes first commanded attention as carcinogens when they were found to produce liver cancers after incorporation into the diet of rats. The best-known member of the group is dimethylaminoazobenzene, also called "Butter Yellow"

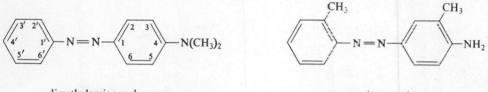

dimethylaminoazobenzene   o-aminoazotoluene

because of its former use as a food coloring. Numerous studies of the structure-activity relationships in this group have provided a body of empirical data about the requirements for carcinogenicity. As with the polycyclic hydrocarbons, modifications that alter the coplanar configuration abolish carcinogenicity. Methylation of the nitrogen atom at position 4 is essential for activity, but the monomethyl and dimethyl derivatives are equally effective; in any case, metabolic demethylation occurs in vivo. Substituents are tolerated (and sometimes increase potency) in position 3 (ortho to the amine nitrogen), as in the potent carcinogen o-aminoazotoluene. But substitution of any kind in position 2 (meta to the amino group) abolishes activity. Alkyl groups larger than methyl on the amine nitrogen decrease potency.

Although it seemed obvious that these compounds were transformed metabolically in the liver to active carcinogens, so many reactions occurred that it was uncertain which ones might be involved in carcinogenesis. Dimethylaminoazobenzene, for example, is demethylated to the monomethyl compound and to the primary amine, which is then acetylated. Ring hydroxylation at position 4' and also reductive cleavage of the azo linkage occur. Aromatic azo compounds are known to undergo benzidine rearrangements, so it was even possible to imagine a compound like 2,2'-azonaphthalene transformed by a series of steps to 3,4,5,6-dibenzcarbazole, a polycyclic hydrocarbon related to 1,2,5,6-dibenzanthracene. It now appears that the azo dyes, like other aromatic amines, are metabolized to N-hydroxy derivatives. These, in turn, are further metabolized to N-hydroxy esters, as shown earlier in Figure 11-3. Sulfate esters appear to be especially potent proximate carcinogens.[70-72]

Nitrosamines.   This is an interesting group of very potent carcinogens, of special significance because they may be formed in the stomach after ingestion of nitrites,[73-75]

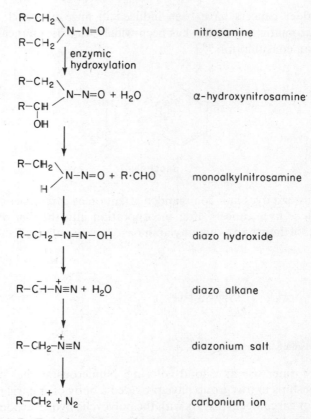

FIGURE 11-7. Transformation of nitrosamine to an active carcinogen. *A general scheme for the probable in vivo metabolic transformation is shown. The active alkylating agent may be the diazoalkane, the diazonium compound, or the carbonium ion. The R groups represent alkyl groups, usually methyl or ethyl. Dimethylnitrosamine is a potent carcinogen in vivo; the ultimate metabolic products would be methylating agents. (From Brookes, Chart 3.[46])*

and are present in tobacco smoke.[76] These agents are converted by hydroxylation reactions to alkylating agents. Figure 11-7 shows the probable scheme of metabolic transformation, but it is not certain if the actual alkylating intermediate is the diazoalkane (e.g., diazomethane from dimethylnitrosamine), or the diazonium salt, or carbonium ion. When dimethylnitrosamine was fed to rats, tumors of the liver, kidney, and lung were produced. The degree of methylation of tissue DNA and protein paralleled the carcinogenic potency for various tissues. A naturally occurring carcinogen, cycasin, found in certain nuts (Cycad nuts), alkylates by a similar mechanism.[77]

$$glucosyl-O-CH_2-N=N-CH_3$$
$$\downarrow$$
$$O$$

cycasin

The compound is a glucoside of methylazoxymethanol. In vivo it breaks down to diazomethane, and its methyl group is transferred to the 7-position of nucleic acid guanine.[78] It has also been shown to be mutagenic in bacteria.

N-hydroxy derivatives are formed in the pathway of transformation of amino-quinolines to proximate carcinogens. Thus 4-aminoquinoline-1-oxide is oxidized (and 4-nitroquinoline-1-oxide is reduced) to 4-hydroxyaminoquinoline-1-oxide. The proximate carcinogen is thought to be a further oxidation product, 4-nitroso-quinoline-1-oxide.[78a]

Urethane.   Urethane is another chemically inert compound known to be carcino-genic. It is now known that urethane is converted to an alkylating agent by N-hydroxylation in vivo.[79] This conversion is known to occur in rats, rabbits, and man.

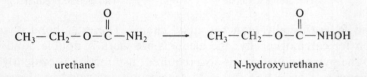

urethane   N-hydroxyurethane

Alternative modes of alkylation are indicated by isolation of two types of product from tissues. The urethane ethyl group may be transferred to form ethylmercapturic acid or S-ethylglutathione, both of which have been isolated after urethane administration. On the other hand, the entire N-hydroxyurethane moiety may be transferred; in this way, for example, N-acetyl-S-carbethoxycysteine is formed.

Alkylating Agents

The chemical reactivity of the alkylating agents was described in Chapter 1 and their mode of action as mutagens was discussed in Chapter 10. It was shown that the prin-cipal point of attack in the nucleic acids is the 7-position of guanine and that numerous groups in proteins can be alkylated, such as the imidazole nitrogen atom of histidine, the sulfhydryl group of cysteine or methionine, the carboxyl groups of the dicarboxylic acids. The bifunctional alkylating agents can cross-link the strands of the DNA duplex (Figure 1-2). That alkylating agents as a group are carcinogenic strengthens the analogy between carcinogenesis and mutagenesis. The most widely studied carcino-genic alkylating agents have been mechlorethamine (nitrogen mustard, Table 1-1), sulfonyl esters such as 1,4-dimethanesulfonoxybutane (busulfan, Table 1-1), and epoxy compounds like the cyclohexane derivative shown below:

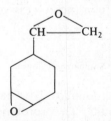

1-ethyleneoxy-3,4-epoxycyclohexane

Certain plant alkaloids (from *Senecio* species) are of great interest because they are alkylating agents with a pyrrolizidine structure.[67,80] If added to the diet, they pro-duce liver cancer in rats. Since plants containing them are used in folk medicine or to prepare bush teas in Africa and India, they might contribute to the high incidence of hepatoma in certain geographic areas. The general structure is given below:

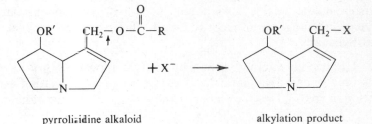

pyrrolizidine alkaloid   alkylation product

Both R and R' are usually branched alkyl chains. The ester bond is an absolute requirement for carcinogenecity; the alcohols are inert. A double bond in the 1,2-position of the pyrrolizidine ring is also required; its function is evidently to labilize the bond between oxygen and the methylene group, indicated by the small arrow. The reaction shown represents the alkylation of any nucleophilic receptor anion, such as a sulfhydryl group.

Ethionine, the ethyl analog of the amino acid methionine, is a liver carcinogen

$$CH_3-CH_2-S-CH_2CH_2CHCOOH$$
$$\underset{NH_2}{|}$$

ethionine

when it is fed to the rat.[81] The body's normal mechanism for methylation, in which methionine acts as a methyl donor, becomes a means of ethylation in the presence of ethionine. Normally, S-adenosyl-methionine participates in the normal methylation of purines in transfer-RNA. When S-adenosylethionine is formed, the ethyl group (shown below in bold type) is transferred to purines and other acceptors:

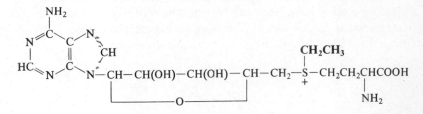

S-adenosylethionine

A number of lactones have been found to have carcinogenic activity and some of these occur in fungi and higher plants.[82] The prototype of the group is β-propiolactone.

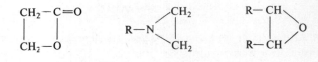

β-propiolactone   ethyleneimine   epoxide

The basis of the alkylating action of this compound is its strained ring structure, a feature common to such typical alkylating compounds as ethyleneimines and epoxides. β-Propiolactone is subject to two kinds of nucleophilic attack. Nonionized nucleophiles form addition products at the ester bond, ionized nucleophiles at the $-CH_2-O-$ bond, yielding carboxyethyl derivatives. For example, S-(2-carboxyethyl)-cysteine and 7-(2'-carboxyethyl)guanine have been isolated from organisms treated with β-propiolactone. In the same way, after exposure to the simple epoxide ethylene oxide, 7-(2'-hydroxyethyl)guanine could be isolated. That the intact lactone ring is essential to carcinogenesis was indicated by the finding that sarcomas were produced by subcutaneous injection of β-propiolactone in rats, whereas its hydrolysis product β-hydroxypropionic acid was inert.

Penicillin contains a β-lactam ring, which is essential to its antibacterial action, and which is opened in vivo when hapten-antigen complexes are formed (cf. Chapter 7). This suggests the possibility that the drug might be carcinogenic; at very high doses, it has indeed produced sarcomas in rats, although there is no evidence of carcinogenicity under conditions of therapeutic use. Other naturally occurring lactone carcinogens include parasorbic acid, from the berries of the mountain ash, and a fungal product, aflatoxin, to be discussed later (p. 692):

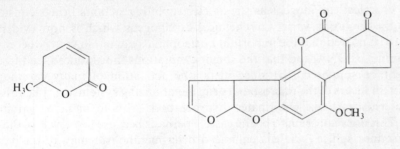

parasorbic acid   aflatoxin B$_1$

Another interesting carcinogen found in plants is safrole, present in oils of sassafras, nutmeg, and cinnamon. It is ingested in sassafras tea, and it was used as a flavoring agent in root beer until 1960, when it was banned in the United States following the demonstration of its hepatocarcinogenic properties in the rat. It is converted in vivo to a highly reactive electrophilic product, 1'-hydroxysafrole.[83,84]

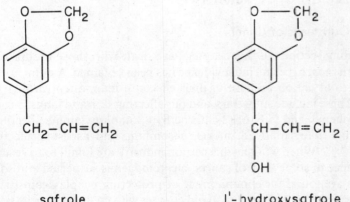

safrole   1'-hydroxysafrole

Alkylation and Arylation in the Carcinogenic Process

Advances in our understanding of drug metabolism are leading to a unitary view of the biochemistry of carcinogenesis. Some years ago, when such compounds as the polycyclic hydrocarbons the aromatic amines, and the azo dyes were thought of as rather nonreactive molecules, it was difficult to discern any common pathway that could account for the carcinogenic effects of such diverse chemical structures. The position has changed completely as a result of these developments, discussed earlier in detail: (1) the discovery of the carcinogenic properties of alkylating agents and the relationship between their carcinogenic and mutagenic properties; (2) the elaboration of a theory that stressed the chemical reactivity of a particular region in the polycyclic hydrocarbon molecule, and the proof of that reactivity by isolation of complexes with tissue proteins and nucleic acids; (3) the demonstration that all the seemingly unreactive carcinogens undergo extensive metabolic transformation in vivo, that some of the metabolites are more carcinogenic than the parent compounds, that metabolites are often active locally whereas the parent compounds are not, and that electrophilic metabolites are mutagenic although the parent compounds are not; (4) the fact that metallic carcinogens—beryllium, cadmium, cobalt, nickel, and lead—are also, in their ionic forms, electrophilic reactants.[85,86] "The characterization of ultimate chemical carcinogens as strong electrophilic reactants brings considerable order to the confusing variety of chemical carcinogens which is now evident."[5] It remains to be proved that the important nucleophilic reactant in vivo is a component (e.g., guanine) of DNA, and that the somatic mutations thus induced lead to cancer.

It might be supposed that since metabolic activation of many carcinogens is important, inducers of the microsomal drug metabolizing system (e.g., phenobarbital, aromatic hydrocarbons chlorinated hydrocarbons) should enhance carcinogenic potency. This does not seem to be the case,[87] perhaps because low levels of the microsomal enzymes suffice, whereas enhanced drug metabolism may result in further degradation of the proximate carcinogens to inert derivatives. Thus, phenobarbital has been reported to diminish rather than increase the carcinogenic effects of aflatoxin in the rat.[88] Likewise, workers exposed occupationally to DDT appear to have a lower incidence of cancer than expected.[89]

CARCINOGENIC HAZARDS IN THE HUMAN ENVIRONMENT

Epidemic Outbreaks of Cancer

The preceding sections of this chapter have dealt with those groups of carcinogens about which most experimental evidence has been obtained. A number of carcinogens first came to attention because of their effects in man, often through occupational exposure. These include soots, tars, and oils affecting skin and lungs, 2-naphthylamine, 4-aminodiphenyl, and N,N-bis(2-chloroethyl)-2-naphthylamine affecting the urinary bladder, and sulfur mustard, nickel, chromium, and asbestos affecting primarily the lungs.[5,90,91] When workers in a certain industry are found to have an inordinately high incidence of some kind of cancer, a carcinogen is suspected and soon identified, and means are found for eliminating it or protecting people against it. In this way, measures have been developed to avoid contact with coal tars, special precautions are taken in the dye industry, and azo dyes have been eliminated from use as food colorings.

In the same way, exposure to ionizing radiation is carefully controlled, now that its carcinogenicity is appreciated.[92] The incident of the watch dial painters who moistened their brushes alternatively with a solution of radium salts and with saliva and died of osteogenic sarcoma is not likely to be repeated. And the exposure of miners to radon-contaminated dust is now carefully regulated following the recognition of lung cancer as an occupational hazard. Nevertheless, we are still unexpectedly confronted from time to time by outbreaks of cancer on an epidemic scale—outbreaks that reflect the introduction of new carcinogens into our environment.[93,94] Fortunately, these episodes often affect animals first, so that precautionary measures may be taken in time to protect the human population. Two epidemics of liver cancer in animals will illustrate the effects of a sudden increase in the intake of a carcinogen in the diet. The production of lung cancer by cigarette smoking in humans will illustrate the effects of a gradually increasing exposure of the population to a carcinogen.

Several years ago, an epidemic of liver cancer afflicted the domestic trout population of the United States.[95] The suddenness with which the disease appeared and the very large numbers of fish involved were remarkable. It so happens that essentially all the trout living in rivers and lakes of this country are raised in hatcheries, and there they are fed on stock commercial diets. Since hepatoma is the characteristic form of cancer that develops when a carcinogen is eaten, it appeared likely that something was contaminating the fish diet. Experimental studies soon revealed that a control test diet could be devised that produced no tumors whatsoever. Extraction of the stock commercial diet with lipid solvents yielded an extract that was carcinogenic when added to the control diet. This finding led to a general survey of potential carcinogens administered to trout by addition to the diet. Table 11-1 presents results of feeding tests carried out for 20 months. Especially provocative was the finding that the insecticide DDT was carcinogenic, in view of the known widespread exposure of fish

TABLE 11-1. Production of trout hepatoma by substances fed in the diet.
Each substance was fed for 20 months at the concentration shown, and the number of hepatomas were then recorded. Of special interest is the carcinogenic activity of the insecticide DDT. (From Kraybill and Shimkin,[95] Table VIII.)

Chemical	Dose in diet (mg/100 g)	Frequency No.	%
Control test diet	—	0/300	0
Dimethylnitrosamine	480	38/46	82
Aminoazotoluene	120	22/43	52
Aminoazotoluene	30	3/49	6
Dichlorodiphenyltrichloroethane (DDT)	8	4/11	36
2-Acetylaminofluorene	30	9/45	20
Thiourea	480	7/38	18
p-Dimethylaminoazobenzene	30	6/46	13
Tannic acid	120	6/48	13
Urethane	480	5/55	11
Carbon tetrachloride	120	4/44	10
Carbarsone	480	5/50	10

to insecticides used agriculturally on a wide scale and carried into rivers and streams by runoff from the contaminated land.

Another extraordinary outbreak of cancer on an epidemic scale in animals was the turkey hepatoma that ravaged turkey flocks in England a few years ago.[95] In this instance, the causative agent was tracked down and isolated. The turkeys had been fed on spoiled pearut meal contaminated with a fungus, *Aspergillus flavus*, that produced the carcinoger (named aflatoxin), a polycyclic lactone whose structure was shown on p. 689. Aflatoxin is an extraordinary potent carcinogen. In the rat, for example, it produced hepatomas experimentally when fed at a daily dose of only 6 μg, whereas dimethylaminoazobenzene had to be given at a dose 500 times larger to obtain the same high incidence of liver tumors.

The discovery of aflatoxin and the circumstances of the turkey hepatoma epidemic have raised the general question whether mycotoxicoses present any hazard of carcinogenesis for human populations. Especially provocative are the statistics on the incidence of hepatic cancer in various populations. In Denmark, the incidence of this disease per 100,000 population is only 0.18; in the white population of the United States it is 1.7, nearly 10 times higher. Among Bantus in South Africa, the incidence reaches 14, and this one disease comprises 68% of all cancers in this ethnic group. The Bantus are known to eat moldy corn. The Japanese, who also have a high rate of hepatic cancer, may eat fungus-infected rice. It is possible that these characteristic dietary habits may account for the unusual prevalence of hepatoma among these groups. What dietary peculiarity accounts for the fact that the hepatoma rate is so much higher in the United States than in Denmark remains to be discovered.

Another striking example of geographic influence is the case of esophageal cancer. In certain parts of Iran, as many as 20% of all people who die after age 50 are killed by this disease, which is very rare in other parts of the world. Similarly, this disease is extraordinarily common in some parts of Africa but rare in others.[96] The specific environmental factors have thus far eluded identification.

Demographic-epidemiologic investigations can sometimes implicate environmental factors that would otherwise be lost in the mass of population statistics.[97] A sequential space-time cluster analysis in the United States for the years 1950–1967 found sufficient nonrandomness to suggest the influence of 11 different carcinogenic factors, each responsible for two or more tumor types.[98] Only two of them, cigarette smoking and solar radiation, could be identified with certainty. It has been estimated that at least one-third of all cancer deaths are attributable to unknown environmental agents and are, therefore, probably preventable. Since there are presently about 335,000 deaths per year from cancer in the United States, the importance of identifying and controlling carcinogenic factors in our environment is obvious.[99]

Smoking and Lung Cancer

The connection between smoking and lung cancer was first observed in retrospective studies reported in 1939.[100] An increase in the frequency of primary carcinoma of the lung was noted in routine autopsies on males, and an inquiry was initiated into the smoking habits of patients with lung cancer and of an equal number of healthy subjects matched as to age. A significant difference was found between the groups with respect to the frequency of heavy smoking. Since then, many more elaborate retrospective studies have been conducted, always with the same result. In addition, prospective studies have established beyond question that cancer of the lung is associated with cigarette smoking and that the incidence of this cancer is directly related to the extent and duration of smoking. Most significant, the incidence of lung cancer decreased in a group of heavy smokers after they stopped smoking.[101]

The growing concern about the high and increasing incidence of lung cancer led to the appointment by the Surgeon General, in 1962, of an advisory group of scientists to review all the available evidence about the relationship between smoking and health. The extensively documented reports of this committee were published in 1964, 1967, and 1972.[102,103] Conclusions about lung cancer were summarized as follows:

"Cigarette smoking is causally related to lung cancer in men: the magnitude of the effect of cigarette smoking outweighs all other factors. The data for women, though less extensive, points in the same direction. The risk of developing lung cancer increases with duration of smoking and the number of cigarettes smoked per day, and is diminished by discontinued smoking. In comparison with non-smokers, average male smokers of cigarettes have approximately a 9- to 10-fold risk of developing lung cancer and heavy smokers at least a 20-fold risk. The risk of developing cancer of the lung for the combined groups of pipe smokers, cigar smokers, and pipe and cigar smokers is greater than for non-smokers, but much less than for cigarette smokers."

With regard to cancer at other sites, the report states:

"Pipe smoking appears to be causally related to lip cancer. Cigarette smoking is a significant factor in the causation of cancer of the larynx."

The report goes on to indicate the presence of an association between tobacco use and cancer of the urinary tract or esophagus, but the data did not permit a decision as to whether these relationships are causal or not.

Table 11-2 presents some data of this report. These are pooled results of seven prospective studies initiated at various times between 1951 and 1960. The populations surveyed included British physicians, war veterans in Canada and the United States, and randomly chosen males in various parts of the United States. At the time a subject was enrolled in a study, his then-current smoking habits were recorded, as well as data about his age, occupation, and so on. More than 1 million usable questionnaire replies were obtained. Then, over a period ranging from about 2–10 years, the cause of death was ascertained for every enrolled person who died. Since death rates are obviously related to age, it was necessary to adjust the mortality rates thus determined to take account of the age distributions in the smoker and nonsmoker groups. When this adjustment had been made, it was found that the overall mortality was considerably higher in the smoker group. On the average, it was about 70% higher, and this difference was observed in all age groups. It was then asked whether the higher mortality for smokers applied uniformly to all causes of death, or whether certain specific causes of death were principally responsible.

The tabular data show that the mortality (expressed as the ratio of observed deaths in the smoker group to expected deaths if the death rate had been the same as in the nonsmoker group) was 11 times higher for cancer of the lung. It is especially noteworthy that whereas the mortality ratios were high for cancers of the lung, larynx, oral cavity, esophagus, bladder, and certain other tissues, elevated ratios were not observed for all kinds of cancer. Nor, in general, was there a comparably high mortality ratio for other causes of death. However, the mortality ratio for cardiovascular

TABLE 11-2. Mortality for specific causes of death among smokers and nonsmokers in prospective studies.

The data are from prospective studies on more than one million men. Subjects were categorized as to their smoking habits at the time of enrollment in the study. In the entire group, there were 37,391 deaths at the time the data were compiled (11,168 nonsmoker deaths and 26,223 smoker deaths). Column showing expected deaths was obtained by applying the death rate for nonsmokers to the number of smokers, making appropriate adjustment for the age distribution. If smokers and nonsmokers had the same death rate for a specific cause of death, the mortality ratio would be 1.0. (From *Smoking and Health*,[102] Table 19, p. 102.)

Underlying cause of death	Deaths (smokers)		Mortality ratio
	Expected	Observed	
Cancer of lung	170.3	1833	10.8
Bronchitis and emphysema	89.5	546	6.1
Cancer of larynx	14.0	75	5.4
Cancer of oral cavity	37.0	152	4.1
Cancer of esophagus	33.7	113	3.4
Stomach and duodenal ulcers	105.1	294	2.8
Other circulatory diseases	254.0	649	2.6
Cirrhosis of liver	169.2	379	2.2
Cancer of bladder	111.6	216	1.9
Coronary artery disease	6430.7	11,177	1.7
Other heart diseases	526.0	868	1.7
Hypertensive heart disease	409.2	631	1.5
General arteriosclerosis	210.7	310	1.5
Cancer of kidney	79.0	120	1.5
All other cancer	1061.4	1524	1.4
Cancer of stomach	285.2	413	1.4
Influenza, pneumonia	303.2	415	1.4
All other causes	1508.7	1946	1.3
Cerebral vascular lesions	1461.8	1844	1.3
Cancer of prostate	253.0	318	1.3
Accidents, suicides, violence	1063.2	1310	1.2
Nephritis	156.4	173	1.1
Rheumatic heart disease	290.6	309	1.1
Cancer of rectum	207.8	213	1.0
Cancer of intestines	422.6	395	0.9
All causes	15,653.9	26,223	1.68

diseases, although only 1.7, accounts for such a large proportion of all deaths, that the role of smoking may be very important in terms of actual numbers of deaths, despite the relatively low ratio. It is also interesting that the mortality ratio is rather low for deaths due to accidents, suicide, and violence, suggesting that differences in temperament do not play a significant role in relation to the higher mortality of smokers than of nonsmokers.

The quantitative relationship between the amount smoked and the death rate due to various diseases was ascertained in one of the most carefully conducted prospective studies.[101] In this investigation, questionnaires were sent to all members of the medical profession in the United Kingdom (59,600 men and women). Complete replies were received from 34,494 men, who were enrolled in the study. Four years and five months later, there had been 1714 deaths from all causes among men over 35. Of these deaths, 84 were due to lung cancer, 220 to other forms of cancer, 126 to other respiratory diseases, 508 to coronary thrombosis, and 779 to all other causes. Figure 11-8 shows the relationship between the death rates due to the various causes and the

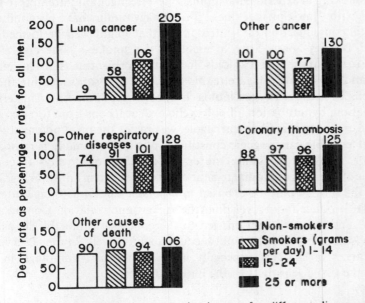

FIGURE 11-8. Relationship between death rates for different diseases and amount of smoking. *Smokers are classified according to the grams of tobacco smoked each day (one cigarette contains about 1 g). The rates shown for each cause of death are the death rates as percentages of the death rate due to that cause for all men. For example, the death rate due to lung cancer among nonsmokers was only 9% of the rate among all men (smokers and nonsmokers). If smokers and nonsmokers had the same death rate, the figure shown would be 100 for both. (From Doll and Hill, Table V.[101] By permission of the British Medical Association.)*

amount smoked. These data did not distinguish between cigarette, cigar, and pipe smokers; but further analyses showed a significantly higher death rate due to lung cancer among the cigarette smokers as compared with the other smokers. The figure as a whole shows that there was a striking positive correlation between the amount smoked and the death rate for lung cancer, and a weak positive correlation for other respiratory diseases and for coronary thrombosis, but not for other causes of death.

Most of the available data relate to males because the high incidence of lung cancer in men (but not in women) forced attention to males. It should not be concluded, however, that the sexes differ in sensitivity to tobacco carcinogenesis. Historically, women began smoking much later than men; and currently the incidence of smoking and the amount of tobacco consumed are much greater for men than for women. Moreover, the incidence of lung cancer among women is rising at a rate that reflects the increasing frequency of smoking among women.

Tobacco smoke contains various substances that could account for the carcinogenicity. The coal tar hydrocarbons are certainly present.[102-104] 3,4-Benzpyrene is the most potent carcinogen and is found in the largest amount, about 16 μg per 1000 cigarettes smoked. Dibenzpyrene and 1,2,5,6-dibenzanthracene are present in smaller amounts but are also potent carcinogens. Tobacco smoke condensates are certainly carcinogenic when painted on mouse skin and have also produced cancers in the lungs of rats.[104a] It has been difficult, however, to produce conditions analogous to human cigarette smoking in experimental animals, despite ingenious attempts to force smoke inhalation with "smoking machines." Pulmonary tumors have been induced in mice by subcutaneous injection of a nitrosamine that might well be formed in tobacco smoke.[105] Besides about 5 mg of nicotine, the smoke of one cigarette contains 100 μg of secondary amine alkaloids, including nornicotine. This compound reacts with NO and NO_2 found in cigarette smoke to form nitrosonornicotine, the postulated carcinogen. Bronchogenic carcinoma has been produced in hamsters by direct administration, by intubation, of polycyclic hydrocarbons from tobacco tar condensates. One compound, a dibenzcarbazole, was by far the most potent studied.[106]

Another possible carcinogenic constituent of cigarette smoke is radioactive polonium-210.[107] This isotope is an α emitter with a half-life of 138 days. Its concentration in the urine of smokers was found to be about six times that in nonsmokers. The amount to which the lungs would be exposed in a person smoking 40 cigarettes daily was estimated to produce about seven times the background radiation. Computations based on several uncertain assumptions led to the conclusion that the deposition of the polonium isotope in the lungs could account quantitatively for the observed incidence of lung cancer in smokers, especially if cocarcinogens (promoters) in the smoke increased the tissue sensitivity to the local radiation.

The Problem of Eliminating and Excluding Carcinogens from the Environment

Guidelines for the protection of the population against the hazards of environmental carcinogenesis are very difficult to formulate. The course of the controversy over smoking is very revealing of the economic, political, and psychologic barriers that impede action even after the scientific determination has been made. Certainly the evidence implicating cigarette smoking as a prime cause of cancer in humans is as thorough and convincing as one can expect to obtain. Nevertheless, cigarette consumption has continued at a high level among young people, in whom the risk is greatest because their total exposure will be longest. And although in the United States some minor modifications of cigarette advertising techniques have been enforced, no major regulatory action by government has been forthcoming. Many argue, indeed, that the principle of personal liberty includes liberty to indulge in a pleasure like smoking at the expense of future illness and premature death.

What, then, of drugs, food additives, insecticides, industrial wastes, and air pollutants, about which there may be only indecisive evidence of carcinogenicity?[69,108-112] Suppose such a substance proved to be carcinogenic at some particular dosage and route of administration in laboratory animals. How is one to extrapolate the result to man? We do not even know if there is a threshold of dosage below which no cancers would occur, regardless of the size of the exposed population.[94,113,114] And suppose a food additive or air pollutant were tested in 100 animals, or even 1000, and yielded no cancers. It might then be asserted that the substance was not a strong carcinogen. But might it be capable, nevertheless, of causing an unacceptable cancer rate in a large exposed population? If only one person in 1000 were affected, there would be 200,000 new cases of cancer in the United States. This result would be the more appalling because, unlike cigarette smokers, these victims would be exposed to the carcinogen through no choice of their own. This problem has been dealt with legislatively in the United States in the most conservative way possible. The so-called Delaney Amendment[115] to the Food and Drug Act prohibits the use, in foodstuffs, of any substance that has been shown (at any dose) to produce cancer in any experimental animal.

A tragic example of carcinogenesis in the human as a result of drug administration is the surprising appearance of vaginal adenocarcinoma in young women aged 15 to 19, reported in various parts of the United States in 1971. Because this type of cancer was virtually unknown in young women, intensive investigation was stimulated. In every case, it developed, the mothers of the victims had taken doses of the synthetic estrogen, diethylstilbestrol, during pregnancy. For a short time in the 1950's, this drug was popular for "threatened abortion," but fortunately, its use never became widespread. Obviously, initiation of these cancers had taken place in utero; only after a latent period of 15–20 years had the cancers developed.[116,117]

Unlike most drug toxicities, which are manifested fairly soon after exposure so that timely action is demanded by the public and can be taken by the authorities, the long-delayed effects of carcinogens rob the issue of urgency. Air pollution in our cities illustrates the contrast. Epidemics of smog-induced respiratory disease occur periodically, as recounted in Chapter 5. These episodes may be characterized by a high mortality rate and therefore may have a high "visibility" in the arena of public affairs. As a rule, urgent measures are then called for to institute more rigid control measures. But considerable evidence indicates that the same air pollutants contain carcinogens, whose effects are potentiated by respiratory viruses.[118–120] Yet this ever-present hazard appears too remote to engender demands for immediate action, especially when drastic controls might be expensive or disrupt an accustomed way of life. The position adopted by regulatory agencies is necessarily a compromise between the desire to eliminate all carcinogenic hazards and the necessity of weighing the magnitude of each hazard against the benefits derived from the hazardous substance or environment.

REFERENCES

1. G. WOLF: *Chemical Induction of Cancer*. London, Cassell and Co., Ltd. (1952).
2. K. YAMAGIWA and K. ICHIKAWA: Experimental study of the pathogenesis of carcinoma. *J. Cancer Res.* 3:1 (1918).
3. D. B. CLAYSON: *Chemical Carcinogenesis*. Boston, Little, Brown and Co. (1962).
4. G. E. W. WOLSTENHOLME and M. O'CONNOR, eds.: *Ciba Foundation Symposium on Carcinogenesis*. Boston, Little, Brown and Co. (1958).
5. J. A. MILLER: Carcinogenesis by chemicals: an overview. G. H. A. Clowes Memorial Lecture. *Cancer Res.* 30:559 (1970).
6. Twentieth Annual Symposium on Fundamental Cancer Research, 1966: *Carcinogenesis: A Broad Critique*. The Williams and Wilkins Co., Baltimore (1967).

7. H. V. GELBOIN: Carcinogenesis, the environment, and gene action. *Radiology* 99:251 (1971).

8. H. J. P. RYSER: Chemical carcinogenesis. *New. Eng. J. Med.* 285:721 (1971).

9. E. C. MILLER and J. A. MILLER: Mechanisms of chemical carcinogenesis: nature of proximate carcinogens and interactions with macromolecules. *Pharmacol. Rev.* 18:805 (1966).

10. G. PINCUS and E. P. VOLLMER, eds.: *Biological Activities of Steroids in Relation to Cancer.* New York, Academic Press (1960).

10a. O. V. ST. WHITELOCK, ed.: Genetic concept for the origin of cancer. *Ann. New York Acad. Sci.* 71:807 (1958).

11. F. BIELSCHOWSKY and E. S. HORNING: Aspects of endocrine carcinogenesis. *Brit. Med. Bull.* 14:106 (1958).

12. O. MÜHLBOCK and L. M. BOOT: The mechanism of hormonal carcinogenesis. In *Ciba Foundation Symposium on Carcinogenesis*, ed. by G. E. W. Wolstenholme and M. O'Connor. Boston, Little, Brown and Co. (1958), p. 83.

13. M. M. COOMBS, T. S. BHATT, and C. J. CROFT: Correlation between carcinogenicity and chemical structure in cyclopenta [a]phenanthrenes. *Cancer Res.* 33:832 (1973).

14. W. R. BRYAN and M. E. SHIMKIN: Quantitative analysis of dose-response data obtained with three carcinogenic hydrocarbons in strain C3H male mice. *J. Nat. Cancer Inst.* 3:503 (1943).

15. I. BERENBLUM and P. SHUBIK: A new, quantitative, approach to the study of the stages of chemical carcinogenesis in the mouse's skin. *Brit. J. Cancer* 1:383 (1948).

16. D. GAUDIN, R. S. GREGG, and K. L. YIELDING: DNA repair inhibition: a possible mechanism of action of co-carcinogens. *Biochem. Biophys. Res. Comm.* 45:630 (1971).

17. E. T. OPPENHEIMER, M. WILLHITE, I. DANISHEFSKY, and A. P. STOUT: Observations on the effects of powdered polymer in the carcinogenic process. *Cancer Res.* 21:132 (1961).

18. J. C. WAGNER: Asbestos cancers. *J. Nat. Cancer Inst.* 46:v (1971).

19. M. KANNERSTEIN and J. CHURG: Pathology of carcinoma of the lung associated with asbestos exposure. *Cancer* 30:14 (1972).

20. N. G. MAROUDAS, C. H. O'NEILL, and M. F. STANTON: Fibroblast anchorage in carcinogenesis by fibres. *Lancet* :807 (1973).

21. F. BISCHOFF and G. BRYSON: Carcinogenesis through solid state surfaces. *Prog. Exp. Tumor Res.* 5:85 (1964).

22. F. M. BURNET: The concept of immunological surveillance. *Prog. Exp. Tumor Res.* 13:1 (1970).

23. R. J. HUEBNER and G. J. TODARO: Oncogenes of RNA tumor viruses as determinants of cancer. *Proc. Nat. Acad. Sci. U.S.A.* 64:1087 (1969).

24. H. J. IGEL, R. J. HUEBNER, H. C. TURNER, P. KOTIN, and H. L. FALK: Mouse leukemia virus activation by chemical carcinogens. *Science* 166:1624 (1969).

25. B. C. CASTO, W. J. PIECZYNSKI, and J. A. DIPAOLO: Enhancement of adenovirus transformation by pretreatment of hamster cells with carcinogenic polycyclic hydrocarbons. *Cancer Res.* 33:819 (1973).

26. C. E. WHITMIRE and R. J. HUEBNER: Inhibition of chemical carcinogenesis by viral vaccines. *Science* 177:60 (1972).

27. Z. M. BACQ and P. ALEXANDER: *Fundamentals of Radiobiology*, 2nd ed. London, Pergamon Press (1961).

28. H. S. KAPLAN: Some implications of indirect induction mechanisms in carcinogenesis: a review. *Cancer Res.* 19:791 (1959).

29. W. M. COURT-BROWN: Nuclear and allied radiations and the incidence of leukaemia in man. *Brit. Med. Bull.* 14:168 (1958).

30. The effects on populations of exposure to low levels of ionizing radiation. Report of the Advisory Committee on the Biological Effects of Ionizing Radiations. Division of Medical Science, National Academy of Sciences—National Research Council, Washington, D.C. (1972).

31. W. L. MC GUIRE, K. HUFF, A. JENNINGS, and G. C. CHAMNESS: Mammary carcinoma: a specific biochemical defect in autonomous tumors. *Science* 175:335 (1972).

32. M. H. SALAMAN: The use of cocarcinogens in the study of carcinogenesis. In *Ciba Foundation Symposium on Carcinogenesis*, ed. by G. E. W. Wolstenholme and M. O'Connor. Boston, Little, Brown and Co. (1958), p. 70.

33. Y. BERWALD and L. SACHS: In vitro transformation of normal cells to tumor cells by carcinogenic hydrocarbons. *J. Nat. Cancer Inst.* 35:641 (1965).

34. E. BORENFREUND, M. KRIM, F. K. SANDERS, S. S. STERNBERG, and A. BENDICH: Malignant conversion of cells in vitro by carcinogens and viruses. *Proc. Nat. Acad. Sci. U.S.A.* 56:672 (1966).

35. C. HEIDELBERGER and P. T. IYPE: Malignant transformation in vitro by carcinogenic hydrocarbons. *Science* 155:214 (1967).

36. T. S. HAUSCHKA: The chromosomes in ontogeny and oncogeny. *Cancer Res.* 21:957 (1961).

37. F. K. ZIMMERMANN: Genetic aspects of carcinogenesis. *Biochem. Pharm.* 20:985 (1971).

38. P. BROOKES: On the interaction of carcinogens with DNA. *Biochem. Pharm.* 20:999 (1971).

39. J. A. MILLER and E. C. MILLER: The metabolic activation of carcinogenic aromatic amines and amides. *Prog. Exp. Tumor Res.* 11:273 (1969).

40. V. H. MAHER, E. C. MILLER, J. A. MILLER, and W. SZYBALSKI: Mutations and decreases in density of transforming DNA produced by derivatives of the carcinogens 2-acetylaminofluorene and N-methyl-4-aminoazobenzene. *Mol. Pharmacol.* 4:411 (1968).

41. T. H. CORBETT, C. HEIDELBERGER, and W. F. DOVE: Determination of the mutagenic activity to bacteriophage T4 of carcinogenic and noncarcinogenic compounds. *Mol. Pharmacol.* 6:667 (1970).

42. E. HUBERMAN, L. ASPIRAS, C. HEIDELBERGER, P. L. GROVER, and P. SIMS: Mutagenicity to mammalian cells of epoxides and other derivatives of polycyclic hydrocarbons. *Proc. Nat. Acad. Sci. U.S.A.* 68:3195 (1971).

43. B. N. AMES, P. SIMS, and P. L. GROVER: Epoxides of carcinogenic polycyclic hydrocarbons are frameshift mutagens. *Science* 176:47 (1972).

43a. E. BOYLAND: Polycyclic hydrocarbons. *Brit. Med. Bull.* 20:121 (1964).

44. P. O. P. TS'O and P. LU: Interaction of nucleic acids. I. Physical binding of thymine, adenine, steroids, and aromatic hydrocarbons to nucleic acids. *Proc. Nat. Acad. Sci. U.S.A.* 51:17 (1964).

45. T. A. HOFFMANN and J. LADIK: A possible correlation between the effects of some carcinogenic agents and the electronic structure of DNA. *Cancer Res.* 21:474 (1961).

46. P. BROOKES: Quantiative aspects of the reaction of some carcinogens with nucleic acids and the possible significance of such reactions in the process of carcinogenesis. *Cancer Res.* 26:1994 (1966).

47. H. C. PITOT and C. HEIDELBERGER: Metabolic regulatory circuits and carcinogenesis. *Cancer Res.* 23:1694 (1963).

48. C. HEIDELBERGER: The relation of protein binding to hydrocarbon carcinogenesis. In *Ciba Foundation Symposium on Carcinogenesis*, ed. by G. E. W. Wolstenholme and M. O'Connor. Boston, Little, Brown and Co. (1958), p. 179.

49. G. R. DAVENPORT, C. W. ABELL, and C. HEIDELBERGER: The interaction of carcinogenic hydrocarbons with tissues. VII. Fractionation of mouse skin proteins. *Cancer Res.* 21:599 (1961).

50. E. WEILER: Loss of specific cell antigen in relation to carcinogenesis. In *Ciba Foundation Symposium on Carcinogenesis*, ed. by G. E. W. Wolstenholme and M. O'Connor. Boston, Little, Brown and Co. (1958), p. 165.

51. T. KUROKI and C. HEIDELBERGER: Determination of the h-protein in transformable and transformed cells in culture. *Biochemistry* 11:2116 (1972).

52. International Union of Pure and Applied Chemistry. Definitive rules for nomenclature of organic chemistry. *J. Am. Chem. Soc.* 82:5545 (1960).

53. A. PULLMAN and B. PULLMAN: Electronic structure and carcinogenic activity of aromatic molecules. New development. *Adv. Cancer Res.* 3:117 (1955).

54. A. PULLMAN: The theory of chemical carcinogenesis and the problem of hydrocarbon–protein interactions. In *Biopolymers, Symposia No. 1* (1964), pp. 47–65.

55. V. T. OLIVERIO and C. HEIDELBERGER: The interaction of carcinogenic hydrocarbons with tissues. V. Some structural requirements for binding of 1,2,5,6-dibenzanthracene. *Cancer Res.* 18:1094 (1958).

56. E. CAVALIERI and M. CALVIN: Molecular characteristics of some carcinogenic hydrocarbons. *Proc. Nat. Acad. Sci. U.S.A.* 68:1251 (1971).

57. M. J. COOKSON, P. SIMS, and P. L. GROVER: Mutagenicity of epoxides of polycyclic hydrocarbons correlates with carcinogenicity of parent hydrocarbons. *Nature New Bio.* 234:186 (1971).

58. A. L. WALPOLE and M. H. C. WILLIAMS: Aromatic amines as carcinogens in industry. *Brit. Med. Bull.* 14:141 (1958).

59. G. R. PROUT: Current concepts: bladder carcinoma. *New Eng. J. Med.* 287:86 (1972).

60. C. A. VEYS: Two epidemiological inquiries into the incidence of bladder tumors in industrial workers. *J. Nat. Cancer Inst.* 43:219 (1969).
61. D. B. CLAYSON: The aromatic amines. *Brit. Med. Bull.* 20:115 (1964).
62. E. BOYLAND: The biochemistry of cancer of the bladder. *Brit. Med. Bull.* 14:153 (1958).
63. J. L. RADOMSKI and E. BRILL: Bladder cancer induction by aromatic amines: role of N-hydroxy metabolites. *Science* 167:992 (1970).
64. J. H. WEISBURGER and E. K. WEISBURGER: Biochemical formation and pharmacological, toxicological, and pathological properties of hydroxylamines and hydroxamic acids. *Pharmacol. Rev.* 25:1 (1973).
65. G. M. BONSER, D. B. CLAYSON, and J. W. JULL: Some aspects of the experimental induction of tumours of the bladder. *Brit. Med. Bull.* 14:146 (1958).
66. E. C. MILLER, J. A. MILLER, and H. A. HARTMANN: N-Hydroxy-2-acetylaminofluorene: a metabolite of 2-acetylaminofluorene with increased carcinogenic activity in the rat. *Cancer Res.* 21:815 (1961).
67. J. A. MILLER and E. C. MILLER: Natural and synthetic chemical carcinogens in the etiology of cancer. *Cancer Res.* 25:1292 (1965).
68. J. A. MILLER and E. C. MILLER: Metabolism of drugs in relation to carcinogenicity. *Ann. N.Y. Acad. Sci.* 123:125 (1965).
69. G. T. BRYAN, E. ERTURK, and O. YOSHIDA: Production of urinary bladder carcinomas in mice by sodium saccharin. *Science* 168:1238 (1970).
70. J. R. DEBAUN, E. C. MILLER, and J. A. MILLER: N-Hydroxy-2-acetylaminofluorene sulfotransferase: its probable role in carcinogenesis and in protein-(methion-S-yl) binding in rat liver. *Cancer Res.* 30:577 (1970).
71. J. A. MILLER: Carcinogenesis by chemicals: an overview. *Cancer Res.* 30:559 (1970).
72. L. A. POIRIER, J. A. MILLER, E. C. MILLER, and K. SATO: N-Benzoyloxy-N-methyl-4-aminobenzene: its carcinogenic activity in the rat and its reactions with proteins and nucleic acids and their constituents in vitro. *Cancer Res.* 27:1600 (1967).
73. P. N. MAGEE and R. SCHOENTAL: Carcinogenesis by nitroso compounds. *Brit. Med. Bull.* 20:102 (1964).
74. I. A. WOLFF and A. E. WASSERMAN: Nitrates, nitrites and nitrosamines. *Science* 177:15 (1972).
75. M. C. ARCHER, S. D. CLARK, J. E. THILLY, and S. R. TANNENBAUM: Environmental nitroso compounds: reaction of nitrite with creatine and creatinine. *Science* 174:1341 (1971).
76. D. E. JOHNSON and J. W. RHOADES: N-Nitrosamines in smoke condensate from several varieties of tobacco. *J. Nat. Cancer Inst.* 48:1845 (1972).
77. D. W. E. SMITH: Mutagenicity of cycasin aglycone (methylazoxymethanol), a naturally occurring carcinogen. *Science* 152:1273 (1966).
78. H. DRUCKREY and A. LANGE: Carcinogenicity of azoxymethane dependent on age in BD rats. *Fed. Proc.* 31:1482 (1972).
78a. A. MATSUYAMA and C. NAGATA: Detection of the unstable intermediate, 4-nitrosoquinoline 1-oxide. In *Topics in Chemical Carcinogenesis*, ed. by W. Nakahara, S. Takayama, T. Sugimura, and S. Adashima. Tokyo, University of Tokyo Press (1972).
79. E. BOYLAND and R. NERY: The metabolism of urethane and related compounds. *Biochem. J.* 94:198 (1965).
80. C. C. J. CULVENOR A. T. DANN, and A. T. DICK: Alkylation as the mechanism by which the hepatotoxic pyrrolizidine alkaloids act on cell nuclei. *Nature* 195:570 (1962).
81. E. FARBER: Ethionine carcinogenesis. *Adv. Cancer Res.* 7:383 (1963).
82. F. DICKENS: Carcinogenic lactones and related substances. *Brit. Med. Bull.* 20:96 (1964).
83. P. BORCHERT, P. G. WISLOCKI, J. A. MILLER and E. C. MILLER: The metabolism of the naturally occurring hepatocarcinogen safrole to 1'-hydroxysafrole and the electrophilic reactivity of 1'-acetoxysafrole. *Cancer Res.* 33:575 (1973).
84. P. BORCHERT, J. A. MILLER, E. C. MILLER, and T. K. SHIRES: 1'-Hydroxysafrole, a proximate carcinogenic metabolite of safrole in the rat and mouse. *Cancer Res.* 33:590 (1973).
85. D. B. CLAYSON: *Chemical Carcinogenesis*. Baltimore, William and Wilkins (1962).
86. F. W. SUNDERMAN, JR.: Nickel carcinogenesis. *Dis. Chest* 54:527 (1968).
87. W. F. BENEDICT, N. CONSIDINE, and D. W. NEBERT: Genetic differences in aryl hydrocarbon hydroxylase induction and benzo[a]pyrene-produced tumorigenesis in the mouse. *Mol. Pharmacol.* 6:266 (1973).

88. A. E. M. MC CLEAN and A. MARSHALL: Reduced carcinogenic effect of aflatoxin in rats given phenobarbitone. *Brit. J. Exp. Pathol.* 52:322 (1971).
89. E. R. LAWS: Evidence of antitumorigenic effects of DDT. *Arch. Environ. Health* 23:181 (1971).
90. A. MUNN: Assessment of industrial bladder cancer hazards from experimental data. *J. Nat. Cancer Inst.* 43:277 (1969).
91. F. P. LI, J. F. FRAUMENI, N. MANTEL, and R. W. MILLER: Cancer mortality among chemists. *J. Nat. Cancer Inst.* 43:1159 (1969).
92. J. B. LITTLE: Environmental hazards: ionizing radiation. *New Eng. J Med.* 275:929 (1966).
93. Epidemiologic approaches to cancer etiology. Symposium sponsored by the American Cancer Society. *Cancer Res.* 25:1271 (1965).
94. E. BOYLAND: The biological examination of carcinogenic substances. *Brit. Med. Bull.* 14:93 (1958).
95. H. F. KRAYBILL and M. B. SHIMKIN: Carcinogenesis related to foods contaminated by processing and fungal metabolites. *Adv. Cancer Res.* 8:191 (1964).
96. Editorial: Oesophageal cancer in Africa. *Lancet* 2:1178 (1969).
97. Metropolitan Life: Regional variations in mortality from cancer. *Statistical Bulletin* 54:3 (1973).
98. F. BURBANK: A sequential space-time cluster analysis of cancer mortality in the United States: etiological implications. *Am. J. Epidem.* 95:393 (1972).
99. National Cancer Institute: *Etiology Annual Program Review Document, Fiscal Year 1972.* U.S. D.H.E.W., Public Health Service, N.I.H. (1972).
100. F. H. MÜLLER: Tabakmissbrauch und Lungencarcinom. *Z. Krebsforsch.* 49:57 (1939).
101. R. DOLL and A. B. HILL: Lung cancer and other causes of death in relation to smoking. *Brit. Med. J.* 2:1071 (1956).
102. *Smoking and Health.* Report of the Advisory Committee to the Surgeon General of the Public Health Service, U.S. Public Health Service Publication No. 1103. Washington, D.C., U.S. Government Printing Office (1964).
103. U.S. Department of Health, Education, and Welfare: *The Health Consequences of Smoking, A Public Health Service Review: 1967.* Public Health Service Publication No 1696, Washington, D.C. (1968). See also the 1972 report.
104. E. L. WYNDER and D. HOFFMANN: Experimental tobacco carcinogenesis. *Adv. Cancer Res.* 8:249 (1964).
104a. M. F. STANTON, E. MILLER, C. WRENCH, and R. BLACKWELL. Experimental induction of epidermoid carcinoma in the lungs of rats by cigarette smoke condensate. *J. Nat. Cancer Inst.* 49:867 (1972).
105. E. BOYLAND, F. J. C. ROE, and J. W. GORROD: Induction of pulmonary tumours in mice by nitrosonornicotine, a possible constituent of tobacco smoke. *Nature* 202:1126 (1964).
106. P. SHUBIK: Current status of chemical carcinogenesis. *Proc. Nat. Acad. Sci. U.S.A.* 69:1052 (1972).
107. E. P. RADFORD, JR., and V. R. HUNT: Polonium-210: a volatile radioelement in cigarettes. *Science* 143:247 (1964).
108. W. C. HUEPER: Environmental carcinogenesis and cancers. *Cancer Res.* 21:842 (1961).
109. R. TRUHAUT, ed.: *Potential Carcinogenic Hazards from Drugs.* UICC Monograph Series, Vol. 7. Berlin, New York, Springer-Verlag (1967).
110. R. L. BRENT: Protecting the public from teratogenic and mutagenic hazards. *J. Clin. Pharmacol.* 12:61 (1972).
111. F. J. C. ROE: The relevance of preclinical assessment of carcinogenesis. *Clin. Pharmacol. Therap.* 7:77 (1966).
112. M. KUSCHNER and S. LASKIN: Experimental models in environmental carcinogenesis. *Am. J. Pathol.* 64:183 (1971).
113. N. MANTEL: The concept of threshold in carcinogenesis. *Clin. Pharmacol. Therap.* 4:104 (1963).
114. T. F. HATCH: Thresholds: do they exist? *Arch. Environ. Health* 22:687 (1971).
115. "Delaney amendment" is a clause of the Food Additive Amendment of 1958 to the Federal Food, Drug, and Cosmetic Act of 1938. Reference can be found under Title 21 USC 348(c)(3)(A).
116. P. GREENWALD, J. J. BARLOW, P. C. NASCA, and W. S. BURNETT: Vaginal cancer after maternal treatment with synthetic estrogens. *New Eng. J. Med.* 285:390 (1971).
117. A. L. HERBST, R. J. KURMAN, R. E. SCULLY, and D. C. POSKANZER: Clear-cell adenocarcinoma of the genital tract in young females. *New Eng. J. Med.* 287:1259 (1972).

118. P. KOTIN and D. V. WISELEY: Production of lung cancer in mice by inhalation exposure to influenza virus and aerosols of hydrocarbons. *Prog. Exp. Tumor Res.* 3:186 (1963).
119. H. L. FALK and P. KOTIN: Chemistry, host entry, and metabolic fate of carcinogens. *Clin. Pharmacol. Therap.* 4:88 (1963).
120. E. SAWICKI and K. CASSEL, JR., eds: Symposium on Analysis of Carcinogenic Air Pollutants. *National Cancer Institute Monograph No. 9* (1962).

CHAPTER 12
Chemical Teratogenesis

Certain chemical agents can affect the somatic cells of a developing embryo in such a way that defects of one or another organ system are produced. If the embryonic germ cells escape damage, only the individual will be affected; thus, most congenital anomalies are not hereditary. Substances that cause abnormalities of fetal development are called *chemical teratogens*.[1-17]

A more remarkable process than embryogenesis is hard to imagine. The finely balanced interplay of cell proliferation, differentiation, migration, and finally organogenesis represents a precisely programmed sequence of events, repeating itself in each detail for every zygote of a species.[18-20] Underlying the morphologic development of the embryo is a progressive unfolding of biochemical potentialities, a temporally regulated transcription and translation of genetic messages, the details of which we are only beginning to understand. Embryogenesis involves complex interactions in both time and space. In the earliest stages, rapid cell multiplication is the rule. The numerous products of these early cell divisions have different potentialities, depending upon their relative positions in the embryonic mass. Differentiation begins very early, in some species as early as the 2- or 4-cell stage. Subsequent development of primordial tissue components and organ precursors depends strongly upon mutual interactions of adjacent cell groups, apparently through chemical mediators or modifiers.[21] Migration, infolding, interpenetration, and encompassing of one cell group by another characterize a later stage of organogenesis. These spatial rearrangements account for the ectodermal origin of many internal viscera, the encapsulation of the nervous elements of the adrenal medulla by the mesodermally-derived cortex, the segregation of germ cells in the gonads, and so on. Still later, midline closures of bilaterally symmetric tissues occur, such as the facial structures (lip and palate), the cranium, vertebrae, and anterior body wall. Final morphologic and functional development occurs at various times in different organs and is sometimes completed only after birth.

Two predictions could be made, a priori, on the basis of our knowledge of embryonic development: first, that so complicated a series of events could be interfered with in very specific ways; and second, that the result of such interference could depend strongly upon the timing. Because each step in embryogenesis may depend upon a previous one and because numerous tissues and organs are developing in parallel, even a temporary delay in the development of one group of cells may throw it out of phase with the rest of the embryo and thus lead to an eventual malformation. This has been shown quite clearly to be the case for reno-ureteral defects induced by folic acid deficiency in rats. Here the vitamin deficiency disturbed the migration of primordial cell groups so that later, after the brief vitamin deficiency was terminated, they could no longer attain their correct anatomic position.[22]

Teratogenic research was greatly stimulated on three occasions by the accidental discovery of an external agency capable of producing congenital malformation in man. With increasing awareness of the biologic effects of radiation came the finding, about half a century ago, that pelvic x-irradiation during pregnancy can result in the birth of a malformed child. More surprising was the discovery in Australia[23] in 1940 than an unusually large number of blind or deaf children were born following an epidemic of the mild virus disease rubella. Even if the symptoms of the disease in the mother were mild, seriously defective offspring were sometimes produced when the infection occurred during the first trimester of pregnancy. The experience served as an important stimulus to experimentation with chemical teratogens in animals. Finally, the thalidomide disaster of 1960–1962 (p. 717) showed that an ordinary drug can also produce fetal malformations on a large scale in human populations.

EXPERIMENTAL TERATOGENESIS

Methods

Animal experiments have chiefly employed mice, rabbits, and rats, but primates have also been used.[23a] Like humans, these mammals have a placenta, so that drugs are exposed to maternal tissues and subjected to maternal metabolism before entering the fetus. Moreover, the gestation period is conveniently short (only 3 weeks in a rat or mouse), multiple births are the rule (so that each treated female yields a large amount of experimental data), and housing and maintenance of large numbers of animals is simple because of their small size and low cost. The most serious limitation in the use of rodents is the different structure (and possibly function) of their placentae as compared with that of the human. Rhesus monkeys and other primates have therefore also been used.[24] Placental structure and function, as well as the pattern of embryologic development, are like those in the human. And although primates are very expensive so that large-scale studies are impractical, they respond to the known teratogens that affect humans, such as thalidomide, rubella virus, and androgenic steroids.

Chick embryos are useful when the purpose of an experiment is to study the action of a proximate teratogen (cf. proximate carcinogen, p. 668), which acts directly, without the necessity of prior metabolic transformation. The teratogen can be placed in direct contact with the developing embryo. A good correlation was found for the teratogenic effects of diverse compounds in chick embryos and in rodents.[25] The presence of a yolk sac in both species may explain why some agents that are teratogenic in chicks and rodents are less active in primates, as is the case with trypan blue (p. 713).

Experiments on teratogenesis in rodents begin with isolation of virgin females and determination of the estrous cycle by vaginal smears. Matings can then be arranged at the time of ovulation. Since the timing of teratogenic treatments is extremely critical, it is essential to know precisely when conception occurs. After mating, the females are isolated again, treated as desired with a teratogen, and sacrificed just before term. Since cannibalism is frequent among rodents, the offspring must be obtained by caesarean section in order to obtain reliable data. This procedure permits all implantation sites to be examined and every product of conception to be accounted for as a resorbed, dead, malformed live, or fully developed normal fetus. Gross examination will reveal the most obvious malformations; microscopic examination will reveal others. To be certain all anomalies are detected, an exhaustive gross and microscopic analysis of each fetus is required. Hitherto in investigations of teratogenesis, the emphasis has been almost exclusively upon morphologic abnormalities; now increasing attention is paid to effects of teratogens on biochemical processes in the developing and mature fetus.[26–28] Agents that block DNA synthesis,[28a] RNA synthesis, or protein synthesis may certainly be teratogenic, if the timing is right and the fetus as a whole survives.

Selectivity of Action in Teratogenesis

Of principal interest are teratogens that interfere directly with fetal development at doses that do not disturb placental function or cause serious maternal toxicity. A great many teratogenic agents meet this criterion of selective toxicity for the fetus. There is often a considerable range between the dose that induces fetal malformation and the dose that causes maternal death. Indeed, the most dangerous teratogens may be just those that are well tolerated by the mother in a dose range that is selectively damaging to fetal organogenesis but is not seriously toxic to the fetus as a whole. An agent that is selectively toxic to the mother, or one that is so toxic to the fetus that fetal death and resorption (or abortion) occur, would not present much hazard as a teratogen.[29] It has been shown that even such maternal disorders as severe hemorrhagic anemia and liver damage do not have teratogenic consequences.[30] Most teratogens do not impair placental function, and the most convincing experiments on teratogenesis include a morphologic demonstration of placental integrity. That experimental fetal malformations are so easy to produce without significant harm to the mother is consistent with the effects of rubella and of thalidomide in humans, and points up the risk that drugs and other environmental agents, innocuous otherwise, might be responsible for unexplained human malformations.

All teratogens, when administered at high dosage or very early in embryonic development, can cause fetal death followed by abortion or resorption of the fetus. For example, actinomycin D (which inhibits DNA-dependent RNA synthesis) was administered once intraperitoneally to pregnant rats at various times in gestation.[31] On the 20th day of gestation, the rats were sacrificed and all fetuses and implantation sites were examined. The peak effects occurred when the drug was given between the seventh and tenth day. Fetal death and the incidence of malformations among survivors ran a parallel course. Both effects were dose related, and the sensitivity to both was maximum at the same time in gestation.

Many substances can kill fetuses selectively but are not necessarily teratogenic for survivors. The mitotic poisons colchicine and podophyllotoxin are good examples. Lipopolysaccharides from *Brucella abortus* kill all rat fetuses when administered on the 11th day of gestation and display the same sharp dependence on time of administration as do compounds with teratogenic action. Lipopolysaccharides from several enteric bacteria are teratogenic in rats, and they are known to cause abortion in humans. Aminopterin, at a dose that kills most rat fetuses, is not teratogenic for survivors; yet aminopterin in the human, if it fails to produce abortion, results in fetal malformations. These observations, taken together with the significant statistical association between intra-uterine death, spontaneous abortion, stillbirth, and congenital malformation in the human, indicate a close relationship between teratogenesis and the more general problem of reproductive wastage.

Genetic Influences

If embryogenesis is a programmed sequence, the essentials of the program must be recorded in the genes. Although we do not yet understand what controls the timing of gene expression or repression during embryogenesis, nor exactly how the enzymic products of gene expression intervene in embryonic differentiation, it is nevertheless obvious that genetic defects could derange the process in very selective ways. It is therefore not surprising to find many examples of a genetic role in congenital malformations. Mongolism and chondrodystrophy (a defect in the formation of bone from cartilage) are malformations whose causes appear to be primarily genetic, one associated with trisomy for chromosome 21, the other caused by a gene mutation. Such malformations do not fall under the heading of teratogenesis, since the basic defect was presumably present in the zygote and will affect the germ cells as well as all the somatic cells of the affected individual.

The distinction between genetic and purely phenotypic abnormalities is not completely sharp, however. If a mutagenic agent acted at an early enough stage in fetal development to affect germ cells and somatic cells alike, and if the alteration were compatible with survival, the phenotypic manifestations could occur in the affected individual. Experimentally it has been shown, for example, that when a vitamin antagonist, 6-aminonicotinamide, was injected into pregnant mice on the 13th day of gestation, cleft palate was produced in the offspring. Chromosome abnormalities were also produced (polyploidy and fragmentation), not only in the region of the deformed palates but also in other cells throughout the body of the fetus. Furthermore, similar chromosome changes were observed in the maternal bone marrow after treatment but never in untreated controls.[32]

In the experiment with 6-aminonicotinamide, the teratogen was administered fairly late in fetal development; therefore, the induced chromosome abnormalities must all have arisen during faulty mitoses. However, if such an agent were administered to a female at about the time of fertilization, the result could be a similar disturbance of meiosis in the ovum about to be fertilized. The consequent changes in chromosome number or morphology might be indistinguishable from those regarded as having been inherited from earlier generations. This may really happen in human populations.[33] A "run" of sex chromosome aberrations was noted among infants born in one city during a particular 5-month period. The study began as a routine systematic examination of the sex chromatin in human newborns. The sex chromatin is material with distinctive staining properties that is associated with one of the X chromosomes.[34] It is easy to establish, therefore, by staining and microscopic examination of cells from the amniotic membrane or the infant's buccal mucosa, whether the genetic constitution is normal XX or XY, or whether abnormalities such as XXY, XXX, or XO are present. During the first 18 months of the study, there were no abnormalities out of 1541 infants. In the next five months, there were 6 out of 1009. Finally, in the next 4 months there were none out of 817. Although the actual number of abnormalities was very small, the clustering of these few in a particular short period of time was most unlikely to have occurred by chance. Most interesting, during the same 5-month period, there was an increase in the number (also small) of cases of mongolism in this same community. The implication of the findings is that some mutagenic or teratogenic factor, perhaps a drug or virus, may have been at work in this community during the relevant period.

That certain agents have mutagenic and carcinogenic as well as teratogenic activity is hardly surprising.[35,36] At the right time in embryonic development, induced mutation or chromosomal abnormality, if it did not cause fetal death, might well cause abnormal fetal development. Alkylating agents, for example, are well known to be mutagens and carcinogens, and some (but not all) are potent teratogens. However, such associations are by no means the rule, and numerous teratogens are neither mutagenic nor carcinogenic. This is entirely reasonable, since all that is required for teratogenesis is a significant transient disturbance of cell function during a short critical period of organogenesis, whereas a *heritable* alteration in a cell line is absolutely required in mutagenesis and carcinogenesis.

Thus, most congenital malformations are not associated with any obvious abnormality of the chromosomes and are not heritable. The nonheritable nature of the abnormalities has been demonstrated by brother-sister matings of malformed animals and also on a large scale in human populations. Genetic factors, however, may play an important part in determining sensitivity to teratogens as well as the probability of spontaneous malformation.[37] One indication of the role of genetic factors is the considerable difference in sensitivity between species and between strains of the same species. In three rat strains, the azo dye trypan blue produced exencephalic offspring at wholly different frequencies, 17, 50, and 97%, respectively. Cortisone produced cleft palate in all mouse fetuses of one strain but in only 20% of another; this difference was traced to earlier midline fusion of the palate in the more resistant strain. Cortisone also produced cleft palate in rabbits but no malformations whatsoever in rats. Yet cortisone strongly potentiated the actions of another teratogen, vitamin A, in rats. Such genetically determined differences are not necessarily due to differences in metabolism or transplacental passage of teratogens, as shown by similar findings in chick embryos. As Table 12-1 reveals, injection of a teratogen into the yolk sac of various strains on the 4th day produced micromelia (short upper extremities) at frequencies varying from 5% to 100%.

Findings like those described above have led some investigators to the view that chemical teratogens act by bringing out "concealed weaknesses" of the developmental processes, which have a genetic basis. It has been suggested that many induced defects are really phenocopies, i.e., phenotypic changes of exactly the same kinds as are produced by faulty genes, brought about through the same biochemical disturbances. Supporting evidence was obtained in experiments with 6-aminonicotinamide in chicks.[38] This vitamin antagonist produces skeletal anomalies, principally micromelia and parrot beak, which also occur as mutations. Specially bred stocks heterozygous for these defects had increased sensitivity to the teratogen. Conversely, in a stock possessing modifying alleles that reduce the frequency of mutant defects of the skeleton (chondrodystrophy), the teratogen had reduced efficacy.

TABLE 12-1. Strain differences in sensitivity of chicks to a teratogen.
On the 4th day of embryonic life, 0.05 ml of propanediol-1,3 was injected into the yolk sac. Percent malformations (micromelia) are given for various strains. (From Gebhardt, Table 1.[25])

Strain	Number of eggs	Percent malformed (micromelia)
White Leghorn type 111	20	5
White Leghorn type 988	25	12
Araucano	24	16
North Holland White	17	18
White Leghorn type A	18	72
New Hampshire buff	12	89
Scheikuiken Leghorn	15	93
New Hampshire	16	100
Nederlands Landhoen	13	100

An intriguing finding in experimental teratogenesis with multiparous animals is the regularity with which some fetuses escape unscathed while others in the same litter suffer severe and even multiple malformations. A particularly striking example is afforded by trypan blue.[39] Administered uniformly to more than 200 pregnant rats on the 7th, 8th, and 9th days of gestation, it caused death and resorption of nearly one-half the fetuses, numerous malformations in one-half the survivors, but apparently no effects at all in the remaining one-quarter of the original group. The response differences could not be ascribed to differences between mothers, inasmuch as dead, malformed, and normal fetuses appeared to be randomly admixed in the individual rats and even in the same uterine horn. Such findings, which are quite common with all sorts of teratogens, suggest that the genotype of the fetus plays an important role in determining its susceptibility to a teratogen. Whether the surviving normal offspring in such an experiment could be interbred to produce a teratogen-resistant line is not known.

Sensitive Periods

Perhaps the most interesting finding in experimental teratogenesis is that there are special times during fetal development when malformations can be induced and sharply limited critical periods for the various specific malformations. During the early phase of cell proliferation, no malformations can be induced. At this time, all teratogens have nonspecific all-or-none effects; the embryo may be killed, but if it survives, it becomes a normal individual. All cells at this stage may be so much alike that no selectively toxic action is possible upon those that will eventually form particular organ systems. Alternatively, damaged cells that have undergone partial differentiation may still be replaceable by others that escaped injury. Very late in fetal development, it is also difficult to produce abnormalities, since the processes of organogenesis have been largely completed. In each species there is, therefore, a relatively short period of sensitivity to teratogens, when early organogenesis is in progress. In the rat and mouse, this sensitive period extends from about the 5th to the 14th day of the 23-day gestation period. In the human, there is only meager experimental evidence, but the timetable of embryologic development[9] suggests a period extending roughly from the 3rd week through the 3rd month of pregnancy. At the 20th day after fertilization, the cephalocaudal segmentation of the embryo into somites is just beginning. These segments are the precursors of the axial skeleton and musculature. At about 30 days, the limb buds make their appearance; and by 60 days, organ differentiation in the fetus (now 30 mm long) is well under way. Accordingly, rubella-induced malformations of the eye, ear, and heart occur principally between the 4th and 8th weeks. Thalidomide interference with limb formation is chiefly a hazard of the same period, the second month of pregnancy.

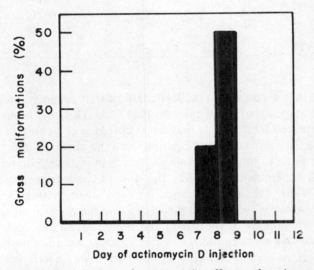

FIGURE 12-1. Critical timing of teratogenic effects of actinomycin D in the pregnant rat. *Actinomycin D was given intraperitoneally in a dose of 75 µg kg[-1] once during pregnancy, at various times after copulation in different animals. The percent of gross malformations among fetuses that survived to term is shown. Not shown are fetal resorption, high when the drug was given early in pregnancy, low in late pregnancy. (From Tuchmann-Duplessis and Mercier-Parot, Figure 2.[40] By permission of Little, Brown.)*

Figure 12-1 illustrates these timing effects quite dramatically in the rat treated with actinomycin D, which presumably disrupts organogenesis by blocking the synthesis of RNA. A fixed dose of this antibiotic caused resorption of nearly all fetuses when administered during the first few days of pregnancy. The frequency of resorptions (not shown) fell to about 10% when the drug was given as late as the 13th day. The incidence of malformations among surviving fetuses showed an extremely sharp peak when the drug was given between the 7th and 9th days.

Specific critical periods for various malformations in the rat, caused by a single teratogen, vitamin A in excessive dosage, are shown in Table 12-2. The sensitive periods correlate well with the known sequence of organogenesis in this species. In general, if it is known with certainty at what time in gestation a particular organ completes its

TABLE 12-2. Critical timing of teratogenic effects of excessive vitamin A administration in the rat.
60,000 International units of vitamin A were given by mouth for 3 days, beginning at different times in pregnancy. Figures are percentages of all surviving fetuses displaying the particular malformation. Plus sign indicates some defects (not more exactly enumerated) of the specified kind. (Data of Giroud and Martinet, cited by Kalter and Warkany.[42])

	Day of pregnancy				
	5–7	8–10	11–13	14–16	18–20
Anencephaly	9	53	0	0	0
Eye defects	4	73	0	0	0
Cleft palate	4	22	92	49	0
Spina bifida	0	3	0	0	0
Limb defects	0	0	+	0	0
Cataract	0	0	0	+	+

differentiation, then a congenital malformation of that organ could only have been caused by a teratogen that acted prior to that time. This rule often enables one to eliminate a suspected teratogen or unusual occurrence as a cause of human malformation because the timing is not compatible with the observed effect.

The need for exact timing of teratogenic treatment imposes two technical requirements upon all experimentation. First, the time of conception must be known accurately. This is not difficult in rodents, for even when matings are not arranged according to the estrous cycle, the presence of a seminal plug in the vagina effectively dates the event. In humans, on the other hand, numerous factors, including irregularities of ovulation and menstruation, conspire to make accurate timing very difficult. Second, the onset and cessation of teratogen action must be well defined and abrupt. With physical treatments such as x-ray or anoxia,[41] the situation is ideal because the exposure can be limited to a period of seconds or minutes. When chemical teratogens are used, the situation is complicated by the time courses of absorption, metabolism, and excretion. Moreover, the actual proximate teratogen may be a metabolite rather than the administered compound. The most successful experiments have employed a systemic route of administration for rapid onset and an antagonist for rapid termination. In an investigation of the teratogenicity of 6-aminonicotinamide, for example, rats were given the compound on the 11th day of pregnancy, followed 2 hr later by the vitamin nicotinamide at a dose known to overcome acute deficiencies caused by the antagonist. This extremely brief teratogenic treatment sufficed to produce cleft palate in the offspring.[43]

Specificity and Variety of Teratogens

It might be imagined that all deleterious influences operating at a particular critical time in organogenesis would produce the same pattern of malformations, i.e., that there would be timing specificity but no teratogen specificity. This is not true. Table 12-3 shows that when rats were subjected to four different vitamin deficiencies at the same time in pregnancy, the resulting malformations were very different. Teratogen-

TABLE 12-3. Teratogen specificity in the rat.
(From Wilson,[37] Table VIII.)

Agent	Most frequent defects	Other defects
Vitamin A deficiency	Coloboma of retina, ectopic ureters, diaphragmatic hernia	Hermaphroditic tendency, fused kidneys, postlental fibroplasia, various cardiovascular defects
Riboflavin deficiency	Shortened long-bones and mandible, fused ribs and toes, cleft palate	Open interventricular septum, hydronephrosis, hydrocephalus, microphthalmia, hernias
Folic acid deficiency	"Universal teratogen"	Affected virtually every organ and system in body, varying considerably with time of treatment
Irradiation	Anophthalmia, encephalocele, etc., renal agenesis	Microphthalmia, various spinal cord and cardiovascular defects, facial clefts, micromelia

specific effects were also obtained in the chick, where maternal and placental factors are excluded. Presumably, the active forms of all the vitamins are required by all growing cells. It must be assumed, therefore, that quantitative differences in these requirements at critical stages of development of each organ must underlie the differential effects of the teratogenic treatments, so that at a given moment one organ is more sensitive to riboflavin deficiency, another to vitamin A deficiency, and so on.

A considerable number and variety of chemical teratogens have been investigated, many of which are listed in Table 12-4. The frequent production of fetal malformations by nutritional deficiency is of interest because of its possible relationship to human congenital malformations. The earliest published data on chemical teratogenesis of any kind dealt with vitamin A deficiency in pigs;[44] when the diet was deficient in this vitamin throughout pregnancy, all the young were abnormal and a variety of malformations occurred. Subsequent matings of the same sows yielded normal offspring, as did brother-sister matings between the malformed animals. In the 35 years since that investigation, the teratogenic effects of other vitamin deficiencies have been established, as shown in the table. Contrary to the long-held view that the fetus has first claim on available nutrients, vitamin deficiencies are selectively damaging to the fetus; teratogenic effects are manifested at degrees of vitamin deficiency too slight to injure the mother. This may well reflect the high requirement of the growing fetus and its lack of stored reserves such as are contained in maternal tissues. On the other hand, general malnutrition, in contrast to specific vitamin deficiency, has only rarely been found to be teratogenic.

The list (Table 12-4) indicates that hormone deficiencies and excesses can prove teratogenic of themselves. Hormones can also potentiate or antagonize the effects of other teratogens. Thus, cortisone increases the incidence of malformations caused by vitamin A, whereas insulin has the opposite effect. Thyroxine antagonizes the teratogenic action of vitamin A, and the antithyroid compound methylthiouracil increases that teratogenic effect. Moreover, thyroxine can reduce the incidence of a spontaneous genetically-determined anomaly, cleft lip, in mice. Such findings suggest that disturbances of hormonal balance might play a role in the etiology of

TABLE 12-4. Some chemical teratogens in rats, mice, rabbits, or chicks.
(Data compiled from Kalter and Warkany,[42] Cahen,[45] Woollam,[46] Carter,[46a] and Kalter.[20])

DIETARY DEFICIENCY: protein, vitamins A, D, and E, ascorbic acid, riboflavin, thiamin, nicotinamide, folic acid, panthothenic acid, trace metal deficiency (Zn, Mn, Co).

VITAMIN ANTAGONISTS: antifolic drugs, 6-aminonicotinamide, 3-acetylpyridine.

VITAMIN EXCESS: vitamin A, nicotinic acid.

HORMONE DEFICIENCY: pituitary, thyroid, insulin (alloxan diabetes).

HORMONE ANTAGONISTS: thiouracil derivatives.

HORMONE EXCESS: thyroxine, cortisone, hydrocortisone, insulin, vasopressin, androgens, estrogens, epinephrine.

ALKYLATING AGENTS: nitrogen mustard, chlorambucil, and others.

PURINE AND PYRIMIDINE ANALOGS: azaguanine, 6-mercaptopurine, fluorodeoxyuridine, and others.

AMINO ACID ANALOGS: azaserine, diazo-oxo-norleucine (DON), hypoglycin-A.

CARBOHYDRATES: 2-deoxyglucose, galactose, bacterial lipopolysaccharides.

ANTIBIOTICS: tetracyclines, penicillin, streptomycin, actinomycin D.

SULFONAMIDES: sulfanilamide, certain antidiabetic sulfonamides.

AGENTS CAUSING ANOXIA: carbon monoxide, carbon dioxide, etc.

AZO DYES: trypan blue, Evans blue, Niagara Sky Blue 6B.

HEAVY METALS: phenylmercuric acetate, methyl mercury, inorganic mercury salts, strontium, lead, thallium, selenium also chelating agents (EDTA).

MISCELLANEOUS: trypaflavin (acriflavin), urethane, colchicine, nicotine, eserine, quinine, pilocarpine, saponin, ricin, chlorpromazine and derivatives, thiadiazole, triazene, boric acid (chick only), salicylate, acetazolamide, hydroxyurea, meclizine, chlorcyclizine, thalidomide, vinca, rauwolfia and veratrum alkaloids, serotonin, triparanol (MER 29), imipramine, 2,3,7,8-tetrachlorodibenzo-p-dioxin, nitrosamines.

PHYSICAL AGENTS: radiation, hypoxia, hypo- and hyperthermia.

INFECTIONS: 10 viruses known, including rubella and cytomegalovirus.

---

malformations in the human. There is a persistent belief among some clinicians that "concealed endocrinopathies" such as prediabetic states or incipient hypothyroidism may account for reproductive wastage and infertility in some women, and it is claimed that hormone treatment improves matters; but there is no convincing evidence to support these opinions.

Deficiency of a trace element can also be teratogenic, as has been demonstrated for zinc, manganese, and cobalt.[35] The effect of zinc deficiency was shown by feeding the chelating agent EDTA (p. 11) to pregnant rats from day 6 to 21; malformations were prevented by simultaneous feeding of zinc carbonate.[47]

One of the earliest indications that a drug or toxic agent could cause congenital malformation was the "monkey-face" syndrome in sheep. In the western United States it was common knowledge that ewes feeding upon plants of the lily family (*Veratrum californicum*) give birth to lambs with facial malformations. Several active teratogens were isolated; they proved to be complex alkaloids, of which cyclopamine is representative.

That growth inhibitors should be teratogenic is not surprising. Actinomycin D is a potent teratogen. In the rat, it causes disorganization of development of the optic nerve, anencephaly, spina bifida, cleft palate and lip, extrusions of the viscera, ectocardia, and dextrocardia.

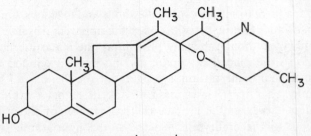

cyclopamine

A few of the antidiabetic sulfonamides have proved to be teratogenic. But the effect is probably unrelated to the lowering of the blood glucose level, inasmuch as some drugs of this class have no teratogenic action at doses that lower blood sugar to the same degree. Likewise, some antibacterial sulfonamides (e.g., sulfanilamide) are teratogenic but not others.

Phenylmercuric acetate administered intravaginally at a dose of 1.1 mg to pregnant mice on the 7th day of gestation caused major abnormalities of the brain, eye, and tail in 15 % of the offspring.[42] This compound is included at very low concentration in some contraceptive jellies and creams to which women may be exposed periodically.

Boric acid is teratogenic in chicks, causing a pattern of deformities that appears to be identical with that produced by riboflavin deficiency.[48,49] Riboflavin prevented these teratogenic effects. The implication is that boric acid produces riboflavin deficiency, but how it does this remains obscure.

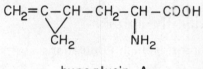

hypoglycin-A

Hypoglycin-A is an unusual leucine analog found in the unripe fruit of a Jamaican plant. Ingestion leads to a severe, often fatal, toxic reaction characterized by persistent vomiting, severe abdominal pain, and hypoglycemia. The compound is teratogenic in rats.[50] The teratogen effect is not prevented by leucine, but it is antagonized by riboflavin. As with boric acid, the mechanism is obscure.

One of the most interesting teratogens is the azo dye trypan blue.[39,51] Administered subcutaneously to rats in a dose of 10 mg between the 7th and 10th days of gestation, it

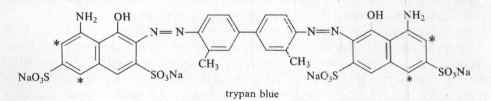

trypan blue

regularly causes malformations of the brain (hydrocephalus secondary to maldevelopment of the aqueduct) and also of the eyes, vertebral column, and cardiovascular system. Similar malformations are caused in rabbits and in chicks. One of the puzzling aspects of trypan blue teratogenesis has been the apparent absence of dye granules from the rat embryo, although they are plentiful in the maternal reticuloendothelial system and also in the placenta. Apparently the dye is excluded by the yolk sac membrane that envelops the rat embryo at about the 9th day of gestation. When the dye was injected directly into the yolk sac in embryo explants, teratogenic effects were obtained even on the 11th day.[52] In the rabbit, on the other hand, trypan blue gains access to the embryonic blastocyst throughout the gestation period. There is evidence of localization of the dye in lysosomes of the yolk sac, and inhibition of several lysosomal enzymes has been reported. It has been proposed that this inhibition interferes with the hydrolytic digestion of the yolk, thus impairing fetal nutrition. Since yolk sac function is of little importance in primates, this theory would explain the greater teratogenicity of trypan blue in chick embryo and rodents than in primates.[53]

The structural requirements for teratogenic activity among the azo dyes are extraordinarily exacting. In the closely related dye Evans blue, all four sulfonate groups are shifted to new positions, marked by asterisks in the formula given above. This change suffices to reduce the teratogenic potency considerably although the pattern of malformations remains the same. If the only change introduced into the trypan blue structure is the substitution of methoxy groups for methyl in the central part of the molecule (Niagara Blue 4B, Niagara Sky Blue 6B), teratogenic activity drops to an even lower level but is still demonstrable. No other azo dye tested was teratogenic, but many possible small changes were not explored. A close relative, azo blue, is wholly inactive.

TERATOGENESIS IN MAN

Congenital Malformations in Human Populations

Infertility, spontaneous abortions, stillbirths, and neonatal deaths are major tragedies of human life, but more tragic by far is the birth of a seriously malformed infant. Congenital malformations have been recognized since prehistoric times, and were once attributed to divine or satanic intervention, to hybridization with other species, or to frightening experiences of the pregnant woman. The birth of a malformed child was early regarded as a portent of future events, whence the term "monster," from the Latin root meaning "to show, to indicate." The long history of irrational attitudes toward congenital deformity still conditions much present-day thinking among uninformed people.[54]

The tendency of a mother to attribute the birth of a deformed child to some unusual event during her pregnancy greatly complicates objective investigation. Many retrospective studies are suspect on this account. A retrospective study begins with the birth of the malformed child and seeks clues to causative factors that may have operated during the preceding 9 months. Controls are normal infants born at about the same time and place. The basic difficulty is that the mother of a malformed child is more likely to remember, exaggerate, or even imagine extraordinary events during pregnancy than is the mother of a normal child.

In the prospective study, all pertinent information about a pregnancy is recorded before delivery, before it is known whether or not the child is normal. Whereas restrospective investigations can deal intensively with small numbers of individuals, the prospective investigation, by its very nature, must deal with extremely large groups in order to include a significant number of congenital malformations. Consequently, data are collected by many physicians, nurses, midwives, and other health personnel, and reliability tends to decrease as the numbers become larger. Only a few prospective studies have ever been carried out, and it is from these that we have most of the meaningful statistics about congenital malformations in humans.

A 5-year investigation dealt with about 6000 pregnancies that were followed in the clinics of teaching hospitals in New York City.[55] Of these pregnancies, 5% terminated in fetal death after the third month. No information was obtained about earlier terminations. Another 2% ended in stillbirths, and a further 2% in live-born infants who died within the first month of life. Thus, the total reproductive loss amounted to no less than 9%. Of all infants alive at one month of age, 7% bore some congenital malformation. Of those who had died earlier, 14–30% were malformed. And out of all who died during the first year of life, 71% were malformed. These findings show that congenital malformations are associated with a high infant mortality rate. It is also known that fetal malformation is common in cases of intra-uterine death or stillbirth. It is really not surprising that major malformations of the vital organs should be incompatible with life. But it is also evident that relatively minor malformations (e.g., of the musculoskeletal system) may reduce life expectancy, especially when survival rates are examined for the first 5 years of life.[56] It may be that the obvious malformations apparent to the examiner are accompanied by related but occult functional derangements elsewhere.

Deleterious genes throughout the biologic world are eliminated by the poorer survival of carriers to the reproductive age, but no such eugenic purpose is served by the premature death of congenitally malformed individuals. In most cases, such people are not suffering from a genetic defect, and if they live to reproduce, their children are likely to be quite normal. Moreover, history affords many examples of congenitally malformed people who have made notable contributions to society.

In the New York study cited above, great care was exercised to record every manifest malformation, no matter how trivial. Accordingly, such conditions as super-numerary breast and pilonidal sinus accounted for a considerable part of the total. A prospective study conducted in Birmingham, England,[56] covered a population 10 times larger and excluded malformations considered unimportant. The incidence of stillbirths was the same as in the New York study, but the total frequency of individuals classed as malformed was only about 2%. This figure is also in good agreement with that observed in a Japanese population of about the same size.[56] In all these large-scale investigations, the principal serious deformities affected the nervous system, but malformations were found in all organ systems. The principal ones (in order of decreasing frequency) were: talipes (clubfoot), cardiac anomalies, spina bifida and associated vertebral defects, hydrocephalus, anencephalus, and cranioschisis (failure of midline closure of the skull), cleft lip or palate, mongolism, hip dislocation, pyloric stenosis, and polydactylism. It should be noted that in surveys like this one some of the malformations observed are known to be genetically determined and thus not relevant to the problem of teratogenesis.

There were significant differences in the frequencies of some conditions between the Japanese and the English populations, between the English and the New York groups, and even between the New York sample and an earlier population surveyed retrospectively) in Philadelphia.[57] A number of these differences cannot be rationalized on the basis of inconsistent diagnostic criteria or different likelihoods of missing a malformation entirely. Clubfoot, for example, which could hardly be overlooked, occurred with frequencies (per 1000 total births) of 1.4, 4.4, 5.3, and 0.3 in the Japanese, English, New York, and Philadelphia groups, respectively. For hydrocephalus, the corresponding figures were 0.5, 2.6, 0.9, and 1.4; and for spina bifida, 0.3, 3.0, 1.6, and 0.9. In the Japanese group, hip dislocations occurred at an incidence of 7.1 per 1000, in the English group at 0.7 per 1000. Such large differences may, of course, be related to genetic differences among the several populations, but they also suggest the possibility that environmental influences may have played a considerable role in causing the malformations.

Curious seasonal variations in the incidence of the more common congenital malformations have been noted.[58] A survey of all births in Birmingham, England, during 1950 revealed that anencephaly tended to occur in infants born in December and January, hare lip in March, patent ductus arteriosus in August. These clustered to a degree that differed significantly from the variations to be expected by chance. It was postulated that a chemical teratogen in food or environment, or virus infections might have been responsible.

In a large-scale study of 24 maternity centers in 16 countries, the frequency of malformations was noted in over 400 thousand pregnancies.[59] Again, large differences between countries were observed. There was a strong association between parental consanguinity and stillbirths or early neonatal deaths related primarily to neural tube defects. A high concordance rate for such defects in twins was also observed suggesting a genetic component; but this finding does not exclude environmental teratogens as the primary causative agents.

Accidental Human Exposure to Teratogens

Only rarely has it been possible to observe directly the result of an experiment on teratogenesis in the human. A few cases have been reported in which acute anoxia caused by carbon monoxide or morphine, taken with suicidal intent early in pregnancy, was followed by the birth of a malformed child, but cause-and-effect relationships in such episodes are uncertain. After the discovery that the antifolic drug aminopterin could cause abortion, it was occasionally taken for this purpose. Some fetuses that survived such attempts were grossly malformed.[4] Progestational steroids, used in the treatment of habitual abortion, have produced abnormalities of the genitalia (masculinization) in the female fetus.[60] For this reason the oral contraceptives that contain progesterone-like steroids are contra-indicated in pregnancy or suspected pregnancy. Toxoplasmosis and syphilis during pregnancy may also cause fetal malformations by direct invasion and destruction of fetal tissue.[4]

Ingestion of methyl mercury compounds by pregnant women, as in Minamata disease (p. 372),[61,62] has caused cerebral palsy in the infant, even though the women themselves remained symptom free. Although technically this must be classified as teratogenesis, a distinction has to be made. Here the fetus is more sensitive to a toxic agent than its mother, but manifests the typical organ toxicity—in this case the same type of neurologic damage seen in adults. On the other hand, in most instances of teratogenesis the causative agent acts in a specific way to disrupt organogenesis, but may be entirely innocuous in the adult.

A dramatic outbreak of congenital malformations was the Australian experience associated with rubella epidemic in 1940.[23] A variety of effects not previously attributed to any exogenous agent were clearly associated with this virus infection. These included cataract and other abnormalities of the eyes, deafness, cardiac defects, and mental retardation. When rubella occurred during the first or second month of pregnancy, the heart and eye defects predominated, but hearing defects were most common when the disease occurred in the third month. Rubella contracted after the third month of gestation was without effect. Early estimates based upon the retrospective method of data collection led to the impression that three-quarters or more of pregnant women who contracted rubella during the first trimester of pregnancy would give birth to a defective child. Subsequent prospective studies have yielded a much lower figure, about 17%.

The experience with rubella, the experimental evidence for teratogenesis by various chemical agents, and the isolated instances of congenital abnormality in humans caused by antifolic drugs should have alerted the medical community to the likelihood that increasing drug use would sooner or later result in unexpected teratogenic actions. But it required a major catastrophe to demonstrate that what happens in experimental animals can also happen in humans.[63] Thalidomide was introduced in the late 1950's in West Germany, England, and other countries, as a tranquilizing agent and hypnotic. It was effective and seemed remarkably nontoxic. Although a typical therapeutic dose was about 100 mg, patients recovered from ingestion of as much as 14 g

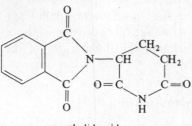

thalidomide

taken with suicidal intent. About 1960, some scattered reports indicated that patients receiving this drug for a long time sometimes developed neurologic disturbances.

Shortly after the introduction of thalidomide into therapy, there was an increase in the number of infants born with phocomelia, a shortening or complete absence of the limbs.[64] The data are interesting. At the University Pediatric Clinic in Hamburg, for example, not a single case of phocomelia was seen in the decade 1949–1959. In 1959, there was a single case; in 1960, 30 cases; and in 1961, 154 cases. Comparable increases in the frequency of this anomaly, previously almost unknown, occurred simultaneously in many parts of the world where thalidomide was in use. Finally, in November 1961, an astute pediatrician[65] suspected an association between phocomelia and the ingestion of thalidomide by the pregnant mother. Subsequent investigations in several countries[66,67] indicated that in virtually every case of phocomelia the mother had taken thalidomide between the third and eighth weeks of pregnancy. Sometimes only a few doses during the critical period sufficed.

The critical period for each kind of malformation produced in the human fetus has been established by careful retrospective analysis.[68] When thalidomide was taken 35–36 days after the last menstrual period (approximately 21–22 days of gestation), absence of the external ears and paralysis of the cranial nerves resulted. Three to 5 days later (about 24–27 days of gestation), the phocomelia effect was at its maximum, affecting principally the arms. A day or two later, similar defects of the legs occurred. The sensitive period terminated 48–50 days after the last period (34–36 days of gestation) with the production of hypoplastic thumbs and anorectal stenosis.

That thalidomide was responsible for the outbreak of phocomelia is beyond reasonable doubt. But it is still uncertain what exact degree of risk is attached to the ingestion of this drug by a pregnant woman. If a large number of pregnant women were given thalidomide during the critical period, what fraction of the infants would be malformed? Some investigators believe that practically all would be affected, since it was difficult to find well-authenticated instances of thalidomide ingestion followed by the birth of normal infants. Others place the risk very much lower, believing that the retrospective method of investigation exaggerates such an association to an extreme degree.[46] Thus, a woman who has given birth to a malformed child will readily recall (or even imagine) taking thalidomide, especially when the effects of the drug have been publicized; but a woman with normal child, who may also have taken thalidomide during pregnancy, has no particular interest in recalling that fact.

Thalidomide was withdrawn from the market at the end of 1961, and the outbreak of phocomelia subsided promptly. In the United States, the drug had not been approved by the Food and Drug Administration and was therefore never in general use. The total number of infants throughout the world that were deformed by thalidomide must be around 10,000. Although phocomelia is the most obvious and directly disabling abnormality, congenital malformations of the internal organs are also common in the affected children.

Lessons of the Thalidomide Catastrophe

A major consequence of the thalidomide experience was the institution of improved procedures for screening new drugs. Teratogenic effects had not been examined routinely in the past, partly because the potential seriousness of the problem had been underestimated, but also because effective methods had not been developed. As had been shown for numerous other teratogenic agents, thalidomide displays a strong species specificity. In rats, for example, congenital abnormalities could not at first be produced by this drug. In certain strains of white rabbits, it was found that carefully timed administration of thalidomide between the 8th and 16th days of pregnancy led to typical limb malformations.[69] Subsequent work with rats showed that this species was sensitive after all, but only on the 12th day of gestation.[70] Eventually, a syndrome of thalidomide-induced malformations was produced in monkeys, which is very much like that seen in humans.[71]

A possible cause of species differences in the teratogenicity of thalidomide, and of differences in sensitivity among humans, may be variations in metabolic pathways. Thalidomide is extensively metabolized; evidently, a metabolite, rather than thalidomide itself, is the proximate teratogenic agent.[72] Hydrolysis of amide bonds and ring hydroxylation alone could account for more than 100 metabolites, of which a dozen or so have been identified in vivo.[66] When the piperidine ring is opened, a glutamine or glutamic acid derivative is formed, as shown:

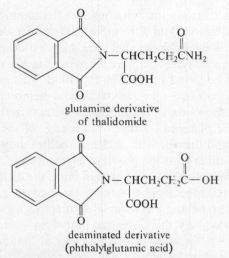

glutamine derivative
of thalidomide

deaminated derivative
(phthalylglutamic acid)

Decarboxylation of phthalylglutamic acid yields a monocarboxylic acid, which is the most abundant metabolite.

Early studies showed that none of the metabolites were teratogenic when injected into pregnant rabbits under the same conditions in which thalidomide showed its characteristic actions. It was discovered, however, that this was due to the inability of the metabolites to pass from maternal plasma into the fetus in appreciable quantity. Figure 12-2 shows that when thalidomide was administered, it was all converted to

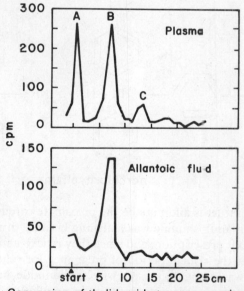

FIGURE 12-2. Conversion of thalidomide to a monocarboxylic acid derivative in the rabbit fetus. *Samples of plasma (above) and allantoic fluid (below) were subjected to paper electrophoresis 4 hr after administration of radioactive thalidomide to a pregnant rabbit. Anodal migration is toward the right; distance is shown on x-axis. Radioactivity in the paper is shown on y-axis. Peak A, thalidomide; peak B, monocarboxylic acid derivative; peak C, dicarboxylic acid derivative. Neither carboxylic acid passed from plasma into allantoic fluid if injected into the rabbit. (From Keberle et al., Figure 10.[72])*

the monocarboxylic acid in the fetus.[72] Radioactive thalidomide was used, and samples of the plasma and of allantoic fluid were subjected to paper electrophoresis. Localization of the radioactivity peaks shows that after 4 hr thalidomide itself, the monocarboxylic acid, and a dicarboxylic acid were all present in plasma; but only the monocarboxylic acid could be found in the allantoic fluid. This experiment, and the previously demonstrated inability of the carboxylic acid metabolites to pass the placental barrier in the rabbit, shows that thalidomide is metabolized in the fetus, or at least on the fetal side of the placenta. Without knowledge of the teratogenic potency of the monocarboxylic and dicarboxylic acid metabolites, however, it was impossible to conclude which (if either) was the proximate teratogen.

Subsequent experiments showed[73,74] that in mice, the dicarboxylic acid (phthalyl-L-glutamic acid) was teratogenic when administered to the pregnant female on days 7 to 9 of gestation. The D isomer was completely inactive, as were various products of further metabolism. It is likely, therefore, that phthalyl-L-glutamic acid is a proximate teratogen in thalidomide teratogenesis. An analog of thalidomide, in which one of the CO groups in the phthalyl moiety has been reduced to CH_2, is also a potent teratogen.[75]

In the aftermath of the thalidomide episode there was intensified investigation of various drugs, both established ones and new ones, with respect to teratogenicity. An antihistaminic, meclizine hydrochloride, and a related compound, cyclizine, were found to cause skeletal abnormalities in rats.[76] Both compounds yield the same metabolite, norchlorcyclizine,

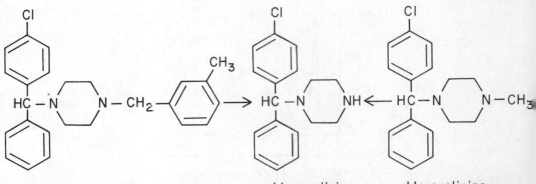

meclizine   norchlorcyclizine   chlorcyclizine

which is found in the rat fetus and may be the proximate carcinogen.[77] The finding of teratogenicity by an antihistamine was alarming because drugs of this kind were widely available without prescription, and since they relieve nausea, they were likely to be used precisely at the critical period of pregnancy for relief of "morning sickness." This, indeed, was a major reason why thalidomide had such devastating effects.[46] However, extensive prospective studies in populations of pregnant women have not revealed any abnormal frequency of malformations or abortions in women taking these drugs.[78,79] Anti-inflammatory steroids have been shown to cause cleft palate in the mouse,[80–82] but their possible teratogenicity in humans remains an open question. Even caffeine, probably the most widely used of all drugs, has been reported to produce fetal abnormalities in mice,[83] although at doses (per kg) at least 50 times higher than those taken by people. Other drugs in common use that have been shown to be teratogenic in laboratory animals include diphenylhydantoin,[84] griseofulvin,[85] and tetracycline.[86,87]

Widespread use of LSD among youth beginning in the 1960's coincided with increased concern about chemical teratogenesis, and early studies with mammalian cells in culture suggested that LSD, at least in high concentrations, could act as a chromosome breaker. In rats, mice, hamsters, rabbits, and rhesus monkeys, malformations could not consistently be produced. A few birth defects were observed among the children of young women who admitted to using LSD during pregnancy. However, proper investigations in humans may well be precluded. Prospective experiments, involving deliberate administration of LSD, are obviously out of the question. And retrospective studies with users of illicit LSD are virtually impossible to evaluate because of multiple drug use, uncertain purity of the LSD, unknown dosage and timing, inadequate nutritional status of many drug abusers, and the biases associated with all retrospective studies and discussed elsewhere in this chapter. Thus, there is no convincing evidence to implicate LSD as a teratogen in humans, yet the possibility cannot be excluded.[88,89]

Certain pollutants to which people may be exposed in the general environment or through occupational contact have proved to be teratogenic in animal experiments. A potent mutagen, carcinogen, and teratogen is dioxin (2,3,7,8-tetrachlorodibenzo-p-dioxin, p. 463), which is found as a contaminant in the herbicide 2,4,5-trichloro-phenoxyacetic acid (2,4,5-T), formerly widely used both in agriculture and as a defoliant for military purposes.[90–93] The fungicide captan (N-trichloromethylthio-4-cyclohexene-1,2-dicarboximide) is also teratogenic.[94] Organic mercurials have already been discussed (p. 716); lead, which is a major environmental pollutant in urban areas, may also be teratogenic.[95]

Drugs with known teratogenic effects should obviously not be used by pregnant women, but these same drugs might well be effective and harmless in men, in women beyond the menopause, and in children. A practical question is whether pregnancy can be recognized soon enough to avoid inadvertent administration of teratogens during the time of fetal sensitivity. The problem is presented schematically in Figure 12-3. We know that the sensitive period for teratogenesis coincides with the phase of organ differentiation. In the human embryo, the period of organogenesis begins at about the 20th day of gestation (the first somite stage) and continues most vigorously through the third month.[18] A continuing process of finer morphologic and bio-chemical differentiation goes on throughout the second trimester; and even premature infants born in the seventh or eighth month are incompletely developed in some respects. In the women with regular menses, ovulation occurs approximately 14 days (12–16 days) prior to the onset of the next menstrual period, and fertilization takes place within a day or two after ovulation.[96,97] Thus, at fetal age 20 days, the missed period is more than a week overdue, and most pregnancy tests are already positive.[98] This hypothetical woman with perfectly regular menstrual cycles will know she is pregnant just in time to discontinue potentially teratogenic medications. Unfortunately, however, the length of the menstrual period varies widely, not only between women, but also in the individual woman.[99] Fully one-third of all women have a range of 13 days or more between their shortest and longest cycles, whereas only 1 women in 10 varies less than 5 days. The greater the irregularity of past periods, the longer will be the time needed for the missed period to be noted and for the woman to consider herself pregnant. It follows that for the population as a whole, if

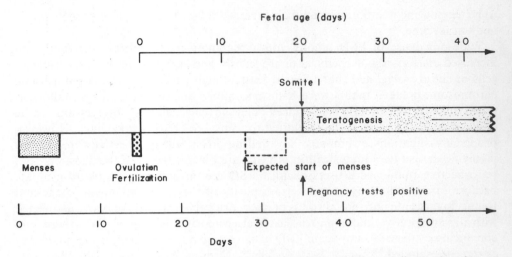

FIGURE 12-3. Relationship of teratogenic susceptibility to diagnosis of pregnancy. *The diagram applies to a hypothetical, perfectly regular 28-day menstrual cycle. Pregnancy will be recognized before the earliest time the fetus is susceptible to teratogenic action; before fetal age 20 days, abortion will be the likely result of damage to the fetus. Variability in the time of ovulation will delay recognition of pregnancy until beyond fetal age 20 days.*

women of child-bearing age are permitted access to medications that are potentially teratogenic, an unacceptably large proportion of them will have exposed their embryos to the risk of malformation before pregnancy is recognized. Clearly, then, the only safe course is to set up special safeguards for the administration of drugs to all women of child-bearing age.

It is clear that the risks of chemical teratogenesis, like those of chemical mutagenesis (cf. Chapter 10), are accentuated during the first trimester, although the risk of the fetus being damaged remains through the gestation period. Until much more information becomes available, the very diversity of known teratogens and mutagens should dictate caution.[100,101] Whenever a drug is being administered to a woman of child-bearing age, the possibility of pregnancy should be kept in mind. A woman who is known to be pregnant should not be exposed to drugs at all during pregnancy (especially during the first trimester), unless the need is pressing. Moreover, since self-medication has been found to be very common among pregnant women,[102] positive warnings should be given by the physician. At least until experimental or statistical investigations show them to be harmless, caffeine, nicotine, and alcohol, to which people are so frequently exposed, should be regarded as possibly hazardous to the fetus. Even aspirin may be capable of causing blood clotting disorders in the neonate when administered to mothers during the week prior to birth.[102a]

The thalidomide experience served to bring drug-induced teratogenesis out of the realm of laboratory curiosities and into the social arena. It focused attention throughout the world upon the need for more thorough testing of all possible adverse drug effects in many animal species before drugs are approved for human use. Because exhaustive animal testing is time consuming and expensive, and because new techniques often have to be devised, one consequence is a slowing of the rate at which new drugs are introduced into therapeutics.[103] Another lesson of the thalidomide tragedy has not yet been learned well. An effective system for the gathering of data on adverse drug reactions and a method for data analysis on a national or international scale are urgently needed.[104-108] When the unexpected happens, as when a very promising and apparently safe drug begins to produce rare congenital anomalies, it is imperative that the association of drug with adverse effect be established with all haste so that preventive measures can be taken. A centralized system of data collection and analysis would have signaled the association of thalidomide with phocomelia much sooner than the means by which it was finally recognized, and the epidemic could have been aborted sooner.[109] The important general problem of protecting society from adverse drug effects is discussed in Chapter 14.

The problem of congenital malformation in the human is similar in some respects to the problems of mutation and cancer. All three occur spontaneously, and can also be produced by external physical or chemical treatments. In none have the causes of the spontaneous events been ascertained. Deliberate experiments are for the most part confined to laboratory animals, while human data must be largely of a statistical nature. More prospective statistical investigations in humans might bring to light associations, as yet unsuspected, between environmental influences during pregnancy (including exposure to drugs) and the subsequent birth of a malformed child.

Chemical teratogenesis, like chemical mutagenesis and chemical carcinogenesis, is a challenging new area of pharmacologic investigation. Our present understanding of mechanisms of action in this field is pitifully primitive. We do not know how any teratogen really acts, nor whether chemical teratogens play any significant part in spontaneous human malformations. With increasing knowledge about the biochemical events in normal embryogenesis should come better understanding of teratogenesis. Eventually, therefore, as with other diseases of man, practical means may be developed for the prevention of congenital malformations.

REFERENCES

1. A. P. NORMAN: *Congenital Abnormalities in Infancy*, 2nd ed. Oxford and Edinburgh, Blackwell Scientific Publications (1971).
2. G. E. W. WOLSTENHOLME and C. M. O'CONNOR, eds.: *Congenital Malformations. Ciba Foundation Symposium*. Boston, Little, Brown and Co. (1960).
3. M. FISHBEIN, ed.: *Birth Defects*. Philadelphia, J. B. Lippincott (1963).
4. J. WARKANY and H. KALTER: Congenital malformations. *New Eng. J. Med.* 265 993, 1046 (1961).
5. M. FISHBEIN, ed.: *Second International Conference on Congenital Malformations*. New York, The International Medical Congress, Ltd. (1964).
6. J. G. WILSON: Experimental teratology. *Amer. J. Obstet. Gynecol.* 90:1181 (1964).
7. D. A. KARNOFSKY: Drugs as teratogens in animals and man. *Ann. Rev. Pharmacol.* 5:447 (1965).
8. J. M. SUTHERLAND and I. J. LIGHT: The effects of drugs upon the developing fetus. *Pediat. Clin. North Am.* 12:781 (1965).
9. H. NISHIMURA, J. MILLER, and M. YASUDA: *Methods for Teratological Studies in Experimental Animals and Man*. Tokyo, Igadku Shoin (1969).
10. A. BERTELLI: Teratology. International Congress Series No. 173, Amsterdam, Excerpta Medica Foundation (1969).
11. Pharmacology Society Symposium: Developmental pharmacology. *Fed. Proc.* 31:43 (1972).
12. American Society for Experimental Pathology Symposium: Teratology. *Fed. Proc.* 30:102 (1971).

13. Editorial: Teratology. *Lancet* 2:530 (1969).
14. M. N. RUNNER: Comparative pharmacology in relation to teratogenesis. *Fed. Proc.* 26:1131 (1967).
15. A. RANE and F. SJÖQVIST: Drug metabolism in the human fetus and newborn infant. Symposium on Pediatric Pharmacology. *Pediat. Clin. North Am.* 19:37 (1972).
16. G. M. MC KHANN and S. J. YAFFE, eds.: *Drugs and Poisons in Relation to the Developing Nervous System*. Proceedings of the Conference on Drugs and Poisons as Etiological Agents in Mental Retardation. Washington, D.C., Public Health Service Publication No. 1791 (1968).
17. D. H. M. WOOLLAM, ed.: *Advances in Teratology*. New York and London, Academic Press (1966–1972). Vol. 1–5.
18. W. J. HAMILTON, J. D. BOYD, and H. W. MOSSMAN: *Human Embryology*, 3rd ed. Baltimore, Williams and Wilkins (1962).
19. W. FUHRMANN: Genetics of growth and development of the fetus. *Pediat. Clin. North Am.* 12:457 (1965).
20. H. KALTER: *Teratology of the Central Nervous System*. Chicago and London, University of Chicago Press (1968).
21. Symposium on Specificity of Cell Differentiation and Interaction. *J. Cell. Comp. Physiol.* 60:suppl. 1, 1 (1962).
22. M. M. NELSON: Teratogenic effects of pteroylglutamic acid deficiency in the rat. In *Congenital Malformations. Ciba Foundation Symposium*, ed. by G. W. E. Wolstenholme and C. M. O'Connor. Boston, Little, Brown and Co. (1960), p. 134.
23. N. M. GREGG: Congenital cataract following German measles in the mother. *Trans. Ophthalmol. Soc. Australia* 3:35 (1941).
23a. L. R. AXELROD: Drugs and nonhuman primate teratogenesis. *Adv. Teratol.* 4:217 (1970).
24. J. G. WILSON: Use of rhesus monkeys in teratological studies. *Fed. Proc.* 30:104 (1971).
25. D. O. E. GEBHARDT: The use of the chick embryo in applied teratology. *Adv. Teratol.* 5:97 (1972).
26. P. S. LIETMAN: Pharmacologic effects on developing enzyme systems. See ref. 11, p. 62.
27. B. L. MIRKIN: Ontogenesis of the adrenergic nervous system: functional and pharmacologic implications. See ref. 11, p. 65.
28. S. B. SPARBER: Effects of drugs on the biochemical and behavioral responses of developing organisms. See ref. 11 p. 74.
28a. R. D. SHORT, K. S. RAO, and J. E. GIBSON: The in vivo biosynthesis of DNA, RNA and proteins by mouse embryos after a teratogenic dose of cyclophosphamide. *Teratology* 6:129 (1972).
29. G. B. WEST: Teratogenic activity of drugs. *J. Pharm. Pharmacol.* 16:63 (1964).
30. J. G. WILSON: Influence on the offspring of altered physiologic states during pregnancy in the rat. *Ann. N.Y. Acad. Sci.* 57:517 (1954).
31. J. G. WILSON: Embryological considerations in teratology. *Ann. New York Acad. Sci.* 123:219 (1965).
32. T. H. INGALLS, E. F. INGENITO, and F. J. CURLEY: Acquired chromosomal anomalies induced in mice by injection of a teratogen in pregnancy. *Science* 141:810 (1963).
33. A. ROBINSON and T. T. PUCK: Sex chromatin in newborns: presumptive evidence for external factors in human nondisjunction. *Science* 148:83 (1965).
34. M. A. FERGUSON-SMITH: The techniques of human cytogenetics. *Amer. J. Obstet. Gynecol.* 90:1035 (1964).
35. J. A. DiPAOLO and P. KOTIN: Teratogenesis oncogenesis: a study of possible relationships. *Arch. Pathol.* 81:3 (1966).
36. H. KALTER: Correlation between teratogenic and mutagenic effects of chemicals in mammals. In *Chemical Mutagens: Principles and Methods for Their Detection*, ed. by A. Hollaender. New York and London, Plenum Press (1971), vol. 1.
37. J. G. WILSON: Experimental studies on congenital malformations. *J. Chron. Dis.* 10:111 (1959).
38. W. LANDAUER: Gene and phenocopy: selection experiments and tests with 6-aminonicotinamide. *J. Exper. Zool.* 160:345 (1965).
39. J. G. WILSON: Teratogenic activity of several azo dyes chemically related to trypan blue. *Anat. Record* 123:313 (1955).
40. H. TUCHMANN-DUPLESSIS and L. MERCIER-PAROT: The teratogenic action of the antibiotic actinomycin D. In *Congenital Malformations. Ciba Foundation Symposium*, ed. by G. E. W. Wolstenholme and C. M. O'Connor, Boston, Little, Brown and Co. (1960), p. 115.

41. C. T. GRABOWSKI: Embryonic oxygen deficiency—a physiological approach to analysis of teratological mechanisms. *Adv. Teratol.* 4:125 (1970).

42. H. KALTER and J. WARKANY: Experimental production of congenital malformations in mammals by metabolic procedure. *Physiol. Rev.* 39:69 (1959).

43. F. C. FRASER: General discussion. In *Congenital Malformations. Ciba Foundation Symposium*, ed. by G. E. Wolstenholme and C. M. O'Connor. Boston, Little, Brown and Co. (1960), p. 282.

44. F. HALE: Relation of vitamin A to anophthalmos in pigs. *Am. J. Ophthalmol.* 18:1087 (1935).

45. R. L. CAHEN: Evaluation of the teratogenicity of drugs. *Clin. Pharmacol. Therap.* 5:480 (1964).

46. D. H. M. WOOLLAM: Principles of teratogenesis: mode of action of thalidomide. *Proc. Roy. Soc. Med.* 58:497 (1965).

46a. C. O. CARTER: Incidence and aetiology. In *Congenital Abnormalities in Infancy*, ed. by A. P. Norman. Oxford and Edinburgh, Blackwell Scientific Publications, 2nd ed. (1971).

47. H. SWENERTON and L. S. HURLEY: Teratogenic effects of a chelating agent and their prevention by zinc. *Science* 173:62 (1971).

48. W. LANDAUER: On the chemical production of developmental abnormalities and of phenocopies in chicken embryos. *J. Cell. Comp. Physiol.* 43:suppl. 1, 261 (1954).

49. W. LANDAUER and E. M. CLARK: On the role of riboflavin in the teratogenic activity of boric acid. *J. Exper. Zool.* 156:307 (1964).

50. T. V. N. PERSAND: Teratogenic effect of hypoglycin-A. *Adv. Teratol.* 5:77 (1972).

51. C. GILBERT and J. GILLMAN: The morphogenesis of trypan blue induced defects of the eye. *S. African J. Med. Sci.* 19:147 (1954).

52. M. M. TURBOW: Teratogenic effect of trypan blue on rat embryos cultivated in vitro. *Nature* 206:637 (1965).

53. F. BECK, J. B. LLOYD, and A. GRIFFITHS: Lysosomal enzyme inhibition by trypan blue: a theory of teratogenesis. *Science.* 157:1180 (1967).

54. J. WARKANY: Congenital malformations in the past. *J. Chron. Dis.* 10:84 (1959).

55. R. MCINTOSH, K. K. MERRITT, M. R. RICHARDS, M. H. SAMUELS. and M. T. BELLOWS: The incidence of congenital malformations: a study of 5,964 pregnancies. *Pediatrics* 14:505 (1954).

56. T. MC KEOWN and R. G. RECORD: Malformations in a population observed for five years after birth. In *Congenital Malformations. Ciba Foundation Symposium*, ed. by G. E. W. Wolstenholme and C. M. O'Connor, Boston, Little, Brown and Co. (1960), p. 2.

57. D. P. MURPHY: *Congenital Malformations*, 2nd ed. Philadelphia, J. B. Lippincott (1947).

58. J. H. EDWARDS: The epidemiology of congenital malformations. In *Second International Conference on Congenital Malformations*, ed. by M. Fishbein. New York, The International Medical Congress Ltd. (1964), p. 297.

59. A. C. STEVENSON, H. A. JOHNSTON, M. I. P. STEWART, and D. R. GOLDING: Congenital malformations. *WHO Bul.* 34:Supplement (1966).

60. H. JACKSON: Antifertility substances. *Pharmacol. Rev.* 11:135 (1959).

61. H. MATSUMOTO, G. KOYA, and T. TAKEUCHI: Fetal minamata disease. *J. Neuropath. Exp. Neurol.* 24:563 (1965).

62. R. D. SNYDER: Congenital mercury poisoning. *New Eng. J. Med.* 284:1014 (1971).

63. G. W. MELLIN and M. KATZENSTEIN: The saga of thalidomide. *New Eng. J. Med.* 267:1184, 1238 (1962).

64. H. B. TAUSSIG: A study of the German outbreak of phocomelia. The thalidomide syndrome. *J. Amer. Med. Ass.* 180:1106 (1962).

65. W. LENZ: Kindliche Missbildungen nach Medikament-Einnahme während der Gravidität? *Deutsche med. Wochenschr.* 86:2555 (1961).

66. R. T. WILLIAMS: Teratogenic effects of thalidomide and related substances. *Lancet* 1:723 (1963).

67. W. G. MC BRIDE: The teratogenic action of drugs. *Med. J. Australia* 2:689 (1963).

68. W. LENZ: Epidemiology of congenital malformations. *Ann. N.Y. Acad. Sci.* 123:228 (1965).

69. V. LARSEN: The teratogenic effects of thalidomide, imipramine HCl and imipramine-N-oxide HCl on white Danish rabbits. *Acta Pharmacol. Toxicol.* 20:186 (1963).

70. G. BIGNAMI, D. BOVET, F. BOVET-NITTI, and V. ROSNATI: Drugs and congenital abnormalities. *Lancet* 2:1333 (1962).

71. C. S. DELAHUNT and L. J. LASSEN: Thalidomide syndrome in monkeys. *Science* 146:1300 (1964).

72. H. KEBERLE, P. LOUSTALOT, R. K. MALLER, J. W. FAIGLE, and K. SCHMID: Biochemical effects of drugs on the mammalian conceptus. *Ann. N.Y. Acad. Sci.* 123:252 (1965).

73. H. OCKENFELS and F. KOHLER: Das L-isomere als teratogenes prinzip der N-phthalyl-DL-glutaminsaure. *Experientia* 26:1236 (1970).

74. F. KOHLER, W. MEISE, and H. OCKENFELS: Teratologische prufung einiger thalidomid-metabolite. *Experientia* 27:1149 (1971).

75. H. J. SCHUMACHER, J. TERAPANE, R. L. JORDAN, and J. G. WILSON: The teratogenic activity of a thalidomide analogue, EM12, in rabbits, rats, and monkeys. *Teratology* 5:233 (1972).

76. C. T. G. KING: Teratogenic effects of meclizine hydrochloride on the rat. *Science* 141:353 (1963).

77. S. A. NARROD, A. L. WILK, and C. T. G. KING: Metabolism of meclizine in the rat. *J. Pharmacol. Exp. Therap.* 147:380 (1965).

78. J. YERUSHALMY and L. MILKOVICH: Evaluation of teratogenic effect of meclizine in man. *Am. J. Obstet. Gynecol.* 93:553 (1965).

79. G. W. MELLIN: Drugs in the first trimester of pregnancy and the fetal life of *Homo Sapiens*. *Am. J. Obstet. Gynecol.* 90:1169 (1964).

80. B. E. WALKER: Cleft palate produced in mice by human-equivalent dosage with triamcinolone. *Science* 149:862 (1965).

81. L. PINSKY and A. M DI GEORGE: Cleft palate in the mouse: a teratogenic index of gluco-corticoid potency. *Science* 147:402 (1965).

82. F. D. ANDREW, D. BOWEN, and E. F. ZIMMERMAN: Glucocorticoid inhibition of RNA synthesis and the critical period for cleft palate induction in inbred mice. *Teratology* 7:167 (1973).

83. H. NISHIMURA and K. NAKAI: Congenital malformations in offspring of mice treated with caffeine. *Proc. Soc. Exp. Biol. Med.* 104:140 (1960).

84. R. D. HARBISON and B. A. BECKER: Relation of dosage and time of administration of di-phenylhydantoin to its teratogenic effects in mice. *Teratology* 2:305 (1969).

85. M. F. KLEIN and J. R. BEALL: Griseofulvin: a teratogenic study. *Science* 175:1483 (1972).

86. J. BERGMAN: Tetracycline and neonatal deformites in fish. *New Eng. J. Med.* 282:225 (1970).

87. E. B. FEEHAN: More on mollies and tetracycline. *New Eng. J. Med.* 282:1048 (1970).

88. S. Y. LONG: Does LSD induce chromosomal damage and malformations? A review of the literature. *Teratology* 5:75 (1972).

89. I. EMERIT, C. ROUX, and J. FEINGOLD: LSD: no chromosomal breakage in mother and embryos during rat pregnancy. *Teratology* 6:71 (1972).

90. W. T. JACKSON: Regulation of mitosis: cytological effects of 2,4,5-trichlorophenoxyacetic acid and of dioxin contaminants in 2,4,5-T formulations. *J. Cell Sci.* 10:15 (1972).

91. D. SHAPLEY: Herbicides: AAAS study finds dioxin in Vietnamese fish. *Science* 180:285 (1973).

92. G. L. SPARSCHU, F. L. DUNN, and V. K. ROWE: Study of the teratogenicity of 2,3,7,8-tetra-chlorodibenzo-*p*-dioxin in the rat. *Cosmet. Toxicol.* 9:405 (1971).

93. B. A. SCHWETZ, G L. SPARSCHU, and P. J. GEHRING: The effect of 2,4-dichlorophenoxy-acetic acid (2,4-D) and ester of 2,4-D on rat embryonal, foetal and neonatal growth and development. *Cosmet. Toxicol.* 9:801 (1971).

94. M. J. VERRETT, M K. MUTCHLER, W. F. SCOTT, E. F. REYNALDO, and J. MC LAUGH-LIN: Teratogenic effects of captan and related compounds in the developing chicken embryo. *Ann. N.Y. Acad. Sci.* 160:334 (1969).

95. J. SCANLON: Fetal effects of lead exposure. *Pediatrics* 49:145 (1972).

96. C. F. FLUHMANN: *The Management of Menstrual Disorders*. Philadelphia, W. B. Saunders (1956).

97. D. L. GUNN, P. M. JENKIN, and A. L. GUNN: Menstrual periodicity; statistical observations on a large sample of normal cases. *J. Obstet. Gynecol.* 44:839 (1937).

98. K. E. PASCHKIS, A. E. RAKOFF, and A. CANTAROW: *Clinical Endocrinology*, 2nd ed. New York, Hoeber-Harper (1958).

99. L. B. AREY: The degree of normal menstrual irregularity. *Am. J. Obstet. Gynecol.* 37:12 (1939).

100. V. APGAR: Drugs in pregnancy. *J. Am. Med. Ass.* 190:840 (1964).

101. J. L. MARX: Drugs during pregnancy: do they affect the unborn child? *Science* 180:174 (1973).

102. W. A. BLEYER, W. Y. W. AU, W. A. LANGE, and L. G. RAISZ: Studies on the detection of adverse drug reactions in the newborn, I. fetal exposure to maternal medication. *J. Am. Med. Ass.* 213:2046 (1970).

102a. W. A. BLEYER and R. T. BRECKENRIDGE: Studies on the detection of adverse drug reactions in the newborn, II. the effects of prenatal aspirin on newborn hemostasis. *J. Am. Med. Ass.* 213:2049 (1970).

103. F. C. FRASER: Experimental teratogenesis in relation to congenital malformations in man. In *Second International Conference on Congenital Malformations*, ed. by M. Fishbein. New York, The International Medical Congress, Ltd. (1964), p. 277.

104. A. G. MAC GREGOR and W. L. M. PERRY: Detection of drug toxicity. *Lancet* 1:1233 (1962).

105. C. R. GREEN: The frequency of maldevelopment in man. *Am. J. Obstet. Gynecol.* 90:994 (1964).

106. T. H. INGALL and M. A. KLINGBERG: Implications of epidemic embryopathy for public health. *Am. J. Public Health* 55:200 (1965).

107. I. LECK: Examination of the incidence of malformations for evidence of drug teratogenesis. *Brit. J. Prevent. Social Med.* 18:196 (1964).

108. J. J. MULVIHILL: Congenital and genetic disease in domestic animals. *Science* 176:132 (1972).

109. F. O. KELSEY: Problems raised for the FDA by the occurrence of thalidomide embryopathy in Germany, 1960–61. *Am. J. Public Health* 55:703 (1965).

CHAPTER 13
Drug Development

INTRODUCTION

Through the ages, there have been societies in which medicine men performed the functions of both physician and priest, gathering herbs or animal organs, processing and mixing them according to sacred rituals, and employing them in ceremonial rites. Ancient and medieval prescriptions blended a multiplicity of natural products with religious and astrologic lore. A 10th-century prescription reads: "Against dysentery, a bramble of which both ends are in the earth, take the nether root, delve it up, cut nine chips with the left hand and sing three times the Miserere Mei Deus and nine times the Pater Noster; then take mugwort...."[1] The traditional symbol ℞, still employed in some modern prescriptions, may stand for the Latin *recipe* ("take"), but there are scholars who believe it to be derived from the symbol of the planet Jupiter, ♃, under whose auspices the healing arts were conducted. Even today there persists among many people a belief in the magical powers of medications, in the potency of herbal mixtures, and in other practices of folk medicine.[2,3]

Until fairly recent times, few questioned the efficacy of the traditional remedies. One who did was Paracelsus (1493–1541), professor at the University of Basel, who regarded much of the contemporary practice of medicine as fraud. Rejecting the authority of Galen (ca. 130–ca. 200), he spoke out in condemnation of the herbal mixtures, contending that useful drugs were diluted to impotent concentrations by the abundance of inert ingredients. He recognized the dose relationship between the desirable action of a drug and its toxic effects. Attacked for using "poisons" when he tried to administer potent single substances, he replied that any active drug could be toxic if given at excessively high dosage. He introduced heavy metals into therapy and used volatile agents to anesthetize animals. But he made acceptance of his views virtually impossible by his open disdain for the leading physicians of his time. The era of scientific medicine was not yet at hand, and Paracelsus had little lasting impact upon the established traditions.[4]

The 18th century saw major advances in therapeutics. The cinchona alkaloids were imported from South America to Europe, where it became obvious that they were highly effective in the treatment of malaria. Withering (1741–1799) identified the leaf of the purple foxglove (*Digitalis purpurea*) as the active principle in a folk remedy for "dropsy" (i.e., edema caused by congestive heart failure), and thereby introduced into therapeutics one of the most important of all pharmacologic agents. Jenner (1748–1823) expounded the principle of vaccination, foreshadowing the prevention of virus infections by specific immunization.

But it was the scientific revolution in medicine during the 19th century, led by men like Claude Bernard (1813–1878), that laid the basis for a rational therapy. With the development of experimental methods for testing actions of drugs in animals and man came the possibility of separating the useless from the efficacious remedies. At about the same time, there began the explosive development of organic chemistry. The first isolation and crystallization of an active drug from a natural source was the accomplishment of a pharmacist's assistant, Sertürner (1783–1841), who obtained pure morphine from natural opium in 1803. Pure quinine was isolated from cinchona bark in 1820. In the latter part of the century, the German dye industry led the way toward the deliberate synthesis of new drugs and the molecular modification of existing ones.

At the beginning of the 20th century, there remained voluminous pharmacopeias containing many drugs of unproved worth. This gave rise to a school of nihilism in therapeutics, exemplified by Osler (1849–1919), who adopted an attitude of skepticism toward all drugs and stressed the overriding importance of diagnosis. "Patients are more often damaged than helped," he wrote, "by the promiscuous drugging which is still only too prevalent." A less rational reaction produced the doctrines of *homeopathy*, which held that drugs become more effective as the dose is reduced.

But nihilism was already doomed by the ever-growing number of dramatic successes achieved by new pharmacologic agents. Morton (1819–1868) had changed the character of all surgery and childbirth by the introduction of ether as an anesthetic. Lister (1827–1912) and Semmelweis (1818–1865) had made surgery and obstetrics tolerably safe by using antiseptics to prevent infection. Ehrlich's (1854–1915) victory over syphilis by the use of an entirely new synthetic compound ushered in the era of modern chemotherapy, and Behring's (1854–1917) successful preparation of antitoxins opened the way to specific immunologic attack on infectious diseases. Still later, the isolation of insulin and the dramatic demonstration of its efficacy in diabetes[5] showed incontrovertibly how specific pharmacologic therapy could transform a uniformly fatal disease into a mere inconvenience of life. By this time, the synthesis of barbiturates, salicylates, and procaine by the German chemical industry made it apparent to physicians and to the public that manufacturers could readily keep pace with demand, once the value of a drug had been demonstrated.

Since World War II there has been an unprecedented expansion of basic research in the biomedical sciences, accompanied by a vast program of research and development in the pharmaceutical industry.[5a] The tangible effects have been a remarkable increase in the kinds and number of new drugs available for clinical use and a continuous expansion in the list of disease conditions that can be cured, ameliorated, or prevented by drugs. In the years 1939–1957, for example, total drug sales in the United States increased 10 times, from 149 million to 1677 million dollars, and to 7211 million by 1970.[6,5a]

The beneficial changes have brought new problems. Not so very long ago, the physician compounded for his own patients whatever few medicinal agents he required. Thus, courses in botany, pharmacognosy (the study of crude drugs), and the preparation of medicines were a regular part of the medical curriculum. Today, the physician prescribes drugs but rarely dispenses them, and he must choose among a myriad of commercially available preparations. The pharmacist's role has also changed. He is rarely called upon to compound a medication; usually he dispenses drugs already made up in the appropriate dosage forms.

Drugs are produced today almost exclusively by large industrial firms. Some drugs are for sale directly to the public ("over the counter"), while others are available only on prescription. Conflicts have sometimes arisen between economic interests of the manufacturer and the interest of the medical profession and the public concerning the safety, efficacy, and cost of new drugs. It has been a matter of some controversy whether the production, promotion, pricing, and sales procedures that are appropriate to other commodities in the consumer market are necessarily also suitable for products that are essential to the practice of medicine and that directly affect public health. The rapid growth of this relatively young industry has provoked legislative inquiry and periodic revision of the legal basis of governmental control over the introduction, promotion, and distribution of new drugs.[7,8,8a]

From the business point of view, the uncertain outcome of research and development creates an urgent necessity for the industry to capitalize upon promising pharmacologic agents, often before their full effects and scope of usefulness have been worked out thoroughly, and before their adverse effects in man have been adequately evaluated. It has been typical to first overestimate the merit of a new drug and underestimate its toxicity before initial overenthusiasm gradually gives way to a balanced perspective on the drug's proper place in therapy. This pattern has been exemplified in recent years by the antihistamines, chloramphenicol, the tetracycline antibiotics, the various types of tranquilizers, and the "psychic energizers."

The modern pattern and pace of drug development create a serious problem for physicians and others who wish to keep informed about the efficacy and safety of new drugs. Especially difficult is the task of choosing from among a variety of agents, each one claimed by its manufacturer to be superior to the others. Textbooks cannot keep abreast of current progress, and there is not sufficient time for one person to read and appraise all the medical literature. In this chapter we shall explain, with detailed illustration, how new drugs are developed, tested, and made ready for clinical trial prior to their introduction into medical use. In the following chapter, we shall describe the procedures that are used to evaluate drugs in man and the guidelines for the selection and prescription of drugs.

QUALITATIVE AND QUANTITATIVE ESTIMATION OF DRUG ACTION

The ideal drug would have a perfectly selective biologic action, with no side effects and no toxicity. There is no such drug, but the aims of drug development are to approach this ideal. The desired effect must be well defined, and a procedure is needed that can determine whether or not a particular drug has the specified effect. If it has, a quantitative method is needed to estimate its potency and its selectivity of action. Related drugs can then be compared to see which is most selective for the desired pharmacologic effect. The initial steps in drug development for determining whether or not a compound possesses the desired actions are sometimes referred to as *screening*, and the procedures themselves as *screens*.[8b–8e,9] Quantitative determinations of potency and toxicity by means of dose-response relationships are known as *bioassays*.

Screening

A pharmacologic screen consists of a specified set of procedures to which a series of compounds can be subjected.[10] The screen may employ animals or it may consist of procedures carried out in vitro. In general, since the dosage is completely unknown at the outset, one administers various doses up to the "maximum tolerated dose," i.e., the range in which toxicity occurs. The question, then, is whether or not the desired therapeutic effect is obtained at nontoxic doses. The earliest example of a large-scale screening program was that carried out in the original search for a chemotherapeutic agent to cure syphilis.[11] The spirochete *Treponema pallidum* is pathogenic for rabbits, so potentially useful drugs could be screened in this species. Only the 606th compound tested, arsphenamine ("salvarsan") showed a decisive margin between curative and toxic doses; this drug was eventually introduced into clinical use.

A prototype that illustrates the general organization of a mass screening program is the Malaria Survey conducted during World War II in the United States.[12] Seventeen university and commercial laboratories participated and over 15,000 compounds were screened. The problem was to find an antimalarial agent to replace quinine, the sources of which had fallen into enemy hands. The human malaria parasite of main interest, *Plasmodium vivax*, does not infect other species. Canaries, chicks, and ducks have specific forms of malaria, and these were chosen as convenient screens. This illustrates a general difficulty about animal screens—even with infectious diseases the conditions are not exactly the same in animals and in man; with non-infectious human diseases, it may be extremely difficult to find any suitable animal model. Here the behavior of certain known antimalarial drugs gave some assurance that the avian malarias could be expected to respond to at least some agents that were also effective in man. The birds were infected under specified conditions, parasite counts were performed at regular intervals, and the reduction of parasitemia was specified as the criterion of response. A concrete example of one of the testing procedures exemplifies the general scheme.

Chicks 7–8 days old and about 50 g in weight were inoculated via the jugular vein with heparinized chick blood infected with *Plasmodium gallinaceum*, 16 million parasitized red blood cells being administered. The parasitemia in untreated birds reaches its peak on the fourth to seventh day, when 60–90% of the red cells are parasitized; over 99% of the birds die. Treatment with a test drug was given twice daily by mouth, beginning just before the birds were infected, and continuing 4 days. Five birds were used for each test group, and a series of 50–120 birds were used for appraisal of a single drug. An untreated control group was included in each series. The maximum tolerated dose of the drug was first determined by administering it on the same schedule to uninfected birds in a preliminary trial. The test doses then began with the maximum tolerated dose and decreased geometrically by a divisor of 2. Each series also included groups of birds on standard doses of quinine, the drug of reference. The count of parasitized red cells was determined on the day after the last drug dose. Quinine, at a dose of 32 mg kg^{-1} daily, given as described, reduced the parasitemia to below 25% of the control. This extent of reduction was chosen as criterion of drug effect, and if it was not achieved at the maximum tolerated dose, then the drug under test was considered to be unpromising. The lowest dose that achieved the criterion was expressed as a "quinine equivalent," the ratio of the dose of quinine to the dose of the test drug for this specified effect. Thus, if the test drug were effective at a dose of 3.2 mg kg^{-1} daily, the quinine equivalent would be 32/3.2, or 10. Toxicity tests were also carried out routinely in mice, rats, dogs, and monkeys. All groups of animals in which parasite counts gave evidence of drug activity, according to the criteria described here, were followed to see if the drug had any curative activity.

Table 13-1 is a typical extract from the final voluminous report of the Malaria Survey.[12] It deals with Survey Number 7618, the 4-amino-quinoline derivative chloroquine, which became the drug of choice for the suppression of vivax malaria as a result of these screening studies. The coded information is interpreted as follows: A-1, A-2, and A-2a are screening procedures conducted at the National Institutes of Health. A-1 is the procedure described above, using chicks. The other procedures employed sporozoites from mosquitoes, rather than infected red cells, in a test for prophylactic action that would prevent the establishment of infection. The quinine equivalent for the suppressive test was 15, as indicated by the symbol Q 15. In the prophylactic tests, since quinine has no such activity, the reference drug was sulfadiazine (D), and the data show that even at the maximum tolerated dose (mtd) the sulfadiazine equivalent was rather low. The remaining entries refer to tests conducted at other laboratories. They show that high quinine equivalents were the rule whenever

TABLE 13-1. Sample data from the Survey of Antimalarial Drugs

The extract shown for Survey Number 7618, chloroquine, the suppressive antimalarial that became the drug of choice as a result of the mass screening conducted in the years 1941–1945. Meaning of symbols is explained in text. (From Wiselogle,[12] vol. II, p. 1145.)

Drug tested	Screening procedures and results		
SN 7618. $C_{18}H_{26}ClN_3$. *chloroquine.*	A-1	Q	15
(structure: 7-chloro-4-aminoquinoline with side chain HN—CH(CH$_3$)—(CH$_2$)$_3$—N(C$_2$H$_5$)$_2$)	A-2	D	< 6 (at mtd)
	A-2a	D	< 0.8 (at mtd)
	B-4	Q	15
	B-9	active	
	D-1	Q	10
	D-1	Q	15
	D-2	Q	60
	Q-4	Q	15
	Q-8	Q	30
	S-1	Q	15
	S-2	inactive	
	1-A	Q	10
	1-B	Q	5
	1-D	Q	5
	1-U	Q	5
	1-U	Q	10

suppressive activity was tested. The only other inactive outcome was in S-2, a prophylactic test on canaries. The information grouped at the bottom refers to toxicity tests. Here the quinine equivalents were lower, on the whole, than for the antimalarial effects, signifying the possibility that chloroquine might have a wider margin of safety than quinine. Consider, for example, the outcome in the chick, of studies A-1 and 1-A, conducted in the same laboratory. In A-1, as we have seen, the desired reduction of parasitemia was accomplished with $\frac{1}{15}$ the dose of quinine. In 1-A, the maximum dose that did not cause suppression of growth over a 4-day period was taken as criterion, and here chloroquine was toxic at $\frac{1}{10}$ the dose of quinine. If the toxicity equivalent is significantly lower than the suppressive equivalent, the therapeutic ratio (cf. Chapter 5) of chloroquine is greater than that of quinine.

Out of more than 15,000 compounds tested in the antimalarial survey, two were clearly superior to other drugs then available. One of these, chloroquine, was superior to quinine as a suppressive antimalarial. As it turned out, chloroquine had been synthesized previously and tested in 1934 by the German pharmaceutical industry under the name "resochin." However, information about it did not become available in other countries until after World War II. The other outstanding product of the Malaria Survey was primaquine (SN 13,272), superior to any drug then known in its ability to eradicate the tissue forms of the malaria parasite and thus bring about radical cure of the disease.

It is curious that the two major drugs to emerge from the Malaria Survey were quinolines, and that both are so closely related to the 4-amino- and 8-aminoquinolines that had been in clinical use as antimalarials for many years. Perhaps something about the design of the antimalarial survey led to this outcome. It is known now that not all antimalarials are quinoline derivatives. A program conducted in Great Britain at the same time as the Malaria Survey in the United States yielded a completely new class of antimalarials, namely, antifolic compounds with antimalarial activity. Here the follow-up of initial observations on sulfadiazine led to deliberate molecular modifications such as those described later in this chapter.

Screening has been very useful, in general, for finding anti-infective agents. Of the antibiotics, penicillin was discovered by complete accident, but all the others have been obtained through exhaustive screening of soil samples from various parts of the world. For these agents, the "screen" consists of determination, in vitro, of antibacterial and antifungal activity. The common antibiotics, such as streptomycin, are rediscovered again and again, at great expense. The probability of discovering a new antibiotic of value through repetitive application of the same screening procedure obviously diminishes year by year.

Apart from infectious diseases, the analogy between human illness and animal models may be tenuous, and drug screening in animals may fail to reveal a useful action or may falsely suggest great utility. Some human illnesses have no discernible animal counterpart; examples are mental depression and idiopathic epilepsy. There is great incentive to find effective anticancer drugs, and large-scale screening has been conducted for many years, using transplantable rodent tumors. But it is not at all certain that these are biologically equivalent to spontaneous cancer in man. Often, although an exact counterpart of a human disease is not known in animals, enough is known of the mechanisms of the human disease so that an artificial equivalent can be produced in animals, or a meaningful screen can be devised for some specific drug effect. Even though a disease analogous to essential hypertension may not exist among ordinary laboratory animals, reduction of blood pressure can nevertheless be sought in an animal screen. In the same way, empirical "analgesia" tests can be conducted in animals, even though it is not certain that they feel pain in the same way we do. A screen based on abolishing the "tail flick" of a rat subjected to a thermal stimulus (cf. p. 599) does serve to identify the known analgesic drugs; similar screens have been employed successfully to find new analgesics.

Occasionally drugs are subjected to "blind screening,"[13] in which specific criteria for particular desired actions have not been established in advance. The aim is to see if a new compound or group of compounds has useful pharmacologic activity of any sort. Such screens can be standardized so that they are neither too cumbersome not too expensive. For example, in searching for effects of neuropharmacologic interest, very detailed observations of animal behavior, motor activity, coordination, state of the righting reflex, and so on, may be made according to carefully compiled checklists. The simple procedures for observing and handling mice are standardized so that all technical personnel are able to produce reliable data. An arbitrary scoring system is used for each type of behavior observed. Table 13-2 presents a score card used in this type of screening. The scale of scores runs from zero to 8. For normal signs, the reference score is 4; subnormal responses are scored less than 4; supernormal, more than 4. The reference score for abnormal responses is zero. Since a normal mouse grooms itself, the normal score under "grooming" is set at 4; at a dose of 1 mg kg^{-1}, the mice are seen to have engaged in excessive grooming activity, so a score of 5 was assigned. Vocalization does not normally occur, so the normal score is zero; at a dose of 3 and 10 mg kg^{-1}, the mice evidently vocalized slightly, for scores of 1 were assigned. The general pattern of dose-related effects is often quite characteristic of a given drug, and the method can serve to detect potentially useful kinds of neuropharmacologic action. The drug portrayed in the table, for example, at doses that produced certain autonomic effects but that were not lethal, had generally sedative action. The mice became less alert, more uncoordinated, and passive (tranquilized). Muscle tone was greatly relaxed, and at the higher doses, the animals were in the prone position, with decreased respiratory rate.

Thus far, we have talked about techniques of screening. As for the extent of screening, it is difficult to formulate criteria for terminating a screening program. If a potentially useful compound turns up early in a series, is it worth trying to improve on it by extensive molecular modifications? If no promising compound turns up, how long should the search continue? There is some evidence that marketable drugs tend to be found fairly early in a series. For example, 16 pharmaceutical manufacturing firms responded to a questionnaire sent out to a total of 70 firms in Switzerland, the United Kingdom, and the United States.[14] With respect to 79 useful drugs that had been developed in their laboratories, they indicated that if every series had been terminated at the 40th compound synthesized, only 18 % of the useful drugs would have been missed. Yet the average series length was 147 compounds. It seems, therefore, that nearly three-fourths of the synthesis and testing was useless. One reason for increased yield early in a series is probably that the best efforts and rationale go into the first few compounds and the congeners related to them. Some of the "excess" synthesis and screening may be related to a desire to secure patents on related compounds in order to reduce competition. Some also may be attributable to unavoidable time lag between synthesis and screening. On the other hand, examples are plentiful of important drugs that are perfected only after hundreds of others have been synthesized, tested, and discarded.

TABLE 13-2. Profile checklist for "blind" neuropharmacologic screening.

Arbitrary scores are assigned to the various categories of behavior, as described in text. The tests are conducted with groups of three mice, at various doses increasing by a factor of 3. Normal score for each category is shown at top; higher score is increase, lower score is decrease in the particular behavior. (From Irwin, reproduced in Turner,[13] Figure 5.)

Header information:
Test — CNS activity and acute toxicity screen | Perphenazine | Test No. P-3 | Chemist
Species: Mouse | Sex: Male | Weight (gm): 18–24 | Route: Oral | B.F. = 1.18
Vehicle: H₂O | pH = 5, pH = 3 | 0.2%, 2.0% | ☒ Sol., ☒ Sol. | ☐ Insol., ☐ Insol.

Category	Behavior	Normal score	0.01	0.03	0.10	0.30	1	3	10	30	100	300	1000
Awareness	Alertness	4					1	1	0	0	0	0	
	Visual placing	4			3	2	2	1	1	0	0	0	
	Passivity	0							5	8	8	8	
	Stereotype	0											
Mood	Grooming	4				5							
	Vocalization	0					1	1					
	Restlessness	0											
	Irritability (aggression?)	0											
	Fearfulness	0											
Motor activity	Reactivity (envir.)	4			3	2	2	1	0	0	0	0	
	Spontaneous activity	4			3	2	2	1	0	0	0	0	
	Touch response	4			3	3	1	1	0	0	0	0	
	Pain response	4				1	1	1	1	0	0	0	
CNS excitation	Startle response	0											
	Straub tail	0											
	Tremors	0						1	2				
	Twitches	0										1	
	Convulsions	0											
Posture	Body posture	4								P	P	P	
	Limb position	4			3	3	2	1	0	0S	0S	0S	
Motor Incoord.	Staggering gait	0						2	1				
	Abnormal gait	0											
	Righting reflex	0					2	3	4	7	8	8	8
Muscle tone	Limb tone	4			3	3	1	1	0	0	0	0	
	Grip strength	4				3	2	1	1	1	0	0	
	Body sag	0					2	3	8	8	8		
	Body tone	4			3	3	2	1	0	0	0	0	
	Abdominal tone	4			3	3	2	1	0	0	0	0	
Reflexes	Pinna	4					2	2	0	1	0	0	0
	Corneal	4					3	2	1	1	0	0	0
	IFR	4					2	2	1	1	1	0	0
	Writhing	0											
Autonomic	Pupil size	4											
	Palpebral opening	4					3	2	2	1	1	1	
	Exophthalmos	0											
	Urination	0					1	1	1	2	2	2	
	Salivation	0											
	Piloerection	0											
	Hypothermia	0										1	
	Skin color	4										3	
	Heart rate	4											
	Respir. rate	4								3T	3T	2T	1T
	Lacrimation	0								1		1	
Misc.													
Dead	No. acute	0											
	No. delayed	0											

Bioassay

A bioassay is a procedure for determining the quantitative relationship between the dose (or concentration) of a drug and the magnitude of biologic response it evokes. One purpose of bioassay is to ascertain the potency of a drug, or more usually, the comparative potencies of two or more drugs. In this use, the bioassay serves as the quantitative part of any screening procedure. An example already presented is the determination of quinine equivalents of potential antimalarials.

Another purpose of bioassay is to standardize preparations of impure drugs, so that each contains the same specified pharmacologic activity. In this use, bioassay serves as a guide in the commercial production of drugs when chemical analyses will not suffice. This is especially important before the exact chemical structure of a drug is known, as with most antibiotics shortly after their discovery. Penicillin exemplifies the usual course of events. This antibiotic was used very widely in the form of impure extracts of the culture media in which the *Penicillium* mold was grown, and the pharmacologic activity was expressed in arbitrary *units*. A unit is always defined at first in terms of biologic activity. The unit of penicillin was the amount required to inhibit completely the growth of a test organism, *Staphylococcus aureus*, Oxford strain, in 50 ml of a defined culture medium. Eventually, when penicillin was crystallized and its chemical structure worked out, it turned out that one unit was equivalent to 0.6 μg of pure penicillin G. When that stage has been reached, the bioassay procedure and the unit serve no further purpose and should be dropped.

Standardization of impure drugs is essential if dosage is to have any meaning. The physician has to be able to prescribe a dose that will always, as nearly as possible, represent the same pharmacologic activity. And the bioassay procedures are rigorously defined by appropriate public agencies. In the U.S., the standards for "biologics" (vaccines, serums, and toxins) are set by the Division of Biologics Standards of the National Institutes of Health. Standards for antibiotics are set by the Food and Drug Administration. Standards for other drugs are defined in the United States Pharmacopeia.[15] International standards are also available.[16] Other drugs still standardized by bioassay include hormones such as corticotropin, glucagon, insulin, oxytocin, and vasopressin, and natural products such as digitalis, heparin, and tubocurarine. Bioassays of hormones are required even though the chemical structures of the active principles may be known. Because it may not yet be practical to package and sell the chemically pure substance, preparations pure enough for clinical use are made instead from the endocrine glands of animals. The hormone content of such preparations may vary from batch to batch.

Three different approaches may be employed in bioassays:[17]

1. The threshold dose is measured for obtaining a specified biologic end point. For example, an extract of digitalis is infused into a pigeon's vein at a prescribed rate. The threshold dose is the amount that has been infused at the moment of cardiac standstill. This is the standard procedure for the assay of powdered digitalis. It is interesting that what is assayed is not the desired pharmacologic action but a related toxic effect. Also, since the drug is given intravenously in the assay procedure but orally in its usual therapeutic use, a substance that was poorly absorbed from the gastrointestinal tract might nevertheless show high activity in the assay.

2. A graded biologic response is measured at several doses, and the potency of the unknown is compared with that of a standard preparation of the same drug. In the testing of new antihistamine drugs, each unknown might be compared with a standard

antihistaminic agent, such as diphenylhydramine, with respect to its relative potency in antagonizing the effect of histamine on the guinea pig ileum in a tissue bath (cf. Figures 1-71 and 1-82). Another example is the official procedure for standardizing insulin, described below.

3. A quantal response is measured, the percentage of positive effects at each dose being recorded. The unknown is then compared with a standard with respect to potency in causing the quantal effects. The commonest application of this approach is the testing of toxicity (e.g., LD50 determinations), as described in Chapter 5.

The United States Pharmacopeia contains an excellent working summary of the procedures of bioassay, and of the statistical analysis of bioassay data (U.S.P. XVIII, pp. 867–882).[15] The reader is referred elsewhere for fuller treatment of the principles and mathematics of bioassay.[18-20] We choose here, for illustration, the standardization of insulin by bioassay (U.S.P. XVIII, p. 882). *Insulin Injection* is defined as "a sterile, acidified solution of the active principle of the pancreas which affects the metabolism of glucose." It "possesses a potency of not less than 95% and not more than 105% of the potency stated on the label, expressed in U.S.P. Insulin Units." Long before the chemical structure of insulin was known, the unit of insulin activity was defined as the amount of insulin that reduces the blood sugar level of a 2-kg rabbit to 45 mg per 100 ml in 5 hr. Today, the unit is expressed in terms of a U.S.P. Zinc-Insulin Crystals Reference Standard, containing about 22 units per mg. Two solutions are prepared from the standard: standard dilution 1, containing 1.0 unit per ml, and standard dilution 2, containing 2.0 units per ml. Two solutions of the unknown are also prepared, to contain, as nearly as can be estimated, the same activities as the two standard dilutions.

Rabbits of a specified weight are maintained on a prescribed feeding schedule. They are divided into four equal groups of at least six animals, and the same volume (usually 0.30 to 0.50 ml) of each of the four solutions is injected subcutaneously into the rabbits according to the following design:

Group	1st injection	2nd injection
1	Standard dilution 2	Sample dilution 1
2	Standard dilution 1	Sample dilution 2
3	Sample dilution 2	Standard dilution 1
4	Sample dilution 1	Standard dilution 2

The second injection is made at least 24 hrs after the first. At 1 hr and 2.5 hrs after each injection, blood is drawn from the marginal ear vein and the blood sugar levels are determined. For purposes of computation, the blood sugar levels at both times are given equal weight. This bioassay exemplifies the simplest design capable of yielding reliable confidence limits for the estimated relative potencies of the standard and the unknown. It is known as a 2 × 2 *assay* because two dose levels of unknown are compared with two dose levels of standard (cf. Figure 5-12). The design incorporates several important features whose purpose is to reduce variability and therefore to improve the reliability of the result. The use of six or more rabbits in each group ensures that an aberrant response of one animal will not unduly influence the outcome. The *crossover*, in which each rabbit is used twice, once for a standard injection and once for an unknown injection, ensures that differences between rabbits will not be falsely ascribed to a difference between standard and unknown, as might happen if the standard were tested on one group of animals and the unknown on another. The plan of the crossover also ensures that differences between responses on different days will not be ascribed to potency differences between solutions, for all four solutions are tested on each day. Finally, measurement of blood sugar level at two times after an injection ensures that minor differences in the rate of onset or offset of the insulin action will not unduly influence the assay.

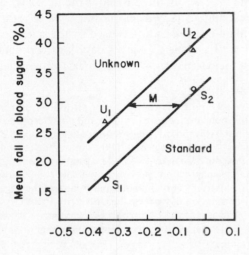

FIGURE 13-1. Bioassay of insulin. *2 × 2 assay as described in text. Each point is the mean response of a group of rabbits given one dose of standards (S_1, S_2) or unknown (U_1, U_2). Dose is expressed in units per rabbit. The "unknown" potency was known to be 1.41 times that of the standard. (From Bliss and Marks, Figure 1.[21])*

An illustration of this assay is presented in Figure 13-1. In this demonstration experiment, the "unknown" was actually another solution of the standard; two dilutions of "unknown," U_1 and U_2, each contained 1.41 times as much insulin as the respective dilutions of standard, S_1 and S_2. The mean responses are plotted as percent fall in blood sugar against log dose. The best parallel lines are drawn through the points. The potency difference is given by horizontal distance M between the two lines. Since the x-axis is logarithmic, M is a difference in logarithms, corresponding to a *potency ratio*. Here M was found to be 0.179, and antilog 0.179 is 1.51. Naturally, the experimentally determined value of M is not likely to correspond precisely with the true value. But the confidence limits of M should include the true value; and in this example the true value, 1.41, was well within the computed 95% confidence interval. The computations for obtaining the confidence interval may be found elsewhere.[19,20] In the usual bioassay, of course, there will be a solution containing an unknown amount of insulin. In such an assay, M will represent the potency ratio for the dilutions employed in the assay (i.e., U_1/S_1 or U_2/S_2), whence the potency of the unknown stock solution will have to be determined. In the best conducted assay, the two lines would be superimposed and the value of M would be zero. This would simply mean that the unknown had been diluted successfully to match the standard. The potency ratio of the dilutions would be 1.0. The dilutions of the unknown would contain 1.0 and 2.0 units ml^{-1}, exactly as the dilutions of the standard. The insulin content of the original unknown solution could then be obtained by correcting for whatever dilution had been made.

A bioassay does not necessarily employ as criterion of biologic response the same effect that is made use of in the clinical application of a drug. A corollary effect may be employed, as when insulin is sometimes assayed by its convulsant effect in laboratory animals. Inasmuch as the convulsions are a direct consequence of the blood sugar lowering action, results may be obtained without the necessity of determining blood sugar levels. Side effects may usually be employed for a bioassay, provided they are inseparable from the main drug effect and caused by the same compound rather than by a contaminating impurity. Table 13-3 gives data for the potencies of the posterior pituitary hormones oxytocin and vasopressin, assayed by five different procedures.[22,23]

TABLE 13-3. Bioassay methods for posterior pituitary hormones.
Shown are the relative potencies of pure oxytocin and pure vasopressin, in terms of the U.S.P. Posterior Pituitary Standard. Figures are potencies in U.S.P. units per mg of substance. Oxytocic activity was measured by the contractile response of the isolated rat uterine horn; avian depressor activity, by blood pressure lowering in the fowl; milk-ejecting activity, in the female rabbit; pressor activity, by rise of blood pressure in the rat; and antidiuretic activity, by reduction of urine volume in the dog. (From Van Dyke et al.,[22] Table I. By permission of Rockefeller University Press.)

	Potency by assay method (units/mg)				
Hormone	Oxytocic (rat uterus)	Avian depressor (fowl)	Milk-ejecting (rabbit)	Pressor (rat)	Anti-diuretic (dog)
Oxytocin	500	500	500	7	3
Vasopressin	30	85	100	600	600

The reference standard was an extract of pituitary glands containing both kinds of activity. The table shows three methods yielded the same result for pure oxytocin, even though only the rat uterus assay is directly related to the therapeutic action of this drug in the human. Similarly, two methods yielded the same result for pure vasopressin, although only the antidiuretic action in the dog is directly related to the therapeutic action in man. These findings justify the prescribed U.S.P. assays for these hormones,[15] both of which employ side effects rather than a main therapeutic effect. Oxytocin is assayed by the avian depressor procedure; its potency is compared with the standard in causing fall of blood pressure when injected intravenously in the chicken. Vasopressin is assayed by the rat pressor procedure rather than by anti-diuresis, the effect of interest in man; yet this hormone does not have significant pressor effect in man. The table shows, incidentally, that each hormone has a small amount of activity ordinarily associated with the other, as noted in the discussion of structure-activity relationships in this group of compounds (cf. Chapter 1).

Sometimes it is even possible to use a lethal effect as an appropriate assay. A good example is the standardization of digitalis. Digitalis is the dried leaf of the foxglove plant. The reference standard is a mixture of many preparations of powdered dried leaves, representing an average composition of the several glycosides contained in the plant. The U.S.P. Digitalis Unit is the activity contained in 100 mg of this standard powder. The assay of unknown preparations of powdered leaf is conducted as follows : An alcoholic extract (a *tincture*) is prepared and diluted with physiologic saline solution. A fixed volume of this solution is administered repeatedly to an anesthetized pigeon, by the intravenous route, at 5-minute intervals, until the animal dies of cardiac arrest. Six pigeons are used for the standard and six for the unknown. The reason cardiac arrest can be used as an end-point for digitalis assay is that, as with all the cardiac glycosides studied thus far, the therapeutically effective dosage is a constant fraction of the lethal dosage. Another effect invariably associated with cardioactive glycosides is emesis; formerly, emesis in the pigeon was the basis of standardization of digitalis preparations.

METHODS OF DEVELOPING NEW DRUGS

Purification of Drugs from Natural Sources

Natural products were once the source of all drugs, and the purification of medicinal substances from the plants became a major concern of medicinal chemistry during the 19th century. In recent years, progress in analytic and preparative methods stimulated a resurgence of interest in this field.[24] Natural products and their derivatives still represent nearly half of all drugs in clinical use; antibiotics constitute the major fraction of these.[25]

Occasionally, native lore provides clues to plants with pharmacologic activity.[26] Digitalis, opiates, and the *Cinchona* alkaloids (quinine and quinidine) came into modern medicine by this route. Curare was obtained from a South American plant long used by natives to prepare arrow poisons. Cardiac glycosides from *Strophanthus* seeds and physostigmine from Calabar beans exemplify useful drugs employed as poisons in the native habitat. *Rauwolfia serpentina* was used for centuries in India as a native remedy for a variety of illnesses; only in recent years were its tranquilizing properties recognized in Western medicine and the active principle, reserpine, isolated. Atropine, pilocarpine, nicotine, ephedrine, cocaine, theophylline, and numerous other drugs were obtained first by purifying extracts of plants alleged to have medicinal qualities. But despite these useful contributions to the modern pharmacopeia, folk medicine is a notoriously unreliable guide in the search for active products. There has been intensive interest, for example, in discovering antifertility agents. According to the natives of certain Pacific islands, about 200 different local plants are efficacious in reducing male or female fertility. Extracts made from 80 of these were fed at high dosage levels to rats for periods up to four weeks without any effect upon pregnancies or litter sizes.[27]

Antibiotics.   The purification of antibiotics offers a good illustration of the essential procedures. The work begins with the discovery of antibacterial or antifungal activity in the culture medium in which the organisms under investigation have grown. The earliest deliberate search for antibiotics was initiated on the rational basis that soil organisms might have evolved that are capable of attacking and destroying competing microorganisms in the soil.[28] Soil samples were incubated in the presence of pathogens in the hope of producing an enrichment with respect to any antibiotic-producing organism that might be present. From such a culture was obtained a gram-positive spore-forming bacterium, *Bacillus brevis*, which produced antibacterial substances. The crude material, called *tyrothricin*, could be dissolved in alcohol and then separated into two crystalline products by adding ether. The material precipitated under these conditions was called *gramicidin*; the soluble material, crystallizable from acetone, was called *tyrocidine*. Table 13-4 shows the differences in antibacterial and hemolytic

TABLE 13-4. Antibacterial and hemolytic activity of crude gramicidin and tyrocidine. Bacteria were grown on meat infusion peptone agar in the presence of the amount of each antibiotic shown in 3 ml of bacterial suspension. Hemolysis was determined by incubating the amount shown with 1 ml of a 10% suspension of washed erythrocytes; results were the same for all incubation times from 15 min to 24 hr. Symbols: — = no bacterial growth or no hemolysis; + + + + = abundant bacterial growth or complete hemolysis. (From Dubos and Hotchkiss,[29] Tables I and III.)

	Amt. of antibiotic (mg)	Bacterial growth		Hemolysis
		E. coli	Staphylococcus	
Gramicidin	0.500	+ + + +	—	
	0.400			—
	0.200			—
	0.100	+ + + +	—	—
	0.050			—
	0.020			—
	0.010	+ + + +	—	
	0.005	+ + + +	—	
	0.002	+ + + +	+	
Tyrocidine	0.500	—	—	
	0.400			+ + + +
	0.200			+ + + +
	0.100	—	—	+ + +
	0.050	—	—	+
	0.025	+ + +	—	
	0.020			—
	0.010	+ + + +	+ + + +	

activities of the two antibiotics. Gramicidin is seen to be highly selective against the test organisms, preventing growth of the gram-positive staphylococci but not the gram-negative *Escherichia coli*. This agent was found to be effective also against pneumococci, streptococci, diphtheria bacilli, and the aerobic sporulating bacilli. Tyrocidine, on the other hand, was equally active against gram-negative and gram-positive organisms. Gramicidin produced no hemolysis, whereas tyrocidine was hemolytic within the concentration range of its antibacterial activity. Because of its toxicity, the crude mixture, tyrothricin (about 1 part gramicidin to 4 parts tyrocidine), is employed only for topical application as a solution or ointment.

More powerful methods of separation soon showed that neither gramicidin nor tyrocidine is a single compound; both are mixtures of closely related cyclic polypeptides. In the representation of a cyclic peptide arrows indicate the polarity of the peptide bonds, $-CO \rightarrow NH-$.

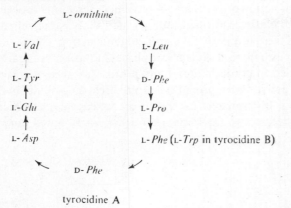

tyrocidine A

By the procedure of countercurrent distribution (cf. p. 232) tyrocidine, for example, was resolved into three pure products. That complex polypeptides as nearly identical as tyrocidines A and B should be completely separable well illustrates the resolving power of this technique. Once pure compounds were obtained, the usual methods of protein chemistry for determining amino acid composition and sequence could be applied.[30] In this instance, it was important to establish the steric configuration of each amino acid, for two phenylalanine residues turned out to be of the unusual D type.

The successful isolation of these antibiotics from soil microbes was followed by an extensive search for others. Indeed, the "rediscovery" and practical development of penicillin were apparently stimulated in part by these "interesting studies on the acquired bacterial antagonism of a soil bacterium which have led to the isolation from its culture medium of bactericidal substances active against a number of gram-positive microorganisms."[31] Other antibiotics discovered by screening procedures, isolated, crystallized, identified chemically, and introduced into clinical use include bacitracin (1943), streptomycin (1944), polymyxin B and chloramphenicol (1947), chlortetracycline (1948), neomycin (1949), oxytetracycline (1950), erythromycin (1952), vancomycin and novobiocin (1956), paromomycin (1959), gentamycin (1963), ampicillin and cephalothin (1964), lincomycin (1965), cephaloridine (1968), and rifampin (1971). The rate of introduction of new and significant antibiotics into clinical use continues at about one per year.

Vinca Alkaloids.   The isolation and identification of the active alkaloids in the leaves of the periwinkle plant (*Vinca rosea*) afford an example of the application of modern analytical chemistry to the problem of separation and complete chemical identification of very complex compounds. Crude preparations of plants of this species enjoyed a reputation in some parts of the world for being useful in diabetes. Extracts of the plant were therefore assayed for hypoglycemic activity. No such hypoglycemic activity was ever observed in tests with plant extracts, but in the course of the work, it was noticed that treated rats frequently suffered a fatal fulminating infection. Investigation showed that the fatal septicemia was secondary to a massive leukopenia. Depression of the white cell count was then adopted as bioassay criterion, permitting the isolation of one of the responsible alkaloids, vinblastine, in 1958.[32] In another laboratory, routine screening of the crude plant materials in an anticancer program revealed activity against a transplantable lymphocytic leukemia of mice.[33] This antileukemic action proved to be a convenient screening tool, and by 1963 over 30 different alkaloids had been purified, four of which (vinblastine, vinleurosine, vincristine, and vinrosidine) were found to have antileukemic activity.[34]

We can distinguish three characteristic phases of these investigations. First, biologic activity is detected in crude material and a bioassay system is set up to permit the identification of active fractions and the rapid discarding of inactive ones. Second, the crude material is fractionated by the most appropriate chemical procedures, all fractions are tested, active fractions are further fractionated, and so on, until pure

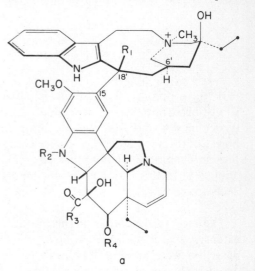

a. Two-dimensional representation of vincristine methiodide as determined by x-ray crystallographic methods. Vinblastine and vincristine have no methyl group on the 6'-position; they are tertiary amines. Carbon atoms are shown as dots *joined by bonds. Heavy* lines *are meant to indicate bonds projecting toward the reader,* broken lines *indicate bonds projecting away from the reader. The bond between the 15- and 13'-positions can rotate freely in solution.* R_1 *COOCH$_3$;* R_3, *OCH$_3$;* R_4, *COCH$_3$. In vinblastine,* R_2, *CH$_3$; in vincristine,* R_2, *CHO*

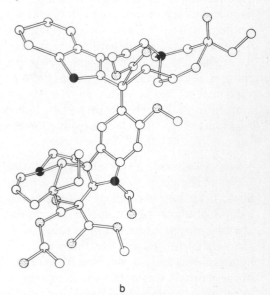

b. The vincristine methiodide molecule as it actually appears in the crystal. Carbon atoms are open circles, *nitrogen atoms are* solid black circles, *oxygen atoms are* stippled circles. *Hydrogen atoms are not shown.* (Drawing by courtesy of W. N. Lipscomb.)

FIGURE 13-2. Conformational structure of vinblastine and vincristine. *(From Moncrief and Lipscomb, Figure 3.[36] By permission of Munksgaard.)*

crystalline compounds are obtained. Third, the chemical structures of the pure compounds are determined. Nowadays, the second and third phases may be carried out with astonishing speed by large teams of chemists. Only about 3 years were required to isolate the more than 30 *Vinca* alkaloids, although they are very much alike in chemical structure. The techniques employed were generally similar to those described for the isolation of drug metabolites (cf. Chapter 3). Differential extraction into organic solvents was the first step; with proper pH control, this permitted separation of the alkaloids according to their degree of basicity. The second procedure used was chromatography on columns of alumina gel. Chemical identification was carried out more or less concurrently with isolation.[35] Here the powerful techniques of infrared spectroscopy, nuclear magnetic resonance, and mass spectroscopy were combined with the older methods of degradation and elemental analysis. By 1965, the molecular structures, stereochemistry, and absolute configuration of two of these molecules were reported, based upon x-ray diffraction analysis of the crystalline material (Figure 13-2).

Other *Vinca* alkaloids are quite closely related to the compound shown in Figure 13-2; they are monomers or dimers containing indole or dihydroindole residues. The conclusive determination of so many complex structures within only a few years after the compounds were first isolated is a truly extraordinary achievement. In contrast to this rapid progress, it may be noted that the structure of the far simpler morphine alkaloid, which had been isolated from crude opium in 1803, was only tentatively established in 1925 and not confirmed until many years later; and its spatial configuration was only worked out about 20 years ago.

Curiously, it now seems that the original notion about hypoglycemic activity in *Vinca* extracts may not have been entirely without merit. Several of the highly purified alkaloids (not the cytotoxic ones described above) can indeed lower the blood sugar of fasting rats.[37] This activity was not readily discernible in crude extracts, probably because of the severe reactions caused by the cytotoxic alkaloids also present.

Steroids.   Steroid hormones can be isolated from animal sources, but not in sufficient amounts or at low enough cost to supply a mass market. The practical advances in the therapeutic use of anti-inflammatory glucocorticoids and the introduction of oral contraceptives rest entirely upon the systematic purification of steroids from various natural sources and their use as starting materials for new organic syntheses.

The first practical impetus to research in this area came during World War II when a rumor circulated that Germany had perfected an adrenal cortical hormone capable of protecting airmen from the effects of high altitude. As a result, American pharmaceutical firms were requested by the government to investigate the possibility of large-scale production of steroid hormones. Eventually, a complicated 31-step process was developed for producing the adrenal hormone cortisone from deoxycholic acid (Figure 13-3). Following the discovery in 1949 of a dramatic therapeutic effect of cortisone in patients with rheumatoid arthritis,[38] there began an intensive competitive search on the part of drug manufacturers for an inexpensive way of producing synthetic steroid hormones.[39] At that time, the possible starting materials consisted of cholesterol, the bile acid deoxycholic acid, the plant sterols like stigmasterol (from soy beans), the sapogenins like diosgenin or hecogenin, or the closely related aglycone sarmentogenin. (When the sugar residues are removed from a glycoside, what remains is known as an *aglycone*, also called *genin*.) The structures of all these compounds are given in Figure 13-3. Cortisone and progesterone are typical of the adrenal cortical hormones and sex hormones, respectively, which were to be end-products of the desired synthesis.

Of the naturally occurring steroids, cholesterol is plentiful and inexpensive; but, unfortunately, the cleavage of its side chain is difficult, so that an efficient economic synthesis was not possible. Deoxycholic acid was far easier to handle; furthermore,

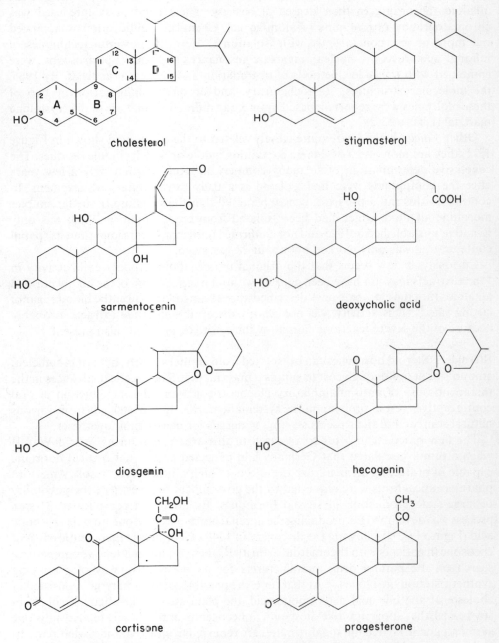

cholesterol

stigmasterol

sarmentogenin

deoxycholic acid

diosgenin

hecogenin

cortisone

progesterone

FIGURE 13-3. Structures of some naturally occurring steroids.

it already has an oxygen atom in position 12, which could be shifted (although with some difficulty) to position 11. But deoxycholic acid, derived from ox bile, was itself expensive and limited in amount. In the early days, when supplies of cortisone were derived from deoxycholic acid, a one-week supply of cortisone for one arthritic patient would have cost about $6000.

Stigmasterol also seemed to be a promising starting material, especially because of the double bond in its side chain, which made it easier to modify than cholesterol. But stigmasterol, too, was in relatively short supply and expensive. The situation precipitated an almost frantic search for plant sterols that would be cheap, plentiful, and readily modified in the chemical laboratory. The years 1949 and 1950, for example, were marked by a "great *Strophanthus* search,"[26] an effort to find a reputed source of sarmentogenin in a variety of *Strophanthus* in Africa. Sarmentogenin was especially sought after because it already contained an oxygen atom at position 11, as in cortisone and hydrocortisone. This sterol was known to exist, for it had been isolated from a batch of *Strophanthus* seeds in 1915, but no one knew where they had come from or exactly what variety of the plant produced them. Sarmentogenin might well have provided a satisfactory starting material, but an adequate source was never discovered.

At last, Mexican yams (*Dioscorea*) were found to contain the sterol diosgenin (Figure 13-3), which could be converted by an economic process to progesterone.[40,41] Within less than 10 years of the discovery of this source, the price of progesterone, which had been selling at about $80 per gram, fell to $1.75 per gram. The final breakthrough was the discovery in 1952 of a way to use progesterone in the synthesis of adrenal cortical hormones. This required introduction of an oxygen atom in position 11. A strain of *Rhizopus* was isolated that could carry out an enzymic hydroxylation of progesterone to 11α-hydroxyprogesterone.[42] The price of progesterone now fell to 48 cents per gram, and the production of low-cost adrenal cortical hormones became a reality. Nowadays, progesterone sells for less than 15 cents per gram.

A curious by-product of the developments recounted above was the accidental discovery that halogenated steroids were highly potent with respect to glucocorticoid activity, with relatively little mineralocorticoid (sodium-retaining) action. In the conversion of 11α-hydroxy steriods produced by the microbial reaction to biologically active 11β-hydroxy compounds, halogen was introduced in the 9-position. Partly because biologic testing was a routine procedure and partly to help determine that the substitution had the correct configuration, the halogenated intermediates were tested; they proved to be surprisingly potent.[43] If was found, for example, that 9α-fluorohydrocortisone was more than 10 times as potent as cortisol with respect to anti-inflammatory effects.[43a] It thus became evident that steroids with greater selectivity of action than the natural hormones could be synthesized. The end result was the introduction into clinical use of such fluorinated anti-inflammatory steroids as dexamethasone, triamcinolone, and fluocinolone acetonide.

Cardiac Glycosides.   In this important group of drugs, synthetic alternatives to the naturally occurring agents have not yet been found. Plants of the genera *Digitalis* (foxglove), *Strophanthus* (dogbane, related to oleander and periwinkle), and *Urginea* (squill) contain pharmacologically active sugar derivatives of sterols, which are known collectively as cardiac glycosides. Their most important actions are to improve the contractility of the failing heart and to produce partial heart block in atrial fibrillation. These effects were originally obtained by the oral administration of extracts of dried powdered digitalis leaves.[44] Standardization by means of bioassay made it possible for the physician to rely upon the potency of such crude material; indeed, powdered digitalis leaf is still widely used as an inexpensive and effective agent for routine maintenance in congestive heart failure.

The impetus for purification came principally from a hope that compounds with lower toxicity relative to their cardiac activities might be discovered. This hope has not materialized. Although differences in potency have been found, it has also become apparent that the major toxic effects (cardiac arrhythmias, emesis, visual disturbances) are inseparable from the therapeutically useful actions on the heart. But the extensive programs of purification, identification of chemical structures, and biologic testing have yielded important practical dividends of another kind. By careful selection of the right plants as starting materials in order to exploit the differences in types of glycoside between one plant and another and by fractional crystallization and other methods of chemical separation, it has been possible to obtain in pure form several new drugs with useful therapeutic properties.

The unique cardiac activity depends upon the presence of a 5- or 6-membered unsaturated lactone ring at position 17, and a hydroxyl group at position 14, both in the β configuration. Rings C and D must be *cis*. These requirements are exemplified in the structure of digitoxigenin, the aglycone of digitoxin, which is the principal

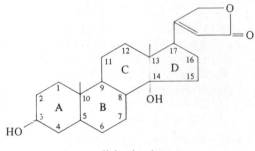

digitoxigenin

glycoside in Digitalis purpurea. Although these compounds are found in nature as glycosides, with various sugars attached in the β configuration at position 3, the sugar residues are not essential to the pharmacologic activity. Each kind of plant produces its own characteristic mixture of glycosides. The aglycones (genins) differ from one another in the lactone moiety or in the number and position of substituents on the sterol nucleus. The glycosides differ with respect to the number and kinds of sugar residues and their state of acetylation.

Table 13-5 illustrates with selected data from a large-scale investigation that both the aglycone and the sugar residues influence potency. Potency was determined by intravenous infusion in cats, using cardiac standstill as end-point. Strophanthidin, purified from seeds of *Strophanthus Kombé*, differs from digitoxigenin in having a hydroxyl group at position 5, and also –CHO instead of –CH$_3$ at position 10.

Purified glycosides have been useful for two reasons. First, it is often desirable to digitalize a patient by a parenteral route. For this purpose purified glycosides are obviously better than extracts of dried leaf, and several preparations are now available for this use. Second, the various glycosides have been found to differ with respect to rate of onset and duration of action. These important differences are exemplified by a

TABLE 13-5. Relative potencies of various aglycones and glycosides.

The pure substances were tested by slow intravenous infusion in cats, to determine the amount required to produce cardiac standstill. Ten cats were used for each compound. (Recalculated from Chen et al.,[45] Figures 1 and 2.)

	Aglycone					
	Digitoxigenin			Strophanthidin		
Sugars	Compound	M.W.	Lethal dose (μ moles)	Compound	M.W.	Lethal dose (μ moles)
None	digitoxigenin	374	1.25	strophanthidin	404	0.83
Cymarose	somalin	519	0.59	cymarin	549	0.20
Glucose	digitoxigenin glucoside	555	0.23	strophanthidin glucoside	576	0.15
(Digitoxose)$_3$	digitoxin	765	0.43			

comparison of digitoxin with digoxin. Digoxin is obtained by mild hydrolysis from lanatoside C, which is the main glycoside of *Digitalis lanata* leaf. Both compounds are triglycosides with identical sugar residues, and the genins differ only by the presence of a hydroxyl group in position 12 of digoxin. The fate of the two glycosides has been studied by means of radioactive labeling.[46,47] Digitoxin is excreted very slowly by the kidneys and is further conserved by the mechanism of an enterohepatic cycle. It is largely metabolized in the body, with a biologic half-life of about 5 days. Digoxin is much more readily excreted than digitoxin; its biologic half-life is only about 34 hr. Moreover, the onset of action of digoxin after intravenous administration is much more rapid than that of digitoxin. Rapid onset and short duration of action appear to be related, in general, to the presence of polar substituents on the sterol nucleus. The glycoside with the most rapid onset of action (a few minutes) is ouabain, from *Strophanthus gratus* seeds.[48] Its aglycone, ouabagenin, has hydroxyl groups at positions 1, 5, and 11 and a primary alcohol group at position 10, in addition to the usual hydroxyl groups at positions 3 and 14.

Modification of Chemical Structure

There are various reasons for modifying the chemical structure of existing drugs to obtain new ones. Usually the aim is to improve the selectivity of action by finding molecular changes that will increase a desired biologic action relative to a side effect. Sometimes the aim is to modify absorption, distribution, or elimination in order to obtain more useful properties. Sometimes the aim is to achieve a substantial reduction in the cost of production. Sometimes the aim is simply to find a marketable alternative drug that will compete with an existing one. A large investment of effort and funds may sometimes yield only a trivial modification, producing a drug that offers no real advantage over others already available.

Modification to Improve Selectivity of Action.   The result most frequently sought in molecular modification of drug structures is to eliminate or reduce the intensity of an unwanted side effect and thereby improve the therapeutic ratio for the desired action. A straightforward example is given in Table 13-6, showing a comparison of antihistaminic drugs. The antihistaminic potencies were measured by subcutaneous injection of various doses into groups of 10 guinea pigs, and then 30 min later giving a uniformly lethal dose (0.5 mg kg^{-1}) of histamine intravenously. The ED50 was the dose estimated to protect one-half of all animals from the histamine lethality. The LD50 was determined by intraperitoneal injection in mice, as described in Chapter 5. The therapeutic ratio is given in the last column of the table; the larger this ratio, the safer is the compound estimated to be. The data show that toxicities of the first four compounds (tested in mice) were approximately the same, whereas their potencies varied over a range of more than 100-fold. In this series, therefore, it was possible to separate toxicity from antihistaminic potency by molecular modifications. The poor potency and low therapeutic ratio of hetramine are presumably responsible for its not being employed in man, although its *p*-methoxy derivative, thonzylamine, is a useful and effective antihistaminic drug. The other compounds are all fairly safe in man, so that the large differences between their therapeutic ratios, as revealed by the animal tests, have turned out to be unimportant clinically. All members of the group are useful.

TABLE 13-6. Therapeutic ratios of five antihistaminic drugs.

Molecular modifications were made in the series with the general structure $R-CH_2-CH_2-N(CH_3)_2$. ED50 was determined in groups of ten guinea pigs given a lethal dose of histamine (0.5 mg kg^{-1}) intravenously 30 min after subcutaneous injection of the test drug. LD50 was determined by the intraperitoneal route in mice, except as noted. (Data of Winter[49] and Roth and Govier.[50] By permission of Williams and Wilkins.)

Compound	R	ED50 (μmole kg^{-1})	LD50 (μmole kg^{-1})	LD50/ED50
Diphenhydramine		0.21	480	2300
Hetramine		0.51	260	500
Tripelennamine		0.012	230	19,000
Pyrilamine		0.0037	250	68,000
Chlorpheniramine racemic		0.47	680*	1400
(+)		0.20	620*	3100
(−)		19.	450*	24

* By mouth in guinea pigs.

TABLE 13-7. Potency, irritancy, and lethal toxicity in a series of local anesthetics.
The upper part of the table compares oxygen and sulfur analogs in a series of the general formula:

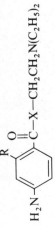

The threshold concentration for local anesthesia was determined by the intracutaneous wheal method in the guinea pig, irritancy by the trypan blue method in rabbits, and lethal toxicity as LD50 values after intravenous injection in mice. Therapeutic ratios for irritancy/local anesthesia and lethal toxicity/local anesthesia were computed, and each of these ratios was expressed relative to procaine. Thus, the higher the relative therapeutic ratio, the greater the spread between toxic and local anesthetic dose, relative to that for procaine. The lower part of the table gives the same data for four local anesthetics belonging to other series. (From Luduena and Hoppe,[52] Tables 1 and 2.)

Compound	R	X	Local anesthesia (mM)	Tissue irritancy (mM)	Relative therapeutic ratio	Lethal toxicity μMols kg^{-1}	Relative therapeutic ratio
Procaine	H	O	8.8	176	1.0	220	1.0
Thiocaine		S	1.26	23	0.9	31	1.0
(V) (# 3260)	OCH$_3$	O	4.66	156	1.7	250	2.1
		S	0.85	73	4.3	20	0.9
Propoxycaine (# 3766)	O(CH$_2$)$_2$CH$_3$	O	0.81	75	4.6	22	1.1
		S	0.09	15	8.4	1.7	0.8
Sympocaine (# 3800)	O(CH$_2$)$_3$CH$_3$	O	0.312	39	6.2	11.5	1.5
		S	0.087	4.7	2.7	1.7	0.8
(IX) (# 4510)	O(CH$_2$)$_5$CH$_3$	O	0.116	5.4	2.3	5.5	1.9
		S	0.051	1.5	1.5	0.9	0.7

Lidocaine	2.69	62	1.2	85	1.3
Cocaine	1.16	79	3.4	62	2.1
Tetracaine	0.69	12	0.9	27	1.6
Dibucaine	0.45	5.6	0.6	14	1.2

Chlorpheniramine is particularly interesting because it was resolved into $(-)$ and $(+)$ stereoisomers, which were tested separately.[50] The toxicities, determined in guinea pigs, were about the same. The antihistaminic action, on the other hand, was highly stereospecific; nearly all the potency was accounted for by the $(+)$ isomer. Thus, from the standpoint of safety, a 2-fold improvement was accomplished by resolving the racemic mixture; and the more active isomer had a therapeutic ratio more than 100 times greater than the less active one.

The local anesthetics have been explored very thoroughly to see what advantages can be gained by molecular modification. Cocaine (Table 13-7), a complex ester alkaloid obtained from cocoa leaves, was introduced as a topical anesthetic in 1884 by Sigmund Freud (1856–1939). Its central stimulant and addictive properties were soon recognized, and in 1905 several synthetic dialkylaminoalkyl aminobenzoates were discovered to have local anesthetic properties. One of these, procaine, displaced cocaine (except for topical ophthalmologic use) and became the standard local anesthetic.[51] Of the hundreds of other compounds with similar activity that have been synthesized and tested in the past 60 years, a few have been preferred to procaine because of greater stability or longer duration of local anesthesia. But it is not really clear that they are superior to procaine from the standpoint of central nervous system toxicity or local tissue irritancy.

Some comparative structure-activity data are summarized in Table 13-7 for a series of oxygen and sulfur analogs, and also for cocaine and three of the newer and widely used synthetic agents.[52] Local anesthesia was determined in guinea pigs by injecting a fixed volume containing different concentrations of a drug and then testing the response to pinpricks in the area of the wheal formed by the drug solution; an arbitrarily defined threshold anesthetic concentration was thus determined.[53] Irritancy was estimated in the rabbit by injecting the drug at various concentrations subcutaneously and giving trypan blue intravenously; capillary damage in the vicinity of the injected drug causes visible dye leakage into the tissues, and a threshold irritant concentration can thus be estimated. Finally, lethal toxicity was determined by measuring LD50 in the mouse by intravenous injection. Therapeutic ratios were computed as irritancy dose/anesthetic dose and LD50/anesthetic dose. Then, for ease of comparison, these therapeutic ratios were expressed relative to those for procaine, set equal to unity. Compounds with relative therapeutic ratios greater than one are therefore safer than procaine with respect to irritancy or lethal toxicity in this assessment.

The data illustrate several interesting points. For the series in the upper part of the table, as the alkyl portion of the R group becomes longer, the absolute potency shows a regular increase, both in the oxygen series and in the sulfur series. This is true, with few exceptions, for all three pharmacologic actions. Moreover, every sulfur compound is more potent than its oxygen analog. These findings are consistent with the general relationship between lipid/water partition coefficient and potency among drugs that act upon the nervous system, for the lipid solubilities of these compounds undoubtedly follow the same trend (cf. Chapter 2). Despite the wide range of potencies, the relative therapeutic ratio with respect to lethal toxicity remains within very narrow limits. Some compounds, on the other hand, do show an unusually favorable relative therapeutic ratio with respect to tissue irritancy, up to 8 times better than procaine in the most favorable case.

The four agents at the bottom of the table are used widely for local anesthesia in man. From the standpoint of these animal testing procedures, cocaine would seem to have the most favorable properties, with a therapeutic ratio 2 or 3 times that of procaine. Lidocaine, tetracaine, and dibucaine, by the same criterion, seem no better than procaine. These data illustrate a practical point of some importance in drug development. It is impossible to predict a priori whether molecular modifications will be capable of producing substantial improvement in the therapeutic ratio. Sometimes, as in the antihistamine series, the most troublesome side effect proves to be unrelated to the therapeutic action; then molecular modification can be fruitful. But in the local anesthetic series, as Table 13-7 shows, no important improvement in therapeutic ratio could be achieved. Nevertheless, in the course of structure-activity studies advantages of other kinds may be found. Thus, procaine was adopted initially for infiltration anesthesia, not because it was less toxic than cocaine but primarily to avoid the addiction liability of cocaine. Tetracaine, dibucaine, and to some extent lidocaine are preferred for topical anesthesia of mucous membranes because they have a much longer duration of action than procaine.[54] Lidocaine is more stable than procaine and therefore has a longer duration of action after subcutaneous injection. None of these important favorable properties would have been evident from the potency and toxicity tests alone.

Modification to Alter Absorption, Distribution, or Elimination. Although much effort is being expended to develop rational and effective drug delivery systems (cf. Chapter 2), the oral route is still the only convenient one for drugs that have to be given on a continuing basis. Much effort has been devoted, therefore, to the modification of drug structure to improve absorption from the gastrointestinal tract. In the most elementary case, the water solubility has to be improved; salts of some drugs are so insoluble that they pass through the intestinal tract essentially unchanged. This happened with calcium salts of the tetracyclines.[55]

An interesting example of water solubility as a limitation to oral absorption is seen with the phenylbutazone analogs shown in Table 13-8. Of the numerous agents studied, only the first three were soluble enough at pH 7.0 to permit effective absorption by the oral route; yet all the compounds listed were effective anti-inflammatory agents when tested intravenously in experimental animals.

One of the most successful molecular modifications leading to orally active preparations concerns the estrogenic and progestational steroids. The natural hormones estradiol and progesterone are quite ineffective by mouth. In a standard assay procedure, for example, using the rabbit, progesterone is wholly inactive by the oral route at 40 times the dose that elicits a moderate effect when given intramuscularly. It is not completely clear why these steroids should be inactive by mouth. Nothing about their structures suggests that absorption would be poor. It is known from studies with radioactive estradiol and progesterone that after intravenous administration their biotransformation to metabolites occurs within a few minutes.[57,58] It is likely, therefore, that rapid metabolism as they pass from the portal circulation through the liver, and possibly also degradation within the intestinal tract, reduce the amounts that reach the systemic circulation to less than effective levels. Several modified steroids, chiefly 19-nor derivatives, on the other hand, are highly effective by mouth;[59] norethindrone (19-nor-17α-ethynyltestosterone), for example, was found to be equally active by the oral and intramuscular routes of administration.[60] These modifications, leading to orally effective progestational hormones, have produced the oral contraceptive agents.[61-63] It is noteworthy that the entire impact

TABLE 13-8. Water solubilities and oral absorption of phenylbutazone analogs. Solubilities were determined at pH 7.0. (From Brodie and Hogben,[56] Table VII.)

Compound	Structure	Solubility (mg ml^{-1} at pH 7.0)	Absorption after oral administration to man
	$C_6H_5-N-C=O$ $\quad$ $HC-R$ $\quad$ $C_6H_5-N-C=O$		
Phenylbutazone	R = $CH_2CH_2CH_2CH_3$	2.2	rapid and complete
p-Hydroxyphenylbutazone	R = $CH_2CH_2CH_2CH_3$	10.0	rapid and complete
G-1	R = $CH_2CH_2SC_6H_5$	1.6	rapid and complete
G-3	R = $CH_2CH_2CH_2C_6H_5$	0.14	slow and incomplete
G-8	R = $CH_2CH_2SC_6H_3op(CH_3)_2$	0.13	slow and incomplete
pp-Dichlorophenylbutazone	R = $CH_2CH_2CH_2CH_3$	0.09	slow and incomplete
pp-Dimethylphenylbutazone	R = $CH_2CH_2CH_2CH_3$	0.12	slow and incomplete
G-23	R = $\overset{O}{\overset{\|}{C}}-CH_2CH_2CH_3$	0.12	slow and incomplete

of this new field of drug action depended here upon the development of compounds that would be effective when taken by mouth.

Molecular modifications that alter the distribution of a drug within the body can have profound effects upon its pharmacologic properties. Often such modifications involve changes in the lipid/water partition coefficient (cf. Chapter 2). Thiopental was developed from pentobarbital by replacement of an oxygen atom by a sulfur atom. This simple replacement was found, on a purely empirical basis, to convert an anesthetic with moderate duration of action to an ultrashort-acting one. As already explained (p. 196), the rapid entry of thiopental into the brain after intravenous injection, and its equally rapid efflux from the brain, account for its very fast onset and offset of action; this rapidity of passage across the blood-brain barrier is due to the drug's very high lipid/water partition coefficient. The same property accounts for the eventual sequestration of thiopental in fat depots, prolonging the persistence of drug in the body. Certain N-alkyl thiobarbiturates are even more fat soluble.[64] N-Methyl-thiopental, for example, has so high a lipid/water partition coefficient that fat depots continue to act as a sink for it, even after repeated anesthetic doses have been given. In principle, this is a useful improvement. With thiopental, recovery from anesthesia after repeated doses becomes slower as the fat depots become equilibrated. With N-alkyl barbiturates, it may be possible to maintain fast recovery after injections of a larger total amount of anesthetic because of the greater capacity of the body fat to sequester these drugs.

Lipid solubility and storage in body fat also play a role in the duration of action of steroid sex hormones. Women being treated for menopausal symptoms with the orally effective estrogen ethinyl estradiol 3-cyclopentyl ether showed a much more persistent drug effect after discontinuance of therapy than did women receiving the parent compound, ethinyl estradiol.[65] Direct determination of drug levels in body fat after oral administration of these drugs to experimental animals showed that the cyclopentyl ether accumulated in fat, forming a depot from which slow release continued, but the parent compound did not. A similar phenomenon has been observed with methyltestosterone and its 3-cyclopentyl enol ether.[66] Here again, although both compounds were absorbed well from the intestine, only the ether accumulated significantly in fat, thus providing low but effective hormone levels for a long time. Administered by the oral route, therefore, the ether appeared to be more effective than methyltestosterone itself.

The recognition that ionized compounds are, in general, excluded from the brain (cf. Chapter 2) has led to deliberate molecular modifications for the purpose of promoting or hindering the ability of a drug to pass the blood-brain barrier. An example is the cholinesterase reactivator pralidoxime (p. 409), a quaternary compound. Since inhibition of acetylcholinesterase within the central nervous system is important in the toxicity of organophosphate insecticides and nerve gases, attempts have been made to develop nonionic reactivators of the pralidoxime type. Such agents include diacetylmonoxime (DAM) and monoisonitrosoacetone (MINA) (Figure 5-17). On the other hand, tertiary amines like atropine and physostigmine, which enter the brain readily, have been modified by producing quaternary derivatives in order to secure peripheral autonomic effects without the complication of central actions. Examples are atropine methyl nitrate and neostigmine.

Finally, structural modification can alter the metabolic fate of a drug to shorten or prolong its duration of action. A good example is the development of procainamide from procaine. Procaine was known to have useful properties as an agent that could abolish certain cardiac arrhythmias; but it is an ester and rapidly hydrolyzed by plasma and liver esterases. Simple substitution of the amide linkage for the ester group produced procainamide. The useful cardiac actions were not lost but the hydrolysis rate in vivo was greatly reduced.[67] Another example, discussed in Chapter 3,

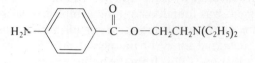

procaine

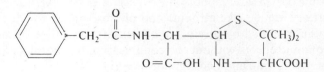

procainamide

is the mild antipyretic analgesic acetanilid. The production of aniline in vivo by deacetylation leads to methemoglobinemia. Modification of the acetanilid structure by hydroxylation in the para position yielded a compound that was not subject to significant deacetylation, and, therefore, was less toxic. In the barbiturate series, the principal effect of substituent modification is to alter rates of metabolism and thus duration of action. Barbital is essentially not oxidized at all, phenobarbital very slowly, pentobarbital and secobarbital more rapidly; and the durations of hypnotic action throughout the series closely parallel the rates of drug metabolism.

The structure of penicillin can be modified to prevent its degradation by pathogenic bacteria, as discussed already in Chapter 8. The usefulness of the penicillins in staphylococcal infections was compromised by the fact that strains of this pathogen produce and secrete a β-lactamase (penicillinase), and thus resist the bactericidal action of the antibiotic by destroying it. The enzyme attacks the internal peptide bond, which forms the essential β-lactam ring; thus, penicillins are converted to inactive penicilloic acids:

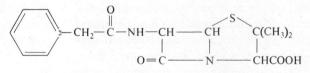

penicillin G

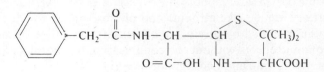

penicilloic acid

In an effort to combat this problem, semisynthetic penicillins were sought, which might be resistant to cleavage by penicillinase. It was known that antibacterial activity is found in numerous penicillins with different acidic substituents. The first step was to use an amidase to remove the phenylacetate residue from penicillin G. The resulting 6-aminopenicillanic acid could then be used as a starting material to be coupled with various organic acids. When the compounds thus formed were assayed for resistance

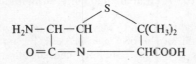

6-aminopenicillanic acid

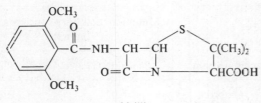

methicillin

to penicillinase, several suitable drugs were obtained.[68] One of these was methicillin, the structure of which is shown above.

The resistance of methicillin to hydrolysis by the penicillinase of *Staphylococcus pyogenes* and of *Bacillus cereus* is shown in Table 13-9. compared with penicillin G. The staphylococcal enzyme did not degrade methicillin at all in the 60-min. incubation

TABLE 13-9. Resistance of methicillin to penicillinase. Penicillinase from *S. pyogenes* and from *B. cereus* was incubated in buffer at 37° with added penicillin G or methicillin. The course of the hydrolytic degradation of the penicillin was followed. (From Rolinson et al.,[69] Tables VII and VIII.)

Time (min)	Penicillin G (μg ml^{-1})	Methicillin (μg ml^{-1})
S. pyogenes penicillinase		
0	1000	1000
5	330	1000
10	0	1000
60	0	1000
B. cereus penicillinase		
0	2000	2000
1	0	1740
2	0	1610
3	0	1500
4	0	1400
5	0	1330

period, and the *B. cereus* enzyme degraded it much more slowly than penicillin G. Table 13-10 shows the comparison of antibacterial activity against a number of strains of *S. pyogenes*, some sensitive and others highly resistant to penicillin G.

TABLE 13-10. Antibacterial activity of methicillin and penicillin G.

Methicillin and penicillin G were assayed for growth inhibition against several strains of *Staphylococcus*, by a tube dilution method. The minimum inhibitory concentrations are given. Strains of bacteria are identified by code number. The sensitive Oxford strain of *S. aureus* was the one originally used to assay penicillin. (Selected data from Rolinson et al.,[69] Table II.)

Bacterial strain	Minimum inhibitory concentration (μg/ml)	
	Penicillin G	Methicillin
Oxford	0.02	1.25
No. 1083	125.0	2.5
1089	125.0	2.5
1112	125.0	1.25
1091	62.5	2.5
1111	50.0	2.5
1095	25.0	2.5
1104	12.5	2.5
1098	5.0	2.5
1096	5.0	1.25
1108	2.5	1.25
1084	1.25	1.25

Although methicillin was much less potent against the Oxford strain of *S. aureus* than was penicillin G, the important finding was that all the penicillinase-producing penicillin-resistant strains were moderately sensitive to methicillin. Subsequent research has led to the production of several other penicillinase-resistant semisynthetic penicillins.

Modification to Reduce Cost. Because drugs are only useful if they are widely available to meet the need, cost is an important factor in drug development. Some molecular modifications have yielded drugs that are better than the parent primarily because they are cheaper. Diethylstilbestrol is a good example. It was introduced in 1938 at a time when the natural estrogenic hormones were both scarce and extremely expensive.[70] It is a synthetic, orally active compound with estrogenic activity, apparently as useful as the natural estrogens and widely used today. Curiously, it is not even a steroid; but its 3-dimensional structure does have certain features in common with the steroid hormones:

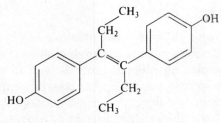

diethylstilbestrol

A similar case involves the narcotic analgesics. Methadone is an uncomplicated synthetic compound seemingly unrelated to the structure of the opiate narcotics, but its acute pharmacologic effects are almost indistinguishable from theirs. It was developed during World War II in Germany, when shortage of supplies of morphine made it imperative to develop new and inexpensive substitutes. Now it is clear that the conformational structure of methadone is closer to that of the opiates than had been realized by the chemists who made it (cf. p. 33).

Chloramphenicol was first isolated from cultures of *Streptomyces venezuelae* in 1948.[71] For a few years, the antibiotic was in short supply and very expensive. When the structural formula was elucidated, it turned out to be a relatively easy compound to synthesize, so it was no longer necessary to depend upon cumbersome fermentation and isolation procedures. Although no change in molecular structure is involved here, this is an example of reduction in cost of a natural product through chemical synthesis.

The insect sex attractant produced by female gypsy moths is extremely potent; 10^{-7} μg is effective in attracting males in field trials. The substance has been useful in insect control and eradication programs carried out by the United States Department of Agriculture. The structure of the active agent was determined on 20 mg of material isolated from a half-million female moths.[72] Unfortunately, synthesis of the natural attractant proved very difficult. However, a closely related compound, two carbon atoms longer, could be derived readily from ricinoleic acid, abundant in castor oil. The artificial attractant, named *gyplure*, is as potent as the natural substance.[73]

natural attractant

(+)-10-acetoxy-*cis*-7-hexadecen-1-ol

gyplure

Synthesis of New Drugs

Invention of Drugs De Novo. The inventive pharmacologist or medicinal chemist is sometimes pictured as devising unprecedented drug actions de novo, predicting the requisite chemical structures on rational grounds, and then actually synthesizing effective drugs to fit the specifications. This has certainly happened, but rarely. The history of the development of dimercaprol as an antidote to the arsenical war gas lewisite (cf. p. 402) approaches this ideal. So does the development of the cholinesterase-reactivating agent pralidoxime (PAM), tailored on rational grounds to the inferred structure of the acetylcholinesterase active center (p. 409). Perhaps the synthesis and trial of some antimetabolites used in cancer chemotherapy could be attributed to rational design, but serendipity also played a part. For example, the introduction of folic acid antagonists for the treatment of childhood leukemia was based on the chance observation that folic acid seemed to exacerbate the disease process.[74] Folic acid analogs, including aminopterin, were being developed concurrently as an outgrowth of nutrition studies with microorganisms. The partial success achieved in inducing remissions of leukemia with aminopterin led to the synthesis of numerous structurally related compounds, of which methotrexate (p. 426) has been the most useful. The principle having been established, a great variety of antimetabolites were synthesized—analogs of the amino acids (e.g., ethionine, p-fluorophenylalanine), purines (e.g., 6-mercaptopurine), pyrimidines (e.g., 5-fluorouracil), and so on, as detailed in Chapter 1.

The diuretic agent ethacrynic acid was developed as part of a deliberate attempt to synthesize inhibitors of sulfhydryl enzymes that would not contain heavy metals.[75] The rationale for this approach was the belief that the highly effective organic mercurial diuretics owed their effects to inactivation of sulfhydryl groups in essential –SH enzymes of the renal tubule cells. Mercurials are toxic, so there was sound motivation for developing a new class of drugs. An aryl oxyacetic acid derivative containing an α, β-unsaturated ketone was found to react with –SH groups in vitro and to be a potent diuretic. The structure of this compound, ethacrynic acid, is shown below:

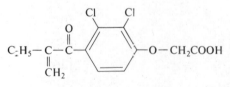

ethacrynic acid

Curiously, ethacrynic acid is less active as an inhibitor of sulfhydryl enzymes in vitro than are the organic mercurials. Moreover, its diuretic action, unlike that of the mercurials, is not antagonized readily by dimercaprol. Its mechanism of action is still unknown; it would not be surprising if it turned out to have nothing to do with sulfhydryl groups. It can interfere with the concentrating ability of the kidney, possibly by an effect on the loop of Henle, and it can also cause excessive potassium loss.[76–76c]

Some drugs are developed primarily to influence the pharmacologic behavior or disposition of other drugs. Examples are SKF 525A (p. 267), which inhibits the metabolism of many drugs, and disulfiram (p. 268), which inhibits a step in the oxidation of ethyl alcohol. The monoamine oxidase inhibitors also fall into this category. Another such drug is probenicid. This compound was originally developed for the purpose of conserving penicillin by blocking its renal tubular secretion. For some

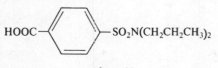

HOOC—⟨ ⟩—SO₂N(CH₂CH₂CH₃)₂

probenecid

time after penicillin was introduced into therapy it was very scarce, and its rapid clearance by the kidneys was a real handicap. It was found that the same active transport system was responsible for penicillin excretion as for the tubular secretion of numerous other anions like phenolsulfonphthalein, p-aminohippurate, and p-aminosalicylate. Probenecid, which could be administered by mouth, competed with penicillin for this secretory mechanism and thereby effectively prolonged the duration of penicillin action.[77] During its use for this purpose, it was observed to increase the excretion of uric acid,[78] although at low doses it decreased urate excretion, probably by inhibiting the same transport system in the renal tubules. Large doses evidently inhibit the reabsorption of urate from the glomerular filtrate, probably by blocking a specific transport system for reabsorption of this anion. Thus, the major use of probenecid is as a uricosuric agent in the treatment of gout, a disease characterized by high urate levels in the body. Curiously, its original use to maintain high penicillin levels is again becoming important in the treatment of gonorrhea due to penicillin resistant organisms.

The history of the development of the antifolic-type antimalarial drugs illustrates the roundabout path that is often followed before a new kind of drug is perfected. When the screening of possible antimalarials began during World War II it was known that the sulfonamides suppressed the erythrocytic phase of avian malaria, although they were not effective in the human disease. Since sulfadiazine was one of the most effective compounds in the series, attention was focused on the pyrimidine

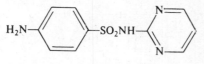

sulfadiazine

ring. Simple pyrimidine derivatives were ineffective. But since a diethylamino alkylamino side chain was an important component of the then-known antimalarials (e.g., quinacrine, pamaquin), an attempt was made to link such a moiety to an aromatic pyrimidine compound.[79] This eventually yielded an active drug, code number 2666, shown below:

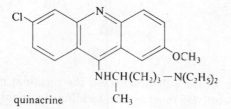

quinacrine

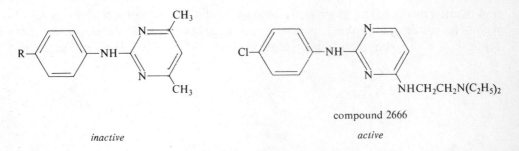

compound 2666

inactive   *active*

Further modification of the structure of compound 2666, guided by a bioassay of activity against avian malaria, led to the finding that introduction of a guanidinium group between the benzene ring and the pyrimidine ring increased the potency greatly. Compound 3349 was thus obtained:

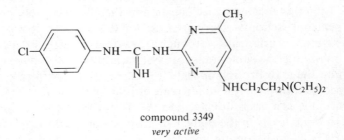

compound 3349
very active

It now appeared that the biologic activity might well arise in a system of conjugated alternating carbon and nitrogen atoms, of which the pyrimidine ring was a part. This proved to be a fruitful lead, for when the pyrimidine ring was opened, high activity was retained, even when the typical antimalarial side chain had been discarded:

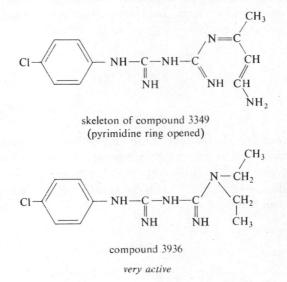

skeleton of compound 3349
(pyrimidine ring opened)

compound 3936

very active

Finally, manipulation of the substituents on the terminal nitrogen atom revealed that the isopropyl group was most active, yielding the highly effective antimalarial chloroguanide.[80] Remarkably, no part of the rationale that guided these syntheses survived intact; chloroguanide is not a sulfonamide, does not contain a pyrimidine ring, and lacks the quinacrine side chain.

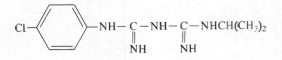

chloroguanide

The subsequent development of the antifolic antimalarial pyrimethamine makes an even more extraordinary story. It was observed in the course of investigations on antagonists of folic acid in *Lactobacillus casei* that 2,4-diaminopyrimidines were highly effective, and it was noted that one of the most potent could be considered, in a formal sense, to be a structural analog of chloroguanide:[81]

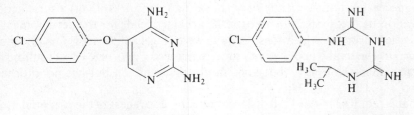

2,4-diamino-5-*p*-chlorophenoxypyrimidine   chloroguanide

This relationship led to the testing of the 2,4-diaminopyrimidines for antimalarial activity and of chloroguanide for antifolic activity, both with a positive outcome. Further, it was found that chloroguanide was completely inactive when added to serum in an in vitro test using exoerythrocytic forms of *Plasmodium gallinaceum*, whereas serum taken from an animal that had been treated with the drug was active.[82] Thus, the antimalarial action of chloroguanide must be due to a metabolic product of the drug. The active metabolite was subsequently isolated and identified.[83] It turned out to be a triazine, the very one that had been proposed as a formal analog

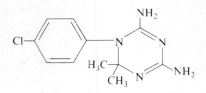

active metabolite of chloroguanide

of the 2,4-diaminopyrimidines. This active metabolite, interestingly, is less useful as an antimalarial than is chloroguanide itself because it is excreted too rapidly.

Finally, a large number of diaminopyrimidines were tested in avian, mouse, and monkey malaria, and the best of these compounds, pyrimethamine, was introduced into clinical use.[84] It is clear, therefore, that the essential structure for antimalarial

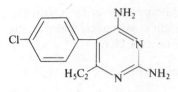

pyrimethamine

activity of the antifolic type is, after all, a pyrimidine ring (or the closely related triazine ring), with amino, alkyl, and aryl substituents. This structure may be regarded as an analog of the pteridine portion of the folic acid molecule.

Exploitation of Side Effects of Existing Drugs. The commonest pattern in the development of new drugs is not invention de novo but rather the exploitation of side effects of existing drugs. An action seen as undesirable in one therapeutic context may become the primary drug action in another. Phenylbutazone, for example, was developed as an antirheumatic drug, but it had considerable uricosuric action too. Studies on its metabolism in vivo (p.248) provided leads for the development of two wholly new drugs in which these actions were largely separated. Oxyphenbutazone retains antirheumatic activity with greatly reduced uricosuric effect; sulfinpyrazone is more potent than phenylbutazone in uricosuric action but has no antirheumatic activity.

What is required in this kind of development is awareness of the potential usefulness of a side effect, a bioassay for following potency as chemical structure is modified, and an imaginative and flexible approach to the possibilities of chemical synthesis. This pattern of perfecting new families of drugs is nowhere better illustrated than in the sulfonamide series. These drugs were introduced into medicine as antibacterial agents in 1935. The astute exploitation of their side effects has led to wholly new and useful drugs of three kinds—diuretic, antidiabetic, and antithyroid.

Diuretic sulfonamides. Carbonic anhydrase inhibitors and thiazide diuretics have their origin in the early days of sulfonamide chemotherapy. Patients receiving sulfanilamide tended to develop metabolic acidosis with an alkaline urine. Investigation revealed that this side effect was due to inhibition of renal carbonic anhydrase. This enzyme catalyzes the hydration of dissolved carbon dioxide in the kidney cells:

$$CO_2 + H_2O \underset{\text{carbonic anhydrase}}{\rightleftharpoons} H_2CO_3 \rightleftharpoons H^+ + HCO_3^-$$

The carbonic acid thus formed dissocates very rapidly to yield hydrogen ions and bicarbonate. The rate at which hydrogen ions are made available for secretion into the lumen of the renal tubules is limited by the rate of hydration of CO_2, a relatively slow process in the absence of the enzyme. Thus, inhibitors of carbonic anhydrase cause a decrease in the rate of acidification of the urine, and this accounts for the alkaline urine and metabolic acidosis. Since K^+ as well as H^+ normally exchanges for Na^+ across the tubular epithelium, potassium excretion tends to increase as proton excretion decreases. Therefore the urine, in the presence of a carbonic anhydrase inhibitor, contains more sodium and potassium ions than usual, together with bicarbonate and chloride anions. The additional salt excretion is accompanied by an osmotic equivalent of water; hence the increased urine volume.

Sulfanilamide itself was too toxic for use as a diuretic, and it was soon displaced from use as an antibacterial agent by safer sulfonamides. These newer derivatives of sulfanilamide all had substituents on the sulfonamide nitrogen atom, as shown below:

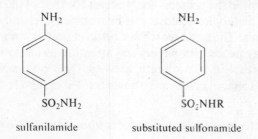

sulfanilamide   substituted sulfonamide

Of all the sulfonamides, only unsubstituted sulfanilamide itself was a carbonic anhydrase inhibitor and diuretic. Thus, a requirement for this action was evidently a free primary amine group in the sulfonamide moiety. Contrasting requirements are found with respect to the amino group para to the sulfonamide moiety. Here free $-NH_2$ is essential for the antibacterial action, but not for the diuretic effect.

Deliberate modification of structure to improve potency with respect to carbonic anhydrase inhibition led to heterocyclic sulfonamides like benzothiazole-2-sulfonamide, hundreds of times more potent than sulfanilamide when tested against the

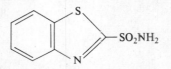

benzothiazole-2-sulfonamide

enzyme in vitro. But this compound had no diuretic action when administered orally to dogs. The inactivity in vivo was probably related to rapid metabolism. An ethoxy derivative proved effective as a diuretic in animals and man.[85-88] Further study

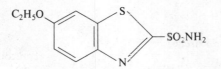

6-ethoxybenzothiazole-2-sulfonamide

showed that acetylation of the free amino substituent of a thiadiazole compound further enhanced enzyme inhibition. Thus, acetazolamide was selected as the best of the heterocyclic sulfonamides. This drug, 300 times more potent than sulfanilamide

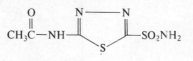

acetazolamide

as a carbonic anhydrase inhibitor, soon became established as a clinically useful oral diuretic agent.

Acetazolamide, however, was not an ideal diuretic. For one thing, the maximum diuresis possible was limited by the amount of hydrogen ion that would normally be excreted, since only as much sodium could be lost as would ordinarily have exchanged for protons in the tubules—only about 10–15 % of the total filtered electrolyte. Moreover, the metabolic acidosis can be troublesome, and excessive potassium loss can be dangerous. Thus, the search for better diuretics continued. The next step was to alter the assay procedure, paying less attention to carbonic anhydrase inhibition and more to actual in vivo diuretic activity. Data obtained in dogs with compounds related to acetazolamide are shown in Table 13-11, in comparison with

TABLE 13-11. Development of diuretic agents from sulfanilamide by molecular modifications.
Studies were carried out under standard conditions in dogs. Carbonic anhydrase inhibition was determined in vitro with enzyme derived from beef erythrocytes. Doses were given intravenously by infusion at the rates shown; a dose very nearly equivalent to the amount infused per hour was given initially as a priming dose. (From Beyer and Baer,[89] Table 3.)

Compound	50% Inhibition of carbonic anhydrase ($\times 10^6 M$)	Intravenous dose (mg/kg·hr)	μEq/min excreted			
			Na	K	Cl	pH
H_2NSO_2—⬡—NH_2 Sulfanilamide	13	control	14	14	3	6.8
		30	51	25	13	6.9
H_2NSO_2–C(N–N, S)C–NH–COCH₃ Acetazolamide	0.07	control	43	22	21	6.3
		3.0	186	128	53	8.0
H_2NSO_2—⬡(SO₂NH₂)(Cl) 1,3-disulfonamido-6-chlorobenzene	0.14	control	42	24	15	5.9
		3.0	468	101	303	7.4
H_2NSO_2—⬡(SO₂–NH–CH=N)(Cl) Chlorothiazide	1.7	control	11	11	7	6.1
		0.05	20	24	7	6.6
		0.25	115	34	80	6.7
		1.25	308	65	236	6.9
H_2NSO_2—⬡(SO₂–NH–CH=N) Dechloro-chlorothiazide	9.9	control	26	40	3	6.4
		7.5	150	43	18	7.6

Compound	50% Inhibition of carbonic anhydrase ($\times 10^6 M$)	Intravenous dose (mg/kg·hr)	μEq/min excreted			
			Na	K	Cl	pH
Flumethiazide	42	control	55	19	6	6.4
		0.05	143	20	62	6.9
		0.25	262	40	197	6.9
		1.25	321	57	241	7.0
Hydrochlorothiazide	23	control	62	34	43	6.5
		0.01	126	32	122	5.9
		0.05	265	33	291	5.5
		0.25	414	39	427	5.9
Hydroflumethiazide	170	control	5	8	2	5.6
		0.05	74	43	43	7.1
		0.25	363	66	309	7.0
		1.25	459	77	453	6.7
Benzhydroflumethiazide	310	control	25	22	18	5.9
		0.002	94	36	124	5.5
		0.01	321	53	318	5.9
		0.05	493	61	455	6.4

acetazolamide itself and with sulfanilamide. The first column shows the chemical structure, the second column gives the concentration required for 50% inhibition of carbonic anhydrase in vitro. The next column gives the intravenous dose administered, and the subsequent columns show the excretion of the principal cations (Na^+ and K^+) and of Cl^-. The bicarbonate ion excretion can be approximated by the difference between total cations and chloride ion and by the pH, according to the Henderson–Hasselbalch equation.

During the course of the studies that led to the development of acetazolamide, the chlorobenzene derivative shown just below it in Table 13-11 was tested. Although it was only half as potent as acetazolamide in inhibiting carbonic anhydrase, it proved to be highly effective in enhancing the excretion of sodium and chloride, and to a lesser extent, potassium and bicarbonate. This suggested that compounds of the acetazolamide type might have diuretic properties not attributable to carbonic anhydrase inhibition, and a concerted attempt was made to find such compounds which would selectively promote sodium and chloride excretion. Chemical manipulation of one of the two sulfonamide groups of the chlorobenzene compound led to chlorothiazide. This agent was less than $\frac{1}{20}$ as potent an inhibitor of carbonic anhydrase as acetazolamide (although still 10 times more potent than sulfanilamide), but was 5–10 times more potent than acetazolamide in promoting the loss of sodium and chloride; yet it was less potent in promoting potassium and bicarbonate loss. Nevertheless, some effect on potassium excretion remained, so efforts were made to develop still better agents.

Omission of the chloride group from chlorothiazide abolished the enhancement of chloride ion excretion. On the other hand, introduction of a trifluoromethane group in place of chlorine at the same position led to a compound, flumethiazide, with full diuretic potency but a pronounced further reduction in carbonic anhydrase inhibition. The reduced analogs, hydrochlorothiazide and hydroflumethiazide, were more potent than their parent molecules, with even less enzyme inhibitory activity. Finally, benzhydroflumethiazide, an extremely potent diuretic, was essentially devoid of activity as a carbonic anhydrase inhibitor.

The diuretic potency of various thiazides varies over a range of 10,000 fold. But there is a biologic limit to the amount of diuresis that can be achieved. If log dose-response curves are plotted for various thiazide diuretics, it is found that they are essentially parallel, as expected when the mechanism of action of different drugs is the same (cf. p. 90). The maximum diuresis produced by large doses of the weakest member of the group cannot be exceeded at any dose of the most potent member. The important feature of the molecular modifications, therefore, is not the increase in absolute potency achieved. The unimportance of absolute potency is indicated clearly by a comparison of chlorothiazide and hydrochlorothiazide, both of which are promoted for clinical use. Advertisements for the two drugs, made by the same firm, as well as descriptions prepared by experts for the guidance of physicians[90] are identical except with regard to the recommended dosage, 500 mg–1 g for chlorothiazide, 25–200 mg for hydrochlorothiazide.

The value of molecular modifications in this series has been the significant increase in therapeutic ratio that results from the complete separation of carbonic anhydrase inhibition from the promotion of electrolyte excretion. It is thought that the thiazides interfere with sodium chloride reabsorption in the renal tubules, but their exact mechanism of action is not yet known.

In retrospect, the important turning points in the development of the thiazide diuretics can be recognized. First came the decision to exploit a toxic side action of sulfanilamide. This could not really be done effectively until progress in renal physiology led to better understanding of the mechanism of hydrogen ion excretion. Indeed, the recognition of the diuretic effects of carbonic anhydrase inhibitors helped to disclose the role of this enzyme in normal proton secretion by the renal tubules. Further fruitful developments were stimulated by dissatisfaction with the limited diuretic capability of carbonic anhydrase inhibitors and the astute observation that, in sulfonamides of the thiazide type, diuretic action seemed not to correlate well with enzyme inhibitory potency.

Antidiabetic sulfonamides. The antidiabetic sulfonylureas also had their origin in a chance observation. Patients with typhoid fever under treatment with an isopropyl-thiadiazole derivative of sulfanilamide (below) became weak and dizzy. Investigation revealed varying degrees of hypoglycemia in those who received the drug. Further study showed that the effect could be produced in animals (although larger dosage

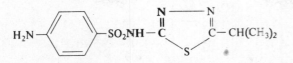

sulfanilamidoisopropylthiadiazole

was required) and that it was mediated by the release of insulin from the pancreatic islets.[91] In other words, this orally effective drug stimulated insulin release. In the absence of functional islets, it was ineffective.

The deliberate search for orally effective antidiabetic agents was not undertaken for several years, even though it was recognized that the ineffectiveness of insulin by mouth makes the maintenance therapy of diabetes troublesome. Perhaps it was felt that a drug requiring functional islet tissue for its action would be useless in diabetes. As it turned out, however, there are mild cases of the disease that are benefited by drugs of this kind. Systematic screening was eventually conducted,[92] using as assay the reduction in blood sugar level of normal animals, as described earlier (p. 738). These studies led to the conclusion that the hypoglycemic action depended primarily upon the urea-like structure formed by a nitrogen and carbon atom of the thiadiazole ring and the nitrogen atom of the sulfonamide grouping (shown in boldface in the structural formula). Thus, it became clearly evident that the basic structure for this activity was $Ar-SO_2NHCONH-R$, where Ar is aryl and R is an alkyl group. Changes within the urea moiety did not prove advantageous, but modification of the aryl and alkyl groups yielded compounds of greater potency and also greater duration of action. In carbutamide, the aryl group is unchanged p-aminobenzene, but the R substituent is n-butyl instead of isopropyl. Tolbutamide has the same R group as carbutamide but the aryl moiety is p-toluene. This compound is oxidized in the body, the methyl group being converted to $-COOH$, and the duration of action is accordingly rather brief. Replacement of methyl by chlorine and

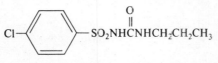

chlorpropamide

n-butyl by n-propyl yielded chlorpropamide, most potent of the series, with a long duration of action.[93,94]

Antithyroid sulfonamides. The antithyroid drugs of the thiouracil type had their origin in the accidental observation, in 1941, that rats receiving sulfaguanidine developed goiters.[95] The original purpose of the investigation had been to study the

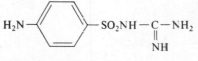

sulfaguanidine

role of intestinal bacteria in the biosynthesis of essential nutrients, and sulfaguanidine was being used to sterilize the gut. Other investigators observed similar goitrogenic effects in rats given phenylthiocarbamide (PTC) for an entirely different purpose.[96]

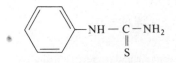

phenylthiocarbamide (PTC)

The bitter taste of this substance (cf. p. 470) was being exploited in experiments on free-choice diets; hypertrophy and hyperemia of the thyroid gland developed when the drinking water contained quite low concentrations of PTC.

In the systematic screening investigations that followed, it was found that thiourea itself was a potent goitrogen, and that among the sulfonamides sulfadiazine was most active.[97,98] Since sulfadiazine contains a pyrimidine ring, it was logical to

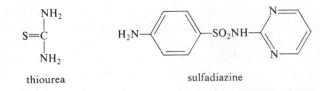

thiourea   sulfadiazine

incorporate the thiourea moiety in a pyrimidine, and thus thiouracil was obtained. This drug proved satisfactory for clinical use in the treatment of hyperthyroidism.[99] The mechanism of action of this family of drugs is to produce a blockade of thyroid hormone synthesis. The resulting goiter was due to overstimulation of the gland by

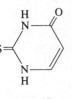

thiouracil

pituitary thyroid-stimulating hormone in response to low circulating levels of thyroid hormone.

Thiouracil produced toxic reactions, particularly agranulocytosis, at a rather high frequency; in one study, the incidence was 13% in a population of 2490 treated patients. Modifications of the thiouracil structure were studied in an attempt to find

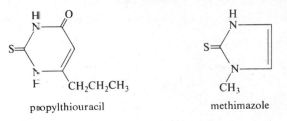

propylthiouracil   methimazole

a safer compound with the same antithyroid action.[100] Two superior drugs emerged. Propylthiouracil in effective clinical dosage caused toxic reactions in only 3% of a large group of patients. Methimazole, a closely related compound, which is no longer a pyrimidine, also has a very low toxicity.

REFERENCES

1. C. H. LA WALL: *Four Thousand Years of Pharmacy*. Philadelphia, J. B. Lippincott (1927).
2. W. G. BLACK: *Folk-Medicine; A Chapter in the History of Culture*. London, Elliot Stock (1883).
3. D. C. JARVIS: *Folk Medicine*. New York, Holt (1958).
4. J. M. STILLMAN: *Paracelsus: His Personality and Influence as Physician, Chemist and Reformer*. Chicago, The Open Court Publishing Co. (1920).
5. F. G. BANTING and C. H. BEST: The internal secretion of the pancreas. *J Lab. Clin. Med.* 7:251 (1922).
5a. E. J. ARIËNS, ed.: *Drug Design*. Vols. I–III, New York, Academic Press (1971).
6. L. LASAGNA: The Drug Industry and Medicine Avenue. In *The Doctor's Dilemma*. New York, Harper & Row (1962). p. 131.
6a. Statistical Abstract of the United States, U.S. Dept. of Commerce, Bureau of the Census, Table 91 (1972). p. 66.
7. Hearings before the Subcommittee on Antitrust and Monopoly of the Committee on the Judiciary, United States Senate, 86th Congress, First Session, Pursuant to Senate Resolution 57: Part 14. *Administered Prices in the Drug Industry (Corticosteroids)*. Publication No. 35621, Washington, D.C., U.S. Government Printing Office (1960).
8. Federal Food, Drug, and Cosmetic Act. As amended: *Code of Federal Regulations*, Title 21. Washington, D.C., U.S. Government Printing Office (1963).
8a. M. TISHLER: The role of industry in national science policy. The people's welfare: Health and Medicine. *Perspec. Biol. Med.* 13:528 (1970).
8b. R. A. TURNER and P. HEBORN: *Screening Methods in Pharmacology* New York, Academic Press (1965). Vol. II.
8c. R. A. TURNER: *Screening Methods in Pharmacology*. New York, Academic Press (1965). Vol. I.
8d. A. BURGER, ed.: Drugs affecting the peripheral nervous system, Drugs affecting the central nervous system, Selected pharmacological testing methods. *Medicinal Research Monographs*. New York, Marcel Dekker, Inc. (1968). Vols. 1–3.
8e. S. IRWIN: Drug screening and evaluative procedures. *Science* 136:123 (1962).
9. G. ZBINDEN: The problem of the toxicologic examination of drugs in animals and their safety in man. *Clin. Pharmacol. Therap.* 5:537 (1964).
10. A. BURGER: Approaches to drug discovery. *New Eng. J. Med.* 270:1098 (1964).
11. P. EHRLICH and S. HATA: *Die experimentelle Chemotherapie der Spirillosen*. Berlin, Springer (1910).
12. F. Y. WISELOGLE, ed.: *A Survey of Antimalarial Drugs*. 1941–1945. Ann Arbor, J. W. Edwards (1946).
13. R. A. TURNER: The organization of screening. In *Screening Methods in Pharmacology*. New York, Academic Press (1965). pp. 22–41.
14. J. R. VANE: A plan for evaluating potential drugs. In *Evaluation of Drug Activities: Pharmacometrics*, Vol. 1, ed. by D. R. Laurence and A. L. Bacharach. New York, Academic Press (1964). pp. 23–45.
15. *The Pharmacopeia of the United States of America*, 18th Revision. Easton, Mack Publishing Co. (1970).
16. *Pharmacopoea Internationalis* (International Pharmacopoeia), 1st ed. vol. I, 1951; vol. II, 1955; Supplement, 1959; Geneva, World Health Organization.
17. A. S. V. BURGEN and J. F. MITCHELL: *Gaddum's Pharmacology*. 7th ed., New York, Oxford University Press (1972). pp. 211–227.

18. J. H. GADDUM: Simplified mathematics for bioassays. *J. Pharm. Pharmacol.* 5:345 (1953).

19. D. J. FINNEY: *Statistical Method in Biological Assay.* New York, Hafner (1952).

20. A. GOLDSTEIN: *Biostatistics: An Introductory Text.* New York, Macmillan (1964).

21. C. I. BLISS and H. P. MARKS: The biological assay of insulin. II. The estimation of drug potency from a graded response. *Quart. J. Pharm. Pharmacol.* 12:182 (1939).

22. H. B. VAN DYKE, K. ADAMSONS, JR., and S. L. ENGEL: Aspects of the biochemistry and physiology of the neurohypophyseal hormones. *Rec. Progr. Hormone Res.* 11:1 (1955).

23. M. SCHACHTER and J. MORLEY: Biologically active polypeptides. In *Evaluation of Drug Activities:Pharmacometrics*, vol. 2, ed. by D. R. Laurence and A. L. Bacharach. New York, Academic Press (1964). pp. 627–648.

24. N. BOHONOS and H. D. PIERSMA: Natural products in the pharmaceutical industry. *BioScience* 16:706 (1966).

25. R. A. GOSSELIN: The status of natural products in the American pharmaceutical market. *Lloydia* 25:241 (1962).

26. M. B. KREIG: *Green Medicine.* Chicago, Rand McNally (1964).

27. J. R. PRICE: Antifertility agents of plant origin. In *A Symposium on Agents Affecting Fertility*, ed. by C. R. Austin and J. S. Perry. Boston, Little, Brown and Co. (1965). pp. 3–17.

28. R. J. DUBOS: Studies on a bactericidal agent extracted from a soil bacillus. I. Preparation of the agent. Its activity in vitro. *J. Exp. Med.* 70:1 (1939).

29. R. J. DUBOS and R. D. HOTCHKISS: The production of bactericidal substances by aerobic sporulating bacilli. *J. Exp. Med.* 73:629 (1941).

30. T. P. KING and L. C. CRAIG: The chemistry of tyrocidine. V. The amino acid sequence of tyrocidine B. *J. Am. Chem. Soc.* 77:6627 (1955).

31. E. CHAIN, H. W. FLOREY, A. D. GARDNER, N. G. HEATLEY, M. A. JENNINGS, J. ORR-EWING, and A. G. SANDERS: Penicillin as a chemotherapeutic agent. *Lancet* 2:226 (1940).

32. R. L. NOBLE, C. T. BEER, and J. H. CUTTS: Role of chance observations in chemotherapy: *Vinca rosea. Ann. N.Y. Acad. Sci.* 76:882 (1958).

33. I. S. JOHNSON, H. F. WRIGHT, G. H. SVOBODA, and J. VLANTIS: Antitumor principles derived from *Vinca rosea* Linn. I. Vincaleukoblastine and leurosine. *Cancer Res.* 20:1016 (1960).

34. I. S. JOHNSON, J. G. ARMSTRONG, M. GORMAN, and J. P. BURNETT, JR.: The vinca alkaloids: a new class of oncolytic agents. *Cancer Res.* 23:1390 (1963).

35. N. NEUSS, M. GORMAN, W. HARGROVE, N. J. CONE, K. BIEMANN, G. BÜCHI, and R. E. MANNING: Vinca alkaloids. XXI. The structures of the oncolytic alkaloids vinblastine (VLB) and vincristine (VCR). *J. Am. Chem. Soc.* 86:1440 (1964).

36. J. W. MONCRIEF and W. N. LIPSCOMB: Structure of leurocristine methiodide dihydrate by anomalous scattering methods; relation to leurocristine (vincristine) and vincaleukoblastine (vinblastine). *Acta Crystallographica* 21:322 (1966).

37. G. H. SVOBODA, M. GORDON, and M. A. ROOT: Alkaloids of *Vinca rosea* (Catharanthus roseus). XVIII. A preliminary report on hypoglycemic activity. *Lloydia* 27:361 (1964).

38. P. S. HENCH, E. C. KENDALL, C. H. SLOCUMB, and H. F. POLLEY: The effect of a hormone of the adrenal cortex (17-hydroxy-11-dehydrocorticosterone: compound E) and of pituitary adrenocorticotropic hormone on rheumatoid arthritis. *Proc. Staff Meetings Mayo Clin.* 24:181 (1949).

39. N. APPLEZWEIG: *Steroid Drugs.* New York, McGraw-Hill (1962/1964). Vols. I, II.

40. L. S. FEISER and M. FEISER: *Steroids.* New York, Van Nostrand Reinhold (1959). p. 547.

41. R. E. MARKER and N. APPLEZWEIG: Steroidal sapogenins as a source for cortical steroids. *Chem. Eng. News* 27:3348 (1949).

42. D. H. PETERSON, H. C. MURRAY, S. H. EPPSTEIN, L. M. REINEKE, A. WEINTRAUB, P. D. MEISTER, and H. M. LEIGH: Microbiological transformations of steroids. I. Introduction of oxygen at carbon-11 of progesterone. *J. Am. Chem. Soc.* 74:5933 (1952).

43. L. H. SARETT, A. A. PATCHETT, and S. L. STEELMAN: The effects of structural alteration on the anti-inflammatory properties of hydrocortisone. *Fortschr. Arzneimittelforsch.* 5:11 (1963).

43a. J. FRIED and E. F. SABO: 9α-Fluoro derivatives of cortisone and hydrocortisone. *J. Am. Chem. Soc.* 76:1455 (1954).

44. W. WITHERING: *An Account of the Foxglove, and Some of its Medical Uses; with Practical Remarks on Dropsy, and Other Diseases. Medical Classics.* 2:305 (1937).

45. K. K. CHEN, F. G. HENDERSON, and R. C. ANDERSON: Comparison of forty-two cardiac glycosides and aglycones. *J. Pharmacol. Exp. Therap.* 103:420 (1951).

46. G. T. OKITA, P. J. TALSO, J. H. CURRY, JR., F. D. SMITH, JR., and E M. K. GEILING: Metabolic fate of radioactive digitoxin in human subjects. *J. Pharmacol. Exp. Therap.* 115:371 (1955).

47. J. E. DOHERTY and W. H. PERKINS: Studies with tritiated digoxin in human subjects after intravenous administration. *Am. Heart J.* 63:528 (1962).

48. H. GOLD: The choice of a digitalis preparation. *Connecticut Med. J.* 9:193 (1945).

49. C. A. WINTER: A study of comparative antihistaminic activity of six compounds. *J. Pharmacol. Exp. Therap.* 90:224 (1947).

50. F. E. ROTH and W. M. GOVIER: Comparative pharmacology of chlorpheniramine (chlortrimeton) and its optical isomers. *J. Pharmacol. Exp. Therap.* 124:347 (1958).

51. S. WIEDLING and C. TEGNER: Local anesthetics. *Progr. Med. Chem.* 3:332 (1963).

52. F. P. LUDUENA and J. O. HOPPE: 2-Alkoxy benzoate and thiolbenzoate derivatives as local anesthetics. *J. Pharmacol. Exp. Therap.* 117:89 (1956).

53. E. BÜLBRING and I. WAJDA: Biological comparison of local anesthetics. *J. Pharmacol. Exp. Therap.* 85:78 (1945).

54. J. ADRIANI, R. ZEPERNICK, J. ARENS, and E. AUTHEMENT: The comparative potency and effectiveness of topical anesthetics in man. *Clin. Pharmacol. Therap.* 5:49 (1964).

55. W. P. BOGER and J. J. GAVIN: An evaluation of tetracycline preparations. *New Eng. J. Med.* 261:827 (1959).

56. B. B. BRODIE and C. A. M. HOGBEN: Some physico-chemical factors in drug action. *J. Pharm. Pharmacol.* 9:345 (1957).

57. J. ZANDER: The chemical estimation of progesterone and its metabolites in body fluids and target organs. In *Progesterone. Brook Lodge Symposium,* ed. by A. C. Barnes. Augusta, Mich., Brook Lodge Press (1961). p. 77–89.

58. W. H. PEARLMAN: Circulating steroid hormone levels in relation to steroid hormone production. In *Hormones in Blood. Ciba Foundation Colloquia on Endocrinology,* vol. 11, ed. by G. E. W. Wolstenholme and E. C. P. Millar. Boston, Little, Brown and Co. (1957). pp. 233–251.

59. R. HERTZ, W. TULLNER, and E. RAFFELT: Progestational activity of orally administered 17α-ethynyl-19-nortestosterone. *Endocrinol.* 54:228 (1954).

60. D. A. MC GINTY and C. DJERASSI: Some chemical and biological properties of 19-nor-17α-ethynyltestosterone. *Ann. N.Y. Acad. Sci.* 71:500 (1958).

61. V. A. DRILL: *Oral Contraceptives.* New York, McGraw-Hill (1966).

62. G. PINCUS: The Control of Fertility. New York, Academic Press (1965).

63. C. DJERASSI: Steroid oral contraceptives. *Science* 151:1055 (1966).

64. E. M. PAPPER, R. C. PETERSON, J. J. BURNS, E. BERNSTEIN, P. LIEF, and B. B. BRODIE: Physiological disposition of certain N-alkyl thiobarbiturates. *Anesthesiology* 16:544 (1955).

65. A. MELI, A. WOLFF, and W. L. HONRATH: The mechanism by which 3-etherification with cyclopentyl alcohol enhances the oral activity of ethynylestradiol. *Steroids* 2:417 (1963).

66. A. MELI, W. L. HONRATH, and A. WOLFF: Mechanism by which 3-enol etherification enhances the oral activity of methyltestosterone in rats. *Endocrinology* 74:79 (1964).

67. L. C. MARK, H. J. KAYDEN, J. M. STEELE, J. R. COOPER, I. BERLIN, E. A. ROVENSTINE, and B. B. BRODIE: The physiological disposition and cardiac effects of procaine amide. *J. Pharmacol. Exp. Therap.* 102:5 (1951).

68. A. V. S. DE REUCK and M. P. CAMERON, ed.: *Resistance of Bacteria to the Penicillins. Ciba Foundation Study Group No. 13.* Boston, Little, Brown and Co. (1962).

69. G. N. ROLINSON, F. R. BATCHELOR, S. STEVENS, J. C. WOOD, and E. B. CHAIN: Bacteriological studies on a new penicillin—BRL 1241. *Lancet* 2:564 (1960).

70. E. C. DODDS, L. GOLDBERG, W. LAWSON, and R. ROBINSON: Oestrogenic activity of alkylated stilboestrols. *Nature* 142:34 (1938).

71. Q. R. BARTZ: Isolation and characterization of chloromycetin. *J. Biol. Chem.* 172–455 (1948).

72. M. JACOBSON: Insect sex attractants. III. The optical resolution of *dl*-10-acetoxy-*cis*-7-hexadecen-1-ol. *J. Organ. Chem.* 27:2670 (1962).

73. M. BEROZA: Agents affecting insect fertility. In *Agents Affecting Fertility,* ed. by C. R. Austin and J. S. Perry. Boston, Little, Brown and Co. (1965). pp. 136–158.

74. S. FARBER, L. K. DIAMOND, R. D. MERCER, R. F. SYLVESTER, JR., and J. A. WOLFF: Temporary remissions in acute leukemia in children produced by folic acid antagonist, 4-aminopteroyl-glutamic acid (aminopterin). *New Eng. J. Med.* 238:787 (1948).

75. K. H. BEYER, J. E. BAER, J. K. MICHAELSON, and H. F. RUSSO: Renotropic characteristics of ethacrynic acid: a phenoxyacetic saluretic-diuretic agent. *J. Pharmacol. Exp. Therap.* 147:1 (1965).

76. M. D. MILNE: Renal pharmacology. *Ann. Rev. Pharmacol.* 5:119 (1965).

76a. E. J. LANDON and L. R. FORTE: Cellular mechanisms in renal pharmacology. In *Ann. Rev. Pharmacol.* 11:171 (1971).

76b. P. J. CANNON, H. O. HEINEMANN, W. B. STASON, and J. H. LARAGH: Ethacrynic acid: Effectiveness and mode of diuretic action in man *Circulation* 31:5 (1965).

76c. D. E. DUGGAN and R. M. NOLL: Effects of ethacrynic acid and cardiac glycosides upon a membrane adenosinetriphosphatase of renal cortex. *Arch. Biochem. Biophys.* 109:388 (1965).

77. K. H. BEYER, H. F. RUSSO, E. K. TILLSON, A. K. MILLER, W. F. VERWEY, and S. R. GASS: "Benemid" p-(di-n-propylsulfamyl)-benzoic acid: its renal affinity and its elimination. *Am. J. Physiol.* 166:625 (1951).

78. J. H. SIROTA, T. F. YÜ, and A. B. GUTMAN: Effect of benemid (p-(di-n-propyl sulfamyl)-benzoic acid) on urate clearance and other discrete renal functions in gouty subjects. *J. Clin. Invest.* 31:692 (1952).

79. F. H. S. CURD, D. G DAVEY, and F. L. ROSE: Studies on synthetic antimalarial drugs. II. General chemical considerations. *Ann. Trop. Med.* 39:157 (1945).

80. F. H. S. CURD, D. G. DAVEY, and F. L. ROSE: Studies on synthetic antimalarial drugs. X.— Some biguanide derivatives as new types of antimalarial substances with both therapeutic and causal prophylactic activity. *Ann. Trop. Med.* 39:208 (1945).

81. E. A. FALCO, G. H. HITCHINGS, P. B. RUSSELL, and H. VANDER WERFF: Antimalarials as antagonists of purines and pteroylglutamic acid. *Nature* 164:107 (1949).

82. F. HAWKING and W. L. M. PERRY: Activation of paludrine. *Brit. J. Pharmacol.* 3:320 (1948).

83. A. F. CROWTHER and A. A. LEVI: Proguanil—the isolation of a metabolite with high antimalarial activity. *Brit. J. Pharmacol.* 8:93 (1953).

84. E. A. FALCO, L. G. GOODWIN, G. H. HITCHINGS, I. M. ROLLO, and P. B. RUSSELL: 2:4:Diaminopyrimidines—a new series of antimalarials. *Brit. J. Pharmacol.* 6:185 (1951).

85. J. M. SPRAGUE: Some results of molecular modifications of diuretics. In *Molecular Modification in Drug Design. Advances in Chemistry*, Series No. 45. Washington, D.C., American Chemical Society (1964). pp. 87–101.

86. R. O. ROBLIN, JR. and J. W. CLAPP: The preparation of heterocyclic sulfonamides. *J. Am. Chem. Soc.* 72:4890 (1950).

87. W. H. MILLER, A. M. DESSERT, and R. O. ROBLIN, JR.: Heterocyclic sulfonamides as carbonic anydrase inhibitors. *J. Am. Chem. Soc.* 72:4893 (1950).

88. R. V. FORD, C. L. SPURR, and J. H. MOYER: The problem of bioassay and comparative potency of diuretics. II. Carbonic anhydrase inhibitors as oral diuretics. *Circulation* 16:394 (1957).

89. K. H. BEYER and J. E. BAER: Physiological basis for the action of newer diuretic agents. *Pharmacol. Rev.* 13:517 (1961).

90. Council on Drugs, American Medical Association: *Drug Evaluations*, Chicago, American Medical Association (1971). p. 47.

91. A. LOUBATIÈRES: The hypoglycemic sulfonamides: history and development of the problem from 1942 to 1955. *Ann. N.Y. Acad. Sci.* 71:4 (1957).

92. H. FRANKE and J. FUCHS: Ein neues antidiabetisches Prinzip; Ergebnisse klinischer Untersuchungen. *Deut. Med. Wochensch.* 80:1449 (1955).

93. W. M. MC LAMORE, G. M. FANELLI, S. Y. P'AN, and G. D. LAUBACH: Hypoglycemic sulfonylureas: effect of structure on activity. *Ann. N.Y. Acad. Sci.* 74:443 (1959).

94. J. A. SCHNEIDER, E D. SALGADO, D. JAEGER, and C. DELAHUNT: The pharmacology of chlorpropamide, *Ann. N.Y. Acad. Sci.* 74:427 (1959).

95. J. B. MAC KENZIE, C. G. MAC KENZIE, and E. V. MC COLLUM: The effect of sulfanilylguanidine on the thyroid of the rat. *Science* 94:518 (1941).

96. C. P. RICHTER and K. H. CLISBY: Toxic effects of the bitter-tasting phenylthiocarbamide. *Arch. Pathol.* 33:46 (1942).

97. C. G. MAC KENZIE and J. B. MAC KENZIE: Effect of sulfonamides and thioureas on the thyroid gland and basal metabolism. *Endocrinology* 32:185 (1943).

98. E. B. ASTWOOD, J. SULLIVAN, A. BISSELL, and R. TYSLOWITZ: Action of certain sulfon-
     amides and of thiourea upon the function of the thyroid gland of the rat. *Endocrinology* 32:210
     (1943).
99. E. B. ASTWOOD: Treatment of hyptherthyroidism with thiourea and thiouracil. *J. Am. Med. Ass.*
     122:78 (1943).
100. W. P. VANDERLAAN and V. M. STORRIE: A survey of the factors controlling thyroid function,
     with especial reference to newer views on antithyroid substances. *Pharmacol. Rev.* 7:301 (1955).

CHAPTER 14
Drug Evaluation in Man

THE CLINICAL TRIAL

Introduction

The systematic procedure for the evaluation of drugs in groups of people is known as the *clinical trial*.[1-4] One might wonder why special techniques should be required at all. Certainly many drugs (e.g., opium for pain, quinine for malaria) earned an established place in therapy long before the days of modern experimental science. But experience has shown that "clinical impressions" can be misleading. Many a therapeutic regimen has ultimately been proved useless despite traditional and unquestioning employment. Especially when a drug's alleged effect is less than dramatic, one cannot accept without decisive proof that there has been any therapeutic effect at all. Ascorbic acid, flavinoids, other vitamins, antihistamines, and antibiotics, for example, have at one time or another enjoyed wide popularity for preventing or aborting the common cold, but no properly designed experiments have ever borne out their reputation.

The persuasiveness of personal experience is very strong. If a person who has experienced frequent colds begins taking a medication and finds after a time that the colds seem less frequent or less severe or stop entirely, he is very likely to attribute that result to the medication. In so doing, he may overlook entirely a number of other variables, such as change of residence, change in emotional stresses, change in exposure to inclement weather, change in prevalence of colds in the immediate environment, and so on. One variable—the taking of a given medication—is defined as the critical one and other variables are simply ignored. This tendency to attribute anything that happens to a particular medication is very widespread and must be controlled if useful information about drug effects is to be obtained. In methadone maintenance programs, for example, patients blame methadone quite regularly for all physical and emotional ills they experience, overlooking the fact that concurrent disease may exist and that the symptoms complained of may have antedated the first dose of methadone[5].

Rigorous methods of drug evaluation in man were slow to be accepted, even after controlled animal experimentation had been on a firm basis for many decades. In part, this reluctance reflected a feeling of helplessness in the face of the vast number of variables encountered in studies with human beings. Each person, it was argued, is unique; the expression of disease processes is so individualized that no valid comparisons are possible, objective criteria fail, and only "clinical judgment" will suffice. But on the contrary, it is precisely because of the variability between people that sound experimental design, unbiased observation, and valid statistical analysis of data are indispensable.[6–15]

Placebo Controls and Concurrent Comparisons

Except in an unconscious patient, every drug administration consists of more than the mere introduction of a particular chemical substance into the body. The act of prescribing or actually administering a drug is an integral part of the total relationship between physician and patient. The physician wishes the drug to produce a certain effect and expects it to do so, or he would not have given it. The patient wishes desperately for the drug to be effective, and if he has confidence in the physician, he shares the latter's expectations. Thus, drug administration often occurs in a situation characterized by biased expectations and enhanced suggestibility on both sides.

Health and disease are greatly influenced by psychic and emotional factors. Symptoms and disease complexes of psychosomatic origin are just as "real" as those arising from simple organic causes. In the same way, psychic responses to drugs and psychic modifications of drug actions are real phenomena to be reckoned with. All those reactions to drug administration that arise from the very act of taking the drug and that are unrelated to the pharmacologic actions of the drug are known as *placebo effects*. An inert substance masquerading as a drug is called a *placebo*. The Latin word means "I shall please"; it referred originally to medications given merely to placate the patient when no specific remedy was available. All drugs may produce placebo effects. If the physician is aware, for example, that certain toxic manifestations may occur and warns the patient, or if the patient himself has heard (rightly or wrongly) about untoward reactions, the patient may then anticipate effects other than the desired beneficial ones. This complicates the interpretation of drug responses in man and necessitates special controls to enable one to distinguish between pharmacologic and placebo effects of drugs.[16]

Placebos are still occasionally prescribed as medication quite apart from their use as controls in human experimentation. A physician may employ a placebo diagnostically to assess the psychic component of a patient's symptom complex, which may be amenable to relief by suggestion. When a placebo is used therapeutically, the physician has usually decided to his own satisfaction that no better course of treatment is indicated and that some benefit may result from the placebo effect. With improvements in diagnosis and with greater understanding of the need for psychiatric treatment of anxiety and other emotional states, this frank use of placebos in medicine is rightly falling into disfavor. Placebo medication carries with it the danger that thorough diagnosis and more appropriate treatment may be neglected. And sometimes placating the patient with lactose capsules may be too easy a way to temporize in a difficult situation.

Some investigations have suggested that approximately 30% of all people are suggestible and tend to give positive responses of various sorts to placebos. These so-called placebo reactors, if they could be identified in advance of an experiment, could be excluded from it. Other studies have shown, however, that the frequency of placebo responses differs widely from experiment to experiment, that the same individuals may react more or less readily to a placebo at different times, and that circumstances can be found in which nearly all people respond to placebos. It is impractical, therefore, to identify and exclude placebo reactors.[17] The only alternative, if we are to gain meaningful information about drug actions, is to take account of placebo responses within each experiment, to whatever extent possible. The problem is really one of establishing a control group that is identical to the experimental group in all respects except for the one variable (i.e., the drug) that is under study. Even in animal experimentation we follow the same principle. Animals subjected to a surgical procedure are compared with sham-operated controls. Animals injected with a drug are compared with others injected with the drug-free vehicle (e.g., saline solution). Thus, if we wish to test a drug in humans in the simplest kind of design, we would compare drug administration with placebo administration, all other conditions being identical in the two groups.

Placebo controls are not always necessary or desirable. If a useful drug is already available and the question is whether or not a new drug is superior, a placebo control would be inappropriate. Moreover, there would be no justification for withholding an effective drug from some patients merely for the sake of scientific curiosity. The appropriate clinical trial in such a case would be a comparison between the old drug and the new.

A large part of the variability in biologic experimentation arises from individual differences between subjects. This part of the total variability can be minimized by arranging matters so that each subject acts as his own control. A comparison between drug and placebo (or between two drugs) might be carried out as follows: All subjects receive placebo, and on a different occasion they all receive the drug. Then instead of comparing all drug responses with all placebo responses, each subject's response to the two treatments is noted on an individual basis. A group of differences is thus generated between drug and placebo responses for individual subjects, and such data can be tested for significance by standard statistical methods.[13,14] This crude design has a serious flaw, however. There is no way to tell how much of the observed difference between drug and placebo might have been due to differences in conditions on the occasions of the respective drug and placebo administrations. Moreover, it is possible that the prior administration of a placebo might in itself modify the subsequent response to a drug.

The design usually adopted to circumvent this difficulty is called a *crossover*. The subjects are divided randomly into two groups, one to receive the placebo first, and drug later, the other to receive placebo and drug in reversed order. Crossover is an elementary example of the more general principle of balancing experimental designs so that all variables (drugs, order of administration, dosage, route of administration, etc.) appear systematically in all possible configurations. This is often accomplished by means of a Latin square, as shown in Table 14-1.[18] Here a drug is being tested at three dose levels, designated *a*, *b*, and *c*; and a placebo is also being employed. Four days are allotted for the experiment, and the subjects are assigned randomly to four groups, as shown. The Latin square provides a framework for ensuring a proper balance. Each dose and the placebo are tested on every day; each group receives every treatment; *a* precedes *b* half the time and follows *b* half the time; and so on. The data obtained in a balanced design of this kind are readily subjected

TABLE 14-1. A Latin-square design.
The conduct of the experiment is prescribed by the Latin square. This is one of many possible 4×4 Latin squares. Here a, b, and c represent different dosages of a drug under test. Subjects are assigned randomly to the four groups.

	Day 1	Day 2	Day 3	Day 4
Group 1	a	b	c	placebo
Group 2	b	a	placebo	c
Group 3	c	placebo	b	a
Group 4	placebo	c	a	b

to an analysis of variance, to determine which effects differ significantly from one another.

Even the simple crossover design may prove inadequate, as when prior treatment with one drug significantly affects the response to (or the metabolism of) a comparison drug. Suppose drug A induces enzymes that greatly accelerate the metabolism of B, but that B has no such effect on the metabolism of A. Then, in addition to other chronologic variables that would ordinarily be controlled in the crossover procedure, it would now be found that B given after A is inferior to A, whereas A given after B might be inferior to B. The design might better include groups that receive only A or only B without crossover.

Implicit in the concept of balanced experimental design is the principle that the various treatments must be compared at the same time. It is only rarely possible to evaluate a new drug or other treatment properly in comparison with previous experience. The severity of the illness being treated may have been different in the past, as with virus infections due to different strains. The populations compared may be quite different in ways not apparent to the investigator; without purposeful matching and randomization there can never be assurance of equivalence. Ancillary treatments change with time, hospital and nursing care improve, medical and surgical techniques are perfected, accessory new drugs come into use, general progress occurs in sanitation and in living standards.

It is true, of course, that if a previously fatal disease is cured by a new drug, the event is so markedly different from all past experience that it may usually be accepted without elaborate controls. This was the case when subacute bacterial endocarditis was first cured by massive penicillin infusions. Table 14-2 presents a summary of results in a large number of patients with miliary tuberculosis or tuberculous meningitis, conditions that were uniformly fatal prior to the introduction of streptomycin into therapy in 1946. There is no question about the efficacy of chemotherapy in these conditions. The data also show better results when streptomycin was supplemented with p-aminosalicylate than when it was used alone, and still better results when isoniazid was added.

Usually, treatment effects are less dramatic than the reduction of mortality from 100% to 5% shown in Table 14-2. The question then arises whether the improved outcome would have occurred even without the drug. The introduction of penicillin for the treatment of syphilis, for example, appeared to change the incidence of that disease considerably; but the use of the drug was accompanied by mass education

TABLE 14-2. Effect of chemotherapy on mortality from miliary and miliary-meningeal tuberculosis.
Patents were male adults treated in Veterans Administration hospitals between 1946 and 1959, and followed for 5–10 years. (From Falk,[19] Tables 3 and 8.)

Drug treatment	Type of tuberculosis	No. of patients	Mortality (%)
None (retrospective; patients before 1946)	miliary	—	100
	miliary-meningeal	—	100
Streptomycin only	miliary	63	47
	miliary-meningeal	114	94
Streptomycin + PAS[a]	miliary	102	18
	miliary-meningeal	51	78
Streptomycin, PAS, and isoniazid	miliary	138	5
	miliary-meningeal	52	23

[a] p-aminosalicylate.

and public health measures that would have contributed to the control of venereal diseases even if penicillin had not been introduced. As a rule, clinical trials are meaningless unless they embody concurrent comparisons.

Randomization

A very important aspect of the design of a clinical trial is the method used to assign subjects to experimental groups. It is essential that at the outset of the experiment the various groups be as nearly equivalent as possible in every way. It might be supposed that any essentially haphazard procedure would work, provided subjects were not selected deliberately for one group or another on the basis of their disease state or likely response to drug treatment. But experience has shown that haphazard methods are very unreliable. The investigator may unconsciously allocate the more seriously ill patients to the treatment he believes will be most beneficial. It is well known in animal experimentation that inadvertent selection can bias the experimental outcomes. If a large group of mice, for example, is to be divided into two groups, one to receive a drug, the other to serve as control, then merely removing one-half the mice to another cage will not suffice. Heavier, more sluggish, and more docile mice are easier to catch, and therefore the two groups will not be equivalent. Since we cannot really know what complex physiologic differences may be associated with ease of capture in this situation, it must be concluded that no valid experiments whatsoever could be performed with groups of mice selected in this way.

The literature on human experimentation offers numerous examples of inadvertent selection. All patients on one hospital ward, for example, may be given one drug, all patients on a different ward receive another drug or a placebo. But what were the circumstances that led to a particular patient being placed on one ward or the other, and might these circumstances have selected inadvertently for qualities that will affect the response to the drugs? In an investigation of the efficacy of drugs that prevent blood clotting in the treatment of coronary thrombosis, drugs or placebos were assigned according to the day of admission to hospital. After the experiment was well under way, it was discovered that the purpose of the investigation and the method of assigning medications had become known to the physicians in the community. If a physician believed that treatment with the untried drug would be beneficial, he would arrange, if possible, to have his patients admitted on the appropriate day for admission to the drug group; in this way the equivalence of the groups was destroyed and conclusions about the merit of the drug were invalidated.[10] Even assigning patients to groups on an alphabetical basis according to surnames may be hazardous, since names often connote ethnic, national, religious and other characteristics possibly related to the variables under study.

For all these reasons, it is the invariable rule to assign medications *randomly*. A random design is not the same as a haphazard one; randomness must often be planned very carefully. The criterion of random assignment to groups is that no characteristic of a subject whatsoever shall play any part in determining to what group he is assigned. The simplest way of accomplishing this is by the use of chance devices: coin tossing for two groups, die throwing for up to six groups, drawing lots, and so on. The most versatile chance device is the table of random numbers,[18] illustrated in Table 14-3. Such a table consists of a sequence of digits generated by

TABLE 14-3. Random digits.
A selection of 400 random digits from a very large sequence. (Extracted from the table published by The Rand Corporation,[20] p. 89.)

95523	16893	48247	03407	31665	66917	98339	69569
62477	35693	90285	00994	74594	90414	80392	86873
57327	96854	12771	31236	89768	32495	67307	16957
41636	48701	55198	93603	58155	89862	55728	80036
69743	71852	38521	70835	21981	20370	40829	38049
27583	54945	40301	09374	64651	87504	46483	54700
43193	77444	60036	96246	56872	23543	71399	46681
74121	08564	82161	68832	23596	93906	44956	42941
32155	01757	32402	01704	13312	93761	79236	70219
24415	95858	89258	11388	42821	07595	90003	02631

some procedure that ensures equal probability for any digit to appear at any point in the sequence. The sequence is tested exhaustively by statistical procedures, to make sure there was no malfunction of the device (e.g., a computer) that generated the sequence. The table is used as follows: If there is a known number of subjects to be assigned to a certain number of experimental groups, every subject is given a serial number. Then the table is entered at an arbitrary point and the first group is filled by taking numbers in sequence. Let us assume there are 60 subjects to be allocated equally to 4 groups. The subjects will be numbered serially from 01 to 60. Now to fill the first group we enter Table 14-3 at upper left and read out 2-digit numbers. Numbers greater than 60 are ignored, as are numbers already assigned. The first number, 95, we ignore. Subject 52 is the first subject assigned to the first group. Following the same procedure, the first group also receives subjects 31, 48, 24, and so on, until 15 assignments have been made. Then the second and third groups are filled in the same way. The remaining 15 subjects are placed in the fourth group.

No characteristic of any subject will have played any part in his assignment to a group.

Often, in a clinical trial, the patients cannot be identified at the outset. A drug is going to be tested, perhaps, on patients who will be reporting to a clinic over a period of months. The procedure for making group assignments is exactly as described, by table of random numbers, except that the serial numbers picked from the table refer to the sequence in which patients will present themselves at the clinic. Using the same example as above, the assignment of 60 patients to 4 treatment groups, the procedure would be as follows. First, the sequence numbers 1 to 60 are listed; these represent patients, in the order in which they will be admitted to the study. These patients are assigned to the 4 treatment groups, a priori, by drawing numbers from the table of random numbers. Thus the 52nd, 31st, 48th, 24th patient, and so on, would be assigned to the first treatment group. After 15 such assignments had been made, filling that group, the second and third treatment groups would be filled in the same way. The remaining 15 unassigned sequence numbers would form the fourth treatment group. In this way, all members of the sequence would be pre-assigned, before they present themselves, in a randomized manner and by a procedure that establishes groups of equal size. Then when each patient actually enters the clinic, assigning him to a treatment group simply means referring to the prepared list of assignments.

Blind Designs

If at all possible, the subjects should be unaware of what medication they are receiving. The importance of this requirement depends somewhat upon the magnitude of the drug effect. If a drug were developed that cured leukemia, a disease now uniformly fatal, it would probably not influence the outcome of the test if treated patients knew they were receiving that drug. But usually, because of the influence of expectations upon an experimental outcome, such knowledge by the subjects would throw most of the conclusions into doubt. Especially if one wishes to assess the frequency or severity of side effects it is important that the nature of the treatment be concealed from the patients. Obviously, all medications (including placebo) must be identical in appearance and should, if possible, be administered on the same schedule. Such a design, in which the subjects are unaware of the nature of the medications, is called blind.

It may not be easy or practical to maintain blind conditions. The drug may produce unmistakable side effects that are not produced by a placebo. Antihistaminics, for example, produce drowsiness, whereas placebos presumably do not. Any subject receiving an antihistaminic and becoming drowsy may conclude that he has been given a potent drug, and this knowledge may well influence his expectations about whatever other pharmacologic action is under test. Another example is propranolol, a β-adrenergic blocking agent used as an adjunct in the treatment of angina pectoris. Here the response of the heart to exercise is muted by the drug, so that the subject soon realizes he is getting an agent that affects this response. In a placebo-controlled study,[21] it was found that patients treated with propranolol took fewer nitroglycerine tablets (i.e., presumably had fewer angina attacks) than those on placebo, but the reassuring knowledge that a drug with obvious cardiovascular actions was being given could well have influenced this outcome. Much controversy has been engendered over experiments with propranolol yielding conflicting results.[22-24] If a medication is being administered by mouth, the drug may have a characteristic taste; in this case, one may try to match the taste by adding appropriate inert materials to the placebo. Even when the material is contained in a capsule there may be an aftertaste that identifies the drug to the subject.

It is equally important, but not so obvious, that the investigators who deal with the subjects in the course of the experiment, and who evaluate the results, must be unaware of which medications have been assigned to which subjects. The personnel who actually administer the medications often cannot deceive the subjects; if they know what drug is being administered or that a placebo is being given, their behavior will betray their knowledge in numerous ways. And when the results of an experiment are being evaluated, subjective bias comes strongly into play if the assignment of medications is known. This is true not only for evaluations in which the criteria are subjective (e.g., assessment of improvement in schizophrenic patents),[25] but even for objective criteria such as size of lesions on an x-ray plate or the sedimentation rate of erythrocytes. No procedure is immune to distortion by an observer's bias. Blood cells can be counted inaccurately, spectrophotometers can be misread, pathologic changes in a tissue specimen can be detected or overlooked, roentgenographic anomalies can be exaggerated or discounted, psychotic patients can be adjudged more tractable or more hostile. The only sure way to eliminate bias of this kind is to arrange matters so that not only the subjects but also the investigators directly involved in the experimental procedures and evaluations remain unaware of the allocation of drugs or placebos from the beginning to the end of the experiment. Such a design is called *double blind*.

In practice, the conduct of a double-blind clinical trial is not as difficult as might be imagined. Once the decision has been made how the random assignments of subjects to groups is to be carried out, the medications are coded by serial number (see below), and the code is locked away securely. Safeguards are provided so that in case of adverse reaction, or for any reason involving the welfare of a patient, the code can be broken for that patient, who is then removed from the study. In the pioneering clinical trials organized by the British Medical Research Council, for example, the coding of the medications for assignment to patients all over the United Kingdom was done by a person who was to have no personal contact with the subjects. The code was retained in a safe in London, and only after all the final evaluations had been completed was the code consulted to identify each subject's medication.[26]

The labeling of medications must convey no information about their nature. Some early trials were conducted in the following simple way. On a hospital ward, capsules of drug were kept in a jar labeled *A* and capsules of placebo, identical in appearance to the drug capsules, were kept in a jar labeled *B*. No one could decide from these letters which was the drug, but enough information was conveyed, nevertheless, to invalidate the results. Because of the two jars, both the medical personnel and the patients deduced that two different medications were being compared. More serious, the conditions were present for a spread of subjective bias across the whole experiment. A few subjects, experiencing real or fancied effects of either medication, would spread the word to other patients; whereupon biased expectations concerning *A* or *B* would soon develop throughout the subject groups. The medical personnel, likewise, observing some apparent effect of one or the other drug, would soon generalize this effect unconsciously to all *A* or to all *B* patients. Therefore, the only admissible procedure is to label every subject's medications individually by a serial number or by subject's name. If serial numbers are used, care must be taken to avoid assigning any distinctive pattern of numbers to particular medications, such as odd numbers for drug and even numbers for placebo.

Two Trials with Antihistamines: An Illustrative Contrast

Two studies on the effects of antihistamine drugs on the course of the common cold, conducted within two years of each other, present an interesting contrast between a poorly designed and a well-designed clinical trial. In the first investigation [27] a total of 572 patients were treated between October 1, 1947 and May 1, 1948 in dispensaries at military bases. The subjects were those who reported that they had colds, provided that the examining physicians found "no evidence to disprove it." The group included military personnel, their dependents, and civilian employees. Therapy was started at any stage of the illness. Five different antihistamines and a placebo were used. "An effort was made to give various drugs to patients in succession and without selection," but apparently no rigorous randomization procedures were followed. Thus there was no assurance that the treatment groups would be matched with respect to age, sex, time of onset of illness, or severity of symptoms. Amphetamine was "frequently given" with the first dose of an antihistamine to counteract the sedative effects. Double-blind procedures do not appear to have been followed. "Cure" was defined as eradication of symptoms within 24 hr and absence of symptoms during the subsequent 48 hr. Of 319 patients with no history of allergy, 262 were treated with antihistamines, and 105 of these were cured. Of 57 such patients given placebo medication, only 5 were cured. From a statistical standpoint this difference is highly significant. Remarkably, 19 of 21 patients treated with an antihistamine drug within 1 hr of onset of their colds were cured. Unfortunately, only 2 patients in the placebo group were treated as early as this, as a result of the failure to randomize or to match groups with respect to duration of symptoms. If one wonders about the criteria for diagnosis that permit treatment to be instituted "within 1 hr of onset," the principal investigator comments: "When one has been unusually susceptible to colds all his life as the writer has been, and then lives an entire year without a cold as he has done by the simple expedient of taking one or two doses of an antihistaminic drug at the first hint of a cold, the problem of diagnosis becomes academic."

Poorly designed studies of this kind, conducted by investigators who were strongly biased toward a certain outcome and took no precautions to eliminate that bias, led to the widespread promotion and sale of antihistamine drugs for the treatment of the common cold. Despite recognition by experts that the evidence was unsatisfactory,[28] it was only with the carrying out of proper trials that justifiable action could be taken to protect the public against false claims of efficacy of these drugs.

A large-scale, well-designed trial of the usefulness of one antihistamine drug, thonzylamine, was carried out in Great Britain and Northern Ireland in the winter and spring of 1950, under the direction of the Medical Research Council.[29] Subjects over 15 years of age who met the following criteria were admitted to the trial: "A catarrhal inflammation of the upper respiratory passages usually without pyrexia but with watery or mucous discharge from the nose and associated with sneezing, fullness in the head and nose, and sometimes with cough, headache, sore throat, hoarseness and running eyes." People who had recently taken antihistamines or who had evidence of other infectious disease were excluded.

Subjects were assigned randomly to drug or placebo groups. The nature of the tablets given to each patient was not known to the patient or to the dispensing physician. Each box of tablets for each subject was marked with a serial number. Subjects in the drug group received three tablets daily of the antihistamine, 50 mg each, for three days. The placebo group received three similar tablets daily of an inert substance containing an insignificant amount (5 mg) of quinine sulfate. Immediate swallowing of the medication was encouraged so that taste would not help identify the drug. A standard form was provided upon which the medical officer was to record pertinent data upon admission of each subject to the trial and during the progress of the trial.

A total of 775 subjects received the antihistamine and an equal number received the placebo medication. The final analysis omitted 394 records (196 from the drug group, 198 from the placebo group) because they were incomplete. The results therefore concern 579 subjects who had received the drug and 577 who had received the placebo. The effectiveness of the randomization procedure may be judged by the data of Table 14-4, which shows the frequency of presenting symptoms at the first

TABLE 14-4. Frequency of presenting symptoms at first visit.
These symptoms were recorded by the medical examiners at subject's entry into the study, *before* he was assigned randomly to drug or placebo group. (From Medical Research Council,[29] Table IV. By permission of the British Medical Journal.)

Symptoms	Persons given antihistaminic treatment		Persons given placebo treatment	
	No.	%	No.	%
Watery nasal discharge	359	62.0	337	58.4
Mucoid nasal discharge	114	19.7	118	20.5
Purulent nasal discharge	49	8.5	42	7.3
Blocked nose	321	55.4	307	53.2
Fullness in the head	385	66.5	390	67.6
Sneezing	413	71.3	408	70.7
Sore throat	217	37.5	231	40.0
Hoarseness	183	31.6	177	30.7
Cough	242	41.8	226	39.2
Headache	196	33.9	207	35.9
Feeling ill	44	7.6	46	8.0

visit, as recorded by a medical officer. The nearly identical figures in the two groups are noteworthy. The duration of symptoms before treatment (not shown here) also showed a nearly identical distribution in the two groups.

For evaluation of drug effect two criteria were established. The term "cured" referred to those persons who were completely free of symptoms and who were found to be without objective signs on examination. The term "improved" referred to those persons who on questioning and examination were found to be improved but not cured since the previous examination. Table 14-5 gives the percentages of subjects

TABLE 14-5. Percentages of subjects cured or improved by treatment.

"Cured" and "improved" are defined in text. Numbers of patients are given in parentheses under each category. Figures are percentages. Differences are given with standard errors. D = Antihistaminic drug; P = placebo. (From Medical Research Council,[29] Table V. By permission of the British Medical Journal.)

		Duration of cold before treatment										
		Under 1 day			1 Day			2 Days			3 Days or more		
Day of observation		D (201)	P (173)	Difference	D (180)	P (213)	Difference	D (96)	P (84)	Difference	D (102)	P (107)	Difference
First day	improved[a]	47.8	45.1	2.7 ± 5.2	47.2	38.5	8.7 ± 5.0	50.0	40.5	9.5 ± 7.4	48.0	45.8	2.2 ± 6.9
Second day	cured	13.4	13.9	−0.5 ± 3.6	7.8	6.6	1.2 ± 2.6	3.1	4.8	−1.7 ± 2.9	6.9	6.5	+0.4 ± 3.5
	cured or improved	68.2	64.7	3.5 ± 4.9	58.3	55.4	2.9 ± 5.0	59.4	57.1	2.3 ± 7.4	57.8	62.6	−4.8 ± 6.8
One week	cured	48.8	46.8	2.0 ± 5.2	42.2	37.1	5.1 ± 5.0	31.3	33.3	−2.0 ± 7.0	29.4	36.4	−7.0 ± 6.5
	cured or improved	80.6	74.6	6.0 ± 4.3	77.8	77.5	0.3 ± 4.5	70.8	79.8	−9.0 ± 6.5	70.6	78.5	−7.9 ± 6.0

[a] Includes the few patients (9 on drug and 5 on placebo) who said they were cured on the first day.

cured or improved after 1 day, 2 days, or a week categorized according to the duration of their colds before treatment. The data as a whole give little indication of any drug effect as compared with placebo. When all the results were combined, regardless of duration of cold before treatment, 48.0% of the drug group and 42.1% of the placebo group were cured or improved at the end of the first day's treatment. The small difference in favor of the drug was just significant in a technical, statistical sense, according to the investigators, "but even if it be real it is so small that it clearly has no practical importance." Even this small difference vanished on the second day, when the combined data showed cumulative percentages of 8.8 and 53.0 in the drug group and 8.5 and 51.3 in the placebo group, for "cured" and "improved," respectively. It was concluded that thonzylamine had little or no value in the treatment of the common cold. It was felt that the minor difference in favor of the drug on the first day might have been attributable to a slight sedative effect, or possibly to the unwitting inclusion of some subjects suffering from hay fever or allergic rhinitis. Table 14-6 gives

TABLE 14-6. Side effects attributed to treatment.
Figures are numbers of subjects in each group reporting the various side effects at some time during the trial. (From Medical Research Council,[29] Table VIII. By permission of the British Medical Journal.)

Main symptoms	Persons given antihistaminic treatment	Persons given placebo treatment
Drowsiness, lassitude, listlessness	26	35
Dizziness, giddiness, vertigo	21	13
Headache	21	16
Headache combined with other nervous symptoms	11	6
Depression with or without other nervous symptoms	2	5
Insomnia	3	1
Gastrointestinal	13	12
Combined gastrointestinal and nervous symptoms	8	7
Miscellaneous	16	16
Total	121	111

the frequencies of side effects attributed to treatment. Here there were no significant differences between drug and placebo. The large number of side effects reported in both groups may have been symptoms due to the infection but erroneously attributed to the medication.

Sequential Trials

The conventional type of controlled clinical trial described above, in which subjects are assigned randomly to treatment groups of predetermined size, can be inefficient. If one treatment were very much superior to another, this might be revealed decisively before all the members of all the groups have been treated. Especially when not all the subjects are at hand initially but will be placed in groups and treated as they present themselves over a period of time, it is not reasonable to go on with the trial after the results become clear. Moreover, in addition to the economic disadvantage of continuing an unnecessary trial, there is the ethical objection that after a certain point in the trial, some subjects will necessarily be treated with a medication or regimen already shown to be inferior. The same general argument applies when there is no important difference between treatments under test. It should be possible to decide this as soon as possible, and discontinue the trial without necessarily completing the treatments and observations on all the members of all the groups. The designs developed to permit such efficient and timely termination of drug evaluations are known as *sequential trials*.[30]

In sequential trials, observations are paired so that the alternative treatments (e.g., drug and placebo) are represented in each pair. A pair might consist of two observations on the same patient, one after each treatment, or actually of a pair of patients, each receiving a different treatment. By some criterion adopted in advance, one treatment will be rated as better than the other in a given pair. This outcome is called a *preference*. Let the alternative treatments be designated A and B, and suppose that relief of symptoms in a chronic disease is the criterion of evaluation. Then if a patient receives A for one week and B for another, and A is judged superior, a preference is recorded for A. If prolongation of life is the criterion, patients having been matched and paired at the outset with respect to age, sex, and severity of disease, then whenever a patient dies a preference is recorded for the treatment being received by the surviving member of his pair. Pairs within which no preference can be assigned do not enter the analysis at all.

The design is shown schematically in Figure 14-1. The total number of preferences is indicated on the x axis. Every preference for A is plotted by moving a path 1 unit diagonally up and to the right; every preference for B, by moving diagonally down

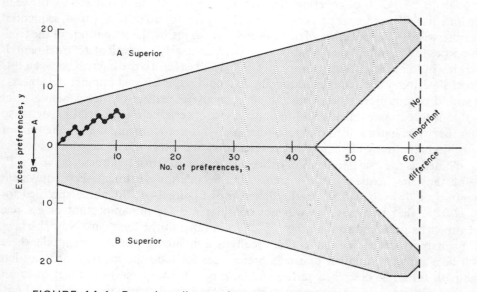

FIGURE 14-1. Boundary diagram for a sequential trial. *Here* $2\alpha = 0.05$, $1 - \beta = 0.95$, *and the specified value of* θ_1 *is 0.75. The values of* α *and* β *at the boundaries are approximate. See text for explanation. (Plotted from specifications of Armitage.[30])*

Drug Evaluation in Man

and to the right. In the example illustrated, there were 3 preferences for A, then 1 for B, then 3 more for A, and so on. Obviously, if A is better than B, the line will continue indefinitely upward; and if B is better than A, it will move indefinitely downward. The aim is to terminate the trial as soon as one of the following conclusions can be drawn: (a) that one treatment is superior to the other; or (b) that there is no important difference between the treatments. These terms require a priori definition. In deciding that one treatment is superior to the other, we declare the null hypothesis false; as in any statistical procedure. we do this at a certain level of significance. If the level of significance (here designated 2α) is 0.05, then we will accept a chance of 1 in 20 of being wrong when we declare a superiority of one treatment over the other, i.e., we shall say there is a difference 5% of the time when none really exists. In the diagram, the choice of a level of significance determines the positions of the upper and lower boundaries, for when either of these boundaries is reached, we shall declare one treatment superior and terminate the trial. It might be supposed that these boundaries would be given directly by the binomial probabilities, but the sequential nature of the decision-making process complicates the computation of probabilities.[31] From a practical point of view, the boundary specifications for $2\alpha = 0.05$ and $2\alpha = 0.01$ may be obtained from appropriate tables.[30] Figure 14-1 depicts upper and lower boundaries for the significance level most often adopted, $2\alpha = 0.05$.

The next thing that has to be specified is the power of the procedure, i.e., the probability with which a specified difference between the treatments will be detected if it exists. Usually one wishes to be fairly sure of finding a real difference, so the power (designated $1 - \beta$) is usually chosen to be a large fraction, commonly 0.95. This means that a real difference of a specified magnitude will be found 95 times out of 100 trials, on the average.

Finally, the *specified difference* referred to above has to be decided upon. This will be the degree of superiority of one treatment over another considered important enough to be worth discovering. The point here is that small differences between treatments will require very large numbers of subjects to prove. In any trial, sequential or otherwise, the importance of the objective has to justify the magnitude of the trial. Suppose, for example, that treatment A were so nearly equivalent to treatment B that it would be judged superior in only 51% of all cases. To distinguish between this slight superiority and complete equivalence would require a vast number of subjects; it would obviously not be worth the effort. A useful feature of the sequential trial is that it forces an explicit decision about these criteria before the trial is begun, so that the investigator is forced to recognize both the minimum and maximum number of subjects that may be required. The term used to express the specified difference is θ_1, defined as the true frequency of preference for the superior treatment, $\theta_0 = 1 - \theta_1$ being the true frequency of preference for the inferior treatment. For equivalent treatments, $\theta_1 = \theta_0 = 0.50$. In the diagram of Figure 14-1, the value specified for θ_1 is 0.75; that is to say, we will not consider a difference important unless one treatment is preferred to the other 75% of the time, in the long run. Now the laws of probability determine that if there really is a difference of that magnitude, there will be a sufficient number of excess preferences for the superior treatment so that the path traced as described earlier will be expected to intersect an upper or lower boundary before the total number of preferences exceeds a certain limit. That limit, for the parameters chosen here, is 62. In other words, if a superiority of A (or B) is not demonstrable with a sample size of 62 preferences, we can declare (with 95%

probability of being correct) that it does not exist. Or, in terms of the boundary diagram, if the path crosses the vertical broken line at $n = 62$ before it crosses an upper or lower boundary, there is no important difference between the treatments, and the trial can be terminated.

The wedge-shaped indentation of the right boundary has a simple explanation. Because the path traced by the sequential preferences cannot rise or fall at more than a 45-degree angle, it follows that there are certain positions at the right of the diagram from which the path could no longer intersect an upper or lower boundary within the total permissible number of preferences. Thus, if the path were at $y = 0$ by the 44th preference, the trial would be over because even if every subsequent preference were in favor of one treatment, an upper or lower boundary could not be reached.

Figure 14-2 presents a boundary diagram for a higher value of the specified difference ($\theta_1 = 0.85$) and for the 0.01 level of significance as well as the 0.05 level. It is

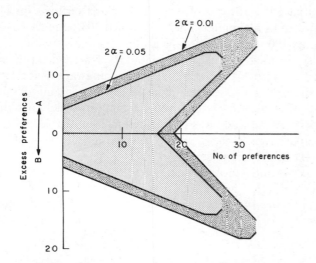

FIGURE 14-2. Boundary diagram for a sequential trial. *Here* $1 - \beta = 0.95$, *as in Figure 14-1; but* $\theta_1 = 0.85$. *Two boundary diagrams are shown, one for* $2\alpha = 0.05$, *the other for* $2\alpha = 0.01$. *Values of* α *and* β *at the boundaries are approximate. See text for explanation. (Plotted from specifications of Armitage.[30])*

of interest to note the effect of these changes on the shape of the diagram. The main result of insisting that a treatment difference be greater in order to be defined as "important" is that the right boundary moves to the left. Thus, the maximum number of preferences necessary to conclude that there is no important difference has diminished here from 62 to 27. The result of using a more rigorous level of significance for the decision that there is a difference, i.e., for the path to intersect an upper or lower boundary, is a need for a greater excess of preferences in favor of one treatment.

The specifications for drawing boundary diagrams for different chosen values of θ_1, at $2\alpha = 0.05$ or $2\alpha = 0.01$, and $1 - \beta = 0.95$ are given elsewhere.[30]

A trial of anticoagulant therapy was conducted to see if it would reduce the risk of myocardial infarction in patients with angina pectoris or previous infarction.

The trial was started in 1957 as a conventional design with two groups to be filled randomly as patients presented themselves. One group was to receive an anticoagulant, phenindione, at sufficiently high dosage to reduce the plasma prothrombin level to 20% of normal. The other group was to receive the same drug, but at lower dosage, sufficient to reduce the plasma prothrombin level to 50% of normal. These were called the "20% group" and "50% group," respectively. A control group was considered unjustified, since there was already evidence of a beneficial effect of anticoagulant therapy in preventing recurrences of myocardial infarction. But since no information was available about optimum dosage, and since overdosage carries a risk of hemorrhage, it was considered proper to conduct a trial of high versus low dosage. The published description of this study[32] exemplifies the adoption, in advance, of rigorous criteria for admission of patients to the study, establishment of subgroups according to sex, history, and plasma cholesterol level, and random assignment of patients within each subgroup to one or the other treatment. Of 394 patients with a history of angina pectoris or previous myocardial infarction, 191 did not meet the initial criteria; most of these had angina pectoris for longer than the two years established as maximum. There remained 203 patients, 103 assigned to the high dosage group, 100 to the low dosage group. The patients were followed closely throughout the study, their plasma prothrombin levels were determined periodically, and twice a year all were examined by physicians unaware of the treatment group to which they belonged. Episodes of myocardial infarction and all deaths occurring during the study were subjected to careful scrutiny in order to obtain as exact a diagnosis as possible. The study was terminated in 1960. Table 14-7 shows the data on myocardial infarctions in the groups. The difference in favor of the high dosage ("20%") group was highly significant.

In 1959, the newly introduced sequential method came to the attention of the investigators. Accordingly, the subjects were followed by this procedure too. The result is shown in Figure 14-3. Each time there was a death or myocardial infarction,

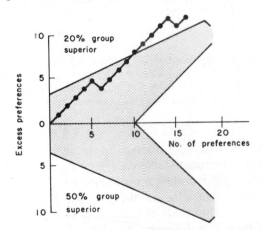

FIGURE 14-3. Result of sequential trial: Myocardial infarction or death in two treatment groups. *This graph is for the same experiment summarized in Table 14-7. Patients were paired, one from the 20% group (high dosage of phenindione) and one from the 50% group (low dosage). If a patient developed a myocardial infarction or if he had a cardiovascular death, a preference was given to the group to which the other patient in the pair belonged. Here $2\alpha = 0.05$, $1 - \beta = 0.95$, $\theta_1 = 0.90$. (From Borchgrevink, Figure 11.[32])*

TABLE 14-7. Rate of myocardial infarction in two treatment groups.
Patients with angina pectoris or a previous myocardial infarction were maintained on the anti-coagulant phenindione at 2 dosage levels. The higher dosage reduced the prothrombin levels to 20% of normal, on the average; on the lower dosage, prothrombin levels were 50% of normal. The infarction rate in the 20% group was significantly lower than in the 50% group ($P < 0.01$). (From Borchgrevink,[32] Table 17.)

	No. of patients	Observation period in patient years	Infarctions		Infarction rate (% per year)
			No.	%	
20% Group					
Women	21	32	0	0.0	0.0
Men	82	110	2	2.4	1.8
Total	103	142	2	1.9	1.4
50% Group					
Women	18	25	1	5.6	4.0
Men	82	98	12	14.6	12.2
Total	100	123	13	13.0	10.6

a preference was given to the treatment group to which the other patient of the pair belonged. The upper boundary was crossed by the tenth event. The study could have been closed at this time, seven months before the prearranged termination. During those final seven months, six more patients had attacks of myocardial infarction and two of these died, both of them in the low dosage ("50%") group. It is not known, of course, whether raising the dosage for all patients, as soor as the superiority of the high dosage had been demonstrated, would have been timely enough to alter the outcome for those six patients,[33] but these results certainly demonstrate vividly a principal advantage of the sequential method.

Critical Appraisal of Reports on Clinical Trials

Physicians and others concerned with drug actions in man are increasingly called upon to examine critically the experimental evidence on which claims of drug efficacy are based. Three fundamental questions should be asked about any published report describing the outcome of a clinical trial.

1. *Was the experimental design adequate?* Was the drug compared with a placebo or with an established standard drug in a double-blind design? Were the patients assigned randomly to the various treatment groups? Is it stated explicitly what precautions were taken to exclude subjective bias at every stage of the experiment, especially during the evaluative procedures? Were the patients included in the trial typical of those for whom the drug is now recommended, or did the conditions of selection for the trial or of nonspecific treatment during the trial favor the new drug? Were the trials conducted by reputable independent investigators, qualified by experience in the design and conduct of such trials? Were the trials carried out, for

example, under the aegis of an independent academic or research institution? If there is any serious doubt that these questions can all be answered affirmatively, there is usually no point in proceeding further, for the most elegant statistical analysis cannot salvage meaningful data from a poor experiment.

This first question is the most important, and failure to consider it is the most common cause of error in interpreting clinical trials. Even scientists are not immune to this error, which is commonly associated with a strong conviction about what the outcome of the experiment ought to be, based on personal experiences (e.g., "ascorbic acid prevented *me* from catching cold").[34] It is indeed interesting to see how the story of the antihistaminic agents as cold cures, detailed earlier in this chapter, was played out again with ascorbic acid 10–20 years later. Several investigators claimed favorable results, so that one could readily, though uncritically, find confirmation of one's beliefs in this vitamin. But every investigation that meets the basic criteria for sound clinical trials has yielded clearly negative results. Ascorbic acid, in doses 3 to 30 times the recommended daily dietary allowance, is not superior to a placebo in preventing or curing colds.[35–38]

2. *Are the results claimed for the new drug statistically significant?* If the experimental design was adequate, then the next question to be settled is whether observed differences between the treatment groups are likely to have been due to the treatments or to chance fluctuations unrelated to the treatments employed. The published results should contain enough of the raw data to permit the reader to make his own statistical analysis, should he wish to do so.[14,15] And the investigators, when making statements about statistical significance, should always indicate what procedures were used. If the groups do not differ significantly (at the chosen level of significance), then the drug's proponent has failed to prove his point, for the results might well have come about by chance. This does not mean, of course, that the drug is worthless. A better experimental design, which reduces the variation between subjects, a larger number of subjects, or a different schedule of drug administration are some of the changes that might, in a new trial, reveal a positive drug effect.

Most clinical trials have been based upon group comparisons. It should be borne in mind, therefore, that unusual individual results may be obscured by the group trend. A result showing no difference between two drugs (or between a drug and a placebo) in groups of patients may conceal a real and significant effect in some patients. Special techniques have been developed for evaluating drugs on a variety of different criteria in the same patient, or making repeated assessments within individual patients over a period of time.[39,40] However, for a group or for an individual, if enough independent criteria are chosen, some are bound to yield "significant difference" at whatever level of probability has been chosen. At the 5 % level, one out of every 20 criteria on the average, will yield a positive result on a purely chance basis, even when the drug under test has no value.

3. *Are the benefits claimed for the drug in comparison with an established treatment or placebo of practical significance in the context of the proposed use of the drug?* If the superiority of the drug over alternative treatment is real, then the next question is whether the drug offers any important advantage. A small advantage in favor of the drug under test may indeed be real (i.e., not due to chance) yet not important enough to matter. "A difference, in order to *be* a difference, has to *make* a difference."

If a drug is only slightly better than the established treatment, has it been tried in enough patients to reveal uncommon side effects? Has its toxicity been studied thoroughly enough under the conditions in which it will actually be used? It must be assumed that new risks, as yet unrecognized, may emerge, and this likelihood has to be weighed against the better-known efficacy and toxicity of the established drug[41]. Will the new drug be substantially more expensive for the patient than equivalent medications that have been in use for a long time? Finally, has the drug's relative value been assessed by competent independent professional groups charged with the function of evaluating new drugs?

Ethics of Human Experimentation

Well-designed and properly executed clinical trials are essential for gaining valid information about drugs. But all experimentation with human beings is subject to ethical restraints. A fundamental distinction is recognized between research in which the aim is therapeutic for the individual patient and research in which the aim is purely scientific and may be without therapeutic value to the person who is the subject.[42] As for the first kind of research, the doctor must be free to use a new drug or other therapeutic measure "if in his judgment it offers hope of saving life, reestablishing health, or alleviating suffering."[43] If it is possible and consistent with the patient's welfare, a full explanation should be given and his consent should be obtained.

If a wholly new drug of unknown value is being tested in a clinical trial with patients whose condition, there is reason to hope, may be benefitted by it, is it ethically justifiable to assign some of these patients to a placebo group? The answer seems reasonably clear. To conduct such a trial in an uncontrolled fashion would really be unethical; for, since no valid information would then be obtained, risks would be assumed without any possible benefit.

An investigator, however, has no inherent right to conduct experiments on other human beings at all, regardless of the potential benefits to humanity. In every experiment, the *informed consent* of the subjects (or their guardians) must be secured.[44] This "means that the person involved has legal capacity to give consent, is so situated as to be able to exercise free power of choice, and is provided with a fair explanation of pertinent information concerning the investigational drug, and/or his possible use as a control, as to enable him to make a decision on his willingness to receive said investigational drug. This latter element means that before the acceptance of an affirmative decision by such person the investigator should carefully consider and make known to him (taking into consideration such person's well-being and his ability to understand) the nature, expected duration, and purpose of the administration of said investigational drug; the method and means by which it is to be administered; the hazards involved; the existence of alternative forms of therapy, if any; and the beneficial effects upon his health or person that may possibly come from the administration of the investigational drug."[45]

In the typical situation postulated earlier, in which a new drug of unknown value is to be tested, the patients would be told: (*1*) that a new drug has been developed that might be beneficial to them; (*2*) that it can only be tested properly in a controlled way, so that some patients will receive the drug whereas others will receive different treatments; (*3*) that these assignments will be made by chance; (*4*) that certain risks are likely; and (*5*) that other unanticipated risks may materialize. Consent should then be obtained in writing. This is in essence the procedure that was followed in setting up large-scale trials of the killed-virus poliomyelitis vaccine before its effectiveness was known, except that parents had to give consent for their children.[46] It is obvious that certain children contracted the disease and died or were paralyzed because they were in the placebo group instead of the vaccine group. But the risk to the control group was not greater than before the trial of the vaccine, which had potential hazards of its own; and the controlled trial was the only way to determine whether or not the vaccine was effective.

No patient may justifiably be denied the benefits of the best treatment available. Certainly, therefore, placebo controls are not permissible if an effective drug is already known. Therefore any new drug must be evaluated in a comparative trial against the best existing one. This was how isoniazid and p-aminosalicylate were tested for the treatment of pulmonary tuberculosis in extensive clinical trials after streptomycin was in wide and effective use.[47] The anticoagulant studies described earlier were based on the same principle of comparative evaluation without a placebo control. In order to deny no one the benefits of an improved therapy, investigators have the obligation to conduct every trial efficiently, not to accept any unnecessary risk, and to arrive at a conclusion and terminate a trial as soon as possible, so that the benefits, if any, can be extended promptly to all who are in need.

More difficult questions arise with research of the second kind, when those who are to be subjects of a clinical trial, whether patients or normal volunteers, are unlikely to benefit in any direct way from the experiment—at least no more than humanity as a whole. The history of medicine affords fine examples of contributions made by heroic volunteers toward the eventual understanding and control of disease. One such was the deliberate infection of human volunteers with yellow fever for the purpose of establishing the mode of transmission of this illness by mosquitoes.[48] Another was the infection of prisoner volunteers during World War II with malaria parasites in order to test the efficacy of new and much-needed antimalarial drugs.[49] Trials of this sort are exceedingly important, and they need to be carried out. But they can only be conducted with subjects who freely give their informed consent in the fullest sense of the term. A responsible adult, in full command of his reason, may wish to serve as an experimental subject and to suffer a certain degree of discomfort or minor risk for remuneration, or in the hope of helping others. Altruistic motivation may be especially strong in patients who know they are victims of an incurable disease. Prisoners may feel sincerely that they can atone for past antisocial behavior by making a contribution to the progress of medical research, and there may also be the more selfish hope of more favorable consideration by a parole board. In all cases, the investigator is obliged not only to explain fully what is proposed, including the possible hazards, but also to avoid exerting undue pressure or exploiting a relationship of dependency or trust between the subject and himself. The subject, in short, must choose freely and without coercion.

Some investigators, unfortunately, have sought to belittle or even ridicule the requirement for informed consent. One argument has been that the procedures are too technical for the average patient or volunteer to understand. This misses the point. It is not the procedural details but the essentials of the experiment that are at issue here. A patient giving consent for a therapeutic pneumonectomy for lung cancer has to be told whatever the surgeon knows about the danger of the operation, the relative risks of not having it as compared with having it, and the probable kinds and extent of disability consequent to the operation. An understanding of the procedures for cutting, hemostasis, suturing, and so on is not required in order to give informed consent. Exactly the same principles apply to experimental procedures, except that the reasons for participating in the experiment are never as strong as for consenting to a therapeutic procedure of known value.

The willingness of the investigator or his relatives to participate has been offered as a seal of approval on the legitimacy of the experiment, thereupon avoiding the necessity of obtaining each subject's individual consent. But no person can make such a decision for another. Indeed, the history of science offers examples of investigators with more courage than prudence, or even with a degree of reckless bravado that should be allowed to endanger no one other than himself.

Psychological experimentation has special hazards. What may seem an innocuous procedure to the investigator could cause serious psychic harm to the subject. And whereas many kinds of physical harm become healed with time, this is not always true of psychological harm. Experiments that involve terror, fear, deception, loss of self-esteem, and the use of mind-altering drugs may not be admissible at all—and if they are admissible, certainly only after truly informed consent has been obtained. Harm done in the course of an experiment cannot necessarily be undone at a "debriefing session." Deception of a subject is categorically inadmissible under all circumstances. This means that experiments in which deception is a crucial part can only be done in the course of a very long association with the subjects, in which the general nature of the deceptions has been explained and consented to, but the specifics of when and how would not be known in advance. This would be analogous to placebo controlled experiments, in which the subject consents to receive either a medication or a placebo (without knowing which), or sometimes a medication and sometimes a placebo (without knowing when).

Many potentially informative experiments simply cannot be carried out. Sometimes the optimal design would be transparently unethical because it would cause harm needlessly. It has been asserted, for example, that women who contract mumps at a critical stage of pregnancy may give birth to congenitally malformed infants. Obviously, the most decisive proof of whether or not this is true would be obtained by infecting large numbers of women with mumps during pregnancy. Just as obviously, such an experiment would be unthinkable, so that less direct means of attacking this problem are called for. Often the prospective epidemiologic approach is appropriate. By this means, i.e., by recording the occurrences of infectious disease in pregnant women and then observing the outcome of pregnancy, the question of teratogenesis by mumps was fairly well settled. In a prospective study in which the well-known anomalies after rubella was observed, there was no evidence of any fetal malformations caused by mumps, nor by measles or chickenpox.[50] On occasion, a proposed experiment may seem important and justifiable to the investigator, yet he cannot obtain the consent of truly informed subjects. Then such an experiment is also unthinkable. *The needs of scientific research do not supersede the rights of individuals.*

The ghastly "experiments" carried out by doctors on unwilling prisoners under the Nazi regime in Germany led to the formulation of standards for human experimentation, first in the so-called Nuremberg Code,[51] and later in the *Declaration of Helsinki* of the World Medical Association.[43] This document codifies the ethical principles that should guide investigators working with patients or other human subjects. Since the obligations and ethical responsibilities of clinical investigators have not been universally understood and accepted,[52] it seems appropriate to reproduce this statement verbatim, except for the omission of three introductory paragraphs of a rather general nature:

DECLARATION OF HELSINKI

In the field of clinical research a fundamental distinction must be recognized between clinical research in which the aim is essentially therapeutic for a patient, and clinical research the essential object of which is purely scientific and without therapeutic value to the person subjected to the research.

I.   BASIC PRINCIPLES

1. Clinical research must conform to the moral and scientific principles that justify medical research, and should be based on laboratory and animal experiments or other scientifically established facts.
2. Clinical research should be conducted only by scientifically qualified persons and under the supervision of a qualified medical man.
3. Clinical research cannot legitimately be carried out unless the importance of the objective is in proportion to the inherent risk to the subject.
4. Every clinical research project should be preceded by careful assessment of inherent risks in comparison to foreseeable benefits to the subject or to others.
5. Special caution should be exercised by the doctor in performing clinical research in which the personality of the subject is liable to be altered by drugs or experimental procedure.

II.   CLINICAL RESEARCH COMBINED WITH PROFESSIONAL CARE

1. In the treatment of the sick person the doctor must be free to use a new therapeutic measure if in his judgment it offers hope of saving life, re-establishing health, or alleviating suffering.
   If at all possible, consistent with patient psychology, the doctor should obtain the patient's freely given consent after the patient has been given a full explanation. In case of legal incapacity consent should also be procured from the legal guardian; in case of physical incapacity the permission of the legal guardian replaces that of the patient.
2. The doctor can combine clinical research with professional care, the objective being the acquisition of new medical knowledge, only to the extent that clinical research is justified by its therapeutic value for the patient.

III.   NON-THERAPEUTIC CLINICAL RESEARCH

1. In the purely scientific application of clinical research carried out on a human being it is the duty of the doctor to remain the protector of the life and health of that person on whom clinical research is being carried out.
2. The nature, the purpose, and the risk of clinical research must be explained to the subject by the doctor.
3a. Clinical research on a human being cannot be undertaken without his free consent, after he has been fully informed; if he is legally incompetent the consent of the legal guardian should be procured.
3b. The subject of clinical research should be in such a mental, physical, and legal state as to be able to exercise fully his power of choice.
3c. Consent should as a rule be obtained in writing. However, the responsibility for clinical research always remains with the research worker; it never falls on the subject, even after consent is obtained.

4a. The investigator must respect the right of each individual to safeguard his personal integrity, especially if the subject is in a dependent relationship to the investigator.

4b. At any time during the course of clinical research the subject or his guardian should be free to withdraw permission for research to be continued. The investigator or the investigating team should discontinue the research if in his or their judgment it may, if continued, be harmful to the individual.

USE AND MISUSE OF DRUGS

The existence of potent drugs in great variety poses new dangers to the public health. Ill-advised self-medication can be more harmful than in former times. Drug ingestion has become a major method of suicide, and drugs are a principal cause of accidental poisoning among children (cf. Chapter 5). Even when prescribed by a physician, medication is more dangerous nowadays than formerly. The irrational mixtures of old were ineffective, on the whole, but they were also usually innocuous. Today, even when they are administered correctly, drugs carry a certain risk of untoward adverse effects and even of fatal reactions, as described in earlier chapters.

Legal Controls over Drug Availability

There are obvious differences between drugs and most ordinary commodities. Incorrect use of drugs may endanger the consumer's health, yet he has no simple way to judge the efficacy of a drug or its hazards. In virtually all societies, therefore, these judgments are made for him by others, who are technological experts, and such judgments are embodied in laws that are enforced by the state. This arrangement, which restricts the rights of citizens to do as they wish with their own bodies, has been contested on philosophic grounds.[53] Certainly a system can be imagined, which depends more heavily upon education, in which the medical profession enjoys no monopoly on the distribution of drugs, but devotes more effort to explanation and persuasion, with all drug sales conducted on an over-the-counter basis. Obviously, there are possible alternative systems. Our aim here is to explain how the existing system works.

For all drugs, as for other commodities, truthful information must be furnished by the manufacturer about what the medication contains, what it is alleged to do (its efficacy) and what harm it can cause (its safety). For over-the-counter drugs, this information is supplied directly to the consumer. Prescription drugs are unique in that the consumer exercises no choice whatsoever but depends upon the physician's judgment; for this class, the information is supplied only to the physician. For both classes of drug, procedures are specified in law for the securing and furnishing of this information, upon which the regulatory agency will decide whether to permit over-the-counter sale or whether to classify it a prescription item. "Any drug limited to prescription use ... shall be exempted from the prescription-dispensing requirements when the Commissioner (of Food and Drugs) finds ... that the drug is safe and effective for use in self-medication as directed in proposed labeling."[45] Throughout most of the world, these procedures are embodied in legislation and regulated by governmental agencies entrusted with control over the manufacture, export, import, sale, advertising, and prescription of drugs. Some of the regulatory mechanisms are international in scope, as for addicting drugs. A brief description of the regulatory mechanisms in the United States will be given; the procedures in other countries usually differ only in detail.

The first national legislation establishing controls over drugs in the United States was the pure food and drug law of 1906. The present legislative basis of such controls is the Federal Food, Drug, and Cosmetic Act of 1938, as amended. This act, including amendments adopted in 1962 and 1965, establishes the authority of the government to safeguard the public health against certain potential hazards, and to protect the consumer's interest.[54-55] The *Food and Drug Administration* (FDA) is the regulatory agency charged with enforcing these laws. The main provisions of the legislation require:

1. that foods, drugs, and cosmetics be labeled accurately to show all ingredients and their amounts;
2. that drugs deemed unsafe for unsupervised use not be sold except on prescription;
3. that wholly unsafe drugs not be marketed at all, even for prescription use;
4. that physicians be informed fully by the manufacturer about toxic potentialities and side effects of prescription drugs;
5. that false and misleading claims not be made either in advertising or in the labeling of drugs;
6. that advertisements and promotional brochures describe all adverse effects and contraindications; and
7. that drugs acting on the central nervous system and liable to abuse be subject to especially rigorous controls.

Technically, in the United States, the authority of the federal agencies extends only to drugs shipped in interstate commerce. From a practical standpoint this covers nearly all manufacturers and nearly all drugs. But there are, in addition, state laws that extend similar controls to drugs manufactured and sold entirely within a state. Moreover, through the licensing of pharmacists, physicians, dentists, and veterinarians, states can exercise special authority over the prescribing and sale of drugs.

The first step in preparing a prospective new drug for the market is for the manufacturer to file with the FDA a "Notice of Claimed Investigational Exemption for a New Drug" (IND) application.[57] Accurate information must be furnished about the chemical structures of all components, the quantitative composition of the preparation, the sources and methods of production including quality control procedures. All preclinical and any preliminary clinical data already obtained must be furnished, including the names and qualifications of the investigators, in sufficient detail to permit objective scientific review. All informational material to be given to the investigators, as well as the exact labeling of the drug must be disclosed; and the names, qualifications, and previous experience of the proposed investigators must be communicated. The proposed investigations must be described in detail, according to three phases. *Phase 1* is close study in a few patients or volunteers, to determine the human toxicity, metabolism, absorption, elimination, safe dosage range, and pharmacologic actions. *Phase 2* consists of initial trials on a limited number of patients. *Phase 3* is a full-scale clinical trial "to produce well-controlled clinical data." Adequate and complete records are required to be kept, including indications of adverse effects as well as of useful results. All the studies in humans must be approved and monitored by a local institutional review committee, comprising representatives of the medical profession, scientists, lawyers, and laymen. Informed consent procedures are explicitly required. During the investigational use of the drug, no promotion or commercial distribution is permitted. After 30 days have elapsed following the filing of an IND application, if FDA has made no objection, the investigations may proceed. If FDA denies the application or requires termination of the investigation after it has begun, appropriate appeal procedures are available. Regular reports are required, especially the prompt reporting of any adverse reactions attributed to the drug. Special rules apply to drugs with stimulant, depressant, or hallucinogenic action on the central nervous system if there appears to be potential for abuse.

Following the investigational period, if the drug still appears to merit general distribution, a New Drug Application (NDA) may be filed. This will contain, in greater detail, the basic information called for in the IND application and in addition will communicate in full the results of the investigational studies. In particular, the clinical trials are required to conform essentially to the principles outlined earlier in this chapter, in order to be considered valid evidence of the efficacy and safety of the drug. The various claims of efficacy must be stated and supported by evidence, and the verbatim text of the package insert and certain promotional materials must be submitted. Upon final approval by FDA, the drug may be distributed and marketed in accordance with the approved claims, with appropriate warnings and contraindications stated. If the application is for a drug to be sold over-the-counter, safety for general unsupervised use must be shown. Surveillance by the regulatory agency continues, with collection of data designed to uncover any long-term adverse effects. At any time after a drug is in use, the FDA may require a change in the labeling, in advertising claims, or in the information furnished to physicians; or it may even order the drug withdrawn. The Kefauver–Harris amendments of 1962 required, for the first-time, that the efficacy of drugs be established as well as their safety.[55] As a result, the FDA engaged the National Academy of Sciences National Research Council to evaluate the efficacy of many drugs already in use prior to 1962. This review resulted in withdrawal of approval for a number of such products. In addition, a continuing review of over-the-counter preparations was initiated, resulting in withdrawal of some of these.

The implementation of much stricter regulations by FDA during the decade following passage of the 1962 legislation engendered much controversy, as might be expected. At issue is the question whether or not the public interest is best served by a system that increases greatly the cost of developing and introducing a new drug. Opponents of the new procedures assert that incentives for the pharmaceutical industry are diminished, and therefore, that new drug research and development are bound to slow down. The great costs usually mean that only the largest corporations can afford to introduce new drugs. Certainly, the number of "new drugs" introduced declined sharply. However, since in the previous era a great many so-called new drugs were in reality combinations or minor chemical modifications of existing products, it is difficult to assess the true impact on the development of significant new pharmacologic agents.

Other governmental agencies are concerned in the control of drugs. A special agency of the National Institutes of Health, the *Division of Biologics Standards*, is responsible for licensing serums, vaccines, and other biologic products, including human blood and its derivatives. Standards are established for safety and potency, and each batch manufactured must be standardized by bioassay (p. 737). Periodic inspection of manufacturing facilities is carried out by agents of the Division. The *Federal Trade Commission* has general authority to prevent dissemination of false claims with respect to drugs (as to any other commodity) in interstate commerce. Advertising of proprietary "over the counter" drugs comes under its special purview. Remedies are sold for widespread ills like arthritis, the common cold, headaches, "nervous tension"; and vitamins and food supplements are recommended widely for conditions not likely to be improved by them. It was reported that in a single year (1963), 396 million dollars were spent for products claimed to be beneficial for the common cold or cough.[58] The *Federal Communications Commission* has authority to act against false advertising on radio and television. The *Postal Service* can deny the use of the mails for fraudulent claims or illegal shipments of useless medicines and therapeutic devices

Every government exercises special control over drugs that are subject to abuse, especially the addicting drugs upon which dependence may develop (cf. Chapter 9). In the United States, legal controls over narcotics were established by the *Harrison Narcotic Act* of 1914.[59] This law, ostensibly a revenue measure, vests control in a *Bureau of Narcotics* (now called *Bureau of Narcotics and Dangerous Drugs*) in the Treasury Department. It regulates the importation, marketing, and prescribing of specified drugs, principally opium and its derivatives (including synthetic opioids), coca leaf and its derivatives, and marijuana. To keep the law abreast of new developments, the Secretary of the Treasury is empowered to place new drugs under the Act. The importer, manufacturer, distributor, pharmacist, and practitioner are all required to keep exact records accounting for all narcotic drugs. The pharmacist must account for his stock of narcotics, keep his records open for inspection, and retain narcotic prescriptions on file for two years. He is forbidden to supply narcotics except on valid prescription for legitimate medical use. When he dispenses a narcotic, he is required to label the container with his name and registry number, the serial number of the prescription, the name and address of the patient, and the name, address, and registry number of the prescribing practitioner. The physician, dentist, or veterinary surgeon must register, pay a yearly fee, and obtain a registry number to be shown on all his narcotic prescriptions. He is then permitted to prescribe narcotics for legitimate medical use. Certain preparations (e.g., cough mixtures) containing narcotics in small amounts are excluded from the provisions of the Act; these are called *exempt preparations*. A record must be kept by the pharmacist who dispenses them showing the name and address of each purchaser, the date, and the name and quantity of the exempt preparation. In some states, the dispensing of exempt preparations is no longer permitted.

The *Comprehensive Drug Abuse Prevention and Control Act of 1970*[60] codified the regulations covering drugs subject to abuse. Unlike the original *Harrison Act*, which purported to be a tax measure and therefore placed enforcement under the Treasury Department, this act gave central authority to the Attorney General, often in consultation with the Secretary of the Department of Health, Education, and Welfare. Five schedules of controlled substances were established, according to a twofold criterion: legitimacy of medical use and potential for abuse. Schedule I contains substances without currently accepted medical use, which have a high potential for abuse. Strictest controls were imposed upon the drugs in this schedule, which form a strange array indeed. Schedule I contains heroin and a large variety of synthetic opiates not used in medical practice; these do indeed have a high abuse potential (except for the erroneously included L(+) opioid, dextrorphan, which has no narcotic actions). Schedule I also contains marijuana, mescaline, peyote, and LSD, none of which can be said to have a very high abuse potential. Alcohol, which has virtually no legitimate medical indication and has a very high abuse potential, was not defined as a controlled substance at all. Schedules II to V contain substances that have legitimate medical uses; assigned to Schedule II are those said to have the greatest abuse potential and greatest danger of severe dependence, with the remaining schedules containing progressively less hazardous drugs. Again, however, the assignments lack objective scientific validity. Schedule II, for example, contains opium and the opiates used in medical practice: whereas barbiturates and amphetamines, which produce a more severe type of dependence than the opiates, are relegated to Schedule III. Schedule IV contains a small number of long-acting depressants such as phenobarbital, with low abuse potential. Finally, Schedule V contains dilute preparations containing codeine or other opiates in low concentration, such as are used for antitussive effect.

The principal effect of the act was to regularize and standardize on a national basis the procedures for control of drugs subject to abuse. Possession of drugs in Schedule I was made entirely illegal (except for legitimate scientific purposes), and possession of drugs in the other categories was prohibited except for legitimate medical use on prescription. Manufacture and shipment were controlled and regulated through a system of registration and record keeping. The act also dealt with prescribing. Schedule I substances, of course, cannot be prescribed; Schedule II substance prescriptions cannot be refilled; and refilling of prescriptions for Schedule III and IV substances is restricted to a maximum of five times and to a total period of six months.

A large part of the act was devoted to law enforcement provisions and penalties. Noteworthy is the controversial "no-knock" section 509(b), which authorizes the issuance of special search warrants "at any time of the day or night," permitting an officer to break open a door or window without warning, in order to enter premises.

The act established a Commission on Marijuana and Drug Abuse, to conduct a study on the use of marijuana, the efficacy of existing marijuana laws, the pharmacology of marijuana, the relationship of marijuana use to aggressive behavior and crime, and to the use of other drugs, and the international control of marijuana. This commission submitted its report in 1972.[61]

The Bureau of Narcotics, soon after its inception in 1914, adopted the position that prescribing for a narcotic addict in order to satisfy his needs is not legitimate medical use within the meaning of the Harrison Act. It also held that treatment of the addict by gradual withdrawal (prescribing decreasing doses of a narcotic) could be carried out only in a closed institution. These doctrines, the punitive approach of the Bureau toward the addiction problem, and the severe penalties for violations, led the medical profession as a whole to disengage itself from the treatment of narcotic addiction. Addicts were sentenced to confinement in federal hospitals to be withdrawn from narcotics. The high rate of relapse of addicts after return to their home environments,[62] however, and the modern tendency to view deviant behavior less emotionally than in former times, reopened the question of what our approach to addiction should be. Opiate addiction is clearly both a medical and a social problem. The total number of addicts is estimated at nearly half a million, now involving not only minority ethnic groups in our urban ghettoes but also large numbers of middle-class white youth. The past decade has brought significant reinvolvement of the medical profession and of para-professional and community groups in dealing with this disease. An important catalyst was the introduction of methadone maintenance as an aid to the rehabilitation of narcotic addicts on an ambulatory basis in their own communities.[63,64]

It is now recognized that the problem of drug abuse is much larger than that of addiction to opiates. Although attended by much publicity, the numerical significance of opiate addition remains relatively small. The most important drug of abuse, both from the standpoint of numbers and of personal and social consequences, is certainly alcohol. In 1972, it was estimated that there were nine million alcoholics in the United States, "a number far exceeding all other types of drug abuse combined."[65] Yet alcohol enjoys a pecular social approbation that grants it immunity from the intensified concern over drug abuse in general. Central stimulants and depressants such as amphetamine and barbiturates are also abused by many more people than are heroin or morphine. It has been estimated that one-half of the total output of these agents is sold illegally. The widespread distribution of these drugs rests upon their indiscriminate marketing by unethical manufacturers.

Self-Medication, Prescribing Practices, and Iatrogenic Disease

Excessive self-medication is responsible for many ills. The toxic effects of drug misuse have been documented elsewhere (cf. Chapter 5). Proprietary drugs sold across the counter include cough remedies, analgesics, skin lotions, food supplements, vitamins, laxatives, "tonics," antacids, and many others.[66] Table 14-8 shows expenditures on such home remedies in 1963, amounting to nearly 2 billion dollars in the United States. It is questionable whether the benefits to be derived from most of these preparations outweigh the potential harm they do. They account for poisonings when taken in excess, by accident or with suicidal intent, they cause allergic and other adverse reactions, and their use often delays proper medical attention to serious illnesses.

The physician is often consulted about the remedies purchased by patients for self-medication. The mild analgesics are a good example. Ordinary aspirin is as effective, and safer, for most patients than any of the related drugs (phenacetin, aminopyrine, dipyrone, acetaminophen) marketed as substitutes or in combinations with aspirin. Well-controlled trials have also failed to confirm any advantage of "buffered" aspirin preparations over ordinary aspirin;[67-71] indeed the insignificant quantity of antacid incorporated in the tablet could hardly exert any important effect. Even propoxyphene, which gained a considerable reputation as a moderately strong analgesic without addictive qualities, could not be shown to be superior to aspirin in a double-blind study on pain relief.[72] Despite all such rational findings, physicians continue to prescribe and recommend these analgesics, although their cost to the patient is considerably higher than aspirin.

The misuse of prescription drugs is also a real problem. A drug prescribed for one illness may be saved and used on another occasion, or a drug prescribed for one patient may be used by another member of the family. The physician can exert a measure of control over this abuse by prescribing just enough of a drug to suffice for the current illness, and by educating his patients to discard left-over medications.

TABLE 14-8. Consumer expenditures for home remedies. Data are for proprietary drugs purchased without prescription in the U.S. during the year 1963. (From Mandel,[58] Table 2, originally from *Drug Topics*, July 27, 1964.)

Type of medication	Expenditure (in millions of dollars)
Total packaged medications	1900
Analgesics, internal	414
Cough and cold items	396
Vitamin concentrates, nonprescription	200
Laxatives	170
Analgesics, external	104
Tonics	93
Antacids	76
External antiseptics	51
Diarrhea remedies	41
Suntan lotions and oils	31
Acne aid products	29
Sleeping aids, nonprescription	18
Hemorrhoidal suppositories and ointments	16
Poison ivy remedies	15
Motion sickness preparations	15
Burn remedies	12

Iatrogenic diseases (Greek *iatros* = physician) are those caused by the physician, by prescribing a drug when none is needed or by poor selection of drugs or drug dosage. Several examples have been given elsewhere in this book of severe or even fatal reactions to drugs that were administered needlessly. The history of the use of chloramphenicol illustrates how easily lessons are forgotten. Sales of this antibiotic dropped sharply after the first reports of aplastic anemia in the period 1950–1952 and reached a minimum in 1954. By 1958, however, sales had climbed to 5 times the 1954 level, and by 1960 enough of this drug was being sold in the United States to supply more than 3 million people with a 10-g course of treatment. In a series of 30 cases of aplastic anemia seen in a 3-year period, 8 patients had received chloramphenicol. Most of these patients died; yet they had received the drug for minor infections or other conditions in which this antibiotic is not indicated.[73] And chloramphenicol is still used widely for infections that would respond to safer medications. Antibiotics, in general, seem to be used with less caution than other drugs. In a survey of prescribing practices in hospitals, it was found that they were often used incorrectly. Sometimes no antibiotic whatever should have been used; in other cases the selection of antibiotic was incorrect.[74]

The irrational use of drug combinations exposes patients to several compounds needlessly, each of which can cause toxic or allergic effects. Few drug combinations have any legitimate place in modern medicine, for reasons already explained. Yet such mixtures abound and presumably are being prescribed. One such remedy contains codeine (antitussive), pseudoephedrine (sympathomimetic), chlorcyclizine (antihistaminic), aspirin and phenacetin (analgesic), and caffeine (stimulant). It is a prescription drug recommended for the symptomatic relief of upper respiratory infections.[75] The probability that a patient would have symptoms for which all these drugs are indicated, and for which the doses of all are appropriate, is surely vanishingly small.

A special hazard today is the effect of drugs upon skill in driving a motor vehicle; and since driving is so nearly universal, the physician must keep this in mind when prescribing any drug. A patient's need to drive is an important factor to be considered in deciding if a drug should be given at all. The main effects of tranquilizer and sedative agents and the side effects of numerous drugs of other kinds may all impair driving ability.[76] "Polypharmacy is especially dangerous for motorists because potentiating, additive, and antagonistic drug actions increase the difficulty of predicting effects. This problem is compounded by the use of preparations containing multiple drugs; prescribing each drug separately is less hazardous, an advantage that may outweigh the inconvenience of taking two or more tablets."[77]

Two recent trends of importance in achieving more rational prescribing practices involve the use of computers to obtain quantitative data about the use of prescription drugs, and the involvement of pharmacists in monitoring such use.[78-82] In several large hospitals, all drug orders by physicians have been entered into a computer file at the time the pharmacy dispenses the drug either for use within the hospital or to an outpatient for use at home. Analysis of the data has revealed remarkable differences in the prescribing patterns of various physicians. A few physicians in each institution were found consistently to write orders for an excessive amount of medication. Striking differences were also found in the prescribing of multiple drug combinations. In some hospitals, a computer alerting system has been introduced to warn the pharmacist that a given patient is already receiving other drugs, some of them possibly incompatible with the new drug being prescribed. The hope is that physicians will modify their procedures when unusual or inappropriate prescriptions are called to their attention. A comprehensive health care system could utilize pharmacists in this way as important members of the health care team, vesting them with real responsibility for monitoring prescription medications (both their quality and their quantity). The pharmacist could serve as a drug counsellor, alerting the physician about possible dangers inherent in the prescription and furnishing information and explanation to the patient about the drug, its proper mode of use, and the side effects that should be watched for.

The act of prescribing, it has been pointed out, serves the function of terminating the doctor-patient interview in a way seen as satisfactory by both parties.[83] Physicians' time is very limited; it has been estimated that an average patient contact in the doctor's office takes about 20 min. It is all too easy, therefore, under the pressure of time, for the prescription to take the place of extended diagnostic workup or therapeutic counselling. Moreover, prescription drugs are very big business, which has grown at a remarkable rate. From about 1 billion dollars in 1950, the amount spent for these items grew to over 2 billion in 1960, 4 billion in 1969, and 9 billion in 1971. For every dollar spent on doctors' fees, the patient spends 32 cents for prescription medications. Thus on the one hand, the physician has the obligation to choose for his patients the most effective and least dangerous medications available and often to choose no medication at all. On the other hand, his unique position as prescriber of drugs makes him the target of intense pressures—from patients to "do something" and from pharmaceutical firms to use their particular products. He is bombarded by promotional materials and drug advertisements and by gifts and personal visits from "detail men"—all with the result that excessive prescribing, irrational choices of prescription drugs, and lack of concern for the cost of drugs to the patient are seen far too frequently.[84]

Advertising of prescription drugs is directed at physicians. It takes the form of package inserts, advertisements in medical journals, mailings directly to physicians, and personal visits by agents of the manufacturers (detail men). Package inserts are the small leaflets that are required by law to accompany each package of a drug. They are exceedingly useful sources of information, for they describe the chemical structure of the drug, its pharmacology, clinical use, toxicities, contraindications, and recommended doses. The contents of these inserts are reviewed by the FDA to ensure that they represent a full and accurate disclosure about the drug. Pharmaceutical manufacturers are required to send copies of these inserts to physicians upon request. The wise physician will insist upon studying the package insert for every drug he intends to prescribe.

The quality of advertisements for drugs spans a wide range. The best is informative and educational;[85] the worst is insulting to the practitioner's intelligence. In the most restrained type of advertising, a pharmaceutical firm merely brings its name to the attention of physicians or points out some well-established drugs manufactured by it. In the most insidious kind of advertising, the claims for a new drug preparation are exaggerated or misleading. References to the literature often convey the impression that the claims are substantiated by reputable published research, whereas the articles cited may deal only indirectly with the supposed virtues of the new drug or may consist of poorly designed and uncontrolled clinical trials.[85] Flagrant disregard of the truth may be prevented by alert governmental regulatory agencies. But there is a wide area of advertising claims which, although not actually false, nevertheless fall short of what ought to be required to convince a properly conservative physician. Drug combinations, which should almost never be used (cf. p. 283), are especially prone to be overvigorously promoted. The reason is that although the separate components may be available in competing brands at reasonably low prices, the combination, given a unique name and a higher price, becomes a precious commodity of one manufacturer.

In testimony before a U.S. Senate investigating committee,[87] one large drug company reported that it had 430 detail men, and a subsidiary company was reported to have over 100 detail men. The president of the company estimated that the average salary of a detail man was $7900. At that time, the firm was paying over 4 million dollars per annum for this type of promotion of its products. The president of the Pharmaceutical Manufacturers Association stated: "A key factor in getting medicines off the shelf and into use is the professional service representative, often referred to as a detail man . . . . In a survey by the American Medical Association, approximately two-thirds of the physicians in America rated the detail man as their top source of new product information."[87]

The natural desire of the physician to have all new remedies at his command makes him vulnerable to claims for new wonder drugs. But he should realize that the natural desire of the pharmaceutical manufacturer to sell his products will not always coincide with the best practice of medicine and the best interest of the patient.

The physician need not be and should not be dependent upon industry for information about drugs. Numerous sources of informed and disinterested expert opinion are available to him. The situation, as summarized by a British professor of therapeutics, probably is about the same in most parts of the world:

> ... there is the formidable and skilled promotion of drugs by the pharmaceutical houses, some of which is subject to justifiable criticism in violating truth and good taste. Nevertheless, the cure for this is in the hands of the medical profession, for no ethical drug (that is, no drug which has to be prescribed and cannot be bought over the counter) can reach the public save through its intermediary. . . . Thus the advertising of ethical drugs, on which vast sums of money are expended, is not directed, like the advertising of most commodities, at the population of the country as a whole but at the relatively small number of its duly qualified medical men who are sought after, chased, wooed, and importuned to a fantastic extent. . . . We should stop bemoaning this attack on our professional maturity and begin to realize how justified it must be, for no advertising which does not work will continue to run. In our society the market-place may not be responsive to idealism but it is always sensitive to sales curves. . . . Let us as doctors but withhold our approval of new drugs and preparations until conclusive evidence has been presented in support of the claims made for them and it will cease to be economically feasible to market new drugs without such evidence.[88]

Drug Nomenclature and Drug Prices

Every drug has a nonproprietary name. Before a manufacturer receives approval to market a drug, this name must be agreed upon. *The United States Adopted Names Council* is a collaborative enterprise of the United States Pharmacopeia (*U.S.P.*), National Formulary (*N.F.*), and Council on Drugs of the American Medical Association. This organization receives information about the proposed new drug from the manufacturer, who also suggests a nonproprietary name. That name, or an alternative, is agreed upon with the manufacturer, and is then published as the U.S. Adopted Name (*USAN*) of the drug. It will become the official designation if the drug is admitted to *U.S.P.* or *N.F.*, and international agreement to the same nomenclature will be sought through the mechanisms of the World Health Organization. The FDA has legal authority to designate an official name, but in most cases this will probably be the one recommended by the USAN Council.

Pharmaceutical manufacturers prefer to have their products known and prescribed by trade name. It usually turns out that the trade name is shorter, simpler, more euphonious, and easier to remember than the nonproprietary name.[89] Table 14-9 illustrates this phenomenon by a parallel list of nonproprietary names and trade names selected randomly from *New Drugs*, 1965 edition.[90] The method of selection, decided upon before consulting the volume, was to begin at page 20, selecting the first drug description encountered thereafter, and then to move forward 40 pages at a time, following the same procedure. Thus the list of 12 drugs was generated. Even when salt designations (e.g., hydrochloride) were omitted from consideration, the mean and median syllable contents of the nonproprietary names were significantly longer than those of the trade names. The comparison of euphonic quality of names in the two lists is also revealing, although not subject to quantitative analysis.

TABLE 14-9. Nonproprietary and trade names of a random selection of new drugs.

In *New Drugs*, 1965 edition,[90] the first drug encountered after opening to page 20 was recorded; the same procedure was followed for pages 60, 100, 140, etc. The number of syllables in each drug name is indicated in parentheses following the name; in this computation salt names (also in parentheses) were omitted.

Nonproprietary names		Trade names	
Demethylchlortetracycline (Hydrochloride, *N.F.*)	(8)	Declomycin	(4)
Hexetidine	(4)	Sterisil	(3)
Amitriptyline (Hydrochloride)	(5)	Elavil (Hydrochloride)	(3)
Benactyzine (Hydrochloride)	(4)	Suavitil	(3)
Acetylcysteine	(6)	Mucomyst	(3)
Glycopyrrolate	(5)	Robinul	(3)
Cyclandelate	(4)	Cyclospasmol	(4)
Triamterene	(4)	Dyrenium	(4)
Dydrogesterone	(5)	Duphaston	(3)
Tolbutamide (U.S.P.)	(4)	Orinase	(3)
Cyclophosphamide	(5)	Cytoxan	(3)
(Calcium) Ipodate	(3)	Oragrafin	(4)
Median syllable content	(4.5)		(3.0)
Mean syllable content	(4.8)		(3.3)

It is certainly desirable for the physician to be able to identify the manufacturer of every drug. FDA regulations ensure this by requiring that the manufacturer's identity be indicated on the package, the package inserts, and all drug advertising. There may be good reason why a physician should wish to prescribe (or avoid prescribing) the product of a particular manufacturer; but these considerations do not justify the existence of trade names. For most commodities other than drugs, the brand name indicates the manufacturer, and the names of the products are common nouns, e.g., beans, television sets, cigarettes, etc. When a single drug like digitoxin is called Crystodigin, Purodigin, Digitaline Nativelle, etc., these are really not brand names in the commonly accepted sense but a new category of substitute nomenclature.[91]

There are good reasons why the physician should think about drugs, refer to them, and prescribe them by their nonproprietary names.[92,93] The practice encourages accurate recognition of each drug. The textbooks and current medical literature generally avoid trade names, especially because there are so often multiple trade names for the same drug manufactured by different companies. The burden of name memorizing is greatly reduced if only a single name is remembered for each drug. Sometimes, the same drug is given different trade names when promoted for different uses; the antihistaminic agent diphenhydramine is called Benadryl when it is used to relieve allergies and Dramamine when it is used to prevent motion sickness. Alternatively, a mixture of two or more drugs is usually given a single trade name, making it easier to overlook the fact that more than a single active ingredient is present. Finally, a single drug used for one purpose may masquerade under two trade names because one manufacturer has licensed another manufacturer to produce the drug; the tranquilizer meprobamate is known as Miltown and also as Equanil.

International communication and understanding in the fields of pharmacology and therapeutics also requires uniformity of nomenclature, especially when patients and their medications can move so rapidly from country to country. A dramatic illustration of the chaos that can result unless an international nonproprietary nomenclature is followed is illustrated in Table 14-10. Here, 21 names are listed by which a single common analgesic drug, 1-methyl-4-phenylpiperidine-4-carbonic acid ethyl ester, is known in different parts of the world.

TABLE 14-10. Synonyms of a single drug in various parts of the world.
The list contains trade names and nonproprietary names of one analgesic drug, 1-methyl-4-phenyl-piperidine-4-carbonic acid ethyl ester. The official name of this drug in the U.S. is meperidine.

Alodan	Eudolat
Amphosedal	Isonipecaine
Antiduol	Mefedina
Centralgin	Meperidine
Demerol	Meperine
Dispadol	Pantalgine
Dolantin	Pethidine
Dolantol	Piridosal
Dolopethin	Sauteralgyl
Dolosal	Suppolosal
Dolvanol	

Finally, the question of nomenclature has a direct bearing upon the price of drugs. Consistent use of nonproprietary names in prescribing will, it is agreed, in the long run lower the cost of medications for the patient. Organizations responsible for welfare and medical care on a large scale recognize this and insist on nonproprietary nomenclature because of the substantial savings that result.[94] The conscientious physician will also take an interest in what his patient has to pay for the drugs he prescribes. He will be aware of variations in cost and, whenever possible, will prescribe the cheaper drug if it meets the requirements. Numerous examples can be cited in which expensive preparations offer no advantage over cheaper ones. Thyroid, U.S.P., for instance, is the dried powder of the thyroid gland of cattle. For the ordinary maintenance therapy of hypothyroidism it is entirely suitable, and there is no evidence that a purified form of this hormone offers any advantage.[95] Yet Sodium Liothyronine, U.S.P. (triiodothyronine) is marketed and widely prescribed as a trade name preparation at more than three times the cost. Another typical example concerns the antihistamine drug chlorpheniramine maleate. After exclusive patent rights had expired, several firms began to market this compound. Samples of the drug from 20 different companies were subjected to laboratory analysis of their content and of tablet disintegration time; all were found to conform to U.S.P. specifications. The price paid by the pharmacist ranged from $1.40 to $17.50 per thousand tablets; the highest price was being charged for the brand previously patented and identified by the trade name by which this drug is most widely known.[96]

Whether or not prescribing by nonproprietary name actually results in lower costs depends, of course, upon the pharmacist; he may supply the least expensive brand, but he is also free to supply a more expensive one. When a brand name is specified in the prescription, he has no choice. A recent survey by a nonprofit organization in New York City revealed some remarkable differences in cost for the same drug. At one pharmacy a prescription for reserpine cost $2.95, whereas the same amount and dosage form of the same drug at the same pharmacy cost $8.95 when prescribed under a trade name. In a different neighborhood, the identical supply of reserpine prescribed under its nonproprietary name cost $1 25. The greatest price difference was found for prednisone, which ranged from $1.25 when sold under its nonproprietary name at one pharmacy to $11.50 when sold under a trade name at another.[97] Sometimes, on the other hand, manufacturers' prices appear to have been set at identical levels regardless of brand name. Senate committee hearings, for example, elicited information that three companies, during each of 4 years ending in 1960, sold cortisone acetate, each under its own trade name, at $5.48 per gram, cortisol under three trade names at $7.99 per gram, and prednisone or prednisolone under three names at $35.80 per gram.[98] Another problem is that it may be nearly impossible to find simple, inexpensive drugs on the market, even when these are listed in an official or unofficial compendium. Decavitamin Capsules, *U.S.P.*, for example, are ideal for those conditions in which a vitamin supplement is indicated; their composition meets the known daily requirements for ten vitamins in correct proportions. Yet most manufacturers find it more profitable to market costly, complicated, highly advertised mixtures; consequently, the ordinary *U.S.P.* vitamins are hard to find.

MONITORING OF DRUG USE

Large-scale Surveillance

Continuing surveillance of drugs after their introduction into clinical use is important for several reasons, some of which were already pointed out in Chapter 5:

1. Clinical trials necessarily involve a much smaller number of subjects than will eventually be exposed to a new drug. Consequently, after a drug comes into general use, adverse reactions may occur which, because of their relatively low frequency, were not observed previously. The hematologic toxicity of chloramphenicol, for example, was not discovered for several years. Another example is meprobamate, originally claimed to be a safe and nonaddicting tranquilizer. An intensive promotional campaign led to extremely widespread use, the sales of this drug exceeding 50 million dollars per year in 1956–58.[99] As it turned out, meprobamate had a serious addicting potential and produced dangerous withdrawal effects; it also caused suicidal depression in some psychiatric patients.[100] In 1965 it was dropped from the U.S. Pharmacopeia. Another sedative and hypnotic agent, glutethimide, had a rather similar history.[101]

2. A different population than was tested in the clinical trials may be placed at risk. Thalidomide exemplifies this problem (p. 717). The special effects of drugs upon the

fetus during early pregnancy were not even considered when this drug was introduced into use after clinical trials had indicated a high degree of safety in adults of all ages. Another interesting example concerns an orally active agent capable of interfering with spermatogenesis.[102] Clinical trials were conducted with a group of prisoner volunteers. The drug appeared to be effective and reversible, and there was no indication of adverse side effects. When it was used by nonprisoners, however, it was discovered to act like disulfiram (p. 268). When alcohol was ingested after the drug had been taken, alarming symptoms developed. The enforced abstinence of the prisoner subjects made them a completely nonrepresentative sample, in which the peculiar toxicity of this drug could not have been discovered.

3. Technologic advances may alter the criteria for evaluation after a drug is in general use. This applies to a great many drugs that were introduced into medicine before the modern clinical trial was perfected; consequently, satisfactory evaluations of such drugs were never really carried out. Moreover, if a newer, more effective, and safer drug is developed for some particular medical use, then older and more hazardous drugs should obviously be withdrawn after convincing evidence of their inferiority has been obtained in comparative clinical trials.

4. Chronic toxicity in man may develop only after exposure for a much longer time than could be studied in the clinical trials. Possible carcinogenic actions of drugs fall into this category. The carcinogenic effects of tobacco smoke could not have been discovered except after smoking had been prevalent for many years. Especially with drugs that are to be used on a very large scale, continuing surveillance will be important for detecting possible long-term hazards. There has been concern, for example, about possible carcinogenesis by the oral contraceptives, since some cancers of the female reproductive organs and breasts are hormone dependent. Continuous observation of women receiving these drugs has revealed, thus far, no increase in the incidence of cancer.[103]

If continuous surveillance of drug use is to have any validity, two requirements have to be met. *First*, physicians and hospitals must report all adverse reactions that might possibly be due to drug administration. *Second*, data must be available on the total usage of each drug, so that the number of adverse reactions can be assessed in relation to the total number of people exposed to the drug. An effective national or world-wide system for accomplishing both requirements is within the capacity of present-day computer technology, but no such system yet exists.[104,105] Indeed, it seems unlikely to develop until the total medical care delivery system is better organized. Well meaning attempts to secure the voluntary cooperation of physicians in reporting adverse reactions failed to produce useful data; it could never be ascertained what fraction of all adverse reactions to a given drug were being recognized and reported, nor was it clear what, exactly, was the total usage of that drug.

A different approach to the problem was implemented in the late 1960's, namely, a comprehensive drug surveillance program based on a collaborating group of hospitals[106] or outpatient clinics.[107] The essential feature of these systems, in contrast to the unsuccessful spontaneous reporting schemes, is that they record all drug exposures and all adverse events, without the necessity for the reporter (physician, nurse, etc.) to make any subjective judgment about the relationship between them. Thus, events rather than "adverse reactions" are reported, an event being defined as "a particular untoward happening experienced by a patient . . . irrespective of whether that event is thought to be wholly or partly caused by the drug."[108] The data on drug exposures and events are entered into a computer file, where they can be surveyed automatically and continuously for the appearance of relationships between events and particular drugs. Very large numbers of records can be monitored, so that a small incidence of adverse reaction or small differences in adverse reaction frequency can be recognized. The numbers required for detecting a real difference with confidence are interesting. In a trial of two drugs in 200 subjects, for example, there is only an even chance of demonstrating a difference clearly if the true incidences of adverse reaction are 5 and 11 %, respectively. With 1000 subjects on each drug, rates as different as 1.5 and 3.0 % would only stand an even chance of detection. With 15,000 subjects on each drug, a difference of 0.1 and 0.2 % would have only an even chance of detection, yet such a difference would be highly significant to society if the drug were one to which millions of people were exposed.

The key feature of this approach is the training of specialist personnel as reporters, so that the quality of the data will be high. On each ward a nurse monitor is wholly occupied with the work of the surveillance program, so there is no interference with the patient-care duties of the regular ward personnel.[106] The monitor obtains data from the clinical records, interviews the patient and attending physician, and conducts special tests for genetic traits, including blood tests. All drug starting orders are recorded, together with information on dosage, instructions for administration, and stated indication. Whenever a drug is discontinued, the physician is interviewed, and a statement is entered as to the reason, as well as the physician's evaluation of the drug's efficacy, adverse events, and whether or not the adverse event was thought to be due to the drug.

Accurate statistical information about drug usage emerges from such monitoring programs. Table 14-11 is an illustration of this type of data from over 6000 hospitalized

TABLE 14-11. Drug utilization among medical patients in 6 hospitals.
A drug exposure is the administration of a given drug to a patient, regardless of dosage changes or duration of drug treatment. (From Jick et al., Table 1.[106])

Hospital	No. of patients	Average Hospital stay (days)	Average No. of drug exposures
1	2417	26	8.9
2	1371	14	10.0
3	952	13	8.0
4	1078	15	6.4
5	293	14	5.5
6	201	15	6.4
All	6312	19	8.4

patients in 6 hospitals throughout the world, which collaborated in the monitoring program. The difference in numbers of drug exposures among the hospitals is noteworthy, as well as the large number of drugs to which patients are exposed (each "drug exposure" represents a different drug). The frequency of adverse reactions clearly related to a drug exposure was surprisingly high—nearly 5% of 53,000 drug exposures. The most common adverse events were nausea, drowsiness, vomiting, allergic skin reactions, electrolyte disturbances, and arrhythmias. Reactions considered to be life threatening (0.5 % of drug exposures) involved 4.5 % of the patients, and 0.4 % of all the patients died of causes attributed to drugs.[106,109]

A few examples will be presented to show the power of this type of monitoring system in discovering unsuspected relationships. In the early years of program operation, the data analysis brought to light a consistent deficit of blood group O among women who develop thromboembolic disease while taking oral contraceptives, or during pregnancy, or after delivery.[110] Since there was no abnormal distribution of blood groups among patients using oral contraceptives, it was apparent that women of blood group O have some genetically determined resistance to thromboembolic phenomena. The relative risk for healthy women of other blood groups as compared with those of group O was approximately 2 to 4 times greater. These data were obtained from hospitals in three countries, the same finding being obtained in all. A similar analysis has linked another blood antigen phenotype, ss, to the frequency of breast cancer.[111]

Through such original monitoring, a surmise or hypothesis on the part of an investigator can be verified or disproved quickly. Since binding of drugs to plasma proteins may influence the response to a drug or the duration of its action, the investigators called for a computer printout on the relationship between albumin and globulin levels and physician efficacy ratings and adverse reaction frequency for 52 different drugs. One unusual finding was immediately apparent. Patients with low plasma albumin levels (but not with low globulin) had an unusually high frequency of adverse reaction to the glucocorticoid drug, prednisone (Table 14-12).[112] Most of

TABLE 14-12. Relationship of prednisone side effects to plasma albumin levels. Patients given prednisone were divided into 2 groups, those with very low plasma albumin (less than 2.5 g/100 ml) and those with more normal values. The incidence of side effects was determined in both groups. Data are numbers of patients. Percents are given in parentheses. The difference between the low and normal albumin groups in incidence of side effects is highly significant ($P < 0.01$). (From Lewis et al., Table 4.[112])

Serum albumin (g%)	With side effect (%)	Without side effect (%)	Total
< 2.6	8 (53%)	7 (47%)	15 (100%)
> 2.6	16 (15%)	89 (85%)	105 (100%)
Totals	24	96	120

these reactions were typical of prednisone overdosage, and analysis of the data showed that at all dose levels patients with very low albumin levels had a higher frequency of adverse effects. Presumably, the low albumin (and probably also low transcortin, the specific corticosteroid binding protein) resulted in a lower fractional binding at each given dose level, and thus an excessive concentration of prednisone in the plasma water and tissues.

The same methodology, once established for adverse event monitoring, can also be used for the conduct of large-scale double-blind trials, for the machinery—personnel and procedures—is already in place and working.[72]

Drug Plasma Levels

When patients are given identical doses of a drug, or even identical doses per kilogram of body weight, very large differences in response may be seen. In some patients, the drug may have no therapeutic effect or insufficient therapeutic effect, in others it may work well, and in still others toxicity associated with overdosage may be seen. Theoretically, two sources of this variation between patients may be segregated: differences in plasma level established by a given dose, and differences in effect produced by a given plasma level. For most drugs that have been studied sufficiently, the principal variation is in the plasma level. Thus, it is often possible to specify a fairly narrow range of plasma levels that characterizes a threshold for therapeutic effect and a higher range associated with toxicity. When diphenylhydantoin was used for its antiarrhythmic action, for example, the effect was seen consistently between 9.5 and 9.8 μg ml^{-1}. Toxic effects on the central nervous system were seen[113] above 20 μg ml^{-1}.

Since identical doses produce very different effects in different people, and since identical plasma levels produce reasonably predictable effects, it follows that the same dose of a drug must produce very different plasma levels in different patients. This is proving to be true with all drugs thus far studied, although the degree of variability differs. A well-documented example is shown in Figure 14-4, for the tricyclic antidepressant desmethylimipramine. Patients were given equal daily doses until steady state plasma levels were reached. As seen, these levels differed over a range of more than 30-fold. Similar findings have been obtained repeatedly with the anticonvulsant, diphenylhydantoin.[115,115a] Results like this force a reexamination of the concept of a "standard dose" and of the idea that the physician can easily titrate the individual patient's need. How could individual titration be effective, and how long would it take for an antidepressant or anticonvulsant where the assessment of therapeutic efficacy (improved mood, decreased frequency of seizures) may take weeks or months? If in Figure 14-4, the desired level were 50 ng ml^{-1} and plasma levels were unknown, how many cautious dose increases would the physician try with patient KE before concluding that the medication was useless (assuming KE did not commit suicide before that)?

There are 3 main reasons for plasma level variation. The first is simply that patients frequently fail to follow directions about taking medications. Before concluding, therefore, that a dose change is required, the finding of an abnormal plasma level should be cause for making sure the appropriate dose is being taken. Sometimes this requires hospitalization. The second reason is poor absorption, demonstrated, for example, in a case of low diphenylhydantoin plasma level when the drug was given by mouth; normal plasma levels were established when the same daily dose was given intravenously.[115] Urinary excretion studies confirmed the interpretation. The third and most common reason is difference in drug metabolism or elimination. This is under strong genetic control, as evidenced in twin studies, and there is also significant environmental influence (diet, hormonal status, etc.). In the next section of this chapter, the special influence of one drug upon the metabolism—and, therefore, upon the plasma level—of another drug will be considered.

Evidently, in order to use drugs in an optimal manner, it will be necessary to monitor their plasma levels, so that the dose can be adjusted to whatever is necessary to achieve the desired levels. This need not necessarily be done with all drugs. Certainly,

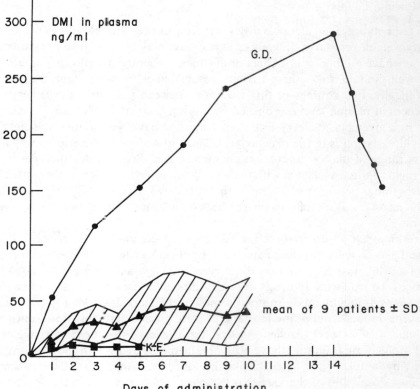

FIGURE 14-4. Plasma levels of desmethylimipramine in eleven patients. *Equal doses (25 mg) were given to all patients by mouth at 6 a.m., 2 p.m. and 10 p.m. Blood samples were taken at 1 p.m. daily. Patients K.E. and G.D. are shown separately. Means and standard deviations are shown for the remaining nine patients. In G.D., dosage was discontinued at day 14 and the decline of plasma level was followed. (From Hammer et al., Figure 1.*[114])

if the therapeutic ratio s very high, the simplest way to ensure adequate therapy is to give a dose that is large enough to establish a sufficient plasma level even in those patients at the low end of the frequency distribution. This is actually the customary procedure with a drug like penicillin, in which there is virtually no dose-related toxicity; gonorrhea, syphilis, and other susceptible infections are treated with large excesses of drug without hazard to the patient. However, if the therapeutic ratio is relatively small, and if the between-patient variation is relatively large, plasma level monitoring would seem to be called for. This is especially important if there is no direct and straightforward therapeutic endpoint. An analgesic agent can probably be titrated well enough by the patient's subjective responses; but an anticonvulsant or antipsychotic agent cannot, and it becomes essential to establish and maintain a suitable plasma level, by whatever dose adjustments are necessary. Another indication for plasma level monitoring is with drugs that have both a narrow therapeutic ratio and very serious toxic actions. Cardiac glycosides fall into this category, it being often difficult to tell whether a patient who is doing poorly, with congestive failure, has too little or too much drug in his system.

Increasing attention has been paid recently to the development of suitable plasma monitoring procedures.[116] For drugs present in the $mg\,ml^{-1}$ or $\mu g\,ml^{-1}$ range, ordinary chemical methods have sufficed, although they are usually cumbersome and costly. In the $ng\,ml^{-1}$ range and below, special techniques are required, such as radio-immunoassay, or "enzyme multiplied immunoassay."[117] Since, ideally, the monitoring should continue as long as a drug is administered, and should also include assays at different times of day and night to measure diurnal fluctuation, fast, inexpensive, reliable, and easy methodology will be desirable. We call such procedures *therapeutic control assays*, for their purpose is to control the therapeutic effectiveness of medication schedules in a more rigorous way than has been customary in the past. It is possible that saliva may be useful instead of plasma for such assays, since saliva is derived from plasma water, and may contain a drug at the same concentration as in plasma.

DRUG INTERACTIONS

This topic concerns the modification of an effect of one drug by the presence of another, whether by direct or indirect means. Interactions may affect absorption, distribution, receptor action, metabolism, or excretion. They may be beneficial or hazardous. They may vary from person to person and from species to species. They may be of major clinical significance or of no clinical significance at all.[118–126]

Absorption

Two substances may complex in the gastrointestinal tract, so that both are poorly absorbed. Some years ago, tetracycline tablets were formulated with calcium carbonate, leading to the formation of an insoluble calcium salt of the antibiotic, and resulting in very poor and erratic blood levels.[127] This interaction was eliminated by changing the tablet formulation. Similar effects are seen with aluminum ion, a matter of some importance in view of the widespread availability of aluminum hydroxide gels as over-the-counter antacids. Serum levels of the antibiotic demethylchlortetracycline, for example, were reduced by simultaneous administration of aluminum salts, in much the same way as tetracycline levels were affected by calcium salts.[128,129] Cholestyramine, which is used in large doses to reduce cholesterol absorption in hypercholesterolemia, also complexes other steroids such as the cardiac glycosides and bile salts, as well as iron salts and thyroxine.[130–132] Neomycin interferes with the absorption of fats and lipid-soluble drugs from the small intestine.[133] Human volunteers were given single 3 gram doses of neomycin by mouth, with a standard 0.5 mg dose of digoxin. The mean peak plasma level of digoxin was $2.01 \pm 0.24\,ng\,ml^{-1}$ in controls, as compared with only $0.73 \pm 0.24\,ng\,ml^{-1}$ in the presence of neomycin.[134]

A surprising example of drug interaction operating on absorption is that of phenobarbital and the antifungal agent griseofulvin. In the presence of phenobarbital, the griseofulvin plasma level is reduced. As already discussed in Chapter 3, phenobarbital is known to increase the metabolism of many drugs by inducing increased formation of liver microsomal enzymes; it is therefore commonly assumed that interactions with phenobarbital must result from this phenomenon. However, when griseofulvin was given intravenously, the plasma levels were the same and declined at the same rate, whether or not phenobarbital had been administered. Griseofulvin is slowly and incompletely absorbed from the gastrointestinal tract; after phenobarbital, absorption was even poorer, but the mechanism was not established.[135]

Gastrointestinal absorption may be hindered by mechanisms other than direct complexing. The intestinal flora, for example, are able to alter many drugs through a variety of biochemical alterations such as hydroxylations, decarboxylations, and ester hydrolysis.[136] Antibiotics, acting upon the intestinal flora, can abolish some of these and thereby alter the ultimate drug levels in the plasma. In theory, microbial alteration of a drug could in some instances decrease, in others increase the drug absorption. For drugs with a low therapeutic ratio, this type of interaction could be responsible for poor therapeutic effectiveness or increased toxicity.[137]

Enzymes involved in transport of essential nutrients across the intestinal wall may be inhibited by drugs, and this in turn may result in rather complex interactions. Folic acid has to be hydrolyzed to the monoglutamate before it can be absorbed. Diphenylhydantoin inhibits this hydrolysis, and thereby diminishes folic acid absorption. (Oral

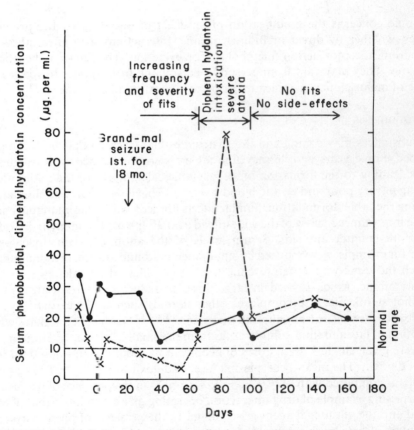

FIGURE 14-5. Folic acid on diphenylhydantoin plasma levels. *An epileptic patient with folate deficiency was given folic acid (5 mg) in addition to the regular daily dosage of diphenylhydantoin and phenobarbital at the start of the record. Solid curve is the plasma level of phenobarbital, broken curve is the plasma level of diphenylhydantoin. At the 60th day, the diphenylhydantoin dose was doubled (to 600 mg daily) and the folic acid dose was reduced to 2 mg daily. Diphenylhydantoin dosage was reduced to 300 mg daily at day 90. (From Baylis et al., Figure 1.[138])*

steroid contraceptives have the same effect.) During long-term therapy of epilepsy with diphenylhydantoin, therefore, folate deficiency is sometimes seen, manifested by megaloblastic anemia. As shown in the case illustrated in Figure 14-5, when folic acid was given to overcome the deficiency, the level of diphenylhydantoin fell sufficiently to cause an increased frequency of seizures. This effect of folic acid may be due to a stimulated metabolism of diphenylhydantoin. When the folic acid intake was reduced, and the daily dose of the anticonvulsant was increased, the diphenylhydantoin level soared into the toxic range.

Effects of one drug upon absorption of another from a subcutaneous or intramuscular depot have already been discussed in Chapter 2. Typical examples are epinephrine and methacholine, which respectively decrease and increase the local blood flow, and consequently alter the entry of another drug into the nearby capillaries.

Distribution

Competition between different drugs for the same binding sites on plasma proteins may have important consequences, especially when one of the drugs has a very high fractional binding at therapeutic plasma levels (cf. Chapter 2).[139] Consider drug A, with a low fractional binding, e.g., 30%. If drug B displaces 10% of drug A from its binding sites, the net result will be merely to increase the amount of drug A that is free in the circulation from 70% to 73%, a negligible change. But if drug A is 98% bound (as is the case, for example, with digitoxin), and 10% is displaced, the result will be to increase the free amount from 2% to 12%, an increase of 6-fold. Since free drug has access to the sites of action (or of toxicity) in the tissues, such displacement can have great clinical significance.[140] In premature infants, the conjugating system responsible for coupling bilirubin with glucuronic acid (cf. p. 289) is deficient. Normally, the rapid excretion of the water-soluble bilirubin glucuronide accounts for most of the elimination of bilirubin, whereas bilirubin itself is very slowly excreted. Thus, the metabolic deficiency leads to a prolonged and elevated bilirubin level. The situation is made worse by the high rate of bilirubin formation during the first few days after birth, attributable to the destruction of excess erythrocytes present in the fetus. A large fraction of the bilirubin in the body is bound by plasma proteins and thereby prevented from entering the tissues. Sulfonamide drugs and vitamin K, which are also bound extensively to plasma proteins, interact at the same sites as do the bilirubin molecules. When these drugs are administered, the competition for binding sites leads to considerable displacement of bilirubin, and the free bilirubin passes into the tissues. The entry of bilirubin into brain causes a grave disturbance known as kernicterus, which is often fatal. The effect was discovered by accident in a clinical trial of the comparative efficacy of tetracycline and of a penicillin-sulfonamide mixture in the management of premature infants.[141] The sulfonamide mixture led to significantly higher mortality, and kernicterus was found frequently at autopsy.

An elegant experimental illustration of the same phenomenon is shown in Figure 14-6. Here a strain of rats was used that lack glucuronyl transferase and therefore have a high level of unconjugated protein-bound bilirubin. After sulfonamide administration, a rising plasma sulfonamide level was associated with a falling plasma bilirubin concentration, as displaced bilirubin diffused out into a much larger volume of distribution in the tissues. As the sulfonamide was eliminated, the plasma bilirubin became bound again to protein. This reduced the free bilirubin concentration in

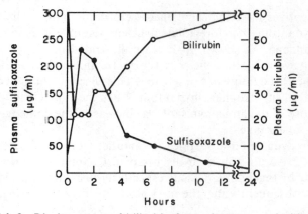

FIGURE 14-6. Displacement of bilirubin from plasma protein binding sites by a sulfonamide. *Sulfisoxazole was administered to rats of the Gunn strain at time zero. These rats are unable to conjugate bilirubin because they lack the glucuronyl transferase. (Data of Johnson et al., from Nyhan, Figure 6.*[142] *By permission of C. V. Mosby.)*

plasma, creating a diffusion gradient for re-entry of bilirubin from the tissues, and finally the initial plasma bilirubin level was restored.

The orally active anticoagulants are prominently involved in this type of interaction.[143] Patients receiving anticoagulants are usually monitored carefully and continuously (or should be), so that any change in blood concentration is noted as a change in the prothrombin clotting time. Among the many drugs that have been observed to interact with the coumarin anticoagulants are barbiturates, analgesics, antibiotics, and diuretics. The interaction of chloral hydrate and warfarin has been analyzed in detail. It is complex. In the early days of a warfarin regimen, the administration of chloral hydrate can produce dangerously high warfarin levels, due to displacement of the anticoagulant from plasma proteins. Eventually, however, chloral hydrate can induce liver enzymes that degrade warfarin, so that dosage adjustment may again be required, but in the opposite direction. Since many variables will influence which of these effects predominates at a given time, conflicting conclusions have been reached concerning the clinical significance of the interaction.[144-147]

It has been known that administration of phenylbutazone to a patient under treatment with warfarin increases the anticoagulant activity. A careful quantitative study demonstrated two consequences of phenylbutazone treatment; increase in anticoagulant action, and an increased elimination rate of the warfarin.[148,149] Phenylbutazone itself was shown to have no effect on the synthesis or degradation rates of the prothrombin complex, but to change the relationship between the prothrombin complex synthesis rate and the total plasma warfarin concentration. This is shown, for a single patient, in Figure 14-7. The upper part of the figure shows that phenylbutazone shortened the plasma half-life of total (bound + free) warfarin. At the same time, as shown in the lower part of the figure, the prothrombin complex activity was reduced in the presence of phenylbutazone, i.e., the warfarin action was potentiated. Thus, at a given concentration of total warfarin, the effect was that to be expected from a higher warfarin concentration[148] This is consistent with a competition between phenylbutazone and warfarin for protein binding sites in the plasma. Presumably, the increased metabolic destruction and elimination of warfarin are consequences of the greater access of free warfarin to the liver drug metabolizing system.

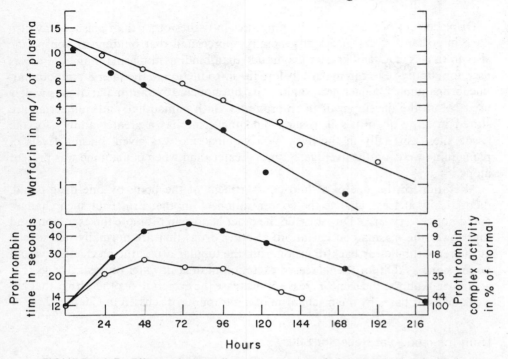

FIGURE 14-7. Effect of phenylbutazone on warfarin plasma levels and effects. *A normal subject was given a single oral dose of warfarin (1.5 mg kg⁻¹). Warfarin plasma levels are shown in upper part of figure (open circles), prothrombin complex activity in lower part of figure (open circles). The experiment was repeated with addition of phenylbutazone (600 mg day⁻¹) given 3 days before and throughout the experiment (solid circles). (From O'Reilly and Aggeler, Figure 1.[149])*

Displacement of a drug from plasma protein binding sites could give the misleading impression that an inert drug has pharmacologic activity. Suppose drug A, which is pharmacologically active, is largely bound to plasma protein, leaving a free concentration below that required for therapeutic action. Suppose drug B, which has no pharmacologic effect, displaces A. It might then be concluded falsely that B is pharmacologically active. Corticosterone, for example, is the major endogenous glucocorticoid in the rat, and is ordinarily bound about 90% to transcortin, a specific steroid binding protein in plasma. Treatment of the rat with a variety of anti-inflammatory agents such as salicylate, phenylbutazone, or indomethacin displaces corticosterone from this binding site. Displacement of the active steroid was shown by preloading the experimental animal with radioactive corticosterone; a 2-fold or greater increase in the free corticosterone occurred after administration of these other drugs. The significance of this phenomenon in man has not been clarified.[150]

The affinity of plasma protein for one drug may be modified by the binding of another. Acetylsalicylic acid, for example, not only binds reversibly to serum albumin, but also acetylates the protein. The acetylated albumin was found to have an increased affinity for phenylbutazone,[151] a decreased affinity for another analgesic, flufenamic acid; and its affinity for an anticoagulant, bishydroxycoumarin, was unchanged. A general implication of this finding is that the effect of an interaction may be manifested long after the drug that is responsible (in this case intact acetylsalicylic acid) has been eliminated.

Displacement of a drug from binding sites in tissues other than plasma may also have important effects. It is not generally appreciated that binding to nonspecific sites in tissues can be of greater magnitude than binding in plasma. Pamaquine was used for curative effect in malaria before the introduction of the safer 8-aminoquino-line, primaquine. Quinacrine, a suppressive but noncurative antimalarial, was widely used before the development of chloroquine. Both pamaquine and quinacrine are stored in large quantites in tissues, but quinacrine has a greater affinity for the tissue sites, especially in the liver. When quinacrine was given, plasma levels of pamaquine were, on the average, 5 times greater than when pamaquine was present alone.[152]

Alteration of the size of a fluid compartment of the body by one drug could, theoretically at least, change the concentration of another drug, but such changes could not be very large. Diuretics, on the other hand, can promote the excretion (and thus lower the plasma concentration) of other drugs that are normally reabsorbed at the renal tubules by back-diffusion from the tubular urine; the mechanism would be the same as that for the increased excretion of urea in water diuresis. Drugs that acidify or akalinize the urine increase or decrease the excretion of other drugs that are weak acids or bases by the mechanism of ion trapping, discussed in Chapter 2.

Drug Interaction at Receptor Sites

This type of drug interaction has been discussed thoroughly, in relation to drug antagonism (e.g., antihistaminics, adrenergic blocking agents, atropine) in Chapter 1, and certain classes of antidotal effect (e.g., narcotic antagonists) in Chapter 5.

Metabolism

It is well known that one drug may inhibit the metabolism of another drug or of a hormone, neurotransmitter, or other endogenous compound. Often this inhibition is the purpose of the drug administration, as when disulfiram causes acetaldehyde accumulation in the presence of ethanol, allopurinol inhibits the oxidation of purine to uric acid in gout, or a cholinesterase inhibitor increases the effectiveness of acetylcholine at neuromuscular junctions in myasthenia gravis. Sometimes enzyme inhibition leads to unexpected adverse effects, as when food containing tyramine is taken in the presence of a monoamine oxidase inhibitor (p. 272). Pyrazole derivatives are inhibitors of alcohol dehydrogenase and have many apparently unrelated pharmacologic actions.[153,154] Patients receiving such drugs should probably be warned of possible adverse effects of ethyl alcohol.

Isoniazid inhibits the hydroxylation of diphenylhydantoin, and simultaneous administration of both drugs can cause toxic reactions to diphenylhydantoin.[155a,b] Patients most likely to show signs of overdosage to diphenylhydantoin when receiving both drugs are the slow acetylators of isoniazid, exemplifying a genetic trait predisposing to a drug interaction.[155c]

Induction of drug metabolizing enzymes has been discussed thoroughly in Chapter 3, and the classes of inducers have been described in detail there. It is obvious that one drug, by this mechanism, may speed the metabolism of another, and thereby lead to a decreased steady state plasma level of the second drug. Clinical studies have produced a wealth of confirmatory evidence that this mechanism of drug interaction can be extremely important. Phenobarbital has been studied most intensively in this respect, probably because it is so commonly used. Thus, phenobarbital increases the metabolism and thereby decreases the plasma level of diphenylhydantoin, the tricyclic antidepressant desmethylimipramine, and the coumarin anticoagulants.[156–158] Ethanol speeds the metabolism of tolbutamide, and alcoholics metabolize tolbutamide unusually rapidly.[159]

The use of phenobarbital to induce bilirubin glucuronide formation in neonatal jaundice by stimulating the synthesis of UDP glucuronyl transferase has been mentioned (p. 283).[160] Since the phenobarbital effect is not limited to induction of this particular enzyme, however, difficulties may arise. By enhancing steroid hydroxylations, for example, phenobarbital may reduce the cortisol level; and it is possible that induction of other enzymes may adversely influence normal developmental processes in the newborn.[161]

Excretion

One drug may block the renal excretion of another, by competing for the same tubular transport system, as when another anion (e.g., carinamide) blocks the excretion of penicillin and thereby prolongs the penicillin plasma level. This type of interaction may be quite complex. The orally active antidiabetic agent acetohexamide is converted in the body to an active metabolite, hydroxyhexamide. When phenylbutazone is given concurrently with the parent drug, the renal excretion of hydroxyhexamide is inhibited, and serious prolonged hypoglycemia may result. Table 14-13 shows that

TABLE 14-13. Effect of phenylbutazone on plasma half-life of acetohexamide and hydroxyhexamide.

Data are mean plasma half-life values in hours ($\pm$ standard error) in 4 to 7 independent experiments, before and after administration of phenylbutazone. The increase in half-life of hydroxyhexamide is highly significant ($P < 0.01$). (From Field et al., Table 1.[162])

Period of test	Acetohexamide	Hydroxyhexamide
Before phenylbutazone	0.93 ± 0.14	5.3 ± 0.9
After phenylbutazone	0.94 ± 0.09	22.1 ± 3.2

although the half-life of the active metabolite is greatly prolonged, that of the parent drug is unaffected.[162] This situation would indeed be difficult to understand if the conversion to an active metabolite had not been discovered.

Blockade of renal tubular reabsorption by one drug could cause more rapid renal elimination of another, which is ordinarily handled by the same transport system. This is the basis of the uricosuric action of phenylbutazone, resulting in increased elimination of uric acid.

Phenobarbital enhances the biliary excretion of many drugs in animals. The effect is due in part to an increased bile flow, and in part to increased synthesis of proteins that function in the biliary conjugation-excretion mechanism. If a drug is conjugated and excreted, its elimination from the body will be speeded by phenobarbital. If it is excreted in bile without conjugation, the increased bile flow may merely increase the amount of the drug that is trapped in the enterohepatic circulation.

Clinical Significance of Drug Interactions

Hundreds of reports about drug interactions have flooded the clinical literature, only a small proportion of which are likely to be of general significance. Many have been assumed to occur in man because they have been demonstrated in experimental animals. But species differences here, as in other aspects of pharmacology, are prominent and unpredictable. Many purported interactions have been poorly documented, usually because it is so difficult to establish rigorous control of variables in clinical experimentation, and because treatment schedules are often very brief. There has been a tendency to overestimate the incidence and severity of drug interactions. Often, even when an interaction is known to occur, its magnitude may not be great enough to contraindicate the simultaneous use of two drugs. Moreover, just as individuals vary greatly in the plasma level established at a given dosage schedule, so do they vary greatly in the extent to which one drug is modified by the presence of another. Consider the much-publicized interaction between phenobarbital and diphenylhydantoin. In many patients, there is no apparent influence of phenobarbital on diphenylhydantoin plasma levels, and in only a few is the effect very large.[163] Moreover, the range of effective but nontoxic plasma levels of diphenylhydantoin is fairly great, probably between 10 and 20 μg ml^{-1}—an ample range for considerable harmless variation. Finally, in this instance, the barbiturate itself contributes to the control of epileptic seizures. Thus, the mere fact that a drug interaction is known to be possible should not preclude the use of an effective combination of drugs.

A few generalizations can be stated with confidence. Certainly, drugs given by mouth should be administered in such a way that no other drug or dietary constituent will block its absorption. When this route is employed, a drug will be especially sensitive to the level of the liver enzymes, since all of it passes through the portal circulation directly upon absorption. Drugs that are highly bound to plasma proteins at therapeutic plasma levels will be sensitive to displacement by other drugs. Drugs that are actively secreted or reabsorbed by the renal tubules may be affected by other drugs that use the same excretory pathway.

An "epidemiology" of drug interactions can be discerned—one can identify groups in the population who are probable candidates for such effects, and be especially watchful in treating them. People who use barbiturates frequently as hypnotics will be subject to unexpected variations in the level of another drug, unless appropriate precautions are taken to discontinue (or to stabilize) the barbiturate intake. Patients with cardiovascular disease, who require carefully controlled levels of cardiac glycosides, possibly also anticoagulants, call for special attention whenever another drug is started or discontinued.[164] Other patients on a long-term therapeutic regimen for a chronic disease fall into the same category—those suffering from hypertensive disease, diabetics, epileptics, psychotics. And the same considerations apply to people who take drugs on a regular basis even though they are not ill, for example, oral contraceptives, antimalarials, and various psychotropic drugs.[165]

The main lesson of all the information amassed thus far about drug interactions would seem to be the need for caution and alertness. If one drug will suffice, two is too many, not only because of the possibility of an interaction, but for other good reasons explained throughout this book. If two drugs are required, no amount of consultation in voluminous uncritical tables listing possible interactions is likely to alter one's decision about therapeutic need. But the knowledge that certain interactions are frequent should make one even more careful than otherwise to titrate the dose to the need of the individual patient. This, indeed, is the crux of the matter. With or without drug interactions, dosage has to be individualized. As pointed out earlier in this chapter and elsewhere in the book, the clinical use of most drugs can become more rational and scientific only through two essential developments. First, adequate routine means must be developed for monitoring drug plasma levels, and such therapeutic control assays must be readily available to every physician. Second, better means must be developed for administering drugs in such a way that constant stable plasma levels can be maintained despite disturbing influences, whatever their origin.

REFERENCES

1. C. G. ZUBROD: General problems in the selection of drugs for clinical trial. Part I. Symposium on Clinical Drug Evaluation and Human Pharmacology. *Clin. Pharmacol. Ther.* 3:239 (1962).
2. E. L. HARRIS and J. D. FITZGERALD: *The Principles and Practice of Clinical Trials.* Edinburgh, E. & S. Livingstone (1970).
3. A. R. FEINSTEIN: *Clinical Judgment.* Baltimore, Williams and Wilkins (1967).
4. A. R. FEINSTEIN: Clinical biostatistics, I–IV. *Clin. Pharmacol. Ther.* 11:135, 282, 432, 595, 755 (1970).
5. A. GOLDSTEIN: Pharmacologic basis of methadone treatment. In *Proceedings of the 4th National Conference on Methadone Treatment,* San Francisco (1972).
6. D. COLQUHOUN: *Lectures on Biostatistics.* Oxford, Clarendon Press (1971).
7. D. MAINLAND: Statistical ward rounds—17, Part I. *Clin. Pharmacol. Ther.* 10:714 (1969).
8. D. MAINLAND: Statistical ward rounds—18, Part II. *Clin. Pharmacol. Ther.* 10:367 (1969).
9. P. ARMITAGE: *Statistical Methods in Medical Research.* Oxford, Blackwell Scientific Publications (1971).
10. L. J. WITTS, ed.: *Medical Surveys and Clinical Trials,* 2nd ed. London, Oxford University Press (1964).
11. M. C. SHEPS: The clinical value of drugs: Sources of evidence. *Am. J. Public Health* 51:647 (1961).
12. Seminar on the clinical evaluation of drugs, in *Clin. Pharmacol. Ther.* 4:255–260, 371–392, 531–547 (1963).
13. A. B. HILL: *Statistical Methods in Clinical and Preventive Medicine.* New York, Oxford University Press (1962).
14. A. GOLDSTEIN: *Biostatistics: An Introductory Text.* New York, Macmillan (1964).
15. J. WORCESTER: The statistical method. *New Eng. J. Med.* 274:27 (1966).
16. S. WOLF: The pharmacology of placebos. *Pharmacol. Rev.* 11:689 (1959).
17. G. HONIGFELD: Non-specific factors in treatment. I. Review of placebo reactions and placebo reactors. *Dis. Nerv. System* 25:145 (1964).
18. R. A. FISHER and F. YATES: *Statistical Tables for Biological, Agricultural and Medical Research.* 6th ed. London, Oliver and Boyd (1963).
19. A. FALK: U.S. Veterans Administration—Armed Forces Cooperative Study on the chemotherapy of tuberculosis. XII. Results of treatment in miliary tuberculosis: a follow-up study of 570 adult patients. *Am. Rev. Resp. Dis.* 91:6 (1965).
20. THE RAND CORPORATION: *A Million Random Digits with 100,000 Normal Deviates.* Glencoe, Ill., The Free Press (1955).
21. R. E. GIANELLY, R. H. GOLDMAN, B. TREISTER, and D. C. HARRISON: Propranolol in patients with angina pectoris. *Ann. Int. Med.* 67:1216 (1967).

22.   W. S. ARONOW and M. A. KAPLAN: Propranolol combined with isosorbide dinitrate versus placebo in angina pectoris. *New Eng. J. Med.* 280:847 (1969).
23.   D. C. HARRISON: New drugs in the treatment of angina. *New Eng. J. Med.* 280:895 (1969).
24.   W. S. ARONOW: The medical treatment of angina pectoris. II. Design of an antianginal drug study. *Am. Heart J.* 84:132 (1972).
25.   L. E. HOLLISTER and J. E. OVERALL: Methodology for the clinical investigation of psycho-therapeutic drugs. *J. New Drugs* 5:286 (1965).
26.   MEDICAL RESEARCH COUNCIL: The prevention of whooping-cough by vaccination. *Brit. Med. J.* 1:1463 (1951).
27.   J. M. BREWSTER: Antihistaminic drugs in the therapy of the common cold. *Ind. Med.* 18:217 (1949).
28.   COUNCIL ON PHARMACY AND CHEMISTRY: Status report on antihistaminic agents in the prophylaxis and treatment of the common "cold." *J. Am. Med. Ass.* 142:566 (1950).
29.   MEDICAL RESEARCH COUNCIL: Clinical trials of antihistaminic drugs in the prevention and treatment of the common cold. *Brit. Med. J.* 2:425 (1950).
30.   P. ARMITAGE: *Sequential Medical Trials.* Springfield, Charles C. Thomas (1960).
31.   A. WALD: *Sequential Analysis.* New York, John Wiley and Sons (1947).
32.   C. F. BORCHGREVINK: Long-term anticoagulant therapy in angina pectoris and myocardial infarction. A clinical trial of intensive versus moderate treatment. *Acta Med. Scand.* 168, Suppl. 359:1 (1960).
33.   MEDICAL RESEARCH COUNCIL: An assessment of long-term anticoagulant administration after cardiac infarction. *Brit. Med. J.* 2:837 (1964).
34.   L. PAULING: *Vitamin C and the Common Cold.* San Francisco, W. H. Freeman and Co. (1970).
35.   G. H. WALKER, M. L. BYNOE, and D. A. J. TYRRELL: Trial of ascorbic acid in prevention of colds. *Brit. Med. J.* 1:603 (1967).
36.   H. E. TEBROCK, J. J. ARMINIO, and J. H. JOHNSTON: Usefulness of bioflavonoids and ascorbic acid in treatment of common cold. *J. Am. Med. Ass.* 162:1227 (1956).
37.   D. W. COWAN and H. S. DIEHL: Antihistaminic agents and ascorbic acid in the early treatment of the common cold. *J. Am. Med. Ass.* 143:421 (1950).
38.   D. W. COWAN, H. S. DIEHL, and A. B. BAKER: Vitamins for the prevention of colds. *J. Am. Med. Ass.* 120:1268 (1942).
39.   A. E. PHILLIPS: A method for analysing assessments of symptom change. *Brit. J. Psych.* 115:1379 (1969).
40.   S. S. SUTHERLAND, A. E. PHILLIPS, and M. S. SUTHERLAND: The response to treatment of individual patients in a drug trial. *Brit. J. Psych.* 115:1383 (1969).
41.   J. CORNFIELD: The university group diabetes program: A further statistical analysis of the mortality findings. *J. Am. Med. Ass.* 217:1676 (1971).
42.   MEDICAL RESEARCH COUNCIL: Responsibility in investigations on human subjects. *Brit. Med. J.* 2:178 (1964).
43.   DECLARATION OF HELSINKI: Recommendations guiding doctors in clinical research. *World Med. J.* 11:281 (1964).
44.   H. K. BEECHER: Consent on clinical experimentation: myth and reality. *J. Am. Med. Ass.* 195:34 (1966).
45.   FEDERAL REGISTER. 32 F.R. 8753, Part 130.37 (h), June 20, 1967.
46.   POLIOMYELITIS VACCINE EVALUATION CENTER: Evaluation of 1954 field trial of poliomyelitis vaccine. *Am. J. Public Health* 45: Number 5, Part 2 (1955).
47.   S. PHILLIPS: VII. Comparison of isoniazid alone with isoniazid-PAS in the original chemotherapy of noncavitary pulmonary tuberculosis. *Am. Rev. Resp. Dis.* 80:641 (1959).
48.   H. A. KELLY: *Walter Reed and Yellow Fever,* 3rd ed. Baltimore, The Norman, Remington Co. (1923).
49.   A. S. ALVING, B. CRAIGE, JR., T. N. PULLMAN, C. M. WHORTON, R. JONES, JR., and L. EICHELBERGER: Procedures used at Stateville Penitentiary for the testing of potential antimalarial agents. Symposium on Malaria. *J. Clin. Invest.* 27:2 (1948).
50.   A. B. HILL, R. DOLL, T. MCL. GALLOWAY, and J. P. W. HUGHES: Virus diseases in pregnancy and congenital defects. *Brit. J. Prevent. Soc. Med.* 12:1 (1958).
51.   Trials of War Criminals before the Nurenberg Military Tribunals under Control Council Law No. 10; Vol. II, p. 181. Washington, D.C., U.S. Government Printing Office (1950).
52.   H. K. BEECHER: Ethics and clinical research. *New Eng. J. Med.* 274:1354 (1966).

53. T. S. SZASZ: The ethics of addiction. *Harper's Magazine*, April 1972.
54. Federal Food, Drug, and Cosmetic Act. As amended. Code of Federal Regulations, Title 21. Publication No. 667340. Washington, D.C., U.S. Government Printing Office (1963).
55. New Drug Regulations under the Federal Food, Drug, and Cosmetic Act. U.S. Department of Health, Education, and Welfare; Food and Drug Administration. Publication No. 691934. Washington, D.C., U.S. Government Printing Office (1963).
56. Fact Sheet. Drug Abuse Control Amendments of 1965. Public Law 89-74, 89th Congress. U.S. Department of Health, Education, and Welfare, Food and Drug Administration. Washington, D.C., U.S. Government Printing Office (1965).
57. New Drug Regulations under the Federal Food, Drug and Cosmetic Act. U.S. Department of Health, Education and Welfare: Food and Drug Administration. June, 1972 amendment. Federal Register #12066.
58. H. G. MANDEL: Therapeutic range and extent of use of home remedies. *Ann. N.Y. Acad. Sci.* 120:902 (1965).
59. U.S. Treasury Department, Bureau of Narcotics. Regulations No. 5, Part 151 of Title 26 (1954), Code of Federal Regulations. Regulatory Taxes on Narcotic Drugs. Opium, Coca Leaves, Isonipecaine or Opiates. Revised October 1964. Washington, D.C., U.S. Government Printing Office (1964).
60. Comprehensive Drug Abuse Prevention and Control Act of 1970, H.R. 18583, Public Law 91-513.
61. NATIONAL COMMISSION ON MARIHUANA AND DRUG ABUSE, FIRST REPORT: Marihuana: A Signal of Misunderstanding. Washington, D.C., Government Printing Office (1972).
62. H. J. DUVALL, B. Z. LOCKE, and L. BRILL: Followup study of narcotic drug addicts five years after hospitalization. *Public Health Rep.* 78:185 (1963).
63. V. P. DOLE and M. NYSWANDER: A medical treatment for diacetylmorphine (heroin) addiction. *J. Am. Med. Ass.* 193:646 (1965).
64. *Proceedings of the Fourth National Conference on Methadone Treatment*, San Francisco (1972).
65. NATIONAL INSTITUTE ON ALCOHOL ABUSE AND ALCOHOLISM: NIMH Publication. D.H.E.W. (H.S.M.) 72–9019. U.S. Government Printing Office (1972).
66. C. S. KEEFER, ed: A symposium on home medication and the public welfare. *Ann. N.Y. Acad. Sci.* 120:807 (1965).
67. J. R. LEONARDS: The absorption of aspirin. *Clin. Pharmacol. Ther.* 4:476 (1963).
68. R. C. BATTERMAN: Comparison of buffered and unbuffered acetylsalicyclic acid. *New Eng. J. Med.* 258:213 (1958).
69. G. A. CRONK: Laboratory and clinical studies with buffered and nonbuffered acetylsalicylic acid. *New Eng. J. Med.* 258:219 (1958).
70. Aspirin, Bufferin and Ecotrin. *Medical Letter* 1:7 (1959).
71. Gastrointestinal disturbances with aspirin. *Medical Letter* 7:75 (1965).
72. H. JICK, D. SLONE, S. SHAPIRO, G. P. LEWIS, and V. SISKIND: A new method for assessing the clinical effects of oral analgesic drugs. *Clin. Pharmacol. Ther.* 12:456 (1971).
73. W. DAMESHEK: Chloramphenicol—a new warning. *J. Am. Med. Ass.* 174:1853 (1960).
74. C. MULLER: Medical review of prescribing. *J. Chron. Dis.* 18:689 (1965).
75. "Emprazil-C" tablets and shotgun therapy. *Medical Letter* 6:24 (1964).
76. Drugs and auto accidents. *Medical Letter* 8:53 (1966).
77. C. J. G. PERRY and A. L. MORGENSTERN: Drugs and driving. *J. Am. Med. Ass.* 195:376 (1966).
78. R. F. MARONDE, P. V. LEE, M. M. MC CARRON, and S. SEIBERT: A study of prescribing patterns. *Med. Care* 9:383 (1971).
79. R. R. MILLER: Drug usage in two Chicago hospitals. *Drug Intelligence and Clin. Pharmacol.* 5:238 (1971).
80. T. D. RUCKER: The role of computers in drug utilization review. *Am. J. Hosp. Pharm.* 29:128 (1972).
81. P. GARDNER and L. J. WATSON: Adverse drug reactions: a pharmacist-based monitoring system. *Clin. Pharmacol. Ther.* 11:802 (1970).
82. E. R. GABRIELI, ed.: The use of data mechanization and computers in clinical medicine. *Ann. N.Y. Acad. Sci.* 161:371 (1969).
83. C. MULLER: The overmedicated society: forces in the marketplace for medical care. *Science* 176:488 (1972).
84. R. BURACK: Burack's Rx. *Harvard Medical Alumni Bulletin* 46:22 (1972).
85. J. G. SEARLE, L. D. BARNEY, F. BOYER, G. R. CAIN, L. C. DUNCAN, R. A. HARDT, D. M. JOHNSON, and E. G. UPJOHN: The pharmaceutical industry. *J. Med. Educ.* 36:24 (1961).

86. C. D. MAY: Selling drugs by "educating" physicians. *J. Med. Educ.* 36:1 (1961).
87. Administered Prices. Hearings before the Subcommitte on Antitrust and Monopoly of the Committee on the Judiciary, U.S. Senate, 86th Congress, First Session. Publication No. 35621. Washington, D.C., U.S. Government Printing Office p. 7901, 10729 (1961).
88. D. DUNLOP: Use and abuse of drugs. *Brit. Med. J.* 2:437 (1965).
89. C. MULLER: Institutional drug purchasing. Factors influencing choices by pharmacists and physicians. *Hospitals* 39 (June 16): 97 (1965).
90. A.M.A. COUNCIL ON DRUGS: *New Drugs, 1965 Edition*. Chicago, American Medical Association, annual.
91. S. GARB: Teaching medical students to evaluate drug advertizing. *J. Med. Educ.* 35:729 (1960).
92. D. G. FRIEND: One drug—one name. *Clin. Pharmacol. Ther.* 6:689 (1965).
93. R. BURACK: *The New Handbook of Prescription Drugs: Official Names, Prices and Sources for Patient and Doctor*, New York, Pantheon Books, 1970.
94. C. MULLER and R. WESTHEIMER: Formularies and drug standards in metropolitan hospitals. *Hospitals* 40 (Jan. 16): 97 (1966).
95. P. H. LAVIETES and F. H. EPSTEIN: Thyroid therapy of myxedema. A comparison of various agents with a note on the composition of thyroid secretion in man. *Ann. Intern. Med.* 60:79 (1964).
96. Chlorpheniramine maleate tablets. *Medical Letter* 7:18 (1965).
97. E. C. BURKE: Drug Prices Here Held Inequitable. In *The New York Times*, Oct. 20 (1965). p. 39.
98. Administered Prices. Hearings before the Subcommittee on Antitrust and Monopoly of the Committee on the Judiciary, U.S. Senate, 86th Congress, First Session. Publication No. 35621, p. 7884, Washington, D.C., U.S. Government Printing Office (1961).
99. Administered Prices. Hearings before the Subcommittee on Antitrust and Monopoly of the Committee on the Judiciary, U.S. Senate, 86th Congress, First Session, p. 8910. Publication No. 35621. Washington, D.C., U.S. Government Printing Office (1961).
100. Meprobamate. *Medical Letter* 2:87 (1960).
101. Doriden. *Medical Letter* 4:61 (1962).
102. J. MAC LEOD: Human seminal cytology following the administration of certain antispermatogenic compounds. In *A Symposium on Agents Affecting Fertility*, ed. by C. R. Austin and J. S. Perry. Boston, Little, Brown and Co. (1965). pp. 93–123.
103. V. A. DRILL: Oral Contraceptives. New York, McGraw-Hill (1966).
104. R. DOLL: Recognition of unwanted drug effects. *Brit. Med. J.* 2:69 (1969).
105. R. DOLL: Unwanted effects of drugs. *Brit. Med. Bull.* 27:25 (1971).
106. H. JICK, O. S. MIETTINEN, S. SHAPIRO, G. P. LEWIS, V. SISKIND, and D. SLONE: Comprehensive drug surveillance. *J. Am. Med. Ass.* 213:1455 (1970).
107. G. D. FRIEDMAN, M. F. COLLEN, L. E. HARRIS, E. E. VAN BRUNT, and L. S. DAVIS: Experience in monitoring drug reactions in outpatients. *J. Am. Med. Ass.* 217:567 (1971).
108. D. J. FINNEY: The design and logic of a monitor of drug use. *J. Chron. Dis.* 18:77 (1965).
109. S. SHAPIRO, D. SLONE, G. P. LEWIS, and H. JICK: Fatal drug reactions among medical inpatients. *J. Am. Med. Ass.* 216:467 (1971).
110. H. JICK, B. WESTERHOLM, M. P. VESSEY, G. P. LEWIS, D. SLONE, W. H. W. INMAN, S. SHAPIRO, and J. WORCESTER: Venous thromboembolic disease and ABO blood type. *Lancet* 1:7594 (1969).
111. Report from Boston Collaborative Drug Surveillance Program. Relation between breast cancer and S blood-antigen system. *Lancet* 1:7694 (1971).
112. G. P. LEWIS, H. JICK, D. SLONE, and S. SHAPIRO: The role of genetic factors and serum protein binding in determining drug response as revealed by comprehensive drug surveillance. In *Drug Metabolism in Man*, ed. E. S. Vessell. *Ann. N.Y. Acad. Sci.* 169:729 (1971).
113. J. T. BIGGER, D. H. SCHMIDT, and H. KUTT: Relationship between the plasma level of diphenylhydantoin sodium and its cardiac antiarrhythmic effects. *Circulation* 38:363 (1968).
114. W. HAMMER, C.-M. IDESTRÖM, and F. SJÖQVIST: Chemical control of antidepressant drug therapy. *Excerpta Medica. Intl. Congr. Series* 122:301 (1966).
115. H. KUTT, J. HAYNES, and F. MC DOWELL: Some causes of ineffectiveness of diphenylhydantoin. *Arch. Neurol.* 14:489 (1966).
115a. O. SVENSMARK and F. BUCHTHAL: Diphenylhydantoin and phenobarbital. *Am. J. Dis. Child* 108:82 (1964).
116. E. S. VESELL and G. T. PASSANANTI: Utility of clinical chemical determinations of drug concentrations in biological fluids. *Clin. Chem.* 17:851 (1971).

117. K. E. RUBENSTEIN, R. S. SCHNEIDER, and E. F. ULLMAN: Homogeneous enzyme immunoassay. A new immunochemical technique. *Biochem. Biophys. Res. Comm.* 47:846 (1972).
118. I. H. STOCKLEY: Basic principles of drug interaction. *Chemistry in Britain* 8:114 (1972).
119. V. M. ROSENOER and G. M. GILL: Drug interactions in clinical medicine. *Med. Clin. N. Am.* 56:585 (1972).
120. Symposium on clinical effects of interaction between drugs. *Proc. Roy. Soc. Med.* 58:943 (1965).
121. Interactions of drugs. *Medical Letter on Drugs and Therapeutics* 12:93 (1970).
122. L. F. PRESCOTT: Pharmacokinetic drug interactions. *Lancet* 2:1239 (1969).
123. S. A. KABINS: Interactions among antibiotics and other drugs. *J. Am. Med. Ass.* 219:206 (1972).
124. H. F. MORRELLI and K. L. MELMON: The clinician's approach to drug interactions. *Calif. Med.* 109:380 (1968).
125. R. BRESSLER: Editorial—Combined drug therapy. *Am. J. Med. Sci.* 225:89 (1968).
126. H. M. SOLOMON, M. J. BARAKAT, and C. J. ASHLEY: Mechanisms of drug interactions. *J. Am. Med. Ass.* 216:1997 (1971).
127. W. M. SWEENEY, S. M. HARDY, A. C. DORNBRUSH, and J. M. RUEGSEGGER: Absorption of tetracycline in human beings as affected by certain excipients. *Antibiotic Med. and Clin. Ther.* 4:642 (1957).
128. J. SHEINER and W. A. ALTEMEIER: Experimental study of factors inhibiting absorption and effective therapeutic levels of declomycin. *Surg. Gynecol. Obstet.* 114:9 (1962).
129. C. W. REES: Avidity of the tetracyclines for the cations of metals. *Nature* 177:434 (1956).
130. G. STROHMEYER: Der enterohepatische kreislauf von Digitoxin. *Der Internist* 13:344 (1972).
131. F. B. THOMAS, F. S. MC CULLOUGH, and N. J. GREENBERGER: Inhibition of the intestinal absorption of inorganic and hemoglobin iron by cholestyramine. *J. Lab. Clin. Med.* 78:71 (1971).
132. R. C. NORTHCUTT, J. N. STIEL, J. W. HOLLIFIELD, and E. G. STANT, JR.: The influence of cholestyramine on thyroxine absorption. *J. Am. Med. Ass.* 208:1857 (1969).
133. S. J. GORDON, E. N. HARO, I. C. PAES, and W. W. FALOON: Studies of malabsorption and calcium excretion induced by neomycin sulfate. *J. Am. Med Ass.* 204:127 (1968).
134. R. M. MAULITZ, J. LINDENBAUM, J. R. SAHA, N. SHEA, and V. P. BUTLER, JR.: Impairment of digoxin absorption by neomycin. *N.Y. Heart Assoc.* 48:1047 (1972).
135. S. RIEGELMAN, M. ROWLAND, and W. L. EPSTEIN: Griseofulvin-phenobarbital interaction in man. *J. Am. Med. Ass.* 213:426 (1970).
136. R. R. SCHELINE: Drug metabolism by intestinal microorganisms. *J. Pharm. Sci.* 57:2021 (1968).
137. D. S. ZAHARKO, H. BRUCKNER, and V. T. OLIVERIO: Antibiotics alter methotrexate metabolism and excretion. *Science* 166:887 (1969).
138. E. M. BAYLIS, J. M. CROWLEY, J. M. PREECE, P. E. SYLVESTER, and V. MARKS: Influence of folic acid on blood-phenytoin levels. *Lancet* 1:62 (1971).
139. E. G. MC QUEENS and W. M. WARDELL: Drug displacement from protein binding: isolation of a redistributional drug interaction in vivo. *Brit. J. Pharm.* 43:312 (1971).
140. M. I. MARCUS, L. BURKHALTER, C. CUCCIA, J. PAVLOVICH, and G. G. KAPADIA: Administration of tritiated digoxin with and without a loading dose. *Circulation* 34:865 (1966).
141. W. A. SILVERMAN, D. H. ANDERSEN, W. A. BLANC, and D. N. CROZIER: A difference in mortality rate and incidence of kernicterus among premature infants allotted to two prophylactic antibacterial regimens. *Pediatrics* 18:614 (1956).
142. W. L. NYHAN: Toxicity of drugs in the neonatal period. *J. Pediat.* 59:1 (1961).
143. J. KOCH-WESER and E. M. SELLERS: Drug interactions with coumarin anticoagulants. *New Eng. J. Med.* 285:489, 547 (1971).
144. Report from the Boston Collaborative Drug Surveillance Program, Boston University Medical Center: Interaction between chloral hydrate and warfarin. *New Eng. J. Med.* 286:53 (1972).
145. L. T. SIGELL and H. C. FLESSA: Drug interactions with anticoagulants. *J. Am. Med. Ass.* 214:2035 (1970).
146. P. F. GRINER, L. G. RAISZ, F. R. RICKLES, P. J. WIESNER, and C. L. ODOROFF: Chloral hydrate and warfarin interaction: clinical significance? *Ann. Int. Med.* 74:540 (1971).
147. Editorial, *Arch. Intern. Med.* 121:373 (1968).
148. R. A. O'REILLY and G. LEVY: Pharmacokinetic analysis of potentiating effect of phenylbutazone on anticoagulant action of warfarin in man. *J. Pharm. Sci.* 59:1258 (1970).
149. R. A. O'REILLY and P. M. AGGELER: Phenylbutazone potentiation of anticoagulant effect: fluorometric assay of warfarin. *Proc. Soc. Exptl. Biol. Med.* 128:1080 (1968).

150. R. P. MAICKEL, F. P. MILLER, and B. B. BRODIE: Interaction of non-steroidal antiinflammatory agents on cortcosterone binding to plasma proteins in the rat, *Arzneimittel-Forschung* 19:1803 (1969).

151. C. F. CHIGNELL and D. K. STARKWEATHER: Optical studies of drug protein complexes. V. The interaction of phenylbutazone, flufenamic acid, and dicoumarol with acetylsalicylic acid-treated human serum albumin. *Mol. Pharm.* 7:229 (1971).

152. C. G. ZUBROD, T. J. KENNEDY, and J. A. SHANNON: Studies on the chemotherapy of the human malarias. VIII. The physiological disposition of pamaquine. *J. Clin. Invest.* 27:114 (1948).

153. R. E. ORTH: Biologically active pyrazoles. *J. Pharm. Sci.* 57:537 (1968).

154. T.-K. LI and H. THEORELL: Human liver alcohol dehydrogenase: inhibition by pyrazole and pyrazole analogs. *Acta Chem. Scand.* 23:892 (1969).

155a. H. KUTT, W. WINTERS, and F. H. MC DOWELL: Depression of parahydroxylation of diphenylhydantoin by antitubercular chemotherapy. *Neurology* 16:594 (1966).

155b. H. KUTT, K. VEREBELY, and F. MC DOWELL: Inhibition of diphenylhydantoin metabolism in rats and rat liver microsomes by antitubercular drugs. *Neurology* 18:706 (1968).

155c. H. KUTT, R. BRENNAN, H. DEHEJIA, and K. VEREBELY: Diphenylhydantoin intoxication: a complication of isoniazid therapy. *Am. Rev. Resp. Dis.* 101:377 (1970).

156. S. A. CUCINELL, A. H. CONNEY, M. SANSUR, and J. J. BURNS: Drug interactions in man. I. Lowering effect of phenobarbital on plasma levels of bishydroxycoumarin (Dicoumarol) and diphenylhydantoin (Dilantin). *Clin. Pharmacol. Ther.* 6:421 (1965).

157. H. KUTT, J. HAYNES, K. VEREBELEY, and F. MC DOWELL: The effect of phenobarbital on plasma, diphenylhydantoin level and metabolism in man and in rat liver microsomes. *Neurology* 19:611 (1969).

158. W. D. DIAMOND and R. A. BUCHANAN: A clinical study of the effect of phenobarbital on diphenylhydantoin plasma levels. *J. Clin. Pharmacol.* 10:1677 (1970).

159. A. H. CONNEY: Microsomal enzyme induction by drugs. *Pharm. Physicians* 3:1 (no. 12) (1969).

160. T. R. C. SISSON: Phenobarbital and neonatal jaundice. *Clin. Ped.* 10:683 (1971).

161. J. T. WILSON: Caution with phenobarbital. *Clin. Ped.* 10:684 (1971).

162. J. B. FIELD, M. OHTA, C. BOYLE, and A. REMERS: Potentiation of acetohexamide hypoglycemia by phenylbutazone. *New Eng. J. Med.* 277:889 (1967).

163. H. E. BOOKER and J. TOUSSAINT: Concurrent administration of phenobarbital and diphenylhydantoin: lack of an interference effect. *Neurology* 21:383 (1971).

164. I. H. RAISFELD: Drug interactions in the therapy of cardiovascular disorders. *Am. Heart J.* 81:709 (1971).

165. D. A. HUSSAR: Factors predisposing a patient to drug interactions. *Am. J. Pharm.* 143:177 (1971).

Index

Physostigmine, 21, 95. *see also* Cholinesterase
  inhibitors
Pilocarpine, 140, local release, 154
Ping-pong reaction, acetylation, 261
Pinocytosis, 167
Piperonylbutoxide, formula, 534
Pituitary hormones, structure-activity
  relations, 39.
  see also Oxytocin; Vasopressin
pK, pKa. *see* individual agents.
  see also Ionization
Placebo controls, 780
Placenta, drug penetration, 198
Plasma cholinesterase, isozymes, 448
Plasma levels, monitoring, 817
Plasma protein binding, drug interactions, 821
Plasma volume, 130
Plasmodium berghei, 527
Plateau principle, derivation, 311
Plutonium, antidotes, 401, 402
Pneumoconiosis, 140
Podophyllotoxin, formula, 649
  spindle poison, 649
Poison control centers, 358, 359
Polonium, antidotes, 402
Polyarthritis, drug allergy, 493
Polycyclic hydrocarbon carcinogens. *see* Hydro-
  carbons
Polyene antibiotics, permeability effects, 183
Polyvinyl pyrrolidone, 112
Posterior pituitary hormones, bioassay, 740
Potassium, in digitalis poisoning, 425
Potency, anesthetic gases, 349
Potency ratio, 89, 739
Pralidoxime, 406, development, 762
  distribution, 757
  formula, 409
Pricing of drugs, 812
Primaquine, formula, 455
  genetic factors, 455
  genetic variation, 442
  hemolytic anemia, 457
  malarial screen, 734
  primaquine sensitivity, 455
  see also Antimalarial drugs
Priming doses, 320
Probenecid, gastric secretion, 148
  hemolytic anemia, 457
  pKa, 148
Probit analysis, 380
Procainamide, development, 757
  formula, 758
Procaine, formula, 257, 754, 758
  metabolism, 257
  therapeutic ratio, 754.
  see also Local Anesthetics
Procaine amide ethobromide, gastric absorption, 147

Procaine amide ethobromide *(continued)*
  pKa, 147
Proflavin, 56, mutagenesis, 639
  permeability, 175
Progesterone, 67, formula, 746
  local release preparations, 153
  receptors, 67
  teratogenesis, 716
Promotion, carcinogenesis, 670
Prontosil, formula, 256
  metabolism, 256
Propanediol-1,3, teratogenesis, 708
β-Propiolactone, carcinogenesis, 675, 688
  formula, 688
Propoxycaine, formula, 754
  therapeutic ratio, 754
Propylthiouracil, development, 772
  formula, 772
Protamine, in heparin toxicity, 405
Protein binding, drugs, 47
  effect on fetal penetration, 202
Protein synthesis, drug metabolism, 278
  genetic code, 553
  mechanism, 552
Proteolipid, acetylcholine receptor, 77
  binding of acetylcholine, 50
Proximate carcinogens, 658, 2-acetylamino-
  fluorene, 575
  N-methyl-4-aminoazobenzene, 675
Pseudocholinesterase. *see* Cholinesterase
Pseudoephedrine, buccal absorption, 150
Psychotropic drugs, genetic factors, 481
PTC. *see* Phenylthiocarbamide
Purine analogs, resistance, 535
  see also Azaguanine; 6-Mercaptopurine;
    Thioguanine
Purine metabolism, 253, regulation, 272
Purine phosphoribosyl transferase, purine meta-
  bolism, 260
Purinethol. *see* 6-Mercaptopurine
Pyramidone, hemolytic anemia, 457
Pyrene, formula, 680
Pyrilamine, formula, 751
Pyrimethamine, development, 765
  formula, 766
  resistance, 524, 545.
  see also Antimalarial drugs
Pyrimidine analogs, resistance, 535
  see also 5-Bromouracil; 5-Fluorouracil

Quinacrine, drug interaction, 824
  plasma protein binding, 159
  priming doses, 323
  see also antimalarial drugs
Quinidine, drug allergy, 502
  hemolytic anemia, 457

Side chain oxidation. *see* Metabolism of drugs
Silica dusts, absorption, 140
Silicon rubber, drug penetration, 153
SKF 525A, development, 762
  drug metabolism, 267
Skin, organization, 137
Smog, toxicity, 364
SN 7618. *see* Chloroquine
Sodium, absorption, 143
Sodium pump, 180
Solubility, anesthetic gases, 338
Solvent extraction, drug metabolites, 230
Somalin, potency, 749
Spare receptors, 101
Specific locus method, mutagenesis, 655
Spectinomycin, resistance, 555
Spectomycin, resistance, 530
Spectrophotometry, drug metabolism, 237
Spermicides, 112
Spin immunoassay, 63
Spindle inactivation, 648
Starvation, drug metabolism, 281
State–dependent learning, 587
Steady states, shifts, 315
Steroid hormone receptors, 66
Steroid hormones, 36, development, 745
  distribution, 757
  mechanism of action, 70
  plasma protein binding, 159
  resistance, 540
Steroids, fetal penetration, 204
  oral absorption, 755
Stibophen, drug allergy, 501
Stigmasterol, formula, 746
Stoke's law, 138
Streptomycin, dependence, 558
  fetal penetration, 204
  formula, 531
  misreading, 557
  plasma protein binding, 159
  resistance, 518, 530, 555
  resistance factors, 521
  subacute bacterial endocarditis, 782
  tuberculosis, 782
Streptozotocin, mutagenesis, 656
Strontium, antidotes, 401, 402
  toxicity, 415
Strophanthidin, 748, potency, 749
Strophanthidin glucoside, potency, 749
Strophanthus, steroid hormones, 747
Subacute bacterial endocarditis, *p*-aminosali-
    cylate, 782
  isoniazid, 782
  penicillin, 782
  streptomycin, 782
Subcutaneous drug administration, 134
Substrate inhibition, 95
Succinylcholine, 31, genetic variation, 442

Succinylcholine *(continued)*
  resistance, 474
Succinylcholine hydrolysis, genetic factors, 444
Succinyldicholine. *see* Succinylcholine
Sugar transport system, 178
Suicides, drugs, 358
Sulfacetamide, binding to albumin, 58
  hemolytic anemia, 457.
  see also Sulfonamides
Sulfadiazine, drug allergy, 504
  fetal penetration, 200
  formula, 45, 763, 772
Sulfaguanidine, brain penetration, 192, 193, 194
  fraction bound, 194
  partition coefficient, 194
  pKa, 194
Sulfamethoxypyridazine, hemolytic anemia, 457
  see also Sulfonamides
Sulfanilamide, fetal penetration, 202
  formula, 45, 256, 261, 767. 768
  hemolytic anemia, 457
  metabolism, 261
  methemoglobinemia, 423.
  see also Sulfonamides
Sulfanilamidoisopropylthiadiazine, formula, 771
Sulfapyridine, drug allergy, 504
  formula, 45
  hemolytic anemia, 457
Sulfates, carcinogenesis, 675
Sulfathiazole, drug allergy, 504
  fetal penetration, 200
  formula, 45
  resistance, 543.
  see also Sulfonamides
Sulfinpyrazone, development, 766
  formula, 249
Sulfisoxazole, elimination, 308
  hemolytic anemia, 457
  see also Sulfonamides
Sulfonamides, allergy, 489
  bilirubin displacement, 292
  carbonic anhydrase inhibition, 65
  drug allergy, 504
  drug interactions, 821
  hepatic porphyria, 463
  hereditary methemoglobinemia, 452
  infant toxicity, 394
  metabolism, 263
  NMR studies, 58
  plasma protein binding, 159
  resistance, 525, 538, 544
  structure–activity relationships, 43
  teratogenesis, 713
Sulfonates, carcinogenesis, 675
Sulfones, hemolytic anemia, 457
5-Sulfosalicylic acid, brain penetration, 192
  gastric absorption, 147
  pKa, 147